Core Curriculum for Pediatric Critical Care Nursing

Margaret C. Slota, RN, MN, CCRN

Adjunct Faculty, University of Pittsburgh
Director, Critical Care Services, Children's Hospital of Pittsburgh
Pittsburgh, Pennsylvania

AMERICAN ASSOCIATION OF CRITICAL-CARE NURSES

AACN
CRITICAL CARE

W.B. SAUNDERS COMPANY

A Division of Harcourt Brace & Company

Philadelphia London Toronto Montreal Sydney Tokyo

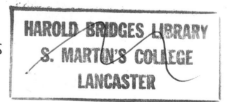

KT-435-905

W.B. SAUNDERS COMPANY
A Division of Harcourt Brace & Company

The Curtis Center
Independence Square West
Philadelphia, Pennsylvania 19106

NOTICE

Nursing is an ever changing field. Standard safety precautions must be followed, but as new research and clinical experience broaden our knowledge, changes in treatment and drug therapy become necessary or appropriate. Readers are advised to check the product information currently provided by the manufacturer of each drug to be administered to verify the recommended dose, the method and duration of administration, and contraindications. It is the responsibility of the treating physician relying on experience and knowledge of the patient to determine dosages and the best treatment for the patient. Neither the Publisher nor the editor assumes any responsibility for any injury and/or damage to persons or property.

THE PUBLISHER

Library of Congress Cataloging-in-Publication Data

Core curriculum for pediatric critical care nursing / [edited by]
    Margaret C. Slota : American Association of Critical-Care Nurses. —
1st ed.
        p.   cm.
    ISBN 0–7216–6114–9
    1. Pediatric intensive care.   2. Pediatric nursing.   3. Intensive
care nursing.   I. Slota, Margaret C.   II. American Association of
Critical-Care Nurses.
        [DNLM: 1. Curriculum.   2. Pediatric Nursing—education.
3. Critical Care—in infancy & childhood.   WY 18 C796848 1997]
RJ370.C67   1997
610.73'62—dc21
DNLM/DLC
                                                              97-9767

CORE CURRICULUM FOR PEDIATRIC CRITICAL CARE NURSING   ISBN 0-7216-6114-9

Last digit is the print number: 9   8   7   6   5   4   3   2   1

With love
to
Katy, Stephen, Michael, and Christopher

Contributors

LISA MARIE BERNARDO, RN, PhD, CEN
Assistant Professor, Health and Community Systems, University of Pittsburgh School of Nursing, Pittsburgh, Pennsylvania
Multisystem Issues: Multiple Trauma

LOUISE CALLOW, RN, MSN, CPNP
Adjunct Faculty, University of Michigan School of Nursing; Clinical Nurse Specialist/Pediatric Nurse Practitioner, Pediatric Cardiovascular Surgery, University of Michigan Hospital, Ann Arbor, Michigan
Cardiovascular System

JANET CRAIG, RN, MS, CCRN
Pediatric Nurse Practitioner, Pediatric Cardiology, Primary Children's Medical Center, Salt Lake City, Utah
Endocrine System

SHARI DERENGOWSKI, RN, MS, CRNP, CCRN
Pediatric Critical Care Nurse Practitioner, University of Maryland Medical Center, Baltimore, Maryland
Gastrointestinal System

PAULA DICKERSON, RN, BSN, CCRN
Burn Nurse Clinician, Burn Intensive Care Unit, Parkland Health and Hospital System, Dallas, Texas
Multisystem Issues: Burns

MARY D. GORDON, RN, MS
Clinical Nurse Specialist, Institute of Surgical Research, San Antonio, Texas
Multisystem Issues: Burns

MARY JO GRANT, RN, MS, PNP
Clinical Assistant Instructor, University of Utah College of Nursing; Pediatric Critical Care Nurse Practitioner, Primary Children's Medical Center, Salt Lake City, Utah
Pulmonary System

CATHERINE L. HEADRICK, RN, MS
Clinical Nurse Specialist, Pediatric Intensive Care Unit, Children's Medical Center of Dallas, Dallas, Texas
Renal System

KAREN M. KILIAN, RN, MN, ARNP, CCRN
Pediatric Nurse Practitioner, Pediatric Cardiac Surgery, Children's Hospital and Medical Center, Seattle, Washington
Pulmonary System

SARAH MARTIN, RN, MS, PCCNP, CCRN
Instructor, Rush University College of Nursing; Practitioner-Teacher, Rush–Presbyterian–St. Luke's Medical Center, Chicago, Illinois
Gastrointestinal System

LINDA L. OAKES, RN, MSN, CCRN
Intensive Care Unit/Pain Clinical Nurse Specialist, St. Jude Children's Research Hospital, Memphis, Tennessee
Hematology and Immunology

CATHY ROSENTHAL-DICHTER, RN, MN, CCRN, FCCM
Teaching Assistant, Doctoral Candidate, University of Pennsylvania School of Nursing, Philadelphia, Pennsylvania
Hematology and Immunology; Multisystem Issues: Septic Shock

MARGARET C. SLOTA, RN, MN, CCRN
Adjunct Faculty, University of Pittsburgh; Director, Critical Care Services, Children's Hospital of Pittsburgh, Pittsburgh, Pennsylvania
Pulmonary System; Cardiovascular System

ROSE ANN GOULD SOLOWAY, RN, MSEd, ABAT
Clinical Toxicologist, National Capital Poison Center; Administrator, American Association of Poison Control Centers, Washington, DC
Multisystem Issues: Toxicology

ELIZABETH C. SUDDABY, RN, MSN, CCTC

Heart Transplant Coordinator, Children's National Medical Center, Washington, DC
Cardiovascular System

PAULA VERNON-LEVETT, RN, MS, CCRN

Family Care Nurse, Pediatric Intensive Care Unit, The Children's Memorial Hospital, Chicago, Illinois
Neurologic System

PAM WALTER, RN, BSN

Unit Manager, Burn Intensive Care Unit, Parkland Health and Hospital System, Dallas, Texas
Multisystem Issues: Burns

HOLLY F. WEBSTER, RN, MS, PNP

Clinical Assistant Instructor, University of Utah College of Nursing; Pediatric Critical Care Nurse Practitioner, Primary Children's Medical Center, Salt Lake City, Utah
Pulmonary System

EILEEN J. WELLS, RN, MSN, CCRN

Clinical Nurse Specialist, Pulmonary Department, Cook Children's Medical Center, Fort Worth, Texas
Caring for Critically Ill Children and Their Families

Reviewers

Tori Adams, RN, MS
Clinical Nurse Specialist, Fort Worth, Texas

P. David Adelson, MD
Assistant Professor of Pediatric Neurosurgery, University of Pittsburgh School of Medicine; Director, Pediatric Traumatic Brain Injury Program, and Director, Trauma Research, Benedum Trauma Program, Children's Hospital of Pittsburgh, Pittsburgh, Pennsylvania

Edward M. Barksdale, Jr., MD
Assistant Professor of Pediatric Surgery, University of Pittsburgh School of Medicine and Children's Hospital of Pittsburgh, Pittsburgh, Pennsylvania

Lee B. Beerman, MD
Professor of Pediatrics, University of Pittsburgh School of Medicine and Division of Pediatric Cardiology, Children's Hospital of Pittsburgh, Pittsburgh, Pennsylvania

Lisa Marie Bernardo, RN, PhD, CEN
Assistant Professor, University of Pittsburgh School of Nursing, Pittsburgh, Pennsylvania

Jean Betschart, MN, RN, CDE
Adjunct Faculty, University of Pittsburgh School of Nursing; Diabetes Program Coordinator, Children's Hospital of Pittsburgh, Pittsburgh, Pennsylvania

Joseph A. Carcillo, MD
Assistant Professor of Anesthesiology and Critical Care Medicine and Pediatrics and Associate Director, Pediatric Intensive Care Unit, Children's Hospital of Pittsburgh, Pittsburgh, Pennsylvania

Lynne A. Cipriani, RN, BSN
Cardiopulmonary Transplant Coordinator, Children's Hospital of Pittsburgh, Pittsburgh, Pennsylvania

Robert S. B. Clark, MD
Associate Director, Pediatric Intensive Care Unit, Children's Hospital of Pittsburgh, Pittsburgh, Pennsylvania

Sarah Day, RN, BSN
Co-Director, Mid South Sickle Cell Center, St. Jude Children's Research Hospital, Memphis, Tennessee

Bonnie S. Dean, RN, MS, ABAT
Director, Training and Education, Children's Hospital of Pittsburgh, Pittsburgh, Pennsylvania

Michele Schaaf Holecek, RN, MSN, CCRN
Pediatric Intensive Care Clinical Nurse Specialist, Children's Hospital of Orange County, Orange, California

Kenneth P. Hopkins, DDS, MS
Director, Dentistry Division, Department of Surgery, St. Jude Children's Research Hospital, Memphis, Tennessee

Edwin M. Horwitz, MD, PhD
Assistant Professor, Department of Pediatrics, University of Tennessee College of Medicine; Assistant Member, Division of Bone Marrow Transplantation and Cell and Gene Therapy Program, St. Jude Children's Research Hospital, Memphis, Tennessee

Walter T. Hughes, MD
Arthur Ashe Chair in Pediatric AIDS Research and Professor of Pediatrics, St. Jude Children's Research Hospital, Memphis, Tennessee

Sherry Johnson, RN, CCRN, CPON
Intensive Care Unit/Bone Marrow Transplant Unit Educator, St. Jude Children's Research Hospital, Memphis, Tennessee

Susan J. Kelley, RN, PhD, FAAN
Professor, School of Nursing, Georgia State University, Athens, Georgia

Arlene Klostermann, RN, MSN
Neuroscience Clinical Nurse Specialist, St. Louis Children's Hospital, St. Louis, Missouri

Samuel Kocoshis, MD
Associate Professor of Pediatrics, University of Pittsburgh School of Medicine; Director of Pediatric Gastroenterology, Children's Hospital of Pittsburgh, Pittsburgh, Pennsylvania

Preface

Much effort is being expended to meet the challenge of providing the high quality of care that every child deserves in the current financial climate of reduced reimbursement and cost containment. How do we continue to respond to the impassioned pleas for help from the many grieving parents who must cope with their child's critical illness or injury?

- We answer with highly skilled, technically competent care delivered by pediatric critical care nursing professionals.
- We answer with compassion blended with courage in playing the hand dealt to us on a daily basis in pediatric intensive care units across the world.
- We answer by integrating the knowledge and contributions of the multiple disciplines required to meet the special and demanding needs of our patient population and by making a strong effort to form a cohesive team from these talented caregivers, who may sometimes be at odds.
- We answer with tears and hugs for the children and families and an affirmation that although we cannot know their pain, we will always be there for them.
- We answer with care focused on the needs of the children, their siblings, their parents, and their extended family because they all hurt so much.
- We answer with extra efforts—bending the rules for the family of a dying child, making sure that impoverished families have enough to eat, pulling numerous team members together to orchestrate one last trip outside or to the beach for a dying child, staying to listen to stories about each precious child, making sure that their favorite stuffed animals or "pieces of home" are always by their side, moving 75+ cards and pictures along with the child to a quieter bedspace, being available to visit with a healed child and family who return to say thanks or with the grieving parents who return alone to bring closure.
- We answer with outcomes-based research and monitoring that validates the essential quality of care issues and documents cost-effective interventions and required financial support.

The *Core Curriculum for Pediatric Critical Care Nursing* is intended to be a reference source for nurses caring for critically ill or injured children in any setting. Contributing authors from across the country have worked to create a comprehensive and relevant source of information. Using a systems approach for easy reference, chapters contain a wide array of information including a review of developmental anatomy and physiology, pathophysiology and defining characteristics of a variety of common pediatric disorders, relevant pharmacology, monitoring and diagnostic testing, and a multidisciplinary approach to the plan of care. Each patient health problem is discussed along the continuum of family-centered care with integration of ethical, legal, and environmental issues within the text of each chapter. Further clinical integration is achieved with the inclusion of a number of case studies in the appendix.

I have learned much from the many children and families I have known and loved over the years and will forever admire for their strength and courage in the face of devastating illness or injury. I acknowledge the caring and dedicated nurses with whom I have had the pleasure of working in five different and challenging pediatric critical care units. I am grateful to the contributing authors for their commitment of time and expertise. I acknowledge the patient copy editor, Mary Espenschied, the editorial staff at W.B. Saunders Company, and the time, effort, and constructive comments from the reviewers.

All of our work as pediatric critical care nurses is dedicated to the memory of all the children and families we have cared for—to those for whom our best technology, knowledge, efforts, and compassion were not enough and to those children who can laugh and play once again.

—*Peggy Slota*

Contents

CHAPTER 1 **Caring for Critically Ill Children and Their Families** 1
Eileen J. Wells

CHAPTER 2 **Pulmonary System** 33
Holly F. Webster, Mary Jo Grant, Margaret C. Slota, and Karen M. Kilian

CHAPTER 3 **Cardiovascular System** 144
Louise Callow, Elizabeth C. Suddaby, and Margaret C. Slota

CHAPTER 4 **Neurologic System** 274
Paula Vernon-Levett

CHAPTER 5 **Renal System** 360
Catherine L. Headrick

CHAPTER 6 **Endocrine System** 387
Janet Craig

CHAPTER 7 **Gastrointestinal System** 424
Sarah Martin and Shari Derengowski

CHAPTER 8 **Hematology and Immunology** 461
Linda L. Oakes and Cathy Rosenthal-Dichter

CHAPTER 9 **Multisystem Issues** 551
Multiple Trauma 551
Lisa Marie Bernardo

Toxicology 595
Rose Ann Gould Soloway

Septic Shock 627
Cathy Rosenthal-Dichter

Burns 652
Paula Dickerson, Mary D. Gordon, and Pam Walter

APPENDIX **Case Studies** 682

INDEX 697

Caring for Critically Ill Children and Their Families

EILEEN J. WELLS

Adam was almost 2 years old and had never been in the hospital before. In the weeks prior to admission, his parents noticed that Adam was holding his head to one side and resisting efforts to straighten it. He also was becoming ataxic. He had difficulty walking at times and seemed to fall often. A few days before Adam was admitted to the hospital, he experienced several episodes of emesis and became lethargic. Adam's parents were frightened when the pediatrician referred them to a neurosurgeon and were in a state of shock when they were told that Adam had a malignant brain tumor. Adam was admitted to the pediatric intensive care unit (PICU) following a craniotomy for the removal of the tumor. He was medically stable and required routine postoperative care. The oncologists had been consulted and were considering the options for treatment of Adam's tumor. The morning after surgery, Adam was awake and looked around but avoided eye contact. He refused to smile or pay any attention to the books and toys offered to him. His head was tilted to one side, and he held his special blanket close to his face. His eyes were huge. With the gigantic white turban of gauze and tape wrapped around his head he appeared so forlorn. While performing Adam's routine care, I also gave him medication for pain. He seemed to relax somewhat but still refused to interact with me in any way. I was not too concerned, thinking that when his parents arrived I would be able to better assess how he was feeling.

Adam initially brightened when his mother came into the room but then showed little interest in her many efforts to beguile him. Since Adam was preverbal, it was impossible for him to tell us why he was so unhappy. We were at a loss to help him to feel better. As his mother and I talked, she told me that Adam was one of four boys. His oldest brother was almost 5 years old. The next boy was 3 years old, and Adam had a twin brother, Noah. Adam's father was at home with the other boys until the grandparents arrived from another state to help with their care.

Adam's mother asked if the other boys could visit Adam. I assured her that the children were welcome to visit and that I would have the child life specialist help them to understand what to expect prior to coming into the unit. When the rest of the family arrived, I observed Adam closely. The sight of his father and older brothers elicited a response similar to his mother's arrival; but when Adam saw his twin brother, a metamorphosis occurred. Noah walked into the unit holding his father's hand. When Noah saw Adam, he broke loose and ran to the bed. I suggested that his mother pick him up and place him on the bed next to Adam. When she did this, Adam became a "new man." He sat up straight, looked around the room, and his beautiful smile was shared with me and his entire family. Adam's twin had brought Mylar balloons. Within minutes, both Adam and Noah were hitting the balloons and laughing out loud. Adam's mother later expressed her feelings to me about the encounter. When she and Adam's father had seen the change in their son, they were able to remain hopeful about their ability to face the future. Their need, at that time, was for their family to be together. Adam's special need was to be with his twin brother.

Caring for children in a health care system that is driven by the needs of the patient and family means being sensitive to the psychosocial and physical needs of the child and family. The admission of a child to the PICU is a highly stressful event for families. Effective pediatric critical care nurses see the child and family as an integral unit and are perceptive to the needs of the entire family as they move through the crisis.

CHILDHOOD DEVELOPMENT: PSYCHOSOCIAL, EMOTIONAL, COGNITIVE

A knowledge of normal growth and development and the ability to assess the child's developmental level is crucial to working effectively with children and parents in any health care setting. Those who view children as small adults are unlikely to be successful in obtaining cooperation from the patients or their families. Those who experience children as individuals at a particular level of development find caring for children a rich and rewarding adventure.

A. **DEVELOPMENTAL STAGES IN INFANCY (0 TO 12 MONTHS)**
   1. **Psychosocial: Trust vs. mistrust:** Infants develop a sense of trust when their basic needs for affection, security, and survival are satisfied.
   2. **Personality: Oral stage:** Sucking provides the major source of enjoyment.
   3. **Cognitive: Sensorimotor stage:** Reflexes are gradually replaced with voluntary behaviors. Infants learn to differentiate themselves from others. Infants begin to develop object permanence at 4 to 8 months. Security objects may alleviate anxiety responses in older infants. Infants use their parents as a social reference. By looking at their mother or father, infants determine how to react to new and unfamiliar situations.

B. **DEVELOPMENTAL STAGES OF TODDLERS (1 TO 3 YEARS)**
   1. **Psychosocial: Autonomy vs. doubt and shame:** Toddlers gradually develop the ability to control their bodies and begin to seek independence. Toddlers express themselves through negativism, temper tantrums, and physical resistance. Older toddlers are eager to please adults. Toddlers learn through sensorimotor experiences.
   2. **Personality: Anal stage:** Toddlers learn bladder and bowel control. Toddlers have an egocentric view of life.
   3. **Cognitive: Sensorimotor stage matures to preoperational stage:** Toddlers exhibit egocentric development and increased use of language. Early memory development and a beginning sense of time occurs in toddlers.
   4. **Concept of death:** Toddlers view death as a temporary event and may continue to ask about the person or pet who has died despite explanations that death has occurred (Whaley and Wong, 1995).

C. **DEVELOPMENTAL STAGES OF PRESCHOOLERS (3 TO 5 YEARS)**
   1. **Psychosocial: Initiative vs. guilt:** Preschoolers begin to develop the superego and learn right from wrong. Preschoolers have a strong need to explore the environment. Preschoolers may feel guilt or fear in response to inappropriate thoughts or actions. Preschoolers are eager to conform to adult expectations.
   2. **Personality: Phallic stage:** Preschoolers develop a beginning gender awareness and identify with the parent of the same sex.
   3. **Cognitive: Preoperational (2 to 7 years)** The preschooler's vocabulary increases, and magical thinking is used. Preschoolers still have a poorly developed concept of time. Preschoolers communicate through play. They are usually unable to see anyone else's point of view at this stage of development.
   4. **Concept of death:** Death is viewed as temporary. Preschoolers may say that someone is "dead" without any understanding of the finality of death. Preschoolers may fear death as a separation from someone they love, as being injured, or as a punishment for misbehavior (Lewandowski, 1992; Whaley and Wong, 1995).

D. **DEVELOPMENTAL STAGES OF SCHOOL-AGE CHILDREN (6 TO 12 YEARS)**
   1. **Psychosocial: Industry vs. inferiority:** School-age children have a need to develop a sense of achievement and competence. School-age children are usually willing and anxious to cooperate.

2. **Personality: Latency period:** Development of the superego continues, and school-age children have serious feelings about what is right and wrong.

3. **Cognitive: Concrete operational (7 to 11 years):** School-age children begin to use logic in thought and can consider another person's point of view. Language and problem-solving abilities improve. School-age children enjoy rules, rituals, and conformity. They expect others, including parents, to obey the rules and will complain if something is "not fair" to them.

4. **Concept of death:** Early school-age children still believe death is temporary and may personify it as a ghost or the devil (Lewandowski, 1992; Whaley and Wong, 1995). Older school-age children understand death as permanent and realize that everyone, including themselves, will die someday (Whaley and Wong, 1995).

E. **DEVELOPMENTAL STAGES OF ADOLESCENTS (12 TO 18 YEARS)**

1. **Psychosocial: Identity vs. role confusion:** Teens are often preoccupied and frequently dissatisfied with their physical appearance. The adolescent years are a time of emotional struggle for independence as the teen searches for a personal identity.

2. **Personality: Genital stage:** This stage begins at puberty with the development of secondary sex characteristics and sex hormones. Teens display frequent mood swings with emotional lability. Teens may fluctuate between wanting to be with their family and avoiding their family.

3. **Cognitive: Formal operational:** The ability to use abstract thinking begins in the early teens. Logical thinking becomes more developed, although teens may retain some magical thinking as well. For example, they may feel that an illness is a punishment for something they did. Use of verbal communication increases.

4. **Concept of death:** Teens understand death as permanent and inevitable but as something that will occur only in the distant future (Lewandowski, 1992).

DEVELOPMENTALLY APPROPRIATE ASSESSMENT OF CHILDREN

Children usually respond well to honesty, gentleness, and respect. Most children want to please their parents and other adults as well.

A. **GENERAL PRINCIPLES FOR WORKING WITH CHILDREN**

1. **Introduce yourself to the child.** Include the child in conversation even if the child does not seem to be responding. Children may not verbally respond but will listen to everything that is said and decide how much comfort or danger the situation holds for them. Assure the child that it is alright not to talk.

2. **Honesty is vital to establishing a trusting relationship with children.** Be honest if a procedure will hurt. To deny that something will hurt and then deliberately cause pain to a child may destroy the possibility of a trusting, cooperative relationship with that child. Admit that you do not know if the child asks a question you cannot answer. Promise to try to find the answer.

3. **Make eye contact and call the child by name.**

4. **Allow the child to see your hands and any instruments you will use.** If possible, allow the child to touch and examine the instruments. Most children are cooperative if they know you are not planning a painful procedure.

5. **Allow the child to make choices whenever possible but avoid giving the child artificial choices.** For example, do not ask permission to measure the child's blood pressure unless you are prepared to respect his or her choice when the

child refuses. Simply state what you need to do in a gentle but matter-of-fact manner and do it.
6. **Allow the parents to participate in the child's care whenever possible.**
7. **Use a calm, soothing voice.**
8. **Encourage the family to bring the child's favorite articles from home.**
9. **Stoop or bend to communicate at the child's eye level when possible.**

B. **PRINCIPLES FOR WORKING WITH INFANTS**
1. Assess affect, color, level of consciousness, and respiratory rate and effort prior to touching the infant, since changes may occur in these parameters when the infant is touched.
2. When possible, perform the assessment while the parent is holding the infant.
3. Warm the stethoscope and other appropriate instruments prior to use.
4. Smile and speak softly to the infant prior to touching.
5. Bright objects may be useful to provide distraction.
6. Avoid restraining the infant as much as possible and assess those areas that require restraint at the end of the examination (i.e., ears, throat, gag reflex) (Vessey, 1995).

C. **PRINCIPLES FOR WORKING WITH TODDLERS**
1. Assess affect, color, level of consciousness, and respiratory rate and effort prior to touching the toddler.
2. Name each body part for the toddler as you examine it.
3. Draw faces on tongue blades or inflated gloves.
4. If possible during the assessment, allow the toddler to sit up and to hold a security item.
5. Allow the toddler to inspect and touch the equipment.
6. Demonstrate the equipment on a doll, a stuffed toy, or the toddler's parent.

D. **PRINCIPLES FOR WORKING WITH PRESCHOOLERS**
1. Explain what you are doing in simple terms as you progress through the assessment.
2. Praise the preschooler frequently.
3. Allow the preschooler to inspect and touch the equipment.
4. Demonstrate the equipment on a doll, a stuffed toy, or the preschooler's parent.
5. Avoid holding your hands behind your back, since preschoolers may wonder what you are hiding.
6. Avoid using words or phrases like "cut," "take," "broken," or "put you to sleep."

E. **PRINCIPLES FOR WORKING WITH SCHOOL-AGE CHILDREN**
1. Speak directly to the school-age child, explaining what you are doing and why you are doing it.
2. Take time to listen to the school-age child.
3. Teach the school-age child about body function (Vessey, 1995).
4. Accord the child respect, privacy, and dignity.
5. Encourage as much mobility as possible to help reduce stress.

F. **PRINCIPLES FOR WORKING WITH ADOLESCENTS**
1. Respect the adolescent's desire for privacy. Adolescents may prefer for their parents to leave during the examination (Vessey, 1995) and for the curtains to be drawn.
2. Avoid unnecessary physical exposure.
3. Explain what you are doing and why you are doing it.
4. Encourage teens to discuss their concerns.
5. Teach the adolescent about normal physical and sexual development.
6. Facilitate visits with peers when possible.

G. **PRINCIPLES FOR WORKING WITH ADOLESCENTS AS PARENTS**
1. Affirm the role of an adolescent parent as "Mom" or "Dad."
2. Discourage grandparents or other relatives from usurping the parent's control.
3. Teach the adolescent parent about normal child development, nutrition, discipline, and care.
4. Assess the parent's level of understanding and teach without condescension.
5. Direct questions and explanations to the parent even when older relatives are present.
6. Treat the adolescent parent with the same respect given to any parent.

STRESS RESPONSES AND COPING BEHAVIORS

Critical illness and admission to a PICU causes both physiologic and psychologic stress in children. Physiologic responses to stress have been well documented and are similar to those of the adult.

A. **PHYSIOLOGIC RESPONSE TO STRESS**
Stress stimulates the sympathetic nervous system and results in the release of stress hormones, causing the following:
1. Tachycardia, tachypnea, and increased blood pressure
2. Peripheral vasoconstriction with cool extremities
3. Inhibition of digestion
4. Inhibition of function of the immune system, which may delay healing (McCarthy et al, 1991)
5. Hyperglycemia in older infants or children; hypoglycemia in young infants
6. Dilated pupils
7. Hyperalert behavior (Kidder, 1989)

B. **ADMISSION TO A PICU**
Admission to a PICU causes the added dimension of psychologic stress and may impair the child's ability to adapt (Kidder, 1989).
1. **Infants:** Infants respond to stress with crying and increased motor activity. Some infants use gaze aversion, refusing to make eye contact with caregivers (Lewandowski, 1992). Infants may throw an arm over the eyes to limit stimulation when stressed. Older infants may throw a blanket or diaper over the head to withdraw or "shut down" when they feel over stimulated. Infants may suck on fingers, pacifiers, blankets, or endotracheal tubes to calm themselves and cope with stress. Older infants may rock themselves or use their arms or legs to make rhythmic movements.
2. **Toddlers:** Toddlers may react to stress with increased physical activity, loud crying, or screaming that may continue to the point of exhaustion. Any fear may cause toddlers to physically resist. Toddlers may think that hospitalization is related to their own misbehavior. They fear abandonment and become distressed when separated from their parents (Lewandowski, 1992). If toddlers feel abandoned, they may become angry and withdraw. Toddlers tend to use regression when hospitalized. Previously toilet-trained toddlers may lose bladder control or revert to thumb sucking. Toddlers are frequently attached to security items and often hold them close to the face.
3. **Preschoolers:** Increased verbal skills allow some preschoolers to cope with stress by seeking information (Corbo-Richert, 1994), asking questions, or repeating phrases over and over such as "Where's my mommy?" "Why?" or "I want to go home!" Preschoolers may visually examine instruments and may offer tense compliance while accepting comfort and support from parents (Ellerton et al, 1994). To gain control in some area, preschoolers may refuse food and not

cooperate with caregivers. Preschoolers continue to hold on to security items. Regression to the toddler stage is common with a return of thumb sucking or increased need for comfort from parents. Preschoolers may project their feelings of sadness, anger, or guilt onto others or onto toys. Preschoolers frequently express their feelings about illness through dramatic play. Preschoolers may withdraw from interaction with others if they are angry, sad, or in pain.

4. **School-age children:** Fear of a loss of control may lead school-age children to deny fears and act "grown up" even when frightened. School-age children may regress to earlier stages of development with a need for security objects or thumb sucking. The children may feel embarrassed about the return of these habits if they are discussed. If feeling out of control, school-age children may withdraw from caregivers, refuse to communicate, and use television or sleep as a means of escape. Regression in school-age children may include physical resistance to treatments or procedures that are feared. School-age children actively seek and process information and accept support from others. They usually attempt to be helpful and cooperative (Bossert, 1994; Corbo-Richert et al, 1993).

5. **Adolescents:** Teens may deny obvious pain and discomfort, especially if peers are present. If feeling out of control, teens may withdraw and refuse to communicate or cooperate. Teens may regress to an earlier stage and become demanding and clinging with caregivers or parents. Some teens may intellectualize their illness to avoid dealing with the emotional issues (Lewandowski, 1992). A sense of invincibility may lead some teens to deny their diagnosis, need for treatment, or prognosis.

ISSUES RELATED TO HOSPITALIZATION

A. **FEAR AND ANXIETY**

Most children experience some fear and anxiety when hospitalized. These emotions may be related to any of the following or to a combination of factors. Fears may be reality based, related to previous procedures or hospitalizations the child has experienced. Information given to the child by friends or relatives may be incorrect. Inadvertently the child may hear comments made by family or caregivers. Children may perceive and react to feelings of fear in parents or others. Children may see or hear things at other bed spaces in the PICU that cause fear and anxiety.

1. **Age-specific fears related to developmental level**

   a. *Infants:* Separation anxiety and fear of strangers begins at 6 to 7 months of age. Crying and clinging to parents is normal behavior and may indicate a healthy parent-child relationship. Infants resist being separated from parents. When parents leave, an infant may exhibit loud and active grief that may continue to the point of exhaustion. Infants may become passive and withdrawn if cries do not cause immediate return of parents. Infants may accept food and comfort from the nursing staff while avoiding eye contact or other interaction.

   b. *Toddlers* may fear separation from parents, large animals, strangers, "the doctor," changes in their environment, or "shots." Toddlers frequently react with temper tantrums or clinging to parents. Toddlers may be attached to security objects.

   c. *Preschoolers* fear bodily injury or mutilation, darkness, separation from parents, loss of control, the unknown, death, or "shots." Preschoolers may regress and act as toddlers or become quiet and withdrawn if they feel out of control. Preschoolers may be able to express their anxiety through play or drawing pictures. Preschoolers may repeat questions over and over because of an immature concept of time or an attempt to gain comfort.

d. *School-age children* may fear bodily injury, loss of control, failure in school, supernatural beings, rejection by others, or death. They may also fear intrusive procedures, particularly injections, and being separated from family and friends (Hart and Bossert, 1994). They may have vague or incorrect ideas about illness, injury, and body function, which lead to increased fear. For example, they may believe that illness is a punishment for bad behavior. Some school-age children may be reluctant to ask questions and feel that they must act "grown up." They may verbalize understanding while still needing additional explanation.

e. *Adolescents'* fear may revolve around social isolation, loss of control, rejection by peers, appearance of being different or dumb, or helplessness. Teens may use denial or regression despite a fear of appearing younger than they are. Teens may tend to dramatize events or may intellectualize illness or injury.

B. Pain

Children in pain frequently receive too little medication or receive no analgesia at all (Eland and Coy, 1990; Rice, 1993). Despite an increase in the emphasis on pain management in children over the past several years, some misconceptions about children and pain persist (Table 1–1).

C. Separation From Family and Friends

Children who are separated from their families may experience a wide variety of symptoms, including tachycardia, sleep disturbances, vomiting, diarrhea, hyperventilation, refusal to eat, bed-wetting, aphonia, regression, and withdrawal (Cataldo and Maldonado, 1987). Young children who have been separated from their families for prolonged periods have shown delayed growth and development with permanent cognitive damage (Cataldo and Maldonado, 1987). Symptoms related

Table 1–1. MISCONCEPTIONS ABOUT PAIN IN CHILDREN

Misconceptions	Truth About Pain
Children do not experience pain the same as adults.	"Pain is whatever the experiencing person says it is . . ." (McCaffrey, 1977) regardless of age.
A child who is not crying is not in pain.	Children express pain in varying ways at different ages.
A child who is asleep is not experiencing any pain.	Some children sleep to try to escape pain, just as adults attempt to do.
Infant nerve pathways are not developed enought to have pain (Schechter, 1989).	Infants may experience harmful physiologic effects from stress responses related to pain (Anand, Phil, and Hickey, 1987).
Children will always tell you if they are in pain.	Children may interpret pain as punishment for misbehavior or believe they are supposed to have pain if nothing is done to relieve it.
Children will become addicted if given narcotics.	Physical dependency is unusual but can occur. These drugs can be weaned just as with adults.
Children always tell the truth about pain.	Children may deny pain to avoid injections. Teens may deny pain in the presence of peers.

to separation may be more severe when a child is ill or in pain. Older school-age children and adolescents may suffer when separated from school and peers (Pederson, 1993).

D. LIMITED UNDERSTANDING

Misconceptions about illness, treatment, and caregiver motives may result from a child's limited understanding. Magical thinking leads children to think an illness is punishment for misbehavior. Words such as "cut" or "take" can be misconstrued by children and increase levels of fear. The vivid imagination of childhood supplies answers to any unanswered questions or unexplained situations. Limited understanding may lead to nightmares and sleep disturbances.

E. LOSS OF CONTROL

Physical restraints may be used to safeguard the child, but they increase the child's levels of fear and anxiety. Children are rarely given much choice in matters of their treatment and have little sense of control when hospitalized. Requests to "go home" or for "Mommy" or "Daddy" may be met with inadequate explanations about "visitor rules" or disregarded entirely. The child's refusal to cooperate is often met with physical force.

ISSUES RELATED TO CRITICAL CARE UNITS

Michelle was 7 months old and had spent most of her short life in the PICU. She had experienced many complications and had been intubated for a long time. She slept in a room that was never dark and listened continuously to the rhythmic swoosh of the ventilator filling her lungs. Intermittent conversation night and day, as well as frequent alarms, became the norm in her world. While the new resident examined her, she made no eye contact with him. To assess Michelle's hearing, he held a metal wash basin next to her tiny ear and struck it forcefully with a metal emesis basin. I gasped, the nurse next to me screamed, but Michelle did not react. "She's deaf!" said the resident. He documented Michelle's diagnosis of deafness in the progress notes despite our attempts to help him understand the world in which she was living.

As the resident left the PICU, I leaned down over Michelle and whispered an apology to her for his insensitive behavior. As I spoke softly to her, Michelle opened her eyes and turned her head toward me.

A. SENSORY OVERLOAD

Sensory overload may lead to confusion, restlessness, anger, agitation, and to ICU psychosis.

1. **Noise** has been associated with lack of sleep, anger, headache, fatigue, release of stress hormones, decreased growth hormone, increased pain, increased need for analgesia, and ICU psychosis (Griffin, 1992; Grumet, 1993).
   a. The Environmental Protection Agency recommends noise levels no higher than 45 decibels (dB) during the day and no higher than 35 dB for sleep. Noise levels interfere with rest when higher than 35 to 45 dB (Grumet, 1993; Slota, 1988).
   b. Noise levels in critical care units range from 50 to 80 dB. Each increase of 10 dB causes sound to be perceived as twice as loud (Grumet, 1993; Table 1–2).
   c. Startle reactions can be caused when an impulse sound, such as an alarm, exceeds the background noise level by 30 dB. Much of this equipment is located next to the child's head in the PICU.
   d. Bedside conversation may be as high as 70 to 90 dB. Bedrails clang at 90 dB, and a stainless steel bowl that is dropped causes an impulse noise at 108 dB (Grumet, 1993).
   e. Research indicates that noise stress may interfere with immune responses and delay wound healing (McCarthy et al, 1991).

Table 1–2. **SOUND LEVELS RECORDED FROM SELECTED NURSING ACTIVITIES**

Activity	dB
Full bottle of formula placed on bedside table	75.3
Storage drawer closed	69.8
Orogastric package opened	71.3
Empty feeding syringe tossed in plastic waste can	55.8
Chair moved across floor	62.0
Running water	54.2
Medication drawer closed	58.9
Medication pump sounding an alarm	57.5
Oxygen disconnected from wall	55.0
Ringing telephone	49.7
Cardiac monitor sounding an alarm at 70% volume	65.8
Cardiac monitor sounding an alarm at 30% volume	55.4

Reproduced with permission from DePaul D, Chambers SE (1995). Environmental Noise in the Neonatal Intensive Care Unit: Implications for Nursing Practice. *Journal of Perinatal and Neonatal Nursing,* 8(4):71–76. Copyright © 1995 Aspen Publishers, Inc.

2. **Constant light** leads to confusion of day and night. Day from night differentiation is difficult if no windows are available. Lights are frequently bright and directly over the child's head.

3. Unfamiliar **tactile and olfactory stimulation** over which the child has little or no control can be disturbing. Children are unfamiliar with hospital food. Medicinal smells may be powerful and unpleasant.

B. SENSORY DEPRIVATION

Although there is an excess of stimulation in most PICUs, there is a lack of the normal types of stimulation beneficial for children. Important bedtime rituals are changed, and there is a lack of familiar blankets, bed, toys, and pajamas. Adults other than parents are directing the child's behavior and schedule. Restricted activity leads to feelings of isolation and boredom and interferes with the child's ability to cope with the stress of hospitalization. Physical activity is a method frequently used by children to cope with stress. Sensory deprivation leads to depression and regression and interferes with normal development (Whaley and Wong, 1995).

C. SLEEP DEPRIVATION

Disruption of normal sleep patterns leads to fatigue, anxiety, increased illness, restlessness, combativeness, disorientation, and ICU psychosis (Slota, 1988). Interaction of noise stress and sleep loss causes a decrease in levels of growth hormone and cortisol, which can affect protein synthesis and leukocyte function (McCarthy et al, 1991). Disrupted sleep while in the hospital leads to sleep disturbances that may continue after discharge (Slota, 1988). The PICU environment is responsible for multiple causes of sleep deprivation (Table 1–3). Interrupted sleep may be related to disorientation and ICU psychosis.

D. LACK OF PRIVACY

1. Many PICUs are large, open units. Children are aware of procedures and crises that occur at beds close to their own. Open areas allow other strangers (other visitors and hospital employees) to see the children and their parents.

2. The need for close observation sometimes leads to physical exposure of the child.

E. TECHNOLOGY DEPENDENCE

The number of technology-dependent patients has increased since the development of mechanical ventilation. Critically ill, unstable children are the highest

Table 1–3.   CAUSES OF SLEEP DEPRIVATION IN THE PICU

Noise levels
Decreased light-dark cycles
Disruption of home sleep rituals
Pain and discomfort
Isolation
Immobilization
Anxiety
Depersonalization
Restraints
Tense atmosphere
Pharmacologic paralysis
REM and NREM suppressant drugs

NREM, non–rapid eye movement (sleep); *REM,* rapid eye movement (sleep).
Reproduced with permission from Slota MC. Implications of sleep deprivation in the pediatric critical care unit. *Focus Crit Care.* 1988;15(3):35–43.

priority in the PICU. Chronically ill but stable children who are technology dependent may receive less developmental and psychosocial support when the PICU is busy or understaffed. Technology may interfere with parental bonding or lead to the parents' emotional withdrawal from their child. Technology-dependent children may experience long periods of separation from their families. Children are aware that alarms are related to them and exhibit fear when any alarm is triggered. Chronic sleep disruption can affect protein synthesis necessary for memory and learning and growth hormone necessary for healing and growing (Warner and Norwood, 1991). A significant number of technology-dependent children are also developmentally delayed (Stutts, 1994).

DEVELOPMENTALLY APPROPRIATE INTERVENTIONS

A. PAIN MANAGEMENT
  1. **Nonpharmacologic management of pain**
      a. Various types of nonpharmacologic measures are useful in the management of children's pain. These techniques work best when combined with appropriate analgesia. (See Table 1–4 for pain behaviors and sources of comfort.)
      b. When possible, tell the child how long the pain will last and be sure to tell the child when the procedure is over. A finger prick hurts but is over quickly.
      c. Encourage the child to express feelings of pain. Assure the child that it is alright if they want to cry when something causes pain.
      d. Tell the child that you want to know when something hurts so that you can try to make it better.
      e. With infants in particular, ask the parents what comfort measures they have found successful at home.
      f. Distractions such as singing, storytelling, reading to a child, listening to music, or watching television may help a child cope with pain.
      g. Positioning may be useful. Infants respond well to swaddling.
      h. The use of motion is helpful. Infants often like to be patted on the back or bottom. Infants, toddlers, and preschoolers like rocking motions.
      i. Some children as young as preschool age can cooperate with imagery (Kachoyeanos and Friedhoff, 1993). Ask the child or parent to identify a

Table 1–4. GUIDELINES FOR AGE-APPROPRIATE ASSESSMENT AND MANAGEMENT OF PAIN

COMMON INDICATORS OF PAIN/DISTRESS*	PREDOMINANT FEARS	POTENTIAL SOURCES OF COMFORT
Infant (0–12 mo)		
Procedural Pain†	Separation from parents	Analgesic as indicated
Moves entire body in response to pain stimulus	Strangers	Consider sedative or amnesic as appropriate for anxiety or repeated painful procedures
Withdraws limb		Presence of primary caregiver or consistent nurses
Cries vigorously		
Facial expression reveals brow bulge		Bundling, holding
Acute Pain‡		Sucking (pacifier or feeding)
Restless, irritable, difficult to comfort		Rocking or other gentle motion
Sleeps fitfully		Comforting sounds, e.g., tape of womb sounds, lullabies, comforting voices (especially familiar voices)
Reluctant to move or be moved if movement increases pain		
Cries quietly or whimpers if vigorous crying increases pain		
Must be coaxed to smile or interact		Security object(s)
Feedings altered in frequency, duration, and/or amount		Peaceful environment§
Toddler (1–3 y)		
Procedural Pain†	Separation from primary caregivers	Analgesic as indicated
Cries, screams		Consider sedative or amnesic as appropriate for anxiety or repeated painful procedures
Struggles against restraint (difficult to distinguish fear of restraint from actual pain)	Immobility and restraint	Presence of primary caregiver or consistent nurses
Acute Pain‡		Staying near, holding, touching
Usually cannot localize pain unless source is visible, e.g., cut, scrape		Rocking or other gentle motion
May verbalize general "hurt" or "owee"		Comforting sounds, e.g., lullabies, familiar voices
Restless, irritable, difficult to comfort		Truthful, age-appropriate explanations and frequent reassurance
Cries frequently if crying does not increase pain		
Cries quietly or just whimpers if vigorous crying increases pain		Security object(s)
Decreased tolerance for frustration		Distraction with short (3- to 5-min) activities
Established sleep patterns disturbed		Encouraging participation in care activities to increase sense of control
May regress behaviorally (e.g., loss of bowel and bladder control)		
Reluctant to move or be moved if movement increases pain		Allowing movement and ambulation as possible
Must be coaxed to smile or interact		Peaceful environment§

*Because pain and the distress it causes are often difficult to distinguish from one another, the behaviors listed in this column may reflect either pain or distress, or some combination of pain and distress.

†Procedural pain is caused by diagnostic technique (e.g., blood draw) or therapeutic intervention (dressing change) and typically diminishes over minutes or hours.

‡Acute pain can be caused by a natural developmental process (e.g., teething), a disease process (e.g., otitis media), or a therapeutic intervention (e.g., surgery). The pain usually diminishes over days or weeks.

§A peaceful environment is one that is (1) safe (all painful procedures should be done in the treatment room, not the child's room) and (2) devoid of stimuli annoying to the ears, nose, eyes, smell, and touch.

Table continued on following page

Table 1–4. GUIDELINES FOR AGE-APPROPRIATE ASSESSMENT AND MANAGEMENT OF PAIN *(Continued)*

COMMON INDICATORS OF PAIN/DISTRESS*	PREDOMINANT FEARS	POTENTIAL SOURCES OF COMFORT
Preschooler (3–5 y) ***Procedural Pain†*** Cries, screams Struggles against restraint (difficult to distinguish fear of restraint from actual pain) Verbal barrage of questions about procedure and pleas to stop it ***Acute Pain‡*** By age 4, can usually localize pain verbally or with markings on body outline Restless, irritable, difficult to comfort Cries frequently if crying does not increase pain Cries quietly or just whimpers if vigorous crying increases pain Decreased tolerance for frustration Voice quality may change; e.g., child becoming very soft-spoken or whiny May regress behaviorally (e.g., clinging to parent, reverting to baby talk) Established sleep patterns disturbed Reluctant to move or be moved if movement increases pain Decreased interest in environment and usual activities	Separation from parents, siblings, home environment Pain as punishment Mutilation	Analgesic as indicated Consider sedative/amnesic as appropriate for anxiety or repeated painful procedures Presence of primary caregiver or consistent nurses; telephone contact with family Being near, holding, rocking Truthful, age-appropriate explanations and frequent reassurance Security object(s) Distraction (10- to 15-min activities) Therapeutic play Encouraging participation in care activities to increase sense of control Peaceful environment§
School-Age (6–12 y) ***Procedural Pain†*** May cry, scream, and protest verbally and with motor behaviors or may cooperate with procedure with only facial grimacing and muscular rigidity Readily verbalizes questions, complaints, protests, instructions May grunt, groan, or sigh, but cries and screams less frequently than younger child ***Acute Pain‡*** Localizes pain verbally or on body outline Describes pain intensity and quality and helps to evaluate pain management interventions Restless, has difficulty finding position of comfort May cry if crying does not increase pain, but cries much less frequently than younger children	Inferiority Separation from peers Loss of peer relationships Mutilation Loss of control	Analgesic (including patient-controlled analgesia [PCA]) as indicated Consider sedative/amnesic as appropriate for anxiety or repeated painful procedures Transcutaneous electrical nerve stimulation (TENS) as indicated Presence of primary caregiver or consistent nurses Telephone contact with family and friends Truthful, age-appropriate explanations and frequent reassurance Security object(s) Distraction Relaxation strategies Therapeutic play Participation in care activities to increase sense of control Peaceful environment§

Table 1–4. GUIDELINES FOR AGE-APPROPRIATE ASSESSMENT AND MANAGEMENT OF PAIN (*Continued*)

COMMON INDICATORS OF PAIN/DISTRESS*	PREDOMINANT FEARS	POTENTIAL SOURCES OF COMFORT
Decreased tolerance for frustration; may be irritable and demanding, especially with family members		
Voice quality may change; e.g., child becoming very soft-spoken or whiny		
May regress behaviorally (e.g., increased dependence on parent)		
Sleep disturbances; e.g., sleeping more or less than usual, awaking frequently		
Reluctant or refuses to move or be moved if movement increases pain		
Decreased interest in environment and usual activities		
Adolescent (13+ y)		
Procedural Pain†	Loss of control	As for school-age, with in-
Usually cooperates with procedure	Loss of independence	creased emphasis on oppor-
Often displays facial grimacing, muscular rigidity	Changes in self-concept and body image	tunities and responsibilities for participating in pain as-
Readily verbalizes questions, complaints, protests, instructions	Loss of peer relationships	sessment and management
May grunt, groan, or sigh, but rarely cries or screams	Complications in future relationships, sexual competency, ability to provide for self	
Acute Pain‡		
Localizes pain verbally or on body outline		
Describes pain intensity and quality		
Adept at evaluating pain management interventions		
Restless, has difficulty finding position of comfort		
May cry if crying does not increase pain, but cries much less frequently than younger children		
Decreased tolerance for frustration; may be irritable and demanding, especially with family members		
Voice quality may change; e.g., child becoming very soft-spoken or whiny		
May regress behaviorally (e.g., increased dependence on parent)		
Sleep disturbances; e.g., sleeping more or less than usual, awaking frequently		
Reluctant or refuses to move or be moved if movement increases pain		
Decreased interest in environment and usual activities		

From Foster R, Stevens B. Nursing management of pain in children. In: Betz CL, Hunsberger MM, Wright S, eds. *Family-Centered Nursing Care of Children*. 2nd ed. Philadelphia, Pa: WB Saunders Co; 1994:892–894.

special place where the child recalls happy experiences. Ask the child to imagine being in that place. Describe the kinds of things the child would see, hear, smell, or feel in that place. Teach children the use of a "pain switch." Ask the child to imagine a pain switch, like a light switch. Teach the child to mentally visualize the switch being turned off in the painful area (Kachoyeanos and Friedhoff, 1993).

2. **Pharmacologic pain management**
    a. *Administration:* Optimal pain relief is provided by maintaining a constant serum drug level. Continuous infusion provides a constant level of analgesia and may be preferable to bolus administration. Administer a bolus dose when the continuous drip is started and each time the infusion rate is increased (Eland and Banner, 1992). Patient-controlled analgesia (PCA) has been used successfully in children as young as 5 years. Parents are most familiar with their children. Ask their opinion about the child's pain (Eland and Coy, 1990).
    b. *Nonnarcotics* are useful for mild to moderate pain and can frequently be given in combination with narcotics for control of more severe pain.
        • Acetaminophen is a mild analgesic frequently used for pain and fever in children. It works well for mild pain or when given in combination with another drug.
        • Aspirin is a useful antiinflammatory drug but has a possible association with Reye's syndrome in children younger than 13 years (Eland and Banner, 1992).
        • Ibuprofen has antiinflammatory and analgesic effects with potential for gastrointestinal side effects.
    c. *Sedatives*
        • *Benzodiazepines* (i.e., diazepam, midazolam, and lorazepam) provide muscle relaxation, amnesia, and relief of anxiety (Eland and Banner, 1992). They are particularly effective when used along with other medications. Taper these drugs slowly and observe for symptoms of withdrawal such as a state of hyperawareness with agitation or seizure.
        • *Ketamine* provides sedation and analgesia. Ketamine raises blood pressure and should not be used in children at risk for increased intracranial pressure. It is a useful drug for children with asthma because of the bronchodilatory effect. Observe for emergence reactions such as excitement, hallucinations, or delirium.
        • *Barbiturates* have anticonvulsant and sedative properties. They should be tapered slowly if used over a long period of time. Observe for seizures.
        • *Chloral hydrate* is easily administered and used frequently in PICU. This drug is a sedative, not an analgesic, and there are side effects associated with long-term use.
    d. *Narcotics:* A wide choice of drugs is available to provide relief of moderate to severe pain (Table 1–5). If a narcotic is used longer than 4 to 5 days, the child should be weaned from the narcotic for a period of time and observed for withdrawal symptoms (Eland and Banner, 1992). Methadone is useful as an oral medication when a child is being weaned from narcotics. Help the family understand that narcotic dependency is a physiologic phenomenon and that the child is not psychologically addicted.

3. **Pharmacologic paralysis:** When intubation is required, neuromuscular blocking agents are frequently used for a variety of reasons. These drugs do not provide analgesia or sedation. In short, they do not affect the child's state of consciousness and should never be used without being accompanied by analgesics and sedatives.

Table 1–5. DOSING AND KINETICS OF NARCOTICS AND SEDATIVES

DRUG	HALF-LIFE	BOLUS DOSE	INFUSION DOSE*
Nalbuphine (Nubain)	Child: 0.5–1.5 h	0.1–0.2 mg/kg (q1–2h)†	0.1–0.4 mg/kg/h
Morphine	Neonate: 11–30 h	0.1 mg/kg/IV (q1–2h)†	0.1 mg/kg/h
	Child: 2–8 h	Caudal/epidural‡ 75– 100 µg/kg	
		Intrathecal‡ 10–20 µg/kg	
Fentanyl	Neonate: 6–32 h	2–5 µg/kg/IV	2–20 µg/kg/h
	Child: 2–4 h	Caudal/epidural‡ 1 µg/kg	Caudal/epidural‡ 0.5–1.5 µg/kg/h
Sufentanil	Neonate: 5–20 h	0.1–3 µg/kg IV	1–1.4 µg/kg/h
	Child: 1.5–4 h		
Methadone	24+ h†	0.1 mg/kg IV	Not recommended
		0.2 mg/kg PO (q6–24h)	
Meperidine (Demerol)	Neonate: 6–39 h	1 mg/kg IV (q2–4h)	Not recommended
	Child: 2–4 h§		
Diazepam (Valium)	24+ h§	0.1 mg/kg IV (q2–4h)	Not recommended
Midazolam (Versed)	Child: 2–8 h	0.05–0.1 mg/kg IV, IM (q1–2h)	0.05–0.2 mg/kg/h
Codeine	Child: 3–4 h	0..5–1 mg/kg PO (q2–3h)	Not recommended

*Rate should be reduced or carefully monitored in preterm babies and in immediate newborn period (<2 wk of age).
†Continuous infusion preferred to intermittent doses.
‡Spinal doses are based on limited data and should be used cautiously.
§Estimated—data limited in pediatrics.
From Eland JM, Banner W. Assessment and management of pain in children. In: Hazinski MF, ed. *Nursing Care of the Critically Ill Child*. St Louis, Mo: Mosby–Year Book Inc; 1992:79–100.

B. COMMUNICATION

Communication is generally considered that interaction we *intentionally* carry out with our patients. In fact, we are *always* communicating with them, although not necessarily those things we had hoped to communicate. The child who is admitted to the PICU, separated from parents, held down or restrained, and undergoes painful, intrusive procedures indeed receives a message from those providing the care. The message, however, is not the one that the caregivers intend to convey.

Critical care nurses can use communication in a positive way to help the children and families as they struggle to cope with the stress of a PICU admission.

1. **Preparation for procedures:** Many procedures can easily be done with a parent present. Children usually cooperate when a parent remains with them. There are exceptions, which need to be addressed individually. If a parent does not feel able to remain with the child, this feeling should be respected. If child life or play specialists are available, their assistance is invaluable in preparing children for surgery or procedures in a developmentally appropriate manner.

   a. *Infancy:* Even infants will quickly learn which cues predict painful events. Infants as young as 6 to 7 months cry when a foot is grasped if they have undergone repeated heel sticks. Awaken the infant prior to any painful procedure so they are not aroused from sleep by pain. Avoid playing familiar music boxes or tapes during procedures such as suctioning or needle sticks so the infant does not learn to interpret them as cues to imminent pain.

   b. *Toddlers:* Use simple words and phrases to explain the procedure immediately prior to performing the procedure. Allow the child to handle the equipment when possible. Use restraints only when necessary. Use phrases like "all done" when appropriate so the toddler knows when the procedure is over.

c. *Preschoolers:* Use pictures, puppets, dolls, or toys during explanations or demonstrations and allow the preschooler to handle them. If time permits, preschoolers may be prepared hours in advance for minor procedures or a few days ahead of time for more serious events (Lewandowski, 1992). Help preschoolers identify safe times when no procedures, vital signs, or other care is planned. Allow preschoolers to keep a security item during procedures. Recognize that the preschooler's bed is his or her "personal space" and keep hands in plain view when approaching or touching the bed.

d. *School-age children:* Allow as many choices as possible. Ask the school-age child to explain what was heard to verify understanding of explanations. Allow time for and encourage questions. School-age children may be prepared weeks prior to a procedure. When advanced planning is not possible, allow the school-age child as much time as possible between the explanation and the event. Teach coping techniques such as imagery and relaxation.

e. *Adolescents:* Give clear, factual explanations and encourage questions. Allow as much control as possible. Allow teens to choose whether they want to have a parent present with them. Teach coping techniques such as imagery or relaxation. Prepare adolescents as soon as it is known that the procedure or surgery is needed.

2. **Communicating with intubated children:** Children in the PICU frequently are intubated and may be physically restrained to prevent dislodgment of the endotracheal tube. Communication is more difficult with these children but no less important than with the child who can respond verbally and interact with caregivers.

    a. Explain why the child cannot make noise or cry out.
    b. Speak to the child prior to and during any procedures.
    c. Use frequent, gentle touching when with the child.
    d. Teach parents how they can safely provide comfort.
    e. Encourage parents to stay with the child and teach them to assist with appropriate care (i.e., diaper changes, bath, oral hygiene, eye care) if they desire to do so.
    f. Picture boards depicting different activities can be used with preschoolers. The child can point to what is needed or desired. Older children can point to words on a board. Educating the children to use these or other communication devices such as electronic spelling boards or computers can be done in advance if a lengthy intubation or tracheostomy is anticipated.
    g. Ask questions that only require a "yes" or "no" answer so the child can shake or nod his or her head.
    h. If the child is not likely to remember being admitted, explain the circumstances in simple language (i.e., "You were hurt in an accident," "You became very sick," or "You are in the hospital—you are getting better"). This may need to be repeated frequently as the child gains awareness.
    i. Referral to a communication specialist prior to or during PICU admission may help.

3. **Communication with children who are sedated and pharmacologically paralyzed**

    a. Even with sedation, those who receive neuromuscular blockers can hear and feel and may remember hearing voices or feeling things being done to them (Davidson et al, 1993; Gross, 1992).

   b. Tell the child what you plan to do even if you think the child might not be able to hear you. Include explanations of vital signs, turning, oral hygiene, suctioning, or bathing.

   c. Attempt to "wake" the child by gentle touch and verbalization prior to painful interventions.

   d. Explain to the child why he or she is paralyzed and that the paralysis is temporary.

   e. Describe things that the child might be hearing or feeling such as ventilators, alarms, suctioning, monitors, chest physiotherapy, cooling or heating pads, restraints, and voices.

   f. Keep the child covered as much as possible. Avoid unnecessary exposure.

   g. Tell the child that he or she will not be left alone. If the family must leave temporarily, inform the child that the family will return.

   h. Encourage parents to touch, stroke, and talk to the child (Davidson et al, 1993). Parents may tell the child about things that family members are doing, read stories, or sing to the child. Family members may record special tapes that can be played in their absence. Suggest that they might want to record the reading of a favorite story for the child.

   i. Ask parents what type of music the child prefers and play tapes periodically. Prior to performing any procedures, turn off the tape and then explain the procedure, so that the child will realize nothing will happen to him while a tape is playing.

   j. Remind others who come to the bedside that the child may be able to hear (Davidson et al, 1993). Place a small reminder sign by the bed so that others remember to speak to the child.

C. INTERVENTIONS FOR SLEEP DEPRIVATION, SENSORY DEPRIVATION, AND SENSORY OVERLOAD

   1. **Minimize noise levels:** Develop an educational program to maintain awareness of those things that cause sound in the unit and look for creative ways to minimize noise and its effects on the children and families (Zwick, 1993). Place noise limitation guidelines on the agenda for staff meetings and seek input from staff. When looking at new equipment, make clear to sales representatives that loud or annoying alarms and noises are unacceptable. Raise and lower bedrails as quietly as possible. Keep alarms at moderate levels with speakers pointed away from the child's head. Beepers can be kept on vibrate mode. Limit conversations around the bedside. Speak in soft, soothing tones. The loudest noises recorded in PICUs are frequently caregiver voices (Slota, 1988). Place sound absorbing pads under telephones and other noise-producing equipment (Griffin, 1992). Have any equipment that squeaks lubricated. Have the children use headphones for watching television or listening to music. Turn music or headphones off periodically so the child can have quiet periods.

   2. **Maintain a day-night cycle:** Dim lights as much as possible at night. Avoid having lights shine into children's faces or shield their faces. Allow sleep periods of at least 90 minutes to normalize sleep cycles as much as possible. Use the child's normal rituals whenever possible (e.g., security objects, tapes of music or family voices, or having a story read before bedtime). Always awaken a child and offer an explanation prior to performing any procedures. Use earphones or ear pads to decrease noise exposure for the children even if they are not listening to music. Place away from the head of the bed any autosyringes and infusion pumps that are likely to alarm.

D. FACILITATION OF PLAY IN THE PICU

Most health care providers who care for children understand the importance of play in the life of a child. Children's hospitals often provide playrooms filled with books and toys for their small patients. But the child who is a patient in the PICU presents a different challenge to caregivers interested in providing play opportunities for their patients.

1. Child life or play specialists, if available, can assist in finding appropriate play activities for children at different levels of development.
2. Encourage parents to bring special toys from home for the child. Even if the child is not able to play with them immediately, they may provide some comfort for both the child and parent by having them in the PICU (Lewandowski, 1992).
3. Caregivers or parents may play for the child who cannot play at all. Puppets and dolls are useful for this type of play.
4. Any child from toddler age or older may benefit from an opportunity for medical play with equipment and supplies.
5. *Infants* enjoy mobiles, pictures of faces, tapes with soothing music or parent's voices, and soft, cuddly toys. Older infants may enjoy watching the caregiver play for them.
6. *Toddlers* enjoy books, security objects, and tapes with music, stories, or recorded family voices. Immobility is difficult for the toddler who may benefit from watching the caregiver play with puppets, cars, or other active toys.
7. *Preschoolers* like to talk and have questions answered. They enjoy water play and having stories read to them. They usually enjoy some television shows and will often take part in medical play if given the tools.
8. *School-age children* often enjoy medical play, coloring, books, and crafts (Lewandowski, 1992). Most enjoy children's movies or television shows. Ask the parents what type of shows the child is allowed to watch at home to avoid conflict related to television.
9. *Adolescents* enjoy books, magazines, and television. Peer visits and telephone calls, if they can be arranged, are helpful to the teenaged patient.

E. **PROVISION OF PSYCHOSOCIAL AND EMOTIONAL SUPPORT FOR THE CHILD**

Johnny was 7 years old and admitted to the PICU in status asthmaticus. He was a bright and cooperative child as I connected the cardiac monitor, pulse oximeter, blood pressure cuff, oxygen cannula, and intravenous (IV) infusion pump. Johnny had never been in the hospital before but was trying hard to be in control and act in a grown-up way despite some obvious anxiety.

As I placed the cardiac leads on his chest, he looked into my face and with a slight quiver in his voice asked, "Are you going to use that machine on me that makes you go like THIS?" As he spoke, he demonstrated a jerking, flailing reaction of his entire body, and I recognized a television portrayal of someone who had been defibrillated. "Have you seen that on TV?" I asked. "Yes," he said, "and the guy died."

I assured Johnny that we had no intention of using that machine on him and that the cardiac leads did not give shocks. I also turned his bed so that he could see the tracing on the monitor, gave him a rhythm strip of his pattern, and demonstrated the alarms for him. By the time his parents arrived, Johnny was breathing more easily and was happily watching the monitor and making it alarm by deliberately changing his breathing pattern.

1. **Recognize that hospitalized children may be angry** about being there, having painful procedures done, having to take medicine, or any number of things that happen to them in the hospital. Ask whether they are angry. Assure them it is all right to be angry. Some children may be unwilling or unable to admit to feelings of anger but may display them by facial expression, withdrawal, or being uncooperative.
2. **Use primary nursing or consistent assignments to limit the number of caregivers** each child and family encounters. Having a familiar nurse helps to allay parental anxiety and may make it easier for parents to leave the child's bedside for periods of time. Nurses who are familiar with a child more easily recognize the child's behavioral cues, responses, and psychosocial needs (Warner and

Norwood, 1991). Children more readily communicate with familiar caregivers. Predictable routines are more easily established by caregivers who are familiar with a child.

3. **Some children do not respond verbally but are willing to nod or shake their heads in response** to a "yes" or "no" question.

4. **Assure children that they did not get sick because of something they thought or did.**

5. **Limit the use of restraints** and remove them whenever someone is able to stay with a child for a period of time.

6. **Offer "tours" for both the child and parents** with planned admissions. Identify equipment that will be used with the child. Explain the purposes of the alarms. Assure the parents and child, when appropriate, that the nurses know which alarms require an immediate response and which do not. Introduce the child and parents to at least one nurse they will see when the child is admitted.

7. **Allow children to wear underwear as soon as possible.** Being able to wear any clothing from home including shoes and socks is helpful for most children.

8. **Respect the child's "space."** Speak when approaching the child. Tell the child what you plan to do prior to touching the bed or the child.

9. **Explain equipment, medications, and procedures in terms of what the child will experience.** Tell children what they can expect to feel, see, hear, smell, and taste. Run a rhythm strip from the monitor and give it to the child to take back to school. If the results are normal, tell the child so. Allow the child to hold the electronic thermometer, remove the blood pressure cuff, and remove old tape. Give as much control to the child as is safely possible.

10. **Recognize regression as a normal defense mechanism** in the hospitalized child and help others to remember it if someone says that a child is " . . . too old to act that way" or "If that was my kid, I would. . . ."

11. **Set limits that a child can understand.** For example, explain that it is all right to feel angry and cry, but it is not all right to bite or kick people. Do not threaten or shame a child. Explain that you are going to help the child hold still, rather than that the child is going to be held down. If parents use threats (e.g., "If you don't hold still, that nurse is going to give you a shot"), explain in a tactful manner, but within the child's hearing, the importance of telling a child the truth and avoiding threats so that the child will trust the caregivers.

12. **Offer whatever comfort the child is willing to accept.** Stroking and hugging may be accepted by some children in the absence of parents. Keep your face at eye level but do not force eye contact with a child who is avoiding it. The use of presence through being physically close, speaking in a soft voice, and using an empathetic touch, conveys a caring atmosphere and strengthens the child's coping ability (Pederson, 1993).

13. **Suggest that the parents bring in family pictures** and place them where the child can see them at all times.

PSYCHOSOCIAL NEEDS OF FAMILIES

Near the Christmas holiday Matthew was admitted to the PICU following a spinal fusion and was expected to transfer to the floor the next day. When his parents came into the PICU I was struck with how familiar they looked. Later that day the nagging feeling continued, and I commented to the parents that I felt I should know them. They quietly reminded me that their other son, Mark, had been a patient in our unit a few years previously and had died just before Christmas that year.

I immediately remembered Mark and turned to the room where I had cared for him. His parents confirmed with a sad smile that Mark had ended his short life in bed space 2. How could I have forgotten,

I thought. Fortunately, I had not admitted Matthew to bed 2 as I had originally planned. I wondered how the parents could tolerate being here again and how they could smile at me.

During the night, Matthew began to have trouble breathing as alveoli collapsed throughout his lungs. Despite vigorous therapy, he developed adult respiratory distress syndrome (ARDS), which required mechanical ventilation. Matthew grew progressively worse as the anniversary date of his brother's death drew close. The strain visibly increased on the parents' faces as they quietly sat by their only child's bedside.

After a few weeks of not knowing whether Matthew would survive, he slowly began to improve and was eventually weaned from the ventilator. When he was transferred out of the PICU, his parents were finally able to begin to smile again. Now when I am tired and tempted to be less than empathetic, I have only to remember these brave parents who could trust us with the life of their only remaining child even though we were unable to prevent the death of their other son.

A. **FAMILY ASSESSMENT**

1. **Sources of stress related to the PICU:** The sight and sound of equipment attached to sick children causes anxiety and fear. Parents often cannot distinguish between alarms that signal life-threatening conditions or those that may indicate something as simple as a completed medication or a false alarm. Parents fear that their child is in pain. Families may fear that the child will die. The presence of other sick, injured, or crying children and their apprehensive parents causes additional stress. Alteration in the parental role occurs (Warner and Norwood, 1991). Parents lose their caregiver role as they watch strangers care for their child. Parents experience loss of control, since they do not know how to care for the child themselves. Feelings of inadequacy may result when parents perceive professionals as better able to care for their child. Parents experience a change in their self image as protector and nurturer of their child and must adjust to a new role as parent to an ill child (Way, 1993). Restricted visiting and being separated from the child causes additional stress. The presence of blood, bruising, bandages, restraints, and tubes on the child increase parental apprehension.

2. **Needs of parents of children in the PICU:**
   a. To be with their child: Recognize that parents' greatest need is to be with their child and develop strategies to support them. Create a partnership with the parents to plan and provide the best care possible for the child (Rushton, 1990)
   b. To receive accurate, current, and consistent information
   c. To speak with the physician caring for their child regularly and when they have questions
   d. To feel that everything possible is being done for their child
   e. To have a place to rest near the PICU
   f. To feel that their child is seen as a unique individual and that the staff care about their child
   g. To participate in their child's care
   h. To feel hopeful about their child's survival
   i. To know that their child is free of pain

3. **Responses to stress and coping behaviors:** Parents generally use coping behaviors they found successful in past crises. These may be helpful behaviors such as talking, praying, or requesting help. Some parents employ unhelpful behaviors such as anger, hostility, avoidance, or drug or alcohol usage.
   a. *Reactions*
      - A shock reaction may occur when parents first see their child in the PICU. Some parents become pale and weak and may faint.
      - Parents may be unable to remember information and may repeat the same question several times.

- The initial response of parents may be to focus on the equipment and monitors and be afraid to approach the bed or their child. Parents may need caregiver "permission" and encouragement to approach the bed and touch their child.
- Some parents demonstrate emotional distancing by minimizing significance through intellectualizing the crisis (Todres et al, 1994).
- Some parents display anger or hostility toward the other parent or toward the caregivers.
- Parents may assist in their child's care with repetitive tasks such as suctioning their child's mouth or draining urine from the tubing into the bag.
- Parents may focus on a detail and repeatedly complain if they feel it is not addressed adequately.

b. *Support systems*
- Grandparents may be close to the child and provide emotional support for parents or may be an additional source of stress if they are unable to cope with the child's illness or injury.
- Other family members, friends, or church members may be part of the family's support group. Parents are often more willing to temporarily leave the hospital if a member of their support system remains with their child or if they have grown comfortable with a staff member caring for their child.
- Parents sometimes ask family members of another child in the PICU to "keep an eye on" their child while they leave the hospital for a rest even if a familiar caregiver is providing care for their child.

c. *Physical needs*
- If their child's admission to the PICU was unexpected, the parents may need assistance with finding a place to rest, to bathe, and to obtain food.
- If the parents live near the PICU, they may want to go home to rest.
- Some parents are not able to cope with leaving the hospital and will need a place to lie down near the PICU.
- Obtain assistance from social services if the parents do not have enough money for food.
- Parents of critically ill children may forget or refuse to eat. Remind them that eating and resting will help them to maintain their own strength so that they will be able to support and care for their child.

d. *Cultural implications*
- Some parents may speak English but have difficulty understanding what is said to them because of stress they are experiencing and the unfamiliar medical language. Obtain the assistance of an interpreter any time you feel that parents are having difficulty understanding. It may be easier for them to ask questions in their own language.
- Be aware that wrist bracelets, ankle bracelets, or objects pinned to the child's clothing may have cultural or spiritual significance for the family. Treat these objects with respect. Consider attaching a patient identification bracelet to them. Do not remove them without parental permission unless absolutely necessary. If objects are pinned to the linen, be sure they do not get lost when the linen is changed.

e. *Spiritual considerations*
- Most parents experience guilt and helplessness when a child is ill or injured because parents feel they must protect their children from harm of any kind.

- Some parents express feelings that God caused the child's illness because of a parent's personal sin or fault.
- If the parents are religious, offer to contact a minister, priest, rabbi, or other religious leader. Offer the assistance of hospital chaplains if they are available.
- Assure privacy by closing a door or curtain when parents wish to pray. Some parents believe that prayer is more effective when several church members are gathered together and lay their hands on the child. Allowances in visiting policies should be made for this type of visit.
- Assess dietary or treatment restrictions related to religion or culture. These may include rules about some foods or a prohibition against certain treatments such as a ban on the use of blood products.

    f. *Financial concerns:* Critical illness usually causes financial stress. Even parents who have insurance may have additional expenses related to hospitalization, which may include the cost of food, travel, baby-sitting for other children, or loss of pay. Parents may have to return to jobs earlier than desired if no vacation time is available or if the employer is unsympathetic to the family's plight.

B. Interventions with Families

Multiple studies have been done to identify family needs when a child is critically ill. All families want reassurance, access to the ill child, and information. We can direct efforts toward interventions to help meet these needs (Dracup, 1993).

  1. **Supporting the parental role**

    a. Recognize that the parents are the experts in caring for their child and treat them as such. Ask how they do things at home and listen carefully to the answers. Document responses in the plan of care. When possible, perform care for the child as it is done in the home.

    b. Avoid taking tasks away from the parents and performing them "better" unless the child will really benefit from the difference in technique.

    c. Tell the parents that although the staff can supply much of what the child needs, no one can take the place of "Mom" or "Dad." Avoid adopting the role of surrogate parent. The role of the caregiver is to support the parent-child relationship, not to usurp that relationship. Caregivers who call a patient "My Baby" or "My Child" may add to the feelings of helplessness, inadequacy, and loss of control that the parents are already experiencing (Warner and Norwood, 1991).

    d. Make the parents feel welcome in the PICU. Provide a place for them to sit without waiting for them to ask. Tell them how their child is doing in words they can understand. If the parents are uncomfortable staying with their child in the PICU, explore the reasons for this feeling. Support their decision if appropriate.

    e. Avoid loud laughter and talking, which may be offensive to families in crisis.

    f. Let the parents know that their child is recognized and valued as a unique individual. Describe individual characteristics and behaviors of the child such as how the child ate, slept, or when the child has been hugging a stuffed toy. Touch the child while the parents are there. Demonstrate a gentle, caring attitude toward the child. Call the child by name. Use the correct pronoun when communicating with the family.

    g. If the child does not "look like himself" because of the severity of the injury or illness, ask the parents to bring pictures taken prior to the hospitalization and place them where all the caregivers can see them.

2. **Communicating with parents**
   a. Make an effort to know the parents' first names so they are not always addressed as "Mom" or "Dad." Ask permission prior to calling them by their first names.
   b. Make an effort to learn how the parents are coping. Asking if they were able to sleep or have been able to eat or drink anything demonstrates an interest in their well-being.
   c. Ask the parents how they think the child is doing. Parents often detect subtle changes. Such questions also help the parents feel they are important in the child's care.
   d. Ask the parents what they were told by the physician in order to evaluate the parents' understanding of their child's condition. Ask the parents if they have questions. After you have responded, explore to be sure they understood the answers or if your responses were adequate.
   e. Consider forming a parent support group for the families. Groups may be facilitated by clinical nurse specialists, nurses from the PICU, or social workers. Personally invite each parent of every child in the PICU to the group. Let the parents know that the group is a safe place and keep everything that occurs in the group confidential (Amico and Davidhizar, 1994).
   f. Assist the parents with physician contact. Plan for a daily meeting with parents, physician, and nurse for information sharing (Dracup, 1993).
3. **Building a relationship of trust:** Parents need to trust the caregivers to feel comfortable enough to leave the bedside for some periods of time. Ask the parents to let you know where they are when not in the PICU and how they can be contacted. Agree about when they want to be called. Some parents prefer to be called with any change at all, positive or negative. If you have agreed to call the parents when their child asks for them, do so. This will enhance a trusting relationship between the nurse and the parents, as well as between the nurse and the child. Consider loaning a pager to the parents so they will know you can easily contact them wherever they are.
4. **Mutual care planning with parents**
   a. Research indicates that parental stress is decreased when the parents are involved in planning their child's care (Curley and Wallace, 1992). Ask the parents how they would like to be involved in their child's care and respect their desires when appropriate (Purcell, 1993). Plan multidisciplinary care conferences that include the parents so that the entire team is moving toward the same goals and the parents are recognized as an important part of the team.
   b. Help the family understand which things they can safely touch and which must remain the caregivers' responsibility. For example, parents like to turn off alarms to be helpful. From their point of view, they are doing the same thing as the nurse who walks into the room, touches a button, and walks away. Take time to explain the unseen assessment that is performed by the nurse as the alarm is silenced.
   c. Share the daily plan for the child. If planning to attempt ventilator weaning or decrease vasopressors, share that information with the family so they know what to expect. If the plan is to observe the child and not make any changes, let them know that too so they are not disappointed by a perceived lack of progress.
   d. Assist the parents in gaining as much control as possible to ease anxiety and maintain the parental role (Schepp, 1992). Offer choices as much as

possible. For example, when possible, let the parents decide when to give a bath or perform oral hygiene.

   e. Offer to be a gatekeeper for the parents. If parents are being stressed by too many visitors who stay too long, let them know that the staff is willing to place limits on visiting so they do not need to do so (Tomlinson and Mitchell, 1992). Suggest that the parents identify a single person to notify the rest of the social network, receive information from the parents, and disseminate it to the rest of the family and concerned individuals (Tomlinson and Mitchell, 1992).

5. **Caring for parents of chronically ill children**

   a. Children with a chronic illness may experience multiple PICU admissions. Avoid making assumptions about the parents' anxiety, since research indicates that having experienced previous admissions does not decrease parental anxiety (Curley and Wallace, 1992).

   b. Parents may be accustomed to performing many procedures at home and have developed their own ways of doing them. Ask how they perform care at home and be open to the possibility that the staff can learn from experienced parents. When possible, assign nurses who cared for the child during previous admissions.

   c. Parents of children with a chronic illness may be reluctant to discipline consistently or at all. Avoid conflicting expectations from the parents and caregivers. Discuss setting limits with the parents when necessary to reach mutual agreement and avoid confusing the child (Wells et al, 1994).

   d. Recognize that the parents may be experiencing chronic sorrow related to having a child with a chronic illness. This may involve feelings of sadness, guilt, failure, and anger. These parents may also feel a lack of closure related to their child's questionable prognosis (Stutts, 1994).

6. **Working with siblings of a child in the PICU**

   a. Child life specialists provide excellent preparation for siblings and help them to know what to expect before they visit in the PICU. Siblings may imagine that a brother or sister is far more seriously ill or injured when they are not allowed to see for themselves.

   b. Siblings may fear that they caused the illness or injury by something they said or did. Siblings may also experience signs of stress such as sleep disturbances or changes in behavior.

   c. Parents may need assistance in making decisions regarding the care of the child's siblings.

7. **Facilitating transfer from the PICU**

   a. When their child is transferred, the parents may experience anxiety related to the following changes:
   - An unfamiliar unit after becoming accustomed to the PICU
   - Unfamiliar staff members caring for the child
   - Changes in how frequently the child is assessed
   - Discontinuation of frequent monitoring
   - No continuous presence of a nurse at the bedside

   b. Tell the family about the plans for transfer prior to the event (Braun and St. Clair, 1994). Prepare families for the changes that will occur. Help them to understand that the transfer means the child is now doing better and no longer needs the PICU. Emphasize the positive aspects of the transfer, such as the more private and quiet environment.

   c. If possible, tour the new unit and introduce the parents to a nurse who works there. Consider a care conference with the family and new unit staff prior to the transfer (Braun and St. Clair, 1994). Plan a follow-up visit to the new unit by a PICU nurse.

8. **"Visiting privileges" in the PICU:** Parents are "visitors" only in the sense that the children are visitors as well and should be treated with respect and dignity. To suggest that parents need our permission to be with their child is the antithesis of a system of health care that is driven by the needs of the patient. The primary need of the parents is to be with their child. The best coping mechanism for the child is to be with his or her parents (Tughan, 1992).

   a. *History of visitation in hospitals:* Health care for sick family members shifted from the home to the hospital around 1920 (Page and Boeing, 1994). Family visits were thought to be detrimental to the patient, disruptive to the staff, and upsetting for everyone in general (Tughan, 1992). By the 1950s, adverse effects of separation on both parents and child began to be recognized (Page and Boeing, 1994). Children separated from their families demonstrate increased anxiety, crying, and grieving. Some refuse to eat and constantly watch the door through which their parents left. Parents also experience increased anxiety along with feelings of helplessness and frustration. In the mid-1990s, many PICUs still have restricted visiting that separates the child from his or her parents.

   b. *Rationale for restricted visiting:* Some caregivers feel that parents become too upset to remain at the child's bedside and that the children "behave better" without their parents. Staff members may feel uncomfortable being watched by parents during procedures. This is more likely to occur if the parents are hostile, critical, or the staff nurse is a novice. Having parents in the unit at all times could be a threat to patient confidentiality. Parents may require staff time that should be spent with the child. Some parents view restricted visiting in a positive way. They feel that the rules allow them to have a break and encourage them to eat and rest. In addition, the rules provide an explanation of why others cannot visit.

   c. *Rationale for open visiting:* Tughan (1992) found many parents felt they should be allowed to stay with their child during emergencies. Even more parents (81.2%) felt they should be able to stay in the PICU and provide support for their child during emergencies involving other children. Adult patients who described the benefits they gained from family visits attribute comfort, relaxation, reassurance, and moral support to the presence of family members (Simpson, 1991). Open visiting is beneficial to both children and parents by decreasing stress and anxiety (Page and Boeing, 1994). Parental involvement in the child's care can be enhanced by open visiting and may assist with discharge teaching and planning (Page and Boeing, 1994).

   d. *Meeting the needs of the children*
      - Encourage an open, supportive atmosphere where parents can come and go around the clock to meet their own needs and those of their child.
      - Make exceptions based on the child's individual needs.
      - Plan for exceptions to rules when a child is dying.
      - Explain to the family if the child's condition does not allow time for the nurse to visit with them just then.
      - Request assistance from the chaplain, social worker, clinical nurse specialist, or child life specialist in working with the family.
      - Close doors or curtains during procedures or admissions so that parents will be asked to leave less frequently.

- Consider the wishes of a parent who does not want to leave a child during a crisis or an arrest.
- Discuss other possible visitors with the parents to develop a plan that meets their needs as a family.

INTERVENTIONS FOR DYING CHILDREN

A. PAIN MANAGEMENT IN THE TERMINALLY ILL
   1. When a child is dying, the focus of care becomes pain relief and promotion of comfort of the child and family. In addition, there is a moral imperative to relieve the pain and suffering of dying children.
   2. As the child develops a tolerance toward the analgesic used, higher doses of narcotics may be required to provide adequate pain relief. High doses of narcotics carry the risk of respiratory depression and hastening the death of the child (Siever, 1994). According to the principle of double effect, when the intended goal is to relieve pain, it is ethically correct to give whatever dose of analgesic is necessary to relieve pain even if life is shortened as a secondary effect (Siever, 1994). Administration of a lethal dose of medication with the intent to cause death as a means of pain relief is not acceptable and is, in fact, active euthanasia (Siever, 1994).
   3. Nonpharmacologic means of pain relief are useful in the dying child but should never be used to the exclusion of medications.
   4. Give analgesics around the clock (ATC) rather than on an as needed (prn) basis to provide better control of pain.
   5. Fear of tolerance or addiction should not be a consideration in the dying child (Siever, 1994).

B. FORGOING LIFE-SUSTAINING MEDICAL TREATMENT
   1. Forgoing life-sustaining medical treatment includes decisions to withhold, withdraw, or limit medical treatment.
   2. Most ethicists feel there is no difference between withholding medical treatment and withdrawing treatment that has already been in use if the treatment is not beneficial to the patient (American Academy of Pediatrics Committee on Bioethics, 1994; Shekleton et al, 1994).
   3. When considering the value of medical treatment in children, the benefits of treatment must be weighed against the burdens of treatment placed on the child.
   4. In most cases, parents are the appropriate decision makers for children. Ideally, parents and caregivers collaborate in making decisions about limiting or withdrawing treatment. The wishes and desires of conscious, coherent children should be given serious consideration (American Academy of Pediatrics Committee on Bioethics, 1994; Frader and Thompson, 1994).
   5. A decision to withhold or withdraw any medical treatment applies only to that specific treatment and should not be generalized to other treatments or care.
   6. A do-not-resuscitate (DNR) order means only that no life-saving measures will be instituted in the event of a cardiac or respiratory arrest unless other measures have been discussed as well. It does not mean that the child should receive any less or different care than another child. It does not necessarily mean that the child is expected to die soon. A care and comfort only policy is written in positive terms and describes the care that will be given to the child such as supportive care and pain management. Limitation of treatment may include the decision to not institute any new therapies or to stop specific therapies already in use or to do both.

7. **Withdrawal of treatment:** Consult parents when planning the time of withdrawal of treatment. There is no urgent need to withdraw support immediately simply because a decision was made. Allow time for parents to gather whatever family members they wish to be with them. Consult the chaplain or social services for assistance. Families may want the clergy from their community to be contacted in addition to or instead of the hospital chaplain. Allow parents all the time they need to say their good-byes to the child both before and after treatment is withdrawn. Parents may wish to hold the child before and after treatment is withdrawn, especially if death is expected to quickly follow withdrawal of support. Parents may wish to play specific music for the child, have certain toys or security objects available, or carry out other rituals that have meaning for them as a family, especially if the child is likely to die when support is withdrawn.

8. Consider discontinuation of monitoring. If the unit has central monitoring capability, consider turning off the monitor in the child's room and continuing monitoring at the central station. Avoid having alarms go off in the child's room if no response to the alarms is planned.

9. Privacy is essential for a family when treatment is withdrawn from a child. Transfer to a private room or provide curtains if no private room is available. Ask parents if they would like to be alone with the child. Assure parents that assistance will be close by.

C. CARING FOR THE POTENTIAL ORGAN DONOR

1. Brain death is defined as the irreversible cessation of function of the whole brain, including the brain stem.

2. Critical care staff are required by law to identify potential organ and tissue donors.

3. Early referral to an organ procurement organization provides for the assistance of skilled professionals to help both caregivers and parents through the process of organ donation.

4. Uncouple the child's death from the idea of organ donation. Allow the family time to be with the child. Assess the family to determine if they are acknowledging the child's death to themselves. Note that acknowledgment is not acceptance. If the family is still asking if there is any chance that the child will recover, they have not acknowledged that the child is dead. Avoid raising the issue of organ donation at the same time the parents are told of the child's death. Allow at least a brief period of time between these events. If possible, allow some time between raising the issue of organ donation and asking for a decision.

5. It may be difficult for parents to believe a child is dead when the child's chest is still moving and a heart rate is visible on the monitor.

6. Parents may need to ask the same questions repeatedly before they are able to hear and remember what they have been told.

7. Assure the parents that organ donation will not disfigure the child's body or preclude an open casket (Yoder, 1994).

8. Offer parents the opportunity to hold the child prior to the time the organs are removed.

9. Some parents may want to leave the hospital before the child's organs are removed, whereas others may need to see the child again following surgery.

10. Be careful to treat the child who is going to be an organ donor with the same respect and dignity afforded to any child still living.

D. CARING FOR THE CONSCIOUS, DYING CHILD

Children who are terminally ill frequently know they are going to die even if they have not been told. Occasionally, families insist that children not be told about their impending death. It is important to help the parents realize that the child probably already knows or suspects and may not talk about it simply because he or she senses the parents' avoidance.

1. Ask the family about the child's understanding of death. Explore their thoughts concerning death to help you understand and support them.
2. Encourage parents to discuss the subject with the child and answer the child's questions.
3. Obtain support from clinical nurse specialists, social services, or chaplains as needed for the family and child.
4. Answer the child's questions openly and honestly.
5. Assure the child that he or she will not be left alone.
6. Allow whatever visitors the child wishes to see.
7. Consider obtaining assistance from a psychiatrist or psychologist for the child, siblings, parents, and caregivers.

E. **CARING FOR BEREAVED FAMILIES**

Grief is the cognitive, emotional, physical, psychologic, and spiritual response to an overwhelming loss. Grief is frequently described in terms of stages, phases, or symptoms. The use of phases is helpful in understanding that grief is a nonlinear process. The bereaved person moves in and out of the phases at various times in the grief process. Symptoms of one phase may overlap with another, and time limits should not be imposed on the individual for completion of this painful process. When a child dies, parental grief is the subjective and individualized response to a hideous loss.

1. **Lindemann** (1944) described symptomatology that was pathognomonic for grief:
   a. Somatic distress: Feelings of tightness in throat or chest, sighing, weakness, shortness of breath
   b. Preoccupation with the image of the deceased: Hearing or seeing the person who has died, inability to focus on anything other than loved one who died, emotional distance from others
   c. Feelings of guilt: Feeling responsible for loved one's death, searching for things that could have been done differently, thinking in terms of "if only"
   d. Hostile reactions: Feelings and expressions of anger
   e. Loss of patterns of conduct: Restlessness, inability to complete things started
2. **Kübler-Ross** (1969) described the stages of death and dying. As with grief, a person may move in and out of various stages at different times prior to reaching acceptance:
   a. Denial: Shock and disbelief
   b. Anger: Angry and hostile reactions expressed
   c. Bargaining: Attempts to delay the death
   d. Depression or despair
   e. Acceptance
3. **Miles and Perry** (1985) identified three phases of parental grief: (1) A state of numbness and shock, (2) a period of intense grief, and (3) a period of reorganization. During the early phase of numbness and shock, parents may use a variety of coping behaviors and display a wide range of emotions.
   a. Some parents may seem to be in a trance and display no emotion at all. They may show concern for others and even try to comfort other family members while expressing little emotion themselves.
   b. Many parents will cry. Some express grief loudly with keening and wailing, whereas others cry quietly. Some parents exhibit inappropriate silliness or euphoria. It is a mistake to judge a parent as unaffected or uncaring because of emotional reactions at the time of a death.

    c.   Although parents are in emotional shock and forget much of what is said to them, paradoxically they often remember verbatim the things that were said to them at the time of their child's death.

    d.   The numbness protects the person from feeling the full impact of their loss. It protects the mind from a grief that is too horrible to be faced at one time.

4. **Interventions with the family at the time of death**

    a.   *Be a presence.* If you are unable to think of something to say, be a silent presence. Being with a family may assist the parents in several ways. Feelings of isolation experienced by the parents may be reduced. Being with the family helps them to know that nothing is being hidden from them. One of the reasons for malpractice suits is that families sometimes feel they are not being told the truth or that information is being hidden. A receptive, nonverbal posture lets people know you are willing to listen if they need to talk. Bereaved parents have described caring people as those who were able to show that they cared by just "being there."

    b.   *Use a gentle touch to express caring and concern.* Be sensitive to those who are not comfortable being touched. This can usually be discerned by a stiffening in the person who was touched. Those who respond to touch will frequently grasp your hand or lean toward you as you touch them.

    c.   *Keep the focus on the family.* This is probably not the best time to share your own experiences, even if you have had a similar loss. Talking about your experiences may take the focus off the parents and put it on you and your own loss (Nelson, 1995). Caregivers who feel compelled to share their own losses may be attempting to meet their own needs rather than those of the parents.

    d.   *Provide opportunity to be with the child.* Go into the room with the parents. Prepare them for what they will see if they were not there at the time of death. Ask the parents if they prefer some time alone with their child. Remain close by and available to them. Offer parents the chance to hold their child. If death is imminent, be sure they understand their child could die while being held. Offer more than once if they seem to be having difficulty processing information given to them. In some circumstances the parents may ask the nurse to hold their child as he or she dies. Parents may wish to help care for the child's body. Offer the chance to bathe and dress the child or brush the child's hair. Provide a rocking chair if possible for parents to rock their child one last time. Siblings may benefit from being able to say good-bye and need to be reassured that they did not cause the illness and death.

    e.   *Consider a referral to a psychiatrist or psychologist* for siblings or parents who are coping poorly and who are beyond the scope of the clinical nurse specialist or social worker.

    f.   *Call the child by name.* Parents need to know that their child was special to others as well as to them.

    g.   *Avoid platitudes* such as "Time heals all wounds," "You wouldn't want him or her to live like that," or "You're lucky, it could have been worse." These phrases, although meant to comfort, tend to minimize a person's loss.

    h.   *Things you can say that are helpful*
- I'm sorry.
- This must be terribly hard for you.
- Is there anyone I can call for you?
- Would you like me to stay with you for a while?

    i.   *Avoid delaying the onset of grief* by offering the parents tranquilizers or sedatives on a routine basis. Medications may ease the situation for caregivers but only delay the inevitable for the parents. Parents may feel they are being told that their grief is not acceptable.

j. *Offer a remembrance packet to the family.* Keep a camera on the unit and offer to take a picture of the child if the parents wish either before or after the child's death. This may be especially important when an infant dies if the parents have few (if any) pictures. Handprints or footprints can easily be made on a card for the family. Parents may wish to have a lock of hair from the back of the child's head. Ask their permission prior to cutting the hair. Baptismal certificates or candles can be provided. Handprints or footprints can be easily made in plaster and provide a special keepsake.

k. *Provide factual information but do not dwell on details that the family has not requested.* Be prepared to answer the same questions more than once.

l. *Allow the family to talk about the child.* Ask questions about the child and listen to the family's answers. Do not be afraid of their tears or your own. Crying is a normal expression of grief for both family and caregivers. There is no need to say, "I didn't mean to remind you"; the parents have not forgotten.

m. *Develop a resource file on the unit* that includes information about grief for families and caregivers, materials to develop a remembrance packet, sympathy cards to be mailed to families, and a list of effective local self-help groups.

n. *A follow-up program is helpful to families.* An index card file system is useful to keep a record of the children who have died. Sympathy cards may be sent to bereaved parents a few weeks following the child's death and again on the first anniversary of the child's death, at Christmas, or any time chosen by the unit staff. Follow-up telephone calls give parents the chance to ask questions and to relate how they are doing. An offer to return to the hospital to visit with physicians or nurses may be helpful for some parents. If an autopsy was done, the parents might have questions and appreciate an opportunity to talk following the autopsy report (Todres et al, 1994).

o. *Consider developing a checklist to guide caregivers at the time of a child's death.* Include those things felt to be most important on your unit for parents.

5. **Take care of each other**

a. Offer emotional support and assistance to the nurse caring for a child who dies.

b. Consider support sessions following a death in the unit. The sessions may be facilitated by a clinical nurse specialist, social worker, or chaplain.
   - Consider attending the funeral or memorial service for a child. This ritual may assist the caregivers and offer support to the family as well.
   - If a child is expected to die, provide a resource person for the nurse who has never cared for a child at the time of death.

REFERENCES

American Academy of Pediatrics Committee on Bioethics. Guidelines on forgoing life-sustaining medical treatment. *Pediatr Nurs.* 1994;20(5):515–521.

Amico J, Davidhizar R. Supporting families of critically ill children. *J Clin Nurs.* 1994;3:213–218.

Anand KJS, Phil D, Hickey PR. Pain and its effects in the human neonate and fetus. *N Engl J Med.* 1987;317:1321–1329.

Bossert E. Factors influencing the coping of hospitalized school-age children. *J Pediatr Nurs.* 1994;9:299–306.

Braun R, St Clair C. Transitional family care: PICU to pediatrics. *Crit Care Nurse.* 1994;14(4):65–68.

Cataldo MF, Maldonado J. Psychological effects of pediatric intensive care on staff, patients, and family. In: Rogers MC, ed. *Textbook of Pediatric Intensive Care.* Baltimore, Md: Williams & Wilkins; 1987:1461–1477.

Corbo-Richert BH. Coping behaviors of young children during a chest tube procedure in the pediatric intensive care unit. *Matern Child Nurs J.* 1994;22:134–146.

Corbo-Richert BH, Caty S, Barnes CM. Coping behaviors of children hospitalized for cardiac surgery: a secondary analysis. *Matern Child Nurs J.* 1993;21:27–36.

Curley M, Wallace J. Effects of the Nursing Mutual Participation Model of Care on parental stress in the pediatric intensive care unit: a replication. *J Pediatr Nurs.* 1992;7:377–385.

Davidson JE, Dattolo JK, Goskowicz RL, et al. Neuromuscular blockade: nursing interventions and case studies from infancy to adulthood. *Crit Care Nurs Q.* 1993;15(4):53–67.

DePaul D, Chambers SE. Environmental noise in the neonatal intensive care unit: implications for nursing practice. *J Perinat Neonat Nurs.* 1995;8(4):71–76.

Dracup K. Helping patients and families cope. *Crit Care Nurse.* August 1993;(suppl):3–9.

Eland JM, Banner W. Assessment and management of pain in children. In: Hazinski MF, ed. *Nursing Care of the Critically Ill Child.* 2nd ed. St Louis, Mo: Mosby–Year Book, Inc; 1992:79–100.

Eland JM, Coy JA. Assessing pain in the critically ill child. *Focus Crit Care.* 1990;17(6):469–475.

Ellerton M, Ritchie JA, Caty S. Factors influencing young children's coping behaviors during stressful healthcare encounters. *Matern Child Nurs J.* 1994;22(3):74–82.

Foster R, Stevens B. Nursing management of pain in children. In: Betz CL, Hunsberger MM, Wright S, eds. *Family-Centered Nursing Care of Children.* 2nd ed. Philadelphia, Pa: WB Saunders Co; 1994:892–894.

Frader J, Thompson A. Ethical issues in the pediatric intensive care unit. *Pediatr Clin North Am.* 1994;41:1404–1421.

Griffin JP. The impact of noise on critically ill people. *Holistic Nurs Pract.* 1992;6(4):53–56.

Gross JP. Recollections of children experiencing pharmacologic paralysis. *Dimens Crit Care Nurs.* 1992;11:326–333.

Grumet GW. Pandemonium in the modern hospital. *N Engl J Med.* 1993;328:433–437.

Hart D, Bossert E. Self-reported fears of hospitalized school-age children. *J Pediatr Nurs.* 1994;9:83–90.

Kachoyeanos MK, Friedhoff M. Cognitive and behavioral strategies to reduce children's pain. *Matern Child Nurs J.* 1993;18:14–19.

Kidder C. Reestablishing health: factors influencing the child's recovery in pediatric intensive care. *J Pediatr Nurs.* 1989;4:96–103.

Kübler-Ross E. *On Death and Dying.* New York, NY: Macmillan Publishing Co Inc; 1969.

Lewandowski L. Psychosocial aspects of pediatric critical care. In: Hazinski MF, ed. *Nursing Care of the Critically Ill Child.* 2nd ed. St Louis, Mo: Mosby–Year Book Inc; 1992:19–77.

Lindemann E. Symptomatology and management of acute grief. In: Parad JJ, ed. *Crisis Intervention: Selected Readings.* New York, NY: Family Service Association of America; 1944:7–20.

McCaffrey M. Pain relief for the child: problem areas and selected nonpharmacological methods. *Pediatr Nurs.* 1977;3:11.

McCarthy DO, Ouimet ME, Daun JM. Shades of Florence Nightingale: potential impact of noise stress on wound healing. *Holistic Nurs Pract.* 1991;5(4):39–48.

Miles MS, Perry K. Parental responses to sudden accidental death of a child. *Crit Care Q.* 1985;8(1):73–84.

Nelson L. When a child dies. *Am J Nurs.* Mar 1995:61–64.

Page NE, Boeing NM. Visitation in the pediatric intensive care unit: controversy and compromise. *AACN Clin Issues Crit Care.* 1994;5:289–295.

Pederson C. Presence as a nursing intervention with hospitalized children. *Matern Child Nurs J.* 1993;21:75–81.

Purcell C. Holistic care of a critically ill child. *Intensive Crit Care Nurs.* 1993;9:108–115.

Rice LJ. Needle phobia: an anesthesiologist's perspective. *J Pediatr.* 1993;122(5; pt 2):S9–S13.

Rushton CH. Strategies for family-centered care in the critical care setting. *Pediatr Nurs.* 1990;16:195–199.

Schechter NL. The undertreatment of pain in children: an overview. *Pediatr Clin North Am.* 1989;36(4):781–794.

Schepp KG. Correlates of mothers who prefer control over their hospitalized children's care. *J Pediatr Nurs.* 1992;7:83–89.

Shekleton ME, Burns SM, Clochesy JM, et al. Terminal weaning from mechanical ventilation: a review. *AACN Clin Issues Crit Care.* 1994;5:523–533.

Siever BA. Pain management and potentially life-shortening analgesia in the terminally ill child: the ethical implications for pediatric nurses. *J Pediatr Nurs.* 1994;9:307–312.

Simpson T. The family as a source of support for the critically ill adult. *AACN Clin Issues Crit Care.* 1991;2:229–235.

Slota MC. Implications of sleep deprivation in the pediatric critical care unit. *Focus Crit Care.* 1988;15(3):35–43.

Stutts AL. Selected outcomes of technology dependent children receiving home care and prescribed child care services. *Pediatr Nurs.* 1994;20:501–507.

Todres ID, Earle M, Jellinek MS. Enhancing communication. *Pediatr Clin North Am.* 1994;41:1395–1403.

Tomlinson PS, Mitchell KE. On the nature of social support for families of critically ill children. *J Pediatr Nurs.* 1992;7:386–394.

Tughan L. Visiting in the PICU: a study of the perceptions of patients, parents, and staff members. *Crit Care Nurs Q.* 1992;15:57–68.

Vessey JA. Developmental approaches to examining young children. *Pediatr Nurs.* 1995;21(1):53–56.

Warner J, Norwood S. Psychosocial concerns of the ventilator-dependent child in the pediatric intensive care unit. *AACN Clin Issues Crit Care.* 1991;2:433–445.

Way C. Parental stress in paediatric intensive care. *Br J Nurs.* 1993;2:572–577.

Wells PW, DeBoard-Burns MB, Cook RC, Mitchell J. Growing up in the hospital, I: let's focus on the child. *J Pediatr Nurs.* 1994;9:66–73.

Whaley LF, Wong DL. *Nursing Care of Infants and Children.* St Louis, Mo: Mosby–Year Book Inc; 1995.

Yoder L. Comfort and consolation: a nursing perspective on parental bereavement. *Pediatr Nurs.* 1994;20: 473–477.

Zwick MB. Decreasing environmental noise in the NICU through staff education. *Neonat Intensive Care.* 1993;6(2):16–19.

2

Pulmonary System

HOLLY F. WEBSTER, MARY JO GRANT,
MARGARET C. SLOTA, and KAREN M. KILIAN

DEVELOPMENTAL ANATOMY OF THE RESPIRATORY SYSTEM

A. EMBRYOLOGY OF THE LUNG
1. **Glandular stage: Conception to 16th week:** The lung begins as a bud on the embryonic gut 28 days after conception. These rudimentary solid tubes grow and divide until the 16th week. By the fourth week of gestation, a lung bud branches from the primitive esophagus to form the airways and alveolar spaces. During weeks 7 through 10 the larynx is developed (Fig. 2–1).
2. **Canalicular stage: 16th to 24th week:** Vascularization of the lung occurs. The first capillaries can be identified in the middle of this phase. Alveolar ducts develop on the terminal bronchioles. Airways are lined with large cuboidal cells filled with glycogen. At about 18 weeks some of the epithelial cells become alveolar epithelial type II cells, which synthesize pulmonary surfactant. The fetus is potentially viable at the end of the canalicular stage of development.
3. **Alveolar stage: 24th week to birth:** Alveolar ducts surrounded by capillaries appear at 26 weeks. Alveoli and alveolar capillaries appear at 30 weeks (Fig. 2–2).
4. **The first breath:** The thorax is compressed as it passes through the birth canal forcing out some of the fetal lung fluid. Chest recoil after the thorax is delivered results in air entry into the lungs. The first inspiratory effort must be large enough to overcome the viscous resistance to movement of the intrapulmonary liquid and overcome the tissue and surface tension. For the first several minutes up to 2 hours, expiration is often incomplete resulting in progressively increasing functional residual capacity. For infants born by cesarean section, it takes longer to establish functional residual capacity. The prematurely born infant has a compliant chest cage, making diaphragmatic function inefficient and limiting the ability to generate a large transpulmonary pressure.

B. POSTNATAL DEVELOPMENT
1. The number of airway branches is fixed at birth, but **airway dimensions and alveolar number** increase until the child is about 8 years of age. The number of alveoli increases approximately tenfold and the air-tissue interface increases to a magnitude 21 times that which exists in the newborn. After birth, the number of alveoli continues to increase dramatically but ceases by 5 to 8 years of age. The smaller alveolar size of the infant predisposes the infant to alveolar collapse; however, alveolar diameter continues to increase until adulthood. Lung volume

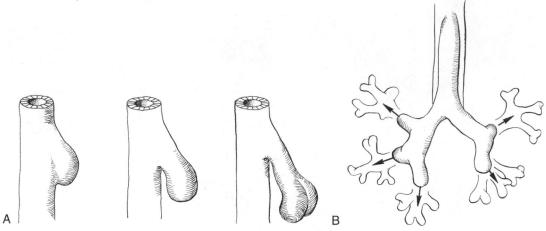

Figure 2–1. Embryologic development of the lungs.

increases fourfold during the first 12 months of life. Collateral ventilation does not develop until after infancy.

2. The infant **chest is cylindric in shape,** with the anteroposterior diameter equal to or slightly greater than the transverse diameter. Following birth there is more rapid growth of the transverse diameter. By about 3 years of age, the adult chest wall configuration is attained, with the transverse diameter greater than the anteroposterior diameter.

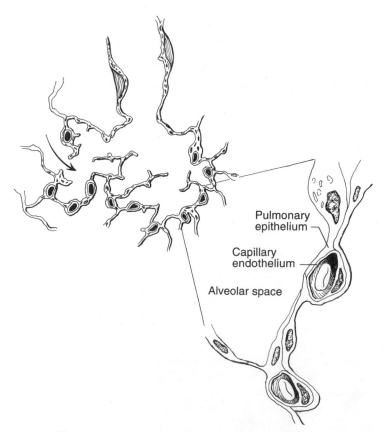

Pulmonary
epithelium

Capillary
endothelium

Alveolar space

Figure 2–2. Epithelial and endothelial development.

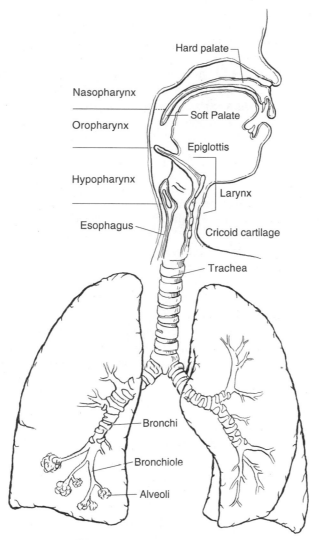

Figure 2–3. Airway anatomy.

C. UPPER AIRWAY DEVELOPMENT

The upper airway is responsible for warming, humidifying, and filtering air before it reaches the trachea (Fig. 2–3).

1. **Nose**
   a. *Embryology:* Nasal cavities begin as widely separated pits on the face of the 4-week-old embryo. At birth the maxillary sinuses are the largest. The ethmoid cells are present and increase in size throughout life. Frontal and sphenoid sinuses do not begin to invade the frontal or sphenoid bones until several years after birth.
   b. Until the age of 6 months, infants are obligatory nose breathers because the elongated epiglottis, positioned high in the pharynx, almost meets the soft palate. However, they are still able to mouth breathe, since blocked nares do not lead to complete upper airway obstruction. By the sixth month, growth and descent of the larynx reduces the amount of obstruction. Nasal breathing doubles the resistance to airflow and proportionately increases the work of breathing.

2. **Pharynx**
   a. *Embryology:* The oropharyngeal membrane between the foregut and the stomodeum begins to disintegrate to establish continuity between the oral cavity and the pharynx in the 4-week-old embryo.
   b. The pharynx is a musculomembranous tube that extends from the base of the skull to the esophageal and laryngeal inlets. The pharynx is the conduit for respiratory gas exchange and vital to the production of speech. The *nasopharynx* is located above the soft palate. The *oropharynx* extends from the soft palate to the level of the hyoid bone. The *hypopharynx* extends from the level of the hyoid bone to the esophageal inlet.

3. **Larynx**
   a. *Embryology:* During the fourth week of embryologic life, the laryngotracheal groove begins as a ridge on the ventral portion of the pharynx. Vocal cords begin to appear in the eighth week. In the newborn infant the larynx is approximately at the level of the second cervical vertebra. In the adult the larynx is opposite the fifth and sixth cervical vertebrae.
   b. The larynx is a funnel-shaped structure that connects the pharynx and trachea. It includes the thyroid cartilage, vocal cords, epiglottis, and the cricoid cartilage. It is important in the production of the cough and protects the airway from aspiration of food during deglutition.
      - Compared with the adult's epiglottis, the child's *epiglottis* is longer and more flaccid. The epiglottis in a newborn extends over the larynx approximately at a 45-degree angle. This more anterior and cephalad epiglottis may make intubation of the airway more difficult in the small infant.
      - In the infant and small child the narrowest portion of the airway is the *cricoid cartilage ring*. This is the only point within the larynx in which the walls are completely enclosed in cartilage. In the rest of the trachea the posterior wall is membranous. Resistance to airflow is inversely proportional to the fourth power of the radius ($R = \frac{1}{r^4}$). Thus, swelling from trauma or infection can lead to additional narrowing in this area, producing large increases in airway resistance.
      - *Vocal cords* must abduct to allow exchange of respiratory gases and close to prevent aspiration.

4. **Trachea**
   a. *Embryology:* The trachea begins to develop in the 24-day-old embryo. At 26 to 28 days a series of asymmetric branchings of the primitive lung bud initiate the development of the bronchial tree.
   b. The trachea is a thin-walled rigid tube. It is characterized by a framework of 16 to 20 cartilages that encircle the trachea, except in its posterior aspect, which is membranous and contains smooth muscle.
   c. The trachea's nervous, vascular, and lymphatic supplies are independent of those to the lungs.

D. **LOWER AIRWAY (LUNG) DEVELOPMENT**
   1. **Lung**
      a. The lungs at birth weigh about 40 g and double in weight by 6 months. By age 2 years, when most of the alveolarization process is completed, they weigh about 170 g. Normal adult lungs weigh approximately 1000 g.
      b. The right lung has three lobes, and the left has two lobes, each further subdivided into bronchopulmonary segments. The surface of the lung is covered with the visceral pleura.

2. **Conducting airways**
   a. *Intrapulmonary airways* may be divided into three major groups: cartilaginous bronchi, membranous bronchioles, and gas exchange units.
      - *Cartilaginous bronchi* are the large airways including 9 to 12 divisions terminating in bronchi having a diameter of approximately 1 mm.
      - *Membranous bronchioles* comprise an additional 12 divisions before ending as terminal bronchioles, the last conducting structure in the lung.
   b. The airways are lined with epithelial membrane that gradually changes from ciliated pseudostratified columnar epithelium in the bronchi to a ciliated cuboidal epithelium near the gas exchange units.
   c. In the largest airways a smooth muscle bundle connects the two ends of the C-shaped cartilage. As the amount of cartilage decreases, the smooth muscle assumes a helical orientation and gradually becomes thinner.

3. **Gas exchange units (alveoli)**
   a. *Alveoli* are a complex network of pulmonary capillaries in which gas exchange takes place. Alveoli are lined by two epithelial cell types. Type I cells cover approximately 90% of the total alveolar surface. These cells are adapted to allow for the rapid exchange of gases. Type II cells, which secrete surfactant material that lowers surface tension and maintains the patency of alveoli during respiration, make up the other 10%.
   b. Two types of *intercommunicating channels* provide collateral ventilation for the gas exchange units. *Alveolar pores of Kohn* are holes in the alveolar wall that provide channels for gas movement between alveoli. These pores are not present until 6 to 8 years of age. *Canals of Lambert* are accessory channels that connect a small airway to an airspace normally supplied by a different airway.
   c. Gas exchange involves the movement of gas between the atmosphere and the alveoli and the pulmonary capillary blood. This movement is by simple passive diffusion where the gases travel from an area of high to an area of low partial pressure.

E. **THORACIC CAVITY**
   1. **Diaphragm**
      a. The diaphragm is the principal muscle of inspiration. If the chest wall is stiff, contraction of the diaphragm during inspiration decreases the pressure within the thoracic cavity and increases thoracic volume. It is innervated by the phrenic nerve (third, fourth, and fifth cervical spinal nerves).
      b. The diaphragm inserts more horizontally in the infant than in the older child or adult.
   2. **The chest wall** in the infant is very compliant when compared to the rigid chest wall of the older child and adult. In the presence of lung disease, contraction of the diaphragm results in intercostal and sternal retractions rather than inflation of the lungs.

F. **PULMONARY CIRCULATION**
   Development closely follows development of the airways and alveoli.
   1. **Embryology:** *Preacinar arteries,* which branch along the airways, develop in utero. Muscular arteries end at the level of the terminal bronchiole in the fetus and newborn but gradually extend to the alveolar level during childhood. Prematurely born infants have less well-developed vascular smooth muscle.
   2. **Pulmonary blood volume:** The lungs receive the entire cardiac output from the right ventricle if there are no intracardiac right-to-left shunts.
   3. **Pulmonary lymphatics:** The lymphatic system is composed of a superficial network in the pleura and the deep network around the bronchi and pulmo-

nary arteries and veins. An increase in the hydrostatic pressure of the pulmonary and systemic circulation can result in effusions by decreasing the rate of pleural fluid absorption.

DEVELOPMENTAL PHYSIOLOGY OF THE RESPIRATORY SYSTEM

A. **PHYSIOLOGIC FUNCTION**

The primary function of the lung is to deliver oxygen to the body and to remove carbon dioxide. During inspiration, the diaphragm contracts, the chest wall expands, and the volume of the lungs increases. Gas flows from the atmosphere into the lung and oxygen diffuses into the blood at the alveolar-capillary interface. During expiration the diaphragm and the chest wall relax, thoracic volume decreases, intrathoracic pressure increases, and gas flows out of the lung. This process is affected by pulmonary compliance and resistance and by pulmonary vascular pressures and resistance.

1. **Pulmonary compliance and resistance**
   a. *Compliance* is the measure of the distensibility of the lungs influenced by surfactant and elasticity of lung tissue.
      - Volume change is produced by a transpulmonary pressure change ($C_1 = \Delta V / \Delta P$). For example, if the volume change produced by a given pressure change is small, the lungs are stiff, or they have a decreased compliance.
      - Compliance of the infant chest wall (especially premature infants) is considerably greater than that of the adult. There is less opposition to lung collapse. Compliance is decreased by pulmonary edema, pneumothorax, pulmonary fibrosis and atelectasis. Compliance is increased by lobar emphysema.
   b. *Airway resistance* is the driving pressure of air divided by the airflow rate determined by airway diameter. It is directly proportional to flow rate, the length of the airway, and the viscosity of the gas and is inversely proportional to the fourth power of the airway radius (Poiseuille's law).
      - The upper airway contributes 70% of the total airway resistance in adults and 50% of total airway resistance in infants. In infants the small peripheral airways may contribute as much as 50% of the total airway resistance as compared to less than 20% for the adult.
      - Resistance is increased by asthma, cystic fibrosis, bronchopulmonary dysplasia, bronchiolitis, tracheal stenosis, and increased respiratory secretions. High resistance increases the work of breathing and creates respiratory distress.

2. **Pulmonary vascular pressures and resistance:** also see Fetal Circulation in Chapter 3.
   a. *Changes in pulmonary circulation at birth*
      - The fetus has low pulmonary blood flow from high pulmonary vascular resistance. This high pulmonary vascular resistance is due to hypoxic vasoconstriction, thicker pulmonary musculature, and smaller surface area. At birth there is a decrease in pulmonary vascular resistance associated with ventilation and the effect of oxygen. In the 6 to 8 weeks following birth there is a further progressive fall in resistance associated with thinning of the smooth muscle layer.

- Pulmonary blood flow is not uniformly distributed throughout the lung. It is gravity dependent related to regional differences in pulmonary vascular pressure and resistance (Fig. 2–4).

b. *Intravascular pulmonary pressure* is measured by placing a catheter in the pulmonary artery and measuring systolic, diastolic, and mean arterial pressures. A balloon-tipped catheter wedged in a pulmonary artery branch approximates the left atrial pressure. Beyond the newborn period, pulmonary artery systolic pressure averages 20 mm Hg, and diastolic pressure is 10 mm Hg with a mean pressure of about 15 mm Hg.

c. *Ventilation-perfusion matching:* Regional differences in lung perfusion are described by West's zones of perfusion. Blood flow is least at the apex and increases at the base of the lung in an upright position.

- Zone I is located in the apexes of an upright adult. Mean pulmonary arterial pressure is less than alveolar pressure.
- Zone II is located in the midlung field. Pulmonary artery pressure is greater than alveolar pressure, which is greater than pulmonary venous pressure.
- Zone III is found in the base of the lung of an upright adult. Pulmonary artery and venous pressure is greater than alveolar pressure.

d. *Pulmonary vascular resistance* is increased by an increase in blood viscosity or a decrease in total cross-sectional area of the resistance vessels related to fewer number of vessels or normal number with narrowing.

- Increased blood viscosity is most commonly seen as a result of a raised hematocrit from cyanotic heart disease. A rise in hematocrit from 40% to 70% approximately doubles blood viscosity.
- A decreased total number of vessels may occur with congenital lung lesions such as hypoplasia or cystic lung changes.

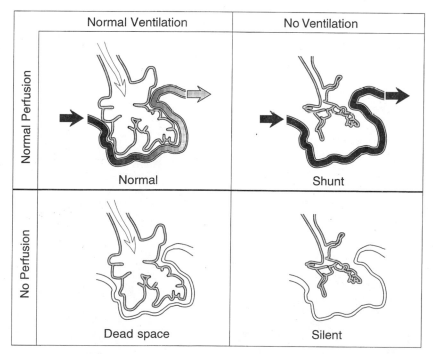

Figure 2–4. Ventilation-perfusion relationships.

- A decreased luminal diameter with a normal number of vessels is more common. Vasoconstriction can be due to biologically active agents (serotonin, norepinephrine) or alveolar hypoxia and metabolic acidemia. Hypoxic pulmonary vasoconstriction occurs when the lungs are ventilated with hypoxic gas. As a result pulmonary arterial pressure increases almost immediately. This process is reversible with the return to ventilation with normal concentrations of oxygen. Hypoxic pulmonary vasoconstriction shunts blood flow away from hypoxic regions of the lung. This minimizes ventilation-perfusion mismatch and optimizes systemic oxygenation.

3. **Control of breathing**
   a. *Central respiratory centers:* The medulla is responsible for the normal rhythm of respiration. The pons contains the apneustic center.
   b. *Peripheral neural reflexes:* Respiratory mechanoreceptors that can affect respiration are located within the upper airways, trachea, and lungs. Impulses are transmitted to the brain stem respiratory centers via the vagus nerve.
   c. *Chemical control of respiration* is mediated by chemosensitive areas in the medulla and through peripheral chemoreceptors (Fig. 2–5).
      - When the medulla is perfused with fluid of a low pH or high P_{CO_2}, it triggers a marked increase in neural discharge. Carbon dioxide freely diffuses from the blood into cerebrospinal fluid. An increase in Pa_{CO_2} quickly increases the hydrogen ion concentration in the cerebrospinal

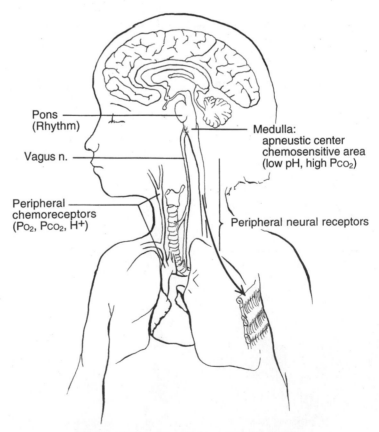

Figure 2–5.   Chemical control of breathing.

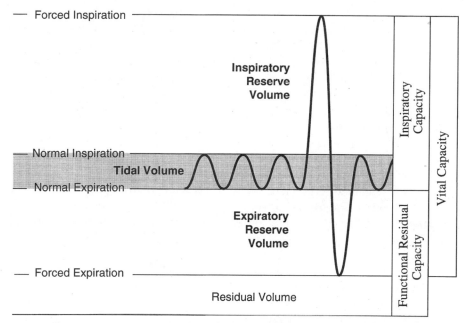

Figure 2–6. Lung volumes.

fluid. This occurs as carbon dioxide combines with water to form carbonic acid (H_2CO_3), which then dissociates into bicarbonate and hydrogen ion. The result is a rise in hydrogen ion concentration and a fall in pH, causing respiratory acidosis.

$$CO_2 + H_2O = H_2CO_3 = H^+ + HCO_3^-$$

- Peripheral chemoreceptors are located at the carotid bifurcation and the arch of the aorta. They respond to changes in arterial Po_2, Pco_2, and hydrogen ion concentration.

4. **Mechanics of breathing:** Elastic properties of the lung come from the elastic tissue and collagen that support the lungs' internal structures. Lung compliance changes with age. The thorax of the infant is much more compliant than an adult. At rest the pressure at the *surface* of the lung is close to atmospheric.

5. **Lung volumes** (Fig. 2–6)
   a. *Total lung capacity* (TLC) is the total volume of the gas contained in the lung at maximum inspiration.
   b. *Vital capacity* (VC) is the maximum volume expired from total lung capacity with maximal expiration.
   c. *Functional residual capacity* (FRC) is the volume of gas remaining in the lungs at the end of a normal expiration.
   d. *Residual volume* is the volume of gas remaining in the lung following a maximal respiratory effort.

B. **GAS EXCHANGE AND TRANSPORT**

Respiratory gas exchange involves the movement of gas from the atmosphere to the alveoli to the pulmonary capillary blood. The alveolar capillary membrane permits the transfer of oxygen and carbon dioxide while restricting the movement of fluid from pulmonary vasculature to alveoli.

1. **Diffusion**
   a. Oxygen diffuses from the alveolus through the alveolar epithelial lining, basement membrane, capillary endothelial lining, plasma, and the red

blood cell. Blood passing through the lung resides in a pulmonary capillary for only 0.75 second. Diffusion of oxygen depends on a difference (gradient) between alveolar and oxygen tension.

b. Carbon dioxide diffuses from the red blood cell to the plasma, through the capillary endothelial lining, basement membrane, and alveolar epithelial lining. The pulmonary capillary mean alveolar carbon dioxide gradient is smaller than that of oxygen.

2. **Oxygen transport**

a. After oxygen passes through the alveolus to the pulmonary capillary, it is carried in two forms:
   - Dissolved oxygen = 0.003 ml O_2/dl $\times$ Pao_2 (Eq. 1)
   - Oxygen bound to hemoglobin (oxyhemoglobin): Hemoglobin concentration (mg/dl) $\times$ 1.34 ml O_2/g Hgb $\times$ Sao_2 (Eq. 2)

b. The total arterial oxygen content is the oxygen bound to hemoglobin plus the dissolved oxygen: Arterial oxygen content = *Equation 1 + Equation 2.*

c. The oxygen capacity is dependent on the oxyhemoglobin dissociation curve.

3. **Oxyhemoglobin dissociation curve** (Fig. 2–7)

a. The oxyhemoglobin dissociation curve is an "S-shaped" curve with percent hemoglobin saturation on the Y axis and Po_2 in millimeters of mercury on the X axis. The release of oxygen to the tissues is facilitated by the proportional relationship of saturation to Po_2. Thus, on the steep portion of the dissociation curve relatively small changes in Po_2 cause large changes in oxygen saturation of hemoglobin.

b. A shift to the right, which facilitates the unloading of oxygen from hemoglobin, is caused by a decrease in pH, increase in Pco_2, elevated temperature, or increase in 2,3-diphosphoglycerate (2,3-DPG). 2,3-DPG decreases the affinity of hemoglobin for oxygen. During hypoxia or anemia, oxygen availability is increased within a matter of hours by an increase in 2,3-DPG.

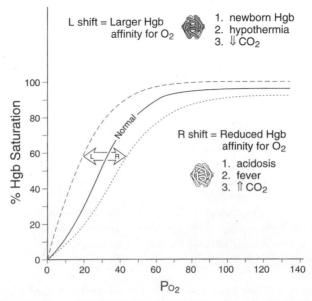

Figure 2–7.   Oxyhemoglobin dissociation curve. *Hgb,* hemoglobin.

    c. A shift to the left, which increases binding of oxygen to hemoglobin, is caused by an increase in pH, decrease in P_{CO_2}, decreased temperature, or decrease in 2,3-DPG.

    d. With fetal hemoglobin the dissociation curve is shifted to the left of the adult hemoglobin curve. Thus, at a given P_{O_2} and hematocrit, fetal hemoglobin is more readily oxygenated than adult blood. Fetal hemoglobin also releases oxygen less readily to the tissues than adult hemoglobin. Fetal hemoglobin is replaced by adult hemoglobin within 4 to 6 weeks after birth.

CLINICAL ASSESSMENT OF PULMONARY FUNCTION

A. HISTORY

1. **Prenatal and delivery** history should include gestational age and Apgar scores, respiratory distress in the neonatal period including oxygen requirement and ventilatory assistance, and length of hospital stay.
2. **Childhood history**
   a. Immunizations and tuberculosis tests: Verify with records
   b. Family history of "asthma," allergies, or other respiratory illnesses
   c. Wheezing episodes with previous illnesses
   d. Frequency of colds and upper respiratory tract illnesses
   e. Environmental smoke in home
   f. Supervision of child (especially if less than 5 years old) to evaluate the risk of foreign body aspiration
   g. Recent illnesses of child or family member
   h. Daily medications and medications used to treat respiratory symptoms
3. **Other significant information**
   a. *Chest pain* (rarely of cardiac origin) is described in quality, timing with respiratory phase, duration (continuous or intermittent), and precipitating factors.
   b. *Growth and development:* Failure to gain weight is often the first sign of chronic pulmonary disease. Activity level or milestones may be delayed with chronic pulmonary dysfunction.
   c. *Gastrointestinal symptoms*
      • Pneumonic processes frequently manifest by generalized abdominal pain in young children.
      • Acute or chronic infection may cause anorexia and occasionally vomiting.
      • Upper airway mucus may impede swallowing and cause gagging, vomiting, or diarrhea in infants and toddlers.
      • Bulky, foul-smelling stools may indicate cystic fibrosis.
      • Gastroesophageal reflux may cause chronic pulmonary aspiration.
   d. *Sleeping habits:* Evaluate duration of sleep at night and causes of interruptions. Nighttime coughing is a frequent symptom of asthma or other lower respiratory tract diseases. Note positioning for sleep (flat or requiring head elevation). If humidifier is used, note care and maintenance of the humidifier.

B. PHYSICAL EXAMINATION

1. **Inspection**
   a. *Anatomic landmarks* of the thorax provide a method for describing physical examination findings (Fig. 2–8).

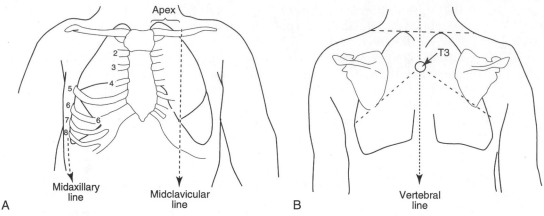

A

B

Figure 2–8. Anatomic landmarks of the thorax. The lower lobes of both lungs have only small projections on the anterior plane on the x-ray film and can be better visualized on a lateral or posterior x-ray film. The midaxillary line, midclavicular line, vertebral line, and intercostal spaces are frequently used landmarks in describing the location of pulmonary findings. **A,** Anterior view: Left lung is divided into two lobes by the left oblique fissure. The right lung is divided into three lobes by the horizontal fissure, with landmarks between the fourth rib medially and the fifth rib laterally. The right oblique fissure is found from the inferior margin (midclavicular line) to the fifth lateral rib. **B,** Posterior view: Fissures dividing upper and lower lobes begin at T-3, medially, extending in a line inferiorly below the inferior tips of the scapula.

b. *Thoracic inspection*
  • Note thoracic contour. A neonate's chest is round with the anterioposterior diameter equal to the transverse diameter. Chest contour is more oval by 2 to 3 years of age. Disproportionate size may be detected by comparing head circumference (occipitofrontal circumference [OFC]) to chest circumference. From birth to 2 years the head and chest circumferences are generally equal. During childhood, chest size is 5 to 7 cm greater than the OFC. Chronic disease may cause enlarged anteroposterior diameter ("barreled" chest similar to the neonate contour) (Fig. 2–9).

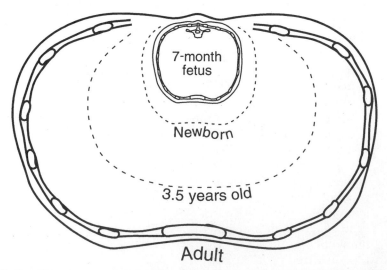

Figure 2–9. Thoracic contours by age. Comparison of the anteroposterior diameter and contour of the chest wall according to age.

- Note skeletal deformities. Anomalies such as sternal depression (pectus excavatum) or protrusion (pectus carinatum) may cause, or be associated with, respiratory abnormalities by altering pulmonary mechanics. Inspect posterior thoracic structures and the spine. Kyphosis and scoliosis can impair pulmonary mechanics (Fig. 2–10).
- Note symmetry of excursion.

c. *Respiratory effort*
- Rate and rhythm is age related. Respiratory rate is approximately one fourth of the pulse rate.
- Evaluate the adequacy of thoracic excursion (depth of respiration).
- Note the effort of breathing. Infants and young children breathe principally with the diaphragm. Infants in respiratory distress may exhibit nasal flaring, head bobbing, expiratory grunting, or head extension.
- Note the use of accessory muscles. Signs of respiratory insufficiency include suprasternal, substernal, intercostal, and subcostal retractions.
- Variations in respiratory patterns are also observed with various neurologic abnormalities (Fig. 2–11).

d. *Note the quality of the voice and breathing,* especially muffled voice, stridor, expiratory wheezing, and barky, loose, congested, or paroxysmal cough.

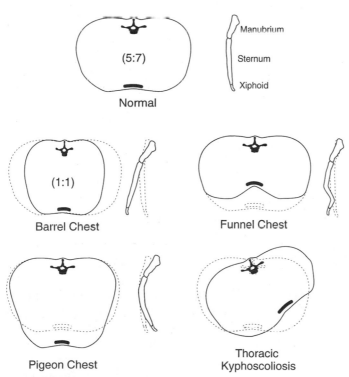

Figure 2–10.   Deformities of chest wall.
- **Barrel chest:** Ratio of anterioposterior diameter to lateral diameter is 1:1.
- **Funnel chest:** Depression in lower portion of Sternum, which may compress the heart and great vessels.
- **Pigeon chest** (pectus carinatum): Sternum is displaced anteriorly. Grooves in chest wall accentuate the deformity.
- **Thoracic kyphoscoliosis:** Spine is curved, with corresponding changes in the thorax.

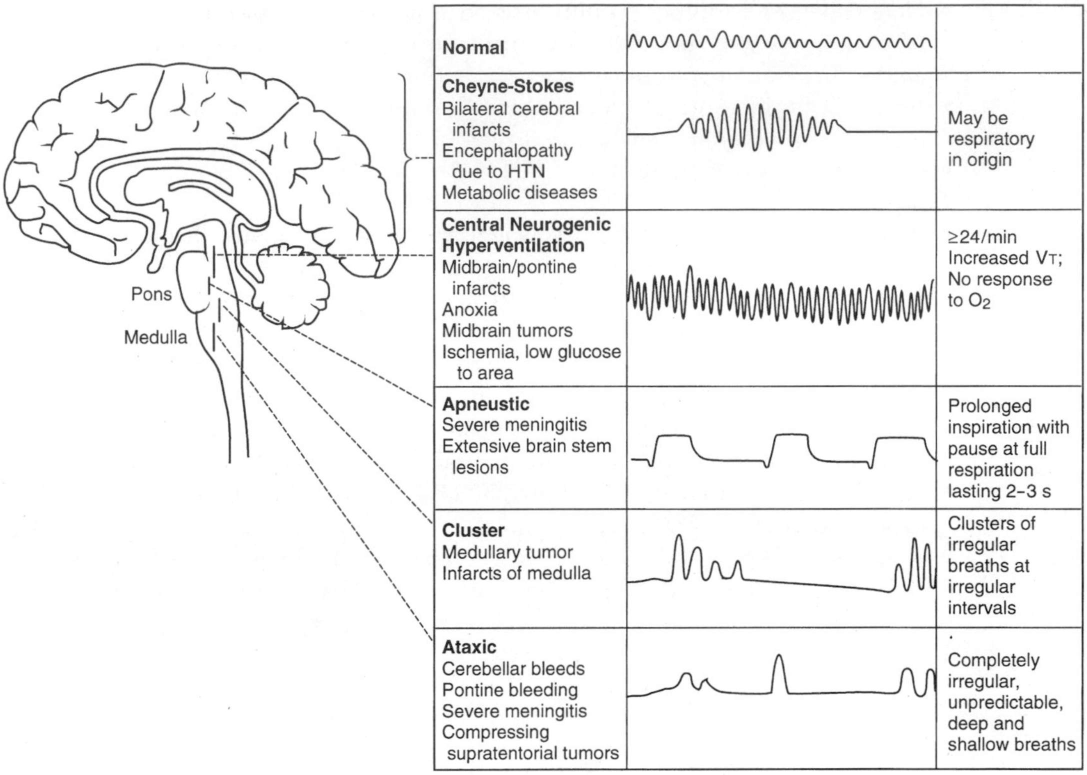
Pons
Medulla
Normal
Cheyne-Stokes
Bilateral cerebral infarcts
Encephalopathy due to HTN
Metabolic diseases
May be respiratory in origin
Central Neurogenic Hyperventilation
Midbrain/pontine infarcts
Anoxia
Midbrain tumors
Ischemia, low glucose to area
≥24/min
Increased VT;
No response to O2
Apneustic
Severe meningitis
Extensive brain stem lesions
Prolonged inspiration with pause at full respiration lasting 2-3 s
Cluster
Medullary tumor
Infarcts of medulla
Clusters of irregular breaths at irregular intervals
Ataxic
Cerebellar bleeds
Pontine bleeding
Severe meningitis
Compressing supratentorial tumors
Completely irregular, unpredictable, deep and shallow breaths

Figure 2–11. Variations in respiratory patterns. Breathing patterns as associated with anatomic regions of the brain. Lesions causing global injury tend to cause an orderly progression of respiratory patterns down to the brain stem. Focal lesions may cause a lower CNS pattern, while higher function is otherwise noted on examination. *HTN,* hypertension; V_T, tidal volume.

e. *Note skin color and appearance.*
- Cyanosis is observed when 3 to 5 g of hemoglobin becomes desaturated. Conditions that may mask or mimic cyanosis include hypothermia, anemia, or polycythemia. If cyanosis persists with oxygen administration, it may indicate an intracardiac shunt.
- Clubbing of fingertips is an indication of chronic hypoxia. The distal phalanx is flat and broad, causing a "club" appearance.

2. **Palpation** is a limited technique in infants but useful in older children.

a. *Expand hands bilaterally and symmetrically across the anterior chest wall and then across the posterior chest wall to evaluate* the following:
- Expansion of the thoracic cage
- Fremitus is conduction of the child's voice while the child says "99." Vibrations should be noted at the trachea and upper airway. Decreased sensation is normally observed centrally near large airways; otherwise, it is associated with occlusions. Increased sensation is associated with solid masses (consolidations). In infants, palpation during crying allows a similar evaluation.
- Palpation of fine vibrations may indicate underlying pleural friction rub.

b. *Palpate the entire thoracic cage for crepitus,* a coarse, crackly feeling (and sound) of air in the subcutaneous tissue.

c. *Evaluate the skeletal structure,* especially clavicles with a history of trauma.

    d. *Palpate the tracheal position* (midline); if shifted, locate the position of maximal impulse (PMI) of the heart. A shift in either or both may indicate fluid or air collection or a collapsed lung.

3. **Percussion**

    a. Percussion is a technique used to determine the presence of air, fluid, or masses in the underlying lung and to determine anatomic landmarks (such as the upper margin of the liver; Fig. 2–12).

    b. *Percuss using the middle finger of one hand flush against the chest wall* in interspaces, noting the quality of sound produced by striking this finger with the middle finger of the other hand.

        • Right side of the anterior chest: Percussion sounds should be resonant in each intercostal space down to the fifth to sixth intercostal space, where the superior liver margin begins. There the sound changes to a dull quality. Farther down where the lung field ends and liver remains, the percussion note becomes flat.

        • Left side of the anterior chest: Percussion of the heart borders can be determined. The superior border is often percussed between the second and third intercostal spaces. The inferior border is at the fourth to sixth intercostal space, and the left border is just lateral to the midclavicular line. At the sixth intercostal space and below, tympany may be observed due to an air-filled stomach.

        • Posterior chest: Percuss side to side to identify abnormal densities.

    c. *Variations in sounds define the density of structures:*

        • Flat: Short, soft; heard over *bone*

        • Dull: Medium pitch; duration heard over liver, spleen, and *mass densities*

        • Resonance: Low, loud, and long; heard over air-filled *lung*

        • Hyperresonance: Deep pitched, loud, and prolonged; heard over *overinflated lung* or air collections such as pneumothorax

        • Tympany: High, musical quality, loud; heard over *gas-filled organs such as the stomach*

4. **Auscultation**

    a. *Evaluate pitch, intensity, quality, and duration of each phase, using the diaphragm of the stethoscope.* For small infants, either a small diaphgram or the bell of a stethoscope may enable localization of sounds.

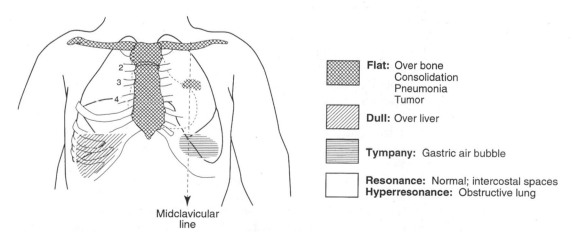

Midclavicular line

Flat: Over bone
Consolidation
Pneumonia
Tumor

Dull: Over liver

Tympany: Gastric air bubble

Resonance: Normal; intercostal spaces
Hyperresonance: Obstructive lung

Figure 2–12.   Percussion of the thorax. Differences in densities are noted to detect the presence of abnormal air, fluid, bone, or mass.

b. *Compare side to side,* starting at the apex and proceeding methodically to the bases. The thin-walled chests of infants create transmitted breath sounds throughout the lung fields. Listen for discreet changes from one location to the next. For emergent situations a quick check under each axilla (rather than upper lobes of the lungs) allows gross determination of the presence of bilateral aeration.

c. *Quality of pitch: Vesicular breath sounds* (I > E) are of long inspiration, low pitch, and soft intensity and are heard over most of the lungs. *Bronchial breath sounds* (I < E) have an equal or longer expiratory phase; are high pitched, loud, and blowing; and are heard over the large airways. Bronchial breath sounds are abnormal when heard over the peripheral lung tissue. *Bronchovesicular breath sounds* (I = E) are high-pitched tubular sounds.

- *Adventitious sounds* are abnormal sounds superimposed on normal breath sounds. Abnormal sounds have classically been defined as rales, rhonchi, and wheezes. However, confusion over definitions has prompted a focus on describing the *quality* and *location* of these sounds, to associate them with common causes. Attention should be given to pitch, timing (inspiratory or expiratory), location, and whether they clear with cough.
  - ○ Fine, high-pitched crackling noises (similar to the sound of rolling hair between fingers) may be heard at end inspiration over peripheral lung fields in pneumonia and pulmonary edema. Medium-pitched crackles are heard in early to mid inspiration with pulmonary edema and with diffuse secretions in the bronchioles. These may partially clear with coughing. Upper airway secretions may cause coarse, bubbling (rhonchi) sounds that clear with cough.
  - ○ Inflamed pleural surfaces may result in a very fine, low-pitched crackle over the focal areas of the chest during both inspiratory and expiratory phases. With cessation of breathing, the crackles are not heard.
  - ○ Wheezing results from narrowed airway lumina. Inspiratory wheezing usually results from high obstruction such as laryngeal edema or foreign bodies. Expiratory wheezing often results from lower obstruction such as with bronchiolitis, severe asthma, or chronic obstructive lung disease.

d. *Diminished or absent breath sounds* are noted as the focal absence of sounds, with occasional crackling, or as an abnormal quality or abnormal location of normal sounds. This may occur in atelectasis, pneumothorax, or with pleural fluid accumulation.

C. **ABNORMAL PHYSICAL EXAMINATION FINDINGS**

1. **Stridor** (Table 2–1)

a. *Description:* Noisy breathing caused by increased turbulence of airflow through a lumen.
- Inspiratory stridor is related to the inward collapse of structures during inspiration. It is most common with supraglottic or glottic lesions because of the negative pressure generated during inspiration.
- Expiratory stridor is most commonly observed with subglottic lesions.
- Fixed lesions (e.g., subglottic stenosis) may cause both inspiratory and expiratory stridor.

b. *Evaluation of the child with stridor includes* nasal patency, size of tongue and mandible, quantity of oropharyngeal secretions and presence of drooling, quality of phonation, head and neck range of motion, evidence of tooth evulsion or oral trauma, presence of fever or infectious symptoms, neurologic status, and the rate of progression of symptoms.

Table 2–1. EVALUATION OF STRIDOR

	SUPRAGLOTTIC	**SUBGLOTTIC**	**TRACHEAL**
Phase of respiration	Inspiratory	Inspiratory or biphasic	Expiratory
Phonation	Muffled	Weak or breathy	Absent or high pitched
Pitch of stridor	Coarse, low pitch	High-pitched, barking or rough cough	

	Differential Diagnosis for Upper Airway Stridor
Intrinsic lesions	Subglottic stenosis
	Web laryngocele
	Tumors such as papillomas
	Laryngomalacia
	Tracheomalacia
	Tracheoesophageal fistula
Extrinsic lesions	Vascular ring
	Cyst hygroma
	Neurologic lesions such as lymphomas
Infections	Epiglottitis
	Laryngotracheobronchitis
	Peritonsillar abscess
	Bacterial tracheitis
	Infectious mononucleosis
Other	Craniofacial abnormalities
	Trauma
	Foreign body aspiration
	Hypertrophic tonsils or adenoids
	Allergic reactions
	Corrosive ingestions

- Note position of preference. Infants with laryngomalacia, micrognathia, or macroglossia often have less distress when placed in a prone position. Children with epiglottitis or croup (laryngotracheobronchitis) often position themselves upright; children with moderate obstruction may exhibit forward extension of the head.

2. **Cyanosis**
   a. *Description:* Central or peripheral blue discoloration of skin tissue caused by desaturated hemoglobin. Cyanosis is usually not appreciated until 3 to 5 g of hemoglobin per deciliter of serum are desaturated, corresponding to an Sao_2 of 80% to 85% in a normal child. Cyanosis is *not* caused by an elevated $Paco_2$. Cyanosis may be caused by other nonpulmonary conditions.
      - Cyanosis may be masked by anemia, causing a more pallid color, or polycythemia, which may create a more "ruddy" color (Fig. 2–13).
   b. *Evaluation of the cyanotic child*
      - Oxygen should be administered before proceeding with the evaluation. Note the response to oxygen and the general degree of distress. If moderate or severe, emergency management should be given before proceeding with further evaluation.
      - Note whether cyanosis is peripheral (nail beds), central (lip and tongue color), or both.

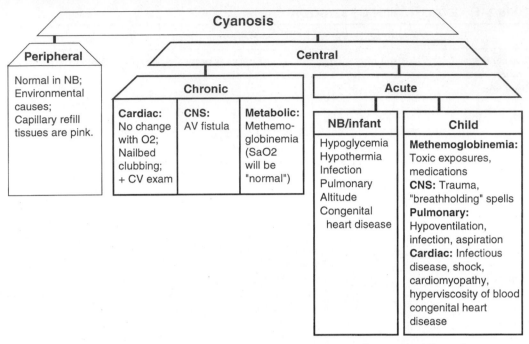

Figure 2–13. Etiology of cyanosis. *AV*, arteriovenous; *CV*, cardiovascular; *NB*, newborn.

Table 2–2. COMMON CAUSES OF COUGH BY AGE GROUPS

Neonates	Infections
	Chlamydia
	Viral: Cytomegalovirus, rubella, pertussis
	Congenital malformations
	Tracheoesophageal fistula
	Vascular rings
	Airway malformations
Infants	Above, plus
	Infections
	Viral bronchiolitis
	Diffuse interstitial pneumonia
	Gastroesophageal reflux
	Cystic fibrosis
Preschoolers	Infections in suppurative disease (e.g., cystic fibrosis)
	Viral infections with or without reactive airway disease
	Foreign body aspiration
	Environmental pollutants
	Gastroesophageal reflux
	Reactive airway disease
School age/adolescents	Reactive airway disease
	Mycoplasma pneumoniae infection
	Cystic fibrosis
	Cigarette smoking
	Psychogenic cough tic
	Pulmonary hemosiderosis

- Assess pulmonary function to identify upper or lower airway causes, including the presence or absence of stridor, phonation, use of accessory muscles, and general state of alertness and activity level.
- Obtain historical information such as the evolution of the cyanosis (sudden or gradual onset) and associated factors (e.g., illness or decreased environmental temperature).

3. **Cough**
   a. *Description:* A cough is an attempt to clear the airway of particulate matter or may result from general tissue irritation. It is produced by a reflex response in cough receptors, found in ciliated epithelium, or may be initiated in higher cortical centers.
   b. *Evaluation*
      - Many causes of cough are age specific. (Table 2–2).
      - Note historical information such as the presence or absence of infectious disease or exposures.
      - Characteristics of the cough may suggest the cause:
        o Loose and productive: Cystic fibrosis, bronchiectasis, asthma
        o Croupy: Viral laryngotracheobronchitis
        o Paroxysmal: Pertussis, mycoplasma, foreign body, chlamydia
        o Brassy: Tracheitis, upper airway drainage, psychogenic
        o Nocturnal: Asthma, sinusitis, gastroesophageal reflux, upper respiratory tract disease
        o During exercise: Asthma, cystic fibrosis, bronchiectasis
        o Loud honking that disappears with sleep: Psychogenic
      - Other associated symptoms: Examine sputum samples for white blood cells or eosinophils. Note hemoptysis. Poor weight gain, steatorrhea, and cough are strongly suggestive of cystic fibrosis.
      - A cough that persists more than 2 weeks or a cough that causes immediate respiratory distress warrants investigation.

INVASIVE AND NONINVASIVE DIAGNOSTIC STUDIES

A. DIAGNOSTIC APPROACH
   1. **Individualization of evaluation:** All sick children are at higher risk for respiratory insufficiency or failure than adults because of the age-related anatomic differences described previously. Monitoring of pulmonary function can be individualized according to the acuity of illness and the age of the child. For a patient with the lowest acuity, clinical examination and serial observations are adequate; but with increasing severity of illness, other monitoring devices should be employed. The options for monitoring include continuous observation and clinical examination, oxygen monitoring, carbon dioxide monitoring, monitoring of pulmonary function, and laboratory and roentgenography studies.
   2. **Immediate assessment and care:** A brief estimation of the severity of distress should be made to determine the immediate need for oxygen or airway assistance.

B. BASELINE RESPIRATORY MONITORING
   1. **Physical examination: All** children who are suspected of having respiratory distress should have their clothing removed for maximum observation, assuring that ambient temperature is controlled. Refer to the clinical assessment

section for details on physical examination techniques. A quick-look observation should be done with all patients for early recognition of respiratory distress requiring emergent management. This 20-second appraisal should include level of consciousness, color, and respiratory effort.

2. **Diagnostic studies for children in respiratory distress from any cause**
   a. Complete history and physical examination
   b. Chest x-ray examination
   c. Sinus x-ray examinations (depending on age)
   d. Complete blood count
   e. Tuberculin skin test
   f. Nasopharyngeal swab for respiratory syncytial virus and viral panel and pertussis, if applicable
   g. Trial of bronchodilator aerosol
   h. Further testing if indicated:
      • Bronchoscopy
      • Sweat chloride test
      • Serology for *Mycoplasma*
      • Tracheal aspirate for Gram stain and culture if intubated
      • pH probe testing for suspected gastroesophageal reflux
      • Quantitative immunoglobulins
      • Pulmonary function testing

C. **LABORATORY STUDIES**

Laboratory testing of blood samples, which can provide invaluable information about pulmonary function, may include arterial blood gases, immunoglobulin assays, α_1-antitrypsin levels, complete blood count, and microbiology evaluation (Table 2–3).

D. **RADIOLOGIC PROCEDURES FOR PULMONARY EVALUATION**

A variety of imaging techniques allow visualization of anatomy, motion dynamics, and identification of abnormalities. Frequently, a patient may require more than one imaging procedure to detail a specific anatomic site.

1. **Chest roentgenography** permits visualization of lung parenchyma and vascular markings.
2. **Fluoroscopy** provides evaluation of thoracic motion, particularly diaphragm movement, which is essential to the infant.
3. **Computed tomography (CT) scan** is the visualization of very thin slices of tissue in a predetermined plane of dimension, enabling identification of masses, fluid accumulation and anatomic definition.
4. **Magnetic resonance imaging (MRI)** uses an external magnetic field around the patient to cause rotation of cell nuclei. Imaging provides well-defined visualization of soft tissues. There is no radiation involved in this procedure.
5. **Ventilation-perfusion scan ($\dot{V}/\dot{Q}$ scan)** is obtained by injecting a radioisotope into a peripheral vein and imaging its flow through the pulmonary vessels. The ventilation-perfusion scan is made following the inhalation of a radioactive gas, which distributes to aerated alveoli. Comparison between *ventilated* areas with *perfused* areas of the lung can be made, looking for "matched" segments. Although many disorders may cause a ventilation-perfusion mismatch, a complete segmental mismatch is a useful clue to the diagnosis of pulmonary embolism.
6. **Pulmonary angiography** involves introduction of a catheter into a peripheral vein; the catheter is guided to the right side of the heart and to the pulmonary artery trunk. Injection of contrast media with serial x-ray examinations of the pulmonary vascular bed allows definitive recognition of the obstruction.

Table 2–3. SUMMARY OF DIAGNOSTIC LABORATORY EVALUATION OF PULMONARY FUNCTION

TEST	SIGNIFICANCE
Arterial Blood Gases pH: 7.35–7.45 Pco_2: 35–45 mm Hg Pao_2: 80–100 mm Hg Sao_2: >94% HCO_3^-: 22–26 mEq/L Base excess (BE): −2 to +2	Evaluation of oxygenation, ventilation, and metabolic processes
Immunoglobulins	Norms are age-related assays. Decreased levels of any immunoglobulin are usually associated with congenital deficiencies and patterns of infections beginning early in life. Increased levels are associated with specific causes as follows. ***Increased Levels Associated With***
IgG: Found in blood, lymph, CSF, pleural fluid, peritoneal fluid, and breast milk; slow response (appears 1 wk after stimulus)	Myeloma Bacterial infections Collagen disorders
IgM: Intravascular; predominant first response to bacterial or viral infection; activates the complement system	Appears early in infectious course but may persist with chronic infection
IgD: Predominant acitivity on the surface of B ells (involving antibody formation)	Increased with chronic infections
IgE: Found in the serum and triggers release of histamine	Increased with allogenic stimulation (e.g., asthma, associated with allergenic stimulus)

Differential White Blood Cell Count
Test total WBC
  <1 y: maximum = 20,000
  1–12 y: maximum = 15,000
Segmented neutrophils (PMNs)
  <12 y = 25–40%
  ≥12 y = >50%
	Infections may cause an elevated or remarkably low ($<4000/mm^3$) WBC count.

Band neutrophils <10%	Increase in bands associated with bacterial infections
Lymphocytes <12 y = >50% ≥12 y = <40% Monocytes 4%–6% Eosinophils 2%–3% Basophils 0.5%	Increased with specific infections such as pertussis, Epstein-Barr virus, hepatitis
Pilocarpine Iontophoresis (Sweat Chloride Test) Sodium <70 mEq/L Chloride <60 mEq/L Potassium <60 mEq/L	Higher levels indicate cystic fibrosis
Sputum or Tracheal Aspirate Cultures Normally should have few if any PMNs and mixed flora Difficult to obtain uncontaminated, deep tracheal secretions Evaluate Gram stain for presence of PMNs Endotracheal tubes and tracheostomy tubes become quickly colonized with existing flora, which may be misleading if microbiology results are interpreted independently from other clinical indicators	PMNs: 3–4+ with dominant organism is more likely to be valid indicator of infection than one with <2+ PMNs and multiple organisms

PMNs, polymorphonuclear neutrophils.

RESPIRATORY MONITORING

A. OXYGEN MONITORING
   1. **Transcutaneous oxygen monitoring ($Ptco_2$)**
      a. *Principles of operation:* A small, heated probe is placed on the skin surface. Localized heating increases capillary blood flow to the site. Oxygen diffuses across the skin and is measured by a thermistor in the probe.
      b. *Uses:* $Ptco_2$ functions well in infants and has shown good correlation with Pao_2 measurements (Gunderson, 1988). It can reduce the quantity of invasive blood gas measurements and provide continuous data for patients who are either being weaned or are otherwise labile.
      c. *Limitations:* With increasing skin thickness, accuracy of measurements diminishes. Poor perfusion, and local skin hypoxia may interfere with measurements. The probe requires site change every 4 to 6 hours with a 10- to 15-minute warm-up time (and a blood gas analysis to verify measurement accuracy). Further, the heated probe may cause blisters in some infants.
   2. **Pulse oximetry**
      a. *Principles of operation:* The device consists of a probe that contains an infrared light source and a photodetector. Both are housed in a wrap-around strip so that the light source is aligned to emit light through tissue (such as a nail bed) to the photodetector. Saturated hemoglobin absorbs little light, whereas desaturated hemoglobin absorbs a large amount of light. The photodetector measures the amount of light that crosses the tissue and with a microprocessor computes the percentage of saturated hemoglobin.
      b. *Uses:* The pulse oximeter requires pulsatile tissue to provide accurate measurements. Fingers, palmar wrap (in small infants), toes, and ear clips are used. The microprocessor unit measures pulse rate and most units have a mechanism to provide a "poor signal" alert if the tissue has an inadequate pulse. It provides a stable, accurate measurement over a wide variety of physiologic conditions.
      c. *Limitations*
         • Severe hypoxemia (<70%) or poor perfusion (low cardiac output states) may interfere with a stable signal (Palve, 1989; Severinghaus, 1987).
         • With elevated carboxyhemoglobin or methemoglobin levels the true oxygenated hemoglobin values are inflated because the pulse oximeter does not distinguish between hemoglobin saturated with oxygen and other bound molecules.
         • A major source of error in children is motion artifact, which causes poor tracking of the pulse.
         • In the neonatal population, where retinopathy is a concern, Sao_2 may not provide any margin of safety because arterial oxygen tension can vary widely when oxygen saturations are greater than 90%.
   3. **Mixed venous oxygen saturation monitoring:** Many pediatric patients are monitored with pulmonary artery catheters for hemodynamic measurements. One type of catheter includes a fiberoptic tip that measures reflected wavelengths of light from saturated hemoglobin in the local (pulmonary artery) blood flow. The mixed venous oxygen saturation ($S\bar{v}o_2$) measurement, which is usually between 65% and 80%, is a global indicator of total oxygen consumption (Vo_2). Either a change in oxygen supply (arterial oxygen saturation) or in oxygen demand (oxygen consumption) will alter this measurement (see Chapter 3 for further information).

B. **CARBON DIOXIDE MONITORING**
   1. **Transcutaneous carbon dioxide monitoring**
      a. *Principles:* A carbon dioxide sensor, housed in a small probe, is mounted on the skin surface and measures diffused carbon dioxide with an electrode similar to that found in standard blood gas machines. Although earlier $Ptco_2$ electrodes used a local heat to "arterialize" the site, recent studies have shown that a predictable linear relationship can be obtained with nonheated electrodes. Typically, the $Ptcco_2$ is 5 to 10 mm Hg higher than the $Paco_2$, but the gradient should remain stable.
      b. *Uses:* Consistent correlations have been documented in neonates (Laptook and Oh, 1991), but less reliability has been demonstrated in older children and adults. After the probe is positioned and the warm-up period is passed, the monitor measurement should be compared to a simultaneous blood gas measurement to establish the gradient. After this point, blood gas measurements can be reduced until the next site rotation (usually every 4 hours).
      c. *Limitations*
         • The sensors appear to be somewhat fragile and prone to discreet alterations, such as inadequate fluid in the sensor. If the gradient between $Ptcco_2$ and $Paco_2$ is unstable, a site change is warranted.
         • Calibration procedures must be exact, necessitating the presence of personnel who are well-trained in the operation of these monitors.
   2. **End-tidal carbon dioxide monitoring ($ETCO_2$):** The measurement of exhaled carbon dioxide gas (termed capnography) provides direct evidence of ventilatory function. An increased carbon dioxide level is an objective parameter for the identification of respiratory failure.
      a. *Principles of operation:* A small device placed in-line with the ventilator circuit, at the proximal airway, measures expired carbon dioxide by mass spectrometry or infrared absorption. Exhaled gas passes through this device, which emits infrared light. A detector measures the light absorption in this sample. The carbon dioxide level is *inversely* proportional to the light absorption.
      b. *Uses:* In the normal subject, $PETCO_2$ is within 1 to 2 mm of $Paco_2$. With any variation in pulmonary blood flow (either ventilation-perfusion mismatch or change in cardiac output) or in metabolism, this gradient is magnified (Anas, 1990). End tidal CO_2, however, can always be used for trending measurements, especially if hyperventilation therapy is being used.
         • End tidal CO_2 monitoring is useful for immediate endotracheal tube placement verification.
         • Weaning patients from a ventilator can be accomplished more efficiently, requiring less blood gas sampling.
         • An estimation of dead space ventilation can be inferred when $Paco_2$ measurements and $ETCO_2$ are compared serially. When the dead space (VDS/VT) increases, the gradient between $Paco_2$ and $ETCO_2$ increases. Conversely, as ventilator adjustments are made in an attempt to improve alveolar ventilation, the gradient should diminish (Yamanaka and Sue, 1987; Table 2–4).
      c. *Limitations:* The choice of sensor for a child must be guided by the sensitivity for smaller exhaled volumes. Clinically, infants weighing less than 5 kg may not be good candidates for this device, but the final decision should be based on comparative measurements with a blood gas. Additional limitations are the warm-up time required and the calibration process, which requires operator competence for its use.

Table 2–4.   COMPARISON OF ARTERIAL AND END-TIDAL CARBON DIOXIDE MEASUREMENTS

P$_{ETCO_2}$	P$_{aCO_2}$	INTERPRETATION
↓	↓	↑ Alveolar ventilation
		Metabolic: Decreased carbon dioxide production
↓	↔ ↑	↓ Cardiac output
		↑ Pulmonary vascular resistance
		Diffusion defect
		Pulmonary embolus
↑	↑	↓ Alveolar ventilation increased
		Metabolic: Increased carbon dioxide production
↑	↔	↑ Mean airway pressure

From Webster HW, Chellis MJ. Physiological monitoring of infants and children. *AACN Clin Issues Crit Care.* 1993;4(1):180–196. Adapted from Levin D, Morris F. *Essentials of Pediatric Intensive Care.* New York: Churchill Livingstone.

C. **DIAGNOSTIC PULMONARY FUNCTION TESTING:** Critically ill children require continuous surveillance of pulmonary function. For those who are not in frank respiratory failure, clinical assessment, including respiratory rate, observation of chest expansion, and use of accessory muscles, provides an estimation of adequacy of minute ventilation. For those in distress, further measurements may be warranted. With children, standard measurements of pulmonary function may not be possible because of lack of patient cooperation.

  1. **Spirometry:** In the cooperative child or one who has had an endotracheal tube placed, lung volumes can be estimated with simple flow spirometers. Flow spirometers, which measure exhaled tidal volumes, can provide an *estimation* of vital capacity (VC), and can be used for trending. In general, 80% of the VC can be exhaled in 1 second and is called the forced expiratory volume, or FEV$_1$.
     a. In *obstructive* disease the patient is unable to breathe out fully and has both decreased VC and FEV$_1$.
     b. In *restrictive* disease, in which the lung cannot fully expand, the VC is low, but FEV$_1$ is still proportionally normal (i.e., greater than or equal to 80% of VC).
     c. In the weakened patient, lower volumes may be observed with a faster respiratory rate (Fig. 2–14).
  2. **Pressure manometers** measure both negative and positive pressure and provide an estimation of muscle condition. A normal school-age child should be able to generate a minimum of −30 cm H$_2$O on *inspiration* (sometimes called negative inspiratory force, or NIF). An infant may generate an NIF of −20 cm H$_2$O, although infant effort is difficult to capture. On *expiration* a school-age child should be able to generate at least +30 cm H$_2$O.
  3. **Measurement of compliance** is the measure of the distensibility of the lung. It is defined as the volume change per unit of pressure change across the lung. This is expressed as:

$$\Delta V/\Delta P$$

     a. *Dynamic compliance* is the relationship of the delivered (tidal) volume to the total pressure required to deliver that volume, calculated by:

$$\frac{\text{Peak Inspiratory Pressure (PIP)} - \text{Positive End-Expiratory Pressure (PEEP)}}{\text{Tidal Volume}}$$

Dynamic compliance includes both elastic recoil and airway resistance factors.

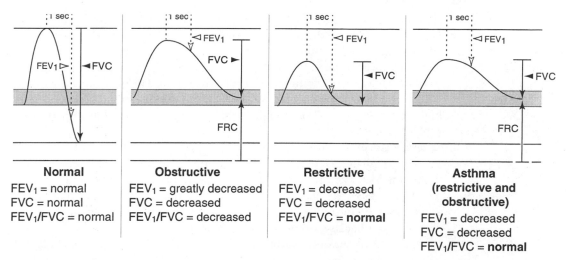

Normal	Obstructive	Restrictive	Asthma

Normal
FEV_1 = normal
FVC = normal
FEV_1/FVC = normal

Obstructive
FEV_1 = greatly decreased
FVC = decreased
FEV_1/FVC = decreased

Restrictive
FEV_1 = decreased
FVC = decreased
FEV_1/FVC = **normal**

**Asthma
(restrictive and obstructive)**
FEV_1 = decreased
FVC = decreased
FEV_1/FVC = **normal**

Figure 2–14. Normal pulmonary function tests and impact of obstructive and restrictive diseases. Normal pulmonary function measurements. Comparison of pulmonary function measurements in the person with obstructive and restrictive pulmonary disease. *FEV₁*, forced expiratory volume in the first second of exhalation; *FRC*, functional residual capacity; *FVC*, forced vital capacity. The ratio of FEV₁/FVC is greater than 80%. Note in restrictive disease that the ratio is normal, but the separate measurements of FEV₁ and FVC are abnormally low.

    b. *Static compliance:* At the end of a breath the ventilator stops moving gas flow. The friction created by that flow disappears, causing the inspiratory pressure to drop slightly. This pressure is the *static* pressure resulting from the stiffness of the lungs and chest wall. In the usual respiratory cycle the static pressure is registered so briefly that it may be difficult to observe. Static compliance is calculated with static pressure (or airway plateau pressure):

$$\frac{\text{Airway Plateau Pressure} - \text{PEEP}}{\text{Tidal Volume}}$$

    c. *Static compliance (or effective compliance)* reflects the elastic properties of the lung (average distensibility of all participating alveoli). The normal range is the same in an infant as in an adult: 60 to 100 ml/cm H_2O. Static compliance decreases with restrictive disease and increases with obstructive disease. Serial monitoring of effective compliance may enable identification of optimal tidal volumes, optimal PEEP, and prediction of weaning readiness.

  4. **Evaluation of volume loops** is a diagnostic tool for evaluating pulmonary function on ventilated patients obtained with an in-line sensor and bedside monitor. Measurements are made of flow, pressure, and volume. Pressure volume loops illustrate the relationship of pressure to volume (thus, compliance). Flow volume loops illustrate the relationship of flow to volume.

PULMONARY PHARMACOLOGY

A. General Principles

Pharmacologic management of pulmonary diseases in children requires understanding of both the pharmacokinetics of the various drugs and the disease conditions for which the drugs are prescribed. Most medications have been studied on adult populations, and application to children has often occurred by extrapolation of data. It is beyond the scope of this text to explore these issues, but there are several ideas that merit consideration by the critical care nurse:

1. **Physiologic differences:** Infants and young children have a greater percentage of total body water, predominately extracellular fluid. The distribution of a drug is determined by the following fluid compartments. In general, drug doses are higher per kilogram of body weight in the infant than in the adolescent or adult (Table 2–5).

2. **Enteral absorption:** Gastric acid secretion and motility appear to be developmentally regulated. The rate of gastric emptying in the normal neonate (less than 10 weeks) is 87 minutes (Blumer, 1992) compared to an adult time of 65 minutes. However, intestinal transit is more rapid in the infant than in the adult. Many medications may not be absorbed as completely as in the older child or adult because of the following factors:

   a. An acidic pH favors absorption of acidic medications; likewise, an alkaline pH improves absorption of alkaline compounds.

   b. The rate of gastric emptying and intestinal transit affects absorption of medications. Delayed gastric emptying or rapid intestinal motility will decrease absorption. Conditions that may decrease absorption include gastroesophageal reflux, respiratory distress syndrome, and congenital heart disease.

   c. In the PICU, many patients receive gastric or jejunal feedings through nasal feeding tubes. Drugs administered through these tubes may bind with proteins in the feedings. Certain drugs that can be monitored by serum assays such as phenytoin (Dilantin), carbamazepine (Tegretol), or theophylline should be administered in a consistent fashion but preferably through a gastric tube that has been rinsed before administration; feedings should be held for a period of time after administration. Adjustment of drug doses (based on serum assay) can only be reliable with consistency in the administration of the drugs.

3. **Protein binding:** Binding of drugs to plasma proteins determines the amount of free drug available for body distribution. Although plasma albumin levels reach adult levels soon after birth, there are differences in the binding properties of infant albumin that influence the dosing of selected medications.

4. **Underlying pathophysiology:** Decreased blood flow to major organs influences absorption, delivery of the drug to targeted site, and elimination. Inflammation may cause an increase in regionalized blood flow with altered capillary permeability. This may result in abnormally high drug delivery to these regions.

Table 2–5. EXTRACELLULAR AND INTRACELLULAR FLUID DISTRIBUTION BY AGE

Age	Total Body H_2O (%)	Extracellular Fluid* (%)	Intracellular Fluid* (%)
Newborn	75	35–44	33
4–6 mo	60	23	37
1 y		26–30	
12 y	60	20	40
Adult	50–60	20	40

*As a percent of body weight.

From Blumer JL. Principles of drug disposition in the critically ill child. In: Fuhrman BP, Zimmerman JJ, eds. *Pediatric Critical Care.* St Louis, Mo: Mosby–Year Book Inc; 1992:1060.

Extravascular fluid collections may provide a protein-rich reservoir for drugs, diverting them from their intended distribution site.

5. **Dosing of medications:** The dosing of medication is frequently based on one of two strategies:

   a. *Target concentration:* Drugs used for chronic or chronically intermittent conditions, such as acetaminophen (Tylenol), antibiotics, or theophylline. The basis for this strategy is that serum concentrations for a given drug have defined therapeutic and toxic ranges. These assays are *guidelines* and not specific to an individual patient. Knowledge of pharmacokinetics is important to the successful use of this strategy.

   b. *Target effect:* A drug is selected with a therapeutic end-point clearly defined before administration. Dosing is titrated to achieve this effect or until toxic effects are observed. Discontinuation of the drug may be necessary if toxicity occurs or if no therapeutic effect is achieved. Medications frequently administered with this strategy include catecholamines, diuretics, and anticoagulants. Many of the medications used in a critical care setting are prescribed in this manner.

B. NEUROMUSCULAR BLOCKING AGENTS

1. **Description:** Muscle relaxants are used in the PICU to facilitate assisted ventilation by intervening within the neuromuscular junction in one of two ways. *Depolarizing agents* cause a continuous release and subsequent depletion of acetylcholine. *Nondepolarizing agents* bind the receptor sites of acetylcholine so that synaptic transmission is blocked.

2. **Indications for use**
   a. Endotracheal intubation procedure
   b. Facilitation of compliance with assisted mechanical ventilation
   c. Reduction of oxygen consumption from muscle movement

3. **Nursing considerations**
   a. The choice of an agent depends on the purpose and intended duration of pharmacologic paralysis. All patients who will receive a paralytic drug should be given adequate sedation.
   b. All children who will be maintained on a muscle relaxant should have electrocardiographic (ECG) monitoring, pulse oximetry (see Respiratory Monitoring), and peripheral nerve stimulation. Monitoring of heart rate (increases from baseline may be caused by pain, fear, or seizures), blood pressure (increased systolic pressure may indicate pain or anxiety), and pupil size (dilation may indicate fear, pain, or other causes of sympathetic nerve stimulation or significant changes in neurologic status) is essential.
   c. Long-term use of muscle relaxants may mask pain, anxiety, and seizures. Whenever possible, withholding of paralytic medications should be scheduled to adequately assess the patient's awareness and condition. (See Acute Respiratory Failure discussion and Table 2–12 for more information on specific agents.)

C. SEDATIVES AND ANALGESICS (Table 2–6)

1. **Benzodiazepines**
   a. *Description:* Benzodiazepines are believed to cause anterograde amnesia through the inhibition of the neurotransmitter γ-aminobutyric acid (GABA) in the limbic system. They have little or no effect on retrograde memory and have no analgesic properties.
   b. *Indications* include short-term general sedation and amnesia for procedures, long-term use for facilitating compliance with assisted ventilation, and acute therapy for seizure management.

Table 2–6. SEDATIVES AND ANALGESICS

DRUG	IV DOSE/ONSET/ DURATION	CONTRAINDICATIONS	COMMENTS
Propofol	Dose: 0.5–2 mg/kg IV push 50 µg/kg/min infusion Onset: 1–2 min Duration: 5–10 min	Allergies to soybean or eggs Liver failure Disorder of lipid metabolism (e.g., pancreatitis)	Helpful with refractory bronchospasm Caution with hypovolemia or congestive heart failure May ↓ ICP Produces green urine Does not provide analgesia
Thiopental	Dose: 2–5 mg/kg Onset: <30 s Duration: 5–30 min	Hypovolemia or hypotension	Produces general anesthesia and amnesia Decreases ICP and cerebral blood flow Monitor for hypotension
Ketamine	Dose: 0.5–2 mg/kg Onset: <30 s Duration: 10–15 min Unconsciousness	Increased ICP	Analgesic, amnestic, hallucinogen Monitor for emergence delirium and nightmares Bronchodilator used for patients with asthma Prevent emergence reaction with benzodiazepines at the end of the procedure
Benzodiazepines			
Midazolam	Dose: 0.05–0.2 mg/kg Onset: 2–4 min Duration: 20–30 min Maximum dose: 0.2 mg/kg	Severe hypotension CNS depression	Sedative-anxiolytic, anticonvulsant Alternate routes of delivery including oral, rectal, and transmucosal (nasal)
Lorazepam	Dose: 0.05–0.1 mg/kg Onset: 2–4 min Duration: 20–30 min	Severe hypotension CNS depression	4- to 12-hour half-life, may be used by intermittent bolus No active metabolite
Diazepam	Dose: 0.05–0.1 mg/kg Onset: 2–4 min Duration: 20–30 min Maximum dose: 0.6 mg/kg in an 8 h period	Not recommended for use by continuous infusion Severe hypotension CNS depression	Prolonged effect because of long half-life and presence of active metabolites
Opiates and Analgesic Agents			
Fentanyl	Dose: 1–2 µg/kg Onset: 3–5 min Duration: 0.5–1 h	Increased ICP Severe respiratory depression	Analgesic, mildly sedating
Methadone	Dose: 0.1 mg/kg Onset: 10–20 min Peak effect: 1–2 h Maximum dose: 10 mg per dose		Half-life 15–29 h Used for managing opiate dependence
Morphine	Dose: 0.1–0.2 mg/kg Peak: 20 min Duration: 4–5 h	Increased ICP Respiratory depression Metabolite accumulation in renal failure	May cause histamine release

CNS, central nervous system; *ICP,* intracranial pressure.

    c. *Nursing considerations*
- Benzodiazepines do *not* provide pain relief. In many situations, use of an analgesic in conjunction with sedation should be considered.
- Patients should be euvolemic before administration of a benzodiazepine to avoid hypotension.
- Prolonged administration may result in physical dependence. Withdrawal symptoms, such as anxiety, sweating, agitation, or hallucinations, may occur with abrupt withdrawal.
- The costs of the individual benzodiazepines vary significantly. The choice of agent should also take into consideration the estimated daily costs after evaluation of the indications and pharmacokinetics.

2. **Morphinelike opioids**
    a. *Description:* Opioid receptors are found in the brain and spinal cord. Five receptors have been described; but three, the mu (M), kappa (K), and sigma (S), are the most clinically recognized targets of opiate binding:
- M = Supraspinal anesthesia; euphoria, respiratory depression, physical dependence
- K = Spinal anesthesia; sedation, miosis, and respiratory depression
- S = Central nervous system (CNS) stimulant; dysphoria, hallucinations, respiratory and vasomotor stimulation
- Most morphinelike narcotics are described as M and K agonists. Other agents work at different receptor sites, such as nalbuphine (Nubain). Nubain is a K and S receptor agonist and M receptor antagonist. Administration of Nubain after morphine may "antagonize" or reverse some of the morphine effects because of its antagonistic effects on the M receptor. Ketamine, another commonly used analgesic/sedative, produces analgesic effects through the S receptors and only minimally the M receptor.
    b. *Indications* for analgesic medications include procedures, relief of pain from underlying disease, and continuous analgesia for facilitating assisted mechanical ventilation. Opioids are *not* a substitute for an anxiolytic and amnestic agent. Although sedation occurs with opioid administration, the mechanisms do not duplicate those found in conventional sedatives such as benzodiazepines.
    c. *Nursing considerations*
- Some opioids, such as morphine, may cause vasodilatory effects from a histamine release. Histamine release is minimal with the synthetic narcotics such as fentanyl. Most opioids, except meperidine, induce a central parasympathetic stimulation and direct depression of the sinoatrial node. All opioids also cause dose-dependent respiratory depression.
- Routes of delivery should be individualized, with the goal of using the lowest possible dosing to provide continuous relief without side effects.
- Fentanyl is a synthetic opioid with approximately 100 times the analgesic potency of morphine. This concentrated solution (unless adequately diluted) may increase the risk for increased intracranial pressure (ICP) (related to increased P_{CO_2} with hypoventilation), increased chest wall rigidity with rapid, high-dose intravenous administration (Benthuysen et al, 1986), and decreased seizure threshold. These side effects can be seen with all opioids and are not necessarily contraindications for their use. Slower administration, lower dosing, and a small dose of pancuronium (0.01 to 0.02 mg/kg) have been shown to attenuate or prevent these side effects (Bailey et al, 1985).

3. **Barbiturates**
   a. *Description:* Barbiturates are among the oldest classes of sedative agents used in PICU patients. They provide good sedation, but are *not* analgesic or amnestic agents. The cardiopulmonary effects are dose dependent and well defined. Several drugs are available and classified according to the duration of activity. In addition to their sedative effect, barbiturates have potent anticonvulsant properties and decrease cerebral metabolism (and may decrease ICP).
   b. *Indications* include short-term sedation for procedures and long-term sedation for ongoing management of assisted ventilation (rarely), increased ICP, and continuous procedures such as extracorporeal membrane oxygenation (ECMO) or intraaortic balloon pump (IABP). Barbiturates are not a substitute for analgesic medications unless the dosing is high enough to produce complete anesthesia.
   c. *Nursing considerations*
      • Cardiovascular effects are dose related. With higher doses, venodilation and depressed myocardial function are observed.
      • Pulmonary effects are also dose related with apnea occurring in the middose ranges. Bag, mask, and oxygen should always be at the bedside.
      • Most barbiturates are in an alkaline solution and, therefore, must be administered separately from other medications and IV solutions.

4. **Ketamine**
   a. *Description:* Ketamine is both an analgesic and amnestic medication. The mechanism of this drug, including S receptor stimulation, is mediated through the sympathetic nervous system and the release of endogenous catecholamines. Increases in heart rate and blood pressure and general stimulation and dysphoria are observed at lower doses (0.5 to 2 mg/kg). Higher doses provide good anesthesia and respiratory depression, but as the patient recovers, the stimulation and dysphoria may reappear.
   b. *Indications:* Ketamine has a minimal effect on cardiopulmonary stability, and, therefore, is a good choice for unstable patients. Bronchodilation occurs (through the release of endogenous catecholamines), which makes ketamine a good agent for patients with bronchospasm. However, ketamine has been shown to increase cerebral blood flow and ICP and, therefore, is not a good agent for patients with altered intracranial compliance (Michenfelder, 1988).
   c. *Nursing considerations*
      • Emergence phenomena are observed more often in older children and adults than in younger children. Administration of a benzodiazepine at the end of the procedure may decrease or prevent this from occurring.
      • Although respiratory depression is dose dependent with ketamine administration, even with normal respiratory function it is unclear whether airway reflexes are completely intact. Therefore, bag, mask, oxygen, and suction should be available at the bedside, particularly if any other sedative agents have been given with ketamine.

5. **Propofol**
   a. *Description:* Propofol is a sedative-hypnotic agent administered intravenously, with rapid onset and short duration of action. The effects are dose dependent. Propofol is provided in a lipid emulsion of soybean oil, glycerol,

and egg phosphates. It has multiple properties, including bronchodilation and rapid recovery (with minimal posthypnotic obtundation), that make it an attractive agent for deep sedation or anesthetic induction.

b. *Indications* include induction of anesthesia, deep sedation for short procedures, continuous sedation for facilitating patient care (e.g., assisted ventilation), and relief of bronchospasm refractory to more conventional agents.

c. *Nursing considerations*
- Before administration, the patient or family should be questioned about possible allergies to eggs or soybeans, because there have been anaphylactic reactions to propofol's lipid emulsion.
- Propofol may produce hypotension by direct vasodilation.
- Propofol decreases cerebral blood flow and metabolic requirements of the brain, which may be an advantage in some patients.
- Propofol increases central vagal tone and may cause bradycardia. If used with other medications known to cause bradycardia (such as fentanyl or succinylcholine), this effect can be cumulative. Sudden death has been reported with a fentanyl, propofol, succinylcholine sequence (Egan and Brock-Utne, 1991).
- Isolated reports of neurologic adverse effects, such as myoclonic movements and convulsions, have raised concern for use of propofol as a long-term therapy (Trotter, 1992).

D. REMEDIAL AGENTS

In providing sedation, analgesia, or pharmacologic paralysis for a child, some agents exhibit predictable, but unwanted, effects that can be prevented or remediated pharmacologically. The following medications may be used to manage the side effects (Table 2–7).

1. **Anticholinergic agents** (atropine-like medications)
   a. *Description:* Anticholinergic agents antagonize the actions of acetylcholine, producing a central vagal blockade (tachycardia, increased blood pressure, mitosis) and specific sympathetic effects in target organs.
   - Atropine crosses the blood-brain barrier and is known to cause CNS stimulation, whereas a newer synthetic agent, ipratropium, does not cross into brain tissue.
   - In addition, the lungs have both cholinergic and adrenergic receptors that regulate bronchomotor tone (see Asthma discussion).
   b. *Indications* include premedication for procedures or medications known to potentiate bradycardia (such as succinylcholine), reduction of salivary secretions, bronchodilation (not as a first-line agent but as an adjunct), and symptom control while using a β-blocker agent.
   c. *Nursing considerations*
   - Pupil size and responsiveness are altered with atropine administration. This is important to note when a neurologic condition is being monitored.
   - Side effects may be bothersome to patients who are awake, including a fast heart rate, dry mouth, and CNS effects (delirium, agitation).
   - Atropine does cross the blood-brain barrier and, therefore, CNS effects such as agitation may be observed.

2. **Naloxone (Narcan)**
   a. *Description:* Narcan is an opioid antagonist, which has an affinity for opiate receptors, blocking them from binding to narcotics. Narcotics attached to the receptor are displaced. Narcan is used to reverse the effects of mor-

Table 2–7.   REMEDIAL AGENTS

SIDE EFFECTS	DRUG	IV DOSE DURATION	COMMENTS
Bradycardia or Bronchospasm	Atropine	*Bradycardia* Dose: 0.02 mg/kg Minimum: 0.1 mg Maximum: 1 mg *Bronchospasm* Dose: 0.05 mg/kg in 2.5 ml NS q6h MDI* or aerosol	Monitor for muscarinic effect: Bradycardia, salivation, broncho-spasm
Pruritus (Epidural opioids)	Naloxone (Narcan)	Continuous infusion 0.001 mg/kg/h	This dose should not significantly reverse analgesia
	Nalbuphine (Nubain)	Continuous infusion 0.01–0.1 mg/kg IV	May improve analgesia May cause increased sedation
(Systemic opioids)	Diphenhydramine (Benadryl)	0.5–1 mg/kg IV q6h	Significant sedation may be observed
Respiratory depression (Benzodiazepines)	Flumazenil Romazicon	*<20 kg:* 0.01 mg/kg (maximum 0.2 mg) Repeat: 0.005 mg/kg (maximum 0.2 mg) *20–40 kg:* 0.2 mg (maximum 1 mg) Repeat 0.005 mg/kg	Caution in patients with seizure history Does not consistently reverse amnesia Used for reversal of conscious sedation May produce convulsions in patients physically dependent on benzodiazepines
(Opioids)	Naloxone (Narcan)	*Mild oversedation* 0.01 mg/kg; repeat 2–3 min *Opiate intoxication* <20 kg: 0.1 mg/kg >20 kg: 2 mg/dose Repeat 2–3 min until response noted May require repeat doses q20–60min	May cause abrupt cessation of pain control; sudden awakening with agitation, nausea and vomiting, and headache
Nausea	Metoclopramide (Reglan)	0.1 mg/kg IV q6h	Low incidence of side effects but extrapyramidal symptoms may occur
	Droperidol (Inapsine)	2–12 y: 0.05–0.06 mg/kg/dose q4–6h >12 y: 2.5–5 mg/dose q4h	Can cause dysphoria, severe hypotension, extrapyramidal reaction
	Ondansetron (Zofran)	0.15 mg/kg IV × three doses at 4 h intervals	No sedation; best used prior to anticipated stimulus (e.g., operating room) Low incidence of bronchospasm, seizures, headaches

*Metered dose inhalers.

phinelike drugs. When given intravenously, it has a duration of only 2 to 3 minutes.

    b. *Indications* include diagnosis and treatment of respiratory depression associated with narcotic use and in research for management of shock.

    c. *Nursing considerations*
- Because of the quick onset of affect with Narcan, the patient may awaken abruptly and be in pain or exhibit nausea and vomiting.
- Because of the short duration of effect with Narcan, there may be a recurrence of the narcotized state, necessitating repeated dosing or continuous infusion. Therefore, the patient requires constant monitoring because the effects of the narcotic may last longer than the effects of Narcan.

3. **Flumazenil (Romazicon)**

    a. *Description:* Romazicon is a reversal agent for the benzodiazepines with a central mechanism of action.

    b. *Indications* include the reversal of benzodiazepine-related side effects, especially respiratory depression.

    c. *Nursing considerations*
- Patients should be monitored continuously with airway equipment at the bedside.
- Use Romazicon with caution in patients with a history of seizures, massive overdoses, or concurrent use of tricyclics.

4. **Other agents:** Nausea and pruritus frequently occur with many of the medications discussed in this section. See Table 2–7 for drug recommendations and dosing to manage these problems.

E. AGENTS THAT AFFECT VENTILATION-PERFUSION MATCHING

  1. **Nitric oxide**

    a. *Description:* Inhaled nitric oxide's potent vasodilator effect is, in theory, limited to the ventilated portions of the lung. It appears to have no effect on the systemic circulation because it binds to hemoglobin and is rapidly inactivated. Studies have suggested that nitric oxide may effectively reduce mean pulmonary artery pressure and intrapulmonary shunting, allowing reduction of FIO_2 in patients with adult respiratory distress syndrome (ARDS) (Day et al, 1996).

    b. *Indications* currently are for protocols or rescue efforts in patients with worsening respiratory failure.

    c. *Nursing considerations*
- Nitric oxide is an inhalational gas delivered through the ventilator circuitry at a flow of 10 to 80 parts per million (ppm).
- Methemoglobin levels should be noted on routine blood gas analysis as methemoglobinemia is a dose-dependent side effect of nitric oxide therapy.

  2. **Surfactant replacement therapy:** In neonates with respiratory distress syndrome, surfactant replacement has been shown to improve oxygenation and survival (Horbar, 1989). This has not been the case in children or adults, however. Although patients with ARDS have both quantitative and qualitative abnormalities in surfactant, trials with both artificial and animal-derived surfactant have been disappointing. In part, this may be true because the alveoli of a patient with ARDS are filled with a proteinase fluid, which may inactivate the surfactant.

F. BRONCHODILATORS

Direct bronchodilation for reactive airway disease (RAD) can be achieved through anticholinergic blockade, direct smooth muscle relaxants, or β-adrenergic stimulation. (See Asthma for further discussion and Table 2-25.) Anticholinergic agents, such as atropine or ipratropium, and smooth muscle relaxants, such as inhalation of halothane, are discussed under Acute Respiratory Failure.

1. **β-Agonist medications**
   a. *Description:* Dilation of the airways can be achieved through the administration of β-agonist agents, specifically the β_2-receptors, found in the smooth muscle of the airways. Epinephrine is the prototype adrenergic medication, but it stimulates β_1-, β_2-, and α-receptors, thus producing a generalized sympathetic response. Agents such as albuterol or terbutaline exhibit primarily β_2-stimulation. When given as an inhalation agent, albuterol has an onset of action approximately 3 to 6 minutes after administration, and its effect may last as long as 4 to 6 hours.
   b. *Indications* include the relief of acute bronchospasm and daily management of RAD.
   c. *Nursing considerations*
      • Adverse side effects include tachycardia, tremors, headache, nausea, and sleep disturbances.
      • Serum potassium should be monitored anticipating a decrease in serum potassium ion levels in patients receiving aerosol treatments more frequently than every 4 hours.

2. **Antiinflammatory agents:** Conditions such as RAD or ARDS are now thought to be mediated by an inflammatory process triggered by environmental or endogenous stimulus. The host inflammatory mechanisms normally provide protection, but in specific settings the process appears to cause injury. Both general antiinflammatory agents (glucocorticoids) and specific agents have been used in the management of respiratory conditions. The drugs described below provide an overview.
   a. *Corticosteroids (glucocorticoids):* Most of these drugs are synthetic preparations of the endogenous hormones. They exert general antiinflammatory effects such as suppression of hypersensitivity and immune responses and metabolic effects with an influence on lipid, protein, and carbohydrate metabolism and sodium retention. *Dexamethasone* is often prescribed to treat upper airway edema, although research is inconclusive as to its efficacy. *Methylprednisolone* is now widely accepted as important therapy for the prevention and management of RAD. Daily aerosols with intermittent "pulse dosing" oral therapy have become the foundation for the treatment of RAD.
      • *Nursing considerations:* Glucocorticoids interact with *many* other drugs; therefore, a medication history is essential before administering these drugs. There are many similar brand names for the various steroid preparations. A careful verification of each drug is important to assure that the patient is receiving a *glucocorticoid* and not a *mineralocorticoid*. Many adverse reactions occur in patients receiving steroids, including sodium and water retention, hyperglycemia, hypokalemia, hypertension, and CNS changes ranging from mood disorders to increased ICP. Patients receiving long-term therapy are at risk for osteoporosis, ulcers, hyperlipidemia, and increased susceptibility to infection with symptoms that may be suppressed by the steroids.
   b. *Nonsteroidal agents:* Although nonsteroidal antiinflammatory drugs have been widely studied in the laboratory with promising data, there are insufficient data and clinical experience to support the use of these drugs for the management of any pulmonary disorder.

ACUTE RESPIRATORY FAILURE

A. DEFINITION/ETIOLOGY

Acute respiratory failure is the inability of the respiratory system to meet the demands of the body for oxygen or provide adequate carbon dioxide elimination, often leading to acidosis.

B. PATHOPHYSIOLOGY

Respiratory failure may be related to pulmonary and nonpulmonary causes. The "respiratory pump" includes the nervous system, airways, and respiratory muscles. Respiratory failure can develop as a result of the failure of any component of the respiratory system. The anatomy of the airway of a child differs from that of the adult in many clinically significant ways (see Table 2–8 and Developmental Anatomy of the Respiratory System). These differences may lead to airway compromise and make airway support more difficult (Fig. 2–15).

1. **Pulmonary causes of acute respiratory failure**
    a. *Impaired integrity of lung tissue*
        - Conditions such as atelectasis, pneumonia, bronchiolitis, and ARDS can lead to low ventilation-perfusion ratios ($\dot{V}/\dot{Q}$).
        - Conditions such as ARDS or cyanotic heart disease can cause mismatches between ventilation and perfusion.
        - Pulmonary edema results from increased pulmonary extravascular water as a result of increased pulmonary capillary permeability or an increase in pulmonary vascular pressure. This causes a diffusion impairment.
    b. *Increased airway resistance*
        - Small amounts of edema can significantly reduce airway diameter and increase resistance to airflow and the work of breathing in the infant or child. High compliance makes the child's airway susceptible to dynamic collapse in the presence of airway obstruction.
        - Congenital upper airway anomalies may restrict flow through upper airways. Aspiration of a foreign body may restrict flow by narrowing the airway.
2. **Nonpulmonary causes of acute respiratory failure**
    a. *Respiratory muscle compromise*
        - The diaphragm is the primary muscle of inspiration for infants. The movement of the diaphragm is limited with abdominal distention or poor diaphragmatic function. Diaphragmatic disorders include diaphragmatic hernia, paralysis, and eventration.

Table 2–8. ANATOMIC DIFFERENCES BETWEEN PEDIATRIC AND ADULT AIRWAYS

ANATOMIC DIFFERENCE	CLINICAL SIGNIFICANCE
Proportionally larger head	Increases neck flexion and obstruction
Smaller nostrils	Increases airway resistance
Larger tongue	Increases airway resistance
Decreased muscle tone	Airway obstruction
Longer and more horizontal epiglottis	Increases airway obstruction
More anterior larynx	Difficult to perform blind intubation
Cricoid ring is narrowest portion	Inflated cuffed tubes not recommended for routine intubation in children <8 y of age
Shorter trachea	Increases risk of right main stem intubation
Narrower airways	Increases airway resistance

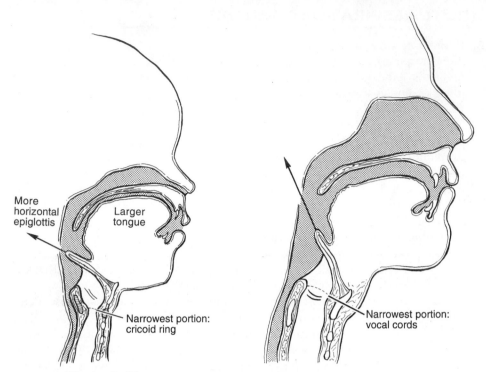

Figure 2–15.   Anatomic differences between child and adult airways.

- The chest wall is extremely compliant, which can further compromise ventilation and lead to chest wall retractions.
- Respiratory muscle fatigue leads to hypoventilation, which may progress to hypoxia and acidosis.

    b. *Alterations in nervous system control of breathing* include immature CNS function, respiratory depression by narcotics, sedatives or anesthetics, and CNS disease such as Guillain-Barré syndrome, head or spinal cord trauma, CNS infection, myasthenia gravis, botulism, or central hypoventilation syndrome.

    c. *Upper airway disorders* include choanal atresia, micrognathia, cystic hygroma, obstruction, and tracheoesophageal fistula.

    d. *Cardiovascular and hematologic disorders* include congenital heart disease, anemia, shock, or sepsis.

C. CLINICAL PRESENTATION

    1. **History** should be evaluated for chronic lung disease and respiratory or nonrespiratory causes of respiratory failure. Evaluate the onset of symptoms, presence of respiratory distress, fever, activity level, and level of consciousness. Determine home use of respiratory medications.

    2. **Physical examination**

        a. *Increased work of breathing* is related to airway obstruction or alveolar disease and results in tachypnea, nasal flaring, and intercostal, subcostal, and suprasternal inspiratory retractions.

        b. Alterations in respiratory mechanics can be related to alveolar collapse and the loss of lung volume associated with pulmonary edema, pneumonia, or atelectasis. Grunting increases end-expiratory pressure, thereby increasing functional residual capacity. Head bobbing, stridor, and prolonged expiration are additional signs of altered respiratory mechanisms.

c. Signs of upper airway obstruction can be related to congenital abnormalities (laryngomalacia, vocal cord paralysis, hemangioma, airway tumor), infections (epiglottitis, croup, bacterial tracheitis), noninfectious upper airway edema (allergic reaction, following intubation, gastroesophageal reflux), or aspiration of a foreign body. Inspiratory stridor and paradoxical chest movement with sternal and intercostal retractions rather than chest and lung expansion may be seen in upper airway obstruction.

d. Lower airway obstruction can be related to bronchiolitis, asthma, pulmonary edema, or intrathoracic foreign body. Prolonged expiration and wheezing are clinical signs of lower airway obstruction.

e. Decreased air entry can be related to hypoventilation, airway obstruction, atelectasis, pneumothorax, hemothorax, pleural effusion, mucous plug, or foreign body aspiration. Breath sounds are diminished unilaterally or bilaterally.

f. Perfusion should be evaluated by examining skin color and temperature. Evaluate mucous membranes, nail beds, palms of hands, and soles of feet for cyanosis, which can be caused by hypoxia or poor perfusion.

g. Changes in the level of consciousness such as irritability, lethargy, or failure to respond to parents may be indications of cerebral hypoxia or hypercarbia and require immediate intervention.

3. **Diagnostic tests to evaluate for respiratory failure**

   a. *$Paco_2$* directly reflects the adequacy of alveolar ventilation. Hypercarbia is an arterial $Paco_2$ greater than 55 mm Hg.

   b. *Oxygenation* is evaluated with the Pao_2. Hypoxemia is an arterial Pao_2 less than 60 mm Hg.

   c. *Acid-base balance* is indicated by the pH. Acidosis is an arterial pH less than 7.35.

   d. *Chest radiographs* are evaluated for areas of consolidation, atelectasis, pneumothorax, effusion, hyperinflation, and edema.

4. **Clinical course:** Determine the cause of the respiratory failure if possible. If spontaneous minute ventilation and oxygenation are effective (evidenced by good air movement in all lung fields, pulse oximetry saturation higher than 90%, and normal mental status), supplemental oxygen may be delivered by cannula or face mask. Intubation is required if respiratory failure (significant hypoxemia, hypercarbia, acidosis, or altered level of consciousness) is present.

D. PATIENT CARE MANAGEMENT

1. **Prevention** of acute respiratory failure includes general principles of management of the infant or child's airway. Encourage coughing and deep breathing in awake patients. Intervene with frequent position changes. Reduce abdominal distention by nasogastric suction if necessary. Use precautions for known reflux.

2. **Noninvasive respiratory monitoring** includes pulse oximetry and end-tidal CO_2 detectors for intubated patients.

3. **Invasive respiratory monitoring** includes arterial blood gas analysis and mixed venous oxygen saturation monitoring via pulmonary artery catheter (see Respiratory Monitoring discussion).

4. **Oxygen delivery systems** provide supplemental oxygen for patients with adequate ventilation (Table 2–9). Bag and mask ventilation is used when a patient's breathing is inadequate. It may be used in conjunction with oropharyngeal or nasopharyngeal airways and allows the administration of PEEP.

   a. *Endotracheal tube airways* are indicated for inadequate respiratory effort (drugs, infections, trauma, chest wall deformities), normal effort but

Table 2–9. OXYGEN DELIVERY SYSTEMS

	INDICATIONS	FIO_2	DESCRIPTION	COMMENTS
Nasal cannula	Nasal breathing; provide oxygen up to 0.5	0.22–0.5	One prong fits into each anterior nares, maximum oxygen flow 4–5 L/min	Least restrictive, FIO_2 unknown, entrains room air
Head hood	Useful for infant or small child	0.21–0.9	Clear plexiglass box placed over patient's head	Less than 10 kg; requires humidification; flows >10 L/min to flush out carbon dioxide
Simple face mask	Useful for delivering aerosols and oxygen; use with mouth breathing	0.44–0.5	Vinyl, fits over nose and mouth; open ports on side of mask to allow exhalation of carbon dioxide Minimum flow rate: 4 L infant, 5 L child	Entrains room air, child cannot eat or drink; high FIO_2 not attainable; FIO_2 is not correlated with high flow rates
Nonrebreathing mask	Useful for patients who require high FIO_2	0.9–1	Vinyl, fits over nose and mouth; reservoir bag attached with one-way gas flow from bag into the mask	No entrainment of room air; oxygen flow determined by patient's minute ventilation
Endotracheal tube with mechanical ventilation	Can deliver positive pressure and high FIO_2; does not require patient respiratory drive when used with a ventilator	0.21–1	Sterile, translucent polyvinyl with radiopaque marker; uniform internal diameter; cuffed or uncuffed	Most effective and reliable method of oxygen delivery; can control inspiratory time, PEEP, and tidal volume when used with a ventilator

PEEP, positive end-expiratory pressure.

overwhelming demand (bronchiolitis, asthma, pneumonia), inadequate CNS control of ventilation, need to maintain a patent airway (loss of protective reflexes, obstruction, edema), need for high peak inspiratory pressure (PIP), and the anticipated need for mechanical ventilatory support (shock, trauma, increased ICP, status post cardiopulmonary arrest, or acute respiratory failure).

Table 2–10. METHODS TO ESTIMATE SIZE OF ENDOTRACHEAL TUBE

Endotracheal Tube Size Calculation

$$\text{Internal Diameter (mm)} = \frac{16 + \text{Age (y)}}{4}$$

Endotracheal Tube Size Estimate
Nares or little finger of patient

Table 2–11.   INTUBATION EQUIPMENT

EQUIPMENT	TYPES	COMMENTS
Laryngoscope	Miller (straight) elevates epiglottis	Size 0–1: Newborns and infants
	MacIntosh (curved)	Size 1–4: Children and adults
Endotracheal tube	Uncuffed	Used in those younger than 8–10 y of age to reduce the risk of subglottic edema and stenosis; an uncuffed tube of appropriate size provides a reasonable seal at the cricoid ring
	Cuffed	Used in those older than 10 y of age and when needed to deliver a significant amount of positive pressure; cuff should be inflated with minimal leak to prevent mucosal ischemia
Monitoring equipment	Pulse oximeter ECG Blood pressure cuff	
Oxygen delivery equipment	Bag-valve ventilation device	
Suction	Large bore (14–18F), disposable tracheal suction Yankauer tonsillar suction	

ECG, electrocardiogram.

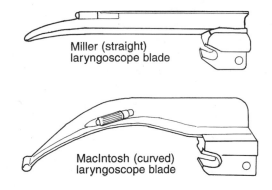

Miller (straight)
laryngoscope blade

MacIntosh (curved)
laryngoscope blade

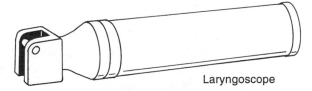

Laryngoscope

Figure 2–16.   Intubation equipment.

Table 2–12. NEUROMUSCULAR BLOCKING AGENTS AND ANTICHOLINERGIC AGENTS

DRUG	DOSE/ONSET/DURATION	CONTRAINDICATIONS	COMMENTS
Neuromuscular Blocking Agents			
Pancuronium	Dose: 0.02–0.1 mg/kg Onset: 120 s Duration: 45–90 min	Renal failure 60–90% renal elimination Tricyclic antidepressant use	Vagolytic: Increased heart rate and blood pressure
Vecuronium	Dose: 0.08–0.1 mg/kg Onset: 120 s Duration: 30–90 min	Liver failure	Renal elimination <25%
Atracurium	Dose: 0.4–0.5 mg/kg Onset: 240–420 s Duration: 30–40 min	Asthma Hypotension Need for rapid onset	Hoffman elimination makes it ideal for kidney or liver failure Very slow onset
Succinylcholine	Dose: 1–2 mg/kg Onset: 30–60 s Duration: 3–10 min	Myasthenia gravis Guillain-Barré syndrome Crush, burn, electrical injuries Open globe injury Increased intracranial pressure	Dysrhythmias Fasciculation Potassium efflux Muscle rigidity
Rocuronium	Dose: 0.6–1.2 mg/kg Onset: 30–60 s Duration: 30–60 min	None	Short duration
Antimuscarinic and Antispasmodic Agents			
Atropine sulfate	Dose: 0.01 mg/kg Minimum: 0.1 mg Onset: 2–4 min Duration: 90 min	Hypersensitivity Narrow-angle glaucoma Tachycardia Thyrotoxicosis Gastrointestinal obstruction Obstructive uropathy	Monitor for muscarinic effect: Bradycardia, salivation, bronchospasm
Glycopyrrolate	Dose to reverse blockade: 0.2 mg IV for each 1 mg of neostigmine or 5 mg of pyridostigmine administered Dose: 2.5–5 µg/kg/dose Maximum: 0.2 mg/dose or 0.8 mg/24 h Onset: 10–15 min after IV administration	Narrow-angle glaucoma Acute hemorrhage Tachycardia Hypersensitivity Ulcerative colitis Obstructive uropathy	Reverses neuromuscular blockade and bronchospasm Controls upper airway secretions Children with Down syndrome, spastic paralysis, or brain damage may be hypersensitive

b. See Table 2–10 for methods to estimate the size of the endotracheal tube and Table 2–11 for intubation equipment (Fig. 2–16).

5. **Medications** such as *neuromuscular blocking agents* (Table 2–12), *sedatives* (see Table 2–6), and *anticholinergics* (see Table 2–12) are often used. See Pulmonary Pharmacology.

6. **Rapid-sequence intubation** is used in patients with a "full stomach" when concern about regurgitation and aspiration is present. Cricoid pressure is used to prevent regurgitation of abdominal contents. BVM ventilation of patients is limited to reduce air entry into the stomach.

7. **Complications** from endotracheal intubation include airway trauma such as tracheal laceration or hematoma of the vocal cords, erosions of posterior vocal cords, loss of teeth, aspiration, hypoxemia from prolonged attempts at intubation, endotracheal tube obstruction, endobronchial intubation from flexion of the head, esophageal intubation, and dislodgment of the endotracheal tube from head and neck extension.

E. OUTCOMES
1. **Extubation** is attempted when the indications for intubation have resolved. Excessive sedation is avoided, the oropharynx is suctioned, and the cuff is deflated.
2. **Postextubation croup** occurs in 1% to 6% of pediatric patients. Most have been intubated longer than 1 hour. Upper airway obstruction occurs acutely up to 3 hours after extubation. Treatment involves cool humidified oxygen, nebulized racemic epinephrine, or a helium-oxygen gas mixture. Steroids may be beneficial.
3. **Other postintubation sequelae** include laryngeal webs, laryngeal and tracheal granulomas, tracheal stenosis, vocal cord paralysis, sinus infections, and tracheomegaly.

MECHANICAL VENTILATION

A. OBJECTIVES OF MECHANICAL VENTILATION
1. **Improve pulmonary gas exchange.**
2. **Relieve respiratory distress** by relieving upper airway obstruction, decreasing oxygen consumption ($\dot{V}O_2$), and relieving respiratory fatigue.
3. **Manage pulmonary mechanics** by aiding upper and lower airway healing, redistributing lung volumes, and facilitating pulmonary toilet.
B. PHYSIOLOGIC PRINCIPLES OF MECHANICAL VENTILATION
1. **Pulmonary volumes** (Table 2–13)
   a. *Tidal volume (V_T):* Volume of air inspired with each resting respiratory effort. A clinical estimation of V_T equals 6 to 8 ml/kg. The calculated tidal volume is the product of inspiratory time and flow rate.

Table 2–13. PULMONARY VOLUMES

Respiratory frequency (RR)	=	Infant: 30–40 bpm
		Child: 20–30 bpm
Inspiratory time	=	Infant: 0.4–0.6 s
		Child: 0.6–1 s
Inspiratory flow	=	Infant: 2–3 L/min
		Child: 8–15 L/min
Tidal volume (V_T)	=	$\dfrac{\text{Inspiratory Time} \times \text{Flow Rate}}{RR}$
Minute ventilation ($\dot{V}E$)	=	$V_T \times RR$
Physiologic dead space (V_{DS})	=	2 ml/kg (40–50% of V_T)
Alveolar ventilation (V_A)	=	$(V_T - V_{DS}) \times RR$
Functional residual capacity (FRC)	=	30 ml/kg
Vital capacity (VC)	=	Infant: 33–40 ml/kg
		Child: 40–50 ml/kg
Total lung capacity (TLC)	=	Infant: 63 ml/kg
		Child: 70–75 ml/kg

   b. *Minute ventilation ($\dot{V}_E$):* Total volume of air moved through the airway (milliliters per liters per minute)
   c. *Alveolar ventilation (V_A):* Volume of air available for gas exchange in the alveoli
   d. *Dead space ventilation (V_{DS}):* Volume of air occupying airway lumina that do not participate in gas exchange
   e. *Functional residual capacity (FRC):* Volume of gas in the lungs at end-expiration (that which maintains alveolar distention)
   f. *Vital capacity (VC):* Volume of gas obtained at maximal expiration after maximal inspiration
   g. *Example:* Clinical estimation of pulmonary volumes in a 10-kg child (resting measurements):
   Respiratory rate (RR) = 25/min
   Inspiratory time = 0.6 s
   Flow rate = 3 L/min
   Airway dead space = 3 ml/kg × 10 kg = 30 ml
   $$V_T = \frac{(0.6 \text{ s} \times 3)}{25} = 72 \text{ ml}$$
   $\dot{V}_E$ = 72 ml × 25 (RR) = 1800 ml/min
   V_A = (72 − 30) × 25 = 1050 ml/min

2. **Inspiratory pressure** is a measurement of the resistance to airflow through the airways. Pressure is directly related to resistance. The higher the resistance, the greater the pressure required to move a given volume of gas.

3. **Resistance** is a force that impedes the flow of energy. Airway resistance is inversely proportional to airway size. The smaller the lumen, the higher the resistance. Resistance is *directly* related to length of the airway, flow rate of the gas, and viscosity of the gas.

4. **Compliance** is the relationship of volume to pressure within a closed space.
   a. *Total lung compliance* is the summation of chest wall compliance and lung compliance.
   b. *Lung compliance* is determined by the elasticity of lung tissue and the presence of surfactant in the alveoli, which prevents collapse.
   c. *Chest wall compliance* is determined by the contour of the thoracic cage and the elastic recoil of the chest wall (Fig. 2–17).

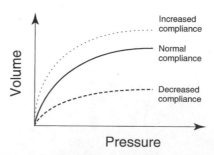

Figure 2–17. Compliance curve. Compliance reflects the amount of pressure required to deliver a given volume of air into an enclosed space such as the lung. Increased compliance of a lung unit indicates that less pressure is needed to distend the lung with a given volume. Decreased compliance indicates that *more* pressure is required to deliver the same volume of air.

5. **Relationship of pressure, volume (flow), and resistance** is expressed by the equation:

$$R \times F = P$$

   a. Ventilator mechanisms allow manipulation of pressure and flow. Resistance is altered by changes in circuit lumina (diameter and length) or by physiologic alterations in the diameter of the child's airways.
   b. In a child with reactive airway disease, resistance *increases* with bronchospasm. To maintain tidal volume, peak airway pressure must increase:

$$\uparrow R \times F \ (V_T) = \uparrow P$$

   With volume ventilation the peak inspiratory pressure (PIP) varies to achieve the same tidal volume.

6. **Physiologic interface between a ventilator and a child:** The physiologic characteristics of a child require specific mechanical performance specifications of a ventilator.
   a. **Airway:** Anatomic, subglottic narrowing of a child's airway creates resistance to exhalation, resulting in inherent or "physiologic PEEP" (approximately 3 cm). Physiologic PEEP provides a mechanism to maintain FRC in small children. Otherwise, alveolar collapse would occur at end-expiration. An artificial airway eliminates innate PEEP (because the airway bypasses the point of subglottic narrowing) evidenced by a slight inspiratory flow leak around an (appropriate size) uncuffed endotracheal tube.
   b. **Respiratory rate (RR):** Children exhibit a faster RR with a shorter inspiratory time. The inspiratory time is determined by lung compliance, airway resistance, and flow rate. A "stiff" lung (decreased compliance) or airway narrowing (increased resistance) may necessitate a longer inspiratory time.
   c. **Tidal volume (V_T):** Small absolute tidal volumes are observed in children (a 10-kg child $V_T = 70$ ml; adult $= 400$ ml). Infants and young children are unable to increase tidal volume effectively because of chest wall elasticity and dynamics. Therefore, respiratory distress in a small child is compensated by an increased respiratory rate.
   d. **Inspiratory flow:** Inspiratory flow patterns are more variable from breath to breath in infants and young children. Constant flow is more typical of the adolescent or adult. Appropriate flow rates through an oxygen delivery system or ventilator must be assured to provide adequate minute ventilation under a variety of clinical conditions.
   e. **Peak inspiratory pressure (PIP):** Lung compliance is an important determinant of PIP. The greater the compliance, the lower the PIP. Inspiratory time and airway size also influence the inspiratory pressure. A change in PIP, alone, reflects a change in lung compliance, airway resistance, or inspiratory time.
   f. **Mean airway pressure (MAP):** MAP is the average airway pressure measured at the proximal airway, from one inspiration to the beginning of the next. MAP can directly affect the PaO_2. It is influenced by a variety of mechanisms, such as tidal volume, PEEP, and PIP.
   g. **Positive end-expiratory pressure (PEEP):** Resting end-expiration lung volume (or FRC) can be increased by applying positive pressure (resistance to patient exhalation) at end-exhalation. In young children, PEEP also appears to "stint" open the airways, which have a natural tendency to collapse at end-expiration.

h. **Synchronization:** Preservation of spontaneous breathing efforts should be maintained whenever possible. Two basic sensing mechanisms allow the patient to trigger the ventilator. *Pressure sensors* measure the amount of negative pressure in the circuit as the patient initiates inspiration. *Flow sensors* measure a change in the flow rate of the circuit when the patient begins inspiration. Placement of these sensors and their sensitivity are important, since respiratory efforts may be difficult to detect. Ideally, a sensor is positioned at the proximal airway and minimizes the respiratory work of the patient.

C. **CLASSIFICATION AND MECHANISMS OF VENTILATORS**

Positive pressure ventilators create a positive pressure at the proximal airway that exceeds alveolar pressure, thus forcing gas flow to the lungs. Negative pressure ventilators create a vacuum around the chest wall, drawing the chest outward with negative pressure and initiating air entry into the lungs.

1. **Conventional positive pressure ventilation**

   a. *Classification:* Current ventilators are versatile and have been classified according to several mechanisms:
      - *Drive* mechanisms (e.g., pneumatic or electric) indicate the power source.
      - *Phase variables* regulate the inspiratory cycle with pressure, volume, and flow.
      - *Modes* describe the level of support provided to each breath and the ease of spontaneous breathing from the ventilator circuit.

   b. *Modes of ventilation*
      - *Controlled mandatory ventilation (CMV)* controls all breaths by the preset ventilator parameters without allowing the patient to breathe spontaneously. Each breath provides the same tidal volume to the patient.
      - *Intermittent mandatory ventilation (IMV)* delivers a preset number of breaths at preset parameters, but the patient can breathe spontaneously from the circuit. The spontaneous breaths are not regulated by the preset parameters; if breaths occur in the IMV timing window, the patient receives an IMV breath in spite of his or her own effort.
      - *Synchronized IMV (SIMV)* delivers a preset number of breaths, but the ventilator incorporates a sensor that can "recognize" spontaneous breaths and retimes the delivery of the next *ventilator* breath. The spontaneous breaths are not regulated by the preset parameters.
      - *Assist-control (A/C)* delivers a preset minimum mandatory rate (CMV breaths) with patient effort. The machine delivers full assistance to each breath, with preset parameters whether it is initiated by the patient or by the machine. *Flow-synchronization* allows the patient to initiate each breath with minimal effort using a flow sensor. The ventilator provides full assistance to each breath with preset PIP. Each breath is terminated by a preset flow cutoff, which is determined by a percentage of the patient's peak flow demand in each breath. A preset IMV rate is set for backup support in the event that the patient is apneic (Donn et al, 1994).
      - *Continuous positive airway pressure (CPAP)* provides positive airway pressure that is sustained throughout the patient's spontaneous respiratory cycles. CPAP should stabilize alveoli while allowing the patient to breathe spontaneously.
      - *Pressure support ventilation (PSV)* allows the patient to breathe spontaneously, triggering ventilator support with a pressure sensor. The ventilator provides a predetermined amount of pressure assistance with each

breath. When spontaneous effort is sensed, gas flow is delivered until the airway pressure reaches a preset minimum limit. The higher the pressure limit, the greater the support for the patient (decreased respiratory work). The patient can continue inspiration with a variable flow rate, while the preset airway pressure is sustained. When the patient begins exhalation and the flow rate decreases, the ventilator releases pressure. PSV can be used with SIMV in preparation for weaning, thus allowing "muscle conditioning" to occur (Fig. 2–18) (Briones & Press, 1992).

    c. *Phase variables* (Chatburn, 1992)
- The **trigger** is the mechanism that *initiates* inspiration. This requires a preset delivery rate (IMV) or a flow or pressure sensor to allow the patient to trigger the ventilator (SIMV or A/C) (Fig. 2–19).
- The **limit** refers to the variables that may *sustain* inspiration.
- The **cycle** is the variable that *terminates* inspiration (can be pressure, flow, or time).
- The **baseline** is the variable that *sustains FRC* (PEEP or CPAP).
- The **conditional variables** allow alternative ventilation modes during the preset variables (e.g., PSV coupled with SIMV). Flow delivery patterns can also be modified to match individual needs (Fig. 2–20).

    d. The choice of mechanisms is guided by the respiratory compliance of the patient, the ability to breathe spontaneously, and predicted clinical course of the underlying disease. Examples of ventilator settings for various pathophysiologic conditions are provided in Table 2–14.

2. **Alternative strategies of positive pressure ventilation**

    a. *Inverse-ratio ventilation (IRV)*
- Conventional modes of ventilation use inspiratory:expiratory (I:E) time ratios of typically 1:2 to 1:4. With IRV, the ratio is reversed. The I:E is greater than 1:1, often 2:1 or more.
- IRV is employed when the usual strategies for enhancing oxygenation have failed. IRV is thought to allow MAP and tidal volume to be maintained at relatively lower levels without increasing PEEP, provided that air trapping does not occur. Patients almost always require sedation and paralysis when receiving ventilation in this mode (Stoller, 1994).

    b. *High-frequency ventilation (HFV): Jet or oscillator delivery*
- *HFV* is a technique of ventilation that delivers ventilatory flow at supra-physiologic frequencies. The tidal volumes delivered by HFV are usually equal to or less than the physiologic dead space. Gas exchange is thought to occur by diffusion, coaxial diffusion, or entrainment. Indications for use include hypoxemia refractory to conventional ventilation, pulmonary air leaks, hypoplastic lungs, diaphragmatic hernia, and for other rescue situations such as persistent pulmonary hypertension of the newborn (Sarnack and Meert, 1996; Venkataraman and Orr, 1992).
- *High-frequency jet ventilation (HFJV)* is used in tandem with a conventional ventilator to provide gas flow, PEEP, and IMV "sighs." Driving pressure assures preset delivery of gas to the jet cannula at a set peak airway pressure. It requires a specific double lumen endotracheal tube. Exhalation occurs passively, and with such short expiratory times, air trapping is a frequent problem (Gordon and High, 1993).
- *High-frequency oscillatory ventilation (HFOV)* requires a specific ventilator with a CPAP circuit that incorporates a piston pump. The pump produces oscillatory flow at a frequency of up to 20 Hz. Exhalation occurs actively allowing carbon dioxide removal, as well as oxygenation. A conventional endotracheal tube can be used. Lung volumes remain stable after

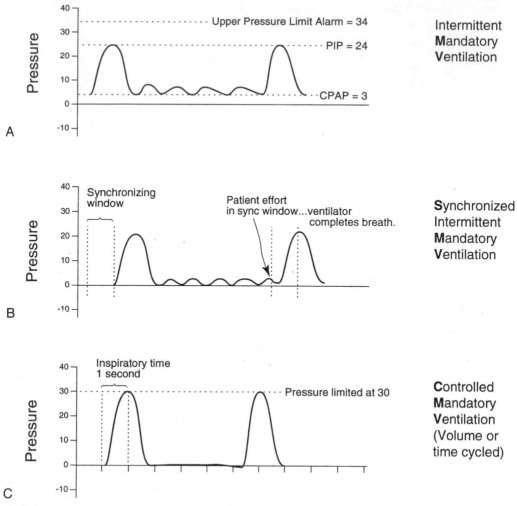

Figure 2–18. Modes of ventilation. A variety of modes of ventilation are available. The choice of ventilation is determined by the underlying disease, the patient's ability to breathe spontaneously, and compliance. *PIP,* peak inspiratory pressure.

- **IMV:** Patient can breathe spontaneously from the circuit, while the ventilator delivers a predetermined frequency of breaths, without regard for the timing of patient's respiratory rate.
- **SIMV:** A timing mechanism is integrated into the circuit to allow the ventilator to deliver a preset number of breaths, which are timed to avoid patient-ventilator competition. At set intervals, the synchronizing "window" is activated: if the patient initiates a breath during this time, the ventilator assists and completes the breath. If no breath is sensed, the ventilator delivers a mandatory breath at a fixed time after the window.
- **CMV:** Ventilator delivers a preset number of breaths with preset parameters. Patient cannot breathe from circuit.
- **Assist-Control (A/C) with flow synchronization:** Ventilator is set, as with CMV, to deliver a preset number of breaths with predetermined parameters, but it allows the patient to determine the timing of each breath. A flow sensor is usually employed to detect patient effort; when the patient initiates a breath, the ventilator assists every breath with the same preset pressure, allowing the patient to determine inspiratory time and flow rate (with upper limits on each).
- **CPAP:** Ventilator circuit can be adjusted to maintain a desired amount of end-expiratory positive pressure throughout the respiratory cycle, with no delivery of positive pressure breaths. This can be done with an endotracheal tube, nasal prongs, or mask delivery. *PEEP* is the term used to describe a method of mechanical ventilation in which a positive pressure above atmospheric pressure is maintained at end-expiration.

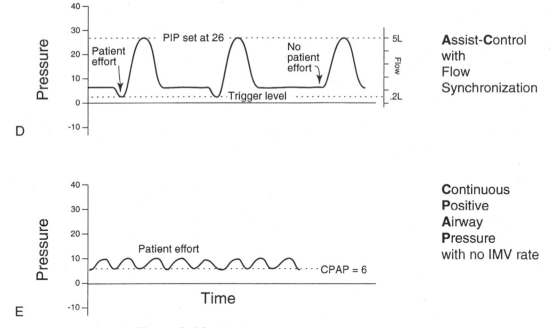

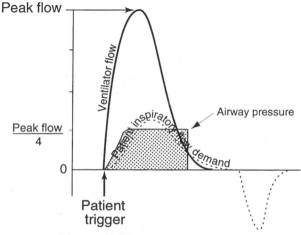

Figure 2–18. *See legend on opposite page*

initiation; therefore, it is important to assure adequate lung inflation at the start of this ventilatory technique to avoid extensive microatelectasis (Arnold et al, 1994).

- *General nursing considerations for HFV:* Pulmonary assessment is altered by the vibration of the chest. Careful observation, palpation, and auscultation allows recognition of problems, especially asymmetric examination findings. Respiratory and ECG monitoring may be difficult and require placement of electrodes on limbs or use of a pulse monitor. Since patient positioning is often limited, pressure-related skin breakdown is a risk. Suctioning procedures for specific HFV techniques should be done by at least two clinicians.

Figure 2–19. Trigger mechanism.

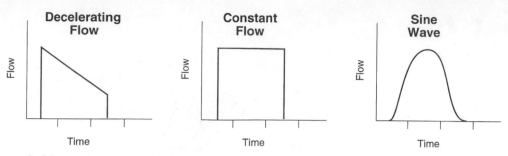

Figure 2–20. Ventilator flow delivery patterns. Many flow patterns are used to match the needs of individual patients. Three of the most commonly used are shown here.

- **Decelerating flow:** Inspiratory flow is maximal early in inspiration, with a gradual fall to zero at end-expiration. This may be useful for a patient with obstructive lung disease, in which a longer, more gradual exhalation is required.
- **Constant flow:** The flow quickly reaches a plateau and is maintained until the moment of expiration. Patients with restrictive lung disease, who have difficulty oxygenating, may benefit from this flow pattern.
- **Sine wave:** Inspiratory flow increases gradually and decreases gradually. This is a more physiologic flow pattern used in patients with mild or no lung disease.

Table 2–14. EXPECTED VENTILATOR REQUIREMENTS ASSOCIATED WITH PATHOPHYSIOLOGIC CONDITIONS

CONDITIONS	PATIENT REQUIREMENTS	VENTILATOR SETTINGS (EXAMPLE)
Upper Airway Obstruction		
Infectious disease (e.g., epiglottitis)	Normal V_T/PIP	Trigger: SIMV
Facial abnormalities	Normal Pao_2/Fio_2	Cycle: Time
Tracheomalacia	Spontaneous breathing, requires little ventilation unless sedated	Limits: None (with upper PIP alarm limit)
		Baseline: PEEP-3
		Condition: Sine-wave flow continuous flow in circuit
Decreased Lung Compliance		
Surfactant deficiency RDS	Ensure adequate V_T and normal FRC	Trigger: IMV or Assist/Control
ARDS	Monitor exhaled V_T and MAP	Cycle: Volume (8 ml/kg)
Pneumonitis	Guard against overdistention (too much V_T)	Limits: Pressure-limited
Fibrosis	May require patient paralysis or heavy sedation	Baseline: Moderate-high PEEP
Pulmonary edema	Severe disease or complications (e.g., air leak syndrome): Faster rates, lower V_T, permissive hypercarbia	Condition: Square wave 1 : 1 I : E ratio
Excessive PEEP		
Neuromuscular Disorders (Usually with Normal Compliance)		
Spinal muscular atrophy	Normal V_T, low to normal PIPs	Trigger: SIMV/flow sensor (for PSV)
Guillian-Barré syndrome	Normal Pao_2/low Fio_2	Cycle: Time
Spinal cord injury	Spontaneous breathing with support is preferable when possible	Limits: IMV: Flow
CNS alterations		PSV: (Upper limits)
Sedation	Monitor exhaled V_T on PSV breaths	Baseline: PEEP-2
Altered consciousness		Condition: PSV 12 cm H_2O
Central apnea		

ARDS, adult respiratory distress syndrome; *FRC*, functional residual capacity; *IMV*, intermittent mandatory ventilation; *MAP*, mean airway pressure; *PEEP*, positive end-expiratory pressure; *PIP*, peak inspiratory pressure; *PSV*, pressure support ventilation; *RDS*, respiratory distress syndrome; *SIMV*, synchronized IMV.

c. *Liquid ventilation with perfluorocarbons*
- *Description:* Perflugon is a chemically inert, high-viscosity liquid. When perflugon is injected into the pulmonary tree, it can provide a medium for gas exchange. In research trials, *full liquid ventilation* using a specialized delivery circuit has been demonstrated to provide sufficient gas exchange during respiratory failure.
- *Advantages:* Liquid ventilation allows recruitment of alveoli with the liquid that may be inaccessible by conventional ventilation. There is further evidence that this liquid may also diminish the inflammatory response.
- *Disadvantages:* The functional problems of full liquid ventilation include the need for a special ventilator for delivery, complicated care and mechanics of the ventilator, and thermal instability.
- *Partial liquid ventilation* is a variation of the above, in which a volume of perflugon, equal to the FRC (30 ml/kg) is instilled through a side lumen of an endotracheal tube. A conventional ventilator is used (positive pressure, time cycled, volume regulated). The perflugon layers to the bottom of the alveoli, recruiting atelectatic alveoli, and pushing alveolar debris to the top, where the debris can be periodically removed by suction (Gauger et al, 1996).

d. *Extracorporeal membrane oxygenation (ECMO)*
- *Principle of operation:* A method of providing gas exchange that bypasses the pulmonary system. Cannulation of either a major artery and major vein (arteriovenous) or one to two major veins (veno-veno) provides an extracorporeal circuit through which blood can pass to provide gas exchange. ECMO has been used in the neonatal population since the 1970s (Nugent, 1993). Pediatric use has been far more limited but early studies are encouraging (Green et al, 1996).
- *Indications:* Currently, ECMO is used as *rescue* therapy for children suffering from intractable respiratory failure (see Chapter 3 for more detail).

e. *Negative pressure ventilation:* Lung expansion can be achieved with a ventilator that delivers negative pressure, rather than positive, to a device that surrounds the chest.
- *Principle of operation:* With the thorax enclosed in the shell or tank, negative pressure is created inside the shell, creating a kind of "vacuum" pressure. The thoracic cage expands outward with this vacuum effect, thus increasing lung volume (and therefore decreasing alveolar pressure). A pressure gradient now exists between the mouth (atmospheric pressure) and the lung (subatmospheric pressure), causing air to fill the lungs. The ventilator is preset to release the negative pressure (an IMV rate) allowing the natural recoil of the lungs to allow exhalation.
- *Clinical application:* Negative pressure ventilators are useful for patients with neuromuscular disorders who have otherwise normal lungs and airways.
- *Limitations:* The seal of the tank or shell must be very tight. Dilation of the great vessels is exaggerated, diminishing cardiac output. Negative pressure ventilation is cumbersome if the child requires 24-hour-a-day ventilation.

f. *Noninvasive positive pressure ventilation:* A simple, positive pressure ventilator is used with an apparatus that is secured to the face and head. The system delivers CPAP and IMV rate (if desired).

- *Principle of operation:* Gas flow is delivered by nasal mask, oral mask, face mask, or mouthpiece according to patient comfort and needs. The ventilators are either volume cycled and deliver a prescribed tidal volume, or they are flow cycled with a pressure boost. The latter augments inspiration and provides an end-expiratory pressure termed *BIPAP* (bilevel positive airway pressure). Patients who have stable breathing patterns and do not require variable flow do well on the volume-cycled ventilators. Patients who exhibit variable flow demands or inspiratory times are more suited for the flow-cycled, pressure-assisted model.
- *Indications:* Patients must have normal airway secretions and adequate cough and gag reflexes. Patients must demonstrate a sustained effort to breathe spontaneously. Noninvasive positive pressure ventilation is becoming more recognized as a viable method for providing support after conventional ventilation. It may allow earlier extubation in some patients (Shala and Madeiri, 1996).
- *Complications* include unrecognized ventilatory insufficiency, skin breakdown, and gastric distention.

D. **PATIENT CARE MANAGEMENT AND MONITORING FOR THE CHILD RECEIVING MECHANICAL VENTILATION**

1. **Airway management:** The goal is to maintain position and patency of the endotracheal tube. Retaping of the endotracheal tube should always be done in the presence of a skilled clinician who can reintubate the patient if necessary. A bag-mask circuit and suction should always be maintained at the bedside.

2. **Assessment of the child receiving mechanical ventilation** (see Clinical Assessment discussion for detailed information)

   a. *General observations* include comfort of the child, synchrony of respiratory effort and ventilator function, chest excursion and expansion appropriate to the size of the child, color and perfusion, level of consciousness, and volume and quality of secretions. Insertion distance of the endotracheal tube should be verified and documented at frequent intervals.

   b. *Auscultation*
   - Note the symmetry of breath sounds and be aware that the thin chest walls of infants transmit breath sounds to the opposite side.
   - Note the quality of breath sounds, noting adventitious sounds, wheezing, or diminished aeration. Absent or severely diminished aeration over one entire lung is an urgent finding, reflecting either a pneumothorax, lung collapse, bronchial obstruction on that side, or malpositioned endotracheal tube.

   c. *Palpation:* Note the presence of crepitus, inspiratory crackles, or bony abnormalities.

   d. Observe for the presence and activation of ventilator and ECG alarms.

3. **Monitoring of the child during mechanical ventilation**

   a. *Arterial blood gases*
   - The conventional approach to verifying adequate oxygenation and ventilation is by periodic sampling of arterial blood with the goal of achieving normal blood gas values. It has been demonstrated that capillary blood sampling provides fairly accurate measurements of pH and P_{CO_2} (Harrison, submitted for publication 1996).
   - *Permissive hypercarbia* is a strategy for guiding ventilator manipulations that allows hypercarbia to exist with normal oxygenation, pH > 7.15, P_{CO_2} 45 to 80 mm Hg, and no evidence of cerebral dysfunction. Over

time, physiologic compensation occurs to balance the pH. The benefit of permissive hypercarbia is that it allows minimal volume ventilation, thereby diminishing the incidence of acute lung injury (Hickling et al, 1994; Martin, 1995).

b. *Pulse oximetry* should be used continuously.

c. *End-tidal Co₂ monitors* are useful in older infants and children for trending, weaning, and monitoring hyperventilation therapy.

d. *Transcutaneous carbon dioxide monitoring* (see earlier discussion).

e. Ensure activation of ECG monitoring alarms. *Appropriate ventilator alarms* should be used according to the cycling mechanisms and modes used.

f. *Serial chest radiographs* are important to verify endotracheal tube position and to evaluate pulmonary processes. The decision for x-ray examinations should be determined by the individual needs of each patient.

g. *Monitoring of neuromuscular blockade ("twitch monitoring")* is used for patients who receive a neuromuscular blocker to assess their level of paralysis. It is performed every 6 to 8 hours to ensure that the minimum amount of medication is used (Murray et al, 1995).

4. **Supportive care**

a. *Equipment function:* The nurse should be knowledgeable about the mode of ventilation, phase variables used including cycling mechanism (flow or volume, time, or pressure), trigger and sensitivity, limits (if any), baseline PEEP, and conditional variables (e.g., PSV). In addition, physiologic variables (tidal volume, PIP, FiO_2, IMV rate, MAP), alarm limits, and humidifier temperature are recognized.

b. *Fluids and electrolytes*
   - Fluid retention may occur because of underlying disease or the syndrome of inappropriate antidiuretic hormone (SIADH), since positive pressure ventilation may be associated with increased levels of antidiuretic hormone (ADH).
   - Calculation of input and output is meticulous for all patients. Fluid restriction may be used in some settings, but urine output should still be maintained at greater than 1 ml/kg/h and hemodynamic stability assured.
   - Alterations in pH affect electrolytes. Permissive hypercarbic acidosis causes bicarbonate retention and chloride excretion.

c. *Nutrition*
   - Early nutrition should be initiated for all patients. Enteral feedings are preferred and can be infused by a nasojejunal tube, even in the presence of hypoactive bowel sounds (Chellis and Sanders, 1996).
   - Formal nutrition screening should be done early and serially. Indirect calorimetry is the preferred method when available. Routine body weight measurements should be scheduled as frequently as the patient's condition allows.
   - Restriction of carbohydrates to less than 30% of metabolic needs may be necessary for patients with ventilatory insufficiency. Excess carbohydrate loads produce excess carbon dioxide (respiratory quotient [RQ] greater than or equal to 1), thus increasing ventilatory work to remove the carbon dioxide. Difficulty in weaning from a ventilator may be attributed to this in some cases (Wesley, 1992).

d. *Skin care:* Patient repositioning is done as often as tolerated at a minimum of every 2 hours. When feasible, the prone position offers significant benefit for lung aeration as well (Erhard, 1995; Stoller, 1994). Use dermal protection on pressure points. High-risk patients, especially those who do not tolerate turning, may require pressure reduction or relief from specialized mattresses. Careful inspection of all pressure points should be documented at least every 8 hours.

e. *Mobilization of pulmonary secretions:* Adequate humidification should be ensured, with proper temperature regulation (32° to 34° C for older children and 34° to 36° C for infants) for all patients.
  - Assess the patient for airway secretions and suction with saline instillation as needed every 2 to 4 hours. Maintain sterile technique for suctioning. Use of an in-line catheter allows quick, uncontaminated suctioning of an endotracheal tube, but children with thick secretions may require hand-bag ventilation with repeated instillation for removal of secretions.
  - Chest physiotherapy may not be beneficial in all patients; however, it may be needed in children with significant airway plugging and poor mobilization of secretions such as in patients with cystic fibrosis (Mackenzie et al, 1978; Martin et al, 1996).

f. *Psychologic needs of the child and family*
  - Communication barriers and sometimes diminished level of consciousness alter the child's expressive language and family relationships. Strategies for minimizing barriers include picture boards for preschoolers, picture or alphabet boards for school-age children, or hand signals described or listed at patient bedside.
  - Provide sedation as needed for comfort but also provide environmental relief through family presence, family voices on tape, or stories or music on cassettes.
  - Balance the needs for patient safety with developmental needs. Restraints are usually necessary but can be removed when there is supervision.

5. **Strategies for weaning from ventilation** (Venkataraman, 1992)
  a. *Indications for readiness:* Many parameters are suggested but must be applied with consideration of individual needs. For most patients these include hemodynamic stability, SaO_2 greater than 90% breathing less than 40% oxygen, less than 4 cm H_2O PEEP, adequacy of respiratory muscles to sustain spontaneous ventilation (tidal volumes greater than 5 ml/kg), $PaCO_2$ in a range acceptable for the patient, presence of an adequate gag and cough reflex, and negative inspiratory force (NIF) greater than 20 to 25 cm H_2O on serial measurements.
  b. *Weaning techniques:* Before weaning, parameters to be monitored for each patient should be clearly identified. They may include SaO_2, PcO_2, respiratory rate, tidal volumes, and general effort and color. *All* patients should have ECG monitoring and pulse oximetry during this process. There are numerous strategies, but the more commonly employed techniques include the following:
    - Trials of spontaneous breathing alternating with IMV support. The spontaneous periods are gradually increased while observing effort, exhaled tidal volume, and when applicable, arterial blood gases.
    - PSV is used initially with IMV. IMV rate is weaned gradually to a predetermined goal, then PSV is weaned, observing trends in exhaled tidal volumes (to be greater than 5 ml/kg) and respiratory rate as support is withdrawn. Be aware that with reduction in PSV, fatigue or atelectasis may not be apparent for 3 to 6 hours or more (Briones and Press, 1992).
    - Weaning from (S)IMV mode involves reducing the IMV rate gradually to CPAP.

- Children can be weaned to noninvasive ventilatory support such as the BIPAP system or a negative pressure shell (Shala and Medeiri, 1996; Udwadia et al, 1992).

6. **Complications of mechanical ventilation**

   a. *Oxygen toxicity:* Patients receiving greater than 50% FIO_2 for prolonged periods of time may develop parenchymal changes from oxygen exposure (Durbin and Wallace, 1993). Oxygen should be treated as a medication, with strict adherence to prescription guidelines. Continuous monitoring of FIO_2 is strongly recommended. The lowest acceptable SaO_2 measurement for the child should be clearly established while FIO_2 is maintained at the lowest possible level.

   b. *Acute lung injury (ALI):* Alveolar overdistention is responsible for the development of pulmonary injury (Martin, 1995). Cyclic opening and closing of lung units with large volumes cause injury by "shearing" forces. Exhaled tidal volumes should be continuously monitored and documented every 1 to 2 hours. Parameters for "acceptable" exhaled volumes should be established for each patient. If the patient is not pressure limited, PIP should be noted; if PIP increases, the patient's condition should be carefully evaluated.

   c. *Barotrauma* has been reported to occur in 13% (N = 100) of patients with ARDS who are receiving mechanical ventilation (Schnapp et al, 1995). High PIPs or distending pressures or sudden changes in either may cause alveolar rupture. Continuous observation of lung volumes and pressures is required to minimize the occurrence of this complication.

   d. *Atelectasis* occurs from nonuniform distribution of tidal volume, inadequate tidal volume, and adsorption atelectasis. Patient positioning may affect the site of atelectasis. Patient repositioning (including head elevation) should be done every 1 to 2 hours. The prone position is useful for lower lobe aeration and should be used when feasible (Erhard, 1995).

   e. *Pneumonia:* Endotracheal tubes become quickly colonized with bacteria, most commonly gram-negative organisms, thus providing entry to the lungs. Some ventilated patients develop nosocomial pneumonia. Aspiration is a constant risk. The presence of an endotracheal tube does *not* guarantee protection for patients. A nasogastric tube is required for drainage. Current research questions the practice of the routine use of gastric acid reduction by such agents as histamine-2 blockers. It is thought that alkaline gastric secretions impose a greater risk for nosocomial pneumonia than acidic (Apte et al, 1992; Craven et al, 1986). The complete blood count with differential and temperature should be evaluated while the endotracheal tube is in place. When a *new* endotracheal tube is placed in a patient with a pneumonic process, tracheal aspirate specimens for Gram stain and culture can be useful. However, the specimens should be interpreted in conjunction with clinical factors, organism, and evidence of inflammatory cell infiltration.

   f. *Decreased cardiac output* caused by elevated intrathoracic pressures (especially high levels of PEEP) is a frequent problem, caused by compression of the great vessels. This can be remediated with adequate volume (preload) expansion. A central vascular line for monitoring CVP or pulmonary pressures is often essential in hemodynamically unstable patients.

   g. *SIADH* may occur because of third spacing or fluid retention. Hourly urine output measurements and serial serum sodium and protein measurements allow early detection.

h. *Complications from intubation* include postextubation edema, tracheal ulcerations, vocal cord injury, granulomas or polyp formation, sinusitis, and airway obstruction due to a plugged endotracheal tube.

7. **Pharmacologic management of the patient receiving mechanical ventilation** Patients requiring mechanical ventilation also usually require a variety of adjunctive medications for either stabilizing pulmonary management or patient comfort (see Pulmonary Pharmacology and Acute Respiratory Failure discussions).

ASPIRATION PNEUMONITIS

A. **DEFINITION**
Pneumonitis is inflammation caused by pulmonary aspiration of fluids. Aspiration of gastric fluid produces direct injury to the mucosal surface of the respiratory tract. Alveolar damage is followed by an interstitial reaction causing acute inflammatory and polymorphonuclear cell infiltration of the alveolus. Common aspirates include gastric irritants and hydrocarbons.

B. **ETIOLOGY**
Any impairment or depression of normal reflexes increases the risk of aspiration. This may be caused by an altered level of consciousness from anesthesia, seizures, or toxic ingestion. Altered anatomy or function of the trachea or esophagus may predispose to aspiration of secretions or stomach contents (Table 2–15).

C. **PATHOPHYSIOLOGY**
Initial parenchymal injury occurs from direct epithelial damage. Indirect damage occurs from generation of toxic radicals, inflammatory cells, and activation of the complement system. Pneumonitis, or inflammation of lung parenchyma, may involve pleura, interstitium, and airways. To be classified as pneumonia, alveolar consolidation must be present.

D. **CLINICAL PRESENTATION**
1. **History:** To appropriately treat the patient it is important to know the nature of the aspirated material. Determine the events surrounding the aspiration episode, such as level of consciousness and feeding history.
2. **Physical examination:** Patients may demonstrate increased cough and fever, acute dyspnea, wheezing, and cyanosis progressing to pulmonary edema. Observe for increased work of breathing, retractions, and increased respiratory rate. Auscultate for absent breath sounds, crackles, or wheezing in the affected lobes. Aspiration of oral secretions presents with signs similar to acute bacterial pneumonia.

Table 2–15.   CAUSES OF ASPIRATION PNEUMONITIS

Altered level of consciousness	Drugs, alcohol, anesthesia, seizures, central nervous system disorders
Altered anatomy of trachea or esophagus	Tracheal or esophageal abnormalities, endotracheal tube, tracheostomy
Altered function of swallow or esophageal motility	Loss of normal reflexes, which prevent aspiration of stomach contents; gastroesophageal reflux, especially when associated with neurologic or anatomic impairment
Inhalation injury	Inhalation of toxic substances such as gastric acids or hydrocarbons

3. **Diagnostic tests**
    a. Chest radiographic changes following aspiration are related to irritation, inflammation, and pneumonia. Aspiration pneumonia characteristically produces patchy opacification in the lung bases and perihilar infiltrations. Radiographs may demonstrate slight hyperventilation to diffuse infiltrates or alveolar densities. Infiltrates are most likely to be observed in the right upper lobe in a patient who was supine at the time of aspiration. Chest radiograph changes may worsen over the first 72 hours and then begin to clear. Radiographic abnormalities may persist for 4 to 6 weeks.
    b. Arterial blood gases should be evaluated if hypoxemia is clinically significant.
    c. Pulse oximetry gives a continuous measurement of hemoglobin oxygen saturation.

4. **Clinical course**
    a. Presentation and management of aspiration pneumonia depends on the nature and quantity of the aspirated material. The degree of lung injury is dependent on the pH of the aspirated material and the presence of bacteria.
    b. Materials with an acidotic pH may produce immediate pulmonary symptoms that worsen over the first 24 hours. Chemical burns increase alveolar capillary membrane permeability with subsequent extravasation of fluid into interstitium and alveoli. Often lung volume decreases, then ventilation-perfusion mismatch and hypoxia occur. Acidotic fluid produces airway irritation, bronchospasm, peribronchial hemorrhage, and necrosis.
    c. Materials with a normal pH can induce hypoxia or pulmonary edema, but generally there is little necrosis.
    d. Irritant gases cause direct injury to the mucosal surface. Epithelial cells become edematous, then necrotic, going through three phases. The acute phase is characterized by pulmonary edema, hypoxemia, and respiratory failure. The delayed phase is characterized by pulmonary edema, airway obstruction, and superinfection. The long-term phase involves reactive airways and interstitial fibrosis.

5. **Differential diagnosis:** Evaluate for foreign body aspiration. Generally cough, dyspnea, and wheezing are seen with foreign body aspiration (see Foreign Body Aspiration discussion). Differentiate between acute bacterial or viral pneumonia by history, chest radiograph, secretions, and tracheal aspirate (if available).

E. **MANAGEMENT**
    1. **Prevention**
        a. An obtunded or tachypneic patient should not receive oral feedings. Patients with CNS injury, those receiving sedation, or those recovering from intraoperative anesthesia are also at risk.
        b. Nasogastric feedings should be monitored closely. Prior to initiation of feedings the patient should be assessed for gastric distention and bowel sounds. Volume of gastric aspirate should be checked periodically to assure adequate emptying of the stomach.
        c. If gastroesophageal reflux is suspected, follow reflux precautions. These include small, frequent feedings and raising the head of the bed after feedings.
        d. Use transpyloric feedings if an endotracheal tube has been placed or if there is a significant risk of gastroesophageal reflux or poor gastric emptying.

    e. In patients who may not have an empty stomach, rapid-sequence intubation techniques (including cricoid pressure) should be employed, and suctioning equipment should be available.

  2. **Supportive care**

    a. High oxygen concentrations, mechanical ventilation, and high PEEP may be necessary.

    b. Choice of antibiotics is dependent on the patient's age and the cause of aspiration. Prophylactic antimicrobials have not been proven to be of benefit and allow for overgrowth of resistant organisms. Antibiotic therapy should be reserved for known or suspected secondary infection.

    c. Reflux aspiration can often be treated medically through elevation of the head and torso while asleep, antacids, gastrointestinal motility–enhancing agents, and small, frequent, thickened feedings.

    d. Bethanechol and metoclopramide are used to increase gastrointestinal motility and lower esophageal sphincter pressure. Cisapride, cimetidine (Tagamet), and ranitidine can be administered to control gastric pH.

    e. Surgical management by a Nissen fundoplication can be done if medical management fails.

F. OUTCOMES

Prognosis is generally good. Mild restrictive or obstructive defects such as bronchiectasis (dilation of the bronchi from bronchial wall damage) and reactive airways disease have been observed.

FOREIGN BODY ASPIRATION

A. ETIOLOGY

Foreign body aspiration is an important cause of accidental death in infants and children. Toddlers younger than 3 years of age are responsible for 60% to 80% of foreign body aspirations. Beginning at 8 to 10 months the curious infant has developed thumb-forefinger grasp, enabling placement of objects into the mouth, and has learned to crawl. By 1 to 2 years of age the toddler is climbing. The foreign body is usually organic, with nuts being the most common. Other small items frequently found in the environment of a child pose a risk for occluding the airway.

B. PATHOPHYSIOLOGY

The severity of lung disease and rapidity of presentation depends on the type of object aspirated and the amount of airway obstruction produced. Less than 5% of inhaled foreign bodies are found in the more distal portions of the tracheobronchial tree. Most lodge in a main stem or lobar bronchus. Laryngeal foreign bodies are more common in infants younger than 1 year of age.

C. CLINICAL PRESENTATION

  1. **History:** Fewer than 40% of patients give a clear history of an aspirated foreign body. The initial episode frequently is associated with choking and coughing. Often the symptoms subside, and the child presents at a later time with diverse symptoms, such as coughing, wheezing, recurrent or protracted pneumonia, and fever. The right bronchus is more often the site of the foreign body than the left bronchus, but the airway may be blocked anywhere from the posterior pharynx to the bronchus (Fig. 2–21).

  2. **Physical examination:** Examination findings may be normal or reveal nonspecific signs, such as decreased air entry, wheezing, rhonchi, or inspiratory stridor. Patients with laryngeal foreign bodies present with stridor, dyspnea, cyanosis, cough, and voice change. Total airway obstruction can occur. Patients with

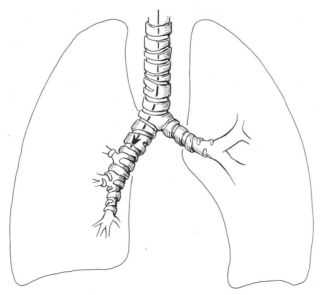

Figure 2–21.   Right main stem bronchus.

bronchial foreign bodies present with cough, asymmetric breath sounds, wheezing, dyspnea, and fever.

3. **Diagnostic tests:** Chest radiographs may show metallic or radiopaque objects. A single foreign body lodged in a single bronchus may present with obstructive emphysema. Chest radiographs may be normal in as many as 38% of cases. A chest radiograph may demonstrate atelectasis, infiltrate, or hyperinflation; however, it is not a reliable indicator of foreign body aspiration. Inspiratory and expiratory radiographs can be evaluated for ball-valve bronchial obstruction. Soft tissue lateral neck x-ray films are used to evaluate for the presence of laryngeal foreign bodies. Endoscopy is used to confirm foreign body aspiration.

4. **Clinical course** depends on the degree of obstruction, location of the foreign body, nature of the object, and availability of equipment or personnel.
   a. For life-threatening airway obstruction follow basic life support emergency measures for the choking child as outlined below. Emergent rigid broncho-scopy should be performed if these maneuvers are unsuccessful.
   b. Prior to removal of the foreign body a quiet environment should be provided and vital signs and respiratory distress must be watched carefully. Monitor for changes in heart rate, respiratory rate, increased retractions, pallor, or cyanosis.
   c. Following removal, respiratory effort should continue to be monitored, observing for signs of airway obstruction from edema at the site of the foreign body removal.

D. PATIENT CARE MANAGEMENT
   1. **Prevention**
      a. Parents should be instructed to limit the availability of nuts, jewelry, small objects, latex balloons, popcorn, and hot dogs to children less than 3 years of age.
      b. Ipecac and poison control phone numbers should be readily available in the child's home.
   2. **Emergency care:** Follow Pediatric Advanced Life Support recommendations. If the child still has adequate air exchange and an effective cough, no attempt is made to dislodge the foreign body prior to definitive management with

a bronchoscopy. If the child has inadequate air exchange, administer five back blows followed by five chest thrusts for a child younger than 1 year of age or the Heimlich maneuver for the older child. Oxygen should be supplied by face mask.

3. **Respiratory care**
   a. Monitor closely for signs of deterioration such as changes in heart rate, respiratory rate, increase in severity of sternal retractions, or increased oxygen requirement.
   b. The most effective intervention for acute aspiration of a foreign body is immediate removal of the object. Laryngoscopy or rigid bronchoscopy may be performed for direct visualization of the airway and removal of the foreign body. Rigid bronchoscopy is performed while the child receives general anesthesia; the procedure is 90% effective in removing a foreign body.

4. **Supportive care**
   a. Administer oxygen as indicated.
   b. Infection can develop in the area of the lung distal to the obstruction and usually resolves rapidly once the foreign body is removed. Antibiotic therapy should be used if a culture of respiratory secretions shows positive results for infection.

5. **Complications and outcome:** There may be pronounced local inflammation or granulation in the airway with long-standing foreign bodies. If the foreign body is not readily removed, obstruction from edema, erosion with infection, perforation, and hemorrhage may develop. Generally, the outcome is good if appropriate and timely management is provided.

AIR LEAK SYNDROMES

A. DEFINITIONS

Pneumothorax is a collection of air in the pleural space (Fig. 2–22).

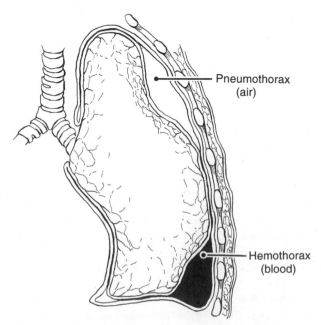

Figure 2–22. Pneumothorax and hemothorax.

B. ETIOLOGY

1. **Postoperative patients** may have air leaks related to pleural space disruption during surgery allowing air accumulation or inadequate air drainage by the chest drainage system.

2. **Air leaks** can occur during chest tube removal, as a complication of mechanical ventilation, or as a complication of respiratory disease.

3. **Upper airway trauma** can cause severe tracheobronchial disruption after high-energy impact injuries. Injuries range from irregular tears to complete transection.

4. **Thoracic trauma** (see Thoracic Trauma and Multiple Trauma discussions) may be blunt or penetrating. A penetrating chest wound allows free, bidirectional flow of air between the affected hemithorax and the surrounding atmosphere.

C. CLINICAL PRESENTATION

1. **History:** Determine the presence of any of the causes just mentioned. Because of the increased compliance of the child's chest wall, tracheobronchial injury may occur without the suggestive chest wall injuries seen in the adult patient.

2. **Physical examination**

   a. Pneumothorax presents with decreased intensity or change in pitch of breath sounds over the involved area, increased PIP (in the child receiving mechanical ventilation), tachypnea, increased respiratory effort demonstrated by the presence of retractions, or a sudden change in color to pale or cyanotic. Referred breath sounds may be heard over the area of the pneumothorax in the infant. Decreased breath sounds are noted over the affected area in the older child.

   b. Tension pneumothorax may present with agitation, hypotension from obstruction of venous return to the heart, severe hypoxemia, unilateral chest wall movement, decreased breath sounds on the affected side, and cardiorespiratory distress. Heart sounds may be shifted away from the pneumothorax. Tracheal deviation and mediastinal shift is away from the side of the pneumothorax. Respiratory failure, distended neck veins, and cyanosis can progress to circulatory collapse (Fig. 2–23).

   c. Tracheobronchial injury may present with subcutaneous emphysema, dyspnea, sternal tenderness, and hemoptysis. Subcutaneous emphysema is noted when gas tracks along the peribronchial and perivascular tissues to the mediastinum and then up into the neck.

   d. Open pneumothorax (sucking chest wound) results from a penetrating chest wound. There can be paradoxical shifting of the mediastinum to the contralateral side with each spontaneous breath (flail chest). Severe respiratory distress with hypoxia can be seen.

3. **Diagnostic tests**

   a. Chest radiographs of pneumothorax demonstrate no pulmonary vascular markings present from the air-tissue interface in the pleural cavity. A pneumothorax is seen as a uniformly translucent area without lung markings. Free pleural air accumulates in the nondependent portions of the chest. A cross-table lateral radiograph may be necessary to detect intrapleural gas in supine patients. This is particularly important in those with noncompliant lungs that do not readily collapse. Multiple broken ribs are generally noted in flail chest. With a tension pneumothorax the diaphragm is flattened, and the heart and trachea deviate to the nonaffected side.

   b. Chest radiographs of tracheobronchial injury demonstrate subcutaneous emphysema, pneumomediastinum, pneumothorax, and air surrounding the bronchus.

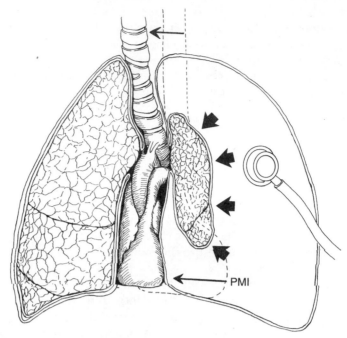

Figure 2–23.   Tension pneumothorax. *PMI,* point of maximal impulse.

  c. Diagnostic bronchoscopy is necessary to confirm the location and the extent of the disruption in tracheobronchial injury.

  d. Transillumination of the chest may enable detection of pneumothorax in newborns and premature infants.

 4. **Clinical course** depends on the size of pneumothorax and the presence or absence of tension.

D. MANAGEMENT

 1. **Prevention:** Care must be taken to avoid reentry of air during chest tube removal. Use ventilatory strategies to minimize barotrauma during mechanical ventilation. Set high pressure alarms on the ventilator to 10 to 15 cm H_2O above PIPs. Avoid excessive peak pressures when manually bagging patient by monitoring with pressure manometer.

 2. **Direct care**

  a. Pneumothorax should be treated with placement of a chest tube. The chest tube is placed in the fifth intercostal space just lateral to the nipple at the point between the anterior and midaxillary line. After placement the chest tube is connected to a water seal and suction system. Multiple tubes may be required depending on the location of air or blood. An emergent needle thoracentesis may be performed if the patient is experiencing significant hemodynamic or respiratory compromise. Needle thoracentesis may be accomplished through the insertion of a 14-gauge needle at the second intercostal space on the midclavicular line, just above the third rib. The catheter may be left in place with a stopcock; some recommend venting to room air until a chest tube is inserted (Fig. 2–24).

  b. Treatment for an open pneumothorax (flail chest) consists of positive pressure ventilation and covering the wound with an occlusive dressing followed by chest tube insertion.

  c. Tension pneumothorax requires prompt evacuation by needle thoracentesis or a chest tube.

3. **Supportive care:** Evaluate for effectiveness of chest tube placement by auscultation and chest radiography. Monitor function of the chest tube drainage system by observing the quantity of air that is evacuated. Monitor the patient for signs of reaccumulation such as tachypnea, hypoxia, or increased respiratory effort. Assess for evidence of erythema or drainage when changing the chest

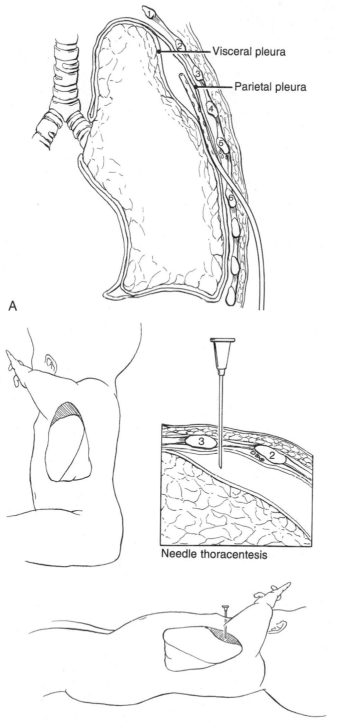

Figure 2–24. **A,** Chest tube placement. **B,** Needle thoracentesis location.

tube dressing. Remove the chest tube when evidence of the air leak has disappeared (no air movement through the water seal chamber of chest tube) and risk of further barotrauma is negligible.

4. **Complications:** Complications of a chest tube placement include hemorrhage, hemothorax, direct bronchial or parenchymal lung injury, infection, and nerve injury.

THORACIC TRAUMA

Thoracic injuries in children are uncommon. There are five major areas of injury in the thoracic area: (1) thoracic space (hemothorax, pneumothorax), (2) large airways, (3) major thoracic blood vessels and heart , (4) pulmonary parenchyma, and (5) the thoracic cage. The injuries most often encountered are pulmonary contusions, pneumothorax, hemothorax, and rib fractures.

A. **ETIOLOGY**

Thoracic trauma may be the result of blunt or penetrating injury. Rib fractures indicate severe chest trauma, and injury to underlying organs, such as the liver, spleen, and lungs, is likely to be present. But serious intrathoracic injury can also be present in the absence of obvious chest wall injury. Therefore, intrathoracic injuries must be suspected and ruled out whenever there is a significant history of blunt or penetrating trauma.

B. **PATHOPHYSIOLOGY**

1. A child's chest wall is extremely compliant, and the mediastinum is mobile. This contributes to a low overall incidence of rib fractures and major vessel or airway injury in children.

2. **Rib fractures**

   a. Half of intrathoracic injuries in children are not associated with rib fractures. The presence of three or more rib fractures in a child reliably identifies him or her in a subgroup of patients with a significant likelihood of intrathoracic, as well as other organ, involvement. Children with rib fractures after trauma have higher mortality compared with children without rib fractures.

   b. In comparison to adults, first and second rib fractures in children do not correlate with the presence of injury to the great vessels; however, great vessel injury should be ruled out. Thoracic spine fractures should increase suspicion of great vessel injury.

3. **Pulmonary contusions** result in hemorrhage and edema in the peripheral alveolar interstitium, as well as focal capillary leaks. Blood in the alveoli leads to ventilation-perfusion mismatch. Contusions may be associated with pneumothorax or hemothorax (presence of blood in the pleural space) (Fig. 2–22). Many cases of pulmonary contusion and other intrathoracic lesions are not radiographically evident until 48 hours after injury.

4. **Tracheobronchial injuries** from blunt trauma can be difficult to diagnose. Half the deaths from tracheobronchial injury occur within 1 hour after the injury. Generally, tracheobronchial injury is the result of blunt trauma to the neck.

5. **Pneumothorax and hemothorax** together account for almost half of childhood intrathoracic injuries. The majority of chest injuries resulting in pneumothorax or hemothorax require only a tube thoracostomy for successful management.

   a. A *tension pneumothorax* produces mediastinal shift with tracheal deviation, which can interfere with central venous return and lead to decreased cardiac output. Tension pneumothorax requires emergency intervention.

    b. *Hemothorax* is a blood collection in the pleural cavity (>20 ml/kg). It presents with ventilatory insufficiency and sometimes hypovolemic shock.

6. **Cardiac injuries** generally result from blunt trauma.

    a. *Myocardial contusion* is a cardiac muscle injury secondary to blunt traumatic forces.

    b. *Cardiac tamponade* is a compression of the heart produced by accumulation of blood under pressure in the confined space of the pericardial sac. This results in decreased filling of the heart and decreased cardiac output. Patients present with a narrow pulse pressure, muffled heart sounds, distended neck veins, and shock (Fig. 2–25).

    c. *Other cardiac injuries* include valvular dysfunction from papillary muscle or chordae tendineae rupture, cardiac rupture, pericardial effusions, and cardiac dysrhythmia. All cardiac injuries demonstrate signs of decreased cardiac output such as poor perfusion and poor pulses.

7. **Aortic and great vessel injuries** most commonly involve traumatic aortic disruption in the older adolescent population.

C. **CLINICAL PRESENTATION**

1. **History** is important to learn the details of the mechanism of the injury to pinpoint possible sites of injury.

2. **Physical examination**

    a. Children with significant intrathoracic injuries may not have suggestive external evidence of these injuries. The primary survey during trauma resuscitation includes a rapid thoracoabdominal examination. Quickly assess airway and breathing. The absence of breath sounds implies the presence of a pneumothorax or hemothorax. However, because of the hyperresonance of the infant's thoracic cavity, breath sounds may be transmitted to the contralateral side. Observe for chest wall ecchymosis, bruising, abrasions, sensation of crepitus, point tenderness over a rib, or a displaced trachea.

    b. *Tension pneumothorax* causes severe respiratory distress, distended neck veins, contralateral tracheal deviation, and poor systemic perfusion. There

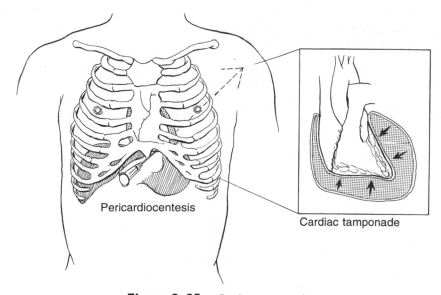

Pericardiocentesis

Cardiac tamponade

Figure 2–25. Cardiac tamponade.

may be hyperresonance to percussion, decreased chest expansion, and diminished breath sounds on the side of the injury (see Air Leak Syndromes discussion).

    c. *Hemothorax* is manifest by signs similar to tension pneumothorax. Tachycardia and hypotension may be a result of decreased venous return to the heart.

    d. In *tracheobronchial injury,* small tears may present with subcutaneous emphysema, dyspnea, sternal tenderness, and hemoptysis. Complete transection presents with severe respiratory distress and failure.

    e. *Rib fractures* may cause palpable crepitus, rib deformity, and asymmetric chest wall movement. Pain leads to splinting of the thorax with impaired ventilation.

    f. *Aortic and great vessel injuries* should be suspected if the patient develops midscapular back pain, unexplained hypotension, upper extremity hypertension, bilateral femoral pulse deficits, large initial chest tube output, sternal fracture, or widened mediastinum demonstrated by chest x-ray examination.

3. **Diagnostic tests**

    a. Radiographic evaluation of the chest is standard in thoracic trauma cases (Table 2–16).

    b. Arterial blood gas monitoring is used to evaluate for hypoxia, hypercarbia, and respiratory acidosis.

    c. CT scan may be a useful adjunct in the evaluation and management of blunt chest trauma.

    d. Bronchoscopy is used to confirm the diagnosis of rupture of the trachea or bronchus.

    e. ECG can be used to evaluate for ischemic changes, premature atrial or ventricular contractions, and other arrhythmias that may occur with myocardial contusion.

    f. Other diagnostic tests for myocardial trauma include serum creatine kinase, CK-MB isoenzyme, radionuclide angiography, and echocardiography.

D. MANAGEMENT

1. **Direct care** involves assessment and establishment of an airway, breathing, and circulation and correction of life-threatening injuries.

    a. Needle decompression is required for tension pneumothorax.

Table 2–16. RADIOGRAPHIC EVALUATION OF THE CHEST IN TRAUMA

Hemothorax	Fluid assumes a dependent position
	Complete opacification of the hemithorax with accumulation of pleural fluid
	The trachea and mediastinum may be shifted away
	A lateral decubitus view may help confirm the presence of free pleural fluid
Pneumothorax	Presents with unilateral hyperlucency
Tension pneumothorax	Underlying lung will collapse
	Trachea and mediastinum will be shifted away from the side of the pneumothorax
Rib fractures	Rib and thoracic spine fractures are evaluated
	Excludes other chest and upper abdominal injuries
Cardiac tamponade, aortic and great vessel injuries	High mediastinal width–to–chest width ratio
	Blurring of the aortic knob
	Tracheal deviation
	Widened peritracheal stripes
	Increased heart size with tamponade

     b. With hemothorax the chest tube is placed more posteriorly if possible. Ideally, the fourth to fifth intercostal space along the midaxillary line is used. This presents little danger to the thoracic nerve and little risk to the liver or spleen. If blood from the chest tube is bright red, the source may be intercostal vessels or the internal thoracic artery. In penetrating injuries the source may be a disruption of the aorta or a hole in the heart. This generally is followed by rapid decompensation and death if early intervention is not accomplished. Thoracotomy is indicated when the thoracostomy tube output is more than 2 to 3 ml/kg/h or greater than 20% of the blood volume.

     c. Myocardial contusion requires an adequate airway and oxygenation, continuous cardiac monitoring, and serial cardiac isoenzymes. Lidocaine infusion may be necessary for dysrhythmias causing hemodynamic compromise.

     d. Cardiac tamponade requires establishment of an airway, breathing, and circulation. Pericardiocentesis is performed, and blood is then aspirated from the pericardium (Fig. 2–25). Thoracotomy is indicated for ongoing hemorrhage to drain the pericardium and repair the bleeding site.

     e. Tracheobronchial injury requires intubation to ensure adequate oxygenation and ventilation and a chest tube for evacuation of air. Surgical intervention is necessary to overcome a large air leak.

     f. Rib fractures may necessitate supplemental oxygen and good pulmonary toilet. Avoid atelectasis and pneumonia by providing analgesia and encouraging deep breathing.

  2. **Supportive care:** Continue with chest tube evacuation of air or blood as long as necessary. Provide rigorous pulmonary toilet to prevent atelectasis (postural drainage, cough). If the patient is receiving mechanical ventilation, provide frequent suctioning and monitor PIP. Use antibiotics only for a confirmed infection. Provide oxygen as necessary.

  3. **Complications** include sudden hypotension after the chest tube is placed and the complications of chest tube placement as defined earlier.

E. OUTCOMES

Most pediatric trauma-related mortality occurs before admission to the hospital, whether in the field or in the emergency department. Initial stabilization of the pediatric trauma victim includes rapid cardiopulmonary assessment, basic airway maneuvers, vascular access skills, and cardiopulmonary stabilization.

BRONCHIOLITIS

A. DEFINITION

Bronchiolitis is an acute inflammatory disease of the lower respiratory tract resulting in obstruction of small airways (Fig. 2–26).

B. PATHOPHYSIOLOGY

  1. The virus replicates in the epithelial cells of the airways, resulting in epithelial damage and proliferation of nonciliated cells. This combined with edema of the submucosal layer causes obstruction of the small airways and diffusion impairment. Multiple areas of atelectasis produce ventilation-perfusion mismatching and abnormal gas exchange.

  2. The principal abnormality in gas exchange is hypoxemia. Most infants are able to maintain normocarbia in spite of ventilation-perfusion mismatch by increasing their respiratory rate. Hypercarbia and respiratory failure develop when the infant becomes fatigued and minute ventilation falls.

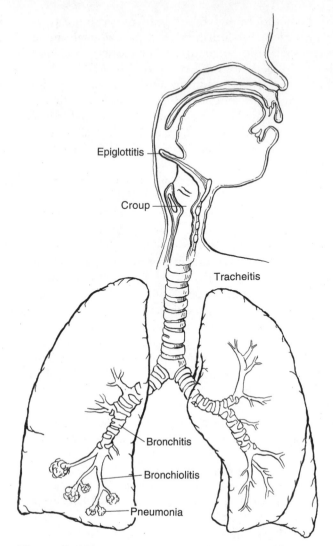

Figure 2–26.   Anatomic location of respiratory infections.

C. **ETIOLOGY**
   1. Bronchiolitis may be caused by a number of viral pathogens depending on the age of the child, immune function, and seasonal and geographic variables. Influenza, parainfluenza, and respiratory syncytial virus (RSV) are most likely. RSV is the most common pathogen.
   2. Peak incidence occurs during midwinter and early spring and typically affects infants approximately 6 months of age.
   3. Infants with bronchopulmonary dysplasia, cyanotic congenital heart disease, prematurity, cystic fibrosis, and other chronic illnesses are at risk for severe bronchiolitis.
D. **CLINICAL PRESENTATION**
   1. **History:** Generally there is a 2- to 5-day history of upper respiratory tract infection with fever and known exposure.
   2. **Physical examination** demonstrates cough, sneezing, rhinorrhea, and respiratory distress with tachypnea, retractions, wheezing, prolonged expiration, rales, and irritability. Infants may also present with poor feeding, low-grade fever, apnea, and cyanosis.

3. **Diagnostic tests:** Diagnosis is based primarily on clinical observations.
   a. Chest radiography demonstrates hyperinflation, atelectasis, and peribronchial thickening in 50% of cases. Partial lobar or patchy involvement in multiple areas of the lung or shifting regional infiltrates may be present.
   b. Arterial blood gas analysis may show hypoxemia or hypercarbia.
   c. Pulse oximetry may demonstrate hypoxemia.
   d. Rapid fluorescent antibody test for RSV may be used to test nasopharyngeal secretions. Direct isolation of the virus may be possible through nasopharyngeal washing but may require up to 2 weeks for positive culture results.
4. **Clinical course:** Bronchiolitis generally peaks in 48 to 72 hours, but may require several days of hospitalization for evaluation and monitoring. Severe cases may require mechanical ventilation for apnea, hypoxemia, or respiratory failure.

E. PATIENT CARE MANAGEMENT
   1. **Prevention:** Nosocomial spread of viral pathogens can be minimized with good hand washing. Influenza vaccine is recommended for children with chronic cardiac, pulmonary, or metabolic disorders.
   2. **Direct respiratory care** involves hospitalization if the patient is younger than 6 months of age or has respiratory distress requiring oxygen therapy. Provide oxygen as needed or mechanical ventilation if respiratory failure, hypoxemia, or apnea develops. Pneumothorax should be considered if a sudden deterioration occurs.
   3. **Supportive care**
      a. Fluids and nutritional requirements are maintained with physiologic maintenance fluids and enteral nutrition if possible. Tube feedings may be considered in infants with tachypnea.
      b. Monitoring is important, since infants can quickly progress to respiratory failure. Vital signs, sensorium, breathing pattern, and skin color are assessed. Noninvasive measurement includes pulse oximetry and end-tidal CO_2 for patients using an endotracheal tube. Invasive monitoring includes arterial blood gas monitoring.
      c. Steroid therapy is generally not indicated, but may be useful in patients with a reactive bronchospastic component to their disease. Because it is usually a viral infection, antibacterial agents are not recommended. If bacterial pneumonia cannot be excluded, antibiotics may be started until appropriate culture results are negative. Ganciclovir is an antiviral with significant activity against cytomegalovirus (CMV) in immunosuppressed patients. RSV chemotherapy (ribavirin) can reduce viral shedding but does not reduce respiratory tract symptoms, so its use remains controversial.
   4. **Complications** include secondary bacterial infection and ARDS.

F. OUTCOMES
   Impaired oxygenation may exist for several weeks after apparent clinical recovery. Studies have shown that between 5% and 50% of children with acute bronchiolitis in infancy develop recurrent wheezing later in life.

ACUTE EPIGLOTTITIS

A. DEFINITION
   Acute epiglottitis is a severe, life-threatening, rapidly progressive infection of the epiglottis and surrounding area (Fig. 2–27).
B. PATHOPHYSIOLOGY
   Thickened epiglottis and aryepiglottic folds lead to narrowing of the airway and turbulent gas flow. Pulmonary edema may occur from an increased transmural

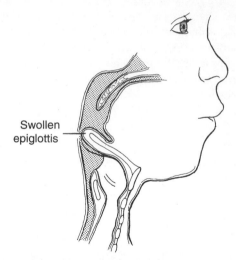

Figure 2–27. Swollen epiglottis in acute epiglottitis.

pressure gradient from pulmonary vasoconstriction due to alveolar hypoxia, as well as the negative pleural pressure generated against the airway obstruction.

C. ETIOLOGY

Acute epiglottitis usually occurs in children 2 to 6 years old, but may occur at any age. Mortality is between 8% and 12% of children admitted to hospitals. The usual cause is *Haemophilus influenzae* type b (Hib) (75% to 80%), β-hemolytic streptococci, or pneumococci. Since most epiglottitis cases in children are caused by Hib, the Hib vaccine has significantly reduced this disease in children.

D. CLINICAL PRESENTATION

1. **History** usually reveals an acute onset of symptoms.
2. **Physical examination**
   a. "Four *D*s and an *S*" describe the symptoms: dysphagia, drooling, dysphonia, distress, and stridor.
   b. Presentation is characterized by an abrupt onset of fever, sore throat, drooling, muffled voice, and inspiratory stridor. Respiratory distress usually is mild to moderate. The child often attempts to maintain a patent airway by leaning forward while sitting and holding his or her head in a sniffing position.
   c. Assess the degree of stridor, color, retractions, air entry, and level of consciousness.
3. **Diagnostic tests**
   a. If epiglottitis is suspected, invasive procedures should be avoided. Avoid direct oral cavity examination as depression of the tongue may force the enlarged epiglottis over the laryngeal opening and agitate the patient.
   b. An anteroposterior radiograph of the neck may not reveal a swollen epiglottis. A lateral neck x-ray examination, however, is diagnostic and is always indicated in the presence of upper airway lesions.
   c. Obtain blood cultures to identify the organism after airway control is established.
4. **Clinical course:** Acute infection usually resolves in 24 to 72 hours with antibiotics.
5. **Differential diagnosis:** Distinguish epiglottis from laryngotracheobronchitis by presentation, lateral neck x-ray examination, or direct visualization in the operating room (Table 2–17).

E. MANAGEMENT
1. **Prevention:** Hib vaccine has significantly reduced the incidence of this disease in children and therefore is strongly recommended for infants.
2. **Direct care:** If epiglottitis is strongly suspected, the patient should be taken directly to the operating room for direct laryngoscopy and subsequent intubation. If respiratory arrest occurs, bag-mask ventilation with 100% oxygen and positive pressure ventilation should be attempted. Keep the child comfortable and disturb him or her as little as possible. Allow the patient to maintain a position of comfort. Supplemental oxygen can be administered while the child is sitting in a parent's lap.
3. **Supportive care** includes admission to the PICU for close monitoring. Use sedation and arm restraints or muscle relaxants to prevent self-extubation and decrease movement of the endotracheal tube in the larynx. Deliver oxygen as necessary. Monitor closely for postobstructive pulmonary edema. Administer a second-generation cephalosporin for adequate coverage. Criteria for extubation may include air leak around the artificial airway or direct

Table 2–17. DIAGNOSTIC FEATURES OF INFECTIOUS CAUSES OF STRIDOR

	LARYNGOTRACHEOBRONCHITIS	EPIGLOTTITIS	BACTERIAL TRACHEITIS
Age range	3 mo–3 y	2–6 y	2–4 y
Etiology	Viral	Bacterial	Bacterial
Pathology	Inflammation of sub-glottic region, trachea, bronchi, bronchioles	Inflammation of epi-glottis, aryepiglottic folds, and surrounding tissue	Acute infectious process in the trachea
Onset	Gradual	Acute	Variable
Signs and symptoms	Hoarseness Barking cough Stridor	High fever Drooling Dysphagia Dysphonia Distress Inspiratory stridor Sniffing position	High fever Inspiratory stridor Drooling May mimic epiglottitis
Diagnosis	History and physical examination	History and physical examination Swollen supraglottis on direct visualization	Thick purulent secretions
Radiographic signs	Subglottic narrowing "Steeple sign"	Increased epiglottic shadow on lateral neck x-ray examination	Subglottic irregularity "Steeple sign" may be present
Treatment	Mist hydration Racemic epinephrine Steroids	Antibiotics Airway management with endotracheal tube	Antibiotics Airway control
Course	Obstructive signs de-crease over a period of 3–4 d	Improvement 36–48 h after antibiotics are initiated	Improvement 36–48 h after antibiotics are initiated May require tracheostomy

examination of the epiglottis. Extubation is performed in the PICU or operating room with intubation and emergency tracheostomy equipment available.

   4. **Complications:** Intubation has been reported to have fewer complications than tracheostomy. These include self-extubation and obstruction from secretions. Patients who underwent intubation, rather than tracheostomy, have been noted to have a shorter period of artificial airway support and hospitalization.

F. OUTCOME

Given appropriate management of the airway during the initial stabilization, there should be no long-term sequelae for this disease.

ACUTE LARYNGOTRACHEOBRONCHITIS (LTB)

A. DEFINITION

Acute LTB is inflammatory swelling of the submucosa in the subglottic area. *"Croup"* is a general medical term that refers to this inflammatory process resulting in stridor, cough, and hoarseness.

B. ETIOLOGY

Croup usually occurs in children 6 months to 3 years of age. There is a tendency for LTB to recur in children who have had one episode. LTB can be either viral or bacterial in origin. Viral LTB accounts for 85% of reported cases. The most common organisms are RSV, parainfluenza virus A, and adenovirus; however, RSV is most common. Nonviral LTB may result from asthma, angioneurotic edema, foreign body aspiration, or subglottic stenosis following endotracheal intubation.

C. PATHOPHYSIOLOGY

In children the cricoid cartilage makes up the narrowest segment of the upper airway. Swelling and secretions in this subglottic region increase resistance to airflow leading to respiratory distress (Fig. 2–28).

D. CLINICAL PRESENTATION

   1. **History:** Characteristically there is a gradual onset and symptoms of a preceding upper respiratory tract infection including rhinorrhea, coryza, and low-grade fever. Symptoms vary over several days, with stridor worsening at night.

   2. **Physical examination:** Clinical manifestations are produced by subglottic obstruction. Clinical signs of respiratory failure are predictive of severity. The onset of LTB is noted by the development of a barking cough and hoarseness. The patient may also demonstrate inspiratory stridor and thin copious secretions. The degree of nasal flaring, tracheal tugging, and retraction of the chest muscles depends on the degree of airway resistance. The larynx is nontender on palpation. A low (rather than high) fever helps to differentiate from bacterial tracheitis and epiglottitis.

   3. **Diagnostic tests:** Chest radiograph (anteroposterior) demonstrates a funnel-shaped narrowing of the glottis and subglottic airway ("steeple sign"). A lateral radiograph of the neck demonstrates a normal epiglottis.

   4. **Clinical course:** Monitor closely for cyanosis, pallor, weakness, or other signs of hypoxemia. Hypoxemia, hypercarbia, tachycardia, and respiratory acidosis may develop if obstruction is severe.

   5. **Differential diagnosis:** See Table 2–17 for comparison of LTB, epiglottitis, and bacterial tracheitis.

E. PATIENT CARE MANAGEMENT

   1. **Direct care**

      a. Although rare, intubation may be necessary for increased work of breathing, pallor, cyanosis, decreased level of consciousness, worsening hypox-

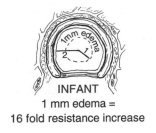

INFANT
1 mm edema =
16 fold resistance increase

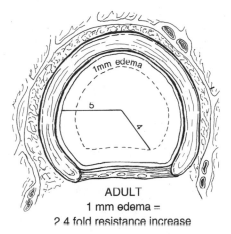

ADULT
1 mm edema =
2 4 fold resistance increase

Figure 2–28. Airway edema in acute laryngotracheobronchitis.

emia or hypercarbia, or respiratory distress unresponsive to treatment. Intubation is necessary if respiratory distress is refractory to medical intervention. Development of an air leak can indicate readiness for extubation.

    b. Racemic epinephrine produces topical mucosal vasoconstriction, thereby reducing mucosal edema. It may be used as frequently as every 30 minutes. Monitor for tachycardia. If no improvement occurs after three doses in 90 minutes, consider intubation.

2. **Supportive care**

    a. Minimize disturbances. Avoid agitation such as obtaining blood gases.

    b. Judge severity using the Croup Score (Table 2–18). The child should be admitted to the PICU for a croup score greater than or equal to 6.

    c. Provide cool humidified oxygen by face mask. Use humidification and adequate hydration to liquefy secretions. Control fever using antipyretics. Administer intravenous fluids to assure adequate hydration. Once epiglot-

Table 2–18.   CROUP SCORE

SYMPTOM	0	1	2
Stridor	None	Inspiratory	Inspiratory and expiratory
Cough	None	Hoarse	Bark
Air entry	Normal	Decreased	Markedly decreased
Flaring and retractions	None	Flaring and suprasternal	Suprasternal, subcostal, intercostal
Color	Normal	Cyanosis in room air	Cyanosis in 40% oxygen

titis and bacterial tracheitis have been ruled out, there is no need for antibiotic therapy.

   d. A helium-oxygen gas mixture (30% oxygen plus 70% helium) may be used for severe croup. The lower density provides less turbulent flow than oxygen alone, and it reduces the work of breathing by decreasing the resistance to turbulent gas flow through a narrowed airway.

   e. The use of a corticosteroid (dexamethasone) is generally accepted but is controversial.

   f. Enteral (transpyloric or gastric) feedings may be considered in patients with respiratory distress.

3. **Complications:** Intubation should be performed by a skilled practitioner to avoid complications of intubation. Endotracheal tube size should be 0.5 to 1 mm smaller than that predicted for the patient's age to aid in passing through the narrowed airway and avoid exacerbating subglottic inflammation.

F. OUTCOME

With appropriate management, the mortality for LTB is low.

PNEUMONIA

A. DEFINITION

Pneumonia is an infection of the lung caused most often by bacteria or viruses.

B. ETIOLOGY

1. The most likely etiologic agent depends on the age of the patient, how the organism was acquired (community or nosocomial), and the presence of underlying disease. Influenza and respiratory syncytial virus (RSV) are most common in young children. See Table 2–19 for the most common viral pathogens and diagnostic tests.

2. The presence of compromised host defenses may predispose a patient to pneumonia. These include the following:
   a. Bypass of nasal defenses from endotracheal intubation or tracheostomy
   b. Pulmonary aspiration from CNS injury or secondary to gastroesophageal reflux or tracheoesophageal fistula
   c. Abnormal airway secretion or mucociliary clearance from infections, bronchopulmonary dysplasia, or cystic fibrosis
   d. Underlying chronic disease or poor nutrition

Table 2–19. SPECIFIC PATHOGENS CAUSING VIRAL PNEUMONIA

PATHOGEN	PREVALENCE	DIAGNOSTICS
Respiratory syncytial virus	Most common	Indirect immunofluorescence antibody test on nasopharyngeal epithelial cells
Parainfluenza virus	Second most common Associated with laryngotracheobronchitis and croup	Indirect immunofluorescence antibody test on nasopharyngeal epithelial cells
Adenovirus	3% of pneumonia More gradual onset	Culture of virus
Influenza	May occur in epidemics	Sudden onset of "toxic" signs Culture of the virus from respiratory secretions

C. PATHOPHYSIOLOGY

1. The invading organism initiates the inflammatory response, which then causes alveolar edema. The edema is a medium for the multiplication of organisms. An inflammatory process of the lungs may involve the interstitial tissue and pleura, leading to lung consolidation, reduced lung compliance, and a decrease in vital capacity and total lung capacity.

2. Mode of transmission of the organism is through inspiration of microorganisms, aspiration of oropharyngeal secretions, or by systemic circulation. The location of the pneumonia on chest radiograph may help differentiate the type of pneumonia. Generally, lobar pneumonia involves one or more lobes of the lung and is observed with bacterial processes. Bronchopneumonia involves terminal bronchioles. Interstitial pneumonia involves the alveolar walls, producing a hazy, diffuse radiographic pattern characteristic of viral pneumonia.

D. CLINICAL PRESENTATION

1. **History:** Prodrome may be of a mild upper respiratory tract infection or sudden fever and cyanosis. Examine for etiologic or precipitating factors.

2. **Physical examination:** Shaking chill followed by a high fever, cough, and chest pain may occur, particularly with bacterial pneumonia. Upper respiratory tract symptoms are characterized by stuffy nose, irritability, and poor feeding. Respiratory distress is manifested by expiratory grunting, flaring of the nostrils, retractions, tachypnea, and tachycardia. Cyanosis may be present. Auscultation of the lungs may reveal fine early inspiratory crackles or bronchial breath sounds heard with lobar pneumonia. Occasionally, infants present with apnea.

3. **Diagnostic tests**

   a. *Chest radiograph:* Pneumonia can initially produce a patchy infiltration with fluffy margins. Later a bacterial pneumonia causes more segmental or lobar disease with more homogenous opacification of the involved area of the lung. Aspiration pneumonia usually develops in the portion of the lung that is dependent at the time of aspiration. Bronchopneumonia produces perihilar congestion from inflammation of terminal bronchioles. Pleural effusion may represent empyema, which most often is associated with bacterial infection.

   b. *Sputum or tracheal secretions* are examined to note the predominant flora and the presence of neutrophils. The presence of a single organism greater than 3+ with 3 to 4 polymorphonuclear neutrophils (PMNs) on the Gram stain may represent infection. RSV enzyme-linked immunosorbent assay (ELISA) and a viral panel may be sent if a viral etiology is suspected.

   c. *Blood cultures* are drawn to evaluate for bacteremia. Results are diagnostic but are positive in only 10% to 25% of cases.

   d. *Quantitative bronchoalveolar lavage* may be indicated to reduce some of the diagnostic confusion that may be created by sputum specimen contamination. However, bronchoalveolar lavage does not always recover the pathogens producing pneumonia.

   e. *Lung biopsy* may be indicated in the child with severe disease or in the immunosuppressed host. This will provide evaluation of lung tissue and a culture obtained under sterile setting to guide more definitive treatment.

   f. *Pleural fluid* is obtained through needle thoracostomy and is sampled for cellular analysis, Gram stain, antigen detection, and culture.

   g. A *white blood cell count* greater than $15,000/mm^3$ is suggestive of infection in older infants and children.

   h. *Bacterial antigen studies* in blood or urine may increase the diagnostic yield.

4. **Clinical course** depends on the cause and presence of an immunocompromised state. Primary bacterial pneumonia is an infrequent cause of admission to the PICU. Occasionally, extrapulmonary manifestations of bacterial pneumonia such as dehydration and obtundation result in patient admission to the PICU.

E. **PATIENT CARE MANAGEMENT**

1. **Prevention:** Immunocompromised patients should receive scheduled trimethoprim-sulfamethoxazole (Septra) as prophylaxis against *Pneumocystis carinii* pneumonia.

2. **Direct care**
   a. Patients are monitored for signs of increasing respiratory distress. Chest radiograph is included in the initial evaluation. Arterial blood gases are monitored at frequent intervals if the pH is low or there is concern of progressive deterioration in respiratory status.
   b. Oxygen delivery should maintain saturations of greater than 90%. Intubate and provide mechanical ventilation for respiratory failure.

3. **Supportive care**
   a. If the patient is dehydrated, a fluid bolus of 10 to 20 ml/kg is administered. Maintenance of hydration can be achieved by intravenous fluids. If the course is prolonged, enteral feedings are initiated.
   b. Antimicrobials are administered for age group and suspected organism and continued for 7 to 14 days. Treatment of nosocomial pneumonia involves the use of antimicrobial agents directed at the identified pathogen or, if unknown, at the most likely etiologic agent based on the clinical setting and available diagnostic information. Treatment of viral infections is supportive.

4. **Complications** from bacterial pneumonia stem from lung injury related to the disease process, high oxygen requirement, or complications of mechanical ventilation.

ASTHMA

A. **DEFINITION**

Asthma is a diffuse, obstructive pulmonary disease characterized by airway inflammation with mucosal edema, thick secretions that cause airway plugging, and hyperreactivity of the tracheobronchial tree that results in bronchospasm of the smooth muscle.

B. **PATHOPHYSIOLOGY**

1. **Cellular mediators:** An extrinsic antigen causes IgE production by plasma cells and lymphoid tissue. IgE binds to mast cells in the bronchial walls. The mast cells then release several mediators, including histamine and bradykinin. The mediators decrease the intracellular levels of cyclic adenosine monophosphate (cAMP, which causes contraction of smooth muscle) and increases the level of guanosine monophosphate (GMP, which increases the release of these mediators) (Fig. 2–29).

2. **Neurogenic factors:** The mediators are thought to stimulate the vagus nerve (cholinergic stimulation), causing bronchial smooth muscle constriction and increased mucus production. β-Adrenergic stimulation, which normally relaxes smooth muscle and decreases vascular permeability, is *inhibited* by the mediators. A relative insensitivity of the β-adrenergic receptors in the smooth muscle may also be responsible for the hyperreactivity observed in this condition.

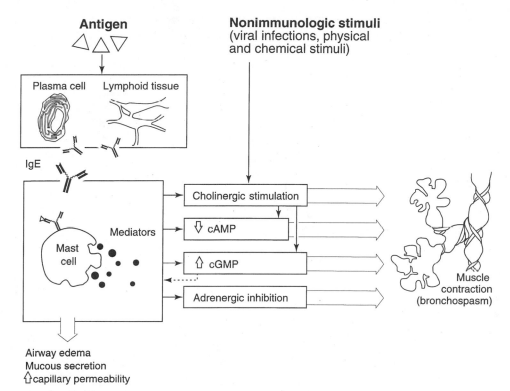

Figure 2–29. Mechanisms of bronchoconstriction in asthma. Cellular mediators and neurogenic mediators. (1) Extrinsic antigen causes IgE production by plasma cells and lymphoid tissue. (2) IgE binds to mast cells, causing release of mediators. (3) Mediators inhibit cAMP production, which normally produces muscle relaxation. Cholinergic stimulation directly inhibits cAMP production.

3. **Pulmonary function:** Airflow obstruction due to decreased airway caliber causes resistance to inspiratory air entry. Mucus plugging of smaller airways causes air trapping and increased residual lung volumes. The diaphragm assumes a flattened position related to hyperinflation rather than the dome-shaped position that allows optimal force of contraction.

4. **Abnormalities of gas exchange in asthma:** Hypoxemia presents early in the course of an asthmatic episode. Copious sticky mucus plugs cause segmental atelectasis, thus creating a ventilation-perfusion ($\dot{V}/\dot{Q}$) mismatch that is worsened by areas of hyperinflation. The degree of hypoxemia correlates well with the degree of airway obstruction in a symptomatic child (Ackerman and Eigen, 1992). Hyperventilation (with a decreased Pa_{CO_2}) is observed in the early phases of the episode in response to hypoxemia. As the disease progresses, Pa_{CO_2} normalizes or rises above 45 mm Hg in spite of tachypnea with a prolongation of expiratory time.

C. CLINICAL PRESENTATION

1. **Initial appraisal** should immediately identify urgent conditions. Symptoms associated with severe respiratory insufficiency in the asthmatic patient requiring *immediate* intervention are summarized in Table 2–20.

2. **History**

   a. First-time episode: Use detailed questioning to identify common triggers including environmental (smoke) and infectious exposures or symptoms (especially respiratory viral symptoms).

Table 2–20.   SYMPTOMS ASSOCIATED WITH SEVERE RESPIRATORY INSUFFICIENCY REQUIRING IMMEDIATE INTERVENTION

Heart rate >170 bpm
Respiratory rate >2 × age
Pulsus paradoxus >30 mm Hg
Diaphoresis
Agitation progressing to lethargy or coma
Marked retractions of accessory respiratory muscles
Cyanosis
Wheezing throughout entire expiratory phase *or* decreased to absent inspiratory breath
   sounds
Metabolic or respiratory acidosis: pH <7.20
$Paco_2$ >50 mm Hg
Pao_2 <70 mm Hg on >100% Fio_2
Pneumothorax
Associated pneumonia

Modified from Levin D, Morriss F. *Essentials of Pediatric Intensive Care.* New York: Churchill Livingstone; 1990:283.

    b.   Episodic: Inquire about historic triggers, known allergies, and clinical profile of previous episodes. List age of onset and previous evaluation and treatments. Attempt to determine general, *daily* severity of asthma, using criteria from the National Association of Emergency Physicians (NAEP) Asthma Guidelines.

    c.   Obtain a complete medication history both for asthma management and other medications used at home.

    d.   Determine the impact of illness on the child and the family.

    e.   Estimate hydration. Inquire about all fluids taken during previous 24 hours and voiding frequency.

3.   **Physical examination findings**

    a.   Evaluate respiratory effort. Patients are typically tachypneic with mild use of accessory muscles *early* in the course. As the episode progresses, a prolonged exhalation time will be observed. End-expiratory wheezing is usually noted early and associated with lower airway narrowing. With progression, inspiratory (upper airway narrowing) and expiratory wheezing may be audible. In some children the wheezing stage may be brief or unappreciated with rapid progression to absent breath sounds segmentally.

    b.   Evaluate cardiovascular status. Color remains normal in early stages but progresses from pale to cyanotic. Tachycardia is observed early in response to increased work of breathing and hypoxemia. Normally, negative intrapleural pressures may reduce cardiac output during inspiration in a spontaneously breathing patient. This causes a reduction in systolic pressure of less than 10 mm Hg during inspiration compared to expiration. With obstructive airway disease, a pronounced negative intrapleural pressure may increase the systolic variance to greater than 15 mm Hg (pulsus paradoxus). Pulsus paradoxus tends to parallel FEV_1 measurements.

    c.   Evaluate arterial blood gases. Metabolic acidosis occurs with increased respiratory work, causing oxygen consumption to be magnified. The acidosis causes pulmonary vasoconstriction, placing a burden on the right ventricle. Left ventricular strain may occur from the demand for increased cardiac output to maintain oxygen delivery.

    d.   Evaluate CNS effects. Level of consciousness is a predictable clinical correlate with severity of disease. Patients who are hypoxic or struggling to maintain normal gas exchange are typically anxious. The use of sympatho-mimetic medications may further aggravate the anxiety. Respiratory fatigue in this setting results in hypoxemia and elevated $PaCO_2$. The patient becomes more sleepy and ultimately obtundent.

4. A **summary impression** of a child during an acute episode is conventionally classified into mild, moderate, or severe acuity. With a mild episode the child's condition can be managed in an outpatient setting. Moderate episodes require hospitalization with close monitoring. Severe episodes require PICU care with intubation equipment at the bedside (Table 2–21).

5. **Differential diagnosis of wheezing**
   a. Bronchiolitis usually presents with viral upper respiratory tract infection symptoms.
   b. Congestive heart failure presents with other supportive evidence on physical examination, such as an enlarged liver and heart murmur.
   c. Foreign body aspiration may have unequal breath sounds or radiologic appearance of foreign body.

Table 2–21. ESTIMATION OF SEVERITY OF ACUTE EXACERBATIONS OF ASTHMA IN CHILDREN

SIGN/SYMPTOM	MILD	MODERATE	SEVERE
PEFR*	70–90% predicted or personal best	50–70% predicted or personal best	<50% predicted or personal best
Respiratory rate, resting or sleeping	Normal to 30% increase above the mean	30–50% increase above the mean	Increase over 50% above the mean
Alertness	Normal	Normal	May be decreased
Dyspnea†	Absent or mild; speaks in complete sentences	Moderate; speaks in phrases or partial sentences; infant's cry softer and shorter, infant has difficulty suckling and feeding	Severe; speaks only in single words or short phrases; infant's cry softer and shorter, infants stops suckling and feeding
Pulsus paradoxus‡	<10 mm Hg	10–20 mm Hg	20–40 mm Hg
Accessory muscle use	No intercostal to mild retractions.	Moderate intercostal retraction with tracheosternal retractions; use of sternocleidomastoid muscles; chest hyperinflation	Severe intercostal retractions, tracheosternal retractions with nasal flaring during inspiration; chest hyperinflation
Color	Good	Pale	Possibly cyanotic
Auscultation	End-expiratory wheeze only	Wheeze during entire expiration and inspiration	Breath sounds becoming inaudible
Oxygen saturation	>95%	90–95%	<90%
PCO_2	<35 mm Hg	<40 mm Hg	>40 mm Hg

Note: Within each category, the presence of several parameters, but not necessarily all, indicate the general classification of the exacerbation.
*For children 5 years of age or older.
†Parents' or physicians' impression of degree of child's breathlessness.
‡Pulsus paradoxus does not correlate with phase of respiration in small children.
From National Asthma Education Program Expert Panel Report. *Guidelines for the Diagnosis and Management of Asthma* (NIH Publication No. 92–3042). Washington, DC: U.S. Department of Health and Human Services, Public Health Service; 1991:105.

    d. Vascular ring presents with progressive symptoms, usually beginning in the first year of life and has a typical appearance on the esophagogram.

    e. Exposure to irritants such as smoke or chemicals may cause a chemical odor to the patient's breath. Cold air may also produce mild wheezing.

    f. Neoplasms of the airway or chest demonstrate characteristic radiologic findings, and in some cases, concurrent anemia.

    g. Infectious diseases such as bronchitis or pneumonia may cause wheezing and are usually identifiable by history of fever, cough, and focal infiltrates on x-ray examination.

    h. Pulmonary hypertension or edema may cause wheezing.

    i. Histrionic behavior reveals dyspnea out of proportion to the physical examination findings, sometimes causing hyperventilation tetany.

D. DIAGNOSTIC EVALUATION

  1. **Laboratory tests**

    a. The *complete blood count* is usually normal but may show evidence of a bacterial process requiring antibiotic treatment.

    b. *Arterial blood gases* may be deferred with mild symptoms, while oxygenation is assessed by pulse oximetry. However, in any patient who appears more compromised, arterial blood gas analysis remains the gold standard for evaluation of pulmonary function. Capillary blood gases provide accurate measurements of $Paco_2$ and pH (Harrison, in press) and may be less traumatic to the child.

    c. *Fluid and electrolyte* measurements may reflect high insensible fluid loss from the pulmonary system. Slight dehydration, evidenced by a high blood urea nitrogen (BUN), may be observed. Since β-agonist medications increase potassium losses, serum K^+ should be periodically evaluated.

  2. **Chest radiographs** are frequently normal but may reveal either a focal infiltrate, hyperinflation, or presence of a foreign body. Small areas of segmental atelectasis may be observed in many patients, which should be differentiated from an infectious infiltrate.

  3. **Pulmonary function tests (PFTs)** (see Fig. 2–14).

    a. *Forced expiratory volume (FEV):* The expiratory volume recorded for an FEV is obtained after a subject inspires maximally and then exhales as hard and as completely as he or she is able. A reduced FEV_1 (the volume of air exhaled in the first second) is observed in subjects with asthma or other obstructive disorders.

    b. *Forced vital capacity (FVC):* FVC is the maximal volume that can be exhaled by forceful and complete exhalation after a maximal inspiration. The subject with asthma has a reduced FVC, although not reduced as much as the FEV_1.

    c. *FEV/FVC ratio:* Normally, the ratio is approximately 80%. In an asthmatic patient this ratio is significantly lower.

    d. Bedside evaluation of pulmonary function and trending of measurements can be performed on cooperative children with a hand-held spirometer. The peak flow rate is relatively correlated with FEV_1. Trending of the FVC can be a useful method of monitoring clinical progression of obstructive disorders such as asthma.

E. MANAGEMENT OF ACUTE EPISODES

  1. The **goal of therapy** is to restore airway patency by reversing the bronchospasm, controlling the inflammatory response, and decreasing secretions. Supportive therapy, including oxygen, ventilation, hydration, correction of metabolic and electrolyte abnormalities, treatment of infections, and management of anxiety should be provided.

2. **Thorough and continuous assessment** of the patient is required to enable early recognition of progressive respiratory insufficiency. A brief bedside assessment tool (Table 2–22) enables swift recognition of risk factors associated with severe episodes and is useful in trending clinical changes.

3. **Intubation and mechanical ventilation** may be required in the presence of decreased respiratory effort with fatigue *or* shallow tachypnea, inability to speak single words, decreased mental status, absence of breath sounds despite respiratory effort, hypercarbia with $PaCO_2$ greater than 50 mm Hg *or* increasing by 5 mm Hg per hour, hypoxemia refractive to oxygen supplementation, or pulsus paradoxus greater than 20 mm Hg.

   a. Prior to intubation the child should receive 100% FIO_2 by nonrebreather mask. Clinicians should assume a "full stomach" in all patients and use a "rapid-sequence" intravenous induction with cricoid pressure. Premedication with atropine is recommended. Some medications are reported to cause a clinically significant histamine release, which could potentially aggravate the bronchial edema. These include morphine, meperidine (Demerol), atracurium, and thiopental (Pentothal). Induction agents may include ketamine, lidocaine (to blunt tracheal reflexes), midazolam (Versed), and propofol. Paralytic agents may include rocuronium, vecuronium, pancuronium, or succinylcholine for a rapid-sequence intubation.

   b. *Modes of ventilation:* Patients usually exhibit thick secretions, mucosal edema, and bronchoconstriction, which cause upper airway resistance. PIPs are therefore elevated. Initially, an A/C or SIMV mode may be used to control the patient's minute ventilation, both modes require heavy sedation and possibly paralysis. Volume-cycled ventilation is usually preferred to assure adequate tidal volumes. Tidal volume should be adjusted to allow delivery of approximately 8 to 10 ml/kg. Respiratory rate is adjusted to allow an I:E ratio of 1:2 to 1:4 and minute ventilation appropriate to individual needs. Initial settings are adjusted to achieve $PaCO_2$ in normal range or a pH within normal range. However, permissive hypercarbia may be necessary in patients with severe asthma. In some cases a peak pressure limit may be used. Exhaled tidal volumes should be monitored to assure adequate volume delivery without aggravating air trapping. Asthmatics have very high FRCs because of air trapping.

   c. PEEP should be used conservatively when conventional modes are inadequate. Although PEEP theoretically increases FRC in a patient who

Table 2–22. CLINICAL ASTHMA EVALUATION SCORE*

VARIABLES	0	1	2
PaO_2	70–100 mm Hg in room air	≤70 mm Hg in room air	≤70 mm Hg in 40% O_2
Cyanosis	None	In air	In 40% O_2
Inspiratory breath sounds	Normal	Unequal	Decreased to absent
Accessory muscles used	None	Moderate	Maximal
Expiratory wheezing	None	Moderate	Marked
Cerebral function	Normal	Depressed or agitated	Coma

*Clinical asthma score for children with status asthmaticus score ≥5 = impending respiratory failure, score ≥7 = plus $PaCO_2$, ≥65 mm Hg = existing respiratory failure.
From Wood DW, Downes JJ, Lecks HI. A clinical scoring system for the diagnosis of respiratory failure. *Am J Dis Child.* 1972; 123:227.

already has air trapping, it has also been shown that PEEP can increase intraluminal pressure to a level greater than intrapleural pressure (Qvist et al, 1982), theoretically "stinting" the airways open. This should minimize small airway closure and thus improve alveolar ventilation.

    d. *Monitoring during ventilation:* An arterial line is useful for periodic arterial blood gas evaluation. Patient goals for each parameter should be clearly defined by the health care team to ensure continuity and to be able to recognize the earliest opportunity for weaning. Continuous noninvasive monitoring is highly recommended but should not be regarded as a substitute for direct arterial measurements of oxygen and carbon dioxide. Pulse oximetry can be used for monitoring of oxygen saturations, and ventilation can be assessed with an end-tidal CO_2 or transcutaneous monitor. With severe air trapping, end-tidal CO_2 measurement may be artificially low.

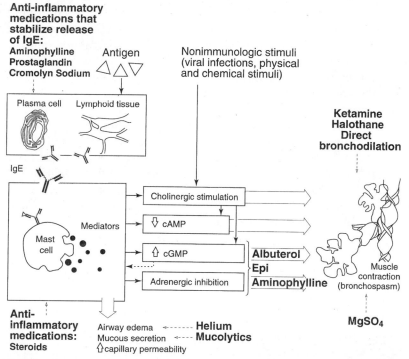

Figure 2–30. Pharmacologic management of asthma based on the mechanisms of disease.

- Antiinflammatory medications such as aminophylline, prostaglandin, and cromolyn sodium are useful for blocking the inflammatory response at the time of antigen stimulation. They are not useful for managing an acute episode.
- Steroids are useful for inhibiting further inflammatory responses, although it takes 24 to 36 hours before their effects are observed.
- β-Adrenergic stimulants such as epinephrine and albuterol enhance β-stimulation and diminish cGMP production, thus producing bronchodilation. Aminophylline is thought to have a weak effect on the beta receptors.
- Halothane and ketamine have direct bronchodilatory effects on smooth muscle.
- Other medications such as magnesium sulfate ($MgSO_4$) appear to enhance bronchodilation, but the mechanism is not well understood.
- Helium is sometimes used as a "carrier" to transport O_2 through the narrowed airways.

    e. *Indications for weaning:* Often weaning and extubation can be done soon after the underlying pathology is clearly resolving. This may be anticipated 36 to 48 hours after institution of steroid therapy in some children. The presence of an endotracheal tube in a hyperreactive airway may aggravate the underlying process; therefore, heavy sedation during the early period of assisted ventilation and accelerated weaning may be required.

  4. The **medications** frequently used to reverse the asthmatic process are directed toward altering intracellular mechanisms, which regulate bronchial reactivity and modulate the inflammatory process (Fig. 2–30).

    a. *Sympathomimetics* cause direct bronchodilation by stimulation of β_2-receptors.

    b. *Anticholinergics* block parasympathetic (vagal) receptors found in the pulmonary tree allowing bronchodilation. They also inhibit cGMP metabolism.

    c. *Antiinflammatory agents* blunt the host response to the stimulus by suppressing either the immune response or the release of mediators, such as histamine. Clinically, this should diminish the secretion of mucous.

    d. *Aminophylline,* methylxanthine, is considered to be a weak bronchodilator, which acts to increase intracellular cAMP. It is also thought to suppress latent response to inhaled allergens, making it more useful in the *prevention* of an acute episode than in reversing *acute* inflammatory responses.

    e. *Mucolytics* thin or reduce mucous secretions. This seems intuitively beneficial, but it is believed that drying of airway secretions may aggravate airway plugging. Furthermore, many mucolytic agents are also known irritants and may cause bronchospasm.

    f. *Antibiotics* may be used for patients exhibiting signs of a bacterial infection but are otherwise not useful.

    g. Other pharmacologic modalities have been shown to cause direct bronchodilation and include ketamine, halothane, prostaglandins, and magnesium sulfate (Table 2–23).

F. SUPPORTIVE CARE

  1. Since patients are often dehydrated from decreased water intake and increased insensible losses, **adequate hydration,** evidenced by appropriate urine output (>1 ml/kg/h), is an important therapeutic goal.

  2. **Metabolic acidosis** occurs in the majority of children with moderate disease because of dehydration and hypoxemia. Rehydration of the patient corrects some of the pH abnormalities, but if acidemia continues, sodium bicarbonate administration may be used. Administration of sodium bicarbonate in the absence of adequate ventilation may cause an adverse increase in Pa_{CO_2} and precipitate respiratory failure.

G. COMPLICATIONS

Complications include secondary bacterial infection, pneumothorax occurring from air trapping and segmental overdistention, sudden airway closure from severe bronchospasm causing respiratory arrest, and chronic illness resulting from malnutrition and medication side effects.

H. PROGNOSIS AND OUTCOMES

  1. **Acute episodes:** Early intervention with medications and supportive care prevents nearly all episodes from progressing to critical states. Up to 5% of patients with acute asthma episodes may progress to respiratory failure (Fuhrman and Zimmerman, 1992). Individual thresholds based on FEV or peak flow measurements should be obtained in the history to determine the need for medical intervention, initiation of steroids, and hospitalization.

Table 2–23. MANAGEMENT OF ACUTE BRONCHOSPASM

DRUGS	DOSING/ADMINISTRATION	COMMENTS
Sympathomimetics		
Albuterol	Aerosol 0.5% solution: <5 y: 0.25–0.3 ml >5 y: 0.5 ml	Use with caution in patients with cardiovascular dysfunction Heart rate and blood pressure should be monitored May decrease serum K^+ levels should be monitored
Terbutaline	IV: Load with 1–2 µg/kg Infusion: 0.1–0.4 µg/kg/min	
Epinephrine	SC: 1 : 1000: 0.01 ml/kg; maximum single dose: 0.3 ml IV: 1 : 10,000: 0.1 ml/kg load Infusion: start 0.1 µg/kg/min	
Anticholinergics		
Ipratropium (Atrovent)	MDI: 18 µg per actuation <12 y: 1–2 puffs q6h >12 y: 2–4 puffs q6h	Can be administered into ventilator circuit
Antiinflammatory Agents Glucocorticoids		
Prednisone	1–2 mg/kg/d PO divided bid × 3–5 d, then taper	May cause Na^+ and water retention; CNS symptoms (e.g., insomnia, nervousness) Hyperglycemia Joint pain
Methylprednisolone (Solu-Medrol)	1 mg/kg q6h or 4 mg/kg/d IV, divided qid × 3–5 d, then taper	Long-term use associated with adrenal suppression and bone demineralization
Aminophylline	IV load: 6 mg/kg for 30 min Then for next 12 h: <1 y: 0.5–0.7 mg/kg/h 1–9 y: 1–1.2 mg/kg/h 9–12 y: 0.9 mg/kg/h	Follow serum levels, which should be 10–20 µg/ml There are *many* drug interactions (see hospital formulary) May cause gastrointestinal symptoms, tremors, tachycardia, agitation Do not infuse single IV dose in less than 30 min
Other Agents		
Ketamine	IV: 1–2 mg/kg per dose	Contraindicated with increased intracranial pressure May cause dysphoria in older children; use benzodiazepine prior to administration
Halothane	Inhalational gas: 0.25–0.5% delivery with oxygen through anesthesia circuit	May cause hypotension
Magnesium sulfate	20–50 mg/kg IV for 20–30 min May repeat q6h	Check Mg levels before redosing Levels >4 mg/dl may cause depressed CNS function, diarrhea, and respiratory depression

MDI, metered dose inhaler.

2. **Morbidity and mortality:** The incidence of asthma has increased in the last decade. There are an estimated 10 million people in the United States with asthma with a disproportionate number of African-American and poor patients. The majority of asthma-associated deaths occur outside of a medical facility. The current mortality rate for infants to 19-year-olds is 3/10,000 population. The death rate increased by 31% per year between 1980 and 1987 (Mansmann, 1994).

ADULT RESPIRATORY DISTRESS SYNDROME (ARDS)

A. **DEFINITION**

ARDS is a condition characterized by acute lung injury and noncardiogenic pulmonary edema. It is initiated by a variety of stimuli that trigger the release of systemic inflammatory mediators. These mediators are *not* specific to the lung but in fact may be responsible for a broader spectrum of multiple organ failure. Therefore, the patient with ARDS may often exhibit signs of single or multiple organ dysfunction, as well as symptoms from the initiating insult. ARDS was first recognized in adult war victims, but the pathology has since been observed in children as well.

B. **PATHOPHYSIOLOGY**

1. **Mechanisms of ARDS**

a. The host response to a local or systemic insult (such as sepsis or trauma), activates a systemic stress response causing the release of proinflammatory mediators that act on the vascular endothelium. The principal mediator of microvascular injury is thought to be the sequestration of neutrophils in the pulmonary vasculature (Fig. 2–31). A local injury or an inciting trigger such as endotoxin causes the activation of the complement pathways. The C5a component is thought to be the principal stimulus for neutrophil activation and aggregation in the pulmonary capillary beds.

b. Neutrophils induce injury by the release of oxygen radicals and the release of proteolytic enzymes. The oxygen radicals appear to directly disrupt the alveolar capillary membrane. The enzymes not only cause direct injury to

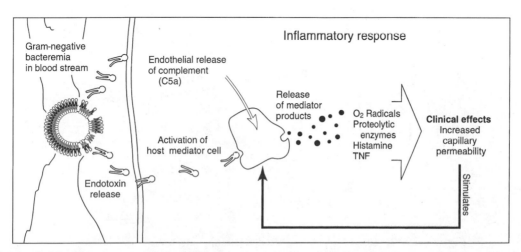

Figure 2–31. Mechanisms of inflammatory responses. Pathogenesis of ARDS: Focal injury or release of an antigenic substance such as endotoxin causes the release of complement and activation of the complement pathway, which stimulates neutrophil aggregation. *TNF*, tumor necrosis factor.

the pulmonary vasculature but also generate additional activated complement. In the host with normal neutrophil counts, aggregation of neutrophils in the pulmonary vasculature creates a cascade of events resulting in pulmonary edema and pulmonary vasoconstriction. In contrast, research has demonstrated that in the neutropenic host a blunted response is observed (Jacobs et al, 1986).

c. The release of other mediators and oxygen radicals, such as histamine, are additive factors in the development of increased alveolar capillary permeability.

d. The collective action of this inflammatory response is the development of pulmonary edema and increased pulmonary vascular resistance (Fig. 2–32).

2. **Pulmonary mechanics and dysfunction**

a. *Pulmonary hypertension* occurs from the action of specific mediators on the pulmonary vasculature, and hypoxemia potentiates this effect because it is a vasoconstrictor.

b. *Bronchoconstriction* often occurs early, although it may be discreet. It may be triggered by the presence of arachidonic acid metabolites derived from cell membranes.

c. *Hypovolemia and increased pulmonary vascular resistance* are thought to cause decreased perfusion to alveolar cells, specifically the type II pneumocytes that produce surfactant. The absence of surfactant creates a greater tendency toward alveolar collapse, thus reducing functional residual capacity (FRC) and compliance.

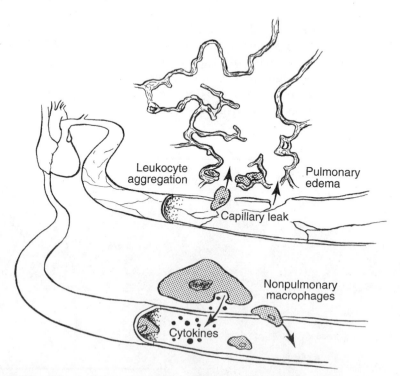

Figure 2–32. Site of injury in ARDS indicating mechanism for pulmonary edema. The inflammatory response within the pulmonary vasculature increases pulmonary permeability, resulting in pulmonary edema.

    d. The lung parenchyma exhibits an abnormal, heterogeneous pattern, with obstructive air trapping interlaced with atelectatic segments, and infiltrates. The net effect of these parenchymal changes is a significant reduction of FRC and decreased lung compliance. The transpulmonary pressure required to open the lower airways to achieve a specific lung volume is greater than normal.

    e. The summation of the inciting injuries to the lung creates a characteristic cascade of effects (Fuhrman and Zimmerman, 1992; Rogers, 1996). Early diffusion defects are caused by mild pulmonary edema. Heterogeneous pulmonary parenchymal tissue is caused by segmental hypoinflation and hyperinflation. Ventilation-perfusion mismatch (shunting of blood flow to nonventilated areas) is progressive and aggravated by hypoxemia, which causes vasoconstriction. Positive feedback loops present at various points in the process to sustain the pulmonary dysfunction, such as the activation of C5a complement $\rightarrow$ neutrophil aggregation $\rightarrow$ C5a activation.

C. ETIOLOGY

1. Direct or focal etiologic injuries include gastric aspiration, near-drowning events, toxic inhalation (smoke, oxygen, chlorine, ammonia), pulmonary infection or contusion, pulmonary embolus, or radiation pneumonitis.

2. Secondary or systemic injuries include prolonged hypotension, trauma, sepsis, multiple blood transfusions, ingestions (associated with aspiration), cardiopulmonary bypass, and head injuries.

D. CLINICAL PRESENTATION

1. **Stage 1 (days 1 to 2):** Symptoms may be subtle such as mild tachypnea, hypoxemia, anxiety, or restlessness.

2. **Stage 2 (days 2 to 3):** Clinical symptoms are clearly apparent and may include cyanosis on room air, tachycardia, increased respiratory effort, and retractions. Parenchymal changes become identifiable on x-ray examination.

3. **Stage 3 (days 2 to 10):** Frank respiratory failure occurs, manifested by diffuse rhonchi or rales, high oxygen requirement, signs of parenchymal consolidation, and a hyperdynamic state. Evidence of multiple organ failure may occur during this time period. Complications from mechanical ventilation such as barotrauma and oxygen toxicity may appear.

4. **Stage 4 (after 10 days):** Stage 3 changes persist with progression of lung restriction. Loculated pneumonia, development of pulmonary fibrosis, and progressive impairment of oxygenation are observed.

E. DIAGNOSIS

The recognition of ARDS in the early stages requires a high index of suspicion, because inciting factors are often nonpulmonary. Presentation always begins with mild tachypnea or dyspnea for which there are many causes. Conventional criteria for defining ARDS include the following (Zaccardelli & Pattishall, 1996):

1. Presence of historical factors.

2. Bilateral, diffuse chest radiographic changes associated with hypoxemia in the absence of cardiomegaly.

3. Altered oxygenation indexes such as PaO_2/FIO_2 ratio less than 180; A-a gradient less than 0.2; or PaO_2 less than 75 mm Hg with FIO_2 greater than 0.5.

4. Pulmonary artery occlusion pressure greater than 18 mm Hg in the absence of any other signs of cardiac insufficiency.

5. Decreased static compliance and increased shunt fraction.

F. GOALS OF THERAPY

Goals of therapy for the precipitating event include the following:

1. Ensuring adequate oxygenation first.

2. Managing the inciting injury (e.g., head injury or sepsis): Early, aggressive management of hypoxemia and infectious processes is essential. Careful hemodynamic resuscitation is initiated to ensure adequate preload without fluid overload. Aggressive management of increased intracranial pressure minimizes the evolution of neurogenic pulmonary edema.

G. PATIENT MONITORING

1. **General monitoring** includes pulse oximetry, ECG, arterial line, pulmonary arterial catheter monitoring for progressive lung disease requiring high PEEP, and monitoring of fluid intake and output. $S\bar{v}O_2$ monitoring with a pulmonary artery catheter can be a useful technique for critically ill patients. (See Chapter 3 for more information.)

2. **Ventilator monitoring:** Exhaled tidal volumes should be observed hourly to detect changes in compliance or ventilator mechanisms. Volume or pressure loop monitoring on the ventilator can be invaluable in determining optimal delivery mechanisms and for detecting alterations in compliance.

H. PATIENT CARE MANAGEMENT

1. **Indications for intubation and mechanical ventilation** include an FIO_2 requirement greater than 60% with an SaO_2 of less than 90% or rapid deterioration with evidence of respiratory fatigue such as decreased effort, decreased mentation, and increasing $PaCO_2$.

   a. *Assisted ventilation modalities:* The principal goal is to increase FRC and minimize potentially traumatic ventilatory mechanisms. Volume ventilation is a conventional choice for initial management of patients with ARDS. Initial ventilator settings may include a tidal volume of 10 ml/kg with an inspiratory time of 0.5 to 1 second according to body size or age, PEEP of 4 to 8 cm H_2O, FIO_2 of 100%, and an adequate rate to ensure minute ventilation.

   b. *PEEP* is instituted *early* to recruit collapsed alveoli and increase FRC; however, because of the heterogeneous pattern of the lungs a tendency to overexpand the "good" alveoli has been observed. After blood gas evaluation, adjust PEEP to allow reduction of FIO_2 to the lowest possible setting (<60% is desirable). Increased distention of the alveoli eventually increases lung volume and intrathoracic pressure. The great vessels may be restricted diminishing blood return to the heart and, therefore, cardiac output (Fig. 2–33).

   c. Pressure control, reverse or 1:1 I:E ratio, and permissive hypercarbia may be tried to minimize tidal volume yet provide adequate MAP and oxygenation.

   d. Nonconventional ventilator management may be necessary for refractive disease and may include high-frequency ventilation, ECMO, or liquid ventilation.

   e. *Chest radiographs* are used for evaluation of disease and identification of evolving pneumothorax or pneumomediastinum. Pneumothorax may cause an acute decompensation or an insidious deterioration of oxygenation.

   f. *Continuous clinical evaluation* of the patient's response to ventilatory assistance includes observation of chest excursion and patient comfort and auscultation of lung fields to assess the adequacy of aeration and the length of inspiratory and expiratory times.

2. **Support of optimal oxygen delivery:** An oxygen delivery capacity (DO_2) of at least 600 ml/min/m^2 is often recommended but individually determined according to oxygen consumption ($\dot{V}O_2$) data and $S\bar{v}O_2$ values. Mechanisms for improving DO_2 include ventilation to improve SaO_2 directed by arterial blood

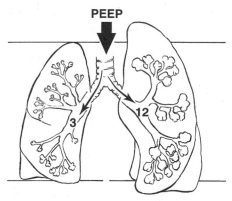

PEEP

Figure 2–33. Effect of positive end-expiratory pressure (PEEP) on functional residual capacity (FRC). In restrictive disease without PEEP, there is increased negative intrapleural pressure at FRC. Alveolar pressures are equal. (Note left side of illustration.) With the addition of 12 cm H_2O PEEP, more pressure is transmitted to the pleural space at the apex, and therefore transpulmonary pressure is increased. Alveolar distention is maintained at end-expiration. Patients with ARDS typically develop patchy atelectasis, requiring higher PEEP to maintain FRC.

gas and oxygenation data and PEEP. **Increase cardiac output** by ensuring normal preload, minimizing afterload, and supporting contractility. At higher levels of PEEP, cardiac output may be compromised. This is easily managed with intravascular volume boluses using the central venous pressure (CVP) measurement as a guide. Pharmacologically, contractility can be increased with a β-agonist medication such as epinephrine or dobutamine. A cardiac index greater than 4 L/min/m² (or greater than 4.5 L/min/m² if the patient is rapidly deteriorating) is often useful to immediately improve Do_2. *Maintain an adequate hemoglobin level* (greater than 12 g/dl is desirable) to ensure optimal oxygen carrying capacity.

3. **Minimize oxygen consumption ($\dot{V}o_2$):** Decrease patient activity and anxiety by providing individual comfort measures, frequent explanations and reassurances, and sedation and analgesia. Maintain normal core temperature.

4. **Provide optimal fluid and nutritional support**
   a. The goal of fluid administration is to maintain normal hemodynamics using the CVP for estimation of fluid requirements (CVP of 4 to 8 mm Hg is usually adequate) and maintain normal renal function (urine output of greater than 1 ml/kg/h).
   b. Fluid retention often occurs because of electrolyte alterations, third spacing, or SIADH. Diuretics may be useful, if indicated, in maintaining euvolemia.
   c. Patients may be hypermetabolic with a specific increase in protein metabolism and may require more than 2 g/kg/d. Indirect calorimetry is the preferred method for estimation of caloric needs, since patients may have caloric requirements greater than, less than, or equal to recommendations for more active children.
   d. Research has supported the use of early enteral nutrition as the preferred method of nutritional supplementation. Twenty-five percent of the intestinal mucosa is lymphoid tissue, and as such, approximately 75% of the body's immunologic secreting cells are found in the intestine (Romito, 1995). Altered circulation (from any cause) decreases splanchnic blood flow, leading to gut mucosal damage and a decrease in gastric barrier function.

Loss of intestinal barriers may result in translocation of endogenous bacteria (generally gram-negative organisms such as *Escherichia coli;* Gianotti et al, 1994). The most important stimulus for mucosal growth and function is a nutrient supply, even in small quantities. Numerous studies have documented a reduced incidence of sepsis and improved wound healing with early enteral nutrition (Heyland et al, 1993; Romito, 1995) compared to parenteral nutrition or no nutrition.

e. Administration of enteral nutrition can be achieved through a gastric tube or one that is positioned in the jejunum. Some experts argue that there is increased risk of aspiration when a patient is fed with a gastric tube, but the evidence is not clear. Montecalvo et al (1992) reported the advantages of jejunal feedings to include the ability to administer a greater percentage of caloric needs and a lower rate of pneumonia. A higher incidence of vomiting has been reported in patients fed with gastric tubes, thus limiting the volume of formula administered to some patients. Bedside placement of nasojejunal tubes is a relatively easy procedure in most children; either pH-guided tubes or less expensive Silastic tubes can be used. Practitioners have successfully placed the Silastic tubes in more than 95% of cases (Chellis and Sanders, 1996).

f. The choice of formulas is guided by nutritional needs; but in general, elemental formulas may be tolerated better than those with complex sugars and proteins.

g. Adverse effects of inappropriate nutritional support may occur. Excessive glucose administration shifts metabolism to lipogenesis, causing increased carbon dioxide production and, therefore, increasing ventilatory demands. Excessive lipid administration *may* aggravate hypoxemia.

5. **Provide infectious disease surveillance,** since patients with ARDS are at risk for nosocomial infections. Risk factors include invasive lines, impaired immunity, decreased nutrient supply, antibiotics, H_2 blockers and antacids (Ben-Menachem et al, 1996), oral and nasal tubes, narcotic administration, and supine positioning, which can cause constipation by inhibiting intestinal motility. Surveillance and preventive measures should include the following:

a. Monitoring of white blood cell count and temperature pattern daily

b. Observance of universal infectious disease precautions, emphasizing strict hand washing by all contacts with patient and restriction of visitors with infectious symptoms

c. Gastric decompression and drainage to decrease the risk of gastric secretion aspiration

d. Decreased use of antacid regimens in patients with an endotracheal tube, since there is evidence that an alkaline pH in gastric secretions may allow bacterial growth normally inhibited by acid (Apte et al, 1992; Craven et al, 1986).

6. **Other therapies** for ARDS have not been demonstrated to be effective in treating ARDS except for the use of nitric oxide (Hudson, 1993). Those in trial include agents that block mediator production or effects (e.g., endotoxin antibodies), protection against oxygen radicals by hemofiltration or oxygen radical scavengers, vasoactive agents for pulmonary dilation (e.g., prostaglandins and nitric oxide [Day et al, 1996]), and surfactant replacement therapy (Weg et al, 1994).

I. COMPLICATIONS AND PROGNOSIS

1. The complications observed in ARDS are related to the precipitating illness and to the therapies employed for treatment. Barotrauma and recurrent pulmonary air leaks are significant and frequent complications. Oxygen toxicity may

occur after 24 hours of FIO_2 greater than 60%. Secondary infections and multiple organ failure are significant markers for outcome, with a higher mortality rate observed in those patients with failure of two or more major organs.

2. Measures to reduce morbidity are first directed toward reducing FIO_2 to less than 60%, using the lowest PEEP setting possible, and guarding against lung injury from overdistention (high tidal volumes and exhaled tidal volumes should be continuously monitored). Infection control measures should be implemented early.

3. Overall mortality of ARDS is approximately 50%. Early deaths are usually associated with the severity of the inciting event. Poor prognosis is associated with gram-negative sepsis, poor response to PEEP, and underlying malignancy. Late deaths (those occurring more than 1 week after diagnosis) usually are due to multiple organ failure.

4. In general, survivors have a good recovery, returning to baseline health in many cases. Pulmonary function test results may be abnormal for 6 to 12 months as indicated by reversible airway obstruction, decreased PaO_2 with exercise, and reduction in lung volumes.

CONGENITAL DIAPHRAGMATIC HERNIA

A. **DEFINITION**

Herniation of abdominal contents into the thoracic cavity occurring prior to birth is called congenital diaphragmatic hernia (CDH). The amount of herniation varies from a small portion of the intestine to extensive herniation involving a majority of the abdominal organs.

B. **EMBRYOLOGY**

1. Diaphragm development occurs during weeks 3 to 12 of gestation from the following four structures:

   a. *Septum transversum:* A portion of mesoderm that forms the central tendon of the diaphragm. This will eventually fuse with the mesenchyma ventral to the esophagus and with the pleuroperitoneal membranes.

   b. *Pleuroperitoneal membranes:* Membranes (pleural and peritoneal) that develop to form the primitive diaphragm. During weeks 3 to 7 of gestation the primitive diaphragm fuses with the dorsal mesentery of the esophagus and septum transversum, completing the separation between the thoracic and abdominal cavities. During formation, pleuroperitoneal canals or openings are present, one on the right (which will close first) and one on the left.

   c. *Dorsal mesentery of the esophagus:* A double layer of peritoneum that forms the medial portion of the diaphragm. Muscle fibers that grow into the dorsal mesentery of the esophagus (during the 9th to 12th week of gestation) form the crura of the diaphragm.

   d. *The body wall:* The body wall is enlarged by the formation of lungs and pleural cavities. Tissue becomes divided into two portions: outer layer, which becomes part of the abdominal body wall, and an inner layer, which becomes the peripheral portion of the diaphragm.

2. At the same time as formation of the diaphragm, the developing abdominal organs have herniated into the base of the umbilical cord to allow room for growth. The gut is returned to the abdominal cavity during the 10th week of gestation. If the pleuroperitoneal membranes are incompletely fused or formed or the gut is returned earlier than usual to the abdominal cavity, the abdominal contents (usually intestines) may herniate into the thoracic cavity via the open canals (Fig. 2–34).

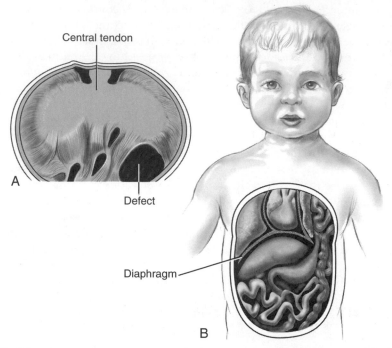

Figure 2–34. **A,** Drawing of a diaphragm with a large posterolateral defect resulting from abnormal formation and/or fusion of the pleuroperitoneal membrane on the left side with the mesoesophagus and the septum transversum. **B,** A "window" has been drawn on the thorax and abdomen to show the herniation of the intestine into the thorax through a posterolateral defect in the left side of the diaphragm, similar to that illustrated in A. Note that the heart is displaced to the right and that the left lung is compressed. (Redrawn from Moore K. *Essentials of Human Embryology.* Philadelphia, Pa: BC Decker, Inc; 1988:71).

C. INCIDENCE, MORBIDITY, AND MORTALITY
 1. This defect occurs in one of every 2000 to 3500 births (Hazinski, 1992; Williams, 1982).
 2. Posterolateral defect of the diaphragm occurs 5 times more often on the left side (foramen of Bochdalek) than on the right (foramen of Morgagni) (Moore, 1988).
 3. Occasionally a diaphragmatic hernia will occur at the esophageal hiatus.
 4. Associated defects, specifically those of cardiac origin, are common (39% in one study) (Fauza and Wilson, 1994).
 5. The mortality rate is high, especially in those infants who present within the first 4 to 6 hours of birth.
 6. Morbidity and mortality are related to the degree of pulmonary hypoplasia and associated anomalies.
D. PATHOPHYSIOLOGY
 Pathophysiology primarily involves the lungs but also has an effect on the heart and gastrointestinal tract.
 1. **Pulmonary involvement**
   a. Abdominal contents present in the thoracic cavity from the 6th to 12th week of gestation compress developing lung buds, producing pulmonary hypoplasia. This results in a decreased number of conducting airways between the trachea and terminal bronchioles. A reduction in the total number and

size of conducting airways leads to a significant decrease in total lung volume.

b. Herniation of abdominal contents after 16 weeks' gestation results in a decrease in the size of the conducting airways but not in the number, as all airways should be formed by this time. Alveoli formed are smaller than normal but are in normal amounts. Alveoli can continue to increase in number until the child is 8 years of age.

c. Fewer type II pneumocytes are present, and a lower than normal lecithin to sphingomyelin ratio may also be present (Composto and Eichelberger, 1992).

d. The ipsilateral lung has decreased compliance and an increase in resistance to ventilation.

e. Pulmonary vasculature develops at the same time as conducting airways and alveoli. Infants with CDH may have fewer conducting airways, alveoli, and blood vessels. The pulmonary microcirculation also has smooth muscle hypertrophy. Generally, the level of arteriolar musculature ends at the level of the respiratory bronchiole. Infants with CDH have increased arteriolar musculature. This reduces the size of the arteriolar lumina, thus increasing resistance to blood flow through the vessels.

f. All these factors may lead to persistent pulmonary hypertension, which can be a difficult problem to manage.

2. **Associated anomalies**

   a. *Heart:* Small ventricular size may result from compression of the thoracic organs during development. Hypoplastic left heart syndrome is one of the more common defects seen in association with CDH (Fauza and Wilson, 1994).

   b. *Gastrointestinal:* Malrotation and nonfixation of the gut is common. Esophageal dilation is found in a high percentage of survivors and may predispose a tendency toward gastroesophageal reflux. These infants are at risk for development of jaundice and biliary obstruction due to common bile duct compression related to malrotation of the bowel.

   c. *Other* anomalies include those of the CNS and renal and skeletal systems and chromosomal abnormalities.

E. GOALS OF PREOPERATIVE NURSING CARE

   1. Preoperative goals include maintaining adequate oxygenation to tissues, ensuring stable acid-base balance, and maintaining perfusion to body organs. Surgery, once done emergently, may be delayed, allowing for a potential decrease in pulmonary vascular resistance and ongoing stabilization of the infant.

   2. **Ensure adequate oxygenation and ventilation.**

      a. Infants in minimal respiratory distress (uncommon) may be managed with supplemental oxygen. Infants in moderate to severe respiratory distress require endotracheal intubation to decrease the work of breathing and to provide adequate oxygenation and ventilation. Endotracheal intubation also lessens the air entry into the stomach and gut normally observed with respiratory distress. Distention of the intestines with gas can cause further pulmonary decompensation.

      b. The goals of mechanical ventilation are to provide adequate oxygenation and carbon dioxide removal, minimize barotrauma, assist in correcting acidosis, and to lessen the work of breathing, thus reducing oxygen demand. Moderately high rates coupled with the lowest peak inspiratory pressure possible are commonly used. Some infants who are nonresponsive to conventional mechanical ventilation may be placed on a high-frequency oscillator or jet ventilator.

c. At some tertiary centers, infants failing mechanical ventilation (conventional and nonconventional) may receive extracorporeal membrane oxygenation (ECMO) life support prior to surgery.

3. **Provide intravenous sedation** in the mechanically ventilated infant via continuous infusions or intermittent bolus, or both. Sedation lessens the stimulus response to noxious stimuli, which can precipitate an increase in pulmonary vasoconstriction, and assists in decreasing oxygen consumption. Muscle relaxants may be used in combination with sedatives to enhance the effects desired with sedative use.

4. Observe for signs and symptoms of **tension pneumothorax** including sudden deterioration for no apparent reason, an acute decrease in blood pressure, and an acute increase or decrease in heart rate. Treat emergently with needle thoracostomy followed by chest tube insertion.

5. **Ensure perfusion** to body organs. Invasive monitoring (arterial line, central venous pressure line) is recommended. Preductal and postductal monitoring of oxygenation allows early intervention should pulmonary shunting occur. The easiest method is simultaneous preductal and postductal oxygen saturation monitoring, but arterial catheters can also be used. One or two peripheral intravenous lines should be placed to ensure adequate venous access.

a. A Foley catheter is used to observe renal perfusion and minimum urine output of 0.5 to 1 ml/kg/h.

b. Intravenous fluid management should consist of one-half to full maintenance fluid requirement. Aggressively treat hypovolemia with fluid pushes of 5% albumin or 0.9% normal saline.

6. **Decrease oxygen demands.** Maintain a neutral thermal environment at all times. Closely monitor glucose levels and treat aggressively with infusions of dextrose and boluses of $D_{10}W$. Minimize noxious stimuli. Cluster the infant's care needs when at all possible. Ear plugs may be placed gently into the external ear canal. Ensure adequate sedation.

7. Observe for signs and symptoms of persistent pulmonary hypertension (PPHN). Increased pulmonary vascular resistance will create multiple levels of shunting related to the increase in musculature around the arterioles. Pulmonary blood flow is shunted past ventilated alveoli, resulting in an increased interpulmonary shunt fraction. High pulmonary vascular resistance shunts pulmonary blood flow away from the lungs via the ductus arteriosus, creating a mixing of desaturated and saturated blood in the aorta. Pulmonary vasoconstriction elevates right ventricular afterload resistance. In an attempt to decompress the right atrium, desaturated blood shunts from right to left via the patent foramen ovale. Hypoxia and acidosis further exacerbate the pulmonary hypertension. If not corrected, the infant eventually succumbs to multiorgan system failure from ongoing hypoxia, acidosis, and ensuing low cardiac output.

a. Vasoactive medications may be used to either increase systemic vascular resistance (which will decrease shunting across the ductus) or decrease pulmonary vascular resistance, or both. Monitor vasoactive infusions meticulously and administer in a dedicated infusion port. Observe closely for side effects of vasoactive medications and treat accordingly.

b. Inhaled nitric oxide may be used either alone or with other vasoactive agents to reduce pulmonary vascular resistance. Meticulous attention to the ventilator circuit is required to identify and minimize leakage. Closely observe the infant to determine the response to therapy.

8. **Provide nutritional support.** If surgery is to be delayed by more than 2 days, intravenous nutrition should be started. A peripherally inserted central catheter (PICC) may be placed to assist in providing high caloric hyperalimentation.

9. **Provide emotional support to the family.** Encourage bonding of the infant with the family as status allows. Allow for religious and cultural rites as requested by the family.

F. **OPERATIVE REPAIR**

1. **Thoracic approach:** An intercostal incision is made in the thorax. The abdominal organs are gently pushed into the abdominal cavity. The drawback to this approach is the inability to do a Ladd's procedure.

2. **Abdominal approach:** A subcostal incision is made in the abdomen. The abdominal organs are gently brought down into the abdominal cavity. The Ladd procedure may then be used to correct malrotation and prevent a volvulus from occurring. This procedure involves rotating the midgut counterclockwise, lysis of Ladd's bands (which adhere the cecum to the abdominal wall), and positioning the duodenum to the right of the abdomen with the cecum and ascending colon positioned in the midline or left of the abdomen.

3. The diaphragm is repaired either primarily or with a patch of varying sizes depending on the size of the diaphragm defect.

4. Occasionally, the abdominal wall will not support complete surgical closure because of insufficient space; thus, a patch may be used.

G. **GOALS OF POSTOPERATIVE NURSING MANAGEMENT**

1. Essentially, preoperative and postoperative management are similar, with the goal of reducing pulmonary vasoconstriction and prevention of PPHN.

2. **Ensure adequate oxygenation and ventilation.** Close observation of blood gases, oxygen saturation, and acid-base balance is imperative. Use relatively high intermittent mandatory rates coupled with low peak inspiratory pressure to lessen the incidence of barotrauma.

   a. Ensure patency of the endotracheal tube with periodic suctioning. Premedication of the infant with a short-acting sedative prior to suctioning may assist in reducing the noxious stimuli associated with this procedure. This bolus of sedation is in addition to the continuous infusion.

   b. Infants receiving ECMO preoperatively may remain on ECMO 1 to 2 weeks postoperatively.

3. **Ensure adequate organ perfusion.** Obtain frequent vital signs. Postoperative third spacing of fluids is common. Fluid boluses in addition to regular maintenance fluids may be required for 24 to 48 hours after surgery. Vasopressors may be used. Minimum required urine output is 0.5 to 1 ml/kg/h. Scrutinize urine output in a patient who has had delayed closure of the abdomen or if the abdomen is tight postoperatively, since ureters may become obstructed from postoperative swelling of organs.

4. **Ensure chest tube(s) function** for decompression and drainage. Generally, the tube is placed to water seal and not continuous suction. Negative intrathoracic pressure created from suction may cause sudden overdistention of the hypoplastic lung, resulting in alveolar rupture and pneumothorax. If the chest tube is to suction, it is to a low amount such as 5 to 10 mm Hg. Observe drainage output; in some instances, replacement fluids may need to be given.

5. **Cluster nursing care to aid in decreasing noxious stimuli** to the infant.

6. **Ensure blood glucose stability** with close monitoring of blood glucose and prompt treatment of hypoglycemia.

7. **Observe for signs and symptoms of PPHN** and report and treat symptoms aggressively. Often, a "honeymoon" period exists postoperatively, where the

infant exhibits low pulmonary vascular resistance, excellent blood gases, and stable hemodynamics.

8. **Observe for other complications.** If a sudden decompensation occurs, a chest x-ray should be obtained to rule out pneumothorax. A tension pneumothorax is diagnosed clinically, not radiographically. If the infant is not responding to conventional therapy (i.e., hand ventilation, medication administration), needling the chest should commence while waiting for the x-ray examination to be taken.

9. **Deliver adequate nutrition.** The infant receives nothing by mouth until the gut begins to function. Nutritional support via hyperalimentation is begun until enteral feedings can be tolerated.

10. **Ensure optimal pain management.** Observe the infant for signs of pain and treat accordingly. Continuous infusion of a narcotic assists in creating a steady state of sedation as opposed to the peaks and valleys of intermittent bolus.

11. **Prevent nosocomial infections.** Infection control is a high priority because of the amount of instrumentation and entry sites for bacteria. Change dressings over the surgical site according to hospital policy, adhering to aseptic technique. Entry into central catheters should be minimal. Observe the infant for signs and symptoms of sepsis such as temperature instability, glucose instability, and rising or falling white blood cell count. Administer antibiotics as prescribed (typically, for the first 2 to 3 days postoperatively).

12. **Provide emotional support to the family** and allow them time at the bedside as the infant's condition allows. The mortality and morbidity rate are quite high for these infants. Be realistic with the family yet do not disallow any hopes they may have. Allow parental grieving, as they have lost their vision of the perfect child. Social services and pastoral support referrals may be helpful.

PERSISTENT PULMONARY HYPERTENSION OF THE NEWBORN (PPHN)

A. **DEFINITION**

PPHN is a newborn syndrome characterized by elevated pulmonary artery pressures and systemic hypoxemia as a result of right-to-left shunting of deoxygenated blood via the patent ductus arteriosus (pulmonary artery to aorta) or via the foramen ovale (right to left atrium) or via both. Most of the affected infants are term or postterm (Walsh-Sukys, 1993).

B. **ETIOLOGY**

1. The etiology is multifactorial and in some cases unknown. Infants with the following conditions should be watched carefully for signs of PPHN: diaphragmatic hernia, respiratory distress syndrome, hypoplastic lungs (i.e., Potter's syndrome), meconium aspiration, and pneumothorax. Rule out sepsis (i.e., β-hemolytic streptococci) and congenital heart defects with high pulmonary blood flow (i.e., anomalous pulmonary venous return, truncus arteriosus).

2. Pulmonary smooth muscle hypertrophy and hyperplasia has been found on postmortem examination of infants with PPHN (Roberts and Shaul, 1993). The presence of increased muscle mass may predispose the infant to pulmonary arteriolar vasospasm. Pulmonary hypertension ensues with the net effect of decreasing pulmonary blood flow. The end result is extrapulmonary shunting of deoxygenated blood via the ductus arteriosus and foramen ovale.

3. Alveolar hypoxia is the most potent and consistent stimulus for pulmonary vasoconstriction, so it must be avoided in infants with pulmonary hypertension.

C. **PATHOPHYSIOLOGY**

1. Any event that disrupts the orderly transition of switching from the placenta to the lung as the major organ of gas exchange results in PPHN (Walsh-Sukys, 1993). Over the first 12 hours of life, the pulmonary vascular resistance declines, reaching 80% of the total decrease at 24 hours of life (Walsh-Sukys, 1993).

2. The neonate's pulmonary blood vessels are very reactive. Additionally, the pulmonary blood vessels easily hypertrophy.

3. An acute injury (meconium aspiration) or hypoplasia of the lung (diaphragmatic hernia) may induce the elevation of pulmonary vascular resistance.

4. Once the pulmonary vascular resistance is elevated, it persists unless recognized and treated aggressively. If untreated, pulmonary vascular pressures exceed systemic pressures. Pulmonary blood flow travels the pathway of least resistance. Deoxygenated blood is shunted out of the lungs via the foramen ovale (right-to-left shunt from the right to left atrium) or via the patent ductus arteriosus (right-to-left shunt from the pulmonary artery to aorta).

5. Postductal blood becomes deoxygenated, resulting in systemic hypoxemia. Preductal blood at first is oxygenated, perhaps even hyperoxygenated; therefore, the infants brain is protected. The right arm also receives oxygenated blood, since the right subclavian artery originates from the aorta preductally.

6. Therapy is aimed toward reducing the elevated pulmonary pressures. If therapy does not alleviate the symptoms, ongoing hypoxemia becomes severe, eventually resulting in deoxygenated preductal blood. Metabolic acidosis ensues from lack of oxygen at the tissue level, and respiratory acidosis eventually occurs. Multiorgan system dysfunction may occur, often resulting in death.

D. **CLINICAL PRESENTATION AND DIAGNOSIS**

1. Observe for signs of shunting of pulmonary blood flow with wide swings in oxygen saturation or arterial Po_2. A right radial arterial blood gas (preductal) will reveal a higher Po_2 (greater than 20 mm Hg difference) than a blood gas taken from a postductal site. Shunting can also be directly monitored by simultaneous oxygen saturation monitoring of a preductal and postductal site.

2. **Echocardiography** is useful to rule out congenital heart disease and to show evidence of right-to-left shunting in a normally structured heart.

E. **GOALS OF PATIENT CARE MANAGEMENT**

1. The key to maximizing success in the treatment of PPHN is early recognition of its presence, followed by aggressive early intervention based on an understanding of pathophysiology. The goal is to interrupt PPHN's characteristic downward spiral of hypoxia and pulmonary vasoconstriction and restore normal circulation (Southwell, 1983).

2. **Reduce elevated pulmonary vascular resistance (PVR).**

   a. *Intubation and mechanical ventilation:* Premedication with sedation or paralytic agents, or both, should be used to accomplish intubation without causing additional undue stress to the infant (which could result in a pulmonary hypertensive crisis). Since high oxygen content and serum alkalosis assist in reducing elevated PVR, hyperoxia (Po_2 over 100 mm Hg) and hyperventilation (Pco_2 25 to 35 mm Hg) are goals of therapy.

   b. *Decrease the infant's response to stimuli.* Sedative or paralytic agents, or both, are used to help decrease the infant's oxygen requirements as well as decrease the response to noxious stimuli. Using ear plugs to decrease auditory stimuli may be advantageous. Cluster nursing care when possible. Placement of the infant in an isolation room helps decrease noise input. Premedication of the infant with a bolus sedative agent prior to suctioning is encouraged to help blunt the infant's response to this noxious stimuli.

    c. *Maximize cardiac output:* Maintain euvolemia. Vasopressors may be used to maintain or increase systemic vascular resistance to the point of overcoming PVR. This may reduce the amount of right-to-left shunting and help break the PPHN cycle.

    d. *Pulmonary vasodilator medications* (i.e., tolazoline, prostaglandin) may be administered in an effort to decrease the PVR. These medications also have a high degree of systemic side effects, the most notable being systemic hypotension.

3. Another method of respiratory treatment is ECMO. Alternate modes of mechanical ventilation such as high-frequency oscillation or high frequency jet ventilation may be used. Use of surfactant may be tried and in some instances may be the first-line medication in infants with a possible deficiency of alveolar surfactant (i.e., infants with RDS). Nitric oxide delivered by endotracheal tube is a potent pulmonary vasodilator and an endogenous agent. Nitric oxide delivered directly to the parenchyma may reduce PVR. Meticulous attention must be given to the ventilator circuit to minimize the chance of leakage.

4. **Infection control:** Infants with PPHN are at high risk for developing infections related to the frequency of invasive procedures. Strict aseptic technique during procedures and ongoing care of invasive lines according to hospital protocol is essential. Observe the infant for signs of sepsis such as temperature instability, glucose instability, and rising or falling white blood cell count.

5. **Nutrition:** Once the infant is stabilized, nutritional support should be started. Enteral feeding is preferred to maintain gut integrity. Intravenous hyperalimentation may be used if the infant's gut is thought to be at risk of developing problems with enteral feedings. Trophic feedings (enteral feedings at 1 to 2 ml/h) may be used in addition to hyperalimentation to assist in maintaining gut integrity.

6. **Assist in providing parental and family support.** Generally, these infants need as little stimulus as possible. Allow parents and family as much time at the bedside as the infant's condition allows and inform them what the infant may or may not accept in terms of stimulus. Social services or pastoral support referrals may be indicated.

TRACHEOESOPHAGEAL FISTULA (TEF)

A. **Definition**

TEF is a congenital defect in which there is incomplete separation of the trachea and esophagus. There are varying types of TEF that may involve esophageal atresia with or without a communicating tracheal fistula.

B. **Embryology and Pathophysiology**

1. The formation of the esophagus, larynx, and trachea takes place during the fourth week of gestation. The laryngotracheal groove evaginates and forms a laryngotracheal diverticulum. The diverticulum is further separated into two lumina by the formation of longitudinal tracheoesophageal folds. This forms a partition known as the tracheoesophageal septum. The septum divides the foregut into a ventral portion, which becomes the laryngotracheal tube, and a dorsal portion, which becomes the esophagus.

2. Incomplete separation results in the formation of a TEF, commonly associated with esophageal atresia (Fig. 2–35).

3. The major types of TEF follow (Kirschner and Block, 1994):

    a. Esophageal atresia with distal TEF (85%)

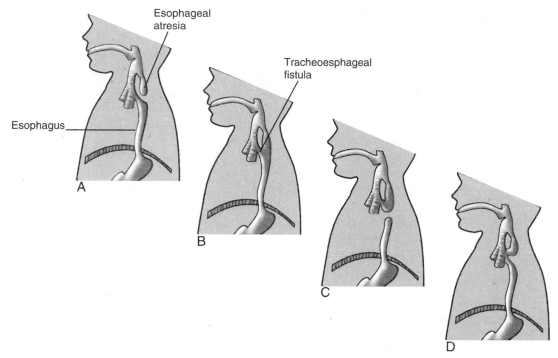

Figure 2–35.   Sketches illustrating the common types of tracheoesophageal fistula. The type shown in **A** occurs in about 90 percent of cases. Note that there is also atresia blockage of the esophagus. (Redrawn from Moore K. *Essentials of Human Embryology.* Philadelphia, Pa: BC Decker, Inc; 1988:71.)

      b. Esophageal atresia with no TEF (8%)
      c. H-type TEF (4%)
      d. Esophageal atresia with proximal TEF (2%)
      e. Esophageal atresia with proximal and distal TEF (1%)
   4. Tracheomalacia is a common associated problem. A structural and functional weakness of the tracheal wall may result in intermittent respiratory obstruction (Beasley, 1991). The abnormality primarily affects the area adjacent to the TEF, but it may extend to involve the lower half of the trachea and, occasionally, the entire trachea (Beasely, 1991).
C. INCIDENCE, MORBIDITY, AND MORTALITY
   1. TEF is the most common congenital malformation of the lower respiratory tract (Moore, 1988).
   2. Forty percent of patients with TEF have associated anomalies (Kirschner and Block, 1994). Cardiovascular anomalies are the most common and include ventricular septal defect (most common), patent ductus arteriosus, vascular ring, and coarctation of the aorta. Associated gastrointestinal anomalies may include imperforate anus, duodenal atresia, and malrotation.
   3. VACTERAL syndrome may be seen in association with TEF:
     V: Vertebral anomalies (hemivertibrae)
     A: Anal atresia
     C: Cardiac defects
     TE: TEF
     RAL: Radial limb dysplasia and renal anomalies
   4. Most neonates with a TEF are diagnosed within the first 24 hours of birth. Neonates with an H-type TEF may not exhibit signs other than frequent choking or recurrent pneumonia.

     5. Survival rate for term infants without other anomalies or complications is more than 90% (Kirschner and Block, 1994).

D. CLINICAL PRESENTATION

    1. **Signs and symptoms**

        a. A significant prenatal sign is that of polyhydramnios (occurring because of the inability of the infant to swallow amniotic fluid into the gut).

        b. Excessive salivation in the infant following birth is an early clinical manifestation. Other postnatal symptoms include frequent choking episodes with feeding associated with cyanosis or coughing.

    2. **Diagnostic procedures:** Diagnosis is made by passing a radiopaque nasogastric or orogastric tube into the blind pouch (most common form of TEF) and obtaining an x-ray examination. The gastric tube appears curled in the blind pouch. The use of contrast dye should be avoided if possible to decrease the possibility of aspiration into the lungs (Shaw, 1990).

E. SURGICAL OPTIONS

    1. Operative management of the infant with TEF is governed by his or her underlying medical condition (prematurity, lung disease, etc.) and the severity of associated congenital anomalies.

    2. Primary repair (end-to-end esophageal anastomosis with ligation of the fistula) is the treatment of choice. Staged repair (initial ligation of the fistula and gastrostomy placement with esophageal reconstruction at a later date) is controversial but may be required, especially with low birth weight (<2000 g; Alexander et al, 1993).

F. GOALS OF PATIENT CARE MANAGEMENT

    1. **Preoperative nursing care**

        a. Preoperative goals include maintenance of the airway, ensuring ventilation, and decompression of the blind esophageal pouch (if present).

        b. Ensure adequate oxygenation and ventilation. An orogastric tube is inserted into the blind pouch and placed on continuous low suction. Prone positioning of the infant with the head of the bed elevated 30 degrees lessens the chance of aspiration of stomach contents into the lungs via the fistula. Observe closely for signs of respiratory distress that may occur from prematurity or gaseous distention of the stomach with impingement on the diaphragm. Should positive pressure ventilation be required, use the lowest inspiratory pressures possible and adjust the rate of ventilation to provide adequate blood gases. Positive pressure ventilation may result in gaseous distention of the stomach when there is no outlet for decompression.

        c. Ensure optimal fluid and electrolyte balance. Since the infant can receive nothing by mouth, intravenous fluids at maintenance requirements are started to achieve adequate fluid balance. The infant's blood glucose should be checked periodically. Observe the urine output closely.

        d. Ensure optimal neutral thermal environment (NTE) to minimize caloric loss from heat expenditure. Infants with a TEF tend to be managed on open bed radiant warmers until they are stabilized postoperatively.

        e. Investigate associated anomalies.

        f. Provide family support and education regarding the postoperative course and plan of care.

    2. **Postoperative nursing care**

        a. The goal of postoperative care is recovery from surgery and anesthesia, ensuring hemodynamic stability, and prevention of infection.

        b. Ensure optimal oxygenation and ventilation. Postoperatively, mechanical ventilation occurs until the infant has recovered from anesthesia. Obtain periodic arterial blood gases, observing for adequate ventilation, oxygenation, and acid-base balance. Mechanical ventilation is weaned as soon as the infant's condition is stable and intrinsic pulmonary function is adequate. The suction catheter is inserted *only to the tip of the endotracheal tube* to lessen mechanical stress on the tracheal suture line.

c. Ensure hemodynamic stability. Observe the infant for signs of hypovolemia, which could occur from blood loss or third spacing of fluids. Administer fluid boluses as indicated. Observe the urine output closely (minimum should be at least 0.5 ml/kg/h). Observe the heart rate and capillary refill time for signs of adequate volume status. Rarely, the infant may require the use of vasopressors depending on other associated anomalies.

d. Monitor drainage output. An extrapleural drain may be in place postoperatively. Monitor output every 1 to 2 hours. Observe for the presence of salivary-like secretions, which could indicate an anastomotic leak. Gastrostomies placed at the time of surgery are initially placed to gravity drainage. When bowel tones are auscultated, the gastrostomy tube is elevated. Placement of a gastrostomy tube is controversial (especially in uncomplicated cases of TEF), as it may lead to an increased incidence of gastroesophageal reflux.

e. Ensure optimal nutritional status. Typically, the infant requires intravenous hyperalimentation until the surgical site is healed. The hyperalimentation should be started as soon as possible postoperatively to provide the infant with calories and healing capability. A peripherally inserted central catheter (PICC) may be placed to achieve high caloric hyperalimentation. A contrast dye study should be performed prior to oral feedings to evaluate the presence or absence of leakage at the anastomosis site. Gastrointestinal reflux is common in infants with TEF. Esophageal dysmotility problems are also common and may be a feature of the anomaly itself, not due to surgical manipulation (Beasley, 1991).

f. Ensure optimal pain management. Observe the infant for signs of pain and treat accordingly. Continuous infusions of a narcotic (i.e., morphine infusion) assist in a steady state of sedation as opposed to peaks and valleys of intermittent boluses. Respiratory depression is infrequent at dose ranges of less than 20 µg/kg/min (Lynn et al, 1993). As with all infants, assess respiratory status carefully while administering any narcotic.

g. Prevent infection. Change dressings over the surgical site according to hospital policy, adhering to aseptic technique. Enter central lines as infrequently as possible. Observe the infant for signs of sepsis such as temperature or glucose instability or a rising or falling white blood cell count. Administer antibiotics as prescribed (typically, for the first 2 to 3 days postoperatively).

h. Provide emotional and educational support to the family. Educate the family to the possible ongoing future issues the infant may sustain (i.e., gastroesophageal reflux, tracheomalacia). Support parental grieving, as they have lost their vision of the perfect child. Social services and pastoral support referrals may be indicated.

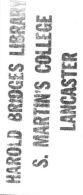

BRONCHOPULMONARY DYSPLASIA (BPD)

A. **ETIOLOGY**

   1. BPD is a chronic lung disease characterized by respiratory distress, oxygen dependency persisting beyond 36 weeks' corrected gestational age, and abnor-

mal chest radiographs. Presentation is variable from minimal symptomatology to significant morbidity, and the incidence varies widely.

2. The most significant risk factors for the development of BPD include birth before 28 weeks of gestational age, respiratory distress syndrome (RDS), birth weight less than 1500 g, male sex, and white race. Contributing factors include high inspired oxygen concentration and positive pressure ventilation with substantial damage to the airways. BPD is most common after treatment for RDS but may also be related to meconium aspiration, persistent fetal circulation, and congenital conditions requiring surgical intervention (McWilliams and Katz, 1993).

B. PATHOPHYSIOLOGY

1. BPD is characterized by increased airway resistance resulting in overinflation and atelectasis, decreased compliance related to fibrosis and decreased alveoli, and limited expiratory flow caused by edema and inflammation in the small airways.

2. Other contributing factors include barotrauma leading to overdistention and remodeling, oxygen toxicity resulting in capillary proliferation, stromal edema, and interstitial fibrosis, abnormal inflammatory responses to injury, poor collateral ventilation, compliant chest walls, prolonged intubation that results in reduced mucociliary function and increased dead space, presence of a patent ductus arteriosus, and persistent fetal circulation with increased pulmonary vascular resistance.

3. Hypercarbia and hypoxemia result from the subsequent ventilation-perfusion mismatch. Initial respiratory acidosis is partially compensated for metabolically with an increase in serum bicarbonate. If diuretics are used simultaneously, increased retention of base may result in metabolic alkalosis. Chronic hypoxemia may cause increased pulmonary vascular resistance, pulmonary hypertension, right ventricular hypertrophy, and cor pulmonale.

4. Infants with BPD also demonstrate dilated lymphatics, interstitial pulmonary edema, and increased accumulation of fluids (McWilliams and Katz, 1993).

5. Respiratory bronchioles and alveoli continue to increase in number and size correlated with linear growth. Therefore, infants tend to improve with normal growth. Significant improvement can occur during the first 3 years of life with the normal rapid lung growth that occurs.

C. SIGNS AND SYMPTOMS

Signs and symptoms include tachypnea, retractions, failure to thrive, increase in ventilatory requirements or inability to wean, hypoxia, hypercapnia, respiratory acidosis, crackling, wheezing, bronchospasm, and fluid intolerance. In the presence of right ventricular failure, tachycardia, hepatomegaly, periorbital edema, and a gallop rhythm are noted. In addition, cardiac output may decrease with signs of inadequate systemic perfusion and decreased urine output. On occasion, "BPD spells" result in irritability, agitation, duskiness, hypercarbia, hypoxemia, and increased respiratory effort. These episodes may be related to bronchospasm or bronchomalacia.

D. INVASIVE AND NONINVASIVE DIAGNOSTIC TESTS

1. **Arterial blood gases** may reveal hypoxemia, hypercarbia, and compensated respiratory acidosis.

2. **ECG** findings may reveal right ventricular hypertrophy resulting from the increased pulmonary vascular resistance, which causes increased right ventricular afterload and right axis deviation.

3. **Chest radiograph** may demonstrate scattered linear infiltrates, atelectasis, patchy areas of hyperinflation, increased interstitial markings, and cardiomegaly.

4. **Pulmonary function studies** may reveal low forced expiratory rates, decreased functional residual capacity, increased minute ventilation, increased work of breathing, high airway resistance, low dynamic compliance, and higher oxygen consumption.

5. **Echocardiogram** is used for estimation of pulmonary hypertension and assessment of right ventricular hypertrophy.

6. **Cardiac catheterization or pulmonary artery catheterization** may be performed (rarely) in children with increasing pulmonary hypertension and failure to thrive who are candidates for vasodilator therapy.

E. NURSING AND COLLABORATIVE DIAGNOSES
    ❖ IMPAIRED GAS EXCHANGE OR HYPOVENTILATION RELATED TO VENTILATION-PERFUSION MISMATCH, HYPERTROPHY OF PERIBRONCHIAL SMOOTH MUSCLES WITH INCREASED BRONCHIAL HYPERACTIVITY AND INCREASED PULMONARY AIRWAY AND VASCULAR RESISTANCE, INFLAMMATION, INTERSTITIAL EDEMA, FIBROSIS, AND ATELECTASIS
    ❖ ALTERED CARDIAC OUTPUT RELATED TO INCREASED PULMONARY VASCULAR RESISTANCE AND SUBSEQUENT RIGHT VENTRICULAR HYPERTROPHY
    ❖ POTENTIAL FOR INFECTION RELATED TO RESIDUAL LUNG DISEASE
    ❖ POTENTIAL FOR ALTERED NUTRITION, LESS THAN BODY REQUIREMENTS, RELATED TO INCREASED WORK OF BREATHING AND INCREASED CALORIC DEMAND
    ❖ POTENTIAL DIFFICULTY WEANING FROM VENTILATORY SUPPORT RELATED TO RESIDUAL LUNG DISEASE
    ❖ LACK OF KNOWLEDGE RELATED TO THE NEEDS FOR CHRONIC HOME VENTILATORY MANAGEMENT OR SUPPLEMENTAL HOME OXYGEN THERAPY AND THE PREVENTION OF INFECTION

F. GOALS AND DESIRED PATIENT OUTCOMES
    1. Arterial blood gases will be within normal limits, or permissive hypercarbia will be accepted to avoid increased barotrauma.
    2. Intubation and mechanical ventilation will produce normal chest movement, adequate saturations, and provide a patent airway.
    3. Systemic perfusion will remain within normal limits as evidenced by capillary refill of less than 3 seconds, warm peripheral skin without mottling or cyanosis, adequate peripheral pulses, normal blood pressure and heart rate for age, urine output of 1 to 2 ml/kg/h, and appropriate sensorium.
    4. Infants will demonstrate evidence of adequate nutritional support including appropriate weight gain.
    5. Eventually the patient will be able to be weaned from ventilatory support with demonstration of adequate spontaneous respiration and the ability to protect and maintain the airway or will be able to maintain an SaO_2 greater than 90% on supplemental oxygen therapy.
    6. Patients will be free from lower respiratory tract infection.

G. MULTIDISCIPLINARY PATIENT CARE MANAGEMENT
    1. **Maintain adequate oxygenation and ventilation.** Maintenance of a patent airway and thorough pulmonary toilet is essential. Weaning from ventilation may be prolonged in these infants and should be done slowly. Tracheostomy or home ventilation may be required. Supplemental oxygen therapy is useful in reducing hypoxemia, decreasing required minute ventilation, providing pulmonary vasodilation, avoiding cardiovascular and pulmonary vascular complications, and possibly enhancing growth. Since oxygen requirements vary depending on activity level, continuous pulse oximetry is used to monitor saturations and prescribe oxygen therapy.
    2. **Provide interventions for complications related to residual lung disease.**
        a. *Bronchodilators* assist in reducing airway obstruction and respiratory effort.
            • β-*Adrenergic agonists* have proven clinically useful in infants with chronic bronchospasm. The preferred route is the inhaled route because of the

rapid delivery and greater bronchoselectivity. Side effects are related to the adrenergic stimulation and include tachycardia, tremors, and gastrointestinal disturbances. Increased dosages may be required in some infants.

- *Inhaled anticholinergics* are also used to treat bronchospasm and may be useful for bronchomalacia where a paradoxic response to β_2-agonists may be seen. Increased dynamic compliance and decreased respiratory effort have been described after administration of nebulized ipratropium bromide (Atrovent).

- *Methylxanthines* (currently less commonly used) such as theophylline or aminophylline decrease airway resistance, promote diuresis, stimulate the CNS respiratory center, and increase diaphragmatic contractility but may also decrease esophageal sphincter tone, potentially resulting in increased gastroesophageal reflux. Many factors, including other drugs, affect metabolism and clearance; therefore, serum levels should be monitored. Adverse effects are common and may increase in severity with higher serum concentrations.

   b. *Antiinflammatory therapy,* such as steroid administration, may not prevent development of BPD but may acutely improve pulmonary function in ventilator-dependent infants and help to reduce bronchial hyperreactivity and bronchospasm in older infants and to facilitate weaning from mechanical ventilation or supplemental oxygen therapy. However, significant complications including infection, hypertension, growth failure, glucose instability, and adrenal suppression may occur (McWilliams and Katz, 1993).

   c. *Diuretic therapy* is often used to aid in the improvement of pulmonary function and decreased respiratory effort through the reduction of excessive fluids. Furosemide is more potent but has been implicated in hypochloremic metabolic alkalosis, secondary hypoventilation, renal calculi, and rickets with long-term use. Thiazide diuretics do not affect calcium excretion in the same way and may be useful for long-term therapy.

3. **Promote normal growth and development.** Adequate nutrition is essential in the recovery of lung function, which often occurs during the first year of rapid lung growth. Nonetheless, many infants with BPD are malnourished related to chronic respiratory distress and repeated hospitalizations. Increased work of breathing necessitates a higher basal caloric requirement and increased oxygen consumption (Kurzner et al, 1988). Calories should not be withheld because of the possibility of fluid overload. If necessary, diuretics can be adjusted. When possible, oxygen consumption should be measured with a metabolic cart to provide accurate caloric requirement calculations. The enteral route is preferred for feedings. Since fluids are often restricted, infant formulas can be modified to increase caloric content, but the high osmotic load of high-calorie formula may cause diarrhea in some infants. Gastroesophageal reflux and poor feeding resulting from long-term mechanical ventilation are complicating factors in providing adequate nutrition. Nasogastric tube feedings are often necessary to supplement oral feedings. Optimal positioning and a calm environment may aid in decreasing caloric demand during feedings. Parenteral feeding is indicated when enteral feedings are not successful.

4. **Monitor for symptoms of recurrent or increasing respiratory distress or imminent respiratory failure.** An increase in the work of breathing and the carbon dioxide level or a decrease in the arterial oxygen level is a sign. The development of acidosis in a child with previously metabolically compensated respiratory acidosis may necessitate reintubation. In addition, increasing pulmonary vascular resistance can precipitate right ventricular failure.

5. **Provide early discharge planning.** Supplemental oxygen therapy or ventilator may be required at home. Caregivers must learn chest physiotherapy, prevention of respiratory infections, signs of respiratory distress (including wheezing, tachypnea, retractions, and feeding difficulties), and use of the equipment needed for home oxygen therapy.

H. COMPLICATIONS AND LONG-TERM OUTCOMES FOR BPD

1. BPD is characterized by exacerbations and remissions. Studies suggest that children with BPD have significant respiratory morbidity after discharge (McWilliams and Katz, 1993). Children with BPD are frequently rehospitalized in the year following discharge, most often related to viral respiratory illnesses. Respiratory syncytial virus (RSV) is a leading cause for readmission. Children at increased risk for RSV include those with concurrent cardiac disease, several siblings, smoking in the home, and the need for supplemental oxygen therapy. Therefore, family caregivers must recognize the implications of smoke and other inhaled irritants. In addition, the significance of good hand washing should be stressed.

2. Long-term outcome studies indicate improvement in the first year of life and later even in severe cases. Late survivors may demonstrate abnormal chest radiographs and mild hypoxemia and hypercarbia or, in some cases, unresponsive obstructive pulmonary impairment. Hyperreactive airways are common in children with BPD. The findings differ from children with asthma, since patients with BPD do not have normal pulmonary function or gas exchange on an ongoing basis (McWilliams and Katz, 1993).

3. Some studies have found developmental delays, significant handicaps, and learning difficulties in certain infants with BPD (McWilliams and Katz, 1993). However, those complications may be related to the overall neonatal course. Nonetheless, early assessment and intervention for developmental delays and movement disorders are recommended.

LUNG TRANSPLANTATION

A. INTRODUCTION AND HISTORICAL CONSIDERATIONS

1. **Definition:** Surgical replacement of one or both lungs or a heart-lung bloc using donor organs for end-stage parenchymal or vascular lung disease.

2. Of the greater than 2200 lung transplants reported to the International Society for Heart and Lung Transplantation Registry as of 1992, less than 10% were performed in patients under the age of 18, and only 4% were in children less than 12 years of age (5% for children less than 16 years).

3. Children have undergone heart-lung, double-lung, sequential bilateral single-lung (using bibronchial anastomoses usually through a "clamshell" procedure [axilla-to-axilla incision under the breast line] or median sternotomy), and single-lung transplantation. Airway anastomosis is frequently done using polypropylene sutures without specific techniques to revascularize the airway. Heart-lung recipients often have an anastomosis just above the carina, whereas double-lung and single-lung recipients often have bronchial anastomoses. The trend is toward heart and bilateral lung transplantation.

B. PATHOPHYSIOLOGY

1. Recipient candidates for lung transplantation have end-stage parenchymal or vascular lung disease with significant impact on activities of daily living (Table 2–24). Generally, school-age children are unable to participate in normal school activities. Often, home oxygen therapy is required prior to transplantation. Rarely, candidates have had ventilator therapy, but it is discouraged.

Table 2–24. INDICATIONS FOR LUNG TRANSPLANTATION

Airway diseases
  Cystic fibrosis
  Chronic bronchitis
  Emphysema
  Bronchiectasis
Pulmonary hypertension
  Primary
  Secondary (related to other heart or lung disease)
Interstitial lung diseases
  Pulmonary fibrosis
  Idiopathic pulmonary
  Desquamative interstitial pneumonitis
Arteriovenous malformation
Graft-versus-host disease
Congenital heart disease, often with Eisenmenger's syndrome
Cardiomyopathy with elevated pulmonary vascular resistance
Retransplantation related to chronic rejection
Rheumatoid lung
Proteus syndrome

Data from Armitage JM, Fricker FJ, Kurland G, Michaels M, Griffith BP. Pediatric lung transplantation: expanding indications: 1985–1993. *J Heart Lung Transplant.* 1993;12(6; pt 2):S246–S254.

2. Candidates with primary pulmonary hypertension (PPH) may have signs of right ventricular failure (increased CVP, hepatomegaly, jugular venous distention, periorbital edema, and pulmonary effusion) and systemic or suprasystemic pulmonary artery pressures.
3. Candidates with congenital heart disease (especially Eisenmenger's syndrome) and pulmonary arteriovenous malformation may demonstrate profound cyanosis, clubbing, polycythemia, and hypoxemia exceeding the child's normal values.
4. Candidates with abnormal airway function have pulmonary function test results (forced expiratory volume in 1 second, forced vital capacity, and forced expiratory flow rates) less than 30% of normal values for age, height, and weight indicating severe obstructive disease (Armitage, 1993b).

C. CANDIDATE EVALUATION
  1. Candidates selected for single-lung transplantation require normal heart function or reversible right ventricular dysfunction and absence of pulmonary infection.
  2. Candidates for double-lung transplantation require normal heart function or reversible right ventricular dysfunction but may have some infectious processes present.
  3. Both heart and lungs must be transplanted in children with a complex, nonrepairable cardiac defect or inadequate cardiac function in addition to end-stage pulmonary disease. Previous thoracotomy or sternotomy is not an absolute contraindication to transplantation.
  4. Patients with cystic fibrosis are difficult to evaluate, since the course of their disease process will wax and wane. Dependence on supplementary oxygen may indicate the need to begin evaluation for transplantation. The presence of *Pseudomonas cepacia* in the airway or sinuses is usually a contraindication to transplantation, but this is dependent on sputum cultures and sensitivity of the *P. cepacia.*

5. **Invasive and noninvasive diagnostic studies** for transplant evaluation may include the following:
    a. Chest x-ray examination
    b. Electrocardiogram
    c. Transthoracic or transesophageal echocardiogram, or both
    d. Multiple unit gated acquisition (MUGA) scan or gated pool study of cardiac function
    e. Pulmonary function studies
    f. Arterial blood gases (in some centers)
    g. Exercise study with pulse oximetry (6-minute walk or bicycle test or none if high risk)
    h. Quantitative ventilation and perfusion scan
    i. Renal function studies and liver function tests
    j. Blood chemistry and hematology studies including viral serology, PRA (percent reactive antibody), and tissue typing if the PRA is greater than 20%. Tissue typing is done at the time of transplantation for everyone.

D. **DONOR EVALUATION**
    1. Criteria for acceptance of donor lungs is continuing to evolve. The opportunity for clinical assessment of the cadaveric donor is helpful in discerning the quality of the lungs for transplantation.
    2. **Desirable criteria for donor lungs** include a clear chest radiograph, arterial oxygen tension of 400 mm Hg on 100% oxygen, negative results from sputum cultures and Gram stain, direct visualization of the lungs through bronchoscopy at the time of procurement, viral serology of the donor, and administration of intravenous antibiotics and steroids and aerosolized gentamicin.
    3. **Relative contraindications to lung procurement** include pulmonary infection (moderate yeast in sputum cultures is an absolute contraindication), pulmonary contusions, chest tubes, tracheostomies, and evidence of significant aspiration.

E. **NURSING AND COLLABORATIVE DIAGNOSES**
    ❖ IMPAIRED GAS EXCHANGE OR HYPOVENTILATION RELATED TO ATELECTASIS, INEFFECTIVE COUGH, INAPPROPRIATE VENTILATION, INCREASED SECRETIONS, AND DECREASED MOBILITY
    ❖ POTENTIAL AIRWAY OBSTRUCTION RELATED TO POSTOPERATIVE EDEMA, ISCHEMIA, OR TUBE DISPLACEMENT
    ❖ ALTERED CARDIAC OUTPUT RELATED TO INCREASED INTRATHORACIC PRESSURE AND COMPROMISED VENOUS RETURN DUE TO VENTILATORY MANAGEMENT
    ❖ POTENTIAL FOR INFECTION RELATED TO IMMUNOSUPPRESSION, VIRAL MISMATCH BETWEEN DONORS AND RECIPIENTS, COMPROMISE IN NUTRITIONAL STATUS, PREVIOUS TRACHEAL COLONIZATION, OR BREAKS IN ASEPTIC TECHNIQUE
    ❖ POTENTIAL FOR ALTERED NUTRITION, LESS THAN BODY REQUIREMENTS, RELATED TO PREEXISTENT DISEASE SUCH AS CYSTIC FIBROSIS
    ❖ POTENTIAL DIFFICULTY WEANING FROM VENTILATORY SUPPORT RELATED TO REJECTION, INFECTION, OR NUTRITIONAL COMPROMISE

F. **GOALS AND DESIRED PATIENT OUTCOMES**
    1. Chest and lung expansion will be equal bilaterally without radiographic evidence of atelectasis.
    2. Arterial blood gases will be within normal limits.
    3. Intubation and mechanical ventilation will produce normal chest movement, adequate saturations, and provide a patent airway.
    4. Systemic perfusion will remain within normal limits as evidenced by capillary refill of less than 3 seconds, warm peripheral skin without mottling or cyanosis, adequate peripheral pulses, normal blood pressure and heart rate for age, urine output of 1 to 2 ml/kg/h, and appropriate sensorium.

5. Child will be without clinical or laboratory signs of infection.
6. Child will demonstrate evidence of adequate nutritional support, including appropriate weight maintenance or gain.
7. Child will be able to be weaned from ventilatory support with demonstration of adequate spontaneous respiration and able to protect and maintain the airway.

G. MULTIDISCIPLINARY PATIENT CARE MANAGEMENT

1. **Provide and monitor immunosuppression:** Cyclosporine or tacrolimus is initiated in the postoperative period intravenously and administered orally when gastrointestinal function resumes. In addition, patients receive another immunosuppressive agent, such as azathioprine, and steroids. Currently, patients with cystic fibrosis receive steroids only intraoperatively and on postoperative day 1. Clinical signs of immunosuppressive therapy toxicities and blood levels are monitored.

2. **Monitor and treat rejection:** Bronchoscopy with bronchoalveolar lavage (BAL) and transbronchial biopsy is performed on a regular basis (at least 2 and 4 weeks after transplantation) to assess graft acceptance. BAL specimens are studied for total cell count with differential, microbiologic assays, and immunologically with a donor-specific lymphocyte test. If no infection is present and clinical and radiographic findings are consistent for lung rejection, patients are treated for rejection based on standardized histologic criteria. Treatment may include increased steroids, total lymphoidal irradiation (TLI) , and courses of lymphocyte immune globulin (Atgam), muromonab-cd3 (Orthoclone OKT3), or mycophenolate. Recipients are also followed closely after discharge for signs of rejection. Outpatient monitoring may consist of clinical evaluation, blood tests, chest radiographs, pulmonary function studies, and bronchoscopy with BAL and transbronchial biopsy. Follow-up visits are individualized based on clinical course and previous history of rejection. All patients with lung transplantation can be taught spirometry for daily home use. When portable spirometers indicate a persistent decrease of 10% in FVC or FEV_1, patients are reevaluated via bronchoscopy.

3. **Monitor for infection and provide infection prophylaxis:** Titers are obtained before transplantation from the donor and recipient to evaluate hepatitis A, B, C, and D viruses, herpesvirus, Epstein-Barr virus, human immunodeficiency virus, toxoplasma, and cytomegalovirus (CMV). Serologic follow-up is performed for patients who have negative results at the time of transplant. Skin testing for tuberculosis and anergy is routine. Sputum cultures are obtained on a routine basis from candidates with cystic fibrosis to guide prophylaxis. During the perioperative period, antibiotic coverage is planned to cover bacterial sensitivities from the donor culture and adjusted if necessary based on surveillance cultures.

   a. Routine postoperative care includes thorough pulmonary toilet using strict aseptic technique. Good hand washing should be emphasized with assurance of compliance from all health care providers and family members. Ventilator tubing and other invasive tubing is changed on a regular basis.

   b. Children are monitored, and cultures are obtained to screen for signs of infection including fever or temperature instability, increasing quantity or a change in the nature of the pulmonary secretions, increasing respiratory distress, worsening arterial blood gases, leukocytosis or leukopenia, or radiographic changes.

4. **Monitor systemic perfusion parameters.**

5. **Monitor nutritional status.** Monitor intake, output, and weight and calculate caloric requirements. Nutritional consults should be sought for patients with

previous malnourishment (e.g., patients with cystic fibrosis). Provide an enteral or parenteral diet as ordered. Monitor the child's wound healing.

H. COMPLICATIONS OF LUNG TRANSPLANTATION

1. The most serious and frequently occurring complications in children include rejection, infection, and posttransplantation lymphoproliferative disease (Table 2–25). Most patients have one to two episodes of **acute cellular rejection** in the first 3 months following transplantation, unrelated to the primary immunosuppressant used. **Chronic rejection** is characterized by **obliterative bronchiolitis** (OB). OB occurs most commonly 1 to 3 years following transplantation but can occur as early as 6 months. OB often causes a significant decrease in small airway function in the second to third year after transplantation and is often refractory to augmented immunosuppression. Treatment for rejection may include intravenous steroids and antilymphocytic therapy. Experimental therapies using augmented immunosuppression (Armitage et al, 1995) have included inhaled cyclosporine, TLI, and photophoresis.

2. Most **infections** that cause death in the non-cystic fibrosis transplant recipient are related to viral and fungal infections. Severe bacterial infection is common in cystic fibrosis. All CMV-positive or mismatched recipients routinely receive intravenous ganciclovir (DHPG) for a minimum of 4 weeks after transplantation. Oral acyclovir has demonstrated poor absorption in pediatric pharmacokinetic studies and has not been shown to be advantageous in most instances. In addition, CMV-negative blood products only are used for transplant recipients. Besides its threat as an infectious process, CMV also increases the risk of subsequent rejection related to upregulation of the immune system. The introduction of ganciclovir, routine screening of both donors and recipients for CMV, the use of CMV-negative blood products only, and routine CMV serology follow-up after the transplantation have helped to reduce these adverse occurrences. The CMV-specific immunoglobulin that recently became available, although costly, may offer promise and is being studied in high-risk pediatric recipients. It may not prevent CMV infection but may decrease the severity of disease (personal communication, University of Pittsburgh Medical Center, 1996).

Table 2–25. COMPLICATIONS OF LUNG TRANSPLANTATION

Infection
Rejection
Posttransplantation lymphoproliferative disease
Postoperative bleeding
Ischemia of the anastomosis site
Phrenic paresis
Bronchial or tracheal stenosis
Pulmonary vein thrombosis
Systemic hypertension*
Hirsutism*
Gingival hyperplasia*
Uterine or nasal bleeding (related to underlying diagnosis, e.g., arteriovenous malformation)
Gastrointestinal problems
Diabetes*
Anemia*

*Drug-related toxicities.
Data from Armitage JM, Fricker FJ, Kurland G, et al. Pediatric lung transplantation: the years 1985 to 1992 and the clinical trial of FK 506. *J Thorac Cardiovasc Surg.* 1993;105(2):338–346.

3. Pediatric organ recipients are at increased risk for **posttransplantation lymphoproliferative disease (PTLD)** especially when the transplanted organ has significant amounts of donor-derived lymphatic tissue such as in lung and small bowel transplantations (Armitage et al, 1995). Patients who test negative for Epstein-Barr virus prior to transplantation and receive donor organs that test positive for Epstein-Barr virus have the greatest risk for PTLD. Most often, the infection occurs in the lung of a recipient and will occur within the first year following transplantation. In some cases, associated infections will occur.

4. Children with **cystic fibrosis** are an ever-increasing percentage of transplant recipients but are high risk and pose several challenges. Their airways are often colonized with organisms that are resistant to antibiotics or difficult to treat. In addition, they are often malnourished, have had long-term intravenous or enteral catheters, and may have chronic sinusitis and osteoporosis. Triple-drug immunosuppression is avoided; aggressive, extended antimicrobial therapy is the norm. In addition, nutritional support and thorough pulmonary toilet postoperatively may improve survival.

5. Complications can occur from the sutured airways, since systemic arterial revascularization is not directly reestablished. Donor airways are dependent on collaterals from the pulmonary circulation until revascularization occurs from ingrowth of surrounding tissues (Griffith, 1993). Ischemia surrounding the anastomosis site has been a problem for some patients, especially those with frequent rejection and infection episodes. It appears that collateral flow to the bronchial level is greater than that to the pericarinal trachea. Hence, bibronchial anastomosis has been more successful. Heart-lung recipients are protected somewhat following transplantation, since there is less interruption of potential collateral channels with transplantation of the heart-lung bloc and surrounding tissues.

I. **SURVIVAL AND MORTALITY**

Results of lung transplantation in children have been promising. Since experimentation with lung grafting in adults occurred first, pediatric patients may have benefitted from the experience. In pediatric patients (as opposed to adults), primary nonfunction of the graft because of preservation injury has been rare. One-year survival rates have been reported to be about 80%. Lower actuarial survival rates at 1 year have been reported for patients with cystic fibrosis as opposed to higher rates in children with congenital heart disease. Infection poses the highest risk for patients with cystic fibrosis. Long-term results for differences (related to type of transplantation) in exercise tolerance, right ventricular function, pulmonary pressures, prevalence of obliterative bronchiolitis, and survival are not yet available.

REFERENCES

Ackerman VL, Eigen H. Lower airway disease. In: Fuhrman B, Zimmerman J, eds. *Pediatric Critical Care.* St Louis, Mo: Mosby–Year Book Inc; 1992:460–461.

Alexander F, Johanningman J, Martin L. Staged repair improves outcome of high-risk premature infants with esophageal atresia and tracheoesophageal fistula. *J Pediatr Surg.* 1993;28(2):151–154.

Alspach JG, ed. *Core Curriculum for Critical Care Nursing.* 4th ed. Philadelphia, Pa: WB Saunders Co; 1991.

Anas NG. End tidal CO_2 monitoring. In: Levin DL, Morris F, eds. *Essentials of Pediatric ICU Care.* St Louis, Mo: Quality Medical Publishers; 1990:869.

Apte NM, Karnad DR, et al. Gastric colonization and pneumonia in intubated critically ill patients receiving stress ulcer prophylaxis. *Crit Care Med.* 1992;20:590–593.

Armitage JM, Fricker FJ, Kurland G, et al. Pediatric lung transplantation: the years 1985 to 1992 and the clinical trial of FK 506. *J Thorac Cardiovasc Surg.* 1993a;105(2):337–346.

Armitage JM, Fricker FJ, Kurland G, Michaels M, Griffith BP. Pediatric lung transplantation: expanding indications: 1985–1993. *J Heart Lung Transplant.* 1993b;12(6;pt2):S246–S254.

Armitage JM, Kormos RL, Stuart RS, et al. Posttransplant lymphoproliferative disease in thoracic organ transplant patients: ten years of cyclosporine-based immunosuppression. *J Heart Lung Transplant.* 1991;10(6):877–886.

Armitage JM, Kurland G, Michaels M, Cipriani LA, Griffith BP, Fricker FJ. Critical issues in pediatric lung transplantation. *J Thorac Cardiovasc Surg.* 1995;109(1):60–65.

Arnold JH, Hanson JH, et al. Prospective, randomized comparison of hi frequency oscillatory ventilation and conventional mechanical ventilation in pediatric respiratory failure. *Crit Care Med.* 1994;22(10):1530–1539.

Bailey PL, Wilbrink J, Zwanikken P, et al. Anesthetic induction with fentanyl. *Anesth Analg.* 1985;64:48.

Benthuysen JL, Smith NJ, Sanford TJ, et al. Physiology of alfentanil-induced rigidity. *Anesthesia.* 1986;64:440.

Beals D, Schloo B, Vacanti J, Reid L, Wilson J. Pulmonary growth and remodeling in infants with high-risk congenital diaphragmatic hernia. *J Pediatr Surg.* 1992;27(8):997–1002.

Beasley SW. Influence of anatomy and physiology on the management of oesophageal atresia. *Prog Pediatr Surg.* 1991;27:53–61.

Ben-Menachem T, McCarthy B, Fogel R. Prophylaxis for stress-related GI hemorrhage: a cost effective analysis. *Crit Care Med.* 1996;24(2):338–343.

Blumer JL, ed. *A Practical Guide to Pediatric Intensive Care.* 3rd ed. St Louis, Mo: Mosby–Year Book Inc; 1990.

Blumer JL. Principles of drug disposition in the critically ill child. In: Fuhrman B, Zimmerman J, eds. *Pediatric Critical Care.* St Louis, Mo: Mosby–Year Book Inc; 1992:1057–1060.

Bonadio WA, Hellmich T. Post-traumatic pulmonary contusions in children. *Ann Emerg Med.* 1989;18:1050.

Bos A, Tibboel D, Koot V, Hazebroek F, Molenaar J. Persistent pulmonary hypertension in high-risk congenital diaphragmatic hernia patients: incidence and vasodilator therapy. *J Pediatr Surg.* 1993;28(11):1463–1465.

Briones TL, Press SV. New ventilatory techniques. *Crit Care Nurse.* 1992;12(4):51–58.

Chameides L, Hazinski MF, eds. *Textbook of Pediatric Advanced Life Support.* American Heart Association; 1994.

Chatburn RL. Classification of mechanical ventilators. *Respir Care.* 1992;37(9):1009–1025.

Chellis MJ, Sanders S. Early enteral feeding in PICU. *JPEN.* 1996a;20(1):71–73.

Chellis MJ, Sanders S. Bedside placement of nasojejunal feeding tubes in the pediatric intensive care unit. JPEN 1996b;20(1):88–90.

Conrardy PA, Goodman LR, Lainge F, Singer NM. Alteration of endotracheal tube position: flexion and extension of the neck. *Crit Care Med.* 1976;4(1):8–13.

Composto R, Eichelberger C. Congenital diaphragmatic hernia: pathophysiology and nursing care. *Neonat Network.* 1992;11(6):57–61.

Craven DE, Kunches LM, Kilinsky, et al. Risk factors for pneumonia and fatality in patients receiving continuous mechanical ventilation. *Am Rev Respir Dis.* 1986;133:792–796.

Day RW, Guarin M, Lynch J. Inhaled NO in children with severe lung disease: results of acute and prolonged therapy with 2 concentrations. *Crit Care Med.* 1996;24(2):215–221.

Demling RH. Adult respiratory distress syndrome: current concepts. *New Horizons.* 1993;1(3):389.

Donn SM, Nicks JN, Becker MA. Flow sync vent of preterm infants with RDS. *J Perinatol.* 1994;14(2):90–94.

Durbin CG, Wallace KK. O_2 toxicity in critically ill patients. *Respir Care.* 1993;38(7):739–747.

Egan TD, Brock-Utne JG. Asystole and anesthesia induction with a fentanyl, propofol, and succinylcholine sequence. *Anesthesia/Analgesia.* 1991;73:818–820.

Erhard M. The effect of patient position on arterial O_2 sat. *Crit Care Nurse.* 1995;10(10):31–36.

Fauza DO, Wilson JM. Congenital diaphragmatic hernia and associated anomalies: their incidence, identification, and impact on prognosis. *J Pediatr Surg.* 1994;29(8):1113–1117.

Finer NN, Stewart AR. Continuous transcutaneous O_2 monitoring in critically ill neonates. *Crit Care Med.* 1980;8(6):319.

Fuhrman BP, Zimmerman JJ, eds. *Pediatric Critical Care.* St Louis, Mo: Mosby–Year Book Inc; 1992.

Garcia VF, Gotschall CS, Eichelberger MR, Bowman LM. Rib fractures in children: a marker of severe trauma. *J Trauma.* 1990;30(6):695.

Gauger PG, Pranikoff T, et al. Initial experience with partial liquid ventilation in pediatric patients with the acute ARDS. *Crit Care Med.* 1996;24(1):16–22.

Gianotti L, Alexander JW, Nelson JL, et al. Role of early enteral feeding and acute starvation post-burn bacterial translocation and host defense: prospective randomized trials. *Crit Care Med.* 1994;22:265–272.

Goldsmith JP, Karotkin EH, eds. *Assisted Ventilation of Neonates.* Philadelphia, Pa: WB Saunders Co; 1988.

Gordon PC, High FV. In: Beachy P, Deacon J, eds. *Core Curriculum for Neonatal ICU Nursing.* Philadelphia, Pa: WB Saunders Co; 1993:170–176.

Green TP, Timmons OD, et al. The impact of ECMO on survival in pediatric patients with acute respiratory failure. *Crit Care Med.* 1996;24(2):323–329.

Griffith BP. Pulmonary transplantation in its various forms—1989. Registry of the International Society for Heart and Lung Transplantation: tenth official report—1993. Compiled by MP Kaye, MD, with the cooperation of the 229 cooperating centers. *J Heart Lung Transplant.* 1993;12(4):117–133.

Gunderson L, Kenner C. Tco_2 monitoring: description and clinical application. *Neonat Network.* 1988;6(6):7.

Harrison M. Comparison of capillary and arterial blood gases in critically ill pediatric patients. Submitted for publication 1996, *Crit Care Med.*

Hazinski MF, ed. *Nursing Care of the Critically Ill Child.* 2nd ed. St Louis, Mo: Mosby–Year Book Inc; 1992.

Heyland DK, Cook DJ, Guyatt GH. Enteral nutrition in the critically ill patient: a critical review of the evidence. *Intensive Care Med.* 1993;19:435.

Hickling K, Walsh J, et al. Low mortality rate in adult RDS using low volume, pressure-limited ventilation with permissive hypercapnia: a prospective study. *Crit Care Med.* 1994;22(10):1568–1578.

Horber JD, et al. A multicenter, randomized, placebo controlled trial of surfactant therapy for respiratory distress syndrome. *N Engl J Med.* 1989;320(15):959–965.

Hudson L. Pharmacologic approaches to respiratory failure. *Respir Care.* 1993;38(7):754–768.

Jacobs RF, Keel DP, Balk PA. Alveolar macrophage function in a canine model of endotoxin-induced lung injury. *Am Rev Respir Dis.* 1986;134:745.

Kirschner B, Black D. The gastrointestinal tract. In: Behrman R, Kliegman R, eds. *Essentials of Pediatrics.* 2nd ed. Philadelphia, Pa: WB Saunders Co; 1994.

Kurzner S, Gars M, Bautiota D, et al. Growth failure in bronchopulmonary dysplasia: elevated metabolic rates and pulmonary mechanics. *J Pediatr.* 1988;112:73.

Laptook A, Oh W. Transcutaneous CO_2 monitoring in the newborn period. *Crit Care Med.* 1991;9:757.

Laskowski-Jones L. Meeting the challenge of chest trauma. *Am J Nurs.* 1995;95(9).

Levin D, Morriss F. *Essentials of Pediatric ICU.* St Louis, Mo: Quality Medical Publishers; 1990:283.

Logvinoff MM, Lemen RJ, Taussig LM, et al. Bronchodilators and diuretics in children with bronchopulmonary dysplasia. *Pediatr Pulmonol.* 1985;1:198.

Lough MD, Doershuk CF, Stern CR, eds. *Pediatric Respiratory Therapy.* 2nd ed. Chicago, Ill: Year Book Medical Publishers Inc; 1982.

Lynn AM, Nespeca MK, Opheim K, Slattery JT. Respiratory effects of intravenous morphine infusions in neonates, infants, and children after cardiac surgery. *Anesthesia/Analgesia.* 1993;77:695–701.

MacKenzie CF, Shum B, McAslen TC. Chest physiotherapy: the effect on oxygenation. *Anesthesia/Analgesia.* 1978;57:28.

McWilliams B, Katz R. Bronchopulmonary dysplasia in the pediatric intensive care unit. In: Holbrook PR, ed. *Textbook of Critical Care.* Philadelphia, Pa: WB Saunders Co; 1993.

Mansmann H. Management of status asthmaticus in childhood. In: Gershwin NE, Hakpin GM, eds. *Bronchial Asthma.* New Jersey: Human Press; 1994.

Manzetti JD, Foust DE. *University of Pittsburgh Lung Transplant Candidate Evaluation.* University of Pittsburgh Medical Center; 1991.

Martin L. New approaches to ventilation in infants and children. *Curr Opin Pediatr.* 1995;7:250–261.

Martin L, Bratton S, Walker L. Principles and practice of respiratory support and mechanical ventilation. In: Rogers MC, ed. *Textbook of Pediatric Intensive Care.* Baltimore, Md: Williams & Wilkins; 1996.

Michenfelder JD. *Anesthesia and the Brain.* New York, NY: Churchill Livingstone Inc; 1988:125–127.

Michols DG, Yaster M, Lappe DG, Buck JR, eds. *Golden Hour: The Handbook of Advanced Pediatric Life Support.* St Louis, Mo: Mosby–Year Book Inc; 1991.

Montecalvo MA, Steger KA, Farber WW, et al. Nutritional outcome and pneumonia in critical care patients randomized to gastric versus jejunal tube feedings. *Crit Care Med.* 1992;20:1377.

Moore K. *Essentials of Human Embryology.* Philadelphia, Pa: BC Decker Inc; 1988.

Moreno C, Iovanne B. Congenital diaphragmatic hernia, I. *Neonat Network.* 1993;12(1):19–27.

Moreno C, Iovanne B. Congenital diaphragmatic hernia, II. *Neonat Network.* 1993;12(2):21–27.

Murray MJ, Coursin DB, et al. Double blind, randomized, multicenter study of doxacurium versus pancuronium in ICU patients who require NBB agents. *Crit Care Med.* 1995;23:450–458.

Nakayama DK, Ramenofsky ML, Rowe MI. Chest injuries in childhood. *Ann Surg.* 1989;210:770.

National Association of Emergency Physicians (NAEP). Asthma Guidelines (June 1991, NIH). *Pediatr Ann.* 1992;21(9):545–553.

Norden M, Butt W, McDougall P. Predictor of survival for infants with congenital diaphragmatic hernia. *J Pediatr Surg.* 1994;29(11):1443–1446.

Nugent J. ECMO in the neonate. In: Beachy P, Deacon J, eds. *Core Curriculum for Neonatal ICU Nursing.* Philadelphia, Pa: WB Saunders Co; 1993.

Palve H, Vuori A. Pulse oximetry during low cardiac output and hypothermia states immediately after open heart surgery. *Crit Care Med.* 1989;17:66–72.

Polgar G, Promedhat V. Peak flow rate. In: *Pulmonary Function Testing in Children: Techniques and Standards.* Philadelphia, Pa: WB Saunders Co; 1971.

Qvist J, Anderson JB, Pemberton M, et al. High level PEEP in severe asthma. *N Engl J Med.* 1982;307:1347.

Reisdorff EF, Roberts MR, Wiegenstein JG. *Pediatr Emerg Med.* Philadelphia, Pa: WB Saunders Co; 1993.

Reyall JA, Levin DL. Adult RDA. I: clinical aspects, pathology, and mechanisms of injury. *J Pediatr.* 1988;112:169.

Roberts J, Shaul P. Advances in the treatment of persistent pulmonary hypertension of the newborn. *Pediatr Clin North Am.* 1993;40(5).

Rogers MC, ed. *Textbook of Pediatric Intensive Care.* 3rd ed. Baltimore, Md: Williams & Wilkins; 1996.

Romito RA. Early administration of enteral nutrients in critically ill patients. *AACN Clin Issues Crit Care.* 1995;6(2):242.

Rudolph AM, ed. *Pediatrics.* 18th ed. Norwalk, Conn: Appleton & Lange; 1987.

Sarnack AP, Meert KL. Predicting outcome in children with severe acute respiratory failure treated with HFV. *Crit Care Med.* 1996;24(8):1396–1401.

Schnapp L, Chin DP, et al. Frequency and importance of barotrauma in 100 patients with ALL. *Crit Care Med.* 1995;23(2):272–278.

Severinghaus JW. Accuracy of response of 6 pulse oximeters to profound hypoxia. *Anesthesiology.* 1987;67:551.

Shala N, Medeiri GO. Noninvasive mechanical ventilation in patients with acute respiratory failure. *Crit Care Med.* 1996;24(4):705–715.

Shaw N. Common surgical problems in the newborn. *J Perinat Neonat Nurs.* 1990;3(3):50–65.

Sibley RK, Berry GJ, Tazelaar HD, et al. The role of transbronchial biopsies in the management of lung transplant recipients. *J Heart Lung Transplant.* 1993;12(2):308–324.

Southwell S. Persistent fetal circulation, III. *Neonat Network.* Feb 1983:14–20.

Stoller JK. Unconventional strategies for ventilator management of ARDS. *Respir Management.* 1994;21:5.

Sturm JT, Hines JT, Perry JF Jr. Thoracic spinal fractures and aortic rupture: a significant and fatal association. *Ann Thorac Surg.* 1990;50:931.

Trotter C, Serpell MG. Neurological sequelae in children after prolonged propofol infusions. *Anesthesia.* 1992;47:340–342.

Udwadia ZF, Santis GK, Steven MH, et al. Nasal ventilation to facilitate weaning in patients with chronic respiratory insufficiency. *Thorax.* 1992;47:715–718.

Venkataraman S, Orr RA. Mechanical ventilation and respiratory care. In: Fuhrman B, Zimmerman J, eds. *Pediatric Critical Care.* St Louis, Mo: Mosby–Year Book Inc; 1992.

Walsh-Sukys M. Persistent pulmonary hypertension of the newborn. *Clin Perinatol.* 1993;20(1):127–143.

Weg JG, Balk RR, Tharratt S, et al. Safety and potential efficacy of an aerosolized surfactant in human and sepsis-induced ARDS. *JAMA.* 1994;272:1433–1438.

Wesley JR. Nutrient metabolism in relation to the systemic stress response. In: Fuhrman B, Zimmerman J, eds. *Pediatric Critical Care.* St Louis, Mo: Mosby–Year Book Inc; 1992.

Williams R: Congenital diaphragmatic hernia: a review. *Heart Lung.* 1982;11(6):532–538.

Wilson RF. *Critical Care Manual: Applied Physiology and Principles of Therapy.* 2nd ed. Philadelphia, Pa: FA Davis; 1992.

Wood DW, Downes JJ, Lecks HI. A clinical scoring system for the diagnosis of respiratory failure. *Am J Dis Child.* 1972;123:227.

Wood EJ, Lynch RE. Fluid and electrolyte balance. In: Fuhrman B, Zimmerman J, eds. *Pediatric Critical Care.* St Louis, Mo: Mosby–Year Book Inc; 1992.

Yamanaka M, Sue D. Comparison of arterial end tidal P_{CO_2} difference and dead space/tidal volume ratio in respiratory failure. *Chest.* 1987;92(5):832.

Zaccardelli DS, Pattishall EN. Clinical diagnosis criteria of the acute respiratory distress syndrome in the ICU. *Crit Care Med.* 1996;24(2):247–251.

3

Cardiovascular System

LOUISE CALLOW, ELIZABETH C. SUDDABY, and MARGARET C. SLOTA

DEVELOPMENTAL ANATOMY AND PHYSIOLOGY

A. **EMBRYOLOGIC DEVELOPMENT OF THE HEART**
 1. **Formation of the heart tube: Days 15 to 23**
    a. The heart is the first functioning organ in the embryo. Although the heart begins as an elongated tube controlled by brain growth, on days 21 through 23 the endothelial tubes fuse to form a single endocardial tube, and the heart begins to beat from a focus in the sinus venosus.
    b. *Cellular units of the developing heart*
       • Central nucleus
       • Sarcoplasm: Intracellular proteinaceous fluid
       • Sarcolemma: The single cell
       • Fiber: Composed of many fibrils, each surrounded by a sarcotubular system
       • Sarcotubular system: A membranous continuation of sarcolemma. The T tubules function to transmit action potential rapidly from sarcolemma to all fibrils in the muscle. Sarcoplasmic reticulum houses calcium ions. Action potentials in the T tubules cause release of calcium from reticulum, resulting in a contraction.
       • Contractile unit: Sarcomere (muscle fiber composed of fibrils). Each fibril is divided into filaments, and each filament is made up of contractile proteins. Contractile proteins consist of actin, myosin, troponin, and tropomyosin. Myosin forms the thick filaments. Actin, troponin, and tropomyosin form the thin filaments.
 2. **Formation of the heart loop: Days 23 to 28** (Fig. 3–1)
    a. The initial straight tube now loops to the right.
    b. The region of tube proximal to the fold becomes the embryonic ventricle.
    c. The atrioventricular (AV) junction moves to the left side of the pericardial cavity.
    d. Cardiac muscle in a mature heart differs from skeletal muscle. It has more mitochondria and can provide more adenosine triphosphate (ATP) and energy for repetitive action. Fibers are connected to each other by intercalated discs forming a lattice arrangement called a functional syncytium. When one fiber is depolarized, the action potential spreads along the syncytium to all other fibers, stimulating them also, and the whole syncytium contracts ("all or none" response).

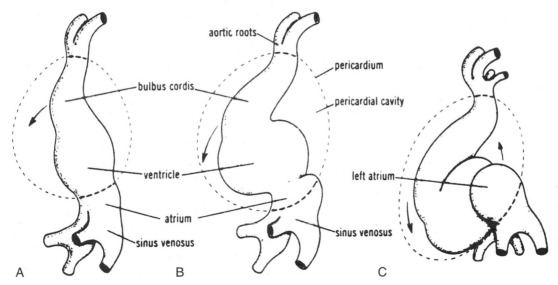

Figure 3–1. Cardiac looping to the right as seen from the left side. **A,** At 8 somites; **B,** at 11 somites; **C,** at 16 somites. The dashed line indicates the parietal pericardium. The atrium gradually assumes an intrapericardial position. (Reprinted with permission from Adams FH, Emmanoulides GC, Riemenschneider TA. *Moss' Heart Disease in Infants, Children, and Adolescents.* 4th ed. Baltimore, Md: Williams & Wilkins; 1989.)

    e. Structure of the cardiac wall in the fully developed heart
- The *pericardium* is a fibroserous membranous sac that encloses the heart. The fibrous pericardium is the outermost layer; the serous pericardium, composed of the parietal layer and the visceral layer, forms the outer surface of the heart.
- The *epicardium* is the visceral layer of the serous pericardium.
- The *myocardium* is the muscular portion of the heart.
- The *endocardium* is the inner membranous surface of the heart, lining the chambers of the heart.
- *Papillary muscles* arise from endocardial and myocardial surfaces of the ventricles and attach to chordae tendineae. *Chordae tendineae* are the tendinous attachments of the tricuspid and mitral valves that prevent eversion of the valves during systole.

3. **Formation of embryologic ventricles: Days 22 to 35** (Fig. 3–2)
    a. After looping, the cardiac tube develops expansions that become chambers, and true circulation begins.
    b. The common atrium divides as two tubes fuse.
    c. Endocardial cushions form from cardiac jelly swelling and later divide to create mitral and tricuspid valves.
    d. Ventricles dilate as cardiac output increases by increased stroke volume.
    e. Trabeculations of the right ventricle form.
    f. The truncoconal portion of the heart moves to lie over the atria.

4. **Formation of cardiac septa: Days 27 to 45**
    a. Active fusion of the cushions or passive expansion of cardiac chambers occurs. Endocardial cushions divide the AV canal into the mitral and tricuspid valves. Conotruncal cushions divide the truncus arteriosus into the aorta and the pulmonary artery. The septum secundum divides the atria.
    b. Expansion of the trabeculated tissue causes the septum primum to form first, followed by the septum secundum.

    c.   The atrial septum forms by the endocardial cushions' fusion of opposing atrial walls.

    d.   Pulmonary veins incorporate into the posterior wall of the left atrium.

    e.   The septum secundum closes with a remaining perforation called the foramen ovale.

    f.   While the medial walls of the expanding ventricles fuse forming the major portion of the ventricular septum, an extension of the endocardial cushions and truncal conus create the membranous septum.

    g.   *Chambers of the fully developed heart*

- The *atria* are thin-walled, low pressure chambers. The right and left atria act as reservoirs of blood for their respective ventricles. Seventy percent of blood flows passively from the atria into the ventricles during early ventricular diastole (protodiastole). The right atrium receives systemic venous blood via the superior vena cava (SVC), inferior vena cava (IVC), and coronary sinus. The left atrium receives oxygenated blood returning from the lungs via the four pulmonary veins.

- The *ventricles* are the "pumps" of the heart. The right ventricle (RV), a low-pressure system, contracts (systole) and propels desaturated blood into the pulmonary circulation via the pulmonary artery (PA) (the only artery in the body that carries desaturated blood). The left ventricle (LV), a high-pressure system, ejects blood into the systemic circulation via the aorta.

5. **Division of the truncus arteriosus: Days 32 to 33:** Outflow tracts divide by fusion of the conotruncal cushions, and spiraling follows the course of cushion development. The conotruncus terminates at the truncoaortic sac forming six pairs of aortic arches.

6. **Formation of cardiac valves: Days 34 to 36**

    a.   The *AV valves* are formed from the endocardial cushion. The mitral valve initially has four cusps; but two cusps grow larger, and papillary muscles fuse into two leaflets (anterior and posterior). The tricuspid valve forms largely from the conus septum, as do the papillary muscles and chordae tendineae.

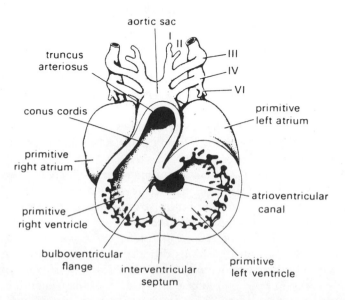

Figure 3–2.   The primitive atria and ventricles are formed and circulation begins. (Reprinted with permission from Adams FH, Emmanoulides GC, Riemenschneider TA. *Moss' Heart Disease in Infants, Children, and Adolescents.* 4th ed. Baltimore, Md: Williams & Wilkins; 1989.)

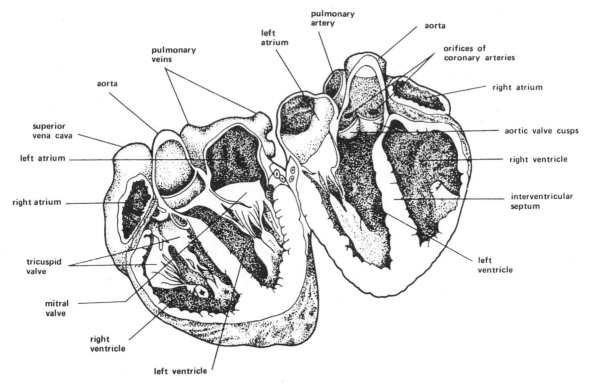

Figure 3–3. Illustration of fully developed intracardiac anatomy, valves, great vessels, and pulmonary veins (Reprinted with permission from Katz AM. *Physiology of the Heart.* New York, NY: Raven Press Publishers; 1992.)

The semilunar valves form at the interface of the truncal cushions and the aorticopulmonary septum.

b. *Cardiac valves in the fully developed heart* (Fig. 3–3)

- *AV valves:* The mitral valve is located between the left atrium and left ventricle, and the tricuspid valve is between the right atrium and right ventricle. The mitral valve is bicuspid, and the tricuspid valve consists of three leaflets (anterior, posterior, and septal). The AV valves allow unidirectional blood flow from the atria to the ventricles during ventricular diastole and prevent retrograde flow during ventricular systole. With ventricular diastole, the papillary muscles relax, the ventricular pressure falls below the atrial pressure, and the valve leaflets open. With increased ventricular pressure and systole, the valve leaflets close completely. Valve closure produces a sound that constitutes the first heart sound, S_1, consisting of a mitral valve and a tricuspid valve component (M_1, T_1). M_1 is the initial and major component of S_1.

- *Semilunar valves:* The pulmonary valve is between the right ventricle and pulmonary artery and consists of an annulus, three commissures, and three cusps. The aortic valve is situated between the left ventricle and aorta and consists of three valve cusps whose base attaches to a valve annulus. The valves allow unidirectional blood flow from the respective ventricle to arterial outflow tract during ventricular systole and prevent retrograde blood flow during ventricular diastole. Opening occurs when the ventricle contracts; the pressure is greater than the arterial outflow tract, and the valve opens. After ventricular systole, pressure in the arterial outflow tract exceeds pressure in the ventricle, and retrograde blood flow causes valve closure. Valve closure produces a sound that constitutes the second heart sound, S_2, consisting of an aortic and pulmonic component (A_2, P_2). A_2 is the initial and major component of S_2.

7. **Formation of the great veins: 4–7th weeks:** Great vein formation is the most variable aspect of cardiac development. Development begins with three pairs of major veins: the cardinal, vitelline, and umbilical veins, which originate in the chorionic villi and return oxygenated blood to the embryo. The right vitelline vein forms the posthepatic IVC. The SVC is formed by the right common cardinal vein and proximal right anterior cardinal vein.

8. **Systemic vasculature in the fully developed heart**

    a. *Systemic vessels* supply tissues with oxygen and nutrients and remove metabolic wastes. The diameter of the vessels (especially the arterioles) and viscosity of the blood create systemic vascular resistance (SVR). Tissue perfusion is controlled via local chemical reactions and nerves that dilate or constrict blood vessels.

    b. *Major components of systemic vasculature*

    - *Arteries* are a high-pressure circuit composed of strong, compliant, elastic-walled vessels carrying blood from the heart to the capillary beds. Elastic fibers within the arterial wall enable the wall to stretch during systole and recoil during diastole.

    - *Arterioles* are the major vessels controlling SVR and arterial pressure. Arterioles are controlled by the autonomic nervous system and by autoregulation. They contain smooth muscle innervated by sympathetic α-adrenergic nerve fibers. Stimulation causes constriction of the vessels, and decreased adrenergic discharge dilates the vessels controlling blood distribution to various capillary beds. Arterioles may give rise to metarterioles (precapillaries) or give rise directly to capillaries where regulation of flow is through constriction or dilation.

    - The *capillary system* allows exchange of oxygen and carbon dioxide and solutes between blood and tissues and permits fluid volume transfer between plasma and interstitium. Capillary filtration is related to hydrostatic and osmotic pressures across membranes. Increased hydrostatic pressure leads to movement of fluid from vessel to interstitium via osmosis. Greater capillary osmotic pressure leads to fluid movement from interstitium into vessels. Capillaries lack smooth muscle. Diameter changes are passive because of precapillary and postcapillary resistance. Because of their narrow lumens, capillaries can withstand high internal pressures without rupturing. Laplace's law states that the tension in the wall of the vessel necessary to balance the distending pressure is lessened as the radius of the blood vessel decreases. Diffusion is the most important process in moving substrates and wastes between blood and tissues via the capillary system.

    - The *venous system* stores approximately 65% of the total volume of blood in the circulatory system. Venules receive blood from capillaries and serve as collecting channels and capacitance (storage) vessels. Veins are capacitance vessels that conduct blood to the heart within a low pressure system. Veins are surrounded by skeletal muscles. When muscles contract, they compress veins, moving blood toward the heart. Valves in veins prevent retrograde blood flow. Under normal conditions the venous pump keeps the venous pressure in the lower extremities at 25 mm Hg or less. Gravity has profound effects on the erect, immobile individual. Pressure can rise to 90 mm Hg in the lower extremities, which results in swelling and a decrease in blood volume because of leakage of fluid from the circulatory system into the interstitium.

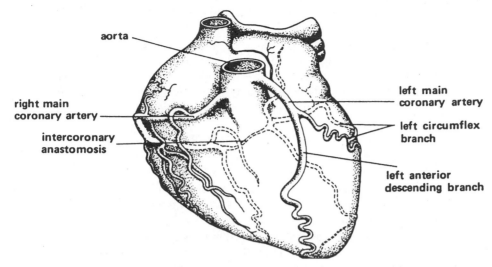

Figure 3–4. Location of coronary arteries and branching from aortic root. (Reprinted with permission from Katz AM. *Physiology of the Heart.* New York, NY: Raven Press Publishers; 1992.)

9. **Coronary vasculature in the fully developed heart** (Fig. 3–4)
   a. *Arteries* branch off the base of the aorta supplying blood to the conduction system and myocardium.
   b. The *right coronary artery (RCA)* supplies the sinoatrial (SA) node (55% of hearts), the AV node (90% of hearts), the right atrial (RA) and right ventricular (RV) muscles, and the inferoposterior wall of the left ventricle. Eighty percent of the time a branch of the RCA called the posterior descending artery is the terminal portion of the RCA, resulting in a right dominant coronary system. Located in the posterior interventricular groove, it supplies the right ventricle, left ventricle, and posterior part of the interventricular septum. The RCA gives off a marginal acute branch that descends from the lateral side of the heart to the apex. It supplies the anteroposterior surface of the right ventricle.
   c. The *left coronary artery (LCA)* branches into the left anterior descending artery (LAD), which supplies the anterior part of the interventricular septum, the anterior wall of the left ventricle, the right bundle branch (RBB), and the anterosuperior division of the left bundle branch (LBB).
   d. The *circumflex artery (CF)*, also branching off from the LCA (into major branches of the CF and one or more obtuse marginal branches [OMBs]), supplies the AV node (10% of hearts), the SA node (45% of hearts), and the posterior surface of the left ventricle via the OMBs.
   e. *Veins* return desaturated blood to the heart. They consist of the great cardiac veins, the small cardiac veins (both drain into the coronary sinus, which drains into the right atrium), and the thebesian veins (which drain blood into the right atrium through the atrial wall).
B. **EMBRYOLOGIC, NEONATAL, AND PEDIATRIC CARDIOVASCULAR PHYSIOLOGY**
   1. **Fetal circulation** (Fig. 3–5)
      a. Gas exchange occurs in the placenta.
      b. Umbilical venous blood (most highly saturated) returns via the umbilical vein from the placenta and accounts for 42% of fetal cardiac output. From the umbilical vein about one half the fetal blood flows through the ductus venosus to the IVC, and the other half enters the hepatic portal system.
      c. There is a preferential flow of more highly saturated blood through the

foramen ovale into the left atrium and left ventricle to the ascending aorta and to the brain and myocardium.

d. The SVC flow is directed to the tricuspid valve and the right ventricle, along with coronary sinus blood. Blood flows from the right ventricle to the pulmonary trunk, and about 8% of RV output perfuses the pulmonary artery. The rest of the RV output flows through the ductus arteriosus to the aorta. Parallel circulation exists in the fetus, since the RV pressure equals the LV pressure.

e. Vascular pressure reflects streaming with RA pressure greater than left atrial (LA) pressure, pulmonary artery pressure (PAP) greater than the aortic pressure, and the umbilical vein pressure higher than that of the IVC.

f. The fetal myocardium is less compliant because of the lower ratio of contractile to noncontractile fibers (30% in fetus; 60% in adult).

2. **Transitional circulation** (Fig. 3–6)

a. Interruption of the umbilical cord creates increased SVR and decreased IVC return to the heart. The primary change in circulation after birth is a shift from gas exchange in the placenta to the lungs.

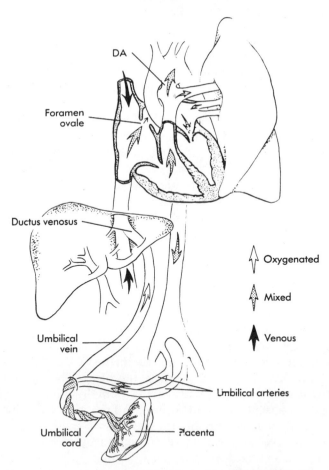

Figure 3–5. Fetal circulation with oxygenated placental blood entering umbilical veins, shunting through the ductus venosus, and entering the right side of the heart. Mixed venous blood shunts through the foramen ovale and ductus arteriosus eventually returning to the aorta and placenta via the umbilical artery. *DA,* ductus arteriosus. (Illustration by Marilou Kundemueller. Reprinted with permission from Hazinski MF. *Nursing Care of the Critically Ill Child.* 2nd ed. St. Louis, Mo: Mosby–Year Book Inc; 1992.)

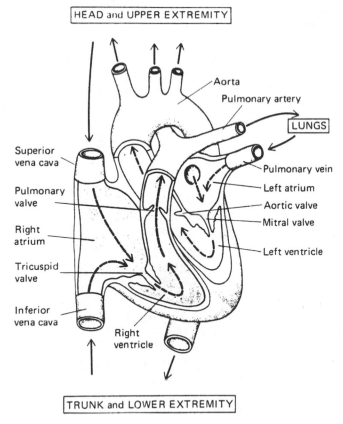

HEAD and UPPER EXTREMITY

Aorta
Pulmonary artery

LUNGS

Superior
vena cava

Pulmonary vein
Left atrium
Aortic valve
Mitral valve

Pulmonary
valve

Right
atrium

Left ventricle

Tricuspid
valve

Inferior
vena cava

Right
ventricle

TRUNK and LOWER EXTREMITY

Figure 3–6. Structure of the heart and course of normal blood flow through the cardiac chambers. (Reprinted with permission from Guyton AC. *Human Physiology and Mechanisms of Disease.* Philadelphia, Pa: WB Saunders Co; 1987.)

    b. Pulmonary vascular resistance (PVR) rapidly decreases in the first 12 to 24 hours of life, and pulmonary blood flow increases. The reduction to normal PVR occurs slowly over 14 to 21 days.

    c. The ductus arteriosus constricts primarily in response to increased arterial Po_2 but may be influenced by the loss of placental prostaglandin. The ductus arteriosus in the mature infant is functionally closed 12 to 24 hours after birth but can be reversed with prostaglandin E_1 (PGE_1). Anatomic closure from fibrosis usually occurs within 2 weeks. The right ventricle ejects all blood into the pulmonary circulation when the ductus arteriosus closes and the PVR decreases. The foramen ovale closes as a result of increased LA pressure from increased pulmonary blood return. The ductus venosus closes soon after birth.

    d. Rapid loss of the low resistance placental circuit increases the SVR and LV pressure, and LV and RV outputs equalize.

3. **Neonatal and pediatric circulation**

    a. The neonatal myocardium functions at near maximum cardiac output. There is a relatively fixed stroke volume in the first weeks. The larger ratio of noncontractile to contractile muscle fibers disappears after about 1 week.

    b. The neonatal myocardium responds to stress by a combination of hyperplasia and hypertrophy. Increased heart rate produces little change in cardiac output because of a high resting heart rate. But because the neonatal myocardium operates high on its cardiac output curve and stroke volume is limited, the cardiac output can be increased by increasing heart rate more so than by increasing contractility. Increased afterload will result in a drop in cardiac output.

c. *Peripheral blood vessel physiology*

- *Local control mechanisms:* The ability of the tissues to control their own blood flow is known as autoregulation. Two major hypotheses exist:
  - *Myogenic response:* As pressure rises, vessels stretch, stimulating the contraction of smooth muscles (feedback mechanism). As tension decreases, smooth muscles relax.
  - *Metabolic hypothesis:* Because of the normal metabolic activity of the tissues, carbon dioxide, potassium, lactate, prostaglandins, and phosphates accumulate and cause vasodilation, which increases the blood flow to the area to flush these waste products away.
  - There may be a delicate balance between these two mechanisms: Myogenic response → vasoconstriction → decrease in blood supply → local increase in metabolites → vasodilation → wastes removed.
- *Autonomic regulation of vessels*
  - *Sympathetic nervous system* fibers secrete norepinephrine at nerve endings, producing vasoconstriction. In arterioles this mechanism helps regulate blood flow and arterial pressure. In veins this mechanism helps vary the amount of blood stored. (Venoconstriction causes an increase in venous return to the heart.)
  - *Parasympathetic nervous system* fibers secrete acetylcholine at nerve endings (cholinergic effect), producing vasodilation.
- *Stretch receptors:* Baroreceptors (pressoreceptors)
  - Receptor sites are located in the aortic arch, carotid sinus, venae cavae, pulmonary arteries, and atria. Sensitive to arterial pressures, the receptor sites are activated by elevated blood pressure or increased blood volume, resulting in stretching of the arterial walls. The impulse is transmitted from the aortic arch and the carotid sinus to the medulla. Sympathetic action is inhibited, and the vagal reflex dominates, resulting in decreased heart rate and contractility, dilation of the systemic vasculature, and normalized blood pressure.
  - In response to decreased blood pressure, the vagal tone decreases, and the sympathetic system becomes dominant, resulting in increased heart rate and contractility and arterial and venous constriction and blood pressure elevated to near normal.
- The *vasomotor center in the medulla* (also called cardioaccelerator center or cardiac center) consists of the vasoconstrictor and vasodepressor areas.
  - Stimulation of the vasoconstrictor area causes increased heart rate, stroke volume, and cardiac output and ultimately, increased arterial blood pressure. Venoconstriction, which decreases stores of blood in the venous system, increases venous return and increases stroke volume.
  - Inhibition of the vasoconstrictor area stimulates the vasodepressor area, which causes vasodilation. An increase in storage of blood in the venous capacitance system occurs, thereby decreasing stroke volume, cardiac output and arterial blood pressure.
  - The vasomotor center works with stretch receptors and chemoreceptors located in the carotid sinus and aortic arch. A rise in blood pressure stimulates the carotid sinus, which inhibits the vasoconstrictor area. This induces vasodilation via stimulation of the vasodepressor area. A fall in oxygen saturation, rise in carbon dioxide, or fall in

pH stimulates chemoreceptors, which then stimulate the vasoconstrictor center and cause a rise in arterial blood pressure.

4. **Neurologic control of the fully developed heart**
   a. *Autonomic nervous system*
      - Sympathetic stimulation initiates the release of norepinephrine. α-Adrenergic fiber stimulation results in arteriolar vasoconstriction. β-Adrenergic ($β_1$) fiber stimulation increases SA node discharge (thereby increasing the heart rate [positive chronotropy]), increases the force of myocardial contraction (positive inotropy), and accelerates AV conduction time (positive dromotropism).
      - Parasympathetic stimulation initiates the release of acetylcholine, which stimulates the action of the right vagus (affecting the SA node) and the left vagus nerves (affecting AV nodal conduction tissue). The rate of SA node discharge is decreased and slows the heart rate (negative chronotropy). It may slow conduction through AV tissue (negative dromotropism).
   b. *Chemoreceptors* are located in the carotid and aortic bodies and are sensitive to changes in Po_2, Pco_2 and pH. They affect heart rate and respiratory rate via stimulation of the vasomotor center in the medulla.
   c. *Stretch receptors* respond to pressure and volume changes. Stretch receptors located in the atria, large veins, and pulmonary artery produce the Bainbridge reflex. An increase in venous return stretches the receptors. Afferent nerve impulses transmit to the vasomotor center in the medulla. The medulla increases efferent impulses, increasing heart rate and cardiac output. This enables the heart to pump out all the blood returned to it.
   d. *Respiratory reflex:* Inspiration decreases intrathoracic pressure, increasing venous return to the heart. Inspiration stimulates stretch receptors in the lungs and thorax. Impulses from the stretch receptors inhibit the vasomotor center in the medulla. This inhibition decreases vagal tone, causing an increase in the heart rate, which allows the heart to pump out the extra blood. This reflex results in "sinus arrhythmia," which may occur in normal children.

5. **Variables affecting the ventricular function of the heart**
   a. *Cardiac Output* (CO) = Stroke Volume (SV) × Heart Rate (HR). *Cardiac index* (CI) is used in children because of the variation in cardiac output by body size. Cardiac index is equal to cardiac output divided by body surface area.
   b. *Stroke volume* is affected by preload, afterload, and contractility.
      - *Preload* is the resting force in the myocardium, which is determined by volume in the ventricles at the end of diastole (left ventricular end-diastolic volume [LVEDV] reflected by left ventricular end-diastolic pressure [LVEDP]). Preload can be related to such variables as fiber length, stretch, and volume of blood returned from veins. An increase in preload stretches myocardial muscle fibers, causing more forceful subsequent ventricular contractions, increasing stroke volume and cardiac output. An increase in preload is accomplished by increasing the volume returning to the ventricles (Fig. 3–7). The Frank-Starling law states that the more the heart is filled during diastole, the greater the quantity of blood pumped into the aorta. The preload or ventricular filling pressure reflects the initial sarcomere length, which influences the development of myocardial force. Muscle fibers reach a point of stretch beyond which contraction is no longer enhanced and stroke volume decreases. In-

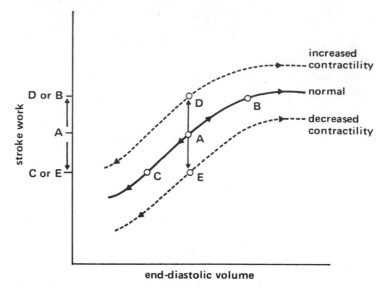

Figure 3–7. The work of the heart varies with changing end-diastolic volume according to the Frank-Starling relationship. The work of the heart can also be varied by changes in contractility. The *solid curve (CAB)* describes normal myocardial contractility, and point A represents the basal state. Changes in cardiac work that result from alterations in venous return shift the work of the heart along this normal curve. Cardiac work can be increased from A to B by enhanced venous return and decreased from A to C by a reduction in venous return. The work of the heart can also be changed by modifications in myocardial contractility. A positive inotropic agent can increase cardiac work from A to D even with constant end-diastolic volume. Cardiac work can be decreased from A to E by a negative inotropic agent without change in end-diastolic volume. (Reprinted with permission from Katz AM. *Physiology of the Heart.* New York, NY: Raven Press Publishers; 1992.)

creased preload may be related to mitral insufficiency, aortic insufficiency, ventricular septal defect (VSD), atrial septal defect (ASD), and patent ductus arteriosus (PDA); fluid overload; and vasoconstrictors. Decreased preload may be related to mitral stenosis (MS), hypovolemia, and vasodilators.

- *Afterload* is the initial resistance that must be overcome by the ventricles to open the semilunar valves and propel blood into the systemic and pulmonary circulatory system.
    - Afterload is clinically measured as SVR (also called peripheral vascular resistance) and PVR. *SVR= [Mean Arterial Pressure (MAP) – Central Venous Pressure (CVP)]/Systemic Blood Flow,* a value measured in resistance units. This number times 80 converts into dynes per second per square centimeter. Normal SVR = $900 - 1400$ dynes/s/cm^2.
    - Factors increasing afterload include fixed anatomic obstruction, peripheral arterial vasoconstriction, hypertension, pulmonary hypertension, polycythemia, and vasoconstrictors. Excessive afterload increases LV or RV stroke work, increases myocardial oxygen demands, and may result in LV or RV failure. Factors decreasing ventricular afterload include vasodilators.
- *Contractility* is the strength and efficiency of contraction (force generated). Positive inotropic drugs, sympathetic stimulation, and hypercalcemia can act to increase the contractile state of the myocardium. Factors that can decrease contractility of the myocardium include negative inotropic drugs; hypoxia; hypercapnia; intrinsic depression due in part to long-standing congestive heart failure (CHF); parasympathetic stimula-

tion; metabolic acidosis, hypocalcemia, hypoglycemia, hypomagnesium, hyponatremia, and hyperkalemia; condition of the myocardium; and intrinsic myocardial disease.

c. *Arterial pressure*

- Factors affecting arterial blood pressure include cardiac output, heart rate, SVR, arterial elasticity, blood volume, blood viscosity, age, body surface area, exercise, and anxiety.
- *Pulse pressure* is a function of stroke volume and arterial capacitance. This difference between systolic and diastolic blood pressure is expressed in millimeters of mercury (Ps – Pd).
- *Mean arterial pressure (MAP)* is defined as (Berne and Levy, 1993) "the average pressure during a given cardiac cycle that exists in the aorta and its major branches . . . . [I]t is dependent on the mean volume of blood in the arterial system and the elastic properties of the arterial walls." This is a function of cardiac output and SVR.
- *Regulation of arterial pressure:* The renin-angiotensin-aldosterone system involves renin, a protease secreted by the kidney that converts angiotensin I to angiotensin II. Release of renin from the kidney is stimulated by stretch receptors in juxtaglomerular cells that are sensitive to changes in blood pressure. Decreased blood pressure, a rise in sympathetic output, or a fall in sodium concentration results in increased renin secretion. Increased blood pressure results in decreased renin secretion. Angiotensin II is the most potent vasoconstrictor known, producing arteriolar constriction and a rise in systolic and diastolic pressures.
- Other mechanisms include capillary fluid shift mechanisms, local control mechanisms, and the renal-fluid volume process. With a rise in arterial pressure, the kidneys excrete more fluid, causing a reduction in extracellular fluid and blood volume; this reduces circulating blood volume and cardiac output leading to normalization of arterial pressure. With a fall in arterial pressure, the kidneys retain fluid, causing increased intravascular volume and cardiac output that may result in normalization of arterial pressure.

ANATOMY OF THE CARDIAC CONDUCTION SYSTEM (Fig. 3–8)

A. **SINOATRIAL NODE (SA NODE)**

The SA node is the pacemaker of the heart because it possesses the fastest inherent rate of automaticity.

B. **INTERNODAL ATRIAL PATHWAYS**

The internodal atrial pathways, consisting of the anterior tract (Bachmann's), middle tract (Wenckebach's), and posterior tract (Thorel's), conduct impulses from the SA node through the right atrium to the AV node.

C. **BACHMANN'S BUNDLE**

Bachmann's bundle conducts impulses from the SA node to the left atrium.

D. **ATRIOVENTRICULAR NODE (AV NODE, AV JUNCTION)**

The AV node delays impulse transmission between atria and ventricles, allowing time for ventricular filling following atrial contraction and prior to ventricular systole. The AV node controls the number of impulses (if the atrial rate becomes excessive) reaching the ventricles, thereby having some control over heart rate.

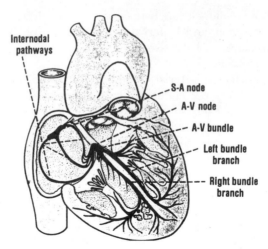

Figure 3–8. Intracardiac conduction system. *A-V,* atrioventricular; *S-A,* sinoatrial. (Reprinted with permission from Guyton AC. *Human Physiology and Mechanisms of Disease.* Philadelphia, Pa: WB Saunders Co; 1987.)

E. **BUNDLE OF HIS**

The bundle of His is composed of thick fibers arising from the AV node that course over the crest of the ventricular septum on its right side to the bundle branch system.

F. **BUNDLE BRANCH SYSTEM**

The bundle branch system is composed of pathways that arise from the bundle of His. The **right bundle branch (RBB)** is a direct continuation of the bundle of His that transmits impulses down the right side of the interventricular septum toward the RV myocardium. The bundle divides into three parts (anterior, lateral, and posterior), dividing further to become parts of the Purkinje system. The **left bundle branch (LBB)** separates into the left posterior fascicle (which transmits impulses over the posterior and inferior endocardial surfaces of the left ventricle) and the left anterior fascicle (which transmits impulses to the anterior and superior endocardial surfaces of the left ventricle).

G. **THE PURKINJE SYSTEM**

The Purkinje system arises from the distal portion of the bundle branches and transmits impulses into the subendocardial layers of both ventricles. It provides for depolarization (from endocardium to epicardium) followed by ventricular contraction and ejection of blood from the ventricles.

ELECTROPHYSIOLOGY

A. **MYOCARDIAL CONDUCTION SYSTEM'S FOUR PROPERTIES**
   1. *Automaticity:* Ability to spontaneously generate impulse
   2. *Rhythmicity:* Regularity of impulse generation
   3. *Conductivity:* Ability to transmit impulses
   4. *Excitability:* Ability to respond to stimulation
B. **RESTING MEMBRANE POTENTIAL (RMP) FOR CARDIAC MUSCLE CELL**

The sodium and unbound calcium ion concentration is greater outside the cell, and the potassium ion concentration is greater inside the cell. The RMP for myocardial muscle fibers is −80 to −90 mV.

C. **STIMULATION OF RESTING MEMBRANES**

Depolarization can result from chemical, electrical, or mechanical stimulation. The stimulus reduces the RMP to a less negative value (depolarization). The threshold potential is the voltage level where an action potential is produced. For all cardiac tissue except the SA and AV nodes, the threshold potential is −60 to −70 mV. For the SA and AV nodes, the threshold potential is −30 to −40 mV. Reaching the threshold causes changes in the membrane. The permeability of the cell membrane is altered, opening specialized channels in the membrane, which permits the passage of sodium and calcium ions into the cell. The action potential (AP) is the graphic representation of this change in RMP.

D. **"GATE" THEORY**

Fast channels of the membrane specific for sodium may be controlled by two gates.

1. The *activation gate* opens the fast channels as the RMP becomes less negative, allowing a rapid influx of sodium into the cell, which causes depolarization (phase 0 of the AP [the upstroke]).
2. The *deactivation gate* closes the channels impeding the influx of sodium into the cell.
3. Closure of the gates is complete in phase 1 of the AP, and sodium ceases to diffuse into the cell.
4. A return to the RMP produces an inward current of calcium (and to a lesser extent, sodium), producing the plateau of the AP phase 0. Potassium ions then diffuse out of the cell.
5. As the slow, inward current of sodium and calcium decreases, the outward current of potassium increases. This causes the cell to rapidly repolarize (phase 3).
6. After repolarization, the sodium-potassium pump regulates the concentration of cations in the cell. The pump, found in the cell membrane, actively pumps excess sodium out of the cell and pumps in the potassium that diffused out during phase 2.

E. **REFRACTORINESS OF HEART MUSCLE**

1. *Absolute refractory period* encompasses phases 0, 1, 2, and part of 3 of the AP. During this period of time the cell cannot respond to another stimulus and produce an action potential.
2. *Relative refractory period* (latter part of phase 3) is a period of time where a strong stimulus can cause depolarization.
3. *Supernormal period* occurs at the end of phase 3. During this time a very weak stimulus that would not normally elicit an AP can evoke a response and cause depolarization.
4. *Vulnerable period* is the point at the very beginning of the relative refractory period. A stimulus at this time (which corresponds to the peak of the T wave on the electrocardiogram [ECG]) can result in myocardial electrical chaos.

F. **CARDIAC PACEMAKER CELLS (SA AND AV NODES) ACTION POTENTIAL**

1. Phase 0 produces a slow, inward movement of calcium and sodium into the cell, producing a slow-response AP curve different from the cardiac muscle cell.
2. Unlike other cells of the heart that require another stimulus to depolarize them once they have been repolarized, the SA and AV nodes spontaneously depolarize in phase 4. This spontaneous depolarization is due to the steady influx of sodium and the efflux of potassium ions raising the nodal tissues back to the threshold potential, initiating an AP. This phenomenon is known as automaticity. The rate of automaticity may be altered by increasing or decreasing the slope of phase 4. Increasing the slope of phase 4 speeds the heart rate and decreasing the slope of phase 4 slows the heart rate.

EXCITATION-CONTRACTILE PROCESS OF MUSCLE

The AP produced during depolarization is transmitted to the interior of the cell via T tubules, which transmit the AP to all myofibrils. Calcium is stored in the lateral sacs of the sarcoplasmic reticulum and is released during the AP. Calcium enters the interior of the cell, causing an interaction between actin and myosin filaments through a complex interaction with enzymes. Actin filaments move progressively inward on myosin filaments as successive electrochemical interactions take place (interdigitation [sliding filament hypothesis]). The result is shortening of sarcomeres and then of muscle fibers and thus myocardial contraction. Relaxation of muscle fibers occurs when free calcium is pumped back into the sarcoplasmic reticulum.

PHYSIOLOGIC RESPONSE TO DEPOLARIZATION AND REPOLARIZATION

The **electroactivity of the heart** produces myocardial contraction.

Electrical depolarization of the atria is represented by the P wave on the ECG. Following atrial depolarization the pressure in the atria rises higher than the diastolic pressure in the ventricles, forcing blood from the atria into the resting ventricles.

Electrical depolarization of the ventricles occurs, producing the QRS complex on the ECG. Isometric or isovolumetric contraction is the first phase of ventricular contraction (systole). Ventricular pressure rises while ventricular volume remains stable because the semilunar valves have not yet opened. The increased pressure in the ventricles closes the AV valves producing the first heart sound or S_1 (mitral and tricuspid closing sounds [M_1, T_1]). As ventricular pressure exceeds great vessel pressure, the semilunar valves open. Blood from the ventricles is rapidly ejected into the great vessels. As the outflow of blood from the ventricles decreases, the pressure in the ventricles also decreases, falling below the pressure in the great vessels. This causes a back flow of blood from the great vessels to the ventricles, which closes the semilunar valves and produces the second heart sound S_2 (aortic and pulmonary closure sounds [A_2, P_2]). The dicrotic notch on the arterial pressure tracing represents closure of the aortic valve.

Repolarization of the ventricles occurs during mechanical systole and produces the T wave on the ECG.

Isometric or isovolumetric relaxation occurs when ventricular pressure falls rapidly following semilunar valve closure. Intraventricular volume remains static before the AV valves open. A "v" wave is produced on the atrial pressure curve during isometric relaxation related to blood flow into the atria from the pulmonic and systemic circuits. As ventricular pressure remains lower than atrial pressure, the AV valves open to initiate the rapid-filling phase.

CLINICAL ASSESSMENT OF CARDIOVASCULAR FUNCTION

A. HISTORY
1. The **chief complaint** is the patient or parents' description of why they are seeking help.
2. **History of present illness:** Determine onset, description, course, and duration. Evaluate exacerbations and remissions of signs and symptoms including the following:
   a. *Feeding pattern:* Duration, associated distress, volume taken, stopping to rest

or breath during eating, caloric supplementation required (earliest sign of CHF)

    b. *Fatigue:* While feeding or playing

    c. *Edema:* Orbital, sacral

    d. *Diaphoresis:* Location, degree

    e. *Dyspnea, tachypnea:* With or without activity

    f. *Cyanosis:* Oxygen saturation with or without activity

    g. *Squatting:* Frequent in children with cyanotic lesions when repairs are delayed

    h. *Growth:* Graph against normal limits for height and weight. With CHF, weight will fall below normal limits before height does.

    i. *Frequency of infections*

    j. *Syncope:* Prodrome, with or without dizziness, time of occurrence

    k. *Palpitations:* With or without chest pain

3. **Past history and family history** includes all previous illnesses, injuries, and family history of similar disease (i.e., history of congenital heart disease [CHD], not coronary artery disease)

    a. *Prenatal and perinatal history*

    b. *Family history* should include evaluation of multifactorial inheritance of environmental, genetic, and unknown factors (see Table 3–1).

      • Environmental factors include drug teratogens, external radiation exposure, systemic diseases, and infections.

      • There is a slightly higher risk (2.5% to 16%) of CHD if one parent or sibling has CHD. CHD can be associated with chromosomal anomalies or syndromes. CHD is also associated with extracardiac anomalies in infants. Musculoskeletal problems, gastrointestinal problems such as tracheoesophageal fistula and congenital diaphragmatic hernia, and renal anomalies may occur. Asplenia is associated with complex cyanotic defects, dextrocardia, abnormal systemic venous return, total anomalous pulmonary venous return (TAPVR), and bilateral symmetry or organs. Polyspenia is associated with ASD, VSD, and TAPVR.

4. **Psychosocial history** includes the use of illicit drugs or alcohol during pregnancy or by the child, daily living patterns, relationships with significant others, recreational habits, educational level of the child and parents, and developmental level of the child.

5. The **medication history** should include all medications prescribed or obtained over the counter, dosages, and reason for use.

B. PHYSICAL EXAMINATION

  1. **Inspection**

    a. *General appearance:* Note size for age (height and weight graphed against normal limits), activity level, level of consciousness, and external signs of chromosomal abnormalities (i.e., Down syndrome).

    b. *Assess skin and mucous membranes*

      • Note pallor, cyanosis, or mottling. Skin color is influenced by vasoconstriction. Cyanosis is evident if saturation is less than 85%, which is equivalent to 5 g of reduced hemoglobin per 100 ml of blood. The degree of visible cyanosis is dependent on total hemoglobin and its saturation. Respiratory cyanosis decreases with crying (improved respiratory effort) and oxygen. In cardiac disease, cyanosis increases with crying (increased resistance to pulmonary blood flow and shunting) and remains unchanged with oxygen administration. Acrocyanosis (cyanosis of the extremities) is normal in the newborn with vasomotor instability. Note the distribution of cyanosis over the body. Peripheral cyanosis (extremi-

Table 3–1.   CARDIAC ANOMALIES ASSOCIATED WITH SYNDROMES AND ENVIRONMENTAL EXPOSURES

	CARDIAC ANOMALY
Syndrome	
DiGeorge	Interrupted aortic arch, TOF
Ehlers-Danlos	ASD, AVC, TOF
Ellis–van Creveld	Large ASD, single atrium
Holt-Oram	ASD, single atrium, TAPVR, pulmonary vascular disease, arrhythmias
Hunter's	Abnormal mitral valve and tricuspid valve, coronary obstruction
Hurler's	Abnormal mitral valve and tricuspid valve, coronary obstruction
Laurence-Moon and Bardet-Biedl	Aortic stenosis, pulmonary stenosis, VSD, TOF
Marfan	Abnormal aortic valve and mitral valve, dissection aortic aneurysms
Neurofibromatosis	Pulmonary stenosis
Osteogenesis imperfecta	Aneurysms, valvular incompetence
Scimitar	PAPVR, dextrocardia
Trisomy 13 (Patau's)	PDA, VSD with pulmonary hypertension, DORV
Trisomy 18 (Edwards')	VSD, PDA
Trisomy 21 (Down)	AVC, VSD, PDA, ASD
Turner's	COA, pulmonary stenosis, TAPVR, AVC
Turner's Mosaic (XO/XY)	Pulmonary stenosis
Williams	Supravalvular AS, PS
Environmental Exposures	
Drugs	
Maternal thalidomide ingestion	Truncus, TOF, VSD, PDA
Fetal alcohol	VSD, ASD, TOF
Amphetamines	VSD, PDA, ASD, TGV
Trimethadione	VSD, TOF
Anticonvulsants	Pulmonary stenosis, arterial stenosis, COA, PDA, TGV, TOF, HLHS
Sex hormones	VSD, TGV, TOF
Lithium	Ebstein's anomaly, TAT, ASD
Retinoic acid	TOF, TGV, DORV, truncus, VSD
Systemic Diseases	
Maternal diabetes	TGV, VSD, hypertrophic cardiomyopathy
Lupus erythematosus	Congenital complete heart block
Phenylketonuria	TOF, VSD, ASD
Thyroid dysfunction	Tachycardias, SVT, cardiomyopathy
Friedreich's ataxia	Cardiomyopathy, complete AVB, PVCs

AS, aortic stenosis; *ASD*, atrial septal defect; *AVB*, atrioventricular block; *AVC*, arteriovenous canal defect; *COA*, coarctation of the aorta; *DORV*, double outlet right ventricle; *HLHS*, hypoplastic left heart syndrome; *PAPVR*, partial anomalous pulmonary venous return; *PDA*, patent ductus arteriosus; *PS*, pulmonary stenosis; *PVC*, premature ventricular contraction; *SVT*, supraventricular tachycardia; *TAPVR*, total anomalous pulmonary venous return; *TAT*, tricuspid atresia; *TGV*, transposition of the great vessels; *TOF*, tetralogy of Fallot; *Truncus*, truncus arteriosus; *VSD*, ventricular septal defect.

ties, perioral [around the mouth]) may represent hypothermia or decreased flow, whereas central cyanosis (inside mucous membranes) indicates reduced hemoglobin saturation. Chronic cyanosis stimulates erythropoiesis and polycythemia, which cause increased blood viscosity and an increased risk of spontaneous cerebrovascular accidents, brain abscess, thrombocytopenia with short platelet survival, reduced platelet aggregation with hemorrhagic abnormalities (which may cause operative bleeding), and vascular sheer stress producing increased PVR even in the face of decreased pulmonary blood flow.

- Note temperature. Skin temperature is influenced by the environment but assists in describing the level of decreased perfusion (i.e., cold to knee, cold to midthigh).
- Note edema, which is more common in periorbital and sacral areas of infants.
- Note presence of diaphoresis.

c. *Observe extremities*
- Note clubbing of nail beds indicated by a flattened angle of the nail base to 180 or more degrees (normal about 160 degrees). Clubbing develops after decreased oxygen saturation persisting more than 6 months (Fig. 3–9).
- Compare both sides for equal growth, particularly length, in children requiring multiple catheterization procedures.

d. *Observe the chest and precordium* for visible pulsations; active precordium (heaves, thrusts over the precordium noted in volume overload such as left-to-right shunts or aortic or mitral insufficiency); shape, contour, and symmetry of chest; breathing pattern; and visible point of maximal intensity of cardiac impulse (point of maximal impulse [PMI]).

e. *Observe the neck for jugular venous distention.*

2. **Palpation**

a. *Precordium*
- Note the PMI, normally found at the fifth left intercostal space (LICS), medial to the midclavicular line after 7 years or at the fourth LICS before 7 years. Lateral displacement of the PMI away from the left sternal border (LSB) indicates elevated diaphragm or left ventricular hypertrophy (LVH). Medial displacement toward the sternum indicates right ventricular hypertrophy (RVH) or an abnormally small left ventricle.

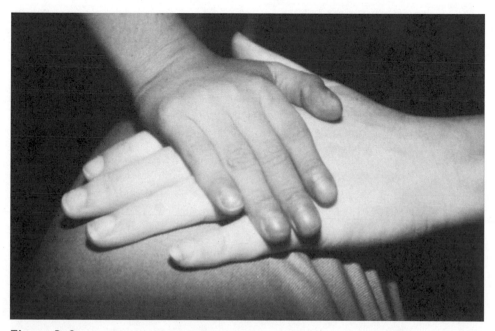

Figure 3–9.   Example of child's clubbed fingers in contrast to normal. (Courtesy of Elizabeth C. Suddaby.)

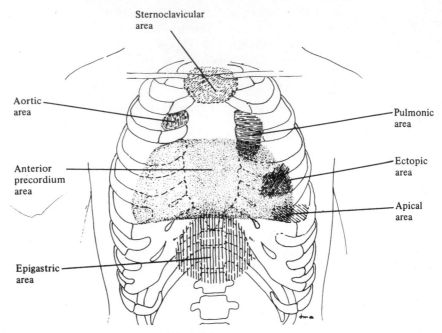

Figure 3–10.   Seven areas to be examined. (Reprinted with permission from Alexander MM, Brown MS. *Pediatric History Taking and Physical Diagnosis for Nurses.* St Louis: Mosby–Year Book Inc; 1979.)

- Seven areas should be palpated (Fig. 3–10), including the supraclavicular (over sternoclavicular notch), aortic (second right intercostal space [RICS] close to the sternum), pulmonary (second LICS close to the sternum), tricuspid (fourth to fifth LICS at the left lower sternal border), mitral (fifth LICS medial to the midclavicular line), epigastric (below the xiphoid process), and the ectopic area (between pulmonic and apical areas).
- *Thrills:* Use the ball portion of the palm of the hand to palpate murmurs (feels like a vibration or a cat purring). Thrills in the aortic area indicate aortic stenosis. Thrills in the pulmonic area with radiation to the left side of neck indicate pulmonic stenosis. In the apical area, thrills during systole indicate mitral regurgitation and during diastole indicate mitral stenosis. Near the suprasternal notch, thrills may indicate aortic stenosis, pulmonic stenosis, or PDA. In intercostal spaces, thrills may indicate coarctation of the aorta with collateral circulation. At the mid to lower left sternal border, thrills may indicate VSD.
- *Lifts* are pulsations noted under the palm of the hand. Pulsation in the pulmonic area indicates mitral stenosis or hypertension. Lifts in the tricuspid area may indicate VSD, elevated RV pressure, pulmonary stenosis, pulmonary hypertension, or ASD.
- *Friction rubs* are similar to the sensation of rubbing two pieces of material together.
  b. *Peripheral pulses* are rated on a scale of 0 to 4.
     0 = absent
     1+ = palpable but thready, easily obliterated
     2+ = normal
     3+ = full
     4+ = full and bounding

- Common arterial sites for palpation include the carotid, brachial, radial, femoral, popliteal, dorsalis pedis, and posterior tibialis.
- Obtain simultaneous assessment of upper and lower extremity pulses to evaluate for coarctation of aorta.
- Describe characteristics of pulses. Strong, bounding pulses are found in PDA, aortic regurgitation, arteriovenous fistulas, and truncus arteriosus. Delayed weak pulses are found in cardiac tamponade, aortic stenosis, mitral stenosis, CHF, shock, and hypoplastic left heart syndrome (HLHS). Pulsus alternans (alternating pulse waves, every other beat weaker than preceding beat) indicates a weak heart muscle as seen in severe hypertension or LV failure. Pulsus paradoxus is an exaggeration of the normal physiologic response to inspiration. Usually on inspiration there is a fall of less than 10 mm Hg in arterial systolic pressure. In pulsus paradoxus the drop exceeds 10 mm Hg during normal inspiratory effort. It can also be found in pericardial effusion, pericardial tamponade, or significant asthma.

c. *Capillary filling time* is evaluated by compressing the extremity with moderate pressure and noting the time required for the blanched area to reperfuse. Normal time is less than 3 seconds.

d. The *liver* is palpated, starting in the lower abdomen and pressing upward at the right costal margin until the liver edge is palpated. The liver edge of an infant is normally 3 cm below the costal margin. The liver edge of a 1-year-old is at 2 cm below; the liver edge of a 4- to 5-year-old is at 1 cm below. By adolescence the edge is not palpable or is at the costal margin.

3. **Auscultation**

a. *Heart rate and rhythm*

b. *Blood pressure:* Use a cuff bladder that is at least two thirds the circumference and two thirds the length of the extremity. Obtain four extremity blood pressure readings during the initial assessment to rule out coarctation of the aorta. Thigh pressure is equal to upper extremity pressure until a child is 1 year old; after that the thigh pressure may be higher. Upper extremity pressures are higher in coarctation. Note the pulse pressure. Low diastolic pressure increases pulse pressure and may indicate PDA or aortic regurgitation. Decreased pulse pressure may indicate aortic stenosis or cardiac tamponade.

c. *Heart sounds*

- S_1 represents closure of the mitral and tricuspid valves and the beginning of systole. The mitral component of S_1 is loudest at the apex. The tricuspid component of S_1 is loudest at the fifth intercostal space (ICS) to the left of the sternum. S_1 is louder than S_2 at the apex. S_1 is increased in intensity from mitral stenosis, anemia, fever, exercise, and hyperthyroidism; S_1 is decreased in intensity from first-degree AV block, mitral regurgitation, shock, cardiomyopathy, hypothyroidism, and left bundle branch block (LBBB). A split S_1 denotes separation of mitral and tricuspid sounds and is normally heard in the tricuspid area. If audible at the anterior axillary line, it is more likely an aortic ejection click.
- S_2 represents closure of the aortic and pulmonic valves at the beginning of diastole. The aortic component of S_2 is loudest at the second RICS. The pulmonic component of S_2 is loudest at the second LICS. S_2 is heard best in the aortic and pulmonic areas. Increased intensity may be normal or may indicate hypertension or coarctation. Decreased intensity (best

heard in the aortic area) indicates aortic stenosis. Decreased intensity (best heard in the pulmonic area) indicates pulmonic stenosis or tricuspid atresia. A split S_2 (best heard in the pulmonic area during inspiration) is physiologically related to the increased venous return to the right ventricle and thus delayed closure of the pulmonary valve. A fixed split of S_2 represents delayed closure of the pulmonic valve from increased pulmonary blood flow through the right ventricle as in ASD and TAPVR. A widely split S_2 may occur with delayed activation of the right ventricle from right bundle branch block (RBBB), LV pacing, or ectopic beats. A single S_2 may be heard in tetralogy of Fallot, pulmonary atresia or stenosis, and transposition of the great vessels (TGV).

  d. *Extra heart sounds*

- S_3 is caused by the rapid entry of blood into the ventricles. S_3 is heard best at the apex with the bell and may be heard in normal children. S_3 sounds like "Ken-tuc-ky." A loud S_3 or ventricular gallop is a pathologic finding caused by resistance to ventricular filling related to increased volume load or decreased compliance. It occurs in mitral regurgitation, CHF, tricuspid insufficiency, left-to-right shunts, and anemia.
- S_4 is produced by atrial contraction, best heard at the apex, and almost never heard in normal children. It sounds like "Ten-nes-see." It can indicate aortic stenosis, pulmonic stenosis, hypertension, heart failure, and anemia.

  e. *Murmurs* are heard because of turbulent flow through an abnormal opening or obstructed area. The following are evaluated:

- *Timing: Systolic murmurs* are heard between S_1 and S_2 (early, mid, or late). Holosystolic murmurs are heard throughout systole. Midsystolic ejection murmurs start after S_1 and end before S_2, usually with a crescendo-decrescendo sound. *Diastolic murmurs* are heard following S_2 (early, mid, or late).
- *Intensity* is based on a scale:
  - I Barely audible (not heard in all positions)
  - II Just easily audible (not heard in all positions)
  - III Heard well in all positions
  - IV Heard well, palpable thrill
  - V Louder, can be heard with stethoscope partly off chest
  - VI Heard with stethoscope off chest
- *Location*
  - Apical area: (with some extension up to the pulmonic area) can hear murmurs of mitral insufficiency or stenosis, subaortic stenosis, aortic insufficiency, aortic ejection click of aortic stenosis, and click or late systolic murmur of mitral valve prolapse.
  - Tricuspid area: (With some extension up to the pulmonic area) can hear murmurs of tricuspid insufficiency or stenosis, pulmonary insufficiency, VSD, and aortic insufficiency
  - Aortic area: Murmurs of aortic stenosis or insufficiency
  - Pulmonic area: Murmurs of pulmonary stenosis or insufficiency, ASD, pulmonary ejection click, and PDA
- *Radiation*
- *Pitch:* High pitch is heard with the diaphragm, and low pitch is heard with the bell.
- *Quality* is described as blowing, rumbling, harsh, or musical.

INVASIVE AND NONINVASIVE DIAGNOSTIC STUDIES

A. LABORATORY STUDIES

Frequently ordered tests include electrolytes, complete blood count (CBC), lipid profile, calcium (total and ionized), and a clotting profile (prothrombin time [PT], partial thromboplastin time [PTT], thrombin time, bleeding time, and platelet count).

B. PULSE OXIMETRY

Pulse oximetry uses changes in infrared light to evaluate the level of saturated hemoglobin, providing an indirect measurement of oxygen saturation (normal 96% to 100%). Pulse oximetry can be used to evaluate or trend cyanosis or to assess tolerance of procedures (suctioning, sedation).

C. CHEST X-RAY EXAMINATION

1. **Heart size** is evaluated by estimation of the cardiothoracic ratio, which is determined by the largest dimension of the heart compared to the widest intercostal diameter of the chest. The normal size is 50%. A large thymus in infants may be mistaken for cardiomegaly.

2. **Cardiac borders** are evaluated on an anterioposterior film (Fig. 3–11). The right border indicates the right atrium. The left lower border indicates the left ventricle; the left atrium blends into the ventricular shadow unless significantly enlarged. The first convexity above the apex is the pulmonary artery. The second convexity above the apex is the aortic arch. Specific defects can be identified from abnormal borders. A boot-shaped heart can indicate tetralogy of Fallot related to RVH with apex upturned. A convex shoulder of the aorta is seen in transposition of the great arteries (looks like an egg with a narrow superior mediastinum).

3. **Pulmonary vascularity:** Increased pulmonary vascularity is indicated by arteries that appear enlarged and extend into the lateral third of the lung field as seen in ASD, VSD, PDA, TAPVR, truncus, transposition, and AV canal (Fig. 3–12). Decreased pulmonary vascularity is noted when the hilum appears small, lung fields are empty and devoid of vessels, and the x-ray image appears black. This

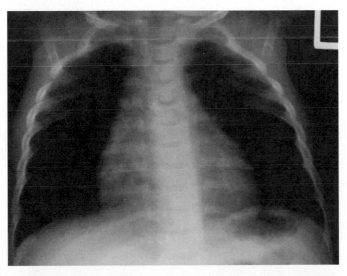

Figure 3–11. Heart borders as seen on anterioposterior chest x-ray film. (Courtesy of Children's National Medical Center.)

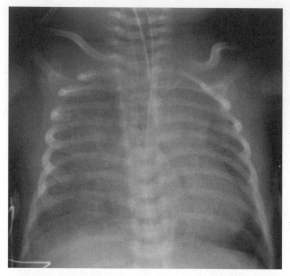

Figure 3–12.   Chest x-ray film with evidence of increased pulmonary vascularity. (Courtesy of Children's National Medical Center.)

may be noted in tetralogy, tricuspid atresia, Ebstein's anomaly, severe pulmonary hypertension, and transposition with pulmonary stenosis (Fig. 3–13).

D. ELECTROCARDIOGRAM (ECG)

1. The **purpose** is to measure electrical activity of the heart by measuring the difference in electrical potential between two points on the body. The recording is used to measure intervals, direction, and amplitudes.

2. **ECG paper**
   a. *Horizontal lines* are divided into a measurement of time with small blocks. Each small block equals 0.04 second, and each larger dark block equals 0.2 second.
   b. *Vertical lines* represent a measurement of voltage with each small block equal to 0.1 mV or 1 mm and each larger block equal to 0.5 mV or 5 mm (if gain of ECG is set to 1 mV = 10 mm).

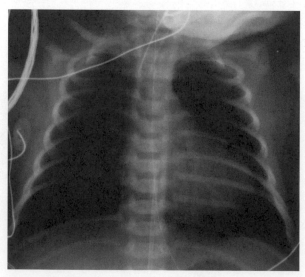

Figure 3–13.   Chest x-ray film with evidence of decreased pulmonary vascularity. (Courtesy of Children's National Medical Center.)

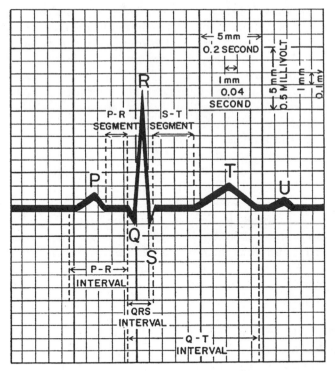

Figure 3–14. ECG paper and waveforms. (Reprinted with permission from Sanderson RG, Kurth CL. *The Cardiac Patient: A Comprehensive Approach.* 2nd ed. Philadelphia, Pa: WB Saunders Co; 1983:129.)

3. **ECG waves and intervals** (Fig. 3–14).
   a. The *P wave* represents atrial depolarization. It is measured from the beginning of the P wave to the end of the wave when it returns to the baseline. Usually it is less than 0.08 second. The normal amplitude is less than 2.5 mm (3 mm in the neonate), and it is usually gently rounded with all waves having the same appearance. Right atrial enlargement is noted by tall peaked P waves greater than 2.5 mm. Left atrial enlargement demonstrates a wide, notched P wave.
   b. The *PR interval* represents atrial depolarization and conduction through the AV node. It is measured from the beginning of the P wave to the beginning of the QRS complex. The normal PR interval is 0.12 to 0.20 second (shorter in younger children with faster heart rates). A prolonged PR interval is an indication of first-degree heart block (Table 3–2).

Table 3–2. MAXIMAL PR INTERVALS

AGE	HR (bpm) <71	HR (bpm) 71–90	HR (bpm) 91–110	HR (bpm) 111–130	HR (bpm) 131–150	HR (bpm) 151
1 mo			0.11	0.11	0.11	0.11
1–9 mo			0.14	0.13	0.12	0.11
10–24 mo			0.15	0.14	0.14	0.10
3–5 y		0.16	0.16	0.13		
6–13 y	0.18	0.18	0.16	0.16		

From Biller JA, Yeager AM. *The Harriet Lane Handbook.* 9th ed. Chicago, Ill: Year Book Medical Publishers Inc; 1981.

c. The *QRS interval* represents ventricular depolarization. It is measured from the beginning of the QRS to the end of the QRS. Normal duration is 0.06 to 0.10 second. Prolonged QRS duration may indicate interventricular conduction delay. Although commonly called the QRS complex, the first initial downward deflection is labeled *Q*, the first upward deflection is labeled *R*, the first downward deflection after the R wave is labeled *S*, and any other deflections are labeled with an accent to indicate "prime" such as rSR'. The size of the wave is indicated by a capital or small letter; waves over 5 mm are in capitals.

d. The *T wave* represents ventricular repolarization and should be in the same direction as the QRS complex. The T wave may change configuration with hypokalemia (flattened) or hyperkalemia (peaked).

e. The *ST segment* represents ventricular repolarization. It is measured from the end of the QRS to the beginning of the T wave. The ST segment should not vary more than 1 mm from the baseline. Elevations may indicate ischemia and inflammation. Depression may indicate strain or ischemia.

f. The *QT interval* represents summation of depolarization and repolarization and varies with the heart rate. It is measured from the beginning of the QRS to the end of the T wave. The QT interval must be corrected for heart rate. The normal is less than 0.45 second.

g. The *12-lead ECG* in children should include a recording of V_{3R} or V_{4R}, or both. These leads are placed on the right side of the chest in the same positions as the V_3 and V_4 leads are placed on the left side of the chest. The purpose of the V_{3R} and V_{4R} leads is to provide an opportunity for analysis of the strong right-sided forces in young children.

4. **ECG analysis**

a. *Rate* is calculated by counting specific wave patterns during a determined time such as 6 seconds. An alternative method (used if the rate is regular with no RR variation) is to estimate the rate by noting the position of one wave on a dark line and then noting the next time the wave falls on a dark line. It is essential to remember the six consecutive numbers: 300, 150, 100, 75, 60, and 50. If it is one large block, the rate is 300/min; two large blocks equal 150/min; and so on. The rate can also be determined in regular rhythm by dividing 1500 by the number of small blocks between complexes. The rate should be determined for both the atrial rhythm (the P wave) and the ventricular rhythm (QRS rate).

b. *Rhythm* is considered regular if the RR interval and PP interval have less than a three-small-block variation. Note if the rhythm is regularly irregular.

c. *P wave relationship to QRS* should be a consistent 1:1 ratio.

d. *PR interval* should be normal for age and heart rate.

e. *QRS interval* should be less than or equal to 0.10 second and have a normal configuration.

f. *QT interval* (corrected) and *ST segment* are evaluated.

E. HOLTER MONITORING

The Holter monitor provides a 24-hour record of ECG activity. It is used to document dysrhythmias at rest and stress and frequency of occurrence in leads II and V_5. Patients and parents use a diary to record activity.

F. EXERCISE STRESS TESTING

1. **Purpose** is to evaluate ECG and simultaneous clinical response to specific stimuli. Exercise stress testing is used to evaluate myocardial oxygen supply and demand, evaluate or provoke arrhythmias, evaluate blood pressure response to exercise, assess aerobic power and "functional" status (or level of conditioning), and evaluate chest pain or syncope.

2. **Technique:** A cycle or treadmill with ECG, blood pressure, oxygen consumption, and cardiac output by rebreathing trend recordings are used. $\dot{V}O_2$ measurements may or may not be included because of the equipment required, technical capabilities, and the ability of the child to wear or tolerate the equipment.

3. **Normal response to dynamic exercise:** Heart rate, cardiac output, and $\dot{V}O_2$ increase. Systolic blood pressure increases with the intensity of the workload, but diastolic blood pressure remains unchanged. Mean blood pressure rises mildly. Stroke volume increases with work, particularly from rest to moderate effort. SVR decreases.

4. **Contraindications to testing** include *acute illnesses* such as myocarditis, pericarditis, asthma, thrombophlebitis, and febrile illness or *chronic illnesses* such as CHF and thyroid, renal, and hepatic dysfunction (relative contraindication depending on patient condition). Special care is required in atrial stenosis, cardiomegaly, hypertension, hypoxemia, anemia, heart blocks, or uncontrolled dysrhythmias.

5. **Complications of exercise stress testing** include arrhythmias (supraventricular tachycardia [SVT], ventricular tachycardia [VT], premature ventricular contractions [PVCs]), hypotension, and syncope.

G. **AUTONOMIC TESTING**

Autonomic testing is used to evaluate vasomotor syncope.

1. **Technique:** Place invasive lines and then test the patient in specific positions (flat, then 60 to 80 degrees) and after drug administration (i.e., isoproterenol [Isuprel], propranolol [Inderal]).

2. **Complications** include dysrhythmias (asystole, bradycardia), hypotension, and collapse.

H. **ECHOCARDIOGRAPHY (ECHO)**

1. **Purpose** is to visualize cardiac structures and measure function.

2. **Technique**

   a. ECHO uses sound waves to measure the density of tissue and elastic properties of the heart.

   b. *M-mode ECHO* gives a graph of lines for each surface seen by probe with space between surfaces. It allows the most accurate measurement of the dimensions of structures.

   c. *2D ECHO* provides a flat picture of structures and is used to identify congenital abnormalities. The *orientation* varies with locations of the probe. The parasternal view reveals left-sided structures including left atrium, mitral valve, left ventricle, and aortic valve. The apical view shows all four chambers of the heart (most similar to drawings of the heart) (Fig. 3–15). The subcostal view demonstrates the right ventricular outflow tract (RVOT), the right atrium, and the right ventricle. The suprasternal view shows the aortic arch.

   d. *Doppler ECHO* measures the velocity of blood flow and is useful to assess the pressure gradient across a valve.

   e. *Transesophageal ECHO* is used to look at atrial structures (specifically for clots) and is also used to assess adequacy of surgical repair during the intraoperative period. It requires placing the ECHO probe orally into the esophagus. To prevent gagging, sedating the patient may be required.

   f. *Contrast ECHO* uses the forceful injection of dextrose and water, saline, or blood into the peripheral or central vein to produce microcavitation, which appears as a cloud of "bubbles" inside cardiac structures visualized by ECHO. Contrast ECHO is used to detect intracardiac right-to-left shunts, identify flow patterns, and validate structures.

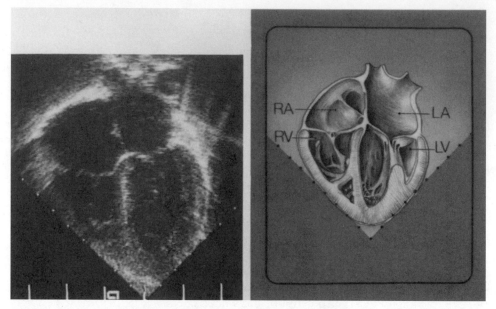

Figure 3–15. ECHO image **(A)** and diagram **(B)** of apical four chamber view of cardiac structures. *LA,* left atrium; *LV,* left ventricle; *RA,* right atrium; *RV,* right ventricle. (Reprinted with permission from Snider AR, Serwer GA. *Echocardiography in Pediatric Heart Disease.* St Louis, Mo: Mosby–Year Book Inc; 1990.)

I. CARDIAC CATHETERIZATION

1. **Purpose** is to evaluate and measure pressures, saturations, and cardiac output and outline anatomy with dye. Cardiac catheterization is also used as a treatment modality for specific cardiac or vascular defects.

2. **Technique**

   a. Pretesting includes an ECHO, ECG, and CBC. The child receives nothing by mouth (NPO) 4 to 6 hours prior to the procedure. Blood should be available, depending on the child's age and the procedure planned. Premedication with sedative, analgesic, or amnestic medications is required.

   b. The catheter is placed in the venous or arterial access and advanced into the heart to obtain oxygen saturation samples, make cardiac chamber pressure measurements (Fig. 3–16), and inject radiopaque dye at selected locations.

   c. Contrast agents have a high sodium concentration and are iodine based (be alert to allergies). Hypertonic solution may result in changes in cellular membrane potentials, producing stimulation that results in heat sensation, pain, and movement. Isotonic agents are available at higher cost and result in less hypocalcemia. They are useful in low cardiac output states, renal failure, or reactions to iodinated compounds. Risks of contrast include acute volume loss, lower blood pressure from vasodilation, and decreased contractility; the risks are lower with the use of low ionic or isotonic contrast.

   d. *Angiography:* The right ventriculogram shows the RV size and structure, RV outflow tract, tricuspid regurgitation, PA anatomy, and pulmonary venous return to the left side of the heart. The left ventriculogram shows the LV size, function, structure, and outflow tract, and left-to-right shunting patterns. The aortogram shows the aortic arch structure, aortic regurgitation, and coronary anatomy. Selective coronary angiography demonstrates coronary blood supply.

    e. *Cardiac output* (CO) is measured by the Fick or thermodilution method.
- CO = SV × HR
- CI = CO/BSA in m²; normal is 2.5 to 4 L/min/m²

3. **Treatment modality**
    a. Balloon dilation of valves includes the pulmonary, aortic, mitral, and tricuspid valves. Balloon dilation of vessels has been used with peripheral systemic arteries, native aorta or recoarctation of the aorta, the pulmonary artery, and pulmonary veins.
    b. Placement of occluding coils is used to embolize an abnormal arterial supply or occlude a PDA, ASD, or VSD.
    c. Devices such as vascular stents are placed.
    d. Other treatments include balloon atrial or blade atrial septostomy and foreign body removal.

4. **Complications** include arrhythmias from catheter manipulation, arterial thrombosis (and emboli), perforation of atria, ventricles, or vessels, allergic reactions to dye, shock, acidosis, or hypotension (from heart failure, stress in a critically ill child, blood loss, or hypoventilation), and death.

J. ELECTROPHYSIOLOGIC STUDIES
1. **Purpose** is to evaluate abnormal rhythms and the medical therapies used to treat them.
2. **Technique:** Pretesting includes an ECHO, ECG, and CBC. The child may also require an exercise stress test and signal averaged ECG. The patient is NPO 4 to 6 hours before the procedure. Premedication with a sedative, analgesic, or amnestic agent is required. Anesthesia and intubation may be used if an extended period of sedation is anticipated. Special precautions similar to those used in surgery are implemented to protect pressure points (occiput, elbows). A large sheath is placed for threading of marked catheters to identify the location of abnormal electrical tissue of the heart.
3. **Treatment modality:** Specific abnormal rhythms (such as SVT, VT) are initiated to test therapeutic medications. Radiofrequency ablation can be used to eliminate abnormal conduction pathways or areas that generate ectopic beats.

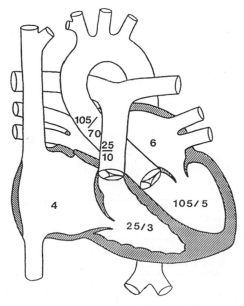

Figure 3–16. Normal hemodynamic measurements (mm Hg) found during cardiac catheterization. 4 and 6 are mean pressures.

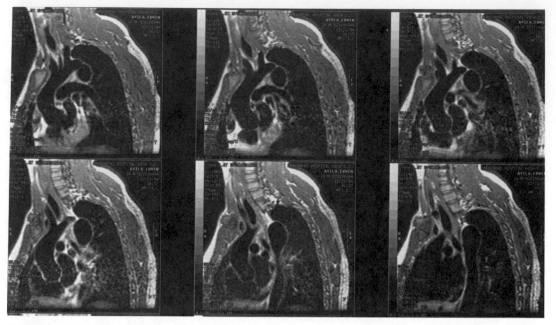

Figure 3–17. MRI showing a coarctation of the aorta. (Courtesy of Children's National Medical Center.)

4. **Complications** (in addition to those related to cardiac catheterization) include uncontrollable arrhythmias, which may result in cardiac arrest and death, varying degrees of conduction disorders, and a higher risk of intracardiac clotting when multiple catheters are used.

K. NUCLEAR MEDICINE TESTING

1. **Perfusion studies** use specific radionuclear materials to evaluate cardiac perfusion. *Thallium-201* detects ischemia (not coronary obstruction) in the myocardium and can be used at rest or with exercise. *Technetium 99m* detects necrotic tissue or infarcted myocardium.

2. **Multiple unit gated acquisition (MUGA)** uses radionuclear materials to obtain images restricted to specific times during the cardiac cycle (gating) such as end-systole and end-diastole. Data from hundreds of beats are stored in the computer to obtain adequate intensity. MUGA is used to assess ejection fraction and LV wall motion abnormalities.

3. **Magnetic resonance imaging (MRI)** uses atomic nuclei subjected to an external magnetic field and stimulated by radio waves to send out energy in the form of radio waves that can be recorded and converted into a map of tissue. MRI is useful in determining structures (Fig. 3–17) and in evaluating tissue health based on different image densities. MRI requires patients to remain perfectly still; in children this may require sedation. MRI cannot be applied in patients with magnetizable material in their bodies (i.e., pacemakers or artificial valves).

CARDIOVASCULAR MONITORING AND INSTRUMENTATION

A. CARDIAC MONITORING

1. **Indications:** Continuous ECG monitoring is useful for detection of dysrhythmias and rapid identification and response to rhythm changes. Continual

monitoring is required in known dysrhythmias, the cardiac surgery postoperative period, and drug overdoses.

2. **Modified chest lead (MCL 1)**
   a. *Lead placement* (Fig. 3–18)
      - Ground lead: Right shoulder midclavicular
      - Negative lead: Left shoulder midclavicular
      - Positive lead: Fourth ICS, right sternal border (RSB)
   b. MCL 1 allows detection of dysrhythmias, bundle branch block (BBB), and differentiation of aberrancy. MCL 1 typical pattern is negative, similar to V_1.

3. **Monitoring rules**
   a. Assess the impact of rhythm on the patient first through assessment of perfusion and blood pressure to determine if the dysrhythmia affects cardiac output.
   b. The following hierarchy represents the most accurate information.
      - 12-lead ECG where all leads are simultaneously recorded with standardized amplitude size
      - Recording on monitor paper
      - Evaluation of monitor screen
   c. Consider the progression and pattern of arrhythmias, impact of surgery on the conduction system, and usual rhythms with the use of specific drugs.

B. HEMODYNAMIC MONITORING
   1. **Arterial pressure monitoring**
      a. *Indications* include situations where a continuous blood pressure reading is desirable, frequent blood sampling is required, or vasoactive medications are in use.
      b. *Insertion sites* can be percutaneous or cut down. The radial site is frequently used. The Allen test can be used to assess ulnar patency or perfusion prior to insertion. The Allen test consists of occluding both the radial and ulnar arteries until the patient's fingers and palm blanch and then releasing only the ulnar artery supply to determine if the alternative blood supply to the hand is adequate should the catheter or clot occlude the radial artery. The

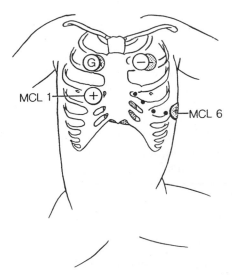

Figure 3–18. MCL I and MCL 6 lead positions. Modified chest leads are useful in identifying aberrant rhythms and bundle branch blocks. *G*, ground lead. (Reprinted with permission from Hazinski MF. *Nursing Care of the Critically Ill Child.* St Louis, Mo: Mosby–Year Book Inc; 1992.)

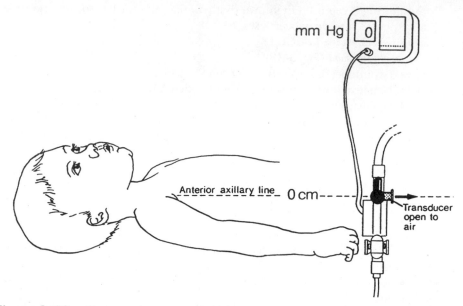

Figure 3–19. Diagram of position of phlebostatic axis. (Modified and reprinted with permission from Hazinski MF. *Nursing Care of the Critically Ill Child.* St Louis, Mo: Mosby–Year Book Inc; 1992.)

dorsalis pedis, posterior tibialis, femoral, temporal, and axillary arteries are alternative sites.

  c. *Monitoring equipment required* includes nondistensible tubing, heparinized infusion fluid, and a transducer.

  d. The *phlebostatic axis* corresponds to the right atrium (Fig. 3–19). The fourth ICS at the midaxillary line is used for zeroing.

  e. *Waveforms* (Fig. 3–20). A normal waveform has a clear dicrotic notch. Fling is related to an unstable catheter. A dampened waveform can be related to occlusion by a clot, absorption by air bubble, a kink, or a loose connection. Absence of a waveform can be related to a displaced or clotted line, equipment malfunction, or spasm.

  f. *Complications* include hemorrhage, ischemia, hematoma, arterial spasm, infection, and inaccurate readings.

2. **Central venous pressure (CVP) monitoring**

  a. *Indications* include assessment of blood volume, assessment of RV function, and infusion of large volume, hypertonic solutions.

  b. *Insertion sites* used include the internal jugular, external jugular, femoral, subclavian, and transthoracic veins into the right atrium.

  c. *Monitoring equipment* includes nondistensible tubing, infusion fluid, transducer, and ECG monitor during placement. Choices involved in the selection of the catheter include nonthrombogenic material, the number of lumens, size of the catheter in relation to blood vessels, and length of the catheter.

  d. *Normal waveform components* (Fig. 3–21)

- a wave: Mechanical atrial systole
- x descent: Reflects the decrease in RA volume during relaxation
- c wave: Reflects the increase in RA pressure from closure of the tricuspid valve
- v wave: Mechanical atrial diastole
- y descent: Emptying of the right atrium into the right ventricle

  e. *Abnormal readings*
- High: RV failure, tricuspid regurgitation, tricuspid stenosis, pulmonary hypertension, hypervolemia, cardiac tamponade, chronic LV failure
- Low: Hypovolemia, increased contractility

  f. *Complications* include arrhythmias, pneumothorax, infection, air embolism or thromboembolism, hemorrhage, vessel perforation, poor venous return, and inaccurate readings.

3. **Pulmonary artery (PA) and pulmonary artery wedge pressure (PAWP) monitoring**

  a. *PA monitoring* is indicated for use in diagnosis of cardiopulmonary failure, management of shock, evaluation of abnormal PVR, and measurement of cardiac output.

  b. *Insertion sites* are percutaneous, cut down, or transthoracic at the time of surgery. The pulmonary artery may be accessed through the femoral, internal jugular, or subclavian veins.

  c. *Monitoring equipment* requirements are the same as for CVP with two pressure lines for the CVP and PA ports. Cardiac lidocaine should be available because of the risk of ventricular arrhythmias from the catheter tip touching the RV wall during passage of the catheter. A defibrillator should be available because of the risk of ventricular arrhythmias deteriorating into a rhythm that requires cardioversion or defibrillation.

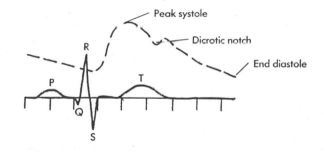

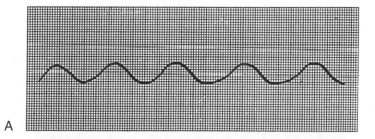

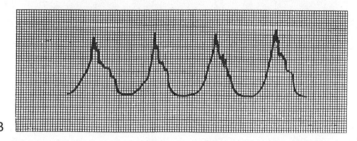

Figure 3–20. Diagram of arterial waveform (dotted line) in relation of cardiac cycle by ECG. **A,** Dampened waveform. **B,** Waveform affected by "fling." (Reprinted with permission from Hazinski MF. *Nursing Care of the Critically Ill Child.* St Louis, Mo: Mosby–Year Book Inc; 1992.)

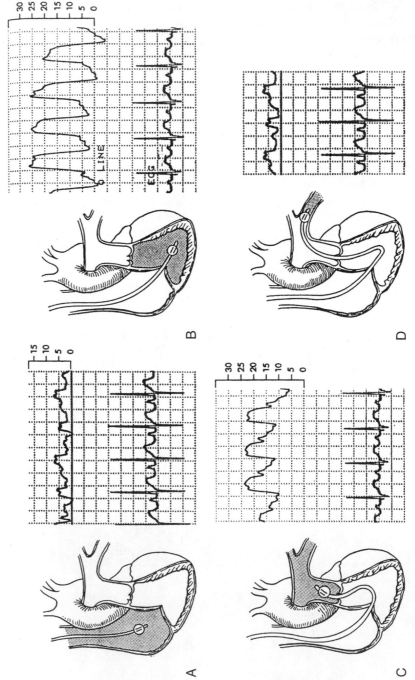

Figure 3–21. Catheter positions and waveforms for pulmonary artery monitoring. (Reprinted with permission from Hazinski MF. *Nursing Care of the Critically Ill Child.* St Louis, Mo: Mosby–Year Book Inc; 1992.)

d. *Normal waveform* (see Fig. 3–21) *components*
  - a wave: LA systole
  - x descent: Decreased LA volume
  - c wave: Closure mitral valve
  - v wave: LA filling (diastole)
  - y descent: Opening of the mitral valve

e. *Pressure readings*
  - RA pressure is the same as CVP. RV pressure normally is 20 to 30/0 to 5 mm Hg, with a mean of 2 to 6 mm Hg. High pressure is related to pulmonary hypertension, pulmonary stenosis, VSD, RV failure, constrictive pericarditis, cardiac tamponade, and chronic LV failure.
  - PA pressure normally is 20 to 30/6 to 10 mm Hg, with a mean of less than 20 mm Hg. High pressure is from increased PVR due to vascular disease, pulmonary parenchymal disease, mitral stenosis, LV failure, or pulmonary vascular changes from increased pulmonary blood flow.
  - Pulmonary capillary wedge pressure (PCWP) usually is 4 to 12 mm Hg. High pressure is related to LV failure, mitral stenosis, mitral regurgitation, cardiac tamponade, hypervolemia, or constrictive pericarditis. Low pressure is related to hypovolemia or vasodilation.

f. *Complications* include arrhythmias, pulmonary infarction, PA rupture, pulmonary embolism, balloon rupture, knotting of catheter, hemorrhage, or infection.

4. **Left atrial monitoring** *is indicated* for direct measurement of LA filling pressure, to measure LVEDP, or for indirect measure of LV compliance. *Monitoring equipment required* includes air filter, nondistensible tubing, transducer, and infusion to maintain line patency *only*. *Waveform* is illustrated in Figure 3–22.

5. **Hemodynamic calculations**
  a. $CO = SV \times HR$; the area under the curve is measured for the change in blood temperature (thermodilution technique)
  b. $CI = CO/BSA$; enter height and weight to calculate body surface area (BSA); *normal: 2.5 to 4 L/min/m²*
  c. $PVR = [mean\ PA\ pressure - PAWP\ (or\ LA\ pressure)]/(CI \times 80)$; *normal: 37 to 250 dynes/s/cm² or 0.5 to 3 Wood units*
  d. $SVR = (MAP - CVP)/(CI \times 80)$; *normal: 900 to 1400 dynes/s/cm² or 11 to 17.5 Wood units*

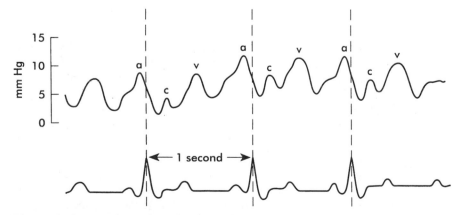

Figure 3–22. Left atrial catheter waveform. (Courtesy of Hewlett-Packard Company.)

C. $S\bar{v}O_2$ MONITORING
  1. **Indications** include the assessment of oxygen supply-demand balance, monitoring of tissue oxygenation, and management of shock states.
  2. **Physiologic basis:** Oxygen content (CaO_2) is determined by PaO_2, SaO_2, and hemoglobin. Oxygen delivery is determined by CaO_2, cardiac output, and tissue demand. Hemodynamic monitoring determines the cardiac output, and blood gas analysis provides CaO_2. Oxygen consumption indirectly reflects tissue demand. $CaO_2 - P\bar{v}O_2 = \dot{V}O_2$
  3. **Monitoring mechanism:** The PA catheter with a fiberoptic tip uses light to reflect off blood saturation (same concept as pulse oximetry). It is floated into place like a PA line or directly placed through the chest wall during surgery. The PA line is used for intermittent analysis of $P\bar{v}O_2$.
  4. **Interpretation**
     a. Values are influenced by the hemoglobin level. Anemia, cyanide toxicity, and increased hemoglobin affinity impair tissue extraction of oxygen and affect $S\bar{v}O_2$ accuracy. Cardiac output, PaO_2, SaO_2, and $\dot{V}O_2$ also influence values. If other factors are stable, $S\bar{v}O_2$ can be used to estimate changes in cardiac output and states of increased oxygen demand or activities that threaten oxygen delivery.
     b. *Normal $S\bar{v}O_2$ ranges from 60% to 80%.* Low $S\bar{v}O_2$ can indicate low cardiac output or increased demand (that the body cannot meet) such as fever, infection, shivering, burns, or suctioning. *High $S\bar{v}O_2$* can indicate low metabolic rate from anesthesia or high-output cardiac failure from sepsis (in which maldistribution of blood flow does not retrieve deoxygenated venous blood from hypoperfused areas).
     c. Continuous monitoring can be used to assess the patient's tolerance of procedures that increase $\dot{V}O_2$.

PHARMACOLOGY

A. INOTROPIC AGENTS
  1. **Mechanism of action:** Inotropic agents work through α- and β-adrenergic receptors on cells. α_1 Receptors are postsynaptic and cause blood vessels to vasoconstrict. α_2 Receptors are presynaptic. β_1 Receptors innervate cardiac muscle and increase AV conduction, heart rate, and contractility. β_2 Receptors innervate vascular smooth muscle in the lungs and cause arterial vasodilation and bronchodilation.
  2. **Amrinone lactate (Inocor)**
     a. *Action:* Decreases preload and primarily afterload by direct relaxation of vascular smooth muscle; increases contractility by affecting the cyclic adenosine monophosphate (cAMP) system and providing energy to muscle
     b. *Uses:* Ventricular failure
     c. *Side effects:* Thrombocytopenia, hepatotoxicity, hypoxemia
     d. *Pharmacokinetics:* Onset 2 to 5 minutes, peak 10 minutes, half-life 4 to 6 hours; requires bolus dose to achieve effective level
     e. *Interactions:* Precipitates with furosemide (Lasix); ineffective over time in dextrose
     f. *Nursing implications:* Mix in normal saline solution (may run with dextrose); assess platelets, liver function tests (LFTs), and cardiac function
     g. *Dose:* Load 0.75 to 2 mg/kg, then 5 to 10 μg/kg/min

3. **Digoxin (Lanoxin):** Cardiac glycoside
   a. *Action:* Inhibits sodium-potassium adenosinetriphosphatase (ATPase), providing calcium for contractile proteins of cardiac muscle
   b. *Uses:* Ventricular failure, tachyarrhythmias
   c. *Side effects:* Dysrhythmias, AV block, hypotension, blurred vision, or yellow-green halos
   d. *Pharmacokinetics:* Onset 5 to 30 minutes, 1 to 5 hours' duration, half-life 1.5 days
   e. *Interactions:* Multiple
   f. *Nursing implications:* Apical pulse prior to administration; adjust dose with renal failure; adjust dose with concomitant use of other antiarrhythmics, e.g., procainamide or quinidine. Follow PR interval for prolongation; assess potassium level; evaluate therapeutic response; teach family signs of toxicity; digoxin immune Fab (Digibind) is the antidote
   g. *Dose:* 15 to 30 μg/kg total digitalizing dose (TDD) divided with half in first dose, one fourth in next two doses q8h for TDD over 24 hours; maintenance: 10 μg/kg/d orally divided twice daily; 5 to 7 μg/kg/d divided twice daily for IV maintenance

4. **Dobutamine (Dobutrex)**
   a. *Action:* Increases contractility, coronary blood flow, and heart rate by acting on β_1-adrenergic receptors of the heart
   b. *Uses:* To improve cardiac output
   c. *Side effects:* Tachyarrhythmias, hypertension
   d. *Pharmacokinetics:* Onset 1 to 10 minutes; duration 2 to 3 minutes.
   e. *Interactions:* Monoamine oxidase inhibitor (MAOI); incompatible in alkaline solutions, $NaHCO_3$
   f. *Nursing implications:* Frequent vital signs, ECG monitoring.
   g. *Dose:* 5 to 20 μg/kg/min

5. **Dopamine (Intropin)**
   a. *Action:* Acts on α-adrenergic receptors to constrict blood vessels and thus increase cardiac output at high doses (greater than 15 μg/kg/min); also selective vasodilation of renal and mesenteric vessels at low doses (less than 5 μg/kg/min); dose specific response
   b. *Uses:* Shock, hypotension, improve perfusion
   c. *Side effects:* Arrhythmias, tachycardia, hypertension, slough of extravasation, decreased renal perfusion (high doses) and increased PVR
   d. *Pharmacokinetics:* Onset 5 minutes, duration less than 10 minutes; metabolized in liver, excreted in liver
   e. *Interactions:* Hypertensive crisis with MAOI; incompatible with alkaline solutions, $NaHCO_3$
   f. *Nursing implications:* Frequent vital signs, ECG monitoring, volume expanders for hypovolemia; careful monitoring of IV site
   g. *Dose:* Low dose 1 to 5 μg/kg/min; can use 1 to 20 μg/kg/min

6. **Epinephrine**
   a. *Action:* Catecholamine, which affects both α- (at higher doses) and β-adrenergic receptors on cardiovascular tissue; low dose (0.01 to 0.02 μg/kg/min) can cause vasodilation via β_2; higher dose can cause vasoconstriction; bronchodilation is caused through stimulation of α and β_1 receptors.
   b. *Uses:* Cardiac arrest, hypotension, acute asthmatic attacks, bronchospasm, severely low cardiac output, and anaphylaxis.
   c. *Side effects:* Dysrhythmias, cerebral hemorrhage if blood pressure is in-

creased significantly, dyspnea, hyperglycemia; increased doses may cause severe vasoconstriction with decreased perfusion.

    d. *Pharmacokinetics:* Onset 1 minute

    e. *Interactions:* Hypertensive crisis with MAOI

    f. *Nursing implications:* Assess perfusion; frequent vital signs; evaluate injection site for tissue sloughing (extravasation is a major concern at high doses)

    g. *Dose:* 0.1 to 1 µg/kg/min

7. **Isoproterenol (Isuprel)** β_1 and β_2 agonist

    a. *Action:* Catecholamine, which increases levels of cAMP to cause smooth muscle relaxation, bronchodilation, and pulmonary vasodilation, which increases heart rate and contractility

    b. *Uses:* Bronchospasm, heart block, bradydysrhythmias, shock, reactive airway disease

    c. *Side effects:* Tachydysrhythmias, ischemic ECG changes, hyperglycemia, decreased diastolic blood pressure, increased myocardial oxygen consumption

    d. *Pharmacokinetics:* Metabolized in liver, lungs, gastrointestinal tract; half life: 2.5 to 5 minutes

    e. *Nursing implications:* Check for tissue sloughing at IV site, evaluate therapeutic effect, ECG monitoring, 12-lead ECG prior to initiation

    f. *Dose:* 0.05 to 2 µg/kg/min

8. **Norepinephrine bitartrate (Levophed)**

    a. *Action:* Catecholamine, which affects both α- and β-adrenergic receptors in cardiovascular tissue causing constriction of blood vessels, increased contractility of the heart, and increased coronary blood flow

    b. *Uses:* Hypotension

    c. *Side effects:* Tachyarrhythmias; tissue slough with extravasation; increases right and left restrictive afterload

    d. *Pharmacokinetics:* Onset 1 to 2 minutes; limited duration; crosses placenta

    e. *Interactions:* Hypertensive crisis with MAOI, ineffective in alkaline solution, $NaHCO_3$

    f. *Nursing implications:* Frequent vital signs, ECG monitoring, volume expanders for hypotension, evaluation of ventricular function

    g. *Dose:* 0.05 to 0.1 µg/kg/min

B. ANTIARRHYTHMICS

  1. **Mechanism of action:** Classified according to effect on cardiac action potential

    a. *Class I:* Act by depressing the fast inward sodium current, thus slowing the conduction and lengthening the refractory period; effective in treating arrhythmias due to reentry or enhanced automaticity

    b. *Class II:* Are competitive β-adrenergic blockers that reduce sympathetic excitation of the heart

    c. *Class III:* Act with uniform lengthening of the action potential duration

    d. *Class IV:* Selectively depress myocardial slow calcium channels in the SA and AV node

  2. **Adenosine (Adenocard)**

    a. *Action:* Slows conduction through the AV node, depresses SA node automaticity

    b. *Uses:* To convert SVT, produce AV block to unmask atrial flutter

    c. *Side effects:* Minimal due to rapidity of action; can see a period of sinus arrest on administration; short-term conduction blocks or hypotension

    d. *Pharmacokinetics:* Action in 10 seconds; need rapid infusion to reach the heart

    e. *Interactions:* Theophylline decreases the activity

    f. *Nursing implications:* IV push as rapidly as possible followed by a rapid flush; documentation of the rhythm

    g. *Dose:* 0.05 mg/kg/dose; double and repeat q2min to a maximum dose of 0.25 mg/kg

3. **Atropine**

    a. *Action:* An anticholinergic agent that blocks acetylcholine at parasympathetic receptor sites, thus blocking vagal stimulation of the heart

    b. *Uses:* Bradycardia

    c. *Side effects:* Urinary retention, headache, dizziness, coma, hypotension, suppression of lactation

    d. *Pharmacokinetics:* Peak 2 to 4 minutes, half-life 2 to 3 hours; excreted by the kidneys, crosses placenta, excreted in breast milk; minimal dosage required to prevent bradycardia

    e. *Interactions:* Incompatible with most drugs

    f. *Nursing implications:* Document response, ECG monitoring

    g. *Dose:* 0.02 mg/kg/dose, minimum dose 0.1 mg, maximum total dose is 1 mg (2 mg for adolescents)

4. **Bretylium** (Class III)

    a. *Action:* Inhibits release of norepinephrine, which increases the action potential duration

    b. *Uses:* Refractory VT, ventricular fibrillation (VF)

    c. *Side effects:* Respiratory depression, hypotension, bradycardia, seizures

    d. *Pharmacokinetics:* Onset 5 minutes, half-life 4 to 17 hours; excreted unchanged by kidneys, unmetabolized

    e. *Nursing implications:* ECG and blood pressure monitoring

    f. *Dose:* 5 to 10 mg/kg/dose slow IV push

5. **Lidocaine** (Class I)

    a. *Action:* Increases electrical stimulation threshold of ventricles, which stabilizes cardiac membrane

    b. *Uses:* VT, dysrhythmias, digoxin toxicity

    c. *Side effects:* Hypotension, bradycardia, heart block, respiratory depression, cardiovascular collapse

    d. *Pharmacokinetics:* Onset 2 minutes, duration 20 minutes; metabolized in liver, excreted in urine, crosses placenta

    e. *Nursing implications:* ECG monitoring with measurement of PR and QRS duration

    f. *Dose:* 1 mg/kg bolus, 20 to 50 µg/kg/min drip

6. **Procainamide (Pronestyl)** (Class I)

    a. *Action:* Depresses excitability of cardiac muscle and slows conduction in the atrium, bundle of His, and ventricles

    b. *Uses:* PVCs, atrial fibrillation, junctional ectopic tachycardia (JET), paroxysmal atrial tachycardia (PAT), VT, and tachyarrhythmias.

    c. *Side effects:* Heart block, cardiovascular collapse, arrest, bone marrow suppression

    d. *Pharmacokinetics:* Need to follow levels of drug and metabolites

    e. *Nursing implications:* ECG monitoring, follow PR and QRS duration, observe for PVCs, blood pressure monitoring

    f. *Dose:* 3 to 6 mg/kg/dose over 5 to 10 minutes loading dose; then 20 to 80 µg/kg/min as continuous infusion; maximum dose 2 g/24 h

7. **Propranolol (Inderal)** (Class II)

    a. *Action:* Nonselective β-blocker with negative inotropic, chronotropic, and dromotropic activity

       b.   *Uses:* SVT, migraine, hypertension

       c.   *Side effects:* Laryngospasm, bone marrow suppression, bradycardia, hypotension, bronchospasm

       d.   *Pharmacokinetics:* Onset 2 minutes, peak 15 minutes, duration 3 to 6 hours; metabolized in liver, crosses placenta and blood-brain barrier, excreted in breast milk

       e.   *Interactions:* AV block with digoxin, calcium channel blockers, less effective with cimetidine

       f.   *Nursing implications:* Monitor ECG and blood pressure; follow liver enzymes

       g.   *Dose:* 0.01 to 0.1 mg/kg over 10 minutes; maximum dose 1 mg

  8. **Quinidine** (Class I)

       a.   *Action:* Increases the action potential duration and effective refractory period, thus decreasing cardiac excitability

       b.   *Uses:* PVCs, PAT, atrial fibrillation, VT

       c.   *Side effects:* Heart block, cardiovascular collapse, thrombocytopenia, respiratory depression

       d.   *Pharmacokinetics:* Metabolized in liver, excreted unchanged by kidneys

       e.   *Interactions:* Multiple, especially with digoxin

       f.   *Nursing implications:* Monitor blood pressure and PR and QRS duration

       g.   *Dose:* 15 to 60 mg/kg/d in 4 or 5 divided doses orally; IV not recommended: 2 to 10 mg/kg/dose q3-6h

  9. **Verapamil (Isoptin)** (Class IV)

       a.   *Action:* Inhibits calcium ion influx across cell membrane, producing slowing of SA and AV node conduction

       b.   *Uses:* Dysrhythmias

       c.   *Side effects:* CHF, bradycardia, hypotension

       d.   *Pharmacokinetics:* Onset 1 to 3 minutes, peak 1 to 5 minutes, duration 10 to 20 minutes; metabolized by liver, excreted in urine

       e.   *Nursing implications:* Monitor ECG and blood pressure; evaluate therapeutic response; use in children younger than 1 year contraindicated because of the high incidence of cardiovascular collapse

       f.   *Dose:* Initial dose 0.1 to 0.3 mg/kg over 2 to 3 minutes; maximum 5 mg per dose; may repeat dose once in 30 minutes; maximum for second dose 10 mg per dose

C. ANTIHYPERTENSIVES

  1. **Captopril**

       a.   *Action:* Renin-angiotensin antagonist, which selectively suppresses renin-angiotensin-aldosterone system; inhibits angiotensin converting enzyme (ACE), resulting in arterial and venous dilation

       b.   *Uses:* Hypertension, afterload reduction

       c.   *Side effects:* Acute reversible renal failure, neutropenia, bronchospasm, hypotension

       d.   *Pharmacokinetics:* Peak 1 hour, duration 2 to 6 hours; metabolized by liver, crosses placenta, excreted in breast milk

       e.   *Interactions:* Increased hypotension with diuretics, adrenergic blockers

       f.   *Nursing implications:* Follow CBC, blood pressure, renal studies, potassium level

       g.   *Dose:* Neonate 0.05 to 0.1 mg/kg per dose q8–24h, can titrate up to 0.5 mg/kg per dose; infant and child 0.5 to 1 mg/kg per dose, maximum 6 mg/kg/d

  2. **Diazoxide (Hyperstat)**

       a.   *Action:* Vasodilates arteriolar smooth muscle

       b.   *Uses:* Hypertensive crisis

   c. *Side effects:* Hypotension, SVT, rebound hypertension

   d. *Pharmacokinetics:* Onset 1 to 2 minutes, peak 5 minutes, duration 3 to 12 hours; crosses blood-brain barrier and placenta

   e. *Interactions:* Increases effect of warfarin (Coumadin), hyperglycemia with diuretics

   f. *Nursing implications:* Frequent vital signs (q5min); give over 30 seconds or less; keep patient recumbent

   g. *Dose:* 2 to 5 mg/kg/per dose (maximum: 100 mg); may repeat in 30 minutes or 1 mg/kg per dose q5–15 min; titrate to blood pressure

3. **Hydralazine (Apresoline)**

   a. *Action:* Decreases blood pressure through vasodilation of arteriolar smooth muscle

   b. *Uses:* Hypertension

   c. *Side effects:* Shock, bone marrow suppression, hypotension

   d. *Pharmacokinetics:* Onset 20 to 30 minutes, peak 1 hour, duration 2 to 4 hours

   e. *Nursing implications:* Frequent vital signs, have volume expanders available

   f. *Dose:* 0.1 to 0.5 mg/kg q4-6h; do not exceed 20 mg per dose

4. **Nifedipine (Procardia)**

   a. *Action:* Inhibits calcium influx across cell membrane during cardiac depolarization, dilates peripheral arteries

   b. *Uses:* Systemic or pulmonary hypertension

   c. *Side effects:* CHF, myocardial ischemia, hypotension

   d. *Pharmacokinetics:* Onset 20 minutes, peak 30 minutes to 6 hours

   e. *Interactions:* Cimetidine increases levels, quinidine decreases levels

   f. *Nursing implications:* Provide a safe environment until the patient's condition is stable on drug; follow blood pressure; difficult to administer, since available only as sublingual capsule that may need to be aspirated to obtain appropriate dose or use long-acting delayed-onset tablet

   g. *Dose:* 0.25 to 0.5 mg/kg per dose, maximum 10 mg per dose

5. **Nitroglycerin**

   a. *Action:* Direct vasodilator; dose-related effect on peripheral vasculature

   b. *Uses:* To decrease preload (venous dilator at 1 to 2 µg/kg/min) and afterload (arterial vasodilator with decreased SVR at 3 to 5 µg/kg/min), selective for coronary circulation

   c. *Side effects:* Hypotension with collapse, headache, flushing, nausea; contraindicated if allergic to nitrates

   d. *Pharmacokinetics:* Onset immediately

   e. *Nursing implications:* Requires nonpolyvinyl chloride tubing, volume expansion available (relative hypovolemia), note therapeutic effect

   f. *Dose:* 1 to 3 µg/kg/min, maximum dose 5 µg/kg/min

6. **Nitroprusside (Nipride)**

   a. *Action:* Directly relaxes arteriolar and venous smooth muscle causing decreased preload and afterload (decreased PVR, SVR, PCWP, MAP, and venous pressure); increases cardiac output by decreasing afterload

   b. *Uses:* Pulmonary or systemic hypertension, afterload reduction

   c. *Side effects:* Hypotension with collapse, coma, cyanide toxicity, ventilation/perfusion ($\dot{V}/\dot{Q}$) mismatch

   d. *Pharmacokinetics:* Onset 1 to 2 minutes, duration 1 to 10 minutes, half-life of thiocyanate 2 to 7 days

   e. *Nursing implications:* Protect from light, mix only in dextrose, follow thiocyanate levels, blood pressure monitoring

   f. *Dose:* 0.5 to 4 µg/kg/min, maximum dose 10 µg/kg/min

ADVANCED CARDIAC LIFE SUPPORT

A. CARDIOPULMONARY FAILURE

1. **Assess pulmonary and cardiovascular function,** its effect on target organs, and the potential for impending arrest. Cardiac arrest in children is most often the result of respiratory failure as opposed to primary cardiac arrest. Therefore, it is essential to recognize and intervene immediately for signs of respiratory distress.

2. **Etiology of respiratory failure:** Respiratory failure is related to inadequate elimination of carbon dioxide or inadequate oxygenation due to intrinsic lung disease or inadequate respiratory effort. (See Chapter 2 for indepth discussion of respiratory failure.)

3. **Assessment of respiratory failure:** Symptoms include increased respiratory rate or effort, diminished breath sounds, diminished level of consciousness or response to pain, poor skeletal muscle tone, and cyanosis.

   a. *Respiratory rate* may be tachypneic, apneic, or bradypneic. Minute ventilation may be low. Increased work of breathing is due to airway obstruction, pulmonary parenchymal disease, or chest wall disorder. *Tachypnea* is usually the first symptom. In the presence of nonpulmonary disease, tachypnea without distress usually results in a normal pH. *Bradypnea* results from fatigue, hypothermia, and central nervous system (CNS) depression.

   b. *Increased work of breathing* is recognized by retractions, flaring, and see-saw breathing.

   c. *Increased carbon dioxide production* eventually causes respiratory acidosis then metabolic acidosis.

   d. *Stridor* is related to upper airway obstruction from the supraglottic space to the lower trachea. Causes include congenital abnormalities, vocal cord paralysis, tumor, infections, or aspiration of a foreign body.

   e. *Prolonged expiration and wheezing* can be due to bronchial or bronchiolar obstruction caused by bronchiolitis or reactive airway disease.

   f. *Grunting* is due to premature glottic closure accompanying active chest wall contraction during early expiration. Infants grunt to increase airway pressure (autoPEEP) to preserve or increase functional residual capacity. Grunting can be caused by pulmonary edema, pneumonia, atelectasis, and adult respiratory distress syndrome (ARDS).

   g. *Cyanosis* is an inconsistent and unreliable sign of distress. It may occur early in polycythemic infants or late in anemic children.

B. CARDIOPULMONARY INTERVENTIONS

1. **Airway and ventilation**

   a. The goal is to anticipate and recognize problems not dependent on diagnosis of the problem. In recognized distress, immediately provide humidified oxygen in high concentrations.

   b. Maintain a patent airway through positioning and suctioning when necessary. Oropharyngeal airways are useful for airway patency in the unconscious child but may stimulate vomiting in a conscious child. Nasopharyngeal airways are better tolerated by conscious patients. The length of the airway should be approximately the same as the measurement from the tip of the nose to the tragus of the ear.

   c. A bag-valve-mask (BVM) device is useful when full endotracheal intubation is not possible or is delayed. The face mask should provide an airtight seal on the face and extend from the bridge of the nose to the cleft of the chin, avoiding compression of the eyes. The mask is held in place with a one-hand head tilt–chin lift maneuver. Avoid hyperextension of the neck to prevent airway obstruction. Use a bag-valve device equipped with an oxygen reservoir to deliver the highest oxygen concentration possible. A pressure-limited pop off valve is available but must be able to be occluded during resuscitation.

    d. Endotracheal airways are necessary for prolonged use or to achieve adequate ventilation when other methods fail. Cuffed tubes are usually used only in children older than 8 years. Placement may be evaluated by symmetric chest movement, equal breath sounds, absence of breath sounds over the stomach, condensation in the endotracheal tube during expiration, skin color, and oxygen saturation.

2. **Circulatory support and vascular access**

    a. *Chest compressions* are performed when the cardiac rhythm is absent or fails to produce a palpable pulse and blood pressure in the child who is unresponsive to oxygenation and ventilation. Compressions are delivered over the lower third of the sternum with the child placed on a rigid surface. The rate is 80 to 100/min at a depth of one third to one half of the child's chest. One hand is used to deliver compressions in children 1 to 8 years of age, and two hands are used for children over 8 years of age. Electrical defibrillation is required when ventricular fibrillation is present. Ideally, paddles should be of a size to be in complete contact with the chest without touching each other. The American Heart Association recommends a starting dose of 2 J/kg. This can be doubled to 4 J/kg and repeated (twice) if ineffective. If child is still unresponsive, epinephrine or antiarrhythmics or both and correction of acidosis should be tried to convert fine fibrillation to coarse fibrillation.

    b. *Central venous vascular access* is essential. The largest and most easily accessible vein is the preferred site. Central cannulation permits infusion of larger volumes of fluid and more direct infusion of medications. Recommended sites include the femoral, internal or external jugular, or subclavian veins.

    c. *Intraosseous vascular access* is an alternative, temporary measure for resuscitation only. It is safe and effective for medications and fluids in children younger than 6 years of age. Access is successful if the needle is placed in the bone marrow as evidenced by lack of resistance after the needle passes through the bony cortex, the needle stands upright without support, there is an ability to aspirate bone marrow, and free flow of infusion occurs.

    d. *Arterial vascular access* permits direct blood pressure measurement and easy blood sampling for oxygen and acid-base analysis. The radial, femoral, posterior tibialis, and dorsalis pedis arteries are often cannulated. The Allen test should be performed to assure adequacy of collateral circulation from the ulnar artery before cannulation of the radial artery.

    e. Until vascular access is achieved, medications should be given via the endotracheal route. Medications should be diluted in 1 to 2 ml saline prior to instillation and injected deeply into the tracheobronchial tree.

3. **Pharmacologic support**

    a. *General guidelines in acute situations:* Medications are preferably given via central venous access. Oxygen should be given in all arrest situations, in hypoxemia, or respiratory difficulty. Delivery should be in the highest concentration possible. Oxygen should not be withheld even if the measured arterial oxygen tension is high, as tissue delivery may be severely compromised.

    b. *Medications* (see Pharmacology section): Epinephrine is used for hemodynamic instability, bradyarrhythmias, and inotropic support and may be helpful in converting fine fibrillation to coarse fibrillation following unsuccessful electrical defibrillation. Isoproterenol is infrequently used to treat hemodynamically significant bradycardia. It may compromise coronary blood flow or decrease diastolic pressure, since it increases myocardial contraction and oxygen demand. Sodium bicarbonate is used to help correct acidosis. Atropine is used to treat bradycardia accompanied by poor perfusion or hypotension. Glucose is given if documented hypoglycemia exists (or in suspected hypoglycemia in infants). Calcium chloride is given only if hypocalcemia is documented. Dopamine is used to treat hypotension or hypoperfusion or to selectively increase renal blood flow at low doses. Dobutamine is used to treat hypotension and hypoperfusion. Other inotropes and antiarrhythmics are used as needed.

4. Parents should be notified as soon as possible after the onset of resuscitation and should be provided with support during the process (such as clinical nurse specialists, social workers, or chaplains).

C. NEONATAL RESUSCITATION

1. **Environment** should protect against excessive heat loss and provide a method to maintain the neonate's body temperature during resuscitation.

2. **Airway and breathing interventions:** The neck should be only slightly extended; the head should be maintained in the sniffing position. Assure a patent airway by suctioning first the mouth and then the nares when necessary. Respiratory effort and rate should be evaluated immediately. Stimulation for maintenance of respiratory effort should not be done more than twice before further methods of respiratory support (intubation) are used. Indications for ventilation include apnea, heart rate less than 100 beats per minute (bpm), and persistent central cyanosis in maximal oxygen environment.

3. **Cardiovascular support:** Bradycardia (heart rate less than 100 bpm) requires respiratory support. Chest compressions should be done if the heart rate is less than 60 bpm or 60 to 80 bpm but not increasing with adequate ventilation. Compressions can be accomplished using both thumbs side by side on the sternum or two fingers placed one finger breadth below the nipple line. The depth of compressions is ½ to ¾ inch at a compression rate of 120 bpm accompanied by ventilation at a rate of 40 to 60 breaths per minute.

D. POSTRESUSCITATION CARE

1. Delivery of oxygen is titrated by arterial blood gas measurement.

2. Continuous ECG monitoring, blood pressure recording, evaluation of peripheral circulation and end-organ perfusion, level of consciousness, evaluation of ventilation, and serial neurologic examinations should be performed frequently, since neurologic sequelae are highly variable.

3. Multiple venous access ports should be secured for ongoing administration of medications and volume requirements.

4. Decompression of the stomach via nasogastric tube improves ventilation and prevents aspiration.

5. Preserve body temperature, especially in infants.

6. Investigate underlying causes for the arrest or respiratory compromise.

EXTRACORPOREAL LIFE SUPPORT

A. INDICATIONS FOR CARDIAC EXTRACORPOREAL LIFE SUPPORT

1. **Congenital heart disease (CHD):** Heart failure occurs more frequently in conditions with increased pulmonary blood flow such as truncus arteriosus hypoplastic left heart syndrome, and single ventricle defects. Obstructions to

blood flow such as aortic stenosis and critical coarctation of the aorta, particularly those causing LV dysfunction and failure, may require time to recover even after surgical intervention. Anomalous left coronary artery (rare) may lead to ischemic damage to the myocardium.

2. **Cardiomyopathy**
3. **Inflammatory diseases** such as myocarditis and Kawasaki syndrome.
4. **Dysrhythmias** can lead to heart failure or produce damage to the heart muscle from myocardial ischemia.
5. **Systemic illness:** Septic shock results in the release of the myocardial depressant factor related to the endotoxin load. Metabolic abnormalities can cause cardiac dysfunction related to hypoglycemia, acidosis, and hypocalcemia. Neonates are particularly susceptible. Toxins such as doxorubicin (Adriamycin; used in the treatment of cancer), snake bites, antiarrhythmics, and heavy metals (iron) can affect cardiac function. Neuromuscular diseases such as Duchenne's muscular dystrophy compromise cardiac activity. Postcardiotomy low cardiac output syndrome can result from dysrhythmias, hypovolemic shock, myocardial injury, electrolyte imbalance, or cardiac stun.

B. CARDIAC ASSIST DEVICES
1. **Intraaortic balloon pump (IABP)**
   a. The pump uses a balloon-inflated counterpulsation to displace blood volume during diastole. This creates increased blood flow and oxygen delivery to the coronary and peripheral circulation. Deflation occurs just before systole and creates a negative aortic pressure to improve ventricular ejection by decreasing the ventricular afterload. Children require a pediatric balloon (smaller French, shorter length, smaller inflation volume) and adaptation of the mechanical console to allow variation in inflation volumes and a faster heart rate. Counterpulsation is timed to the ECG or arterial wave (arrhythmia control is vital). Because of their higher heart rates, children may receive 1:2 or 1:3 pumping rather than support for each beat.
   b. Balloon placement is in the descending thoracic aorta between the left subclavian and mesenteric arteries.
   c. Advantages of counterpulsation include increased coronary blood flow, decreased afterload, and the ease of insertion.
   d. Disadvantages include the need for femoral access, balloon size, technical knowledge required, elasticity of the aorta in children (which may diminish the effectiveness of the pumping), insufficient stroke volume to permit balloon augmentation, and decreased mobility.
2. **Noninvasive assist with external body compression**
   a. Military antishock trousers (MAST) and a pneumatic antishock garment (PASG) increase peripheral resistance in the lower body and redistribute blood flow to increase venous return from the lower body to selectively perfuse the upper body. A noninvasive phasic augmentation device (NIPHAD) has been used following Fontan procedures to increase venous return and thus RA pressure, pulmonary blood flow, left-sided filling pressures, and cardiac output.
   b. Advantages include the ease of applying or removing the garment, noninvasiveness, elevation in blood pressure, decreased heart rate, and clinically improved perfusion.
   c. Pulmonary edema is an absolute contraindication. These devices may also increase intracranial pressure and cause lower extremity ischemia, aortic compression, renal effects or lactate accumulation. In addition, access to the lower extremities is limited.

3. **Ventricular assist devices (VADs)** (Table 3–3)
   a. VADs work with the ventricles to pull blood from the atrium or ventricle and return it to the aorta or pulmonary artery. They provide short-term support for patients with cardiac failure that is reversible or treatable with transplantation.
   b. Advantages: Cardiac rest is provided while allowing the child's heart to remain in place. The pump can provide almost all the cardiac output on a short-term basis, providing more assist than IABP. VADs are relatively easy to insert and represent a lower cost for long-term support.
   c. Disadvantages: One type of VAD is not available for all children because of the variable cardiac output required by children. VADs require anticoagulation. Risks include infection, disconnection of percutaneous access, and the danger of dependence on the device. It is difficult to assess improved cardiac function. The pump is labor intensive requiring constant surveillance.
4. **Extracorporeal life support (ECLS) or extracorporeal membrane oxygenation (ECMO)**
   a. ECMO is a method of gas exchange that provides prolonged cardiopulmonary bypass with membrane oxygenation. The native lungs are not required to participate in gas exchange and can rest with minimal ventilation.
   b. Cannulation can occur emergently through the carotid, jugular, or femoral arteries or as postcardiotomy support in the operating room. Venoarterial ECMO drains blood from the internal jugular vein in most cases. Blood flows through a circuit composed of a pump, oxygenator, heat exchanger, and power source or backup power source using gravity drainage and a roller head pump to return blood to the arterial system (Fig. 3–23).
   c. ECMO is the most commonly used support in children with cardiovascular dysfunction after cardiotomy. Most of these patients have low cardiac output syndrome or severe pulmonary vessel reactivity. ECMO has been used as a

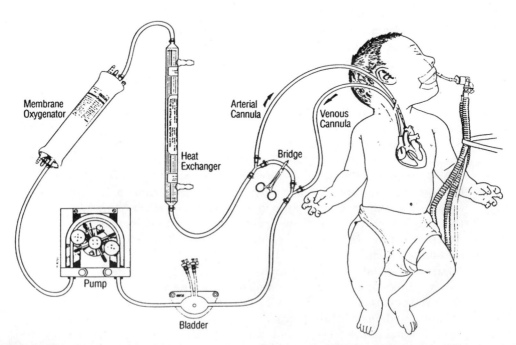

Figure 3–23. ECMO circuit. (Reprinted with permission from Suddaby EC, O'Brien AM. ECMO for cardiac support in children. *Heart Lung.* 1993;22(5):401–407.)

Table 3–3. VENTRICULAR ASSIST DEVICES (VADS)

NAME/TYPE	PATIENT SIZE	INTERNAL/EXTERNAL	CANNULATION SITE	BYPASS	ANTICOAGULATION	MOBILITY
ECMO Nonpulsatile Biventricular support	2 kg and up Variable cardiac output	External	Carotid Femorals Atria Great vessels	No	Continuous heparin	Paralyzed/sedated
Biomedicus Nonpulsatile Biventricular support	Variable cardiac output	External	Femorals Atria Great vessels	No	Heparin once flows <1.5–2 l/min	Paralyzed/sedated
Thoratec Pulsatile Pneumatic LVAD, RVAD	1.5 m^2	External/internal	Great vessels Atria	No/Yes	Heparin ACT 140–160	Ambulation
Heartmate Pulsatile Pneumatic/electric LVAD, RVAD (Bridge to transplant only)	1.5 m^2 83 ml stroke volume	Internal	Great vessels Atria Ventricles	Yes	Aspirin, dipyridamole	Ambulation
BVS 5000 Pulsatile Pneumatic LVAD, RVAD (After cardiotomy only)	82 ml stroke volume	External	Great vessels Atria	No	Continuous heparin ACT 180–200	Limited to bed
Novacor Pulsatile Electric LVAD, RVAD	1.5 m^2 70 ml stroke volume	Internal	Great vessels Atria Ventricles	Yes	ACT >150, antiplatelet Drugs	Ambulation

ACT, activated clotting time; *LVAD*, left ventricular assist device; *RVAD*, right ventricular assist device.

bridge to transplantation in other children with myocarditis or cardiomy-opathy. The duration of ECMO support is usually shorter in children with cardiac failure than in children with respiratory failure.

d. Children requiring ECMO support in the operating room or immediately afterward had an increased mortality (Extracorporeal Life Support Organization, 1990).

e. Bleeding, infection, and vascular injuries are major, serious complications.

5. **Nursing care required for cardiac assist**

❖ DECREASED CARDIAC OUTPUT RELATED TO MYOCARDIAL DYSFUNCTION REQUIRING CARDIAC ASSIST OR RV FAILURE REQUIRING BIVENTRICULAR SUPPORT

a. *Outcome measures:* Adequate cardiac output as evidenced by required assist device flow rates, MAP, urine output, peripheral perfusion, and CNS function.

b. *Nursing actions* include hemodynamic monitoring, assessment of cardiac output to end-organs, monitoring of assist device flow rates, evaluation of volume status and replacement as ordered, assessment for cardiac tampon-ade, titration of inotropic agents and vasodilators, and monitoring of trends in CVP and PA pressures.

❖ BLEEDING RELATED TO BLOOD COMPONENT TRAUMATIZATION, SURGICAL DISSEC-TION, ANTICOAGULATION, ABNORMAL LIVER FUNCTION DUE TO VENOUS CONGESTION, OR DISCONNECTION OF ASSIST DEVICES

a. *Outcome measures:* Normalization of blood clotting factors

b. *Nursing actions* include measurement of blood losses from chest tubes, urine, stool, gastrointestinal tract, and dressings; evaluation of hematology profile including the CBC, PT, PTT, activated clotting time (ACT), fibrino-gen, and fibrin split products (FSP); replacement of clotting factors; and safety measures such as keeping clamps at the bedside.

❖ RISK FOR INJURY FROM THROMBI FORMATION

a. *Outcome measures:* No evidence of thrombi

b. *Nursing actions* include observation of pump head and tubing interfaces, anticoagulation, administration, and monitoring of ACTs.

❖ RISK FOR INFECTION RELATED TO INVASIVE DEVICE CONNECTIONS, INVASIVE MONITOR-ING LINES, OR DEPRESSED IMMUNE RESPONSE

a. *Outcome measures:* Absence of infection as evidenced by absence of redness or drainage, normothermia, and normal white blood cell count (WBC).

b. *Nursing actions* include assessment for signs and symptoms of infection, strict aseptic technique, surveillance cultures, and prophylactic antibiotic admin-istration.

❖ MULTIORGAN SYSTEM DYSFUNCTION (MOSD) RELATED TO LOW CARDIAC OUTPUT STATE OR NONPULSATILE FLOW ASSIST DEVICE

a. *Outcome measures:* Normal function of all organ systems resulting in normal arterial blood gases, LFTs, urine output, creatinine, BUN, and mental state.

b. *Nursing actions* to support other organ systems include ventilation and airway support, hemofiltration, nutrition, skin care, and mobility.

❖ PSYCHOSOCIAL NURSING DIAGNOSES INCLUDE SENSORY ALTERATION, PAIN CONTROL, ANXIETY OR FEAR, SLEEP PATTERN DISTURBANCE, POWERLESSNESS, ALIENATION, DISTUR-BANCE IN SELF-CONCEPT AND BODY IMAGE, KNOWLEDGE DEFICIT, AND LOSS OF PARENTING ROLE

a. *Outcome measures:* Normal sleep, ability to ventilate feelings and cope

b. *Nursing actions* include use of support systems, dark quiet environment at night, schedules, family visitation, rest periods, medications, open commu-nication, answering questions, preparation for procedures, and family participation in care.

CONGESTIVE HEART FAILURE

A. **DEFINITION:** CHF is a condition in which the heart is unable to provide adequate cardiac output or regional blood flow to meet the circulatory and metabolic requirements of the body. CHF may result from structural abnormalities that place pressure or volume loads on the heart muscle or from intrinsic myocardial dysfunction resulting in inadequate cardiac output.

B. **PATHOPHYSIOLOGY**
   1. Hemodynamics that result in cardiac failure are inadequate emptying of venous reservoirs (backward failure) and reduced ejection of blood (forward failure).
   2. Mechanisms of cardiac reserve include increased heart rate and increased stroke volume, increased oxygen extraction, redistribution of blood flow, cardiac dilation, anaerobic metabolism, and cardiac hypertrophy.
   3. *Systemic compensatory response*
      a. Salt and water retention augments preload, causing pulmonary congestion and edema, and results in increased contractility from stretching of the muscle tissue.
      b. Vasoconstriction helps to maintain blood pressure for adequate perfusion but also increases afterload and myocardial energy and oxygen consumption.
      c. Sympathetic stimulation increases heart rate, stroke volume, and energy consumption. Chronic stimulation leads to desensitization.
      d. cAMP release results in calcium uptake to increase contractility. It overloads the system that pumps calcium out of cell during diastole, resulting in decreased relaxation. Overload results in transient depolarizations, causing arrhythmias.
      e. Hypertrophy of the cardiac muscle increases the number of cells to share the workload. Capillary deficit leads to energy and oxygen starvation and myocyte necrosis. Necrosis leads to fibroblast and collagen deposition within the thinned dilated heart. Rapid growth causes variable gene expression of myocardial proteins. Preferential synthesis of "slow" myosin allows increased filling but decreased contractility. Change in the proteins that regulate the calcium channels in the sarcoplasmic reticulum results in rhythm problems.
      f. Desensitization of β-adrenergic receptors decreases energy use and the functioning number of receptor molecules (down regulation), which decreases contractility.

C. **ETIOLOGY (MULTIFACTORIAL)**
   1. **Obstruction of forward flow** can result from defects such as mitral or aortic stenosis or coarctation of the aorta.
   2. **Overload can be due to shunting** (i.e., VSD, AV canal).
   3. **Muscular underdevelopment** may occur such as in hypoplastic left heart syndrome (HLHS) or single ventricle.
   4. **Decreased contractility** may result from ischemia, inflammation, or fibrosis.
   5. **Dysrhythmias** can cause a failure to empty adequately or failure to contract (e.g., bradycardia, conduction disorders).

D. **CLINICAL SIGNS AND SYMPTOMS**
   1. **Sympathetic stimulation** results in increased heart rate, increased dysrhythmias, peripheral vasoconstriction, mottled and cool skin, and diaphoresis.
   2. The **renin-angiotensin-aldosterone mechanism** promotes sodium and water retention, oliguria, peripheral edema, and weight gain (fluid only).
   3. **Systemic venous engorgement** is characterized by increased liver size (hepato-

megaly), jugular venous distention, peripheral or periorbital edema, ascites, pleural effusion, or a combination of these signs.

4. **Pulmonary venous engorgement** results in tachypnea, rales, wheezing that does not clear until the heart failure is treated, increased respiratory effort, retractions, nasal flaring, pulmonary edema, and central cyanosis.

5. **Low cardiac output** is indicated by irritability, lethargy, poor or prolonged feeding with a weak suck, poor weight gain, tachycardia and/or a gallop rhythm, diaphoresis, oliguria, pallor, peripheral cyanosis, decreased capillary refill, pulsus alternans, and pulsus paradoxus. Nonspecific signs include irritability, change in responsiveness, and fatigue.

6. **Redistribution of blood flow** is related to vasoconstricting and vasodilating effects of neurohormonal agents such as norepinephrine, renin-angiotensin-aldosterone, vasopressin, atrial natriuretic factor, dopamine, and paracrine agents. Although protective for the heart and brain, redistributed flow may result in impairment of other organ systems. Long-term redistribution of flow may result in organ impairment (e.g., decreased gut perfusion may result in paralytic ileus; decreased hepatic perfusion results in decreased function; reduced skin or peripheral perfusion may result in necrotic changes; skeletal muscle may atrophy; and decreased glomerular filtration rate can result in acute tubular necrosis).

E. **DIAGNOSTIC STUDIES**
   1. **History and physical examination** are consistent with the above clinical presentation.
   2. **Chest x-ray examination** is useful for recognition of cardiomegaly, increased pulmonary vascular markings, and congestion.
   3. **ECG** will determine associated conduction disorders or dysrhythmias.
   4. **ECHO** establishes the presence or absence of structural defects or pericardial effusion and evaluates contractility.
   5. **PA catheter placement** can help determine cardiac index and evaluate management.
   6. **Cardiac catheterization** is used to evaluate structural defects, quantify cardiac output, and evaluate cause.
   7. **Laboratory studies** diagnose dilutional changes in serum sodium and hemoglobin, anemia, hypoglycemia in infants, digoxin levels, and abnormal results from LFTs related to hepatic venous congestion.

F. **NURSING DIAGNOSES**
   ❖ ALTERATION IN CARDIAC OUTPUT RELATED TO INADEQUATE TISSUE PERFUSION AND INADEQUATE NUTRITION TO TISSUES
   ❖ ALTERATION IN BREATHING PATTERNS
   ❖ ALTERATION IN FLUID AND ELECTROLYTE BALANCE
   ❖ ACTIVITY INTOLERANCE
   ❖ POTENTIAL FOR INJURY FROM MEDICATION THERAPY

G. **GOALS AND PATIENT OUTCOMES**
   1. Establish hemodynamic stability.
   2. Establish positive nutritional state.
   3. Maintain optimal level of activity.
   4. Prevent medication complications.

H. **PATIENT MANAGEMENT**
   1. **Improve cardiac output**
      a. Provide *supportive therapy* to increase oxygen supply (supplemental oxygen, semi-Fowler position, bronchodilators) or decrease oxygen demand (normothermia, reduce activity, digoxin therapy, sedation, gavage feedings to

decrease energy required for eating, increased caloric intake, and mechanical ventilation).

  b. *Pharmacologic therapy: Vasodilators and inotropic agents* alter the determinants of cardiac output (preload, afterload, contractility, and heart rate).

  - *Venous dilators* reduce preload (nitroglycerin).
  - *Arteriolar dilators* reduce afterload (hydralazine, nifedipine).
  - *Mixed dilators* reduce both preload and afterload (nitroprusside, phentolamine, captopril, enalapril, prazosin).
  - *Digitalis glycosides* (advantages: oral; disadvantages: low toxic-therapeutic ratio, increased myocardial oxygen demand, increased arrhythmogenicity)
  - *Catecholamines* stimulate β-adrenergic receptors (norepinephrine, epinephrine, isoproterenol, dopamine, dobutamine). Disadvantages: IV only; side effects: tachycardia, arrhythmogenicity, or vasoconstriction.
  - *Phosphodiesterase inhibitors* provide a positive inotropic effect (nonadrenergically mediated) plus afterload reduction (peripheral vasodilation; amrinone).

2. **Control fluid status** through assessment of edema, weight, and breath sounds. Fluid and sodium restrictions may be used. Measure electrolyte levels for elevated sodium and low potassium levels.

  a. Pharmacologic therapy: *Diuretics*

  - *Loop diuretics* (block sodium and chloride reabsorption in the ascending limb of the loop of Henle) are used most commonly in children.
  - *Furosemide and ethacrynic acid* inhibit sodium chloride transport in the ascending loop of Henle and in the proximal and distal tubule.
  - *Chlorothiazide and hydrochlorothiazide* inhibit reabsorption of sodium in the distal tubule and loop of Henle and inhibit water reabsorption in the cortical diluting segment.
  - *Metolazone* inhibits sodium reabsorption at the cortical-diluting site and in the proximal convoluted tubule.
  - *Spironolactone* is an aldosterone antagonist.
  - *Complications* include electrolyte imbalances, ototoxicity, and elevated values in renal function studies.

3. **Patient and family education** should include teaching about diet, medications, and signs and symptoms of CHF.

4. **Mechanical and surgical interventions**

  a. IABP and ECMO are the last choice of treatment modalities in patients with CHF and cardiogenic shock.

  b. For CHF related to correctable congenital defects, surgery is performed after optimal medical management.

SHOCK

A. DEFINITION

1. Shock is a complex syndrome of decreased blood flow to body tissues resulting in cellular dysfunction and eventual organ failure. Tissue perfusion in shock is inadequate to supply oxygen and nutrients to body cells (Rice, 1991).

2. During compromised cardiac function, compensatory mechanisms enable redistribution of blood flow to vital organs. As shock progresses, the compensatory mechanisms become destructive, and cardiovascular function deteriorates further.

3. Severe heart failure may progress to cardiogenic shock in which forward output of blood from the left ventricle is inadequate to meet the body's metabolic needs.

4. Cardiogenic shock is the final common pathway for *all* advanced forms of shock including hypovolemic, distributive, and septic.

B. ETIOLOGY AND PATHOPHYSIOLOGY

1. **Hypovolemic shock:** Decreased intravascular volume causes decreased venous return and decreased ventricular filling, leads to decreased stroke volume, and decreases cardiac output. As cardiac output falls, the blood pressure falls, and there is decreased blood flow to tissues. Poor blood flow impedes oxygenation and energy delivery to body cells. *Causes* include blood loss related to trauma, surgery, gastrointestinal tract bleeding, and intracranial hemorrhage; plasma loss from capillary fluid shifts in sepsis, thermal injury, anaphylactic reaction, burns, or nephrotic syndrome; and water loss from vomiting and diarrhea, diuretic administration, or diabetes insipidus.

2. **Cardiogenic shock:** Cardiogenic shock is the inability of the cardiac muscle to pump adequately to meet the metabolic demands of the tissues. Decreased stroke volume results in decreased cardiac output. As cardiac output falls, blood pressure falls and blood flow to the tissues is decreased. Decreased coronary perfusion and myocardial ischemia leads to further ventricular dysfunction. *Causes* include ischemic injury, arrhythmias, surgical damage and edema, inflammatory injury, obstruction of outflow, and systemic or pulmonary shunting.

3. **Septic shock** (see Chapter 9)

4. **Cellular changes in shock:** Tissue perfusion is decreased. Lack of oxygen delivery leads to anaerobic metabolism with low energy supply. Pyruvic acid is produced and converted to lactic acid, which accumulates. Acidosis releases lysosome from the cell, which destroys the membrane, resulting in cell death.

5. **Compensatory mechanisms:** The baroreceptor reflex is triggered by decreased stroke volume. This sends impulses to the medulla, which signals the heart to increase heart rate and contractility. The chemoreceptor reflex is triggered by the lack of oxygen and acidosis in the medulla and respiratory center of the brain. This reflex increases the rate and depth of breathing and increases PaO_2, pH, and cardiac output. The CNS ischemic reflex is triggered by ischemia in the vasomotor center of the brain. It stimulates contractility and is intended to increase blood pressure and cardiac output. Low arterial pressure causes lower capillary pressure, which results in fluid shifts based on osmotic pressure changes. This increases the vascular volume to increase blood pressure and cardiac output. Epinephrine and norepinephrine are released in response to low blood pressure. They stimulate heart rate and contractility and also cause arteriolar and venous constriction. Vasoconstriction increases venous return, blood pressure, and cardiac output. The renin-angiotensin mechanism is triggered by low renal blood flow. Renin is released and converted to angiotensin I, which is converted to angiotensin II. Angiotensin II is a potent vasoconstrictor that promotes aldosterone release. Aldosterone secretion is stimulated by low blood pressure and causes vasoconstriction. It acts on the kidneys to retain water and increase intravascular volume. Myocardial depressant factor (MDF) is released in response to tissue ischemia. The resultant decrease in myocardial contractility further impairs tissue perfusion, resulting in a vicious cycle.

6. **Metabolic changes in shock:** Metabolic rate and body temperature decrease. Carbohydrate metabolism is altered. Initially, the child is hyperglycemic in response to epinephrine release; then the child becomes hypoglycemic from

depletion of hepatic glycogen stores and failure of gluconeogenesis. Anaerobic glycolysis results in lactate and pyruvate production. Protein catabolism occurs for additional energy. Plasma catecholamines, 17-hydroxy-ketosteroids, and potassium increase.

C. SIGNS AND SYMPTOMS

    1. **Initially,** there is a deficiency in oxygen and nutrient delivery, resulting in anaerobic metabolism and excess lactic acid.

    2. The **compensatory phase** is characterized by decreased cardiac output and activation of compensatory mechanisms. Vasoconstriction results in cool, pale, or mottled skin with delayed capillary filling time. Diaphoresis results in clammy, moist skin. Urine output decreases. Poor skin turgor, dry mucous membranes, and sunken fontanelles are noted. Heart rate and contractility increase. Increased rate and depth of breathing result in respiratory alkalosis. Decreased level of consciousness is indicated by restlessness, confusion, and lethargy. Pupils may dilate. Infants may demonstrate a weak cry and poor suck.

    3. In the **progressive phase** of shock, compensatory mechanisms fail, leading to multisystem organ failure. Loss of autoregulation in microcirculation increases capillary permeability, leading to third spacing and decreased venous return. Low CVP, blood pressure, and pulmonary capillary wedge pressure (PCWP) occur. Coronary perfusion suffers, resulting in ischemic changes on the ECG. Low blood pressure leads to ischemia to distal extremities with necrosis and ulceration of toes and fingers. Mental status deteriorates. Acute renal failure occurs. Gastrointestinal tract ischemia allows translocation of gram-negative bacteria across damaged mucosa into the circulation, resulting in bowel edema, ulceration, and sepsis. Liver ischemia results in elevated bilirubin, liver enzymes, and jaundice. Alveolar ischemia causes decreased surfactant production, leading to alveoli collapse, atelectasis, and decreased compliance.

    4. In the **refractory phase,** irreversible injury occurs. Bradycardia and profound hypotension occurs with no response to potent vasopressors.

D. DIAGNOSTIC TOOLS

    1. **Chest x-ray examination** demonstrates cardiomegaly and pulmonary congestion.

    2. **ECHO** evaluates the presence of structural disease, systolic function, valvular structure, systolic time intervals, and ejection fraction.

    3. **Laboratory studies:** Arterial blood gases are used to determine hypoxia and respiratory or metabolic acidosis. Electrolytes diagnose hyponatremia, hyperkalemia, hypoglycemia, hypocalcemia. Renal and hepatic function studies determine organ function.

    4. **PA catheterization** measures pressures and cardiac output and evaluates shunting.

E. NURSING DIAGNOSES

    ❖ ALTERATION IN TISSUE PERFUSION
    ❖ ALTERATION IN CARDIAC OUTPUT
    ❖ ALTERATION IN BREATHING PATTERNS
    ❖ IMPAIRED GAS EXCHANGE
    ❖ ALTERATION IN FLUID AND ELECTROLYTE BALANCE
    ❖ FLUID VOLUME DEFICIT
    ❖ POTENTIAL FOR INFECTION

F. GOALS AND PATIENT OUTCOMES

    1. Reestablish hemodynamic stability.

    2. Establish adequate ventilation and oxygenation.

    3. Increase cardiac function by reducing the workload and by improving the efficiency of the heart.

4. Provide adequate nutrition and metabolic state.
5. Prevent complications as a result of shock.

G. **PATIENT MANAGEMENT**

1. **Therapeutic interventions** are aimed at correcting the primary cause of heart failure or altering the adaptive responses that have become damaging.

2. **Cardiovascular supportive care:** *Evaluate cardiovascular function* via an arterial line for continuous blood pressure monitoring, CVP monitoring to assess preload, a PA catheter to assess therapy, and perfusion assessment. Perfusion assessment includes assessment of blood pressure, skin color, temperature, capillary refill, and perfusion to organs. *Support cardiovascular function* with inotropic agents, vasodilators, cardiac rest, and mechanical support when necessary (see Extracorporeal Life Support and Cardiac Assist Devices).

3. **Fluid resuscitation:** *Restore intravascular volume* with fluid resuscitation (10 to 20 ml/kg bolus) until responsive. Isotonic fluids such as normal saline and lactated Ringer's solution can be used until blood is available (if needed). Hypertonic fluids such as 3% normal saline, 50% dextrose, and colloids can be used to pull in interstitial fluid. Blood products and plasma expanders are used as needed. Hetastarch has the same characteristics as 5% albumin, but the effects last up to 36 hours. Dextran has large glucose polymers that draw in water. *IV access* is obtained with large-bore catheters in major vessels. In shock, an intraosseous line can be used to infuse large volumes, blood, and drugs in small children when IV access is unobtainable in a timely manner.

4. **Treat sepsis.**

5. **Support organ function:** Mechanical ventilation provides cardiopulmonary support. Renal support may require diuretics, continuous arteriovenous or venous-venous hemofiltration (CAVH/CVVH), or hemodialysis. Prevent further injury through assessment of organ systems affected by the redistribution of blood flow.

6. **Provide adequate nutrition** through enteral or parenteral nutrition.

H. **COMPLICATIONS** such as renal failure, hepatic failure, sepsis, disseminated intravascular coagulation (DIC), or death may occur.

DYSRHYTHMIAS AND MYOCARDIAL CONDUCTION SYSTEM DEFECTS

A. **PATHOPHYSIOLOGY OF DYSRHYTHMIAS**

A dysrhythmia is an abnormality in the rate, regularity, or site of origin of a cardiac impulse or a disturbance in the conduction of that impulse preventing the normal sequence of activation of the atria and ventricles.

B. **CLASSIFICATION OF DYSRHYTHMIAS**

1. **Dysrhythmias can be classified according to etiology.**

a. Congenital (developmental, congenital complete heart block [CHB], Wolff-Parkinson-White syndrome [WPW], congenital prolonged QT interval syndrome)

b. Secondary to other disease (flutter from the stretched atria of Ebstein's anomaly)

c. Secondary to noncardiac disease (CNS, endocrine or metabolic disease, infectious disease, collagen vascular disorders)

d. Surgically acquired (sick sinus syndrome [SSS], AV block)

e. Primary dysrhythmias (AV nodal reentry tachycardia, reciprocating tachycardia, PVC)

2. Factors that may precipitate dysrhythmias include hypoxia, congenital conduction abnormalities, CHD, pulmonary hypertension, electrolyte or metabolic abnormalities, diseases of the CNS, sepsis, hypotension, viral myocarditis, acute rheumatic fever, procedures (cardiac catheterization, catheter placement), intubation (vagal response and bradycardia), cardiac surgery (damage to conduction from mechanical manipulation, medication or anesthetics, cannulation from cardiopulmonary bypass), transient conduction system injury (edema, inflammation, ischemia, sutures near conduction pathway), hemodynamic changes, electrolyte shifts, and medication interactions.

3. Treatment of the underlying cause may be the most effective therapy.

C. **INTERPRETATION OF DYSRHYTHMIAS**

1. **Rhythm:** Is R-R interval regular (less than 0.12 second variation between intervals)? Is P-P regular? Are there early or delayed beats? Is there a pattern of irregularity? Is it a repeated or chaotic pattern?

2. **Rate:** Is the atrial or ventricular rate normal, decreased, or increased for patient's age and clinical condition? Are atrial and ventricular rates the same (P:QRS ratio = 1:1)?

3. **QRS complex:** Is the QRS duration normal or prolonged (normal less than 0.12 second)? Do all QRS complexes look alike? Does the QRS complex have a fixed relationship with the P wave (measure PR interval)?

4. What is the **atrial activity?** Are there P waves, flutter waves, or fibrillation? Determine the P wave axis (normal axis is 0 to 90 degrees). What is the relationship of atrial depolarizations to QRS complexes? Do all P waves look alike? If atrial and ventricular depolarizations are not related, consider AV dissociation from either slowing of the sinus or atrial rhythm, accelerated junctional rhythm, VT without retrograde conduction, or complete AV block.

D. **SUPRAVENTRICULAR DYSRHYTHMIAS** (Fig. 3–24)

1. **Sinus dysrhythmia:** Normal pause in sinus rhythm

   a. *Sinus dysrhythmia* is related to respiratory variations (heart rate increases with inspiration and decreases with expiration). It may be marked in

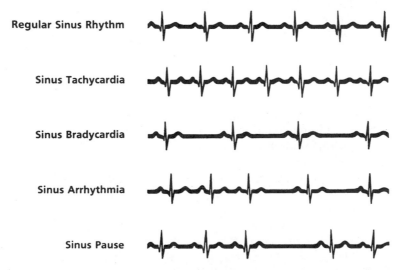

Figure 3–24. Normal and abnormal rhythms originating in the SA node. All rhythms have a P wave in front of each QRS complex with a regular PR interval. (Reprinted with permission from Park MK, Guntheroth WG. *How to Read Pediatric ECGs.* St Louis, Mo: CV Mosby Co; 1992.)

children with airway obstruction, asthma, or increased intracranial pressure and after atrial surgery. This is a normal phenomenon in the fetus and in most children at all ages.

b. Although the history and examination reveal no clinical signs or symptoms, the child has a benign, irregular pulse.

c. *Diagnostic findings:* ECG features include an irregular rhythm, P-P and R-R intervals vary by more than 0.12 second with beat-to-beat variability, upright P waves, one P wave for each QRS complex, and normal PR interval and QRS configuration.

d. *Intervention* is not necessary.

2. **Sinus tachycardia**

a. *Etiology* is related to increased sympathetic tone, pain, fear, anxiety, anemia, exercise, fever, infection, hypoxemia, shock, CHF, and pulmonary edema.

b. *History and examination:* History may reveal the underlying causes (above). Clinical signs and symptoms vary with rate. The child will have a rapid, regular pulse and may also have palpitations or dyspnea or both or may be asymptomatic.

c. *Diagnostic findings:* ECG features include regular rhythm, rate greater than normal, upright P waves, one P wave for each QRS complex, normal PR interval and QRS configuration, and origin of the rhythm in the SA node. Infants may have a sinus tachycardia as high as 220 to 250 beats per minute, overlapping with rates of SVT (Fig. 3–28).

d. *Interventions* include treating the underlying cause. Digoxin is not effective unless the ST is related to congestive failure.

3. **SA node conduction disorders: Pause, block, or arrest:** Period of time of varying length of decreased or absent SA node activity.

a. *Etiology of pause, arrest, or block* can be related to hypoxemia, digoxin toxicity, hyperkalemia, increased vagal tone, or cardiac surgery. In addition, myocardial infarction (MI), ischemia, quinidine, atropine, aspirin toxicity, or infection (myocarditis, rheumatic fever) can be contributing factors.

b. *History and examination* reveal that the patient is usually not aware of the dysrhythmia or may complain of skipped beats. The palpated pulse has a prolonged pause, and CHF and decreased cardiac output may develop if the pauses are frequent.

c. *Diagnostic findings:* ECG features include a varying or irregular heart rate, a prolonged diastolic pause between QRS complexes, absence of one or more expected P waves, QRS complex is absent unless junctional or ventricular escape beat occurs, and the QRS duration is normal (Fig. 3–28). In *SA pause* the diastolic pause is less than twice the underlying sinus interval. In *SA block* the pause is an exact multiple of the underlying sinus interval; the SA node fires but is not conducted. In *SA arrest* the pause is greater than twice the underlying sinus interval.

d. *Intervention* includes treatment of the underlying cause, atropine for frequent episodes, or a pacemaker for symptomatic episodes.

4. **Sinus bradycardia:** The heart rate is low for the patient's age and clinical state, but the rhythm is normal.

a. *Etiology:* The most common causes include surgical disruption of the SA node, use of digoxin or β-blockers, increased vagal tone, increased intracranial pressure, hypothermia, hypothyroidism, hypoxemia, and anorexia. Sinus bradycardia is rarely an isolated finding. More commonly it occurs with severe systemic disease or hypoxemia. It may lead to SA block or an escape rhythm or may allow an irritable focus to take over.

b. *History and examination* reveal a slow, regular pulse. In infants, CHF may occur earlier because of the inadequacy of the rate.

c. *Diagnostic findings:* ECG findings include a P wave before every QRS complex, regular P-P and R-R intervals, normal QRS configuration, normal PR interval, and upright P waves (Fig. 3–28).

d. *Interventions* include 24-hour ECG monitoring to determine the exact degree of bradycardia when the patient is asleep and awake and a stress ECG (if the patient is older than 5 years) to determine the degree of SA node incompetence. Transesophageal pacing can test automaticity and sinus node recovery time. Invasive study of the SA node should include the AV node function. If the conduction system is intact, permanent atrial demand pacing can be used. Treatment of the underlying causes may eliminate the dysrhythmia.

5. **Sick sinus syndrome (SSS, bradycardia-tachycardia syndrome):** The heart rate varies from rates in excess of 180 bpm to severe bradycardia with long sinus pauses. Dysrhythmias may include profound sinus bradycardia, SA exit block, sinus arrest with junctional escape, paroxysmal atrial tachycardia, slow or fast ectopic atrial or nodal rhythm, atrial flutter, or atrial fibrillation.

a. *Etiology:* Causes include disease or ischemia of the SA node and extensive atrial surgery, or it may be of idiopathic origin. SSS may occur following atrial surgery, cannulation for cardiopulmonary bypass, or hypertrophy of an otherwise anatomically normal heart. SSS may also result from fibrosis of approaches to the SA node, AV node, or injury to the sinus node artery.

b. *History and examination:* Infants may experience syncope, seizures, lethargy, poor feeding, or sudden death. Children and adolescents may experience syncope, seizures, dizziness, fatigue, exercise intolerance, palpitations, chest pain, or sudden death.

c. *Diagnostic findings* include an ECG with irregular rhythm, variable rate, and P waves varying in amplitude and morphology.

d. *Interventions* for symptomatic dysrhythmias require a pacemaker for the bradycardia component. Antidysrhythmics are used for the tachycardia component only after pacemaker insertion.

6. **Supraventricular tachycardia (SVT)**

a. *Etiology:* The cause of acute SVT may be rapid firing of a single ectopic focus or reentry mechanism, increased automaticity from hypoxemia, electrolyte imbalance, acid-base abnormalities, myocardial disease, digoxin toxicity, or CHD. Most episodes involve reentry occurring from an accessory AV connection or dual AV node pathways (i.e., AV node reentry).

b. *History and examination:* Acute SVT often precipitates symptoms of shock and CHF, but older children rarely present in heart failure or shock. They may report palpitations, general malaise, and a racing heart with a regular rhythm. SVT is usually well tolerated in the neonate; however, prolonged rates in excess of 200 bpm eventually result in CHF. Chronic SVT is characterized by slower rates, longer lasting episodes, and milder symptoms and is more influenced by the autonomic nervous system.

c. *Diagnostic findings* include ECG features of one P wave per QRS complex, a ventricular rate usually greater than 220 bpm in infants and greater than 150 bpm in children, regular P-P and R-R intervals, abrupt onset and termination of rate, normal QRS configuration, and P waves may be absent, inverted, or superimposed (Fig. 3–25). Chronic SVT may be accompanied by evidence of myocardial dysfunction. Electrophysiology studies may reveal automatic ectopic focus located in the atria or bundle of His,

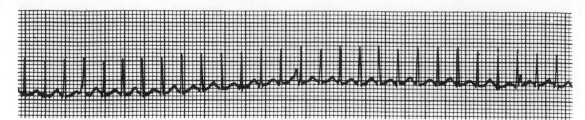

Figure 3–25. ECG tracing of supraventricular tachycardia with normal QRS complex and regular R-R intervals. (Reprinted with permission from Park MK, Guntheroth WG. *How to Read Pediatric ECGs.* St Louis, Mo: CV Mosby Co; 1992.)

　　　　　concealed AV unidirectional retrograde accessory pathway, or permanent form of reciprocating junctional tachycardia.

d. *Interventions* include treatment based on rate, mechanism of tachycardia, degree of myocardial dysfunction, and symptoms.

- For acute SVT, diving reflex and other vagal maneuvers (rarely effective), pharmacologic treatments (digoxin, adenosine, propranolol, and verapamil in children older than 1 year), direct current cardioversion, and overdrive pacing can be used in symptomatic children.

- In chronic SVT, the mechanism of SVT is defined by electrophysiologic catheterization to determine the safety of digoxin use. Vagal maneuvers and pharmacologic treatments (adenosine, verapamil) may be useful. Digoxin improves myocardial performance and slows the rate. Propranolol, quinidine, or flecainide can be added if digoxin alone is not effective in controlling the rate. Surgical or radiofrequency ablation may be performed if the SVT is not responsive to medical treatment, the child develops severe side effects, or the child's lifestyle does not allow effective medication regimens. Accessory connections can be divided surgically or frozen by radiofrequency ablation. SVT may recur if there is only damage to the ectopic focus or pathway and the tissue involved is not destroyed. Pacemakers can be used for automatic overdrive or atrial pacing for control of the rate.

7. **Wolff-Parkinson-White syndrome (WPW)**

a. *Etiology* involves the presence of a congenital accessory connection that conducts electrical activity faster than the AV node. WPW may be an isolated disease or associated with CHD especially Ebstein's anomaly, Pompe's disease, and cardiac myopathies. SVT may occur at any age secondary to reentry. The accessory pathway may disappear in the first year of life but may resurface in the second or third decade of life.

b. *History and examination:* Frequent tachycardia occurs in infancy with reduced episodes in early childhood and resumption of symptoms at puberty. Symptoms may include palpitations, lethargy, decreased activity tolerance, or more rarely syncope, seizures, and sudden death.

c. *Diagnostic findings:* WPW may be diagnosed by surface ECG or, if it is a concealed pathway, by intracardiac electrophysiology study. ECG features include regular rhythm, frequent episodes of SVT or atrial fibrillation, short PR interval, wide QRS complex, and presence of a delta wave.

d. *Interventions* include treatment of frequent episodes of SVT or syncope with quinidine or propranolol, surgical or electrical ablation of accessory pathway (especially if not responsive to medical therapy), and avoidance of digoxin in children older than 6 to 12 months.

8. **Nodal (junctional) tachycardia**
    a. *Pathophysiology* involves an accelerated rate originating in the AV node and the loss of atrial kick (especially harmful if cardiac output is already compromised by heart disease or cardiac surgery). It is the most common dysrhythmia in postoperative patients with cardiac disease.
    b. *Diagnostic findings:* ECG rate varies from 120 to 200 bpm; QRS complex is usually normal and regular, and an inverted P wave may or may not follow the QRS complex (Fig. 3–26). The child may require an electrophysiologic study to determine the exact origin of the tachycardia.
    c. *Intervention* may be required especially in severely compromised patients. Cooling to a temperature of 35° C, sedation, inotropic support, overdrive pacing when able to capture the rate, and medications such as digoxin, procainamide, or quinidine are used. Treatment may not be necessary if the rate is within normal limits and adequate (Table 3–4).

9. **Atrial flutter and fibrillation:** Tachydysrhythmias that originate above the bifurcation of the bundle of His.
    a. **Atrial flutter**
        - *Pathophysiology and etiology* are related to a large stretched atria due to CHD or acquired heart disease, neonates after atrial surgery, hypoxemia, valvular disease, digoxin toxicity, increased sympathetic tone, or infection.
        - *History and examination:* Clinical signs and symptoms of heart failure develop if not treated quickly, depending on the ventricular rate. Children may have palpitations, angina, dyspnea, or decreased cardiac output. Symptoms are more pronounced if there is underlying cardiac disease.
        - *Diagnostic findings* include rapid atrial tachycardia with characteristic flutter waves, normal QRS configuration, rate usually 300 bpm and regular (but may go as high as 400 to 450 bpm), ventricular response from 1:1 to various degrees of AV block, sawtooth configuration P waves, and an unidentifiable PR interval.
        - The most successful *intervention* in symptomatic children is direct cardioversion. Rapid overdrive atrial pacing may be useful through transesophageal or transvenous routes. Medications are given to increase AV block

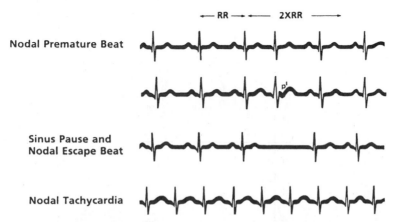

Figure 3–26. Dysrhythmias originating in the atrioventricular node. (Reprinted with permission from Park MK, Guntheroth WG. *How to Read Pediatric ECGs.* St Louis, Mo: CV Mosby Co; 1992.)

Table 3–4. MEDICATIONS FOR MANAGING AV NODAL REENTRY AND ATRIAL FIBRILLATION OR ATRIAL FLUTTER

	Adenosine	Calcium Antagonists	Digoxin	β-Blockers	Class IA	Class IC	Class III
AV nodal reentry	Acute conversion Transient AV block	Acute conversion Prevention	Prevention	Prevention	Prevention	Prevention	Prevention
Atrial fibrillation	Diagnosis Slows AV conduction	Rate control	Rate control	Rate control	Conversion Prevention	Conversion Prevention	Conversion Prevention
Atrial flutter	Diagnosis Slows AV conduction	Rate control	Rate control	Rate control	Conversion Prevention	Conversion Prevention	Conversion Prevention

From Knellen JC, Ramadan D. The patient with recurrent atrioventricular nodal reentrant tachycardia or chronic atrial fibrillation or atrial flutter. *Crit Care Nurs Clin North Am.* 1994;6:41–54.

and decrease ventricular response rate (digoxin, propranolol, verapamil) and to prevent recurrence (quinidine and other antiarrhythmics). Surgical procedures can be used to improve hemodynamics and relieve atrial stretch or for implantation of an automatic atrial antitachycardia pacer.

b. **Atrial fibrillation**
  - *Pathophysiology and etiology* are related to increased sympathetic tone, hypoxemia, valvular disease, structural heart disease with dilated atria, atrial surgery, digoxin toxicity, disease of AV node or lower conduction system, or hyperthyroidism (rare in children). Implications are much greater if the patient has WPW.
  - *History and examination:* Clinical signs and symptoms depend on the ventricular response. Children may have palpitations, angina or dyspnea, decreased cardiac output, CHF, ischemia, atrial emboli, and an irregular pulse.
  - Classic *diagnostic findings* include a wavy baseline with absent P waves and an irregularly irregular ventricular rhythm. ECG features include a rapid and irregular atrial rate (may be over 350 bpm), no discernible P waves, an irregular and slower ventricular rate, immeasurable PR interval, and normal QRS configuration.
  - *Interventions* include digoxin if no WPW is present, propranolol, and cardioversion (in symptomatic patients).

E. **VENTRICULAR DYSRHYTHMIAS**

Ventricular dysrhythmias are rare in otherwise normal hearts but are associated with surgical correction of CHD (Fig. 3–27). They are also found in myocarditis, cardiomyopathies, idiopathic hypertrophic subaortic stenosis (IHSS), cardiac tumors, metabolic disturbances, drug toxicity, CHD, RV hypertrophy, and QT prolongation. PVCs may be found in utero and in normal children. Sudden death following the repair of CHD or sudden death without known heart disease is most likely due to ventricular dysrhythmias. Frequently in postoperative cases the myocardium shows marked fibrosis and fatty infiltrate of sutures.

1. **Ventricular tachycardia (VT)**
  a. *Etiology and pathophysiology* are related to an intramyocardial tumor, metabolic disturbances, cardiomyopathy, drug ingestion, drug toxicity, long QT syndrome, damage to His-Purkinje system or myocardium (MI, myocarditis, surgery), hypoxemia, acidosis, or hypokalemia. Three or more PVCs in a row are considered VT. It is uncommon in children who have not undergone intracardiac surgery. In infants younger than 1 year of age the QRS complex may not be prolonged.

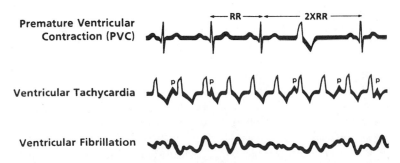

Figure 3–27. Ventricular dysrhythmias. (Reprinted with permission from Park MK, Guntheroth WG. *How to Read Pediatric ECGs.* St Louis, Mo: CV Mosby Co; 1992.)

   b. *History and examination:* Most patients are immediately aware of this dys-rhythmia because of palpitations, dyspnea, dizziness, anxiety, diaphoresis, angina, decreased level of consciousness, syncope, or decreased blood pressure. VT may be asymptomatic in short bursts, but cardiac output may decrease rapidly with prolonged bursts or short bursts in compromised patients. Rhythm may deteriorate to ventricular fibrillation.

   c. *Diagnostic findings* include wide, bizarre, abnormal QRS configuration; a rate usually greater than 100 bpm; P waves not related to the QRS complex; no discernible PR interval; and a sustained or unsustained tachycardia. Diagnosis is confirmed by ECG monitor, surface 12-lead ECG, or intracardiac electrophysiology.

   d. For asymptomatic VT in children with normal hearts, *interventions* may not be warranted. Medical treatment for VT associated with abnormal myocardial function includes lidocaine, propranolol, phenytoin (Dilantin), procainamide, or amiodarone. If present, tumors are excised. Surgical or radiofrequency ablation is used if reentry VT is demonstrated on electrophysiology study. Cardioversion is indicated for acute events.

2. **Ventricular fibrillation (VF)**

   a. *Pathophysiology and etiology* include insults to the His-Purkinje system or myocardium, hypoxemia, electrolyte imbalance, hyperkalemia, electrical shock, drugs, prolonged VT, or long QT syndrome.

   b. *History and examination:* Clinical signs and symptoms include loss of consciousness; no pulse, respiration, or blood pressure; possible seizure, cyanosis, and clinical death.

   c. *Diagnostic findings* include ECG features of repetitive series of chaotic ventricular waves varying in size and amplitude; complete absence of characteristic P wave, QRS complex, and T wave; and no measurable heart rate.

   d. *Interventions* include cardiopulmonary resuscitation (CPR) plus defibrillation. VF not responsive to several defibrillation attempts should be treated with medications such as epinephrine or lidocaine and then defibrillation tried again.

F. **AV NODE CONDUCTION DISORDERS**

Ventricular response depends on the patient's age, clinical state, and physical training. Bradyarrhythmias may be the result of hemorrhage into the conduction tissue (Fig. 3–28).

1. **First-degree AV block**

   a. *Etiology:* Associated with rheumatic fever, CHD, injury to AV node, certain cardiac drugs, surgery, hypoxemia, mitral insufficiency, and ischemia of the conduction system.

   b. *History and examination:* Usually there are no clinical signs and symptoms.

   c. *Diagnostic findings:* ECG features include regular rhythm, a P wave before every QRS complex, regular P-P and R-R intervals, a prolonged PR interval for age and heart rate, a normal QRS configuration, and a constant PR interval (Fig. 3–32).

   d. *Intervention* centers around monitoring, since first-degree AV block may progress to second- or third-degree AV block. Treatment is needed only if the cause is drug toxicity.

2. **Second-degree AV block:** This is a partial AV conduction disorder, since not all P waves are conducted. The ratio of conducted beats varies.

   a. *Pathophysiology and etiology*
   • Wenckebach (Mobitz type I) is found occasionally in normal hearts and is usually of little significance to the ventricles. Wenckebach is a higher AV

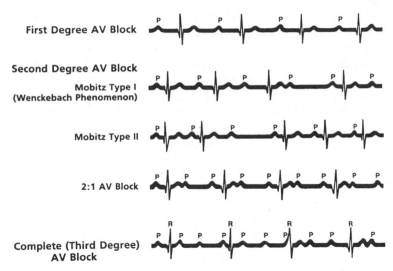

First Degree AV Block

Second Degree AV Block

Mobitz Type I
(Wenckebach Phenomenon)

Mobitz Type II

2:1 AV Block

Complete (Third Degree)
AV Block

Figure 3–28.   Disturbances of atrioventricular conduction. (Reprinted with permission from Park MK, Guntheroth WG. *How to Read Pediatric ECGs.* St Louis, Mo: CV Mosby Co; 1992.)

block. Type I is related to insults to the AV node, inferior MI, hypoxemia, increased vagal tone, and digoxin toxicity.

- Mobitz type II is more serious and due to a block in the distal AV conduction system often related to ischemic changes. Type II is related to insults to the AV node, MI, hypoxemia, cardiac drugs, ischemic disease of the conduction system, CHD, and cardiomyopathy.

b. *History and examination*
- Type I usually has no symptoms. If the rate decreases dramatically, cardiac output may decrease. Usually it does not progress.
- Type II has a slower rate that may diminish cardiac output. Blocks at the level of the bundle of His may progress suddenly and rapidly to complete block with significantly lower rates and signs and symptoms of CHF or syncope (i.e., Adams-Stokes attacks).

c. *Diagnostic findings*
- ECG features of type I include a regular P-P interval, irregular R-R interval, more P waves than QRS complexes; and a PR interval that progressively increases until a QRS complex is dropped and a normal QRS complex resumes (Fig. 3–28).
- ECG criteria of Mobitz type II include a regular P-P interval, a slower ventricular response, normal atrial rate, periodic dropped QRS complexes, P waves upright and normal, fixed PR interval in the conducted beats, more P waves than QRS complexes, and an abnormal QRS complex (usually but not always). With a 2:1 AV block, it is difficult to be certain that it is type I or II (see Fig. 3–28).

d. *Interventions* for type I and II include treatment of the underlying cause, and a pacemaker for symptomatic children.

3. **Complete AV block (CHB):** Complete absence of conduction of atrial impulses to the ventricle related to congenital or acquired disorders.

a. *Pathophysiology and etiology:* CHB may be congenital and occur in otherwise normal hearts. Congenital CHB may be diagnosed antenatally and is associated with maternal connective tissue disorders or antinuclear antibodies. Acquired CHB is relatively uncommon in infants and children.

Associated with structural disease, it also occurs with myopathies, infectious diseases, fibrotic degeneration of the conduction system, CHD, diabetes, collagen disorders or rheumatic fever, interruptive lesions in the bundle of His or lesions in both bundle branches, and tumors. There is higher risk if the ventricular rate is less than 55 bpm and associated with heart failure. This is the most frequent dysrhythmia causing mortality in the first year of life.

b. *History and examination:* Symptoms include syncope (with lower rates), decreased exercise tolerance, associated ventricular ectopy or standstill, slow heart rate, and decreased cardiac output. *Examination* usually reveals normal growth and development, but the child may exhibit signs of CHF if the rate is less than 45 bpm during the first year of life. An evaluation for structural disease should be included.

c. *Diagnostic findings:* ECG features include a regular rhythm, an atrial rate greater than the ventricular rate, regular R-R and P-P intervals, and a variable PR interval (see Fig. 3–28).

d. *Interventions* include an ECG, chest x-ray examination, physical examination, ECHO, and Holter monitor and exercise test every 3 to 5 years beginning at the age of 4 to 5 years. Permanent cardiac pacing is indicated when syncope or heart failure is present, the block is below the bundle of His, in infants with ventricular rates less than 55 bpm, with frequent or complex ventricular dysrhythmias, or with moderate or severe exercise intolerance.

G. **BUNDLE BRANCH BLOCK (BBB)**

1. *Pathophysiology and etiology* are related to damage to the bundle branch from an MI or fibrotic scarring bundle. It is common following some forms of surgical repair for congenital heart defects such as VSD or tetralogy of Fallot.

2. *History and examination:* Usually there are no clinical signs and symptoms. If all three bundles are blocked, the child may develop CHB and asystole.

3. *Diagnostic findings* include ECG features of a QRS width greater than 0.12 second or association with other dysrhythmias. Diagnosis of RBBB or LBBB is determined with a 12-lead ECG.

4. *Interventions* include 24-hour ECG monitoring for patients with bifascicular block to assess development of progressive blocks. Patients are treated with pacing if symptomatic.

PACEMAKERS FOR TREATMENT OF TEMPORARY OR PERMANENT CONDUCTION DISORDERS

A. **INDICATIONS FOR PACEMAKERS**

Pacers are used to deliver an electrical impulse (stimulus) to the heart to initiate depolarization and stimulate a cardiac contraction. SSS, symptomatic bradydysrhythmias, CHB, Mobitz type II, and a denervated heart may require a pacemaker. Overdrive pacing of accelerated tachydysrhythmias may be useful in termination of tachydysrhythmias. Synchronized pacing can restore AV synchrony and the atrial kick.

B. **COMPONENTS OF A PACEMAKER SYSTEM**

The **pulse generator** consists of a battery and circuitry of the pacemaker, most commonly lithium batteries. **Lead wires** conduct impulses from the pulse generator to the heart. An electrode in contact with the heart delivers the impulse. Most leads are bipolar containing active and ground leads. Unipolar leads use the pacemaker generator itself as the ground pole.

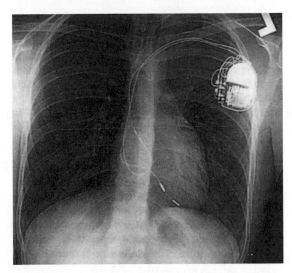

Figure 3–29. Standard transvenous lead position in an adolescent. (Reprinted with permission from Mavroudes C, Backer CL. *Pediatric Cardiac Surgery.* St Louis, Mo: CV Mosby Co; 1994.)

C. **PERMANENT CARDIAC PACEMAKERS**
  1. A **transvenous** pacing catheter is threaded through the subclavian or jugular vein to the right atrium or right ventricle, or both. Transvenous pacers are generally used in children who weigh more than 12 kg. Anatomic variants of CHD may prohibit transvenous lead placement. Generators are placed in the anterior chest wall or abdominal wall (Fig. 3–29).
  2. **Epicardial** leads are placed through a thoracotomy or sternotomy incision on the epicardial surface of the heart by clipping, suturing, or screwing. Younger or smaller patients require transthoracic lead placement, as vessel size prohibits transvenous placement. Epicardial leads may be difficult to place in the presence of scar tissue from repeated operations and resultant adhesions. Generators are placed in the anterior chest wall or abdominal wall.

D. **TEMPORARY CARDIAC PACEMAKERS**
  1. **Bipolar transvenous catheters** are placed through the femoral or upper extremity veins to the right atrium or right ventricle.
  2. **Bipolar epicardial wires** are sutured to the right atrium or right ventricle, or both. Atrial wires exit to the right chest, and ventricular wires exit to the left chest.
  3. An **esophageal** pacing probe passed via the esophagus paces by the impulse traversing tissue between the electrode and the right atrium.
  4. **Transthoracic** pacing is accomplished via electrode pads delivering a stimulus through the chest wall. One pad is placed on the anterior chest, and one is placed on the child's back. Noninvasive pacing is not as reliable and may be uncomfortable. It may be used as support during anesthesia induction for other pacer placement.

E. **PACEMAKER MODES**
  1. **Capabilities** include pacing (ability of pacemaker to deliver an impulse to the heart), capture (effectiveness of the pacing stimulus to cause contraction), and sensing (the ability to detect intrinsic cardiac activity).
  2. **Asynchronous or fixed rate mode:** Pacemaker paces at a continuous set rate without sensing or responding to intrinsic cardiac activity. AV conduction is required for an atrial fixed rate pacing mode.
  3. **Demand (inhibited) mode:** The demand mode allows the pacemaker to sense intrinsic cardiac activity and inhibit pacing when it senses intrinsic activity at a

rate equal to or above the set rate. A pacing stimulus is delivered when the intrinsic rate is inadequate. Demand pacing avoids complications caused by competition between the child's intrinsic rate and the pacer. AV conduction is required for effective atrial demand pacing. AV conduction is not required for ventricular demand pacing, but atrial kick is lost. Synchronous AV demand pacing simulates the normal cardiac cycle.

4. **Triggered and inhibited modes:** In this mode the pacer can trigger and inhibit pacing and can sense intrinsic cardiac activity.

5. **Nomenclature:** The North American Society for Pacemaker Education (NASPE) code is used to communicate pacer functions (Table 3–5). The first letter describes chamber paced, the second letter describes chamber sensed, the third letter describes mode of response to sensing, the fourth letter indicates ability of pacemaker to respond to programming, and the fifth letter indicates the ability of the pacer to respond to tachydysrhythmias by burst pacing or shock.

F. ECG EVIDENCE OF PACERS

A pacer spike is produced on the ECG by pacer only with pacing and not with sensed intrinsic beats. An atrial pacing stimulus is followed by a P wave, and a ventricular pacing stimulus is followed by a QRS complex if the atria and ventricles are captured.

G. COMPLICATIONS OF PACEMAKERS

1. **Insertion** can result in local or systemic infection, pneumothorax, myocardial perforation with transvenous placement, dysrhythmias, and hematoma or bleeding.

2. **Component problems** (Table 3–6): Failure to capture (pacer stimulus does not produce contraction) is related to insufficient pacer output, low battery, disconnection between lead and generator, lead fracture or dislodgment, fibrosis of lead tip, or impulse delivery during refractory period. Failure to sense (generator fails to sense intrinsic rhythm) is related to improper lead placement, generator failure, sensitivity set too low, lead fracture, or a displaced lead. Pacer spikes are present without regard for inherent rhythm.

3. **Bleeding or tamponade** can follow removal of temporary wires.

4. Children with right-to-left intracardiac shunts have an increased **risk of systemic emboli** with transvenous pacing catheters.

5. Children with pulmonary artery hypertension have an increased **risk of pulmonary emboli** with transvenous pacers.

H. NURSING INTERVENTION FOR TEMPORARY PACERS

Assess vital signs as appropriate and assure normal electrolytes and acid-base balance. Patient and family teaching should include indications for pacing and procedures surrounding placement. Pacer wires and equipment should be appropriately grounded to prevent accidental electrocution. Also, properly ground all electrical equipment used by the child, including video and electronic games. Dials should be covered to prevent accidental changes in settings. Stabilize the patient's leg if a transvenous catheter is placed in the femoral vein to avoid leg flexion. Observe catheter site for signs of infection. Monitoring includes continuous telemetry, arterial line, and pulse oximetry to evaluate patients with surgically induced conduction disturbances.

I. NURSING INTERVENTIONS FOR PERMANENT PACERS

Teach the patient and family to assess pacer function and the indications and protocol for transmission of transtelephonic tracings. Teach the patient and family to report dizziness, syncope, weakness, fatigue, increased symptoms of CHF, redness, swelling, drainage at the incision site(s), palpitations, unresolved or frequent hiccups, fever, decreased feeding, or irritability. Provide family with information for medic-alert and stress the importance of always carrying the pacer

Table 3–5. NORTH AMERICAN SOCIETY FOR PACEMAKER EDUCATION IBPEG CODE FOR PACEMAKERS

Position	I	II	III	IV	V
Category	Chamber(s) paced	Chamber(s) sensed	Response to sensing	Programmability, rate modulation	Antitachyarrhythmia function(s)
	0 = None	0 = None	0 = None	0 = None	0 = None
	A = Atrium	A = Atrium	T = Triggered	P = Simple programmable	P = Pacing (antitachyarrhythmia)
	V = Ventricle	V = Ventricle	I = Inhibited	M = Multiprogrammable	S = Shock
	D = Dual (A + V)	D = Dual (A + V)	D = Dual (T + I)	C = Communicating	D = Dual (P + S)
				R = Rate modulation	
Manufacturers' designation only	S = Single (A or V)	S = Single (A or V)			

Pacemaker function is described by the first three letters, and programmability and antitachycardia capability are described in letters IV and V, respectively.
From Bernstein AD, Camm AJ, Fletcher RD, et al. The NASPE/BPEG generic pacemaker code for antibradyarrhythmia and adaptive-rate pacing and antitachyarrhythmia devices. *Pacing Clin Electrophysiol* 1987;10:794.

Table 3–6. DEMONSTRATION OF ABNORMAL PACEMAKER FUNCTION RELATED TO UNDERSENSING, OVERSENSING, OR NONCAPTURE

	SAMPLE ECG APPEARANCE	SOME POSSIBLE CLINICAL CONSEQUENCES	SOME POSSIBLE CAUSES	CORRECTIVE MEASURES
UNDERSENSING Device fails to detect existing cardiac depolarizations, therefore competes with the native rhythm	These native R waves are not detected... ...therefore the pacer emits these unneeded spikes	Competition with a native rhythm Stimulation of dysrhythmias ("R-on-T")	Lead disconnected from pacer or from viable myocardium Sensitivity set too low Lead fracture Low battery	Check connection of lead to pacer Increase sensitivity (turn sensing control to a SMALLER number) Reposition or change lead Change battery
OVERSENSING Device detects noncardiac electrical events and interprets them as cardiac depolarizations, therefore is wrongly inhibited from pacing	Pacing should occur as indicated by the arrows but is inhibited by oversensed non-cardiac electrical noise. When the noise ceases, pacing resumes	Pacemaker-dependent patients receive no stimuli from the pacemaker, producing a pause in rhythm and reduction in cardiac output	Electrical potential caused by non-cardiac muscle contraction (especially pectorals) is detected and misinterpreted by the device Interference from electrical sources (ungrounded equipment, short circuits) is detected and misinterpreted by the device Sensitivity set too high	Decrease sensitivity (turn sensing control to a LARGER number) Remove all ungrounded electrical equipment or have it evaluated by hospital engineers
NONCAPTURE Device emits stimuli which fail to depolarize the myocardium	This dual chamber device paces and captures in the atrium and ventricle for the first two beats. Ventricular capture is then lost; the ventricular pacing spikes are not followed by depolarizations. Fortunately, ventricular escape begins.	Pacemaker-dependent patients receive no stimuli from the pacemaker, producing a pause in rhythm and reduction in cardiac output	Lead disconnected from pacer or from viable myocardium Output set too low in the noncaptured chamber Lead fracture High pacing threshold due to medication or metabolic changes Low battery	Check connection of lead to pacer Increase output in the noncaptured chamber Reposition or change lead Change battery Alter medication regimen, correct metabolic changes

From Witherall CL. Cardiac rhythm control devices. *Crit Care Nurs Clin North Am.* 1994;6:95–102.

identification card with the patient name, physician name, address, phone number, medications, and the pacer type and settings. Teach the patient and family the name, action, side effects, and complications of antidysrhythmic drugs or other medications. If the patient moves out of the area, rapid referral to a new cardiologist is required. Instruct the patient and family on the appropriate timing to return to normal activity including school, driving, and exercise (contact sports are to be avoided). Pregnancy generally is well-tolerated, depending on associated disease.

J. **EVALUATION OF NURSING CARE**
1. Patient is without signs and symptoms of infection.
2. Patient and family verbalize need for pacer and procedure for placement.
3. Patient's ECG demonstrates appropriate sensing and capturing.
4. Patient and family accurately demonstrates technique for checking pacer function.

CONGENITAL HEART DISEASE (CHD)

A. **ETIOLOGIC ASPECTS OF CHD**
1. Cardiovascular diseases of all types are familial. CHD is 10% attributable to primarily genetic factors with little environmental influence and 90% attributable to genetic and environmental (multifactorial) interactions of equal importance. CHD occurs in 8% to 10% of every 1000 live births.
2. **Genetic factors:** Genetic causes are most likely associated with a syndrome (e.g., Down syndrome). The recurrence risk of the heart lesion is related to the recurrence risk of the chromosomal anomaly. A single mutant gene usually causes a syndrome. It may have dominant inheritance (e.g., IHSS, ASD). There are autosomal dominant and recessive forms of conduction defects. With Mendelian inheritance the recurrence risk is high.
3. **Genetic-environmental interaction:** Multifactorial inheritance is responsible for most CHD. Hereditary predisposition to cardiovascular maldevelopment interacts with an environmental trigger at the vulnerable period of cardiogenesis. Generally, the recurrence risk is 1% to 4%. The more common the defect, the more likely it is to recur. Risk increases rapidly with the number of first-degree relatives affected. If two first-degree relatives are affected, the risk recurrence is tripled. If three or more first-degree relatives are affected, the risk is a type C classification with a very high recurrence. Teratogenic exposure in the mother may contribute to the incidence of CHD, although proof is lacking in some cases. Usually the exposure is of short duration.
4. **Risk to offspring of the affected parent:** Risks are higher for offspring if the mother has CHD.
5. **Child at risk for atherosclerosis as an adult:** There is a 1% incidence of single-gene hyperlipoproteinemia. Multifactorial inheritance dominates. The single most important risk factor is early onset of coronary disease in a first-degree relative younger than 55 years (heredity 57% to 63%). Environmental factors such as diet, smoking, and exercise can be manipulated to reduce risk factors.
6. **Essential hypertension:** Usually salt intake and stress compound genetic essential hypertension.
7. **Rheumatic fever** originates with streptococcal infections.

B. **NURSING DIAGNOSES FOR CHILDREN WITH CHD**
❖ HIGH RISK FOR INFECTION RELATED TO CARDIAC SURGERY, INVASIVE LINES, AND IMPAIRED CIRCULATION
1. **Defining characteristics** are temperature above 38.5° C; redness, warmth, and

drainage from insertion or incision sites; elevated leukocyte count with increased neutrophils; cloudy urine (leukocytes); rales and rhonchi present on auscultation of lungs; positive blood or wound culture; chest x-ray examination demonstrating consolidation; temperature and glucose instability; feeding intolerance; and thrombocytopenia.

2. **Expected outcome:** Patient is free of infection as evidenced by temperature less than 38.5° C, wounds dry and without redness, normal leukocyte and platelet counts, clear lungs and chest x-ray examination, and tolerance of feedings.

3. **Interventions:** Inspect skin for redness, extreme warmth, or drainage from incisions and peripheral, arterial, and venous lines. Ensure aseptic handling of all IV lines. Administer antibiotics as prescribed. Report elevation in temperature and changes in laboratory data indicative of infectious process (i.e., increased leukocyte count with increased neutrophils). Change IV tubing and dressings as hospital policy dictates. Remove mucus secretions from the respiratory tract. Encourage deep breathing and coughing, use of incentive spirometer, and blowing bubbles. Assess respiratory status and monitor for adventitious breath sounds. Assist the patient to change position or change the patient's position every 2 hours. Monitor hydration status and administer fluids as ordered. Assess for and provide adequate nutrition. Monitor urine for color, odor, and sediment. Discontinue all catheters, IV lines, and drains as soon as possible. Use body substance precautions. Provide appropriate endocarditis prophylaxis and teach these precautions to the family.

4. **Evaluation of nursing care**
   a. All invasive insertion sites are without signs of infection.
   b. Patient is afebrile.
   c. Patient's lungs are clear to auscultation.
   d. Chest x-ray film is clear without atelectasis or infiltrate.
   e. Leukocytosis and thrombocytopenia are absent.
   f. Patient's skin remains intact with normal turgor.

❖ High risk for knowledge deficit related to diagnosis of congenital heart disease (CHD)

❖ Ineffective management of therapeutic regimen related to insufficient knowledge of CHF

1. **Defining characteristics** are requests for information, incorrectly relating instructions taught to them or incorrectly identifying medications, their uses, dosage, time schedule, and side effects. In addition the patient or family member may incorrectly explain the cardiac diagnosis and therapeutic procedures.

2. **Expected outcomes**
   a. Patient or family member verbalizes understanding of the disease process, causes, treatment regimen, and lifestyle changes that must be taken into account to prevent and control complications.
   b. Patient or family member verbalizes symptoms of complications to be reported.
   c. Patient or family member verbalizes understanding of all medications, their uses, dosage, time of administration, and side effects.
   d. Patient or family member verbalizes understanding of diet regimen and restrictions.
   e. Patient or family member verbalizes impact of growth and development and long-term impact of diagnosis and treatment.

3. **Interventions:** Assess and monitor readiness to learn and support systems and determine best methods for teaching and learning (i.e., structured, unstructured). Incorporate the patient's family when possible. Individualize the plan. Plan periods of time for one-to-one interaction with the patient and encourage

questions. Teach the patient or family member about the disease process and its ramifications. Provide printed instructions to take home regarding medications, signs and symptoms, activity regimens, dietary restrictions, and what to do if questions, problems, and signs and symptoms arise. Provide video and booklet teaching while the child is hospitalized. Have the patient or family member demonstrate all psychomotor skills necessary for home care when appropriate. Initiate community health and social service consultations as necessary for follow-up care. Stress need for lifelong follow-up care and the impact on growth and development. Assess ability to provide necessary transportation for care.

4. **Evaluation of nursing care**
   a. Patient or family member relates appropriate compliance factors to all nursing and medical regimens.
   b. Patient or family member is able to return demonstrate correct procedures regarding home self-care measures.
   c. Patient or family member relates symptoms requiring notification of physician and how to do so.

❖ HIGH RISK FOR ALTERED RESPIRATORY FUNCTION
❖ DYSFUNCTIONAL VENTILATORY WEANING PROCESS

1. **Defining characteristics** are tachypnea, dyspnea, grunting, retractions, and flaring. Arterial blood gases may reflect respiratory alkalosis or acidosis and hypoxemia relative to diagnosis. Bilateral rales and rhonchi, decreased breath sounds, prolonged expiratory phase, and wheezing may occur. Mental status changes such as confusion, restlessness, and irritability may occur. Chest x-ray examination shows pulmonary infiltrates, pulmonary edema, pleural effusions, atelectasis, pneumothorax, or elevated hemidiaphragm. Additional characteristics are increased PA pressure, feeding intolerance, lack of appetite, elevated mean and peak airway pressures on ventilator, oversedation or anesthesia with lack of respiratory drive, and paralyzed diaphragm on ECHO or fluoroscopy.

2. **Expected outcomes**
   a. Patient breathes easier, with normal rate, depth of respirations, and work of breathing.
   b. Arterial blood gases are within normal limits for physiology.
   c. Lungs are clear to auscultation, without adventitious lung sounds.
   d. Patient is developmentally appropriate.
   e. Chest x-ray examination is without effusion, atelectasis, and infiltrates.
   f. Hemodynamic parameters are within normal limits.

3. **Interventions:** Assess the patient for level of consciousness and presence of irritability or restlessness. Maintain a patent airway. Monitor MAP and peak inspiratory pressure (PIP) and minimize positive end-expiratory pressure (PEEP). Expand atelectatic lungs with percussion and postural drainage. Monitor the patient's respiratory status by assessing the lungs for signs of infiltrates and observing the patient's color, respiratory rate, and effort. Institute nursing actions to mobilize secretions (e.g., incentive spirometry, changing positions, chest wall percussion and postural drainage, and delivery of humidified oxygen). Maintain fluid restriction and administer diuretic therapy. Correct acid-base disturbances as ordered. Assist with placement of and maintain chest tubes as needed. Maintain adequate nutrition and provide medium- or low-chain fatty acid diet (e.g., Portagen) for chylous effusion. Use hyperventilation, hyperoxygenation, sedation, paralysis, and pulmonary vasodilators (e.g., nitric oxide) in patients with labile pulmonary resistance and elevated PA pressure and avoid noxious stimuli. Assess for signs and symptoms of pulmonary hypertensive crisis, including hypotension, hypoxemia, brady-

cardia, and elevated PA pressure (which may proceed to cardiac arrest). Monitor PA pressure, blood pressure, and arterial blood gases. Use a small size nasogastric tube in infants, since they are obligate nose breathers.

4. **Evaluation of nursing care**
   a. Patient is hemodynamically stable, and vital signs are within the patient's baseline.
   b. Patient is without pulmonary congestion, effusion, or hypertensive crisis.
   c. Lungs are clear to auscultation.
   d. Arterial blood gases are within normal limits for physiology.
   e. Patient is calm or easily soothed.
   f. Patient is able to tolerate diet.

❖ PAIN IN CHILDREN RELATED TO FEAR OR SURGICAL INTERVENTION

1. **Defining characteristics** include description of pain on objective and subjective scoring scale (e.g., Oucher scale), hypertension, tachycardia, crying, grimacing, guarding of incision, tachypnea, grunting, hyperventilation, restlessness, irritability, and poor feeding.

2. **Expected outcomes**
   a. Patient verbalizes comfort level or low pain scale score.
   b. Patient rests comfortably without restlessness, agitation, tachycardia, or hypertension.

3. **Interventions:** Assess factors that decrease pain tolerance such as age, culture, parental or familial anxiety, child's anxiety, and fear. Determine the child's concept of the cause of pain. Subjectively and objectively assess pain and response to treatment using accepted pain scoring tools and response to treatment. Prepare the patient and family for procedures. Use anesthesia, sedatives, narcotics, or analgesics as necessary and provide accurate information to alleviate the patient's or family's fear of addiction. Provide safe areas and periods of rest using distraction, relaxation, and touch techniques as possible. Reduce or eliminate narcotic side effects (administer stool softeners and antiemetics as needed). Assess ability for patient-controlled analgesia. Consult with the physician about the use of epidural morphine or narcotic. If at all possible avoid the use of intramuscular (IM) pain medications. Identify coping behaviors and observe for these to assist the child in coping with pain. Initiate health teaching and referrals, if appropriate.

4. **Evaluation of nursing care**
   a. Patient remains with normal sleep-awake cycles.
   b. Patient's pain is controlled, and hemodynamic parameters are at baseline.

❖ TISSUE PERFUSION, ALTERED CARDIOPULMONARY

1. **Defining characteristics** are hypotension, tachycardia, oliguria, dysrhythmias, edema evidenced by weight gain of more than 30 g/d, irritability, restlessness, failure to thrive, poor weight gain, cool, mottled extremities, delayed capillary refill, decreased peripheral pulses, excessive volume loss through chest drains, acidosis, hypoxemia, presence of extra heart sounds (S_3, S_4), hepatomegaly, splenomegaly, and fever.

2. **Expected outcome**
   a. Heart rate and blood pressure appropriate for age
   b. Urine output 0.5 to 1 ml/kg/h
   c. Weight gain not in excess of 30 g/d
   d. Dysrhythmia controlled; conduction disturbance resolved
   e. Warm, perfused extremities with palpable peripheral pulses
   f. Weaned from all IV inotropic agents and ventilatory support
   g. Volume status stabilized as evidenced by clear lungs on physical and x-ray examination; balanced intake and output
   h. Laboratory values reflect balanced electrolytes and acid-base balance

3. **Interventions**
   a. Maintain adequate preload: Monitor CVP, and PA and LA pressures and administer volume infusions as ordered (10 ml/kg bolus). Maintain accurate intake and output; record and weigh patient daily. Administer diuretics as ordered. Monitor signs of tamponade from pericardial effusion or surgical bleeding such as increased filling pressures, decreased perfusion, oliguria, acidosis, poor peripheral pulses, cool extremities, muffled heart sounds, decreased mean arterial pressure, and abrupt cessation of chest tube drainage or persistence of bleeding greater than 10% of blood volume per hour for more than 3 hours. Assess coagulation studies and infuse appropriate clotting factors as needed. Monitor for enlarged cardiac silhouette on x-ray examination. Assist with reexploration of the chest in the PICU if necessary or return to the operating room. Maintain chest tube patency.
   b. Reduce afterload: Use vasodilators as ordered to improve ventricular ejection or decrease valvular regurgitation, or do both. Monitor blood pressure. Monitor patient's temperature and assure normothermia.
   c. Assure normal cardiac rate and rhythm: Pace for rate (tachycardia or bradycardia) and AV synchrony or to improve cardiac output. Monitor ECG and institute appropriate antidysrhythmic medications (monitor drug levels).
   d. Support myocardial contractility: Administer positive inotropic drugs. Provide bed rest and rest periods. Observe for changes in level of consciousness, irritability, or restlessness. Obtain arterial and venous oxygen saturations for AV oxygen difference and monitor cardiac output.
   e. Administer pain medication and sedatives as ordered.
   f. Provide nutritional support using high-calorie formula and nasogastric supplementation to maintain calories for hypermetabolic state. Provide total parenteral nutrition if the patient is unable to tolerate gastric feedings. Consult with nutritional support team as needed.
   g. Administer oxygen and ventilation support as needed.
   h. Assess for decrease in hepatomegaly or splenomegaly with treatment.
   i. Monitor laboratory data especially electrolytes, arterial blood gases, hematocrit, hemoglobin, and thyroid functions.
   j. Provide explanations and support to the patient and family.
   k. Assess for changes in level of consciousness, bulging fontanelle, or seizures.
4. **Evaluation of nursing care**
   a. Patient or family member lists symptoms of CHF and actions and side effects of medications.
   b. Patient or family member lists signs and symptoms of tamponade from pericardial effusion and action to take.
   c. Family member relates need for high-calorie formula and is able to provide feedings orally or by nasogastric supplementation.
   d. Patient's heart rate and blood pressure are age appropriate.
   e. Patient is calm and not irritable.
   f. Cardiac rhythm is normal, without dysrhythmia or conduction disturbance.
   g. Blood gases and electrolytes reflect adequate tissue perfusion.
❖ POTENTIAL COMPLICATION: FLUID VOLUME EXCESS
1. **Defining characteristics** are edema (peripheral, facial, periorbital, bulging fontanelle), weight gain in excess of 30 g/d, shiny skin or woody extremities, diaphoresis, shortness of breath, dyspnea, tachypnea, retractions, flaring, grunting, mouth breathing, possible rales, wheezes, prolonged expiratory phase, restlessness, irritability, fatigue, decreased oxygen saturation, dilutional

hypovolemia, resulting in a low hematocrit, sodium, potassium, chloride, and albumin, tachycardia with or without dysrhythmia, hypertension, hepatomegaly, splenomegaly, ascites, elevated filling pressures (RA, CVP, LA), evidence of pulmonary edema (pleural effusion on chest x-ray examination), and immobility due to illness.

2. **Expected outcomes**
   a. Weight gain will be appropriate.
   b. Respiratory functions will be normalized and chest x-ray examination will be clear of edema or effusion.
   c. Vital signs, liver and spleen size, and filling pressures will remain at baseline for age and sex.
   d. Laboratory studies will reflect a normal volume state.
   e. Patient will rest comfortably.
   f. Intake and output will be balanced.
   g. No edema will be present.
   h. Skin will remain intact.

3. **Interventions**
   a. Protect edematous skin from injury. Inspect skin for redness and blanching, breaks in skin, and bony prominence integrity. Reduce the pressure on skin areas by turning the patient at least every 2 hours or by use of a pressure reduction surface. Provide adequate nutrition.
   b. Accurately record intake and output and administer medications (albumin, diuretics, electrolyte replacements) as ordered. Maintain fluid restriction by using high-calorie formula. Administer renal dose dopamine as ordered. Assess weight daily. Monitor serum electrolytes, albumin, BUN, creatinine, and hematocrit.
   c. Assist with chest x-ray examination and abdominal ultrasound.
   d. Assist with ultrafiltration, peritoneal drain, ascites, peritoneal dialysis, hemofiltration, and hemodialysis.
   e. Assist with placement of chest tubes or thoracentesis for pleural effusion. EMLA cream to chest wall prior to procedure may be helpful. Maintain 10 to 15 cm water suction to chest tubes.
   f. Monitor pulse oximetry and arterial blood gases. Provide oxygen and ventilatory support as needed. Monitor peak and mean ventilatory pressures.

4. **Evaluation of nursing care**
   a. No evidence of skin breakdown
   b. Chest x-ray examination free of edema or effusion
   c. Respiratory effort normal
   d. Vital signs normal for age and sex
   e. Balanced intake and output
   f. Normal electrolyte values
   g. Weight gain less than 30 g/d
   h. Patient or family member correctly states reason for edema and treatment course

C. **CONGENITAL HEART DISEASE (CHD) CLASSIFICATIONS**
   1. **Acyanotic lesions** usually are left-to-right shunts. Blood shunts from areas of high to low resistance. These defects generally have symptoms of pulmonary overcirculation from RV and PA volume and pressure loading, which may result in symptoms of CHF.
   2. **Obstructive lesions** produce restrictive blood flow across the stenotic area with hypertensive changes proximal to the obstruction; obstructive lesions may have hypoperfusion states distally.

3. **Cyanotic lesions** usually have obstruction (mechanical [i.e., tricuspid atresia] or anatomic [i.e., total anomalous pulmonary venous return, TAPVR]) to pulmonary blood flow, mandating obligatory right-to-left shunting for blood to enter the pulmonary circulation. This results in intracardiac and extra-cardiac mixing of saturated and desaturated blood and cyanosis. Cyanotic symptomatology is related to the degree and number of right-to-left shunts. Cyanosis may also result from anatomically malposed vessels (i.e., transposition of the great vessels [TGV]).

D. ACYANOTIC PHYSIOLOGY
  1. **Expected outcomes**
     a. Patient or family member will state the need for lifelong cardiovascular follow-up including endocarditis prophylaxis preoperatively and if shunt is placed.
     b. Patient will have no evidence of hemodynamically significant residual shunt on ECHO or examination.
     c. Operative intervention will occur before irreversible pulmonary vascular obstructive disease (PVOD) or severe ventricular dysfunction occurs.
     d. Patient's symptoms of CHF will resolve and growth and development will resume on a normal curve.
     e. Patient or family member can state signs and symptoms of CHF.
     f. Patient's exercise tolerance will be within normal limits for age, or patient or family member will state activity limitations if imposed.
     g. Patient is free of dysrhythmia and conduction disturbances, or the condition will be controlled with medications or with a pacemaker.
     h. Hemodynamic parameters will be normal for age and sex.
  2. **Patent ductus arteriosus (PDA):** Persistence of a normal fetal channel connecting the aorta and pulmonary artery
     a. *Pathophysiology*
        • In fetal life, the ductus arteriosus permits flow to be diverted away from the high-resistance pulmonary circulation to the descending aorta and the low-resistance placental circulation.
        • Closure of the ductus arteriosus normally occurs from contraction of the medial smooth muscle in the wall of the ductus arteriosus in the first 12 to 24 hours after birth, which is initiated by a rise in the perivascular PO_2 and decreased endogenous prostaglandin. This produces functional closure; however, the ductus may be reopened at this point in response to a strong stimulus such as acidosis, hypoxemia, or prostaglandins. Anatomic closure occurs between 2 and 3 weeks and is produced by fibrosis of the ductal tissue with permanent sealing of the lumen to produce the ligamentum arteriosum. Following anatomic closure, the ductus cannot be reopened.
        • In cases where the ductus fails to close normally, blood shunts from left to right into the pulmonary artery and lungs. This occurs as the PVR drops and the pressure in the aorta exceeds that of the pulmonary artery. Pulmonary blood flow increases, thus increasing venous return to the left atrium, and LA and LV volume overload and CHF ensue. Over time, the increased flow and pressure on the pulmonary circulation changes the pulmonary vasculature, resulting in PA hypertension and increased PVR. Once these changes have progressed from medial hypertrophy and intimal hyperplasia to fibrosis of the pulmonary bed, they are irreversible and result in pulmonary hypertension and reversal of the cardiac shunt. Blood is then shunted right to left, causing cyanosis. This reversal of shunt flow due to changes in the pulmonary vascular

bed from pressure and volume overload is known as Eisenmenger's syndrome. Once reversal of shunt flow has occurred, surgical closure of the defect is contraindicated.

- The presence of a large PDA results in a low diastolic pressure. This may adversely affect myocardial function from poor coronary perfusion.

b. *Etiology and incidence:* In preterm infants the response to the vasoconstrictor stimulus of oxygen is not developed, resulting in persistence of the ductus arteriosus. The incidence of PDA in full-term infants accounts for about 5% to 10% of all types of CHD. Failure to close in this population is related to a structural defect in the wall of the ductus. Exposure to rubella during the first trimester of pregnancy is associated with PDA.

c. *Assessment*

- The *presentation* depends on the degree of shunting, compensatory mechanisms, and the stage of lung development. Full-term neonates have elevated PVR, and therefore shunting is not as pronounced. Premature infants may have severe low cardiac output and require emergency closure to restore adequate diastolic pressure and perfusion of the myocardium, as well as other organs. Small PDAs with small shunts rarely produce symptoms, and growth and development are normal. Moderate and large defects produce symptoms of CHF from the left-to-right shunt and LV volume overload.
- *Examination* reveals a machinery like continuous murmur auscultated at the left upper sternal border. Poor feeding, irritability, tachycardia, tachypnea, and slow weight gain are often present. The pulse pressure is wide, and pulses may be bounding.

d. *Diagnostic findings*

- *ECG* shows prominent LV forces, LA hypertrophy, and possibly RVH.
- *Chest x-ray examination* shows enlargement of the cardiac silhouette with LA and LV enlargement. The main pulmonary artery (MPA) segment is prominent. The pulmonary vascular markings are accentuated in moderate to large shunts.
- *Echocardiogram* demonstrates an increased LA diameter, and an estimate of the shunt may be made from the left atrium-to-aorta ratio.
- *Cardiac catheterization* is rarely performed. If done, it will demonstrate a step up in oxygen concentration in the pulmonary artery. The pulmonary artery pressure and resistance can also be evaluated and in large shunts may be elevated.

e. *Intervention*

- Medical therapy involves control of CHF with medications or closure of the ductus with indomethacin once normal kidney function and an adequate platelet count are assured.
- Interventional catheterization can be performed to provide closure with the Rashkind device or Gianturco coils only in a small- or moderate-sized ductus.
- Surgical closure involves division or ligation (or both) of the ductus through a left thoracotomy. Postoperative complications are rare but may include damage to the recurrent laryngeal nerve, chylous effusion, bleeding, infection, paralyzed phrenic nerve, ligation of the left pulmonary artery or descending aorta, or tear in the ductus or aorta.

3. **Atrial septal defect (ASD):** A defect in the atrial septum from improper embryologic formation of the septal wall

a. *Classifications*

- *Sinus venosus:* High in the septum near the junction of the SVC and right atrium associated with partial anomalous pulmonary venous return (PAPVR).

- *Ostium secundum:* Most common; region fossa ovalis cordis; may be associated with mitral valve prolapse (MVP).
- *Ostium primum:* Low in septum, may involve defects of one or both AV valves.
- *Unroofed coronary sinus:* Coronary sinus blood is diverted to the left atrium.

b. *Pathophysiology:* The defect is created by failure of the endocardial cushion tissue to seal the septum primum (ostium primum defect), failure of the valve of the fossa ovalis cordis to close (patent foramen ovale), or failure of closure of the septal fenestration (ostium secundum defect). Defects allow blood to be shunted from the higher pressure left side of the heart to the lower pressure right side of the heart, resulting in RV volume and pressure overload with RA and RV dilation. Pulmonary vascular changes occur in 10% to 20% of patients and are a result of intimal proliferation and medial hypertrophy of the pulmonary vessels. Progression to fibrosis results in reversal of shunt flow, cyanosis, RV failure, and eventual death. This is known as Eisenmenger's syndrome. By the third to fourth decade of life atrial dysrhythmias, CHF, and paradoxical embolus become problems. Endocarditis is uncommon.

c. *Etiology:* Failure of the septum to form in the fetal period results in defects in the atrial septal wall.

d. *Assessment*
- Most patients are asymptomatic but with large left-to-right shunts may exhibit symptoms of fatigue and dyspnea. Growth retardation is unusual.
- *Examination:* Auscultation reveals a systolic ejection murmur at the LSB (pulmonary flow murmur); wide, fixed, split S_2; and a diastolic murmur from large volume flow across the tricuspid valve.

e. *Diagnostic findings*
- *ECG* demonstrates right ventricular and atrial hypertrophy, right axis deviation, RBBB, prolonged PR interval, and possibly evidence of junctional rhythm or a supraventricular tachyarrhythmia.
- *Chest x-ray examination* shows RVH, right atrial enlargement, and increased pulmonary vascular markings, but heart size may be normal.
- *Echocardiogram* confirms the diagnosis in the majority of cases with evidence of right ventricular volume overload, direct visualization of location and size of defect, and identification of associated defects (most commonly anomalous pulmonary veins or pulmonary stenosis).
- Cardiac catheterization is rarely indicated. It demonstrates an increase in oxygen saturation in the right atrium.

f. *Intervention*
- Repair of the defect is low risk and is recommended despite patient age and presentation to prevent long-term problems with pulmonary disease and dysrhythmia. Secundum defects may be closed via a right thoracotomy (if there are no associated intracardiac defects) or through a sternotomy. Both require a short period of cardiopulmonary bypass. The defect may be closed directly or patched.
- Interventional device closure has been successfully performed; however, both devices (clamshell and button) are on hold with the Food and Drug Administration (FDA) at this time.
- Postoperative problems specific to this operation include atrial dysrhythmia, heart block, residual defect, anemia, and AV valve regurgitation in ostium primum defects.

4. **Ventricular septal defect (VSD):** Communication between the right and left ventricle created by an opening in the septal wall
    a. *Classification* (Fig. 3–30)
        • *Perimembranous* is the most common VSD and is located below the crista supraventricularis adjacent to the tricuspid valve. It may be associated with malalignment of the septum.

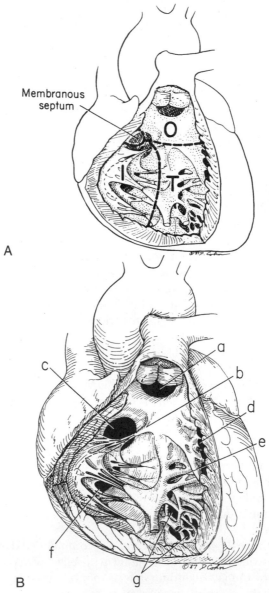

Figure 3–30.   A, Ventricular septum viewed from the right ventricular side is made up of four components: *I,* Inlet extends from the tricuspid annulus to attachments of tricuspid valve; *T,* trabecular septum extends from inlet out to apex and up to smooth walled outlet; *O,* outlet septum or infundibular septum extends up to pulmonary valve and membranous septum. **B,** Anatomic position of defects. *a,* Outlet defect; *b,* papillary muscle of the conus; *c,* perimembranous defect; *d,* marginal muscular defects; *e,* central muscular defects; *f,* inlet defect; *g,* apical muscular defects. (Reprinted with permission from Adams FH, Emmanoulides GC, Riemenschneider TA. *Moss' Heart Disease in Infants, Children, and Adolescents.* 4th ed. Baltimore, Md: Williams & Wilkins; 1989.)

- *Infundibular, subpulmonic, subarterial, conal, and supracristal VSDs* are positioned in the RV outflow tract under the pulmonary valve.
- *Inlet VSD* is a common defect in atrioventricular septal defect (AVSD) located under the AV valve posterior and inferior to the membranous septum.
- *Muscular defects* are located in the muscular septum. If multiple, they are called "Swiss cheese" septum.

b. *Pathophysiology*
- Effects of the VSD depend on the size and number of the defects and resistance to flow through the lungs (flow is also affected by the presence of RV outflow tract obstruction). VSDs may present as small defects with normal pulmonary vascular resistance (PVR), moderate defects with variable PVR, or as large defects with either mild to moderate or marked elevation of PVR.
- Assess size of the defect, magnitude of hemodynamic overload, and status of pulmonary vasculature.
- Children are usually asymptomatic until 2 to 4 weeks of age when PVR drops. The drop in PVR allows shunting from the left ventricle to the right ventricle and creates pulmonary overcirculation. Long-term pulmonary overcirculation causes PA hypertension and vascular changes progressing from medial hypertrophy and intimal hyperplasia to fibrosis and Eisenmenger's syndrome (rarely before 1 year of age).

c. *Etiology and incidence:* Defect results from imperfect embryologic formation of the septal wall. VSD is the most common congenital heart defect (20% of all defects) and is slightly more common in girls.

d. *Assessment*
- *Presentation* is dependent on the size of the shunt and PVR.
- *Examination* reveals a holosystolic murmur at the left sternal border (LSB), normal S_1, split and increased S_2, possible S_3, thrill at the LSB, active precordium, and a diastolic rumble at the LSB in large defects. The murmur decreases as PVR increases.

e. *Diagnostic findings*
- *ECG:* Small defects have normal ECG findings. Moderate to large defects have LA enlargement, LVH with or without RVH, left axis deviation, and bundle branch block.
- *Chest x-ray examination:* Small defects have normal x-ray findings. Moderate to large defects have cardiomegaly, prominent PA segment, and increased pulmonary vascular markings.
- *Echocardiogram* confirms location, size of defect, associated lesions, and LA and LV dilation; ECHO also quantifies the degree of RV and PA hypertension.
- *Cardiac catheterization* demonstrates an elevated pulmonary-to-systemic flow ratio ($Q_p : Q_s$); elevated RV and PA pressures; elevated PVR in large defects; and oxygen step up in the right ventricle and pulmonary artery.

f. *Interventions*
- Indications for intervention include CHF, PA hypertension or evidence for LV volume overload. Some defects close spontaneously. Medical management is used for control of CHF (see Congestive Heart Failure).
- Surgical palliation is rarely done and consists of controlling pulmonary blood flow and protecting the pulmonary vascular bed. It is indicated mainly for large multiple muscular VSDs in the lower septum because these cannot be easily approached surgically in infancy. PA banding via a

left thoracotomy aims to decrease the pressure distal to the band to approximately one half the aortic pressure but may not restrict flow adequately. Surgery poses the risk of chylothorax, phrenic nerve palsy, and damage to the recurrent laryngeal nerve. Complications include migration of the band, distortion of the vessels, failure to adequately protect the other lung, erosion of the band into the pulmonary artery, creation of subaortic stenosis from septal hypertrophy, and damage to the pulmonary valve.

- Device closure is experimental and on hold by the FDA. It is useful in the difficult-to-reach VSD such as apical muscular VSDs. Sometimes, more than one device is required. The device also may not achieve full closure, may pose a risk to the tricuspid valve, and may dislodge.
- For large, hemodynamically important defects, surgical closure is performed at any age to prevent endocarditis and PVOD. A sternotomy on cardiopulmonary bypass is used with circulatory arrest in anatomically difficult lesions or in small patients. Apical VSDs may require limited ventriculotomy (left ventricle). Usually defects are closed by a patch as opposed to suturing. Complications include systemic hypertension resulting from the removal of a large left-to-right shunt, damage to aortic valve, heart block, or pulmonary hypertensive crisis. Repair prior to 2 years usually permits normalization of growth and reversal of developmental delays.

5. **Atrioventricular septal defect (AVSD):** A defect in the atrial and ventricular wall and various degrees of AV valve regurgitation due to deficiency of the endocardial cushion tissue
   a. *Types of AVSD*
      - *Balanced:* Ventricles equal in size
      - *Unbalanced:* One ventricle larger; classified into forms of single ventricular lesions
      - *Incomplete:* Separate AV valve orifices (ostium primum defect)
      - *Complete:* Common AV valve orifice usually with five leaflets
   b. *Pathophysiology:* AVSD is characterized by large ASDs and VSDs and a common AV valve. Physiology is similar to ASD and VSD where shunting of blood is related to the size of intracardiac septal defects, AV valve competency, PVR, and PA pressure. Usually left-to-right shunting occurs once PVR decreases, causing pulmonary overcirculation, elevation in PA pressure, and eventual rise in PVR from long-standing pressure and volume overload. A severely regurgitant AV valve leads to early symptoms of CHF and low cardiac output. This may increase PA pressure and PVR and is difficult to treat medically or surgically.
   c. *Etiology:* Embryologic deficiency of the endocardial cushion tissue results in ostium primum atrial defect, common AV orifice, inlet VSD, malrotation of the aortic valve, elongation and narrowing of the left ventricular outflow tract (LVOT), and abnormal attachment of the AV valve to the ventricular septum. AVSD is often associated with Down syndrome.
   d. *Assessment*
      - *Symptoms* of CHF and pulmonary overcirculation usually occur in early infancy from a large increase in pulmonary blood flow and are associated with elevated PA pressure and complicated by insufficiency of the common AV valve.
      - Usually patients are small and undernourished. Oxygen saturation is normal except in the presence of pulmonary vascular disease in older children or accelerated disease in an infant. Desaturation can result from

ventilation-perfusion ($\dot{V}/\dot{Q}$) mismatch from pulmonary changes secondary to a large left-to-right shunt.

- *Examination:* Auscultation reveals a systolic ejection murmur at the LSB, middiastolic murmur at the lower LSB and apex from AV valve regurgitation, and a split prominent S_2.

e. *Diagnostic findings*
- *ECG* findings are normal sinus rhythm (NSR); prolonged PR interval; right atrial, left atrial, or bilateral atrial enlargement; bundle branch block, and left axis or northwest axis deviation.
- *Chest x-ray examination* shows an enlarged heart, enlarged right atrium, prominent pulmonary artery, and increased pulmonary vascular markings.
- *Echocardiogram* visualizes the VSD and ASD. Both right- and left-sided components of the common AV valve are displaced into the ventricles and are associated with variable deficiency related to the inflow of the ventricular septum. An echocardiogram predicts noninvasive estimates of PA pressure and can quantitate the degree of AV valve regurgitation.
- *Cardiac catheterization* demonstrates an increase in oxygen saturation throughout the right side of the heart; elevated PA pressure and PVR may be present and may or may not be responsive to oxygen.

f. *Intervention*
- Medical treatment of CHF is usually initiated early, and attempts are made to achieve control of the CHF and promote weight gain (see Congestive Heart Failure)
- Surgical repair is recommended for any symptomatic infant to prevent early development of pulmonary vascular disease. Surgery involves a sternotomy and cardiopulmonary bypass with or without circulatory arrest. One or two patches are used, depending on the preference of the surgeon. The VSD is closed, and the AV valve is partially anchored to the patch. The atrial component of the patch is partially sewn in place, the AV valve repair is completed, and the atrial defect is closed.
- Complications include heart block, pulmonary hypertensive crisis (rapid fall in blood pressure and heart rate with concomitant rise in PAP to systemic or suprasystemic levels treated with hyperventilation, hyperoxygenation, pulmonary vasodilators including nitric oxide, sedation, and paralysis), residual shunt, and residual AV valve regurgitation or stenosis (can be detected by left atrial, right atrial, or central venous pressure and tracing on bedside monitor).

6. **Double outlet right ventricle (DORV):** Origins of both great arteries from a morphologic right ventricle
  a. *Pathophysiology*
  - DORV encompasses features of a wide variety of entities including VSD, tetralogy of Fallot, and transposition of the great arteries. Both great arteries arise from the right ventricle; usually a VSD is present, and varying degrees of pulmonary stenosis may exist. The great arteries may be in normal position, side by side, dextroposition, or levoposition. The VSD may be subaortic, subpulmonic (Taussig-Bing syndrome), or doubly committed (a large VSD related to both semilunar valves).
  - Physiology is based on the degree of pulmonary stenosis and the relationship of the VSD to the pulmonary artery and aorta. Blood enters the right side of the heart normally. RV output flows to the lowest resistance circuit. Without pulmonary stenosis blood flow to the lungs is unrestricted, and significant pulmonary overcirculation and PVOD

occur. If pulmonary stenosis is present, blood may exit to the pulmonary artery and aorta. The more severe the obstruction, the greater the flow to the aorta.

b. *Etiology and incidence:* DORV is a rare defect (0.09/1000 live births) in a spectrum of transposed complexes. DORV is related to failure to achieve conotruncal inversion (rotation) and leftward shift of the conal (aortic or pulmonic) segment of both great vessels from the right ventricle.

c. *Assessment* depends on the anatomic variant

- Subaortic VSD with pulmonary stenosis is similar to tetralogy of Fallot: Cyanosis, clubbing, exertional dyspnea, polycythemia, RV impulse at LSB, loud systolic ejection murmur, normal S_1, and single S_2.
- Subpulmonic VSD with or without pulmonary stenosis resembles TGV: Cyanosis early, precordial bulge, high-pitched systolic murmur at the upper LSB, and single S_2.
- Subaortic VSD without pulmonary stenosis is similar to a simple VSD: Active precordium, holosystolic murmur at the LSB, and an apical diastolic rumble.
- Subaortic VSD with no pulmonary stenosis but PVOD is the same as Eisenmenger's syndrome: Cyanosis, clubbing, S_2 loud and single, and a diastolic murmur of pulmonary insufficiency may be heard.

d. *Diagnostic findings*

- *ECG* shows RVH, right axis deviation, normal to increased LV forces, first-degree AV conduction delay, and RA enlargement.
- *Chest x-ray examination:* With pulmonary stenosis, mild cardiomegaly, absent main PA segment, and decreased pulmonary vascularity occur. Without PS, cardiomegaly, increased pulmonary vascularity, and prominent main PA segment are demonstrated. With PVOD, "pruning" of the peripheral pulmonary vascular bed occurs.
- *Echocardiogram* displays mitral and semilunar discontinuity, origin of both great vessels from the anterior right ventricle, absence of LV outflow except through the VSD, associated lesions, and accurate position of the VSD.
- *Cardiac catheterization* results are variable, depending on anatomy. It is helpful in quantitating PAP and PVR.

e. *Interventions*

- Intracardiac repair involves closing the VSD via sternotomy and bypass and sometimes circulatory arrest. Without pulmonary stenosis, early surgery helps to protect the pulmonary vascular bed. Patients may require arterial switch and VSD closure. They may also require an intracardiac baffle to close the defect and route LV flow to the aorta. Neonates may require palliation with PA banding (see Ventricular Septal Defect).
- If pulmonary stenosis is associated, the VSD is closed to reestablish LV-aortic continuity and provide RV-PA continuity. With severe pulmonary stenosis, an RV-PA conduit is required; this conduit will need to be replaced later. If the pulmonary stenosis is mild, it may require only valvotomy or a transannular patch. For infants with a significant degree of pulmonary stenosis, stabilization on prostaglandins followed by palliation with a systemic-to-pulmonary shunt may be necessary.
- Endocarditis is a lifelong risk.

7. **Ebstein's anomaly:** Downward displacement of posterior and septal leaflets of the tricuspid valve with the atrialized portion of the right ventricle.

a. *Pathophysiology*
- Anatomy of the valve is variable, but there is always redundancy of valve tissue and adherence of medial and posterior leaflets to the RV wall. An atrialized right ventricle occurs from downward displacement of the tricuspid valve. The RV function is dependent on the amount atrialized (Fig. 3–31). It is common to have associated anomalies including ASD or patent foramen ovale, VSD, or WPW.
- Physiology depends on the degree of malformation of the tricuspid valve. Mild anomalies may have normal valve function. With severe malformation, cyanosis can occur from right-to-left shunting through the ASD related to massive tricuspid regurgitation and elevated RA pressure. Blood enters the right atrium normally but on entering the right ventricle regurgitates into the right atrium because of tricuspid insufficiency. In rare circumstances, the tricuspid valve may be stenotic and cause RA dilation due to elevated pressure across the stenotic valve.
- Tricuspid insufficiency in newborns may improve, as neonatal elevation of PVR and hence RV hypertension normally regress, thus decreasing cyanosis.

b. *Etiology and incidence:* Ebstein's anomaly constitutes 0.5% of CHD. The perforations that result in the formation of the chordae tendineae and papillary muscles fail to develop, resulting in tissue redundancy. Unusually high incidence occurs in infants of mothers who are taking lithium.

c. *Assessment*
- History varies based on the degree of tricuspid valve deformity. Cyanosis

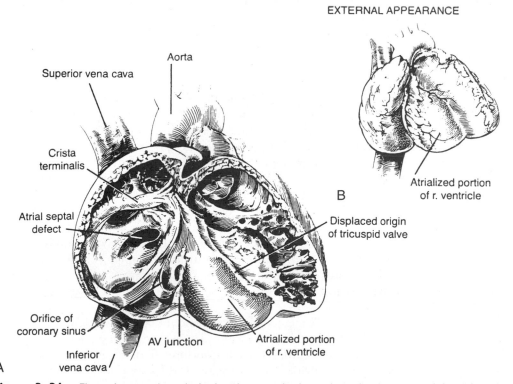

Figure 3–31. Ebstein's anomaly with displaced tricuspid valve and atrialized portion of the right ventricle. (Reprinted with permission from Castaneda AR, Jonas RA, Mayer JE, Hanley FL. *Cardiac Surgery of the Neonate and Infant.* Philadelphia, Pa: WB Saunders Co; 1994.)

may be noted in the neonate; the cyanosis disappears over the next few weeks and returns by age 5 to 10 years. Severe tricuspid insufficiency in neonates involves low cardiac output, hepatomegaly, and cyanosis. After infancy, dyspnea on exertion and fatigue may occur. Dysrhythmias are common (50%). Growth and development are usually normal.
  - *Examination* reveals normal cardiac impulse, variable intensity systolic murmur, normal S_1, and possibly a click. If asymptomatic, the S_2 is normal. If symptomatic, the S_2 is diminished or single and an S_3 or S_4 or both may be heard. Hepatomegaly may be present.
  d. *Diagnostic findings*
  - *ECG* findings are always abnormal. RBBB shows a right axis deviation, right axis enlargement, and a prolonged PR interval. WPW may occur (in 5% to 20% of cases).
  - *Chest x-ray examination* in the symptomatic infant demonstrates at least moderate, if not massive, cardiomegaly with decreased pulmonary vascular markings. Asymptomatic children have normal to slight enlargement of heart size and normal pulmonary vascular markings with RA enlargement of varying degree.
  - *Echocardiogram* demonstrates delayed tricuspid valve closure. Valve displacement is present with a sail-like anterior leaflet of the tricuspid valve. Other anatomic findings, specifically RV size or ASD and eccentric coaptation of the tricuspid valve leaflets, can be defined.
  - *Cardiac catheterization* is not necessary to delineate anatomy. Since dysrhythmias are common, mapping of WPW is warranted. Cardiac catheterization will also demonstrate the portion of the right ventricle that is functioning as the right atrium.
  e. *Interventions*
  - No surgery may be required, or tricuspid valvuloplasty with ASD closure and excision of redundant RA wall may be required to relieve cyanosis and prevent paradoxical embolus. Valvuloplasty is more effective in older patients. Often they require tricuspid valve replacement if valvuloplasty is not effective, usually with plication of the right atrium.
  - For severely symptomatic neonates, prognosis is poor, since stabilization of the newborn is difficult. Sometimes the tricuspid valve is patched to create tricuspid atresia, and a systemic to pulmonic shunt is created. This is done with cardiopulmonary bypass and deep hypothermic circulatory arrest via sternotomy. These patients will go on to single ventricle second stage repair with cavopulmonary shunt and final stage repair with the Fontan procedure. Cardiac transplantation for the neonate with severe Ebstein's anomaly is another option.
  - Ablation (radiofrequency or surgical) of WPW may be required.
  - These patients are at risk for endocarditis. Competitive sports and contact activity are restricted.
E. **OBSTRUCTIVE PHYSIOLOGY**
  1. **Expected outcomes**
    a. Patient or family member will state need for lifelong cardiovascular follow-up, potential reoperation for valvular regurgitation or stenosis, need for endocarditis prophylaxis, and activity limitations of the disease state.
    b. Patient or family member will state ideal PT and side effects of warfarin (Coumadin) where appropriate.
    c. Patient or family member will state action, potential side effects, and complications of all medications.
    d. Patient or family member will state signs and symptoms of CHF.

e. Patient's growth and development will be stable.

f. Intervention will occur before development of severe ventricular dysfunction or pulmonary vascular obstructive disease (PVOD).

g. Systemic hypertension will be controlled to within the 90th percentile for age and sex.

h. Hemodynamic parameters will be normal for age and sex.

2. **Aortic stenosis (AS):** Malformation of the aortic valve that causes obstruction to ejection of blood from the left ventricle.

a. **Valvular aortic stenosis:** Obstruction occurs at the valve annulus.

- *Pathophysiology:* Associated cardiac lesions such as PDA, VSD, or coarctation are common. Valve tissue is thick and rigid with diminished commissural separation of varying degrees, but leaflets are mobile in children. Most often the valve is bicuspid with a single, fused commissure and eccentrically placed orifice. The valve annulus may be hypoplastic (less than 4 to 5 mm). With severe stenosis the left ventricle develops concentric hypertrophy, decreased LV function, compromised myocardial blood flow, elevated LVEDP, and poststenotic dilation of the ascending aorta. Valvular gradients can give some estimation of the degree of stenosis. This number may be misleading in instances of low cardiac output, where output across the valve is already diminished and the gradient may be falsely low. Estimations of valvular gradients used to quantitate severity and guide interventional decisions are (1) mild: 5 to 49 mm Hg, (2) moderate: 50 to 75 mm Hg, and (3) severe: >75 mm Hg. Subendocardial or endocardial fibroelastosis may occur in utero if the stenosis is severe and does not regress after repair. Therefore, despite adequate relief of the stenosis, LV function may be permanently compromised. Complications include endocarditis, sudden death, development of valvular insufficiency, and dysrhythmias.

- *Etiology* and incidence: Aortic stenosis occurs more frequently in boys and occurs in about 3% to 6% of congenital heart defects. It may be associated with nonimmunologic hydrops fetalis.

- *Assessment:* Most children are asymptomatic and grow and develop normally. If symptoms occur, they usually involve fatigue, exertional dyspnea, angina pectoris, and syncope with at least moderate aortic stenosis. Severe aortic stenosis has rapid symptoms of CHF and may even have the presentation of hypoplastic left heart syndrome (HLHS). Examination reveals LV lift, precordial systolic thrill, systolic aortic ejection murmur or ejection click, S_2 delayed or split, S_3, and on occasion a diastolic murmur of aortic insufficiency.

- *Diagnostic findings*
  - *ECG* findings may vary with severity but usually include T wave inversion, deep S wave in V_1, LV strain, LVH, and ST segment depression.
  - *Exercise testing* is used to evaluate blood pressure response and ECG changes with exercise. A fall or a lack of rise in systolic blood pressure suggests the presence of severe obstruction.
  - *Chest x-ray examination* demonstrates normal to minimal enlargement of heart size; rounding of the cardiac apex; LA enlargement if stenosis is severe; pulmonary congestion and enlargement of the pulmonary artery, right ventricle, and right atrium; and poststenotic dilation of the ascending aorta.
  - *Echocardiogram* shows diminished systolic valve movement and demonstrates the anatomy of the valve leaflets, an increase in LV wall

thickness, transvalvular aortic gradients, end-diastolic dimensions to predict LV peak systolic pressure, and associated cardiac anatomy.

○ *Cardiac catheterization* is more important to establish the site and severity of the stenosis, define associated anomalies, measure cardiac output, and assess valve gradients.

- *Interventions:* Congenital aortic stenosis is a progressive lesion, and most affected children require intervention at least once. The earlier the intervention is required, the greater the likelihood that further intervention will be required later in life. Intervention is recommended when severe symptoms or LV strain or syncope is present. Stabilization of the neonate with critical aortic stenosis requires prostaglandin therapy to establish systemic perfusion through the PDA from the pulmonary artery to the aorta.

  ○ Interventional catheterization or balloon valvuloplasty is successful in opening the valve in most patients, and the results in neonates are similar to those of surgical valvotomy. Arterial access is a problem for the small neonate. Risks include inadequate relief of stenosis, creation of aortic insufficiency, perforation, and acute hemodynamic instability during catheterization.

  ○ Surgical valvuloplasty via sternotomy carries the same risks as balloon procedures; however, stabilization on cardiopulmonary bypass during the procedure allows time for the ventricle to rest and resolution of acidosis. It also provides a backup in the instance of ventricular dysrhythmias with valve manipulation (Fig. 3–32).

  ○ For stenosis (initial or recurrent) in patients with limited annulus size, enlargement of the entire aortic root is required. The Konno procedure with aortic root replacement involves enlarging the LV outflow tract and aortic annulus and incorporating an aortic valve replacement

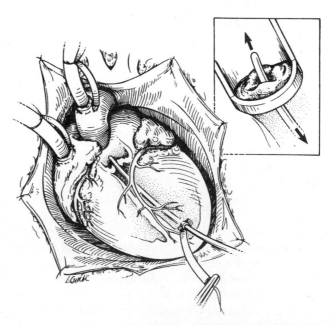

Figure 3–32.   Operative technique demonstrating antegrade transvalvar dilation using blunt dilators through an apical purse-string suture. (Reprinted with permission from Mosca RS, Iannettoni MD, Schwartz SM, et al. Critical aortic stenosis in the neonate. *J Thorac Cardiovasc Surg.* 1995; 109:147–154.)

with a prosthetic valve, homograft, or autograft. This is accomplished through a sternotomy on cardiopulmonary bypass and through incisions made into the RV outflow tract and the ventricular septum and across the aortic annulus. Risks of this operation include heart block from the septal incision, myocardial failure and low cardiac output, patch dehiscence of the ventricular patch used to enlarge the septum and aortic root, and perivalvular leak.

○ Some patients require valve replacement for progressive stenosis or insufficiency but have an adequate aortic annulus size. In this case a decision regarding the best valve for that patient's age, lifestyle, sex, and anatomy is made and replacement performed. In most circumstances these prosthetic valves and homografts require replacement within 10 to 15 years. In patients with aortic and pulmonary roots of the same or similar size, a Ross procedure can be performed. This operation involves translocating the native pulmonary valve into the aortic root (autograft) and replacing the pulmonary valve with a homograft. The proposed benefit is that the autograft will grow and not require further replacement. A moderate degree of pulmonary stenosis or insufficiency is much better tolerated than aortic stenosis or insufficiency. Risks of this operation include bleeding from the many long suture lines, MI from coronary injury during excision of the pulmonary autograft, and low cardiac output.

b. **Discrete subaortic stenosis (sub AS)**
- *Pathophysiology:* Subaortic stenosis includes 8% to 10% of aortic stenosis and occurs more in boys. It consists of a membranous diaphragm or fibrous ring encircling the LV outflow tract beneath the base of the aortic valve. Progressive aortic regurgitation is found and is an indication for surgery.
- *Assessment*
  ○ *Examination:* There may be a systolic ejection sound and a diastolic murmur of aortic insufficiency.
  ○ *Echocardiogram* shows dilation of the aortic root. A fibromuscular ring produces thick echoes from a level near the annular attachment of the anterior mitral leaflet.
- *Intervention:* Surgery is performed through sternotomy on cardiopulmonary bypass. The obstructing membrane or ring is excised along with a small wedge of LV muscle (myomectomy). Myomectomy has been shown to dramatically reduce the recurrence of the stenosis. Risks specific to this procedure include aortic insufficiency, heart block, and creation of a VSD.

c. **Supravalvular aortic stenosis**
- *Pathophysiology:* Congenital narrowing of the ascending aorta may be localized or diffuse, hourglass shaped, membranous type, or hypoplastic type. Coronary arteries are subjected to elevated pressure and may be dilated; the lumina may be narrowed by a thick medial layer. The aortic lumen is constricted, and the distal flow is diminished. It is often associated with Williams syndrome (supravalvular aortic stenosis, PA stenosis, mental retardation, and hypercalcemia in infancy).
- *Assessment: History* is similar to valvular aortic stenosis. *Examination* reveals accentuation of aortic closure sound, prominent transmission of a thrill and murmur, narrowing of peripheral pulmonary arteries producing a continuous murmur, and blood pressure higher in the right arm than in the left arm.

- ○ *ECG* reveals LVH and RVH if peripheral PA stenosis is present.
- ○ *Chest x-ray examination* rarely shows poststenotic dilation.
- ○ *Cardiac catheterization* localizes the site of obstruction and degree of hemodynamic alteration. A pressure gradient is found above the aortic valve. Coronary artery problems can be identified, as well as the presence and degree of PA involvement (peripheral pulmonary stenosis).
- **•** *Intervention:* Via sternotomy and cardiopulmonary bypass, an incision is made into the aorta, and a patch placed to enlarge the area. If there is diffuse hypoplasia of the aorta or accompanying PA hypoplasia, transfer of the gradients further down the aorta or to the pulmonary artery occurs, and the prognosis is poor. Relief of aortic stenosis with significant residual PA stenosis can create a situation of suprasystemic PA and RV pressures postoperatively. The early and late prognosis is not good.

3. **Hypoplastic left heart syndrome (HLHS):** Continuum of CHD characterized by underdevelopment of left heart structures

a. *Pathophysiology*

- **•** Right-sided structures, the pulmonary artery, coronary arteries, and lungs are normal, although the right atrium, right ventricle, and pulmonary artery may be dilated. Left-sided structures have variable levels of underdevelopment. Mitral valve atresia or stenosis occurs frequently. Aortic atresia or stenosis (annulus ≤ 5 mm) occurs. Stenotic valves have a small aortic root with leaflets that are thick, dysplastic, and obstructive. LV hypoplasia occurs in varying degrees (volume <20 ml/m^2). There is a non-apex-forming left ventricle (Fig. 3–33). The endocardium may be thick or sclerotic. The ascending aorta varies in size but is hypoplastic,

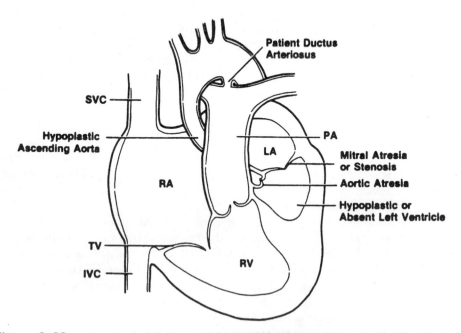

Figure 3–33. Hypoplastic left heart syndrome. *IVC,* inferior vena cava; *LA,* left atrium; *PA,* pulmonary artery; *RA,* right atrium; *RV,* right ventricle; *SVC,* superior vena cava; *TV,* tricuspid valve. (Reprinted with permission from Callow LB. Current strategies in the nursing care of infants with hypoplastic left-heart syndrome undergoing first-stage palliation with the Norwood operation. *Heart Lung.* 1992;20:463–470.)

usually to the level of the transverse arch (usually 2 to 3 mm). Coarctation is present in 80% of patients.

- Associated lesions are not common with classic HLHS but may include AVSD, transposition of the great vessels, and univentricular heart. A PDA and ASD are essential for survival and considered a part of the complex. Occasionally, the ASD is small or restrictive and presents as a newborn with obstructed TAPVR.
- Systemic venous blood returns normally to the right atrium and flows normally out the right side of the heart. Pulmonary venous blood flows across the ASD to the right atrium, since it cannot exit the left side of the heart if aortic atresia is present. Mixing in the right atrium desaturates the blood. All blood flows across the tricuspid valve to the right ventricle to the pulmonary artery. If mitral or aortic stenosis is present, a small amount of forward flow out the left ventricle may occur but not enough to support the cardiac output. Blood flows right to left across the PDA to supply systemic blood flow distally and flows proximally to feed the coronary arteries.

b. *Etiology and incidence:* HLHS occurs in 7% of CHD or 0.163/1000 live births. Research suggests an autosomal recessive transmission. Recurrence risk in siblings is 0.5%; HLHS is more common in boys, and 10% of infants with HLHS have associated extracardiac malformations.

c. *Assessment*
- *History:* Cyanosis is rare at birth; however, as normal involution of the PDA occurs, systemic perfusion is compromised. Symptoms of CHF become evident and, if unrecognized, will progress to vascular collapse. Tachypnea, dyspnea, grunting, cool and poorly perfused extremities, and pallor or gray color will be noted.
- *Examination* reveals auscultation of crisp, loud heart sounds, a single S_2, a pulmonary ejection click, and an S_3; an enlarged liver; a left precordial bulge; a soft systolic ejection murmur; and variable femoral pulses. There may be no gradient with low cardiac output or an open PDA.

d. *Diagnostic findings*
- *ECG* demonstrates sinus tachycardia, peaked P waves, RA enlargement, RVH, and paucity of LV forces and may show ST-T wave changes.
- *Chest x-ray examination:* Levocardia, an enlarged, globular shaped heart, and variable pulmonary vascular markings (severe pulmonary edema and increased markings if ASD is restrictive) are present.
- *Echocardiogram* is a valuable diagnostic tool that defines all anatomic variants of HLHS: the right ventricle and pulmonary artery are enlarged; mitral valve leaflets are not visualized; the LV cavity is hypoplastic; the left ventricle is nonapex forming; the aortic root ≤5 mm; and hypoplasia of the aortic arch is present.
- *Cardiac catheterization* is not required initially except if there is an extreme anatomic variant. It will demonstrate an obligatory left-to-right atrial shunt with increased oxygen saturation in the right atrium, right ventricle, and pulmonary artery; aortic saturation equal to PA saturation; RV pressures elevated and equal to or in excess of systemic arterial pressure; PCWP and LA and RA pressures equal except in the presence of obstructive ASD where PCWP and LA pressure are greater than RA pressure.

e. *Interventions*
- Ductal patency is maintained while the diagnosis is confirmed and decisions are made for interventions. Treatment options include com-

passionate care (death occurs within 1 week 95% of the time), transplantation (requires maintenance with prostaglandin therapy until a donor is found), or staged surgical reconstruction.

- Preoperative stabilization: Balance is maintained between systemic and pulmonary blood flow by manipulating SVR and PVR. If the patient is cyanotic with low pulmonary blood flow, hyperventilation, hyperoxygenation, and relief of pulmonary congestion are used. The patency of the ASD and PDA need to be assured. Pulmonary vasoconstriction and systemic vasodilation are avoided, and the hematocrit is maintained at a level higher than 45 ml/dl. Pulmonary overcirculation can result in poor cardiac output (hypotension, acidosis) with good oxygenation (PaO_2 usually greater than 45 mm Hg). Hypoventilation with a blend of carbon dioxide and nitrogen on ventilator with FIO_2 less than 21% can help to maintain mild metabolic acidosis (pH 7.35). Cardiac output is maintained with medications and volume. Adequate organ function should be present prior to surgical intervention.

- *First-stage palliative reconstructive surgery with the Norwood operation* creates an unobstructed RV outflow tract to prevent ventricular hypertrophy and dysfunction and provide good coronary artery flow (Fig. 3–34). Pulmonary blood flow is controlled to prevent PVOD via use of a nondistorting shunt to allow growth of the central main pulmonary artery. A large ASD (atrial septectomy) is created to allow good mixing of venous blood return at the atrial level and LA decompression and to avoid elevated PA pressure or PVR. The Norwood operation is aimed at maintaining anatomic and physiologic criteria for an eventual Fontan procedure. The Norwood operation is done via sternotomy with cardiopulmonary bypass and hypothermic circulatory arrest. The aortic arch and RV outflow tract are reconstructed using the proximal pulmonary artery and aorta and homograft augmentation. The incision is carried 10 mm past the insertion of the PDA to assure that ductal tissue is excised and to reduce or eliminate the risk of postoperative coarctation formation. Careful reconstruction of the proximal PA-aortic anastomosis is completed to avoid torsion and obstruction to coronary artery flow. Pulmonary blood flow is limited by a systemic-to-pulmonary shunt. Postoperative complications include an unbalanced flow between systemic and pulmonary circulations or severe cardiovascular collapse. The inability to maintain balanced circulation or preoperative obstructed atrial septum may require ECMO for cardiac or pulmonary healing (see Extracorporeal Life Support [ECLS]/Extracorporeal Membrane Oxygenation [ECMO]). Problems with temporary and reversible elevated PVR and severe hypoxemia may be managed by inhalation of nitric oxide. Low cardiac output may respond to blended carbon dioxide or nitrogen inhalation, or both.

- *Second-stage palliation: Bidirectional cavopulmonary shunt (4 to 6 months after initial palliation):* Full hemodynamic and anatomic catheterization to assess the size and stenosis of the pulmonary arteries, PA pressure, pulmonary blood flow, and RV function is necessary prior to cavopulmonary shunt. The purpose of the cavopulmonary shunt is to provide a stable form of oxygenation as the child grows. Removal of the previous systemic-to-pulmonary shunt removes volume overload from the right ventricle, protects the right ventricle from hypertrophy, and preserves long-term function. It is performed via sternotomy on cardiopulmonary bypass and may require hypothermic circulatory arrest. If necessary, PA

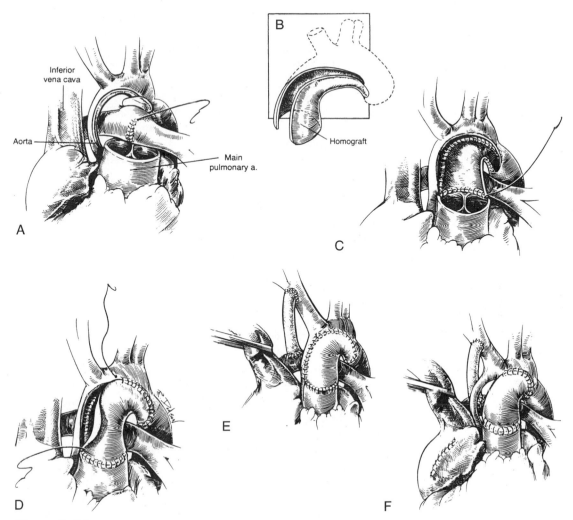

Figure 3–34. Surgical reconstruction in hypoplastic left heart syndrome. Using a homograft patch, the aorta is reconstructed and a systemic-to-pulmonary shunt provides pulmonary flow to the now transected pulmonary artery. (Reprinted with permission from Castaneda AR, Jonas RA, Mayer JE, Hanley FL. *Cardiac Surgery of the Neonate and Infant.* Philadelphia, Pa: WB Saunders Co; 1994.)

stent or arterioplasty is performed to assure unobstructed pulmonary blood flow to permit passive flow without excessively high SVC pressures. The pulmonary arteries are repaired as necessary. The SVC is connected end to side with the right or main pulmonary artery, and flow goes passively to the right and left pulmonary arteries by pressure gradient. A bulging fontanelle, high SVC pressure, irritability, low saturations, and edema of the face, neck, and upper extremities (SVC syndrome) are signs of high venous pressure. PVR is optimized, and early heparin use with conversion to aspirin later may prevent PA clots. Any alteration in PVR will affect pulmonary blood flow, since there is no ventricular pump to overcome this added resistance. Effusions are treated, diuretics are used to reduce volume overload and improve pulmonary mechanics, and appropriate ventilatory support is given. MAP is maintained in a lower range. Early extubation permits physiologic negative pressure, and spontaneous respiration may reduce MAP. Hematocrit should be maintained greater than or equal to 45%. Since IVC blood still flows through the right ventricle, complete unloading of the RV volume overload is not accomplished, and mixing of oxygenated and unoxygenated blood occurs with expected saturations of 80% to 85%.

- *Final-stage physiologic palliation: Fontan procedure (also done for tricuspid atresia or single ventricle hearts of other diagnostic categories than HLHS):* Recommended age is less than or equal to 4 years to prevent ventricular hypertrophy and dysfunction from volume overload and to optimize long-term ventricular function. Full hemodynamic and anatomic catheterization is required prior to a Fontan procedure to assess for suitability. Criteria for adequate outcomes include good PA architecture without stenosis and normal PA pressure, PVR, and ventricular function. Relative criteria include competent AV valve and normal sinus rhythm. The operation is done via sternotomy on cardiopulmonary bypass, possibly with circulatory arrest. The systemic venous return is directed to the pulmonary artery. A bidirectional Glenn procedure directs blood through a baffle from the right atrium to the IVC to the pulmonary artery. An external IVC-PA conduit is used mainly for systemic or pulmonary venous anatomic aberrations prohibiting previous connections. The goal is to achieve passive flow from the systemic veins to the lungs based on the pressure gradient from the SVC or IVC to the main pulmonary artery to the left and right pulmonary arteries to the lungs. Relief of any PA stenosis via arterioplasty or stent placement, or both, is mandatory to prevent a fixed elevation in PVR. Relief of significant AV valve regurgitation is necessary to prevent elevations in atrial pressure transmitted to the lungs.
- Postoperative care may be complicated by ventricular dysfunction, dysrhythmias, elevated PVR, and excessive cyanosis from a baffle leak. Observation of the RA-LA gradient may demonstrate a widening gradient with RA hypertension from increased PVR or a narrow gradient but high LA pressure that may signify LV dysfunction. Ideally, the RA pressure will be less than 15 mm Hg, with transpulmonary gradient not greater than 10. Ventilation should be optimized with low mean airway pressure (use JET ventilation if necessary), and extubation should occur as early as possible. Late complications do exist and are mainly related to the extent of atrial surgery and stretch of the right atrium and to chronically elevated systemic venous pressures. Atrial dysrhythmias, primarily sick sinus syndrome and atrial fibrillation or flutter, can occur. Recurrent pleural effusions, hepatic congestion, protein-losing enteropathy, and exercise intolerance may develop. Long-term ventricular failure requires transplantation. Many Fontan procedures are now fenestrated (controlled hole in intraatrial baffle allowing right-to-left shunting when systemic venous pressures are excessively high). This is felt to decrease the risk to marginal candidates, maintain cardiac output and volume load in the ventricle, and ease transition to passive flow. The right-to-left shunt and cyanosis continue until the fenestration is closed. Fenestration closure is then done following return of hemodynamic stability and may be performed weeks to months after the initial operation. Initially there is a decrease in cardiac output despite normalization of oxygen saturation in patients with fenestration closure.

4. **Coarctation of the aorta (COA):** Narrowing of the aorta causing elevation of pressure proximally and decreased pressure distally
   a. *Pathophysiology:* Classification of coarctation is based on the presence or absence of severe isthmus narrowing and major associated lesions. It is

associated frequently with PDA, VSD, aortic stenosis, aortic insufficiency, bicuspid aortic valve, mitral and tricuspid valve anomalies, and DiGeorge syndrome (usually with interrupted arch). Constriction of the aorta occurs most often at the junction of the ductus and aorta just distal to the left subclavian artery—juxtaductal coarctation. The most severe form of coarctation is the interrupted aortic arch, which is a congenital absence of a portion of the aorta. The types of aortic interruption are based on location. Type A is distal to the left subclavian artery (42%); type B is distal to the left common carotid artery (53%); and type C is between the right and left common carotid arteries (4%) (Fig. 3–35). Evaluation of coarctation is an ongoing process, as the obstruction can worsen over time resulting in increased upper extremity hypertension. Blood exits the left ventricle normally but has varying degrees of difficulty crossing the obstruction. This results in LV hypertension and hypertrophy. In some cases blood cannot cross the constriction. In this case the infant is dependent on right-to-left shunting across the ductus to perfuse the distal aorta and body. As the child grows older, significant aortic collaterals may form to perfuse the aorta distal to the coarctation. Complications of LV failure, long-standing systemic hypertension, stroke, and endocarditis are risks of unrepaired disease.

b. *Etiology and incidence:* Local area intimal thickening and distortion is found distal to the contraductal shelf. It is the fifth or sixth most common CHD and more common in males.

c. *Assessment*
   • *History* depends on the degree of constriction. Neonates with severe obstruction present with severe CHF and cardiovascular collapse and need prostaglandin to maintain ductal patency and reestablish systemic flow until surgical correction. Older children rarely have symptoms but may complain of cramps or pain in calves with exercise.

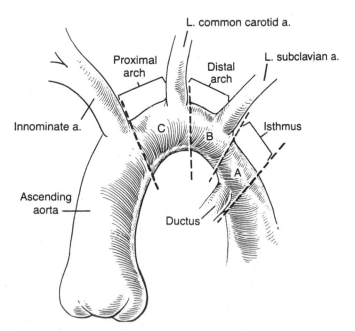

Figure 3–35. Depiction of aortic arch in three segments: proximal arch, distal arch, and isthmus. *Ductus,* ductus arteriosus. (Reprinted with permission from Castaneda AR, Jonas RA, Mayer JE, Hanley FL. *Cardiac Surgery of the Neonate and Infant.* Philadelphia, Pa: WB Saunders Co; 1994.)

- *Examination* of the infant reveals a heaving precordium, equally diminished pulses if the ductus is open, and a nonspecific systolic murmur at the LSB. In the child, a blood pressure differential between the upper and lower extremities, systemic hypertension, a short systolic ejection murmur at the LSB, and a continuous murmur if collaterals are present occur.
  d. *Diagnostic findings in the infant and child*
    - *ECG:* RVH and LV strain in the infant; increased LV forces and strain in the child.
    - *Echocardiogram* defines anatomy, LV function, and associated lesions.
    - *Chest x-ray examination* demonstrates cardiomegaly and possibly increased pulmonary vascular markings in the infant; normal heart size, LV prominence, rib notching, and a prominent descending aorta in the child.
    - *Cardiac catheterization* determines associated lesions, anatomy of coarctation, gradient across the coarctation unless there is low cardiac output or a PDA, and descending aortic saturation less than the ascending aortic saturation (from right-to-left shunting at the ductal level).
  e. *Intervention:* Interventions depend on age, degree of constriction, ductal dependency, and associated lesions. In the neonate, initial stabilization on prostaglandin and correction of any end-organ failure at diagnostic presentation is required. Medical management is not indicated long term. Short-term stabilization of CHF may be necessary.
    - Interventional cardiac catheterization is primarily for older children or residual coarctation after repair. Balloon dilation disrupts the intima. Risks include aneurysm, recurrent coarctation, difficult access in small infants, and inadequate relief. Reduction of collateral vessels following relief of the coarctation by balloon dilation may make operative intervention more hazardous should recoarctation occur. There is increased risk of paraplegia from low perfusion pressure distal to the aortic cross-clamp during surgery when collateral flow is diminished. Cardiopulmonary bypass may be used to prevent this complication.
    - Surgical repair is accomplished via left thoracotomy with one of several methods. Subclavian flap angioplasty, end-to-end anastomosis following resection of the coarcted segment (Fig. 3–36), patch aortoplasty (Fig. 3–37), and interposition graft are surgical options used. Sternotomy and bypass are used if complete arch reconstruction is required or associated lesions are to be repaired (i.e., VSD, subaortic stenosis). Thoracotomy with bypass is used to support the distal aortic pressure during cross-clamp for repair if there is poor collateral flow. Restenosis may occur but is usually amenable to balloon dilation. Specific postoperative complications include paradoxical hypertension, mesenteric arteritis (feed slowly, await return of bowel sounds), and paralysis (bypass is used if distal aortic pressure is less than 40 mm Hg).
  5. **Mitral valve disease or mitral stenosis (MS):** Obstruction of pulmonary venous blood flow from the left atrium to the left ventricle
    a. *Pathophysiology:* Mitral stenosis is classified by the component of mitral valve that is abnormal. Abnormalities include thick rolled leaflet margins, abnormal chordae tendineae, papillary muscle hypoplasia, LV endocardial sclerosis, hypoplasia or atresia of the mitral valve, commissure fusion, excessive tissue, parachute mitral valve, or supramitral ring. Left atrial, pulmonary venous, and pulmonary capillary wedge pressures increase relative to resistance to flow across the mitral valve into the left ventricle. Eventually, mitral stenosis may cause PA hypertension, elevated PVR, and

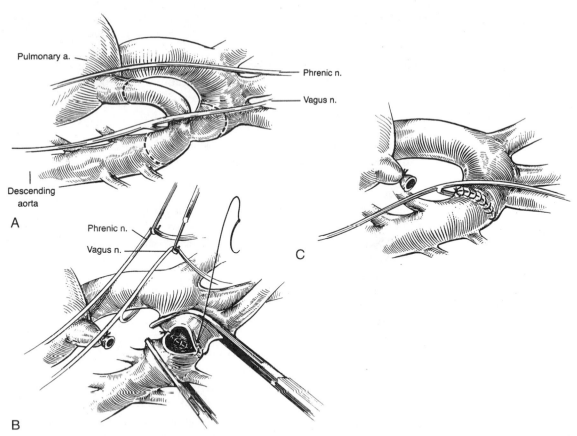

Figure 3–36.   Surgical repair of coarctation with resection and end-to-end anastomosis. (Reprinted with permission from Castaneda AR, Jonas RA, Mayer JE, Hanley FL. *Cardiac Surgery of the Neonate and Infant.* Philadelphia, Pa: WB Saunders Co; 1994.)

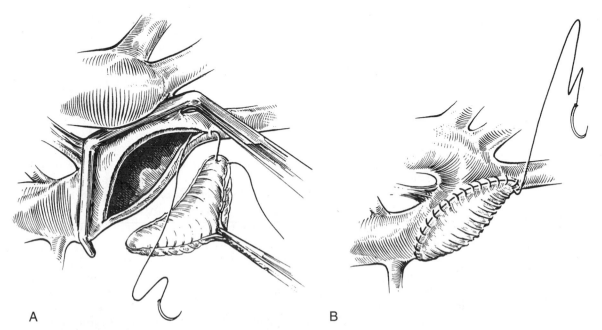

Figure 3–37.   Patch aortoplasty repair of infant coarctation. (Reprinted with permission from Castaneda AR, Jonas RA, Mayer JE, Hanley FL. *Cardiac Surgery of the Neonate and Infant.* Philadelphia, Pa: WB Saunders Co; 1994.)

RV dysfunction from pulmonary vasoocclusive disease. LV volume load decreases, causing ischemia, fibrosis, and further LV dysfunction and decreased cardiac output.

b. *Etiology:* Mitral stenosis is a variable expression of developmental abnormality involving the left ventricle. Excessive or abnormal deposition of tissue occurs embryologically. Deficiency or excess of endocardial cushion tissue is related.

c. *Assessment*
   - *History:* Timing and type of symptoms of mitral stenosis are based on the degree of obstruction to LV inflow. The most severe presentation is similar to the history of HLHS. A history of frequent pulmonary infections, poor weight gain, irritability, tiring with feeding, diaphoresis, tachypnea, chronic cough, and increased work of breathing is noted.
   - *Examination* reveals an active RV impulse with PA hypertension, soft S_1, split S_2, possible S_3 or S_4, and a low frequency middiastolic murmur at the apex.

d. *Diagnostic findings*
   - *ECG:* LA and RA enlargement or RVH suggest PA hypertension and severe mitral stenosis. Diminished LV forces are noted.
   - *Chest x-ray examination* demonstrates LA enlargement, prominence of pulmonary vascular markings, and right-sided enlargement.
   - *Echocardiogram* shows decreased mitral valve opening, abnormal posterior leaflet motion, LA enlargement, reduced aortic wall motion, and diminished LV dimensions. It defines abnormalities of chordae tendineae and papillary muscles and estimates transvalvular gradients, ASD size, and changes in pulmonary vein inflow patterns.
   - *Cardiac catheterization* reveals mild systemic desaturation and hypoxemia, left-to-right atrial shunt with severe mitral stenosis, elevation of PA pressure, PVR, PCWP, and LA pressure, a diastolic pressure gradient from the LA pressure to the LVEDP, and a transpulmonary gradient if PVOD has developed.

e. *Interventions:* CHF is medically managed. Surgical intervention is considered for elevated PA hypertension and PVR. The success of the operation is related to mitral valve and annulus size, LV size, PVR, PA pressure, and age. Older patients have better results if no PVOD is present. The mitral valve orifice must be opened to allow adequate LV inflow and pulmonary vein drainage. Commissurotomy is done via sternotomy and bypass with excision of excess tissue and membranes. Mitral valve replacement is difficult in infants with small annulus size. Postoperative care is directed at PA hypertension, low cardiac output, dysrhythmias, and conduction disturbances.

6. **Congenital mitral insufficiency:** Failure of the valve leaflets to coapt normally, which allows regurgitation of blood into the pulmonary veins

   a. *Pathophysiology:* Congenital mitral insufficiency is associated with or secondary to other cardiac disease such as single ventricle, AVSD, cardiomyopathy, Kawasaki syndrome, connective tissue disorders, metabolic disorder, and mucocutaneous lymph node disease. Classically, there is mitral valve prolapse. Failure of the valve leaflets to coapt normally allows regurgitation of LV volume into the left atrium and, depending on the severity of mitral valve incompetence, into the pulmonary veins, causing PA hypertension and elevated PVR over time.

   b. *Etiology and incidence:* Congenital mitral insufficiency is rare and usually associated with other defects. As with congenital mitral stenosis, consider an isolated cleft in the mitral valve.

c. *Assessment*
- *History* depends on the severity of insufficiency as with mitral stenosis (see Mitral Stenosis).
- *Examination* reveals diffuse apical impulse, active precordium, soft S_1, S_3, split S_2 in the presence of PA hypertension, high-frequency blowing or harsh holosystolic murmur at the apex, and a low-frequency apical diastolic murmur.

d. *Diagnostic findings*
- *ECG* shows LA enlargement and LVH.
- *Chest x-ray examination* shows an enlarged heart with LA and LV enlargement, and increased pulmonary vascular markings and congestion.
- *Echocardiogram* demonstrates an abnormal valve anatomy, increased LA and LV dimensions, normal to increased LV systolic indexes, insufficiency or overlapping of anterior and posterior leaflets, break in leaflet echo suggesting a cleft, and regurgitant flow into the left atrium and pulmonary veins if insufficiency is severe.
- *Cardiac catheterization* reveals elevated PCWP, PA pressure, PVR, LA pressure, and LVEDP, LA opacification to a varying degree with LV injection, and a deceptively normal LV ejection fraction because of the ability to eject retrograde to low pressure atrium.

e. *Interventions:* Treatment may be medical if the child is not in severe CHF. The child must be watched closely for signs of PAH and the development of PVOD. Afterload reduction and diuretics (see Medications) may be used cautiously. Surgical intervention is required in the presence of severe CHF, ventilator dependency or PA hypertension, and vascular changes. Valvuloplasty may be difficult if there is deficient valvular tissue. Prosthetic rings may be used. Cleft or elongated chordae tendineae are repaired. Mitral valve replacement is used as a last resort. Relief of mitral insufficiency producing a competent mitral valve may unmask LV dysfunction. The left ventricle now must eject its entire volume into the high resistance systemic circuit as opposed to allowing leakage into the low resistance left atrium (see Nursing Diagnoses).

7. **Valvular pulmonary stenosis (valvular PS):** Narrowed pulmonary valve causing obstruction to flow from the right ventricle to the pulmonary artery, resulting in RVH (Fig. 3–38).
   a. *Pathophysiology:* The pulmonary valve is conical or domed shaped and is formed by fusion of valve leaflets. It may be bicuspid (20% of cases). Thickened and immobile leaflets provide obstruction to RV outflow. The endocardium of the infundibulum may be thick and endocardial fibroelastosis may develop. In severe cases there is tricuspid valve regurgitation and RA dilation. If an ASD or patent foramen ovale is present, right-to-left shunting can occur, resulting in cyanosis of varying degrees. If pulmonary stenosis is severe and significant right-to-left atrial shunting occurs across the ASD, the right ventricle and pulmonary valve may be hypoplastic. Grading of PS severity is based on transvalvular gradients of (1) mild: 25 to 49 mm Hg, (2) moderate: 50 to 75 mm Hg, and (3) severe: >75 mm Hg.
   b. *Etiology and incidence:* Pulmonary stenosis results from an embryologic error in the formation of pulmonary leaflets. It occurs in 25% to 30% of children with CHD. Dysplastic pulmonary valve is common in association with Noonan's syndrome.
   c. *Assessment*
   - *History* may vary from an asymptomatic presentation to mild exertional dyspnea and cyanosis to severe CHF, depending on the degree of

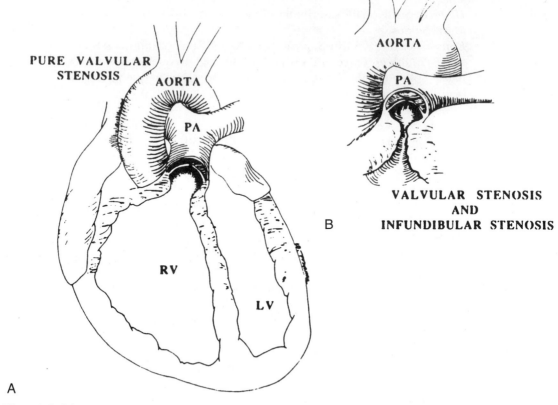

PURE VALVULAR STENOSIS

AORTA

PA

RV

LV

A

VALVULAR STENOSIS AND INFUNDIBULAR STENOSIS

AORTA

PA

B

Figure 3–38. Illustration of valvular and subvalvular PS. *LV*, left ventricle; *PA*, pulmonary artery; *RV*, right ventricle. (Reprinted with permission from Adams FH, Emmanoulides GC, Riemenschneider TA. *Moss' Heart Disease in Infants, Children, and Adolescents.* 4th ed. Baltimore, Md: Williams & Wilkins; 1989.)

pulmonary stenosis. Dyspnea and fatigue with exercise are the most common complaints at first; as stenosis progresses, they occur even at rest. Growth and development are usually normal. The presence of cyanosis from right-to-left atrial shunting indicates moderate pulmonary stenosis.

- *Examination* reveals a normal S_1, pulmonary ejection click, and a diastolic ejection murmur (shorter in milder pulmonary stenosis, longer in severe pulmonary stenosis). The holosystolic murmur of tricuspid insufficiency and soft or absent S_2 are characteristic of severe pulmonary stenosis. In the newborn with severe pulmonary stenosis, S_2 is almost always single.

d. *Diagnostic findings*
- *ECG* is useful to assess the severity of pulmonary stenosis. In mild stenosis, normal RV forces are present. Severe RVH and RAE are present in severe stenosis.
- *Chest x-ray examination* demonstrates a prominent main PA segment, RVH and downward apex, and cardiomegaly in severe pulmonary stenosis only (usually only mild enlargement).
- *Echocardiogram* determines function and anatomy of the pulmonary valve and associated lesions, septal and RVH, prominent valve with restricted systolic motion, poststenotic dilation of the pulmonary artery, and size of the tricuspid valve and right ventricle (small only in severe pulmonary stenosis). It is also used to quantify the PVR and valve gradient.
- *Cardiac catheterization* is not required for diagnosis but it excludes other diagnoses or is used to perform interventional therapy. RV pressure is

elevated. The valve area and gradient and anatomy are defined. Oxygen saturations are usually normal. Cardiac output is quantified to use in determining the accuracy of the valve gradient.

e. *Interventions:* Intervention is required for moderate or greater pulmonary stenosis. Balloon valvuloplasty is the currently accepted treatment providing excellent short-term and long-term results. The balloon catheter is inserted across the pulmonary valve and inflated to a size 10% to 20% greater than the annulus (Fig. 3–39). Valvuloplasty is not as effective for dysplastic valves and neonates with critical pulmonary stenosis although results in this group are improving. Risks include RV perforation, residual stenosis, and creation of insufficiency. Surgical valvotomy may be done in cases where the catheter cannot pass through the pulmonary valve or when associated lesions require surgery. Progressive dilators are inserted through the pulmonary valve via incision in the pulmonary artery to 1 cm greater than the valve annulus. Surgery requires sternotomy and a short period of cardiopulmonary bypass. Dysplastic valves may require excision of excess tissue. Risks include RV failure, creation of pulmonary insufficiency, and inadequate relief of pulmonary stenosis. Endocarditis is a complication of interventional catheterization, and prophylaxis is required at times of predictable risk.

F. **CYANOTIC PHYSIOLOGY**
  1. **Expected outcomes**
     a. Patient or family member will state activity limitations of disease.
     b. Patient or family member will state signs and symptoms of CHF.
     c. Patient or family member will state actions, side effects, and complications of medications.

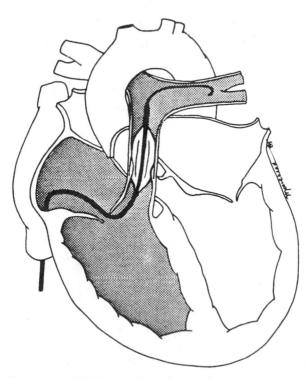

Figure 3–39. Illustration of balloon valvuloplasty catheter positioned across the pulmonary valve. (Reprinted with permission from Adams FH, Emmanoulides GC, Riemenschneider TA. *Moss' Heart Disease in Infants, Children, and Adolescents.* 4th ed. Baltimore, Md: Williams & Wilkins; 1989.)

     d. Patient or family member will state need for lifelong cardiovascular follow-up and endocarditis prophylaxis.

     e. Hematocrit will be greater than 45% and oxygen saturation will be greater than 70%.

     f. Patient's growth and development will be optimized.

     g. Dysrhythmia or conduction disorders will be absent or controlled by medications or pacemaker.

     h. Stenosis or obstruction of prosthetic material will be detected prior to ventricular dysfunction or the development of PVOD.

     i. Patient or family member will state need for staged operative intervention and repeated catheterization.

     j. Caloric intake including nasogastric supplementation will be maximized for growth.

     k. Hemodynamic parameters will be normal for age and sex.

2. **Tetralogy of Fallot (TOF):** Combination of congenital heart defects consisting of a VSD and RV outflow tract obstruction.

     a. *Pathophysiology:* Major features of classic description include a nonrestrictive VSD, RVH secondary to outflow obstruction, aortic override, and pulmonary stenosis of varying degrees but progressive in nature because of the anterior deviation of the infundibular septum (subvalvular or infundibular, valvular, and supravalvular) (Fig. 3–40). Associated anomalies include coronary artery anomalies, AVSD (newborns will present with CHF and cyanosis), absent pulmonary valve (usually dilated pulmonary artery with degrees of respiratory compromise from bronchial compression by dilated pulmonary artery), ASD, or pulmonary atresia.

        • Blood enters the right ventricle normally. RV outflow obstruction causes shunting across the VSD to the aorta thereby mixing systemic venous and pulmonary venous return. The severity of the pulmonary stenosis determines the severity of the cyanosis. As the aorta handles most cardiac output, it is often dilated. Patients are at risk for endocarditis, RV dysfunction, polycythemia, brain abscess, and stroke from cyanosis.

        • Classic hypoxic episodes are marked by increasing cyanosis, hyperpnea, and irritability progressing to unconsciousness, seizures, or cardiac

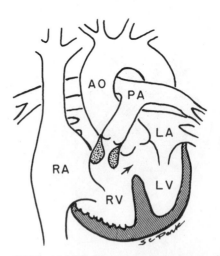

Figure 3–40.   Anatomy of TOF with VSD, PS, and overriding aorta. *AO*, aorta; *LA*, left atrium; *LV*, left ventricle; *PA*, pulmonary artery; *RA*, right atrium; *RV*, right ventricle. (Reprinted with permission from Garson AG, Brecker TJ, McNamara DG. *The Science and Practice of Pediatric Cardiology.* Philadelphia, Pa: Lea & Febiger; 1990.)

arrest. Usually they occur early in the day, probably secondary to a spasm of the infundibulum of the outflow tract or a drop in the systemic resistance, increasing right-to-left shunt and decreasing pulmonary blood flow. The murmur disappears, as no flow occurs across the narrowed pulmonary outflow tract. Patients are treated with sedation, volume (hematocrit ≥45%), bicarbonate, oxygen, knee chest position, and, if necessary, intubation and anesthesia. Morphine sulfate is the drug of choice to relieve agitation. IV propranolol (Inderal) may be used to relax the RV infundibulum and decrease the ventricular response to agitation. Phenylephrine (Neo-Synephrine) IV increases the systolic blood pressure and ideally decreases shunting away from the RV outflow tract. An increasing frequency of spells may indicate a need for earlier repair.

b. *Etiology and incidence:* TOF is the most common form of cyanotic CHD and is possibly related to abnormal septation of the conus. The cause is essentially unknown. It occurs slightly more commonly in boys.

c. *Assessment*
  - *History* depends on the degree of pulmonary stenosis. If severe, neonates are ductal dependent and require immediate surgery. If pulmonary stenosis is not severe, symptoms are mild and include dyspnea on exertion, clubbing, squatting, and cyanosis. Hypercyanotic spells may occur.
  - *Examination* reveals a normal cardiac impulse, normal S_1, single S_2, systolic ejection murmur at the LSB (related to pulmonary stenosis), diastolic murmur (with absent pulmonary vein), and a continuous murmur of collaterals or PDA.

d. *Diagnostic findings*
  - *ECG* shows RA deviation, RVH, normal conduction, and rarely ectopy.
  - *Chest x-ray examination* demonstrates a boot-shaped heart from absence of the PA segment, normal cardiac silhouette, normal or diminished pulmonary vascular markings, and a right aortic arch (25%).
  - *Echocardiogram* is the major diagnostic tool for definition of essential morphology, gradients, and identification of associated lesions (anomalous coronary arteries still difficult).
  - *Cardiac catheterization* is necessary to adequately detail the RV outflow tract. It will show equal pressures in the right and left ventricles. Coronary arteries are difficult to visualize.

e. *Interventions:* Medical intervention is necessary for spells (possibly propranolol), deep cyanosis, or complications of cyanosis. Medical management includes prostaglandins in neonates.
  - Surgical palliation is provided by a systemic-to-pulmonary shunt (usually a modified Blalock-Taussig shunt with Gortex interposition tube between the subclavian artery and ipsilateral pulmonary artery) via thoracotomy (Fig. 3–41). It is usually done for TOF with associated defects or anomalous coronary arteries. Too large of a shunt causes pulmonary overcirculation, symptoms of CHF, and risk of pulmonary vascular disease. Too small of a shunt does not relieve cyanosis. Risks of shunting include chylothorax, damage to phrenic or recurrent laryngeal nerve, infection, and distortion of the pulmonary artery.
  - Corrective operation via sternotomy and cardiopulmonary bypass is done at any age. It consists of VSD closure (Gortex patch) directing LV flow to the aorta, relief of RV outflow tract obstruction, and shunt takedown if one was done previously. Infundibular muscle resection or

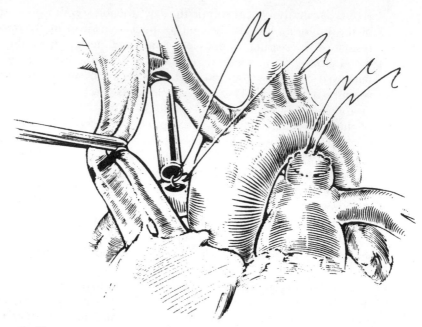

Figure 3–41. Placement of a modified Blalock-Taussig shunt between subclavian and innominate artery junction and right pulmonary artery. (Reprinted with permission from Castaneda AR, Jonas RA, Mayer JE, Hanley FL. *Cardiac Surgery of the Neonate and Infant.* Philadelphia, Pa: WB Saunders Co; 1994.)

       division of muscle bundles with pulmonary valvotomy or transannular Gortex patch results in pulmonary insufficiency. In cases of absent pulmonary valve, anomalous coronary artery, or small pulmonary arteries with narrow outflow tract, an RV-PA conduit is used. Risks include BBB, heart block, residual pulmonary stenosis or VSD, RV dysfunction, pulmonary insufficiency, or damage to the aortic valve.

f.   *Pulmonary atresia with a VSD (PA-VSD)* is considered a more extreme form of TOF. Catheterization is routine at diagnosis to assess the anatomy of the pulmonary artery, which is extremely variable but frequently small and nonconfluent. Patients may not be diagnosed until several months because collateral flow masks cyanosis. Collaterals are frequently stenotic at either the aortic or pulmonary end. Presentation is usually marked by CHF and failure to thrive by 3 to 6 months, occasional cyanosis, continuous murmurs of collaterals, and single S_2. Chest x-ray examination demonstrates mild to moderate cardiomegaly with no main PA segment and increased pulmonary vascular markings. Results and long-term outcome is based on PA architecture and the state of the pulmonary vascular bed at diagnosis. Often, the child requires several surgical interventions. First, the pulmonary arteries are unifocalized, and a RV-PA conduit is placed to promote growth of the proximal and distal pulmonary artery (Fig. 3–42). It may require coil embolization of collaterals once surgical intervention establishes forward flow, since collaterals may create hemodynamically significant left-to-right shunting and CHF. VSD closure (full repair) is accomplished only in those children who have forward RV output and adequately sized pulmonary arteries demonstrated by CHF, increasing saturations, and a left-to-right shunt at catheterization. A postoperative RV:LV pressure ratio of less than 3:4 to 2:3 is necessary to provide good long-term results.

3. **Transposition of the great vessels (TGV):** TGV is a ventriculoarterial discordance in which the morphologic left ventricle gives rise to the pulmonary artery, and the morphologic right ventricle gives rise to the aorta, creating parallel circulations.

   a. *Pathophysiology:* Simple TGV is associated with ASD, VSD, and PDA 80% of the time. Parallel circulation exists, since the systemic venous blood enters the right side of the heart normally but exits through the aorta back to the body. Pulmonary venous blood enters the left side of the heart normally but exits through the pulmonary artery to the lungs. The child requires intracardiac mixing to survive. The degree of cyanosis or acidosis depends on the number, location, and size of intracardiac and extracardiac shunts (ASD, VSD, PDA). Mixing of blood allows systemic saturation of 75% to 90%. LV pressure is maintained at systemic levels for the first 1 to 2 weeks of life. After that, PVR and LV pressure fall. Repair via arterial switch must be done before the fall of LV pressure and mass regression, since the left ventricle will have to handle the systemic pressure load. Early development of PVOD in infants with TGV has been found and is an indication for early repair. PVOD is more common if a VSD is present. PVOD can develop as early as 2 weeks of age and occurs in most patients with TGV by 1 year.
      • Complications include endocarditis, risk of cyanosis, CHF, and PVOD.

   b. *Etiology and incidence:* Although the cause is largely unknown, TGV may be due to a left shift in the pulmonary conus. It is more common in boys of normal birth weight and size. TGV is the most common form of cyanotic CHD to present in the newborn period.

   c. *Assessment*
      • *History* depends on the degree of shunting. Cyanosis within 24 hours of birth is the most common presentation. If a large VSD is present, the infant may present at 2 weeks of age with CHF.
      • *Examination* reveals cyanosis if there is an intact septum; hepatomegaly, tachycardia, tachypnea if with VSD; and clubbing after 6 months. TGV without a VSD reveals a normal S_1, single S_2, continuous murmur of the PDA, and an occasional systolic ejection murmur on auscultation. For

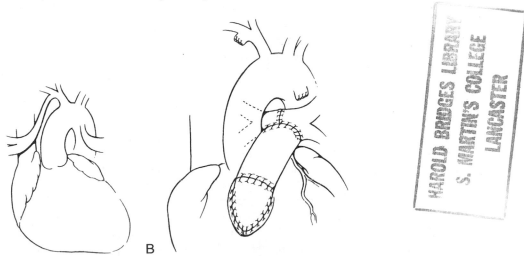

A   B

Figure 3–42. Technique of complete repair with insertion of homograft conduit after primary unifocalization in patients with complete absence of both interpericardial pulmonary arteries. (Reprinted with permission from Shanley CJ, Lupinetti FM, Shah NL, Beekman RH, Crowley DC, Bove EL: Primary unifocalization for the absence of interpericardial pulmonary arteries in the neonate. *J Thorac Cardiovasc Surg.* 1993;106:237–247.)

TGV with a VSD, auscultation reveals a normal S_1, single S_2, and soft systolic ejection murmur at the LSB.

d. *Diagnostic findings: ECG* shows right-axis deviation, RVH, or biventricular hypertrophy, or findings may be normal for age. In the presence of a VSD, the ECG shows biventricular hypertrophy and a normal QRS axis.

- *Chest x-ray examination* demonstrates an oval-shaped "egg on its side" silhouette, narrow superior mediastinum, and moderate cardiomegaly that may be normal for age. With a VSD, the chest x-ray examination demonstrates moderate cardiomegaly, a narrow superior mediastinum, and increased pulmonary vascular markings.
- *Echocardiogram* plays a dominant role in diagnosis by establishing major anatomic features and anatomic variants but may not define coronary anatomy.
- *Cardiac catheterization* is mainly used for balloon atrial septostomy. It demonstrates increased saturation with shunting, LV outflow obstruction, and slight increases in atrial pressure.

e. *Interventions*

- Medical stabilization with prostaglandin therapy is necessary if atrial communication is not sufficient (see Pharmacology). Medications for CHF are used while awaiting operation if there is a large VSD.
- Interventional catheterization is used if the ASD is restrictive or surgery is delayed. Balloon septostomy via catheterization tears the atrial septum. Blalock-Hanlon operation or atrial septectomy via sternotomy on bypass is used to surgically excise the atrial septum, improve mixing and saturation, and reduce acidosis. Because of the early arterial switch operation, this procedure is rarely performed any more.
- Surgical intervention depends on age at presentation, LV pressures, and associated lesions. The Mustard-Senning operation (venous switch) redirects venous inflow via intraatrial baffle so that the pulmonary veins drain via the tricuspid valve to the right ventricle to the aorta and the systemic veins drain via the mitral valve to the left ventricle to the pulmonary artery. The procedure includes closure of the ASD, VSD, and PDA if present. The right ventricle and tricuspid valve remain systemic for life. Complications include early and late atrial dysrhythmias, late RV dysfunction and tricuspid regurgitation, venous baffle obstruction, and late development of PVOD. *Arterial switch* (operation of choice) (Fig. 3–43) provides anatomic correction involving transection of both great vessels. The pulmonary valve becomes the aortic valve with anastomosis of the distal aorta to the proximal pulmonary artery and closure of associated shunts. Coronary arteries with a button of PA tissue are transferred to the new aortic root. The surgery may require circulatory arrest. Criteria for an arterial switch are timing of repair and no fixed pulmonary stenosis, which would become aortic stenosis after the switch. Some forms of coronary artery malformation, primarily intramural coronary artery, are considered a relative contraindication. This procedure leaves the left ventricle and mitral valve as the systemic ventricle and avoids a complex intraatrial baffle, which eliminates the risk of significant atrial dysrhythmias. Early postoperative problems center on LV dysfunction and low cardiac output and myocardial ischemia or infarction from kinking or distorting of the coronary arteries during transfer. Long term, an arterial switch ideally preserves good LV function and growth of the anastomosis. However, patients may have supravalvular aortic or pulmonary stenosis or poor growth of coronary connections. To date, the most

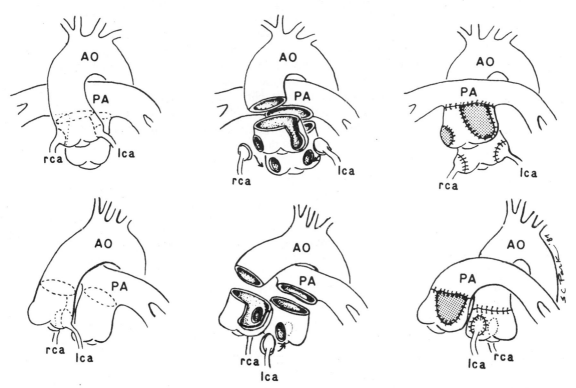

Figure 3–43. Arterial switch operation for transposition of the great arteries. Transection of both great vessels followed by anastomosis to the anatomically correct ventricles with coronary transfer. *AO*, aorta; *lca*, left coronary artery; *PA*, pulmonary artery; *rca*, right coronary artery. (Reprinted with permission from Garson AG, Brecker TJ, McNamara DG. *The Science and Practice of Pediatric Cardiology.* Philadelphia, Pa: Lea & Febiger; 1990.)

common residual defect has been the development of supravalvular pulmonary stenosis.
- Complex TGV includes fixed pulmonary stenosis. Palliation with a systemic to pulmonary shunt occurs in the neonatal period. Correction is completed in 6 months to 1 year with the Rastelli operation, which reestablishes LV-aortic continuity. The VSD is patched to direct LV flow to the aortic valve, and RV-PA continuity is established with an RV-PA conduit. The size of the VSD and location to the semilunar valves determine the degree of surgical difficulty. If the VSD is small and enlargement is necessary, the risk of postoperative complete heart block increases. Problems with the Rastelli operation include dysrhythmia, VSD patch dehiscence, aortic obstruction from improper VSD patch placement, residual pulmonary stenosis from conduit placement, tricuspid insufficiency, and myocardial dysfunction. Operative results and long-term follow-up are good, but the RV-PA conduit requires periodic replacement.

4. **Tricuspid atresia (TAT):** Imperforate tricuspid valve resulting in mandatory right-to-left atrial shunt and eventual single ventricle repair
   a. *Pathophysiology*
      - Agenesis of the tricuspid valve results in no communication between the right atrium and right ventricle. TAT is associated most often with a small right ventricle, ASD, and an aortopulmonary connection (PDA). Physiology and symptoms depend on the degree of pulmonary stenosis or

pulmonary atresia and presence or absence and size of the VSD. As blood cannot exit the right ventricle, blood is shunted right to left at the atrial level, and systemic desaturation occurs. Blood then flows across the left side of the heart to the right ventricle via the VSD and out to the lungs if there is little or no pulmonary stenosis. The result is normal to increased pulmonary blood flow with clinical manifestations of CHF.
- With associated pulmonary stenosis or pulmonary atresia, there will be little or no flow to the pulmonary artery. These infants usually have small right ventricles, are cyanotic early, and are ductal dependent for pulmonary blood flow. With VSD, systemic output may be seriously compromised if the VSD is small or restrictive or becomes so early in life.
- In single ventricle or univentricle hearts, both AV valves empty into one ventricle (known as double inlet). Ventricles are differentiated based on trabeculations. These lesions, as with TAT, may have normal, increased, or decreased pulmonary blood flow based on the degree of pulmonary stenosis. Clinical manifestations, physical examination, diagnostic findings, and interventions are dependent on the degree of AV valve regurgitation, extracardiac or intracardiac shunting, and pulmonary obstruction.

b. *Etiology and incidence:* Etiology is agenesis of the tricuspid valve (TAT) or failure of trabecular components of the ventricle to develop (single ventricle). There is no known cause, but TAT may be associated with polyhydramnios or maternal toxemia and has been reported with use of thalidomide. TAT is an uncommon defect (2.7% CHD).

c. *Assessment*
- *History* is dependent on the amount of pulmonary blood flow (presence of a VSD, degree of pulmonary stenosis or pulmonary atresia). Early cyanosis is common (50%) and expected (78%) by 1 month because of the obligatory atrial shunt. CHF history may occur with VSD and no pulmonary stenosis. Hypoxic spells occur in 16% to 45% of patients younger than 6 months of age. The risk of complications is from cyanosis, stroke, and brain abscess. Patients with CHF from excessive pulmonary blood flow may develop PVOD. All patients are at risk for endocarditis. Atrial dysrhythmias are not uncommon. Delayed growth and development may be seen.
- *Examination* reveals a hyperactive apical impulse, clubbing, left precordial prominence, single S_1 and S_2 (most common unless pulmonary blood flow is increased), systolic ejection murmur at the mid to upper LSB from the pulmonary stenosis, occasional holosystolic murmur at the LSB if a VSD is present, and a continuous murmur of the PDA or collaterals if PVR is normal.

d. *Diagnostic findings*
- *ECG* shows a superior and leftward QRS axis, RA enlargement, absent or diminished RV forces, and increased LV forces.
- *Echocardiogram* demonstrates absence of the tricuspid valve and diminished RV size. ECHO also defines associated defects, increased LV dimensions, size of the VSD and ASD, and the relationship of the great vessels.
- *Chest x-ray examination* with diminished pulmonary blood flow demonstrates normal to mild cardiomegaly, concave main PA segment, and diminished pulmonary vascular markings. Chest x-ray examination with increased pulmonary blood flow demonstrates gross cardiomegaly and increased pulmonary vascular markings.

- *Cardiac catheterization* is not necessary for first-stage palliation but is necessary prior to further surgery. On catheterization, the right ventricle is not entered from the right atrium, and flow of systemic venous blood from the right atrium to the left atrium through the ASD results in decreased saturation of the LA blood. The RA pressure is greater than or equal to the LA pressure. It defines the presence of a VSD, collaterals, relationship of the great vessels, and the degree of pulmonary stenosis. If no pulmonary stenosis is present and there is a VSD, PA pressure and PVR may be elevated.

  e. *Interventions*
  - Medical interventions for the infant with pulmonary stenosis include initial stabilization with prostaglandin infusion to maintain ductal patency until surgery. Initial treatment for patients with nonrestrictive pulmonary flow involves the use of decongestant medications.
  - Surgical interventions include initial palliation for those with decreased pulmonary blood flow. An aortopulmonary shunt is placed via thoracotomy. Initial palliation for increased pulmonary blood flow must be done early to control pulmonary flow and prevent the development of PVOD, which occurs quickly with this diagnosis. One option is via sternotomy and cardiopulmonary bypass to ligate the pulmonary artery and perform an aortopulmonary shunt. A second option is PA banding. Risk particular to this diagnosis is the development of subaortic stenosis in a child who requires a Fontan procedure later. Also, if there are transposed great vessels and a small right ventricle, subaortic stenosis may present a difficult management issue later related to support of systemic blood flow. The third option is a Damus Kaye Stanzel operation in the cohort of patients with transposed great vessels and a hypoplastic systemic outflow chamber. This operation is similar to a Norwood operation, since a systemic outflow is created by aortic-to-pulmonary (off the left ventricle) anastomosis, ligation of the pulmonary artery and creation of a systemic-to-pulmonary shunt. Early palliation is necessary because long-term volume and pressure overload to the left ventricle creates LV failure and dysfunction.
  - Final physiologic palliation for TAT and single ventricle hearts is the Fontan procedure via sternotomy on cardiopulmonary bypass. The ventricle supports systemic output, and the lungs are perfused through direct RA or caval connections to the pulmonary artery.

5. **Truncus arteriosus (TRU):** A single arterial trunk arises from the base of the heart giving rise to pulmonary, systemic, and coronary circulations.
  a. *Pathophysiology*
  - Truncus includes an unrestrictive VSD, single semilunar valve with possible truncal valve abnormalities, and override of the ventricular septum by the truncal valve. Tricuspid truncal valve occurs in 69% of cases. Quadricuspid truncal valve occurs in 22% of cases. Bicuspid truncal valve occurs in 9% of cases. Truncal valve insufficiency is related to thick dysplastic cusps. Truncal valve stenosis is rare.
  - The type of truncus is differentiated by the existence and location of the main pulmonary artery and the PA branches (Fig. 3–44). *Type I* has a short main PA segment, which arises from the trunk then branches into the right and left pulmonary arteries (48%). In *type II* the pulmonary artery arises separately from the trunk but in close proximity to it (29% to 48%). In *type III* the pulmonary artery arises separately from the trunk and at some distance from it (6% to 10%).

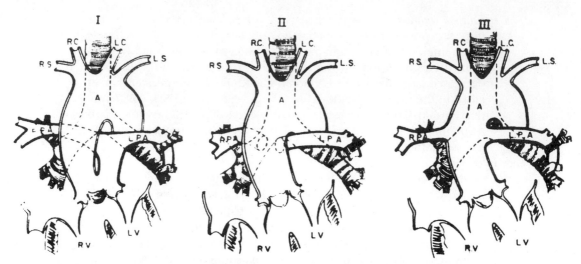

Figure 3–44. Anatomic definition of types of truncus arteriosus. **A,** Small MPA segment. **B,** Separate but close PA origin. **C,** Separate but distant PA origin. *A,* aorta; *LC,* left coronary artery; *LPA,* left pulmonary artery; *LS,* left subclavian artery; *LV,* left ventricle; *RC,* right coronary artery; *RPA,* right pulmonary artery; *RS,* right subclavian artery; *RV,* right ventricle. (Reprinted with permission from Adams FH, Emmanoulides GC, Riemenschneider TA. *Moss' Heart Disease in Infants, Children, and Adolescents.* 4th ed. Baltimore, Md: Williams & Wilkins; 1989.)

- Common associated lesions include coarctation and interrupted aortic arch. Coronary artery anomalies may occur. Extracardiac anomalies occur in about 21% to 30% of children and most often include DiGeorge syndrome, bowel malrotation, and hydroureter. Right aortic arch is more commonly associated with truncus arteriosus than with any other congenital heart defect. Complications of this diagnosis include subendocardial ischemia and PVOD early on from the high pressure and volume of pulmonary flow and progressive truncal valve insufficiency.
- Systemic and pulmonary venous blood returns normally and enters the respective ventricle. Ventricular blood mixes through the VSD and exits the heart through the truncus. Blood then flows to the lungs and body, depending on the respective resistances in each circuit. Symptoms appear when the PVR begins to fall around 2 to 4 weeks of life. In the event of severe truncal valve insufficiency (or more rarely stenosis), low cardiac output and cardiac compromise occur almost from birth.
  b. *Etiology and incidence:* This accounts for 1% to 4% of all CHD. Conotruncal or truncoarterial separation does not proceed normally. Either a deficiency or an absence of conal (infundibular) septum causes a large VSD.
  c. *Assessment*
    - *History:* Symptoms of CHF occur when the PVR drops and pulmonary blood flow increases. In infants with associated DiGeorge's syndrome, hypocalcemia and hypomagnesemia are frequently noted.
    - *Examination* reveals cyanosis only when PVR is increased; this is a concern for eventual repair. Active precordium, normal S_1, loud ejection click, loud and single S_2, and S_3 heard at the apex is common. In addition, a systolic ejection murmur at the LSB and frequently an apical diastolic murmur can be heard. If truncal valve insufficiency exists, a blowing diastolic high-pitched murmur is heard at the LSB.

d. *Diagnostic findings*
- *ECG* shows a normal QRS configuration or minimal right axis deviation, normal sinus rhythm, biventricular hypertrophy, and LAH.
- *Chest x-ray examination* demonstrates moderate cardiomegaly, increased pulmonary vascular markings, right arch in one third of patients, and dilated truncal root. In the presence of PVOD, enlargement of the pulmonary artery and a tapering of the distal pulmonary vascular tree occur.
- *Echocardiogram* confirms the diagnosis, and anatomic features are identified. Origin of the pulmonary arteries, VSD location and size, and anatomy of the truncal valve are accomplished. The pressure gradient across the truncal valve and the degree of insufficiency are quantitated if necessary.
- *Cardiac catheterization* is not necessary except in complex variants. Right and left ventricular pressures are equal, and there is increased oxygen saturation in the pulmonary artery. PVR and PA pressure are elevated to varying degrees and can determine the degree of pulmonary reactivity.

e. *Interventions*
- Repair should not be delayed, since the development of PVOD is rapid. Palliation with a PA band is not frequently performed and may not be successful in protecting the pulmonary vascular bed. Medical management to control CHF is warranted. Irradiated blood should always be used until DiGeorge syndrome can be ruled out because of the high association of T-cell immune compromise with DiGeorge syndrome.
- Surgical repair entails sternotomy and cardiopulmonary bypass with deep hypothermic circulatory arrest. The VSD is closed to the truncal valve, creating left ventricle–to–truncal valve continuity. The pulmonary arteries are connected to the distal end of the RV conduit; the conduit is then connected to the RV outflow tract, reestablishing right ventricle–to–pulmonary artery continuity. Truncal valve insufficiency or stenosis is addressed only if severe. Moderate insufficiency or stenoses often improve when the volume load crossing it is decreased following separation of the circulations. In most neonatal repairs the ASD or PFO is left open to allow bidirectional shunting until RV compliance improves. Increased RV compliance is noted postoperatively as oxygen saturations increase with decreasing oxygen requirements.
- Complications particular to this operation are conduction disturbances, RBBB, heart block, low cardiac output, residual pulmonary stenosis, PA hypertensive crisis, and progressive truncal valve insufficiency.

6. **Total anomalous pulmonary venous return (TAPVR)** occurs when all four pulmonary veins drain anomalously into the right side of the heart. Partial connection (PAPVR) occurs when one to three pulmonary veins drain anomalously.
a. *Pathophysiology*
- Pulmonary veins have no connection to the left atrium. The left atrium is often small and noncompliant. The pulmonary veins may empty in various ways to the right atrium (Fig. 3–45). Supracardiac pulmonary veins drain to the left SVC or right SVC via the vertical vein, forming a confluence posterior to the left atrium (45%). Infracardiac pulmonary veins drain to the IVC via the vertical vein (frequently obstructed at the level of the diaphragm [8%]). Cardiac pulmonary veins drain to the coronary sinus or right atrium and rarely are obstructed or stenotic

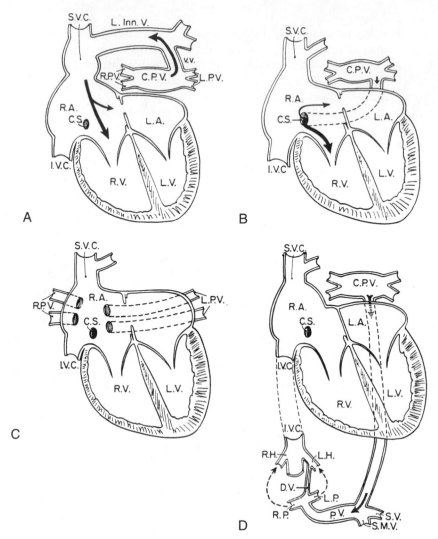

Figure 3–45. Anatomic variations of total anomalous pulmonary venous return. **A,** Common vein to vertical vein to left superior vena cava to right atrium. **B,** Common vein to coronary sinus. **C,** Separate origin pulmonary veins to right atrium. **D,** Common pulmonary vein drains to portal system below the diaphragm. *C.S.,* coronary sinus; *C.P.V.,* common pulmonary vein; *D.V.,* ductus venosus; *I.V.C.,* inferior vena cava; *L.A.,* left atrium; *L.H.,* left hepatic vein; *L.In.V.,* left innominate vein; *L.P.,* left pulmonary vein; *L.P.V.,* left pulmonary vein; *L.V.,* left ventricle; *P.V.,* pulmonary vein; *R.A.,* right atrium; *R.H.,* right hepatic vein; *R.P.,* right pulmonary vein; *R.P.V.,* right pulmonary vein; *R.V.,* right ventricle; *S.V.,* splenic vein; *S.V.C.,* superior vena cava; *S.M.V.,* superior mesenteric vein; *v.v.,* vertical vein. (Reprinted with permission from Adams FH, Emmanoulides GC, Riemenschneider TA. *Moss' Heart Disease in Infants, Children, and Adolescents.* 4th ed. Baltimore, Md: Williams & Wilkins, 1989.)

(35%). Mixed pulmonary veins drain via a combination of the above means (1% to 2%).

- An ASD is considered part of the complex and is mandatory for survival. One third have other cardiac anomalies such as TAT, TGV, pulmonary atresia, or single ventricle. TAPVR is increased in patients with asplenia and other forms of CHD.
- Hemodynamics depend on the distribution of mixed venous blood between the pulmonary and systemic circulation, the size of the ASD, and

the degree of obstruction. All venous blood enters the right side of the heart and exits the pulmonary artery. This creates pulmonary overcirculation and hypertension. For survival, blood must enter the left atrium via the ASD. If the ASD is small, the LV volume will be low and cardiac output will be severely compromised. If the ASD is large and the left atrium is compliant, LV volume will be appropriate. If the pulmonary veins are obstructed, blood cannot exit the lungs. This creates a critical situation of low cardiac output from LV volume underloading, severe pulmonary congestion from the obstruction, hypoxemia, and acidosis. Increased pulmonary venous pressure is transmitted to the pulmonary vascular bed, and reflex PA vasoconstriction occurs to prevent pulmonary edema. The result is decreased pulmonary blood flow, RA hypertrophy, RVH, and RV failure. Even if the veins are not obstructed, the increased pulmonary flow creates medial hypertrophy and intimal hyperplasia, ending with PVOD by the third to fourth decade of life.

b. *Etiology*
   - TAPVR is an embryologic error of incorporation of pulmonary veins into the left atrium.
c. *Assessment*
   - *History:* Patients with obstructed veins present with a history of severe respiratory distress, cyanosis, acidosis and low cardiac output shortly after birth from reduced blood flow to the left ventricle and pulmonary congestion from obstruction of flow through the veins. Patients with unobstructed veins present with CHF after 2 to 4 weeks when PVR decreases and shunting increases.
   - *Examination:* Children with obstructed veins have marked respiratory distress, cyanosis, dyspnea, tachycardia, tachypnea, RV heave, a systolic ejection click, increased S_1, a fixed and split S_2, low cardiac output, and acidosis. With unobstructed veins, there is an increased and split S_2, an S_3, and a systolic ejection murmur at the upper LSB. Although difficult, the diagnosis of obstructed TAPVR must be differentiated from persistent pulmonary hypertension of the newborn.
d. *Diagnostic findings*
   - *ECG* shows RA enlargement, RVH, and right axis deviation (if veins are obstructed).
   - *Chest x-ray examination* demonstrates increased pulmonary blood flow, RA and RV dilation, a prominent PA segment, snowman configuration of the heart in older infants with supracardiac TAPVR, and cardiomegaly if presenting with volume overload and CHF.
   - *Echocardiogram* confirms the diagnosis and localizes the site of venous drainage. Pulmonary venous obstruction is quantified by Doppler. Associated lesions are defined; RV pressure and PA hypertension are noted; and PA, RA, and RV volume overload are noted.
e. *Interventions*
   - Medical treatment for CHF is required for patients with unobstructed veins prior to surgery. Prostaglandin may make the situation worse in cyanotic obstructed veins by increasing even further pulmonary overcirculation.
   - Obstructed veins are almost always surgical emergencies. Unobstructed veins are repaired early to prevent PVOD. Surgical repair is aimed at returning pulmonary vein flow to the left side of the heart, eliminating obstruction, closing the ASD, and preventing PVOD. Repair is done via

sternotomy on cardiopulmonary bypass using deep hypothermic circulatory arrest. The pulmonary vein confluence is anastomosed to the posterior wall of the left atrium or the veins are directed through the ASD by an intraatrial patch, thereby redirecting pulmonary venous return correctly and closing the ASD.

- Postoperative problems include pulmonary hypertensive crisis, sick sinus syndrome and other atrial dysrhythmias, restenosis of the anastomosis, inability to fully relieve the stenosis (temporarily palliated with pulmonary vein stents), or a long ventilator course. ECMO may be required both preoperatively and postoperatively for pulmonary stabilization.

- Long-term prognosis depends on the presence of diffuse pulmonary vein obstruction and the state of the pulmonary vascular bed. Approximately 10% of these children have a second obstruction. LV compliance is poor, and the left atrium cannot easily dilate. Slow volume infusion prevents further increase and transmission of elevated pressure to the lungs. Use of inotropic agents may decrease the amount of volume needed to maintain the blood pressure and thereby decrease extracellular water, edema, and elevated LA pressure.

7. **Pulmonary atresia with intact ventricular septum (PA/IVS):** Complete obstruction of the RV outflow requiring shunting at the atrial and great vessel level for survival.

   a. *Pathophysiology*
      - The defect is characterized by variable size and function of the right ventricle and tricuspid valve. The right atrium may be dilated proportional to the degree of tricuspid insufficiency from lack of RV outflow. An ASD is always present. RV size may be decreased or normal but capable of handling forward cardiac output with relief of obstruction at the pulmonary valve. RV pressure increases related to the outflow obstruction can cause tricuspid insufficiency and increased RA pressure. Shunting can occur across the ASD into the left atrium. Flow into the pulmonary artery and lungs is maintained by the PDA. The left ventricle manages the total cardiac output.
      - Coronary artery anomalies may include fistulous communication between coronary arteries and the right ventricle, which can cause retrograde flow of desaturated blood into the coronary arteries resulting in ventricular ischemia and even death. Coronary arteries may be stenotic.

   b. *Etiology and incidence:* PA/IVS is an uncommon defect (3% of all CHD) associated with complex RV lesions. The cause is essentially unknown but may be an interruption of the neural crest cells or may be viral or infectious agents introduced early in fetal life.

   c. *Assessment*
      - *History* includes cyanosis evident shortly after birth as the PDA physiologically closes. CHF is uncommon unless the defect is accompanied by tricuspid insufficiency.
      - *Examination* reveals an S_1, normal intensity, single S_2, and a continuous murmur of the PDA. When there is significant tricuspid insufficiency, the child may have a holosystolic murmur.

   d. *Diagnostic findings*
      - *ECG* shows LV predominance and RAE. ST-T wave changes reflect major underlying coronary anomalies when present.
      - *Chest x-ray examination* results are normal in most cases (with decreased pulmonary blood flow). Marked cardiomegaly is present with severe tricuspid insufficiency.

- *Echocardiogram* defines an imperforate pulmonary valve, tricuspid valve size and anomalies, and visualization of the ASD and may be able to assess abnormal coronary artery connections.
- *Cardiac catheterization* is essential in full delineation of all anatomic defects. Low systemic venous saturations, decreased LA saturation from right-to-left shunting, and RV pressure are noted. Coronary artery fistulas and stenosis are visualized.

e. *Interventions*
- Ductal patency is mandatory for survival until full diagnostic evaluation and surgical repair is completed.
- The surgical approach depends on multiple factors including predicted RV function, the presence of RV-dependent coronary blood flow or coronary artery stenosis, and the size of the tricuspid valve and ASD. Surgery includes an aortopulmonary shunt via thoracotomy for diminutive right ventricle and eventual single ventricle repair. The RV outflow tract is patched via sternotomy and bypass if the tricuspid valve and RV size are sufficient to handle pulmonary blood flow and if there is no RV-dependent coronary blood flow. Patients with unusable or marginal RV undergo a second-stage palliation with a cavopulmonary shunt. If the RV size is suitable, patients may have SVC-PA (cavopulmonary shunt) and IVC-RV flow established via an RV-PA conduit or RV outflow tract patch in the neonatal period ("1½ ventricle" repair). Cyanosis is not uncommon immediately after surgery while the right ventricle is noncompliant. As compliance increases, volume requirements, tricuspid insufficiency, and cyanosis decrease. The ASD is left open in these infants to provide pressure relief for noncompliant right ventricles (Fig. 3–46).
- Early and late mortality of this defect remains high, and consensus has yet to be reached regarding optimal patient management.

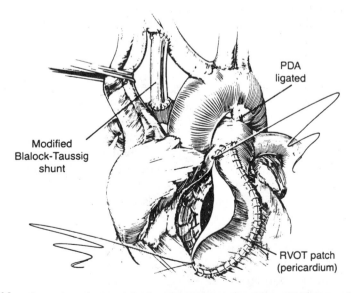

Figure 3–46. A transannular patch is placed to enlarge the right ventricular outflow tract and a right-sided modified Blalock-Taussig shunt is placed from the right subclavian-innominate artery to the right pulmonary artery. (Reprinted with permission from Castaneda AR, Jonas RA, Mayer JE, Hanley FL. *Cardiac Surgery of the Neonate and Infant.* Philadelphia, Pa: WB Saunders Co; 1994.)

HYPERTENSIVE CRISIS

A. **DEFINITION**

An acute, life-threatening elevation in systolic and diastolic blood pressure potentially resulting in end-organ damage or death.

B. **PATHOPHYSIOLOGY**

1. Hypertension poses a risk for generalized vascular disease and other end-organ changes.

2. Normal or abnormal blood pressure should be determined in infancy. Appropriately sized cuffs are vital for accurate measurements. The American Academy of Pediatrics (AAP) recommends that all children age 3 years and older have their blood pressure measured at least yearly. The AAP Task Force established norms taking into account race, ethnic groups, height, and weight for age. Blood pressure varies normally with time of day, physical activity, body position, and emotional state. Hypertension is defined as a blood pressure greater than the 95th percentile for age and sex on at least three different occasions. According to the AAP Task Force, children with elevated blood pressure between the 90th and 95th percentile for age are "at risk" and should be followed more closely.

3. Peripheral vascular resistance and cardiac output determine blood pressure. As total peripheral vascular resistance or cardiac output increase, blood pressure rises. Peripheral vascular resistance is mediated by blood viscosity, arteriolar smooth muscle structure and function, vasoconstrictor substances, renin, angiotensin I, angiotensinogen, vasorelaxants including atrial natriuretic peptide (ANP), and the amount of autonomic discharge.

4. Over time, primary or essential hypertension (multifactorial entity) and secondary hypertension (diagnosed etiology) will produce changes in the arterioles (necrosis and inflammation) that eventually cause decreased blood flow to end-organs. Permanent damage may result.

5. Uncontrolled hypertension may induce a sudden rise in blood pressure, which may lead to accelerated or malignant hypertension. Accelerated hypertension is associated with rapid vascular changes and retinal exudates and hemorrhages (rare in infants and young children). Failure to aggressively treat accelerated hypertension results in malignant hypertension. Malignant hypertension differs minimally from accelerated hypertension in infants. Retinal exudates and hemorrhages, when present, advance to papilledema. Large amounts of renin and angiotensin cause arterial dilation and contraction. This produces turbulent blood flow, which causes microangiopathic hemolytic anemia and intravascular coagulation. The arterial walls swell with fluid, causing fibrinoid necrosis. Hypertensive encephalopathy ensues. Excessive elevation of the blood pressure causes dysfunction of cerebral autoregulation, which in turn causes vasospasms, ischemia, increased capillary pressure and permeability, and cerebral edema and hemorrhage.

6. The frequency of these emergencies is declining because hypertension is detected earlier when underlying disease is diagnosed.

C. **ETIOLOGY**

1. Failure to control essential or secondary hypertension may be related to the inability of medication regimens to control blood pressure or lack of compliance with the regimen.

2. Renal parenchymal disease (acute glomerulonephritis, chronic pyelonephritis, renal vascular disease, renal secreting tumors, chronic renal failure, polycystic disease, Wilms' tumor, hemangiopericytoma) is a major factor in the development of hypertension. Renal vascular diseases also contribute to the incidence

of hypertension. These include thromboembolic phenomena related to umbilical artery catheterization or coagulopathy, fibromuscular dysplasia, neurofibromatosis, vasculitis, arteritis, congenital aneurysms, renal vein or artery thrombosis, or segmental hypoplasia (Ash-Upmark kidney).

3. Other contributing factors include pheochromocytoma, pituitary tumors, coarctation of the aorta, congenital adrenal hyperplasia, Cushing's syndrome, polycythemia, primary aldosteronism, Williams and Turner's syndrome, intraventricular hemorrhage, and obstructive hydrocephalus.

D. ASSESSMENT

1. **History** reveals complaints of severe headache, epistaxis, hypertension (child or family), etiologic factors listed above, known risk factors, or evidence of complications of hypertension (renal dysfunction). Diet history may indicate a high sodium intake.

2. **Clinical presentation** of a hypertensive crisis includes decreased femoral pulses (if coarctation is also present), convulsions, mental status changes or focal neurologic changes, dyspnea, headache, restlessness, epistaxis, tachycardia, rales, S_3, S_4, nonspecific signs of uremia, and blurred vision. A bruit may be auscultated over the femoral area, carotid arteries, abdominal aorta, anterior fontanelle, and anteriorly over the renal vascular area.

3. **Diagnostic findings**
   a. *Laboratory studies*
      - CBC: Hematocrit is decreased in renal failure, and anemia is associated with renal disease.
      - Serum BUN and creatinine clearance values are elevated with renal disease.
      - Serum glucose level is elevated in Cushing's syndrome, pheochromocytoma, and diabetes, all three of which are potential causes of hypertension.
      - Urinalysis determines the presence of proteinuria (indicates renal disease), hematuria (malignant nephrosclerosis), or urinary vanillylmandelic acid (VMA; catecholamines are elevated in pheochromocytoma).
      - Serum uric acid: Hyperuricemia is associated with renal failure.
      - Serum potassium is used to rule out primary aldosteronism, which causes hypokalemia and hypertension.
   b. *Radiologic findings*
      - Renal arteriography is used to show renal artery stenosis, lesions, and dysplasias as causes of hypertension.
      - IV pyelography may indicate the presence of kidney disease but cannot differentiate the type.
      - Chest x-ray examination may reveal cardiomegaly and pulmonary edema.
      - CT scan shows diffuse brain edema in patients with encephalopathy and also demonstrates hemorrhage.
   c. *ECG* may reveal signs of LVH and ischemia.

E. INTERVENTIONS

1. Effectiveness and toxicities of drug therapies vary widely among patients. Therapy is often lifelong when hypertensive crisis occurs in childhood, so doses must be adjusted for growth and maturational changes. Medications include α- and β-blockers, diuretics, vasodilators (including calcium channel inhibitors), and renin-angiotensin inhibitors.

2. Positive pressure ventilation is helpful if pulmonary edema, CHF, and cerebral edema are present.

3. Reduction of anxiety or pain if present aids in reduction of blood pressure.

4. Lifestyle changes may be required for long-term control and avoidance of future crisis. Diet should be low salt, low cholesterol, and low fat. Exercise programs are prescribed with consideration of limitations of the underlying disease.

F. **NURSING DIAGNOSES**
    ❖ EXCESSIVE ELEVATION OF SYSTEMIC BLOOD PRESSURE
    1. **Defining characteristic:** Patient exhibits blood pressure greater than the 95th percentile for age, sex, and ethnic group.
    2. **Expected outcome:** Blood pressure will return to normal limits.
    3. **Interventions**
       a. Continually reassure the patient and family. Maintain a calm, quiet environment.
       b. Assist in the insertion of hemodynamic monitoring lines to monitor patient's response to therapy. Monitor ECG for dysrhythmias.
       c. Administer drugs as ordered: Monitor response and side effects, and titrate to maintain desired blood pressure level. Administer diuretics and monitor intake and output.
    4. **Evaluation of nursing care**
       a. Patient's blood pressure is within prescribed limits.
       b. ECG demonstrates normal sinus rhythm.
    ❖ POTENTIAL FOR HYPOTENSION SECONDARY TO DIURETIC AND ANTIHYPERTENSIVE DRUG THERAPY
    1. **Defining characteristics**
       a. Blood pressure and urine output are below prescribed limits.
       b. Serum electrolyte levels are abnormal.
       c. Child may exhibit hypovolemic shock symptoms.
    2. **Expected outcomes**
       a. Blood pressure is within normal limits.
       b. ECG demonstrates normal sinus rhythm.
       c. Child is normovolemic.
    3. **Interventions**
       a. Monitor hemodynamic pressures closely. Monitor ECG continuously.
       b. Monitor patient's response to the drug therapy and report values that reflect hypotension. Titrate or stop antihypertensive drugs when necessary.
       c. Administer fluids to restore volume. Monitor electrolytes for abnormalities.
    4. **Evaluation of nursing care**
       a. Blood pressure is within prescribed limits.
       b. Hemodynamics reflect adequate filling pressures and cardiac output.
       c. Electrolytes are within normal limits.
       d. ECG demonstrates normal sinus rhythm.

CARDIOMYOPATHY

A. **DEFINITION**
    Myocardial muscle disease of unknown origin
B. **PATHOPHYSIOLOGY**
    1. Cardiomyopathy is characterized by changes or damage to the myocardium producing myocyte degeneration with compensation by hypertrophy, interstitial fibrosis and scarring, endocardial thickening that decreases contractility, and disorganized alignment of cellular structure leading to ineffective depolarization and contraction.

2. Cardiomyopathies are classified as hypertrophic, dilated (congestive), and restrictive.
   a. *Hypertrophic* cardiomyopathy is characterized by varying degrees of myocardial fibrosis and a thick muscle-bound left ventricle with marked increase in myocardial mass (massive ventricular hypertrophy), a decreased ventricular cavity size, and a resistance to LV filling. When it contracts, outflow from the left ventricle is obstructed. Diastolic stiffness of the left ventricle impairs LV filling, producing atrial enlargement. Coronary artery narrowing from intimal and medial vessel proliferation occurs in 80% of children with hypertrophic cardiomyopathy.
   b. *Dilated (congestive)* cardiomyopathy results in massive cardiomegaly as a result of extensive dilation of the ventricles (especially the left), associated mild to moderate ventricular hypertrophy, reduced stroke volume, low ejection fraction, and increased systolic and diastolic volumes. Stasis of blood can occur in the apexes.
   c. *Restrictive* cardiomyopathy is characterized by fibrosis of the ventricle resulting in minimal contractile movement, poor ventricular compliance, and inadequate filling.

C. ETIOLOGY
   1. *Hypertrophic cardiomyopathy* has an autosomal dominant transmission in 60% of cases. There is often a history of sudden death in the family. It can also be secondary to hypertension caused by obstruction to flow such as with aortic stenosis, coarctation, or renal artery stenosis.
   2. *Dilated cardiomyopathy* can be idiopathic or related to viral myocarditis, ischemic damage as with anomalous left coronary artery, metabolic disorders such as hemochromatosis (iron deposition), carnitine deficiency, glycogen storage diseases, drug toxicity (e.g., doxorubicin [Adriamycin]), collagen diseases, or sarcoidosis.
   3. *Restrictive cardiomyopathy* is related to endocardial fibroelastosis (congenital defect of the endocardium) and hypereosinophilic syndrome (infiltration of eosinophils with fibrosis and scarring associated with leukemia and rare in children).

D. SIGNS AND SYMPTOMS
   1. Children may be asymptomatic with murmur, especially until significant disease develops.
   2. Most patients have an enlarged heart resulting in altered cardiac contractility. Dilated cardiomyopathy causes poor contractility; hypertrophic cardiomyopathy causes supercontractility. With restrictive cardiomyopathy there is normal systolic function but decreased diastolic function.
   3. Low cardiac output results in poor perfusion, shock, low urine output, and decreased level of consciousness. Other symptomatology includes CHF (brisk pulses, LV lift, gallop rhythm), systolic ejection murmur, split S_2, gallop, arrhythmias, syncope, thromboembolic events, increased LVEDP by cardiac catheterization, weakness, fatigue, dyspnea on exertion, palpitations, angina, irritability, cough, and anorexia.

E. DIAGNOSTIC STUDIES
   1. **Chest x-ray examination** demonstrates an enlarged heart, normal or increased CT ratio, pulmonary venous engorgement and interstitial edema, and pleural effusions.
   2. **ECG** demonstrates RBBB, LBBB, conduction delays, arrhythmias, LVH with or without ST depression and T wave inversion or other nonspecific T wave abnormalities, and possibly atrial enlargement.

3. **ECHO** is used to assess contractility and rule out CHD. It will define ventricular dilation, disproportionate ventricular septal thickening, possible obstruction of RV and LV outflow tracts, decreased ejection fraction, and poor contractility.

4. **Laboratory studies** rule out metabolic causes and provide viral titers.

5. **Cardiac catheterization** is used to assess cardiac function and obtain an endomyocardial biopsy for myocarditis.

F. NURSING DIAGNOSES

 ❖ ALTERATION IN CARDIAC OUTPUT DUE TO INADEQUATE TISSUE PERFUSION AND AR-RHYTHMIAS

 ❖ ACTIVITY INTOLERANCE

 ❖ POTENTIAL FOR THROMBUS FORMATION

G. GOALS AND PATIENT MANAGEMENT

1. Improve and maximize cardiac output and activity level.

 a. *Pharmacologic therapy:* In hypertrophic cardiomyopathy, β-adrenergic agonists reduce the ventricular workload. Calcium channel blockers provide afterload reduction, decrease myocardial contractility, and thereby improve LV diastolic function. Diuretics are used judiciously, since they may reduce blood volume and increase the risk of obstruction of the left ventricle. Inotropic agents are avoided, since they may burn out muscle by increasing contractility in an already hypercontractile muscle without increasing underlying coronary supply. With dilated and restrictive cardiomyopathy, digoxin and positive inotropic agents (dopamine, dobutamine) are used to improve contractility. Diuretics reduce volume, and vasodilators provide afterload reduction.

 b. *Surgical resection* of hypertrophic septal tissue (ventricular septal myotomy) can be used in hypertrophic cardiomyopathy. Resection of the LV outflow tract is used with IHSS.

 c. *Pacing* can change the timing of ventricular responses, producing an asymmetric right ventricle and septal motion away from the area of the LV outflow tract obstruction during contraction (only in hypertrophic cardiomyopathy).

 d. *Fluid therapy* is aimed at fluid and sodium restriction. Edema, weight, rales, and electrolyte levels are assessed, and diuretics are used.

 e. *Cardiac workload is decreased* through oxygen therapy, intubation or ventilation, rest periods, gavage feedings, and increased caloric intake.

 f. *Thrombus formation* is prevented with medications (e.g., heparin, aspirin, and warfarin [Coumadin]).

 g. *Transplantation* is used for end-stage disease. Although difficult to predict, atrial and ventricular arrhythmias, risk of sudden death, failure to thrive, and thrombus formation are considered.

H. COMPLICATIONS

Complications of cardiomyopathies include arrhythmias, emboli, CHF, and death.

ACUTE INFLAMMATORY DISEASES

A. DEFINITION

Myocardial diseases that produce inflammation of cardiac or vascular tissues including myocarditis, endocarditis, pericarditis, Kawasaki syndrome, and rheumatic heart disease

B. MYOCARDITIS, ENDOCARDITIS, AND PERICARDITIS

1. **Pathophysiology**

 a. *Myocarditis* occurs most commonly as an extension of infective endocarditis especially involving aortic, mitral, or prosthetic valves and results in focal or diffuse inflammation of cardiac muscle or an intramyocardial abscess. It produces temporary or permanent damage to the myocardium. During the acute phase (when the causative organism can be cultured), there is initiation of direct myocardial damage with necrosis of myocardial cells, which includes specialized tissues such as the conduction system as well as muscle. Cellular infiltration of mononuclear WBCs results in disintegration of heart muscle, fibrosis, hypertrophy, chamber dilation, and mural thrombi. The chronic phase is mediated by immune system T cells and natural killer cells that continue to attack the myocardium. The necrotic area of muscle is replaced with scar tissue. Focal hemorrhage, edema, fatty infiltration of the muscle, and fibrosis may also occur.

b. *Endocarditis* is an inflammation of a valve, endocardium, or endothelium that results from a bacteria or fungus in a child with valvular or structural heart disease. Turbulent blood flow results in mural tissue damage with deposition of platelets and fibrin and thrombus formation with entrapment of circulating organisms. Large colonies of bacteria become encased in masses of fibrin-forming vegetations. Vegetations usually occur at the location of jet lesions. In addition, infection may destroy the valve, invade the myocardium to form an abscess, or result in thrombus formation on valves and eventual deformation and valve insufficiency. Portions of the lesions may embolize to other organs, resulting in complement activation and inflammatory responses that may contribute to renal dysfunction.

c. *Pericarditis* is related to inflammation that produces effusion fluid (ranges from serous to thick and cheesy exudate) and fibrin deposits within the pericardial sac. As the volume increases, the pressure rises, cardiac filling decreases, and cardiac output decreases.

2. **Etiology**

a. *Myocarditis* can be caused by any pathogen, including bacteria, viruses, and fungi. Most cases are associated with a viral illness (especially RNA type, e.g., coxsackievirus A and B, influenza A and B), a systemic infection, or active endocarditis. Noninfectious myocarditis may be caused by systemic diseases (e.g., systemic lupus erythematosus).

b. *Endocarditis* is usually bacterial (especially *Streptococcus viridans, Staphylococcus aureus,* and *Staphylococcus epidermidis*) and rarely fungal. It is most likely to affect children with underlying heart disease or intracardiac catheters, especially children with prosthetic valves or those who have undergone surgical interventions (e.g., open heart surgery with foreign patch material or gastrointestinal tract, genitourinary tract, or dental procedures). Fungal organisms are most likely to be identified in infants or immunocompromised children.

c. *Pericarditis* is related to inflammation of the pericardial sac. It implies an active problem, such as trauma, postcardiotomy infection (bacterial, viral, fungal, protozoal), toxic reactions from radiation, drugs, or uremia, and collagen diseases.

3. **Signs and symptoms**

a. *Myocarditis* has a history of bacterial or viral illness, fever, tachycardia, arrhythmias, signs of CHF, lethargy, chest pain, weakness, myalgia, poor systemic perfusion with shock, systolic murmur, pulsus alternans, or pericardial or pleural friction rub.

b. *Endocarditis* is characterized by new or changing murmurs, fever, chills, sweating, fatigue, malaise, anorexia, headache, splenomegaly, valve insufficiency, CHF, and arthralgia. Systemic emboli may produce pain or compromise in the perfusion of extremities, petechiae, splinter hemorrhages of fingernails, hematuria, cerebral infarct, and renal dysfunction. Osler's nodes result in painful intradermal pads. Janeway's lesions result in painless hemorrhages of the palms and soles.

c. *Pericarditis* produces decreased cardiac output and systemic blood pressure, increased intracardiac pressures, pericardial friction rub, accentuated pulmonary component to S_2, muffled heart sounds with effusion, chest pain (worse when lying down or on deep breath) and discomfort. In addition, cough, fever, dyspnea, arrhythmias, and pulsus paradoxus (with effusion) may be noted.

4. **Invasive and noninvasive diagnostic studies**
   a. *Chest x-ray examination* demonstrates an enlarged heart when effusion is present.
   b. *ECG* may show ST changes (elevation or depression), T wave may be inverted, prolonged PR interval, diminished QRS complex and T wave voltage, or arrhythmias.
   c. *Echocardiogram* is used to size the effusion, locate and visualize vegetations and abscesses, rule out structural problems, measure end-diastolic pressures, and evaluate valve function. A transesophageal view may be used for better visualization.
   d. *Laboratory studies* include cultures (minimum of three blood cultures), WBC (leukocytosis may be present), titers to assess for elevated IgM, cardiac enzyme studies, and sedimentation rate (may be elevated).
   e. *Cardiac catheterization* is used to identify restrictive pericarditis or cardiomyopathy, evaluate the severity of constriction, and obtain an endomyocardial biopsy for histologic grading, culture (rarely positive), and polymerase chain reaction (PCR) analysis of tissue for viral genomes.
   f. *Pericardiocentesis* is a needle aspiration used to obtain pericardial fluid for analysis and culture and to relieve tamponade.

5. **Nursing diagnoses**
   ❖ ALTERATION IN CARDIAC OUTPUT
   ❖ ALTERATION IN BREATHING PATTERNS
   ❖ ALTERATION IN COMFORT
   ❖ POTENTIAL FOR EMBOLIC DAMAGE

6. **Goals and desired outcomes**
   a. *Myocarditis*
      • Treat infection.
      • Maximize ventricular function.
      • Provide cardiovascular support.
   b. *Endocarditis*
      • Provide prevention for susceptible patients.
      • Treat infection.
      • Provide cardiovascular support.
      • Treat CHF.
   c. *Pericarditis*
      • Treat infection.
      • Remove fluid collection.

7. **Patient care management**
   a. *Myocarditis:* Provide continuous monitoring (risk of serious arrhythmias and sudden death), bed rest, antibiotics, antipyretics, corticosteroids (controversial), treatment of CHF or shock, and antiarrhythmics. Most children recover with no sequelae. Some develop progressive dilation with decreased ventricular function and AV valve insufficiency. In some, the

primary manifestation is arrhythmias with sudden death.

    b. *Endocarditis* requires appropriate antibiotic therapy intravenously for 6 weeks, neurologic checks, treatment of CHF, and bed rest. Lesions eventually heal following weeks of treatment, although sequela from embolization and renal dysfunction from the inflammatory response may result. Therapeutic antibiotic levels and continuing assessment of effective coverage should be maintained.

    c. *Pericarditis:* Pericardiocentesis is both diagnostic and therapeutic to prevent cardiac tamponade. Antibiotics are prescribed.

  8. **Complications** include CHF, end-stage myocardial damage, tamponade, arrhythmias, valve failure, and microemboli causing infarcts.

C. RHEUMATIC FEVER

1. **Pathophysiology:** Group A β-hemolytic streptococci initiate an autoimmune process that attacks collagen. Streptococcal and myocardial tissue have similar antigenic determinants creating antigenic mimicry (antibodies produced for streptococcal infection react with host tissue producing antibody-induced tissue damage). There is evidence of immunologic cross-reactions: streptococcal carbohydrate and valvular glycoprotein, streptococcal protoplast membrane and neuronal tissue, and hyaluronate produced by streptococci and articular cartilage.

2. **Etiology and incidence:** The cause is unclear, but it usually occurs 1 to 3 weeks after streptococcal pharyngitis, possibly in susceptible individuals with a single recessive gene. Rheumatic fever most often occurs in the age group of 6 to 15 years. It is rare in children younger than 2 years or older than 15 years. The incidence decreased after the introduction of antibiotics. Now it is most common in Third World countries with new outbreaks of resistant strains in the United States.

3. **Signs and symptoms** include recent pharyngitis or upper respiratory tract infection, new murmur, cardiac enlargement, friction rub or effusion, and CHF. Arthritis occurs in 70% of patients and may be the presenting symptom. Children experience migratory heat, redness, and pain that is greater than evidence of involvement. CNS involvement is characterized by chorea resulting in grimacing, slurred speech, weakness, and purposeless movements (Sydenham's chorea [St. Vitus' Dance]). Skin involvement includes painless, firm subcutaneous nodules (0.5 to 2 cm) over the extensor surfaces of joints such as elbows, knuckles, knees, ankles, as well as the scalp and spine. Erythema marginatum rheumaticum is a rash characterized by pink, raised, small irregular macules that are nonpruritic. It usually appears on the trunk and limbs but not on the face.

4. **Diagnostic studies**

    a. *Laboratory studies* include throat culture (positive for group A streptococci), WBC (may be elevated), sedimentation rate (elevated), C-reactive protein (elevated), and antistreptolysin O antibody titer (elevated).

    b. *ECG* may show a prolonged PR interval indicating first-degree AV block, diffuse ST-T wave changes, or T wave inversion.

    c. *Echocardiogram* is used to evaluate for myocarditis, decreased contractility, and valvular insufficiency.

    d. *Jones criteria* are used for diagnosis. The patient needs two major or one major and two minor manifestations to have a high probability of rheumatic fever (Table 3–7).

5. **Nursing diagnoses**

    ❖ ALTERATION IN CARDIAC OUTPUT

    ❖ ALTERATION IN COMFORT

Table 3–7. JONES CRITERIA

MAJOR MANIFESTATIONS	MINOR MANIFESTATIONS
Carditis	Clinical
Polyarthritis	Previous rheumatic fever
Chorea	Arthralgia
Erythema marginatum rheumaticium	Fever
Subcutaneous nodules	Laboratory
	Sedimentation rate
	C-reactive protein
	Leukocytosis
	Prolonged PR interval

6. **Goals and desired outcomes**
   a. Reestablish and maintain hemodynamic stability.
   b. Arrest or control inflammatory processes.
   c. Treat infectious processes.
   d. Optimize cardiac output.
   e. Optimize level of comfort.
7. **Patient care management:** Streptococcal infection is treated with antibiotics. Cardiac workload is decreased with bed rest in a quiet and dark environment, control of arrhythmias, and pain control.
8. **Complications** include valvular and myocardial damage.

D. **KAWASAKI DISEASE (MUCOCUTANEOUS LYMPH NODE SYNDROME)**
   1. **Pathophysiology:** Microvascular inflammation of all vascular tissues occurs. During early stages, generalized microvasculitis is present. Myocarditis develops within 3 to 4 weeks and is associated with WBC infiltration and edema of the conduction system and the myocardial muscle. Occasionally, severe valvulitis and coronary artery dilation and aneurysms develop. Extremely large aneurysms may produce coronary insufficiency leading to myocardial ischemia, CHF, or infarction.
   2. **Etiology** is unclear. It is more prevalent in children of Japanese ancestry and in children younger than 5 years of age. Seasonal outbreaks in winter and spring occur in geographic clusters. Rickettsiae, carpet shampoos, streptococcal toxins, and other agents have been implicated with the disease.
   3. **Signs and symptoms** include high, often spiking, fever (lasting 5 or more days); skin rash; conjunctivitis; injected, fissured lips and erythema of the buccal mucosa; strawberry tongue; cervical lymphadenopathy; and erythema and edema of the hands and feet followed by desquamation 2 to 4 weeks later. Other manifestations have been observed such as arthralgia and arthritis (common), diarrhea, jaundice, urethritis, aseptic meningitis, uveitis, irritability, cranial nerve palsies, abdominal pain, encephalopathy, ataxia, hypertension, pulmonary infiltrates, gallbladder hydrops, ileus, hepatomegaly, and splenomegaly. The child will also experience symptoms of myocarditis and possibly CHF.
   4. **Diagnostic studies**
      a. *Laboratory studies* are done to evaluate anemia, leukocytosis, thrombocytosis, elevated erythrocyte sedimentation rate (ESR), elevated serum amylase, liver function, C-reactive protein, pyuria, and proteinuria.
      b. *ECG* shows nonspecific ST-T wave changes, and there may be a prolonged PR interval.
      c. *Echocardiogram* helps in diagnosing coronary aneurysms (may also need

arteriography or angiography), pericardial effusions, ventricular dysfunction, and valvular insufficiency. Serial studies are done early and at 6 months.

   d. *Cardiac catheterization* is used to assess coronary aneurysms and stenosis (Fig. 3–47).

5. **Nursing diagnoses**
   - ❖ ALTERATION IN CARDIAC OUTPUT
   - ❖ POTENTIAL FOR SHOCK RELATED TO MI
   - ❖ ALTERATION IN COMFORT

6. **Goals and desired outcomes**
   a. Reestablish and maintain hemodynamic stability.
   b. Arrest and control inflammatory processes.
   c. Treat infectious processes.
   d. Optimize cardiac output.
   e. Prevent embolic damage and coronary involvement.
   f. Optimize level of comfort.

7. **Patient care management**
   a. Antiinflammatory agents (indomethacin [Indocin], steroids, salicylate and IV immunoglobulin) reduce inflammation and decrease the incidence of coronary abnormalities.
   b. Serial ECGs and cardiac isoenzymes are evaluated on a regular basis. Tissue plasminogen activator (TPA) is available if symptoms of an infarction develop. A coronary artery bypass graft (CABG) can be used for large aneurysms or significant areas of stenosis.
   c. Recovery is usually complete in those who do not develop coronary vasculitis, although second attacks may occur. Many patients have cardiac involvement, but no more than 10% of those with aneurysms (1% to 2% of all patients) have fatal outcomes (usually within 1 to 2 months of onset).

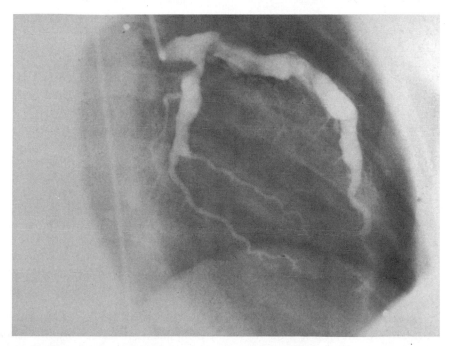

Figure 3–47. Cineangiogram photo of aneurysms created by Kawasaki syndrome. (Courtesy of Children's National Medical Center.)

    d. **Complications** include coronary aneurysms. If greater than 8 mm in size, there is a higher risk of infarct.

CARDIAC TRANSPLANTATION

A. **DEFINITION**
Surgical replacement of the heart used for end-stage, irreversible disease in which no other medical or surgical therapy will be successful

B. **INDICATIONS FOR TRANSPLANTATION**
Indications for transplantation include end-stage cardiomyopathy, complex CHD not amenable to surgical repair, ischemic damage from anomalous left coronary artery, nonmalignant cardiac tumor not amenable to resection, or life-threatening arrhythmias not responsive to medical and surgical therapy.

C. **CLINICAL SIGNS AND SYMPTOMS**
Signs and symptoms are related to the underlying condition (see Cardiomyopathy, Congestive Heart Failure, Congenital Heart Disease).

D. **DIAGNOSTIC STUDIES**
1. **Cardiac evaluation** includes an ECG and ECHO. Cardiac catheterization is performed to assess function and PVR. PVR greater than 4 Wood's units is of concern, and greater than 8 Wood's units is considered a contraindication. Exercise stress testing and Holter monitoring evaluates for arrhythmias as a sign of myocardial dysfunction.
2. Other organ system evaluation includes neurologic examination, liver function studies and renal function analysis by serum laboratory studies, creatinine clearance testing, and glomerular filtration rate renal scan. Serologies determine exposure to viral illnesses (used as baseline for future exposure as well), and cultures rule out current infection. Because of the risk of superinfection with immunosuppression, current infection is a relative contraindication to transplantation until the infection is appropriately treated.
3. The immune system is evaluated with human leukocyte antigen (HLA) testing (HLAs that determine tissue type, used retrospectively to determine degree of matching with donor), percent reactive antibody (PRA; antibodies within blood to other human blood that can produce hyperacute rejection during transplant procedure), and other immune markers used to assess function of immune system cell lines (center specific).
4. Genetic evaluation rules out genetic syndromes that might produce disease or prevent optimum outcome from transplantation.
5. It is preferred that all organ systems have normal function to provide the best possible outcome to transplantation. Surgeons may accept relative abnormalities that can be explained by poor cardiac output and are reversible once transplantation occurs. Active malignancy is avoided. Recent pulmonary embolism or infarction is avoided because of the risk of pneumonia after transplantation.
6. A financial screening interview is used to determine insurance plan coverage for transplantation, to assess the family's ability to provide long-term medical care, and to assess drug coverage needed to provide expensive long-term immunosuppressive medications.
7. Psychosocial evaluation rules out patients and families with problems that might prevent positive outcomes of transplantation; identifies problem issues that may need to be addressed during the stress of waiting, transplantation, and long-term care; and considers drug and alcohol history, psychiatric disorders,

child abuse and neglect history, and evidence of the family's inability to care for the child.

E. NURSING DIAGNOSES
*   ❖ ALTERATION IN CARDIAC OUTPUT DUE TO PREOPERATIVE CONDITION, ISCHEMIC HEART DURING EARLY OPERATIVE RECOVERY, OR REJECTION
*   ❖ ALTERATION IN IMMUNE FUNCTION
*   ❖ RISK OF INFECTION
*   ❖ PATIENT AND FAMILY KNOWLEDGE DEFICIT

F. GOALS AND PATIENT OUTCOMES
1. Establish hemodynamic stability.
2. Prevent cardiac rejection and infection.

G. PATIENT MANAGEMENT
1. Evaluate cardiovascular function as with all postoperative cardiovascular surgery patients. Assess for bradycardia due to denervated heart and prepare for use of chronotropic agents such as isoproterenol (Isuprel) or pacing to maintain cardiac output.
2. Assess for symptoms of rejection including fever, lethargy, malaise, decreased appetite, signs of CHF, decreased ECG voltage, decreased function by ECHO, and grade of rejection by endomyocardial biopsy.
3. Provide immunosuppressive medications such as cyclosporine, FK-506 (tacrolimus), azathioprine, mycophenolate mofetil, methylprednisolone, prednisone, antithymocyte globulin (ATG), antilymphocyte globulin (ALG), and muromonab-cd3 (Orthoclone OKT3). (See Chapter 8 for further discussion of immunosuppression.)
4. Assess for signs and symptoms of infection.

H. COMPLICATIONS
Complications include rejection, infection, lymphoproliferative disease, accelerated coronary artery disease, hypertension, renal failure, primary organ failure, and death.

HEART-LUNG TRANSPLANTATION

See also Lung Transplantation, Chapter 2.

A. DEFINITION
Surgical replacement therapy used for end-stage diseases affecting the cardiopulmonary system.

B. INDICATIONS FOR TRANSPLANTATION
Indications are changing as lung transplantation outcomes improve. They include primary pulmonary hypertension, Eisenmenger's syndrome, CHDs (such as valvular heart disease with pulmonary hypertension), cystic fibrosis, pulmonary parenchymal disease (such as fibrosing alveolitis or pulmonary fibrosis), and bronchiolitis obliterans (chronic lung rejection).

C. SIGNS AND SYMPTOMS
Signs and symptoms are those of the underlying condition (see Cardiac and Respiratory Failure).

D. DIAGNOSTIC STUDIES
Diagnostic studies include cardiac evaluation (see Cardiac Transplantation) and pulmonary function testing (see Chapter 2).

E. GOALS AND PATIENT OUTCOMES
1. Establish hemodynamic stability.

2. Establish respiratory function and stability.
3. Prevent cardiopulmonary rejection.
4. Prevent infection.

F. **PATIENT MANAGEMENT**

See Cardiac Transplantation and Lung Transplantation, Chapter 2.

CARDIAC TRAUMA

A. **PATHOPHYSIOLOGY**

Pathophysiology depends on the mechanism of injury.

1. **Myocardial contusion** may cause bruising, swelling, muscle dysfunction, internal bleeding, and tamponade.
2. **Major vessel or cardiac rupture** can occur by narrowing the anteroposterior diameter of the chest. This results in rapid compression and expansion of vessel structures, which produces shearing forces, tearing the aorta, SVC, IVC, or atrial appendage leading to sudden massive blood loss with shock or tamponade.
3. **Cardiac tamponade** can occur from contusion or penetrating trauma, resulting in blood or fluid accumulation in the pericardial sac. The fluid accumulation impairs ventricular filling.

B. **ETIOLOGY**

1. Compression provides a direct blow when the sternum or ribs impact the heart. This can cause septal defects, wall or valve rupture, and coronary artery occlusion. Direct blows can also cause fatal arrhythmias.
2. Acceleration, deceleration injury may result in avulsion or tears of the aorta, SVC or IVC (Fig. 3–48).

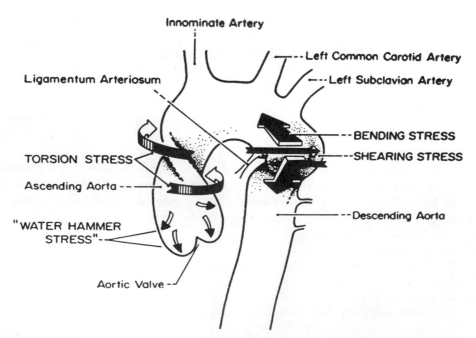

Figure 3–48. Diagram of stresses producing trauma to great vessels. (Reprinted with permission from Synbas PN. *Trauma to the Heart and Great Vessels*. Philadelphia, Pa: WB Saunders Co; 1978.)

3. Changes in intrachamber pressures from crush of the abdomen produces blow out ruptures.

4. Punctures occur from fractured ribs, bullets, or knifes.

C. SIGNS AND SYMPTOMS

1. There should be a high index of suspicion with rib fractures and other chest trauma. A pliable thorax decreases the likelihood of rib fractures in children. With fractures of the first or second rib, look for aortic injury.

2. Symptoms of cardiac injury include widening of the superior mediastinum on chest x-ray examination, deviation of the nasogastric tube from midline, chest pain, arrhythmias (particularly during transport), bruising on chest, jugular venous distention, signs of shock, muffled heart sounds, higher blood pressure in arms than legs, and pulsus paradoxus (less likely to be assessed with rapid respiratory rate).

D. DIAGNOSTIC STUDIES

1. *Chest x-ray examination* may demonstrate changes in the cardiac shadow.

2. *ECG* is relatively insensitive but may show conduction problems such as RBBB.

3. Cardiac enzyme studies are evaluated. If creatine phosphokinase alone is high, it may be from skeletal trauma. Enzyme levels may rise slowly if there is no period without blood flow.

4. *Echocardiogram* is used to identify tamponade and show differential wall motion. A transesophageal ECHO is used to rule out aortic dissection if there is a widened mediastinum.

5. Aortogram defines aortic injuries.

6. Radionuclide angiography delineates vascular injuries.

7. Pericardial tap relieves the pressure of cardiac tamponade.

E. NURSING DIAGNOSES

❖ ALTERATION IN CARDIAC OUTPUT RELATED TO HYPOVOLEMIC SHOCK, INADEQUATE TISSUE PERFUSION, ARRHYTHMIAS, OR CARDIAC TAMPONADE

❖ RISK OF INFECTION RELATED TO EMERGENCY THORACOTOMY

F. GOALS AND PATIENT OUTCOMES

1. Reestablish and maintain hemodynamic stability.

2. Prevent the complications of cardiac tamponade, life-threatening arrhythmias, and infection.

G. PATIENT MANAGEMENT

Treat shock (see Shock). Surgical intervention may be required including pericardiocentesis or emergency thoracotomy. Support cardiac recovery with the use of inotropic agents and afterload reduction.

H. COMPLICATIONS

Complications include exsanguination, cardiac arrest (mortality for traumatic cardiac arrest is very high), arrhythmias, and tamponade. (See also Multiple Trauma in Chapter 9.)

REFERENCES

Adams FH, Emmanouilides GC, Riemenschneider TA. *Moss' Heart Disease in Infants, Children, and Adolescents.* Baltimore, Md: Williams & Wilkins; 1989.

Ahrens T. SvO$_2$ monitoring: is it being used appropriately? *Crit Care Nurs.* 1990;10(7):70–72.

Alspach JG. *Core Curriculum for Critical Care Nursing.* Philadelphia, Pa: WB Saunders Co; 1991.

Anella J, McCloskey A, Vieweg C, et al. Nursing dynamics of pediatric intraaortic balloon pumping. *Crit Care Nurs.* 1990;10(4):24–37.

Apple S, Thurkauf GE. Preparing for and understanding transesophageal echocardiography. *Crit Care Nurs.* 1992;12(8):29–34.

Baker A. Acquired heart disease in infants and children. *Crit Care Nurs Clin North Am.* 1994;6:175–186.

Barragry TP, Ring WS, Blatchford JW, Foker JE. Central aorta–pulmonary artery shunts in neonates with complex cyanotic congenital heart disease. *J Thorac Cardiovasc Surg.* 1987;93:767–774.

Bazil ML. *Basic Pediatric E.C.G.* Marie Bazil; 1991.

Becker AE, Anderson RH. Atrioventricular septal defects: what's in a name? *J Thorac Cardiovasc Surg.* 1982;83:461–469.

Beekman RH, Rocchini AP, Behrendt DM, et al. Long-term outcome after repair of coarctation in infancy: subclavian angioplasty does not reduce the need for reoperation. *J Am Coll Cardiol.* 1986;8:1406–1411.

Bennett B, Singh S. Management of ventricular arrhythmias: then and now. *Am J Crit Care.* 1992;3:107–114.

Benson LN. Dilated cardiomyopathies of childhood. *Prog Pediatr Cardiol.* 1992;1:13–36.

Berne RM, Levy MN. *Physiology.* 3rd ed. St Louis, Mo: CV Mosby; 1993.

Biller JA, Yeager AM. *The Harriet Lane Handbook.* 9th ed. Chicago, Ill: Year Book Medical Publishers Inc; 1981.

Billingsley AM, Laks H, Boyce SW, George B, Santulli T, Williams RG. Definitive repair in patients with pulmonary atresia and intact ventricular septum. *J Thorac Cardiovasc Surg.* 1989;97:746–754.

Blickman JG, O'Connor JF. Imaging pediatric chest trauma. *Emerg Care Q.* 1990;4(1):49–54.

Bolman RM. Pediatric lung and heart-lung transplantation. *Transplant Proc.* 1994;26(1):211–213.

Bove EL. Cardiac surgery for the adolescent with univentricular heart. *Pediatrician.* 1986;13:171–179.

Bove EL. Current technique of the arterial switch procedure for transposition of the great arteries. *J Cardiac Surg.* 1989;4:193.

Bove EL. Senning's procedure for transposition of the great arteries. *Ann Thorac Surg.* 1987;43:678–680.

Bove EL. Transplantation after first-stage reconstruction for hypoplastic left heart syndrome. *Ann Thorac Surg.* 1991;52:701–707.

Bove EL, Beekman RH, Snider AR, et al. Repair of truncus arteriosus in the neonate and young infant. *Ann Thorac Surg.* 1989;47:499–506.

Bove EL, Kohman L, Sereika S, et al. The modified Blalock-Taussig shunt: analysis of adequacy and duration of palliation. *Circulation.* 1987;76(suppl III):III–19.

Bove EL, Lupinetti FM, Pridjian AK, et al. Results of a policy of primary repair of truncus arteriosus in the neonate. *J Thorac Cardiovasc Surg.* 1993;105:1057–1066.

Bove EL, Minich LL, Pridjian AK, et al. The management of severe subaortic stenosis, ventricular septal defect, and aortic arch obstruction in the neonate. *J Thorac Cardiovasc Surg.* 1993;105:289–296.

Bridges ND, Lock JE, Castaneda AR. Baffle fenestration with subsequent transcatheter closure. *Circulation.* 1990;82:1681–1689.

Bromberg BI, Dick M, Snider AR, et al. Tachycardia related cardiomyopathy: response to control of the arrhythmia. *J Interven Cardiol.* 1989;2:211.

Budny J, Anderson-Drevus K. IV inotropic agents: dopamine, dobutamine, and amrinone. *Crit Care Nurs.* 1990;10(2):54–62.

Callow LB. Current strategies in the nursing care of infants with hypoplastic left-heart syndrome undergoing first-stage palliation with the Norwood operation. *Heart Lung.* 1992;20:463–470.

Callow LB. New beginning: nursing care of the infant undergoing an arterial switch operation for transposition of the great arteries. *Heart Lung.* 1989;18:248–257.

Callow LB. Nursing implications of interventional device placement in pediatric cardiology and pediatric cardiac surgery. *Crit Care Nurs Clin North Am.* 1994;6(1):133–153.

Callow LB. Postoperative nursing care of the patient who has undergone the Fontan procedure. *Focus Crit Care.* 1987;14:24–31.

Campbell DB, Waldhausen JA. The Konno procedure for enlargement of the aortic root. *J Cardiac Surg.* 1986;1:69–78.

Carpentier A, Chauvaud S, Mace L, et al. A new reconstructive operation for Ebstein's anomaly of the tricuspid valve. *J Thorac Cardiovasc Surg.* 1988;96:92–101.

Carroll P. Clinical application of pulse oximetry. *Pediatr Nurs.* 1993;19:150–151.

Casale AS, Borkon AM. Penetrating cardiac trauma. *Trauma Q.* 1988;4(2):34–41.

Castaneda AR, Mayer JE, Jonas RA, Lock JE, Wessel DL, Hickey PR. The neonate with critical congenital heart disease: repair: a surgical challenge. *J Thorac Cardiovasc Surg.* 1989;98:869–875.

Chaux A, Gray RJ, Matloff JM, Feldman H, Sustaita H. An appreciation of the new St Jude valvular prosthesis. *J Thorac Cardiovasc Surg.* 1981;81:202–211.

Cobanoglu A, Metzdorff MT, Pinson CW, Grunkemeier GL, Sunderland CO, Starr A. Valvotomy for pulmonary atresia with intact ventricular septum. *J Thorac Cardiovasc Surg.* 1985;89:482–490.

Cohen M, Fuster V, Steele PM, Driscoll D, McGoon DC. Coarctation of the aorta. *Circulation.* 1989;80:840–845.

Cohn JN, et al. Neurohormonal control mechanisms in congestive heart failure. *Am Heart J.* 1981;102(3–2): 509–514.

Crumpley L, Rinkenberger RL. An overview of antiarrhythmic drugs. *Crit Care Nurs.* 1983;3(4):57–63.

Curley MAQ. *Pediatric Cardiac Dysrhythmias.* Bowie, Md: Brady Communications Co Inc; 1985.

Danielson GK, Maloney JD, Devloo RAE. Surgical repair of Ebstein's anomaly. *Mayo Clin Proc.* 1979;54: 185–192.

DePew CL. Furosemide: update on a commonly used drug. *Crit Care Nurs.* 1989;9(2):63–69.

Dunn JM, Donner RM. *Heart Transplantation in Children.* Mt Kisco, NY: Futura Publishing Co Inc; 1990.

Edmunds LH. Why cardiopulmonary bypass makes patients sick: strategies to control the blood-synthetic surface interface. *Adv Cardiac Surg.* 1995;6:131.

Elixson EM. Hemodynamic monitoring modalities in pediatric cardiac surgical patients. *Crit Care Nurs Clin North Am.* 1989;1(2):263–273.

Elkins RC, Knott-Craig CJ, Ward KE, McCue C, Lane MM. Pulmonary autograft in children: realized growth potential. *Ann Thorac Surg.* 1994;57:1387–1394.

Enger EL, Holm K. Perspectives on the interpretation of continous mixed venous oxygen saturation. *Heart Lung.* 1990;19(5–2):578–580.

Engle MA. Growth and development of state of the art care for people with congenital heart disease. *J Am Coll Cardiol.* 1989;13:1453–1457.

Extracorporeal Life Support Organization (ELSO). *National Registry.* Ann Arbor, Mich: ELSO; Oct 1990.

Ferry PC. Neurologic sequelae of open-heart surgery in children. *Am J Dis Child.* 1990;144:369–373.

Fontan F, Baudet E. Surgical repair of tricuspid atresia. *Thorax.* 1971;26:240.

Fowler NO, Gabel M. The hemodynamic effects of cardiac tamponade: mainly the result of atrial, not ventricular, compression. *Circulation.* 1985;71(no 1):154–157.

Frolich ED. Calcium antagonists for initial therapy of hypertension. *Heart Lung.* 1989;18(4):370–376.

Frommelt PC, Lupinetti FM, Bove EL. Aortoventriculoplasty in infants and children. *Circulation.* 1992; 86(suppl II):176–180.

Futterman LG, Lemberg L: Pacemaker update: 1992, I: general remarks and electrocardiographic assessment of pacemaker function. *Am J Crit Care.* 1992;1(3):118–120.

Fyfe DA, Kline CH. Fetal echocardiographic diagnosis of congenital heart disease. *Pediatr Clin North Am.* 1990;37(1):45–67.

Fyler DC. *Nadas' Pediatric Cardiology.* Philadelphia, Pa: Hanley & Belfus Inc; 1992.

Gartman DM, Bardy GH, Williams AB, Ivey TD. Direct surgical treatment of atrioventricular node reentrant tachycardia. *J Thorac Cardiovasc Surg.* 1989;98:63–72.

Gewillig M, Daenen W, Aubert A, Van der Hauwaert L. Abolishment of chronic volume overload. *Circulation.* 1992;86(suppl I):93–99.

Grady KL, Costanzo-Nordin MR. Myocarditis: review of a clinical enigma. *Heart Lung.* 1990;18(4):347–354.

Greenwood RD, Rosenthal A, Sloss LJ, LaCorte M, Nadas AS. Sick sinus syndrome after surgery for congenital heart disease. *Circulation.* 1975;52.

Griffin ML, Hernandez A, Martin TC, et al. Dilated cardiomyopathy in infants and children. *J Am Coll Cardiol.* 1988;11(1):139–144.

Groth MA, Meliones JN, Bove EL, et al. Repair of tetralogy of Fallot in infancy. *Circulation.* 1991;84(suppl II):206–212.

Guyton AC. *Human Physiology and Mechanisms of Disease.* Philadelphia, Pa: WB Saunders Co; 1987.

Hastreiter AR, Vander Horst RL, Chow-Tung E. Digitalis toxicity in infants and children. *Pediatr Cardiol.* 1984;5(2):131–148.

Hazinski MF. *Cardiovascular Disorders in Nursing Care of the Critically Ill Child.* St Louis, Mo: Mosby–Year Book Inc; 1992.

Helton JG, Aglira BA, Chin AJ, Murphy JD, Pigott JD, Norwood WI. Analysis of potential anatomic or physiologic determinants of outcome of palliative surgery for hypoplastic left heart syndrome. *Circulation.* 1986;74(suppl I):70.

Hennein HA, Mosca RS, Urcelay G, Crowley DC, Bove EL. Intermediate results after complete repair of tetralogy of Fallot in neonates. *J Thorac Cardiovasc Surg.* 1995;109:332–344.

Heymann MA. Pharmacologic use of prostaglandin E in infants with congenital heart disease. *Am Heart J.* 1981;101(6):837–843.

Holliday M, Barratt TM, Avner ED. In: Adams FH, Emmanoulides GC, Riemenschneider TA, eds. *Heart Disease in Infants, Children and Adolescents.* 4th ed. Baltimore, Md: Williams & Wilkins; 1989.

Iannettoni MD, Bove EL, Mosca RS, et al. Improving results with first-stage palliation for hypoplastic left heart syndrome. *J Thorac Cardiovasc Surg.* 1994;107:934–940.

Jensen C, Hill CS. Mechanical support for congestive heart failure in infants and children. *Crit Care Nurs Clin North Am.* 1994;6(1):165.

Jonas RA, Lang P, Hansen D, Hickey P, Castaneda AR. First-stage palliation of hypoplastic left heart syndrome. *J Thorac Cardiovasc Surg.* 1986;92:6–13.

Katz AM. Cardiomyopathy of overload. *N Engl J Med.* 1990;322(2):100–110.

Katz AM. *Physiology of the Heart.* New York, NY: Raven Press Publishers; 1992.

Katz AM, Messineo FC. Myocardial membrane function and drug action in heart failure. *Am Heart J.* 1981;102(3–2):491–500.

Keagy BA, Lucas CL, Henry GW, Lores ME, Wilcox BR. Changes in ventricular hemodynamics caused by a systemic-pulmonary shunt. *J Surg Res.* 1985;39:294–299.

Kurer CC, Tanner CS, Norwood WI, Vetter VL. Perioperative arrhythmias after Fontan repair. *Circulation.* 1990;82(suppl IV):190–194.

Kutalek SP, Michelson EL. Cardiac pacing and antiarrhythmic devices: newer modes of antibradyarrhythmia pacing. *Mod Concepts Cardiovasc Dis.* 1991;60:31.

Lauer RM, Ongley PA, DuShane JW, Kirklin JW. Heart block after repair of ventricular septal defect in children. *Circulation.* 1960;12:526.

Lawless S, Burchart G, Diven W, et al. Amrinone in neonates and infants after cardiac surgery. *Crit Care Med.* 1989;17(8):751–754.

LeBoeuf HB. Using vasoactive infusions in pediatric critical care. *Crit Care Nurs.* 1984;4(5):60–63.

Lehrer S. *Understanding Pediatric Heart Sounds.* Philadelphia, Pa: WB Saunders Co; 1992.

Lewis AB, Wells W, Lindesmith GG. Right ventricular growth potential in neonates with pulmonary atresia and intact ventricular septum. *J Thorac Cardiovasc Surg.* 1986;91:835–840.

Lister G, Hellenbrand WC, Kleinman CS, et al. Physiological effects of increasing hemoglobin concentration in left to right shunting in infants with ventricular septal defect. *N Engl J Med.* 1982;306(9):502–506.

Liu PP. New concepts in myocarditis: crossroads in the 1990's. *Prog Pediatr Cardiol.* 1992;1:37–47.

Louis PT, Bricker JT, Frazier OH. Nonpulsatile total left ventricular support in pediatric patients. *Crit Care Med.* 1992;20(4):704.

Lupinetti FM, Kulik TJ, Beekman RH, Crowley DC, Bove EL. Correction of total anomalous pulmonary venous connection in infancy. *J Thorac Cardiovasc Surg.* 1993;106:880–885.

Lupinetti RM, Lemmer JH, Ferguson DW, Stanford W, Behrendt DM. Aortic valve replacement with pulmonary or aortic allografts. *Circulation.* 1991;84(suppl III):89–93.

Lupinetti FM, Pridjian AK, Callow LB, Crowley DC, Beekman RH, Bove EL. Optimum treatment of discrete subaortic stenosis. *Ann Thorac Surg.* 1992;54:467–471.

McGovern BA, Ruskin JN. Ventricular tachycardia: initial assessment and approach to treatment. *Mod Concepts Cardiovasc Dis.* 1987;56:13.

Maron BJ. Cardiomyopathies. In: Adams FH, Emmanoulides GC, Riemenschneider TA, eds. *Heart Disease in Infants, Children and Adolescents.* 4th ed. Baltimore, Md: Williams & Wilkins; 1989.

Martin MM, Lemmer JH, Shaffer E, Dick M, Bove EL. Obstruction to left coronary artery blood flow secondary to obliteration of the coronary ostium in supravalvular aortic stenosis. *Ann Thorac Surg.* 1988;45:16–20.

Mavroudis C, Backer CL. *Pediatric Cardiac Surgery.* St Louis, Mo: Mosby–Year Book Inc; 1994.

Meliones JN, Beekman RH, Rocchini AP, Lacina SJ. Balloon valvuloplasty for recurrent aortic stenosis after surgical valvotomy in childhood: immediate and follow-up studies. *J Am Coll Cardiol.* 1989;13:1106–1110.

Meliones JN, Bove EL, Dekeon MK, et al. High-frequency jet ventilation improves cardiac function after the Fontan procedure. *Circulation.* 1991;84(suppl III):364–368.

Meliones JN, Snider AR, Bove EL, Rosenthal A, Rosen DA. Longitudinal results after first-stage palliation for hypoplastic left heart syndrome. *Circulation.* 1990;82(suppl IV):151–156.

Merl KE, Pauly-O'Neill SJ. Nursing care of the child with a pulmonary artery catheter. *Pediatr Nurs.* 1987;13(2):114–119.

Miller RR, et al. Combined vasodilator and inotropic therapy of heart failure: experimental and clinical concepts. *Am Heart J.* 1981;102(3–2):500–508.

Mosca RS, Iannettoni MD, Schwartz SM, et al. Critical aortic stenosis in the neonate. *J Thorac Cardiovasc Surg.* 1995;109:147–154.

Nakazawa M, Oyama K, Imai Y, et al. Criteria for two-staged arterial switch operation for simple transposition of great arteries. *Circulation.* 1988;78:124–131.

Newburger JW, Burns JC. Kawasaki syndrome. *Cardiol Clin.* 1990;7(2):453–465.

Norwood WI, Dobell AR, Freed MD, Kirklin JW, Blackstone EH. Intermediate results of the arterial switch repair. *J Thorac Cardiovasc Surg.* 1988;96:854–863.

Nunn DB. Thoracic great vessel injuries. *Trauma Q.* 1991;7(4):53–61.

O'Brien P, Elixson EM. The child following the Fontan procedure: nursing strategies. *AACN Clin Issues Crit Care Nurs.* 1990;1(1):46–58.

Olshansky B, Waldo AL. Atrial fibrillation: update on mechanism, diagnosis, and management. *Mod Concepts Cardiovasc Dis.* 1987;56:23.

Owens-Jones S, Hopp L. Viral myocarditis. *Focus Crit Care.* 1990;15(1):25–37.

Park MK, Guntheroth WG. How to read pediatric ECGs. St. Louis, Mo: Mosby–Year Book Inc; 1992.

Perry JC, McQuinn RL, Smith RT, et al. Flecainide acetate for resistant arrhythmias in the young: efficacy and pharmacokinetics. *J Am Coll Cardiol.* 1989;14(1):185–191.

Pridjian AK, Mendelsohn AM, Lupinetti FM, et al. Usefulness of the bidirectional Glenn procedure as staged reconstruction for the functional single ventricle. *Am J Cardiol.* 1993;71:959–962.

Puga FJ. Modified Fontan procedure for hypoplastic left heart syndrome after palliation with the Norwood operation. *J Am Coll Cardiol.* 1991;17:1150–1151.

Puga FJ, Leoni FE, Julsrud PR, Mair DD. Complete repair of pulmonary atresia, ventricular septal defect, and severe peripheral arborization abnormalities of the central pulmonary arteries. *J Thorac Cardiovasc Surg.* 1989;98:1018–1029.

Putnam JB, Lemmer JH, Rocchini AP, Bove EL. Embolectomy for acute pulmonary artery occlusion following Fontan procedure. *Ann Thorac Surg.* 1988;45:335–336.

Quaal SJ. *Cardiac Mechanical Assistance: Beyond Balloon Pumping.* St Louis, Mo: Mosby–Year Book Inc; 1993.

Reedy JE, Schwartz MT, Raithel SC, et al. Mechanical cardiopulmonary support for refractory cardiogenic shock. *Heart Lung.* 1990;19(5–1):514–524.

Rice V. Shock, a clinical syndrome: an update, parts 1–4. *Crit Care Nurs.* 1991;11(4–7):20–27, 28–42, 34–39, 74–85.

Rimar JM. Recognizing shock syndromes in infants and children. *Matern Child Nurs J.* 1988;13(1):32–37.

Rimar JM. Shock in infants and children: assessment and treatment. *Matern Child Nurs J.* 1988;13(2):98–105.

Roach AC. Atenolol. *Crit Care Nurs.* 1982;2(6):21–22.

Rosenthal CH, Susla GM. Medication administration to infants and children. In: Hazinski MF, ed. *Nursing Care of the Critically Ill Child.* St Louis, Mo: Mosby–Year Book Inc; 1992.

Sade RM, Crawford FA, Fyfe DA, Stroud MR. Valve prostheses in children: a reassessment of anticoagulation. *J Thorac Cardiovasc Surg.* 1988;95:553–561.

Schlant RC, Sonnenblick EH. Normal physiology of the cardiovascular system. In: Hurst JW, ed. *The Heart.* 7th ed. New York, NY: McGraw-Hill Information Services Co; 1990.

Scott WA, Rocchini AP, Bove EL, et al. Repair of interrupted aortic arch in infancy. *J Thorac Cardiovasc Surg.* 1988;96:564–568.

Senzaki H, Isoda T, Ishizawa A, Hishi T. Reconsideration of criteria for the Fontan operation. *Circulation.* 1994;89:1196–1202.

Shanley CJ, Lupinetti FM, Shah NL, Beekman RH, Crowley DC, Bove EL. Primary unifocalization for the absence of intrapericardial pulmonary arteries in the neonate. *J Thorac Cardiovasc Surg.* 1993;106:237–247.

Shreve B. Kawasaki disease: early treatment/positive results—one family's story. *Pediatr Nurs.* 1993;19(6): 607–610.

Singleton EB, Morriss MJH. Noninvasive diagnostic methods: plain radiographic diagnosis of congenital heart disease. In: Garson A Jr, Bricker JT, McNamara DG, eds. *The Science and Practice of Pediatric Cardiology.* Philadelphia, Pa: Lea & Febiger; 1990.

Sjogren ER. Lidocaine HCl injection. *Crit Care Nurs.* 1983;3(3):14–16.

Slota MC, Beerman L, Sanchez G. Pediatric electrocardiography overview. *Heart Lung.* 1982;11(1):69–84.

Smith JB. *Pediatric Critical Care.* New York, NY: John Wiley & Sons Inc; 1983.

Snider AR, Serwer GA. Echocardiography. In: *Pediatric Heart Disease.* Chicago, Ill: Year Book Medical Publishers Inc; 1990.

Sole MJ, Liu P. Viral myocarditis: a paradigm for understanding the pathogenesis and treatment of dilated cardiomyopathy. *J Am Coll Cardiol.* 1993;22:99A–105A.

Sommers MS. Cardiac tamponade after nonpenetrating cardiac trauma. *Dimens Crit Care Nurs.* 1986;5(4): 206–215.

Soutter DI, Rodriguez A. Cardiac contusion: diagnosis and management. *Trauma Q.* 1988;4(2):16–23.

Spivey WHL. Intraosseous infusions. *J Pediatr.* 1990;111:639.

Stone KS, Scordo KA. Understanding the calcium channel blockers. *Heart Lung.* 1984;13(5):563–571.

Suddaby EC. Viral myocarditis in children. *Crit Care Nurs.* 1996;16(4):73–81.

Suddaby EC, O'Brien AM. ECMO for cardiac support in children. *Heart Lung.* 1993;22(5):401–407.

Taber's Dictionary. 12th ed. Philadelphia, PA: FA Davis; 1973.

Taylor T. Monitoring left atrial pressures in the open heart surgical patient. *Crit Care Nurs.* 1986;6(2):62–68.

Tripp ME. Metabolic cardiomyopathies. *Prog Pediatr Cardiol.* 1992;1:1–12.

Urcelay G, Dick M, Bove EL, et al. Intraoperative mapping and radiofrequency ablation of the His bundle in a patient with complex congenital heart disease and intractable atrial arrhythmias following the Fontan operation. *PACE.* 1993;16(part I):1437.

Warshaw MP, Winn CW. Pulmonary valvuloplasty as an alternative to surgery in the pediatric patient: implications for nursing. *Heart Lung.* 1988;111:521–527.

Webster HF. Biomedical instrumentation: principles and techniques. In: Hazinski MF, ed. *Nursing Care of the Critically Ill Child.* St. Louis, Mo: Mosby–Year Book Inc; 1992.

Weintraub RG, Brawn WJ, Venables AW, Mee RBB. Two-patch repair of complete atrioventricular septal defect in the first year of life. *J Thorac Cardiovasc Surg.* 1990;99:320–326.

Whipple JK, Medicus-Bringa MA, Schimel BA, et al. Selected vasoactive drugs: a readily available chart reference. *Crit Care Nurs.* 1992;12(3):23–29.

White KM, Winslow EH, Clark AP, et al. The physiologic basis for continuous mixed venous oxygen saturation monitoring. *Heart Lung.* 1990;19(5–2):548–551.

Wiles HB. Imaging congenital heart disease. *Pediatr Clin North Am.* 1990;37(1):115–136.

Worthington de Toledo L. How vasodilators backfire. *RN.* July 1982:41–45.

Yoshizato T, Edwards WD, Albuliras ET, et al. Safety and utility of endomyocardial biopsy in infants, children and adolescents: a review of 66 procedures in 53 patients. *J Am Coll Cardiol.* 1990;15(2):436–442.

Zaritsky A, Chernow B. Use of catecholamines in pediatrics. *J Pediatr.* 1990;105:341.

Ziegler V. Adenosine in the pediatric population: nursing implications. *Pediatr Nurs.* 1991;17(6):600–602.

Zipes DP, Prystowski EN, Heger JJ. Amiodarone: electrophysiologic actions, pharmacokinetics and clinical effects. *J Am Coll Cardiol.* 1992;3(4):1059–1071.

Zweng TN, Bluett MK, Mosca RS, Callow LB, Bove EL. Mitral valve replacement in the first 5 years of life. *Ann Thorac Surg.* 1989;47:720–724.

4 Neurologic System

PAULA VERNON-LEVETT

CENTRAL NERVOUS SYSTEM

A. **DEVELOPMENTAL ANATOMY**
   1. **Embryogenesis:** The nervous system is one of the first organ systems to develop in the embryo (neurula).
      a. All body tissues are derived from three different *germ cell layers:*
         • Mesoderm forms future muscle, skeleton, connective tissue, and the cardiovascular and urogenital systems; assists in the early development of neural tissue; and forms notochord, which is incorporated into the future spinal column.
         • Endoderm forms the future gut and associated organs.
         • Surface ectoderm forms future skin, nails, epidermis, hair, and mammary glands, whereas the neuroectoderm forms future neural tissue.
      b. *Neurulation* is the process of neural tube formation and development (Fig. 4–1).
         • The neural plate is the specialized neuroectoderm cells of the embryo that thicken on either side of the neural groove (on the dorsal surface), forming a flat plate with distinct lateral edges present at approximately 20 days' gestation.
         • The neural groove is the anteroposterior groove in the ectoderm that appears at 2½ weeks' gestation. Development proceeds cranially.
         • The neural crest contains the specialized cells that originate from the neural plate but separate from it to form a parallel band extending the length of the neural plate. The neural crest gives rise to the future peripheral nervous system, spinal and autonomic ganglia, and some nonneural tissue (including the meninges). It is present at 3½ weeks' gestation.
         • The neural tube is formed by the lateral edges (folds) of the neural plate that fold and grow medially until they meet and form a tube. The cavity of the neural tube becomes the future ventricular system of the brain and central canal of the spinal cord. It is closed at 4 weeks' gestation.
         • Epidermal (sensory) placodes are composed of 9 or 10 pairs that arise from separate ectoderm thickening in the head region. Together with the neural crest, they give rise to cranial nerves and cranial sensory organs.
      c. *Brain development:* Further specialization of the neural tube forms three distinct swellings (vesicles) at the rostral end of the tube (Fig. 4–2).

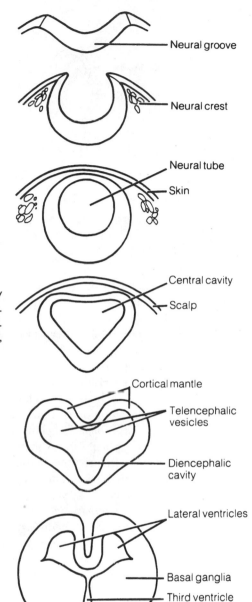

Figure 4–1. Cross sections showing early development from neural groove to cerebrum. (Reprinted with permission from Waxman SG. *Correlative Neuroanatomy*. 23rd ed. Stamford, Conn: Appleton & Lange; 1996.)

- The neural tube forms three bulges (primary brain vesicles) at its cephalic end that develop future parts of the brain (represented at 4 weeks' gestation): prosencephalon (forebrain), mesencephalon (midbrain), and rhombencephalon (hindbrain).
- Early in the second fetal month two of the three primary brain vesicles further subdivide to form secondary vesicles. The prosencephalon forms the telencephalon (future preoptic region and paired cerebral hemispheres of the mature brain) and the diencephalon (future hypothalamus and thalamus of the mature brain). The mesencephalon remains the midbrain (future superior and inferior colliculi; red, reticular, and black nuclei; and cerebral peduncles of the mature brain). The rhomben-

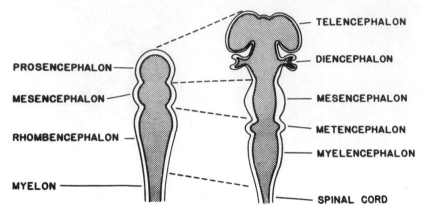

Figure 4–2. Subdivisions of the embryonic human brain. **A,** Primary vesicles. **B,** Secondary vesicles. (Reprinted with permission from Jensen D. *The Human Nervous System.* New York, NY: Appleton-Century-Crofts; 1980.)

cephalon forms the metencephalon (future pons and cerebellum of the mature brain) and the myelencephalon (future medulla of the mature brain).

- Fissure formation begins in the fourth fetal month with development of the lateral sulcus (of the cerebrum) and the posterolateral sulcus (of the cerebellum). The central sulcus, calcarine sulcus, and parietooccipital sulcus are visible in the fifth fetal month. All main gyri and sulci are present by the seventh fetal month.
- Myelinization of the brain begins at 10 months' gestation.

d. *Spinal cord development* begins from the caudal portion of the neural tube. The earliest nerve fiber tracts appear around the second month. Long association tracts appear at the third month. Pyramidal tracts appear in the fifth month. Myelinization begins in the fifth month and is not completed in some tracts for 20 years (Abels et al, 1986).

e. *Neural tissue specialization*
- Neural tissue further differentiates into four concentric zones around the central canal that develop into specific areas of the mature brain. The ventricular zone is located adjacent to the central canal and is a precursor to neurons and macroglia. The subventricular zone generates certain classes of neurons and macroglia and some deep structures of the cerebrum. The intermediate (mantle) zone evolves into gray matter. The marginal zone has no primary cells of its own but evolves into most of the white matter.
- Sensory components of the central nervous system (CNS) develop from further divisions of the neural tube. The basal plate is the ventral portion of neural tube that contributes to the efferent (motor) system. The alar plate is the dorsal portion of the neural tube that contributes to the afferent (sensory) system.

2. **Neuron and associated cells**
a. The *neuron* is the functional and anatomic unit of the nervous system (Fig. 4–3). The cell body (soma) contains the nucleus and gray matter. The perikaryon (neuroplasm) is cytoplasm surrounding the nucleus. The perikaryon contains granular, filamentous, and membranous organelles. Two types of neuronal processes include the dendrites and axons.
- Each neuron usually contains several dendrites that conduct impulses toward the cell body (afferent).

- Each neuron only has one axon. A myelin sheath encases some axons (white matter) and increases transmission of impulses. Nodes of Ranvier are anatomic interruptions in the myelin sheath. Axons conduct impulses away from the cell body (efferent).
- The synapse (Noback et al, 1991) is the site of contact of one neuron with another. The synaptic cleft is the space between the bouton of one neuron and the cell body of another. The neuromuscular junction is the termination of nerve fiber in muscle cell, and the neuroglandular junction is the termination of nerve fiber in glandular cell. The presynaptic membrane is the cell membrane of the axon at the synapse, and the postsynaptic membrane is the cell membrane of the dendrite to cell body, muscle, or glandular cell. The presynaptic vesicle is present in the cytoplasm of the bouton and contains the active neurotransmitter agents.

   b. *Neuroglia* are the supporting and nourishing structures of the nervous system. There are four main types: oligodendrocytes (produce myelin), astrocytes (support, bind, and nourish neurons), microglial (phagocytic properties), and ependyma (line the ventricular system and choroid plexus and produce cerebrospinal fluid [CSF]).

3. **Extracerebral structures** (Fig. 4–4)

   a. The *scalp* is composed of skin, subcutaneous tissue, galea aponeurotica, and pericranium.

   b. The *skull* consists of eight bones: one frontal, two parietal, two temporal, one occipital, one ethmoid, and one sphenoid.

   c. The *sutures* are dense, white, fibrous, connective tissue membranes that separate the bones. The sagittal suture separates the two parietal bones on top of the skull. The coronal suture (frontoparietal) connects the frontal and parietal bones transversely. The basilar suture is created by the junction of the basilar surface of the occipital bone with the posterior surface of the sphenoid bone. The lambdoid suture connects the parietal and occipital bones transversely.

   d. The *fontanelles* are areas where several sutures join together. The posterior fontanelle is formed by the intersection of the sagittal and lambdoid sutures. Two anterolateral fontanelles are formed by the intersection of the frontal, parietal, temporal, and sphenoid bones. The anterior fontanelle is formed by the intersection of the coronal and sagittal sutures. Two posterolateral

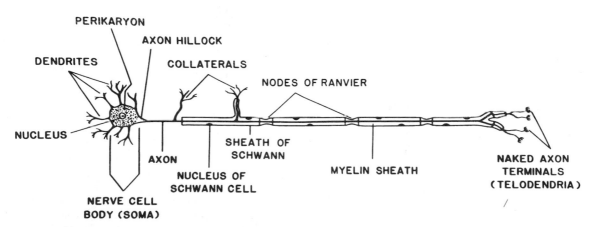

Figure 4–3. The principal morphologic features of a peripheral motorneuron. The total length of the fiber has been shortened considerably. (Reprinted with permission from Jensen D. *The Human Nervous System.* New York, NY: Appleton-Century-Crofts; 1980.)

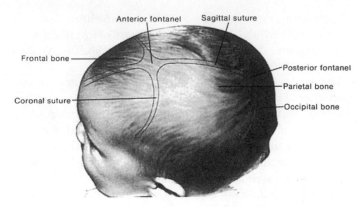

Figure 4–4.   Cranial sutures and fontanelles in infancy. (Reprinted with permission from Betz CL, Hunsberger MM, Wright S. *Family-Centered Nursing Care of Children.* 2nd ed. Philadelphia, Pa: WB Saunders Co; 1994.)

      fontanelles are formed by the intersection of the parietal, occipital, and temporal bones. The posterior and anterolateral fontanelles close at 2 months after birth. The anterior fontanelle closes between 12 and 18 months. The posterolateral closes at 24 months.

    e. *Meninges* are three membranous connective tissue layers that cover the brain. The dura mater is the outermost layer and consists of two layers. The outer periosteum adheres to the inner surface of the skull and vertebrae. The inner layer divides the cerebral hemispheres (falx cerebri), cerebral hemispheres from the cerebellum and brain stem (tentorium cerebelli), and the two cerebellar hemispheres (falx cerebelli). The arachnoid is the middle transparent avascular covering with many fine collagen strands (trabeculae). The pia mater is the inner, delicate, clear membrane that adheres directly to the surface of the brain and spinal cord.

    f. *Ventricular system and CSF circulation*

      • The ventricles are four interconnecting chambers lined by ependyma. The paired lateral ventricles are contained within the cerebral hemispheres, subdivided into four parts: the anterior horn located in the frontal lobe, the body located in the parietal lobe, the inferior horn located in the temporal lobe, and the occipital horn located in the occipital lobe. The third ventricle is connected to the lateral ventricles via the foramen of Monro and connected to the fourth ventricle via the aqueduct of Sylvius. The fourth ventricle communicates with the third ventricle and subarachnoid space around the brain and spinal cord via three exit points. The foramen of Magendie exits to the cisterna magna (central canal of spinal cord) and the spinal subarachnoid space. The foramina of Luschka exit to the cisterna magna and the subarachnoid space around the brain.

      • The choroid plexus is a three layer membrane consisting of the choroid capillary endothelium, pial cells, and the choroid epithelium. It is located in all four ventricles and parenchyma and is responsible for CSF production.

      • CSF is produced by the choroid plexus and to a lesser degree by ependymal cells lining the ventricles and spinal cord (Jensen, 1980). The rate of production of CSF varies by age (Swaiman, 1989). Newborns produce approximately 1 ml/h. Adults produce approximately 30 ml/h. The total volume of CSF in the ventricular system also varies by age (Swaiman, 1989): newborn, 5 ml; adult, 150 ml.

- Circulation of CSF is detailed in Figure 4–5. From the lateral ventricles, CSF passes to the third ventricle via the foramina of Monro. It travels from the third ventricle to the fourth ventricle via the aqueduct of Sylvius. The combined CSF volume passes through two lateral foramina of Luschka and the medial foramen of Magendie into the cisterna magna. CSF travels upward around the cerebrum via the subarachnoid space and downward around the spinal cord via the spinal subarachnoid space.

- Absorption occurs primarily through the arachnoid villi. Fingerlike projections from the arachnoid layer extending into the superior sagittal sinus function as one-way valves allowing CSF to exit the sagittal sinus, but the projections prevent blood from entering the subarachnoid space. The rate of absorption depends on CSF pressure (higher pressures result in more absorption to a certain point) and venous pressure (higher venous pressures can impede absorption).

- Characteristics of normal CSF include the following: CSF is clear and odorless, glucose concentration is one half to one third of the serum glucose concentration, protein concentration is 15 to 45 mg/dl (higher in neonates), white blood cells (WBCs) are usually absent (however, a few may be present, especially in neonates), and red blood cells (RBCs) are absent except during traumatic lumbar tap. The opening pressure is dynamic related to the patient's body position and activities. The normal range is 60 to 180 cm H_2O.

4. The **brain** is divided into the cerebrum, diencephalon, brain stem, reticular formation, and the cerebellum.
   a. **Cerebrum (telencephalon)**
      - The *cerebral hemispheres* consist of four lobes (Fig. 4–6): The frontal lobes hold the primary motor cortex, Broca's motor speech area (written and spoken language), and personality. The temporal lobes are responsible

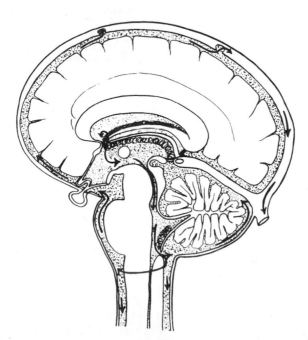

Figure 4–5.   Schematic representation of CSF circulation. (Reprinted with permission from Behrman RE, Vaughan VC. *Nelson Textbook of Pediatrics.* 13th ed. Philadelphia, Pa: WB Saunders Co; 1987.)

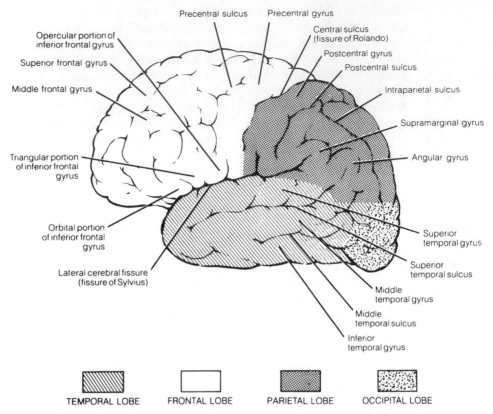

Figure 4–6.   Lateral view of the left cerebral hemisphere illustrating four lobes: temporal, frontal, parietal, occipital. (Reprinted with permission from Waxman SG. *Correlative Neuroanatomy.* 23rd ed. Stamford, Conn: Appleton & Lange; 1996.)

for reception and interpretation of auditory information, emotional and visceral responses, and retention of recent memory. The parietal lobe is responsible for comprehension of language, orientation of spatial relationships, and initial processing of tactile and proprioceptive information. The occipital lobe is responsible for the reception and interpretation of visual stimuli.

- *Basal ganglia* are located deep in the cerebral hemispheres and are composed of four nuclei providing unconscious control of lower motor neurons. The basal ganglia are processing stations, linking the cerebral cortex to specific thalamic nuclei.
- The *corpus callosum* is the largest commissural tract and is composed of a bundle of transverse nerve fibers connecting the two cerebral hemispheres. It transfers information between cerebral hemispheres and makes up the roof of the lateral ventricles and the third ventricle.
- The *limbic system* denotes several structures including the limbic lobe, hippocampus and connections, amygdala, septal nuclei, hypothalamus, anterior thalamic nuclei, and portions of the basal ganglia. This system is primarily responsible for affective behavior and autonomic control (Boss and Stowe, 1983; Jensen, 1980).

b. The **diencephalon** is the rostral end of the brain stem and is located deep within the cerebrum. Sometimes it is classified as part of the brain stem. Anatomically it is divided into the following:

- The *epithalamus* is a narrow band forming the roof of the diencephalon. The epithalamus's exact function is not well understood, but it is associated with the limbic system, optic reflexes, and reproductive activity.

- The *thalami* are the largest subdivision of the diencephalon. Two egg-shaped masses are located deep in each cerebral hemisphere, and their primary function is to be a relay station for sensory input.

- The *hypothalamus* forms the base of the diencephalon and the floor and inferior lateral walls of the lateral ventricles. The primary function of the hypothalamus is physiologic homeostasis by regulating a number of visceral responses, as well as more complex behavioral and emotional responses.

- The *subthalamus* is located lateral to the hypothalamus and is functionally integrated with the pyramidal system (Jensen, 1980).

c. The **brain stem** consists of three continuous structures (Fig. 4–7).

- The *mesencephalon (midbrain)* is located rostral on the brain stem between the diencephalon and metencephalon and is the origin of cranial nerves III and IV. The primary functions of the mesencephalon include serving as a relay center for visual and auditory reflexes and as the center for postural reflexes and the righting reflex (maintains the head in an upright position).

- The *metencephalon (pons)* is located above the medulla and ventral to the cerebellum serving as the origin of cranial nerves V, VI, VII, and VIII. It contains nerve fibers that form the reticular formation and are continuous with other parts of the brain. The metencephalon also contains the medial longitudinal fasciculus (MLF) composed of efferent fibers. The pons helps to regulate respiration.

- The *myelencephalon (medulla oblongata)* is continuous with the pons ros-

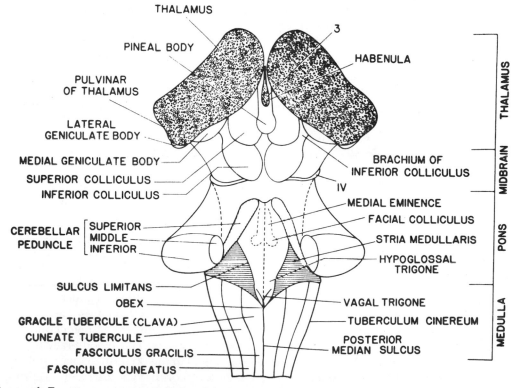

Figure 4–7. Gross anatomic features of the brain stem, dorsal aspect. *3,* Third ventricle. (Reprinted with permission from Jensen D. *The Human Nervous System.* New York, NY: Appleton-Century-Crofts; 1980.)

trally and the spinal cord caudally, and is the origin of cranial nerves IX through XII. Primary functions of the myelencephalon include the primary respiratory and cardiac centers and the vasomotor centers.

d. The **reticular formation** is a diffuse network of neurons located in the brain stem. It begins at the upper end of the spinal cord and extends upward to the hypothalamus and adjacent areas. This formation contains both sensory and motor neurons, nuclei that interact with the extrapyramidal motor control system. The reticular formation is the site of the reticular activating system (RAS), which assists in regulating awareness (sleep-wake cycles).

e. The **cerebellum** is located superior to the fourth ventricle and contains two lobes. It is connected to the brain stem via three pairs of fiber bundles (cerebellar peduncles). Primary functions of the cerebellum include coordination of voluntary movements, control of muscle tone, and maintenance of equilibrium.

5. **Cerebral circulation**

a. *Arterial blood* is supplied by two paired vessels, the common carotid arteries and the vertebral arteries.

- The common carotid arteries are located anteriorly; each bifurcates into two vessels. The internal carotid artery enters the cranial cavity and extends to the circle of Willis, where several major vessels meet. The anterior cerebral arteries supply the medial aspect of the cerebral hemispheres and the frontoparietal regions. The middle cerebral artery supplies much of the lateral aspect of the cerebral hemispheres and basal ganglia. The posterior cerebral arteries supply the lateral, medial, and inferior occipital cortex. The posterior communicating arteries connect anterior and posterior circulation.

- The external carotid arteries supply arterial circulation to the extracerebral structures (skin and muscle of the face and scalp).

- The vertebral arteries are located posteriorly; they originate from the subclavian arteries and join to form the basilar artery. Numerous vessels arise from the vertebral and basilar arteries and include the superior cerebellar artery, anterior inferior cerebellar artery, posterior inferior cerebellar artery, meningeal artery, anterior and posterior spinal arteries, and posterior cerebral arteries. Collectively, all the above vessels supply the cerebellum, brain stem, occipital lobe, and inferior and medial surfaces of the temporal lobes.

b. *Venous blood* is supplied by a network composed of valveless, thin-walled cerebral veins. The superficial veins drain the external surfaces of the brain and include the superior cerebral vein, middle cerebral vein, and inferior cerebral vein, which empty into the dural venous sinuses. The deep veins drain internal areas of the brain and include the basal veins, vein of Rosenthal, and the great vein of Galen. All venous drainage empties at the base of the skull via the internal jugular veins.

c. The *blood-brain barrier* is composed of the anatomic structures and physiologic processes that separate the brain and blood compartments. Brain capillaries are characterized by (Noback et al, 1991) tight junctions between endothelial cells, astrocytes with foot processes that encase capillaries and neurons, and endothelial cells with large numbers of mitochondria (responsible for energy-dependent transport). The blood-brain barrier is believed to be incompletely developed in the preterm neonate (Johnston, 1992). Physiologic properties of the morphologic barrier prevent rapid transport of blood to the brain and maintain a delicate homeostatic balance within the internal brain environment. Chemical barriers restrict some substances such as large serum protein molecules and some chemothera-peutic agents. Substances easily transported across the membrane include water, oxygen, carbon dioxide, glucose, and some lipid-soluble substances such as alcohol and anesthetics.

　　d. The *blood-CSF barrier* is composed of the anatomic structures and physi-ologic processes that separate the brain and CSF compartments (function-ally similar to blood-brain barrier). The morphologic barrier is created by high impermeability of choroid epithelial cells to most substances.

6. **Spinal cord and column**
　　a. The *spinal column* consists of 33 vertebrae: 7 cervical, 12 thoracic, 4 lumbar, 5 sacral, and 4 or 5 coccygeal segments (Fig. 4–8).
　　b. *Vertebrae:* The cylinder body is located anteriorly and increases in size as it progresses downward. The posterior arch has two pedicles and two laminae. The pedicles project posterolaterally from the bodies and form part of the transverse foramen. The two laminae are located posteriorly and are thin and relatively long. The spinous processes are formed by fusion of the two laminae and vary in shape, size, and direction depending on location. The transverse process is located on each side of the arch, providing a lever for muscle attachment. The articular processes (two superior and two inferior) form synovial joints with corresponding processes on adjacent vertebrae. The intervertebral foramina are formed by notches on the superior and inferior borders of the pedicles of the adjacent vertebrae, providing a channel for spinal vessels and nerves. The intervertebral discs are fibrocar-tilage tissue interposed between adjacent vertebrae consisting of an outer concentric layer of fibrous tissue (annulus fibrosus) and a central spongy pulp (nucleus pulposus). The discs provide an elastic buffer to absorb mechanical shocks.
　　c. The *spinal cord* is an extension of the medulla oblongata. It extends downward, tapering (conus medullaris), and terminates at the lower border of first lumbar vertebra in the adult and at the third lumbar vertebra (Moore, 1988) in the neonate. The filum terminale is a slender, median, fibrous thread that extends from the conus medullaris to the coccyx.
　　　• Outer coverings are continuous with the corresponding cerebral meninges. The *dura mater* consists of only one layer, does not adhere to vertebrae, and merges with the filum terminale. The spinal cord is suspended from the dura mater via a series of 22 pairs of denticulate ligaments. The epidural space is located between the dura layer and periosteum of the vertebrae. It contains venous plexuses and fat and is the location for injection of anesthetics. The *arachnoid* is nonvascular and extends caudally to the second sacral level, where it merges with the filum terminale. The subarachnoid space contains CSF and blood vessels and surrounds the spinal cord (spinal or lumbar cistern). The *pia mater* is directly attached to the spinal cord, its roots, and the filum terminale and is vascular.
　　　• The inner core of the spinal cord is composed of gray and white matter. Butterfly- or H-shaped *gray matter* consists of cell bodies and unmyelin-ated fibers. They are anatomically and functionally divided into regions (Fig. 4–9). The anterior (ventral) horns contain the neuronal cell bodies of motor neurons supplying the skeletal muscles. The posterior (dorsal) horns contain the neuronal cell bodies involved in sensory input to the spinal cord. The lateral horns contain preganglionic fibers of the autonomic nervous system.
　　　• *White matter* surrounds the gray matter and consists of myelinated

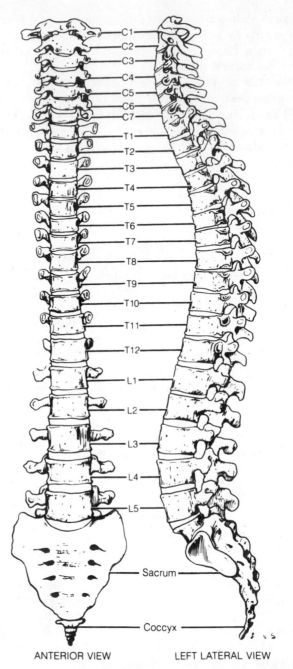

C1
C2
C3
C4
C5
C6
C7
T1
T2
T3
T4
T5
T6
T7
T8
T9
T10
T11
T12
L1
L2
L3
L4
L5
Sacrum
Coccyx

ANTERIOR VIEW   LEFT LATERAL VIEW

Figure 4–8.   The vertebral column. (Reprinted with permission from Waxman SG. *Correlative Neuroanatomy.* 23rd ed. Stamford, Conn: Appleton & Lange; 1996.)

(predominate) and unmyelinated fibers. They are arranged into three pairs of funiculi (columns): posterior, lateral, and anterior. Funiculi are subdivided into bundles of nerve fibers (tracts or fasciculi) that are functionally distinct. Ascending (sensory) pathways transmit sensory information from peripheral receptors to the cerebral and cerebellar cortex and transmit pain, touch, temperature, spatial relationships, vibration, passive movement, and position sense. Descending (motor) pathways contain upper motor neurons, originate from the cerebrum, and descend to the spinal cord (and brain stem). They play a major role

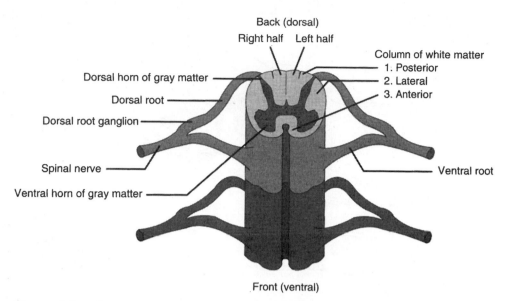

Figure 4–9.   Cross section of spinal cord. (Reprinted with permission from Curley MAQ, Smith JB, Moloney-Harmon P. *Critical Care Nursing of Infants and Children*. Philadelphia, Pa: WB Saunders Co; 1996:345.)

in voluntary motor movement. The central canal is lined with ependymal cells, contains CSF, and is continuous with the fourth ventricle in the medulla oblongata. Tracts are of clinical significance (Table 4–1) and are named based on the column in which the tract travels, origination of cells, and termination of fibers.

   d. The *reflex arc* is an intrinsic neural circuit that, once activated, follows a specific response without conscious control. The *monosynaptic reflex arc* consists of a sensory end-organ (receptor), afferent nerve fibers, one synapse, efferent nerve fibers, and muscle fiber or glandular cell (effector). A classic example is a deep tendon reflex (Fig. 4–10). The *polysynaptic reflex arc* consists of a sensory end-organ, afferent nerve fibers, multiple inter-neurons and synapses, efferent nerve fibers, and an effector. A classic example is withdrawal of an extremity from pain stimuli.

Table 4–1.   COMMON ASCENDING AND DESCENDING SPINAL TRACTS

TRACT NAME	FUNCTION
Ascending (Sensory)	
Dorsal (posterior) spinocerebellar	Proprioception
Ventral (anterior) spinocerebellar	Proprioception
Lateral spinothalamic	Pain, temperature
Ventral (anterior) spinothalamic	Touch, pressure
Descending (Motor)	
Corticospinal (pyramidal tracts)	
Ventral (anterior) corticospinal	Skilled voluntary movements
Lateral corticospinal	Skilled voluntary movements
Rubrospinal	Fine movements, muscle tone
Vestibulospinal	Aid equilibrium, extensor muscle tone
Reticulospinal	Posture, muscle tone
Tectospinal	Mediates optic and auditory reflex movement

From Curley MAQ, Vernon-Levett P. *Critical Care Nursing of Infants and Children*. Philadelphia, Pa: WB Saunders Co; 1996.

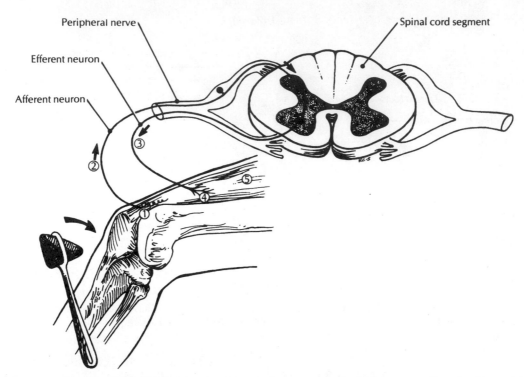

Peripheral nerve

Efferent neuron

Afferent neuron

Spinal cord segment

Figure 4–10. Simple reflex arc (knee-jerk reflex). *1,* The receptor, the sensory nerve fiber that first picks up the impulse as the hammer strikes the tendon; *2,* the sensory transmitter, the afferent neuron that passes the impulse to the spinal cord; *3,* the motor transmitter, the efferent neuron that passes the impulse to the effector (muscle); *4,* the neuroeffector junction, a specialized end-plate of motor nerves; *5,* the effector, a muscle that carries out the actual response (jerking of knee). (Reprinted with permission from Abels L: *Critical Care Nursing: A Physiologic Approach.* St Louis, Mo: The CV Mosby Co; 1986.)

   7. **Spinal column circulation:** Arterial blood is supplied from branches of vertebral arteries and the radicular arteries derived from segmental vessels (i.e., deep cervical, intercostal, lumbar, and sacral arteries). The arteries pass through the intervertebral foramina and divide into two branches: the smaller anterior spinal artery and the larger posterior spinal artery. Venous drainage is via the venous plexus and the veins that parallel arteries.

B. **DEVELOPMENTAL PHYSIOLOGY**
   1. **Impulse conduction**
      a. During the *resting membrane potential (RMP)* (i.e., not conducting a nerve impulse), the intracellular fluid (neuroplasm) of neuron has a more negative electrical charge than extracellular fluid. Na^+ and Cl^- are in higher concentration in extracellular fluid. K^+ is in higher concentration in intracellular fluid. Concentrations are maintained by ionic pumps.
      b. As *depolarization* occurs in response to an electrochemical stimulus, the cell membrane becomes more permeable to Na^+. Na^+ enters the cell, and the membrane becomes less negative internally. Initial depolarization must be greater than a certain threshold value for depolarization to continue.
      c. The *action potential* is the response of the neuron to depolarization. Impulsive flow of ionic current is produced briefly. After a brief delay, the membrane potential shifts back to negative. Na^+ flow is inactivated, and K^+ permeability increases.
      d. *Repolarization* is the reestablishment of negative polarity of the RMP. The cell membrane becomes impermeable to Na^+ and more permeable to K^+. RMP returns to normal via the sodium-potassium pump.

e. The action potential is self-propagating and is an all-or-none phenomenon. The impulse travels as a full-blown force or not at all. The action potential in a myelinated nerve fiber is propagated by saltatory conduction, jumping from one node of Ranvier to the next node of Ranvier. Myelin improves conduction of action potentials.

f. The *presynaptic membrane action potential* activates the release of neurotransmitters contained in vesicles. Neurotransmitters diffuse across the synapse, producing a synaptic delay.

g. The *postsynaptic membrane* contains receptors that combine with neurotransmitters to alter the membrane permeability to specific ions. Excitatory neurotransmitters include glutamate, aspartate, and acetylcholine. The receptor responds with increased permeability for Na^+ and K^+, net influx of Na^+, and cell membrane changes in a depolarizing direction (excitatory postsynaptic potential [EPSP]) and initiates an action potential. Inhibitory neurotransmitters include glycine and γ-aminobutyric acid (GABA). The receptor responds with an increase in permeability for K^+ and Cl^- but not Na^+, an outward flow of K^+, and cell membrane potential shifts in a hypopolarizing direction (inhibitory postsynaptic potential [IPSP]), decreases excitability, and inhibits an action potential.

2. **Intracranial pressure (ICP) dynamics**

a. *Modified Monro-Kellie doctrine:* The rigid skull contains three volume compartments: brain tissue (80% to 90%), CSF (5% to 10%), and blood (5% to 10%). If there is an increase in any one or more of the volume compartments, there must be a reciprocal change in one or more of the other volume compartments to maintain pressure equilibrium:

$$\text{Intracranial Volume} = \text{Vol}_{brain} + \text{Vol}_{CSF} + \text{Vol}_{blood}$$

b. *Pressure-volume relationships*
*   Normal ICP varies in different age groups and is lowest during infancy (Welch, 1980):
    *   Newborn: 0.7–1.5 mm Hg
    *   Infants: 1.5–6 mm Hg
    *   Children: 3–7.5 mm Hg
    *   Adult: Less than 10 mm Hg
*   The volume-pressure curve represents the relationship between changes in intracranial volume and the resulting ICP (Fig. 4–11). Elastance is the change in pressure that occurs with a change in volume ($\Delta P/\Delta V$). Compliance is the inverse relationship of elastance ($\Delta V/\Delta P$). The ICP curve is not linear but a three-phase hyperbolic curve. *Phase 1,* the compensatory phase, is the flat portion of the curve, reflecting good compliance and normal ICP. Temporary increases in ICP are "buffered" by several mechanisms: CSF translocation to the spinal subarachnoid space, venous blood displaced to the extracranial compartment through valveless veins, and decreased production or increased reabsorption of CSF. *Phase 2* is the exponential portion of the curve, representing early decompensation with normal ICP but poor compliance (i.e., slight increases in volume are not tolerated). The critical point when compliance is lost varies and depends on several factors: rate of volumetric change (rapid increases in ICP are not tolerated well), age (younger child has less buffering capacity with acute increases in ICP), and medical interventions. *Phase 3* is the steep portion of the curve, representing the failure of compensation with increased ICP and poor compliance.

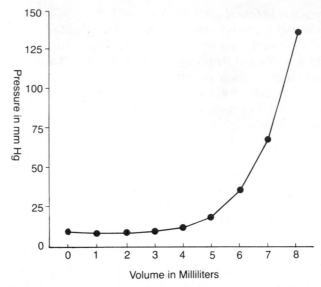

Figure 4–11. The relationship between volume and pressure within the intracranial space. As the volume reaches the point where pressure begins to rise, small increases in volume cause large rises in ICP. (Reprinted with permission from Marshall SB, Marshall LF, Vos HR, Chestnut RM. *Neuroscience Critical Care: Pathophysiology and Patient Management.* Philadelphia, Pa: WB Saunders Co; 1990.)

3. **Brain metabolism**
   a. *Oxygen:* Twenty percent of cardiac output is delivered to the brain, although the brain is only 2% of the total body weight. Brain cells require a constant and consistent delivery of oxygen and are dependent on aerobic metabolism. The cerebral metabolic rate of oxygen ($CMRo_2$) is approximately 3 to 3.5 ml/100 g/min in the adult but is not constant throughout the brain. The exact $CMRo_2$ in the neonate and infant is unknown.
   b. *Glucose:* Glucose stores in the brain are minimal; therefore, cells also require a constant and consistent delivery of glucose. Glucose is associated with significant brain cellular processes including protein synthesis, amino acid metabolism, neurotransmitter release, membrane function, and pH homeostasis. The cerebral metabolic rate of glucose ($CMR_{glucose}$) is 4.5 to 5.5 mg/100 g/min in the adult. The exact $CMR_{glucose}$ in the neonate and infant is unknown. Hypoglycemia and hyperglycemia can cause neurologic damage (Sieber and Traystman, 1992).
4. **Cerebral blood flow (CBF)**
   a. Normal CBF in the brain of the neonate is widely variable with an unknown lower limit (Altman et al, 1988). The actual delivery of oxygen to the tissues is affected by the percent of circulating fetal hemoglobin. The child's CBF is 105 ml/100 g/min (Jensen, 1980). Adolescents and adults have a CBF of 55 ml/100 g/min (Foster and Salter, 1990).
   b. Determinants of CBF
      • The smaller the *arteriolar radius,* the greater the resistance to CBF. Mechanisms that change the caliber of the vessel are cerebral autoregulation and chemical regulation. Autoregulation is a compensatory mechanism that matches CBF to CMR by altering the radius of the cerebral vessels (i.e., vasoconstriction or vasodilation). A constant CBF is maintained when the mean arterial pressure (MAP) is between 50 and 150 mm Hg. $Paco_2$ (pH) affects the cerebral arteriolar radius: low $Paco_2$ (elevated pH) causes vasoconstriction, and high $Paco_2$ (decreased pH)

causes vasodilation. PaO_2, to a lesser extent, affects the cerebral arteriolar radius: PaO_2 less than 50 mm Hg causes vasodilation, and PaO_2 greater than 50 mm Hg causes vasoconstriction but remains constant. Increased *blood viscosity* (polycythemia) decreases CBF. The *length of the vascular bed* is constant at any point in time. Increased length increases resistance to CBF.

- *Cerebral perfusion pressure (CPP)* represents the pressure difference between inflow (arterial) pressure and outflow (venous) pressure across the cerebral vascular bed. Clinically, it is most often calculated by the following equation:

$$CPP = MAP - ICP$$

Normal CPP in the neonate is unknown. The child's CPP should be greater than 50 mm Hg, and the adolescent's CPP should be greater than 60 mm Hg.

PERIPHERAL NERVOUS SYSTEM

A. **DEVELOPMENTAL ANATOMY**
1. **Sensory and motor components**
    a. **Spinal nerves** are connected to the spinal cord via two roots.
    - The *dorsal (posterior) root* carries afferent (sensory) fibers that transmit impulses from sensory receptors in the body to the spinal cord. The fibers supply the innervation for a particular segment of the body called a dermatome (Fig. 4–12). *Afferent fibers* are subdivided according to function. General somatic afferent (GSA) fibers transmit impulses from sensors in the extremities and body wall. General visceral afferent (GVA) fibers transmit impulses from sensors in the viscera.
    - The *ventral (anterior) root* carries efferent (motor) fibers that transmit impulses from the spinal cord. Efferent fibers are subdivided according to function. General somatic efferent (GSE) fibers innervate voluntary striated muscle. General visceral efferent (GVE) fibers innervate involuntary smooth muscles, cardiac muscle, and glands.
    - Fusion of the roots forms 31 spinal nerves: 8 pairs of cervical, 12 pairs of thoracic, 5 pairs of lumbar, 5 pairs of sacral, and 1 coccygeal. Cauda equina (horse's tail) is the long root of lumbar and sacral nerves contained within the spinal cistern (the spinal cord is shorter than the vertebral column). Thoracic, lumbar, and sacral nerves are numbered according to the vertebra just rostral to the foramen through which they pass. Cervical nerves are numbered for the vertebra just caudal to the foramen through which they pass. Fibers are also classified functionally according to conduction velocity.
    b. **Cranial nerves** are the peripheral nerves of the brain. Cranial nerve I originates from the cerebrum, and cranial nerves II through XII originate from the brain stem
    - *Classification* by type and function is described in Table 4–2.
    c. **Autonomic nervous system (ANS)**
    - Components of the ANS are located in the CNS and the peripheral nervous system. The primary (preganglionic) neuron originates in the CNS. The axon of the primary neuron travels outside the CNS to synapse on a secondary (postganglionic) neuron found in one of the autonomic ganglia. The postganglionic fiber terminates in an organ or structure.

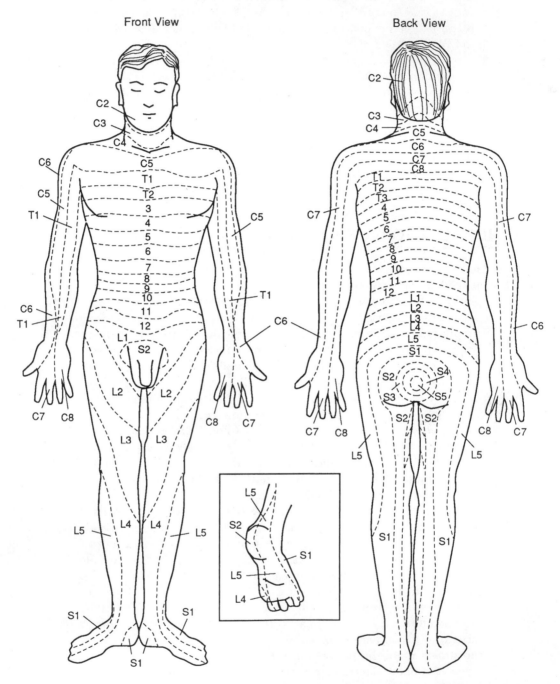

Figure 4–12. Dermatomes. (Reprinted with permission from Cardona VD, Hurn PD, Mason PJB, Scanlon AM, Veise-Berry SW. *Trauma Nursing From Resuscitation Through Rehabilitation.* 2nd ed. Philadelphia, Pa: WB Saunders Co; 1994:444.)

Table 4–2. CLASSIFICATION OF CRANIAL NERVES

CRANIAL NERVE	NAME	TYPE	FUNCTION
I	Olfactory	Sensory	Olfaction
II	Optic	Sensory	Vision
III	Oculomotor	Motor	Pupillary constriction and accommodation, extraocular movements, elevation of upper eyelid
IV	Trochlear	Sensory and motor	Deviation of the eye (inward on adduction, downward on abduction)
V	Trigeminal	Sensory and motor	Muscles of mastication; sensory innervation of the face, nose, and mouth
VI	Abducens	Motor	Lateral deviation of the eye
VII	Facial	Sensory and motor	Muscles of facial expression; sensory components of taste and salivation
VIII	Acoustic	Sensory	Hearing and balance
IX	Glossopharyngeal	Sensory and motor	Motor to pharyngeal region (swallowing); salivation and taste; thermal sensations from posterior tongue, tonsils, and eustachian tubes
X	Vagus	Sensory and motor	Sensory innervation of the larynx and pharynx; motor innervation of the palate and pharynx; and parasympathetic functions
XI	Spinal accessory	Motor	Motor innervation of the sternocleidomastoid muscle and the upper portion of the trapezius muscle (shoulder shrug, turning head)
XII	Hypoglossal	Motor	Movement of the tongue

- In the *sympathetic (thoracolumbar) division* (Fig. 4–13), preganglionic fibers originate in the intermediolateral cell column of segments T-1 through T-12. Fibers emerge from the spinal cord through the ventral roots and branch into the white rami communicants. White rami communicants send fibers to the paired trunk ganglia (located laterally on each side of the thoracic and lumbar vertebrae), where they synapse with postganglionic fibers. The postganglionic fibers exit the trunk ganglia and innervate different organs and structures. T-1 to T-5 are to the head and neck. T-1 and T-2 are to the eye. T-2 to T-6 are to the heart and lungs. T-6 to L-2 are to the abdominal viscera. L-1 and L-2 are to the urinary, genital, and lower digestive systems.
- In the *parasympathetic (craniosacral) division* (Fig. 4–14), preganglionic fibers originate from two areas: brain stem preganglionic fibers (often travel in the cranial nerves, specifically cranial nerves III, VII, IX, and X) and the middle segments of the sacral region. Nerve fibers are distributed exclusively to visceral organs. Most preganglionic fibers have long axons that synapse with a few postganglionic fibers with short axons. The synapse usually occurs in the end-organ. The cranial fibers innervate visceral structures including the head, thoracic cavity, and abdominal cavity. The sacral fibers give rise to the pelvic nerve, which innervates most of the large intestine, pelvic viscera, and genitalia.

B. ESSENTIAL PHYSIOLOGY

1. **Neural transmission** in the ANS occurs via neurotransmitters. Sympathetic division preganglionic nerve terminals secrete acetylcholine (cholinergic), postganglionic nerve terminals secrete norepinephrine (adrenergic), and the postganglionic nerve terminals to sweat glands secrete acetylcholine. Parasympathetic division preganglionic nerve terminals secrete acetylcholine, and postganglionic nerve terminals secrete acetylcholine. Acetylcholine is deactivated by cholinesterase. Norepinephrine is deactivated by monoamine oxidase (MAO) and catechol *O*-methyltransferase (COMT).

2. **Systemic effects of ANS innervation** (Table 4–3): The sympathetic division is organized to exert influences over widespread body regions. Stimulation prepares the body for intense muscular activity "fight-or-flight" response. The parasympathetic division is organized to exert influences in localized discrete

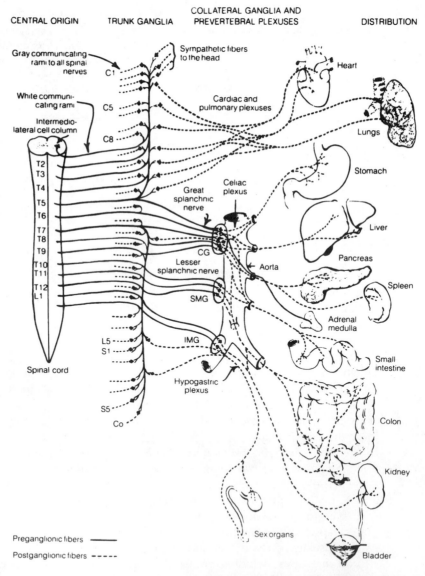

Figure 4–13. Sympathetic division of the ANS (left half). *CG*, celiac ganglion; *SMG*, superior mesenteric ganglion; *IMG*, inferior mesenteric ganglion. (Reprinted with permission from Waxman SG. *Correlative Neuroanatomy.* 23rd ed. East Norwalk, Conn: Appleton & Lange; 1996.)

CENTRAL ORIGIN   PREVERTEBRAL PLEXUSES   DISTRIBUTION AND TERMINAL GANGLIA

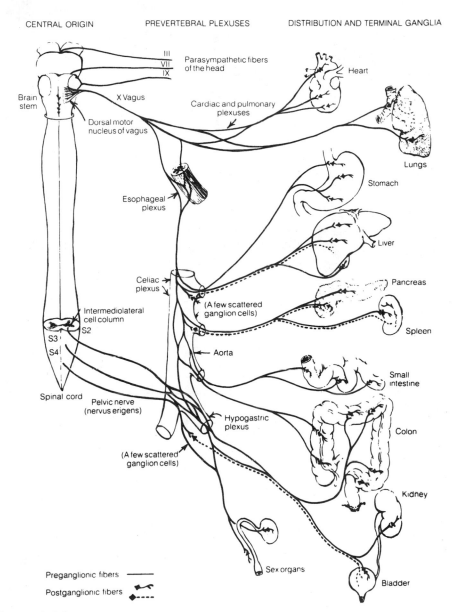

Figure 4–14. Parasympathetic division of the ANS (only left half shown). (Reprinted with permission from Waxman SG. *Correlative Neuroanatomy.* 23rd ed. East Norwalk, Conn: Appleton & Lange; 1996.)

areas of the body. Stimulation prepares the body primarily for "resting" bodily functions.

CLINICAL ASSESSMENT OF NEUROMUSCULAR FUNCTION

The nervous system is incompletely developed at birth and takes several years to mature. Consequently, neurologic assessment of the infant and young child must be individualized to reflect neurodevelopment and temperament of the child.

Table 4–3. EFFECTS OF AUTONOMIC NERVE STIMULATION

ORGAN OR STRUCTURE	SYMPATHETIC (ADRENERGIC) EFFECTS	PARASYMPATHETIC (CHOLINERGIC) EFFECTS	TYPE OF RECEPTOR*
Eye			
Iris: Radial muscle	Contraction; dilates pupil (mydriasis)	Contraction; constricts pupil (miosis)	α
Iris: Circular muscle	—	Contraction; lens thickens, accommodates for near vision (strong effect)	—
Ciliary muscle	Relaxation; lens flattens, accommodates for distant vision (minor effect)	—	β
Smooth muscle: Orbit, upper lid	Contraction	—	—
Heart			
Sinoatrial node	Increased heart rate (tachycardia)	Decreased heart rate (bradycardia); vagal arrest	β
Atria	Increased contractility; conduction velocity	Decreased contractility, some increase in conduction velocity	β
Atrioventricular node, conducting system	Increased conduction velocity	Decreased conduction velocity, atrioventricular block	β
Ventricles	Increased rates of idiopathic pacemakers, contractility, conduction velocity	Decreased contractility (?)	β
Blood vessels			
Cutaneous (skin)	Constriction	Dilatation (minor; doubtful physiologic significance)	α
Buccal mucosa	Dilatation	—	α, β
Coronary	Dilatation, esp. in vivo; constriction (minor effect)†	Constriction (minor); dilatation (strong)	α, β
Skeletal muscle	Dilatation‡; constriction‡	Dilatation§	α
Cerebral	Constriction (minor effect)	Dilatation (minor; doubtful physiologic significance)	α, β
Pulmonary	Dilatation, constriction (minor effects)	Dilatation (minor; doubtful physiologic significance)	α, β
Abdominal, pelvic viscera	Constriction (strong); dilatation§	—	—
External genitalia	Constriction	Dilatation	α
Salivary glands	Constriction	Dilatation	
Lung			
Bronchial muscle	Dilatation	Constriction	β
Bronchial glands	Inhibition (?)	Stimulation	—
Stomach			
Stomach wall, motility and tone	Decrease or increase (variable response)	Increase or decrease (variable response)	β
Sphincters	Contraction (generally)	Relaxation (generally)	α
Secretion	Inhibition (?)	Stimulation (marked)	—

Effector organ	Cholinergic impulses: Response	Adrenergic impulses: Receptor type	Adrenergic impulses: Response
Intestine			
Motility and tone	Increase (marked)	α, β	Decrease (slight)
Sphincters	Relaxation (generally)	α	Contraction (generally)
Secretion	Stimulation	—	Inhibition (?)
Gallbladder, ducts	Contraction	—	Relaxation
Urinary bladder			
Detrusor	Contraction (generally)	β	Relaxation (generally)
Trigone, sphincter	Relaxation	α	Contraction
Ureter			
Motility and tone	Increase (?)	—	Increase (generally)
Uterus			
Nonpregnant	—	β	Inhibition||
Pregnant	—	α	Contraction||
Sex organs	Erection	—	Ejaculation
Skin			
Pilomotor muscles	—	α	Contraction
Sweat glands	General secretion (strong response)	α	Slight local secretion¶
Splenic capsule	—	α	Contraction
Adrenal medulla	Catecholamine secretion (epinephrine, norepinephrine)	—	—
Pancreas, acini	Secretion	α	—
Liver islets	—	β	Glycogenolysis gluconeogenesis
Salivary glands	Copious, watery secretion	α, β	Viscous secretion#
Lacrimal glands	Secretion	—	—
Nasopharyngeal glands	Secretion	—	—

*These receptor types are based on the response of various tissues to the action of various sympathomimetic amines, i.e., compounds which initiate or mimic sympathetic nerve stimulation. In general, α-receptors are most sensitive to epinephrine and least sensitive to isoproterenol and least sensitive to epinephrine, the effect being inhibitory.

†Indirect effects in vivo cause primarily a vasodilatation.

‡In vivo, released epinephrine produces a β-receptor response, i.e., vasodilatation, in blood vessels of skeletal muscles and liver. In other abdominal viscera, an α-response, i.e., vasoconstriction, is elicited by this catecholamine.

§Sympathetic cholinergic nerves induce vasodilatation in skeletal muscle.

||Response variable, depending on stage of menstrual cycle, and levels of circulating sex hormones (estrogen and progesterone) among other factors. Pregnant and nonpregnant uteri differ in their responses.

¶For example, palms of hands (so-called adrenergic sweating).

#The parotid glands are not innervated by sympathetic nerves.

From Jensen D. The Human Nervous System. New York, NY: Appleton-Century-Crofts, 1980.

A. **HISTORY**

1. **Chief complaint:** Use the parents' own words and description and solicit information from school-aged and older children when their condition permits.

2. **Present illness:** Describe onset and development, associated symptoms, and factors that relieve or exacerbate symptoms.

3. **Past history:** Infant and toddler history should summarize antenatal, perinatal, and postnatal courses including maternal infections, medications taken during pregnancy, Apgar scores, gestational age, and birth complications such as meconium aspiration, seizure activity, or respiratory status (oxygen requirements). History should include a chronologic list of developmental milestones, childhood illnesses, immunization status, significant or chronic illnesses (e.g., seizures, diabetes, head injury), and medications.

4. **Family history:** Some neurologic disorders manifest themselves as disturbances in other body systems; therefore, it is important to review the patient's past history.

    a. *Neurologic disorders* may be static or progressive and may be traumatic (acquired) or congenital.

    b. *Endocrine disorders* with neurologic implications include diabetic coma and thyroid disease and hormonal imbalances (growth disorders).

    c. *Cardiovascular disorders* with neurologic implications include cyanotic heart disease (risk for brain infarcts and abscesses) and aneurysms (may have a higher incidence in families with a known history).

    d. *Congenital disorders* with neurologic implications include neural tube defects and metabolic disorders (e.g., phenylketonuria [PKU], cretinism).

    e. *Genetic disorders* may have a neurologic origin or may affect the neurologic system. Most neurodegenerative disorders are transmitted as a recessive gene. Epilepsies and migraine headaches tend to be transmitted as a dominant trait.

    f. *Renal disorders* may produce metabolic imbalances that affect neurologic functioning (e.g., acute renal failure and the increased risk of cerebral edema).

5. **Social history** should include school performance, types of play activities and recreation, substance abuse, and smoking.

B. **PHYSICAL EXAMINATION**

1. **General appearance** evaluation includes behavior, dress, speech and conversation, gait, emotional state, and symmetry of body structures.

2. **Skull examination**

    a. *Inspection* (Bruno, 1995; Curley and Vernon-Levett, 1996) of the skull includes occipitofrontal head circumference, shape and symmetry of head, transillumination (increased with serous fluid [caput succedaneum] and decreased with blood fluid [cephalhematoma]). Extreme downward rotation of the eyes and paralysis of upward gaze (setting sun sign) is often seen with hydrocephalus.

    b. *Palpation* of the *fontanelles* should occur while the infant is upright and quiet. Fontanelles that remain open beyond the usual period of closure may be related to disorders that abnormally increase the intracranial contents (e.g., tumors, hydrocephalus). The anterior fontanelle is usually 4 to 6 cm at its largest diameter at birth, and the posterior fontanelle is usually 1 to 2 cm at its largest diameter at birth. The anterior fontanelle may be full and tense with increased ICP, crying, vomiting, or coughing in the infant. Pulsations of the anterior fontanelle reflect the peripheral pulse and are normally barely palpable. Palpation of sutures reveals overriding sutures, which are common with vaginal deliveries or present with premature closure of the sutures. Widely separated sutures may suggest hydrocephalus.

   c. *Auscultation* of the skull using a bell stethoscope with the child in an erect position is performed over six areas: the temporal fossae, both globes, and the reticuloauricular or mastoid regions. In all cases, a transmitted cardiac murmur should be excluded. Bruit (spontaneous) in the young child may be normal, but an abnormal bruit is often loud, harsh, and asymmetric or accompanied by a thrill, or both.

   d. *Percussion* of the skull is normally dull. A "cracked-pot" sound (Macewen's sign) is heard with separated sutures and increased ICP.

3. **Level of consciousness**

   a. Altered states of consciousness are on a continuum (Plum and Posner, 1982). *Clouding of consciousness* is characterized by reduced wakefulness, confusion, and alternating drowsiness and hyperexcitability. *Delirium* is characterized by disorientation, fear, irritability, visual hallucinations, and agitation. *Obtundation* is characterized by mild to moderate reduction in alertness, reduced interest in the environment, and increased periods of sleep. *Stupor* is indicated by unresponsiveness except to vigorous and repeated stimuli. *Coma* is indicated by no verbal or motor response to environmental stimuli.

   b. Mental status may be assessed in children with minimal alteration in consciousness. In infants, assess the quality of the cry, alertness and level of activity, feeding patterns, language development, presence or absence of primitive reflexes, patterns of sleep and wakefulness, and responses to caregivers. In children, assess attention, alertness, orientation, cognition, memory, affect, and perception.

   c. Coma scales are used to grade the degree of unresponsiveness by standardized assessments. *Glasgow Coma Scale (GCS)* (Table 4–4) assesses arousibility in relation to three responses: eye opening (arousal state), verbal response

Table 4–4. GLASGOW COMA SCALE

Activity	Score*
Verbal response	
None	1
Incomprehensible sounds	2
Inappropriate words	3
Confused	4
Oriented	5
Eye opening	
None	1
To pain	2
To speech	3
Spontaneously	4
Motor response	
None	1
Abnormal extensor	2
Abnormal flexor	3
Withdraws	4
Localizes	5
Obeys	6

*Total score = sum of the score for each of the three components. Score for a fully oriented alert patient = 15. Score for a mute immobile patient with no eye opening = 3.
From Teasdale G, Jennet B. Glasgow Coma Scale. *Lancet.* 1974;2:81–83. © by The Lancet Ltd. 1974.

(content of consciousness), and motor response (arousal state and content of consciousness). Each response is given the best number for a given response. The sum of the numbers range between 3 (least responsive) and 15 (normal). A number of coma scales have been developed to accommodate preverbal children and infants (see Multiple Trauma in Chapter 9). Most scales are scored in similar fashion to the GCS.

4. **Motor function:** Assessment of normal motor development proceeds cephalocaudal and proximodistal.

   a. Assess *primitive reflexes* in infants and toddlers and determine their presence or absence, time of disappearance, and the symmetry of the reflex. The most commonly evaluated reflexes include the following:

   - *Moro:* Elicited by a sudden movement of the body that causes a change in equilibrium. The response is extension and abduction of the upper extremities (fingers fan), followed by flexion and adduction. The reflex appears between 28 to 32 weeks' gestation and disappears by 3 to 5 months after birth.
   - *Palmar grasp:* Elicited by the examiner's placing his or her index finger into the ulnar side of the infant's hand and pressing against the palmar surface. The response is immediate flexion of the infant's fingers around the examiner's finger. The reflex appears at 28 weeks' gestation and disappears between 4 to 6 months after birth.
   - *Parachute:* Elicited by holding the infant in a ventral position. A sudden plunge downward produces extension and abduction of the infant's arms and fingers. The reflex appears at 4 to 9 months after birth and persists throughout life (the response is usually covered up with voluntary movement in older individuals).
   - *Rooting:* Elicited by stroking the perioral skin at the corner of the mouth, moving laterally toward the cheek, upper lip, and lower lip. The infant turns his or her head toward the stimulated side with sucking movements. The reflex appears at 28 weeks' gestation and disappears between 3 to 4 months after birth.
   - *Placing:* Elicited with the infant supported in a vertical position with the dorsum of one foot pressed against a hard surface. The infant's foot will flex and extend, simulating walking. The reflex appears at 35 to 37 weeks' gestation and disappears at 1 to 2 months after birth.
   - *Asymmetric Tonic Neck Response:* Elicited by rotating the infant's head to the side while the infant's chest is maintained in a flat position. The arm and leg extend on the side to which the infant's face is turned, and the opposite arm and leg flex. The reflex appears at birth to 2 months and disappears between 4 to 6 months.

   b. Assess for *developmental milestones* (e.g., sitting, crawling, walking).

   c. If the patient can follow commands, assess *muscle strength and tone, symmetry of movement, and deep tendon reflexes (DTRs)*. Not all DTRs are present in the infant because of the immaturity of the corticospinal tracts. The younger the child, the more common are inequalities in deep tendon reflexes (Menkes, 1990). DTRs are tested based on the segmental level they innervate. The usual reflexes include biceps (segmental levels C-5 and C-6), brachioradialis (segmental levels C-5 and C-6), triceps (segmental levels C-7 and C-8), knee (segmental levels L-2, L-3, and L-4), and ankle (segmental levels S-1 and S-2). The technique for eliciting DTRs is similar to that used for adults; however, the hammer may be replaced with the examiner's semiflexed index finger. The technique includes positioning the limb so that the muscle is slightly stretched, striking the tendon briskly to create an additional sudden tendon stretch, and testing both muscle groups on each side of the body. Reflex responses are usually graded on a scale from 0 (no response) to 4+ (very brisk, hyperactive; may be indicative of disease). Abnormal findings include very brisk or asymmetric responses or deviations from a previous assessment.

   d. *Superficial reflexes* include the Babinski, abdominal, and cremasteric reflexes. The technique for eliciting *Babinski's reflex* includes using a sharp object (thumbnail) to stimulate the plantar surface of the foot. Stimulation begins at the heel and travels along the lateral border of the sole, crossing over the base of the metatarsals to the great toe. A normal response in children younger than 1 to 2 years is immediate dorsiflexion of the great toe and subsequent separation (fanning) of the other toes; this response is abnormal in older children and adults. A normal response beyond the second year is plantar flexion of the toes. The *abdominal reflex* is elicited by lightly, but briskly stroking each side of the abdomen, above and below the umbilicus. A normal response is contraction of the abdominal muscles and deviation of the umbilicus toward the stimulus. The reflex may not be present at birth but is consistently present at 6 months of age. An asymmetric response is abnormal. The *cremasteric reflex* is elicited by lightly but briskly stroking the inner aspect of each of the upper thighs. A normal response is elevation of the testicle on the side stimulated. It may not be present at birth but occurs consistently at approximately 6 months of age. An asymmetric response is abnormal.

   e. *Abnormal motor responses* in the comatose patient include *decorticate posturing* (consisting of flexion and adduction of the upper extremities and extension of the lower extremities with plantar flexion representing dysfunction of the cerebral hemispheres or upper part of the brain stem), *decerebrate posturing* (extensor posturing consisting of extension, adduction, and hyperpronation of the upper and lower extremities and plantar flexion representing dysfunction at the pontomesencephalic level), and *flaccidity* (no motor response to external stimuli representing severe dysfunction of the lower brain stem and vital centers for which spinal cord injury and stroke must be ruled out).

   f. All extremities should be assessed independently. Specific stimuli to solicit a motor response should be documented.

5. **Sensory function**

   a. In infants, sensory testing results are variable and less reliable than in the older child. Light touch is assessed by stroking an extremity (the normal response is to withdraw the limb). Vibration sense is assessed with a tuning fork over bony areas (the normal response is cessation of movement and often a look of surprise). Proprioception cannot be tested in infants or comatose patients because it requires participation of the patient. Pain sensation is assessed with nail bed pressure (at the end of examination).

   b. Light touch and superficial pain is assessed in older children in all four extremities. If abnormalities are noted, a more detailed segmental assessment is done. Proprioception is tested by asking the child to close his or her eyes and move a finger or toe up or down and then asking the child to identify whether the movement is up or down. Pain sensation is tested at the end of the examination by using a pin to test the various dermatomes.

6. **Cerebellar function**

   a. In infants and toddlers, cerebellar function should be assessed by observing the child during play or usual activities. Abnormal findings include tremors, which are rhythmic alterations in movement and, unlike spontaneous seizures, are usually precipitated by a variety of stimuli (e.g., sudden changes in movement) with no alteration in the level of consciousness. Dysmetria (inability to control the range of movement in muscle action) or gait abnormalities (e.g., wide-based or waddling type of gait) may also be noticed.

   b. Maneuvers to assess older children include the finger-to-nose test, the heel-shin test, observation of gait, and toe-to-heel walking. The finger-to-nose test is performed while the child stands erect with arms extended at the sides and is then asked to touch his or her nose with alternating index fingers. An abnormal finding is if the child completely misses his nose. The heel-shin test is done while the child is in a supine position. The child is asked to place one heel rapidly down the shin from the knee to the ankle and repeat on the other side. Movements should be coordinated and accurate. The child can also be instructed to touch each finger to the thumb of the same hand in rapid succession. Each hand is tested, and the response should be symmetric. Observation of gait can be made while the child walks toward and away from the examiner. The child should have good posture and balance. During toe-to-heel walking, the child places the heel of one foot to the toe of the other foot and continues this maneuver for several feet. The child should have good balance.

7. **Cranial nerve function:** The order and specific nerves to be tested depend on the age and condition of the child. The techniques for the assessment of specific cranial nerves are included in Table 4–5.

8. **Fundoscopic examination**
   a. Normal findings include a red reflex that is orange-red and fairly uniform in color, creamy pink optic disc with indented center (physiologic depression) and smooth margins, and veins that are slightly wider than arteries.
   b. Abnormal findings include papilledema, which is characterized by blurring of the nasal and upper margins of the optic disc. Papilledema is seen with increased ICP in the older child or in the infant with acute, rapid increased ICP. Retinal hemorrhage may occur with subarachnoid hemorrhage, severe diabetes, and shaken baby syndrome.

9. **Vital signs**
   a. *Respiratory patterns* (Table 4–6): Respirations are the first of the vital signs to change with neurologic dysfunction. Respiratory patterns are more informative than respiratory rate. Patterns may overlap or change depending on progression of neurologic dysfunction. (See also Chapter 2.)
      • *Cheyne-Stokes respirations* are described as periodic breathing with phases of hyperpnea alternating with apnea. The location of the lesion is bilateral, hemispheric, or diencephalic.
      • *Central neurogenic hyperventilation* is sustained, rapid, and fairly deep hyperpnea. The exact mechanism in the brain (if any) is unknown.
      • An *apneustic respiratory pattern* is characterized by a prolonged inspiration with a pause at full inspiration lasting 2 to 3 seconds. This represents damage to the brain stem near the level of the fifth cranial nerve nucleus.
      • *Ataxic respirations* are a completely irregular breathing pattern with deep and shallow breaths. They are seen in patients with damage to the respiratory centers in the medulla.
   b. *Temperature:* Temperature changes are nonspecific in most patients with neurologic dysfunction. Hyperthermia may result from abnormalities of the brain itself or from toxic substances that affect the temperature-regulating centers. Patients at risk for hyperthermia include neonates (due to immature development of thermoregulation centers), children with

Text continued on page 308

Table 4–5. CRANIAL NERVE EVALUATION

CRANIAL NERVE	FUNCTIONS	METHODS OF TESTING	COMMENTS
Infant*			
I	Olfactory Sense of smell	Assess patency of both nostrils. Hold noxious odor near each nostril separately. Observe for generalized body movement or cry.	Unreliable test for infants. Although smell is intact, the immature myelinization prohibits an integrated, voluntary motor response.
II	Optic Vision	Inspect the fundus with an ophthalmoscope. Test visual fields by introducing a brightly colored object into each visual field from behind the infant. In the infant with a pincer grasp, observe the visual acuity used in spotting and picking up crumbs and small objects.	The optic disc is pale, grey, and poorly developed in the infant. The macula (area of central vision) is not fully developed until 4 mo at which time the infant will notice light contrast and different colors. Infants are capable of binocular fixation at 3 mo and can follow the object for visual field testing.
III	Oculomotor Pupillary constriction, elevation of the upper eyelid, and most of the extraocular movements	Check pupillary responses: shine light directly into each eye from the side and observe the briskness and completeness of the direct pupillary response. Check the consensual response by shining the light into one eye and observing the response in the other eye. Record the size of the pupil in millimeters (mm). Note the shape and equality of the pupils. Note the infant's spontaneous eye opening and any ptosis. Note the presence of doll's eyes (oculocephalic reflex): turn the head to one side quickly and watch the position of the eyes. In an abnormal response, the eyes move in the opposite direction as though still gazing in the initial direction. Check extraocular movements (cranial nerves III, IV, and VI). Test for accommodation noting constriction and convergence as a bright object is brought toward the nose.	Early signs of increased ICP include a sluggishly reactive pupil and incomplete constriction. Infants older than the age of 3 mo are able to accommodate for near vision. The setting sun sign (portion of sclera visible between the iris and upper eyelid) can result from hydrocephalus and brain stem irritation. The oculocephalic reflex (doll's eyes) can result from a lesion of the midbrain or pons or from a deep coma.

*From Slota MC. Neurological assessment of the infant and toddler. *Crit Care Nurse.* 1983;3:87–94.
†From Slota MC. Pediatric neurologic assessment. *Crit Care Nurse.* 1983;3:106–112.

Table continued on following page

Table 4–5. CRANIAL NERVE EVALUATION *(Continued)*

CRANIAL NERVE	FUNCTIONS	METHODS OF TESTING	COMMENTS
IV	Trochlear Downward inward movement of the eye	Check the six fields of gaze: hold a bright object 18 in from the infant and move it from the midline into each of the six fields of gaze (upward outward, laterally, and downward outward) for each eye with someone else holding the infant's head steady. Note conjugate movements of the eyes.	Infants should attempt binocular fixation at the age of 3 mo and be able to follow the object smoothly by the age of one year. Nystagmus is normal in premature infants and neonates. Dysconjugate movements after the age of 6 wk can be indicative of blindness.
VI	Abducens Lateral deviation of the eye		
III	Oculomotor All other extraocular movements		
V	Trigeminal Motor innervation to the temporal and maseter muscles; responsible for jaw clenching and lateral movement. Sensory innervation to the face with three branches: (1) opthalmic, (2) maxillary, and (3) mandibular	Test the strength of the temporal and masseter muscles by assessing the infant sucking hold on the nipple or finger. Note jaw symmetry while the infant is crying. Test for the rooting reflex by stroking the cheek and watching the infant turn to the stimulated side. Test the corneal reflex with a cotton wisp touched lightly to the cornea only. Note the response of blinking and possible tearing.	Jaw weakness and an impaired suck can be present in infants with trigeminal damage. Infants can blink asymmetrically in response to corneal stimulation. Most infants produce tears by the age of 2 to 3 mo. The sensory component of the corneal reflex is the trigeminal nerve, and the motor component is the facial nerve.
VII	Facial Motor innervation to the muscles of the face including the forehead, eyes, and mouth. Sensory innervation to the anterior ⅔ of the tongue where sweet, sour, and salty sensors predominate	Observe facial symmetry during crying and smiling.	While taste is intact at birth, taste testing is not reliable in infants and rarely done. Infants will usually wrinkle their foreheads when crying. Central facial damage will result in paralysis from the eye down, and peripheral damage produces paralysis on the entire side of the face.
VIII	Acoustic Cochlear division: Hearing Vestibular division: Balance	Test acoustic blink reflex by creating a loud noise near infant and noting the blink in response. Create loud noise and note appropriate response for age. Test vestibular branch with doll's eye maneuver (see cranial nerve III) and caloric testing; iced saline is injected into the ear canal with a syringe by the physician after assuring that the tympanic membrane is intact. Note the normal response of nystagmus with the eye jerking away from the irrigated ear.	During the neonatal period, there is a generalized response to noise, usually a cry or Moro reflex. At about 8 to 10 wk, the infant will stop moving to listen to the sound. At about 3 to 4 mo, the infant will turn his head toward the noise. This response is expected by the age of 8 mo at the latest. In coma with an intact brain stem, caloric testing can demonstrate deviation of eyes toward the irrigated ear. With brain stem lesions, there is usually no response.

Table 4–5. CRANIAL NERVE EVALUATION (*Continued*)

CRANIAL NERVE	FUNCTIONS	METHODS OF TESTING	COMMENTS
IX	Glossopharyngeal Sensory innervation to the pharynx and taste on the posterior ⅓ of the tongue	Stimulate a gag. Note hoarse or stridorous crying. Observe swallowing with feedings, and note excessive drooling.	Some drooling is normal in infants. The autonomic system is intact at birth, but infants are particularly sensitive to parasympathetic stimulation. For example, the infant can readily demonstrate bradycardia during gagging or suctioning.
X	Vagus Sensory innervation to the pharynx and larynx Motor innervation to palate and pharynx and parasympathetic functions		
XI	Spinal accessory Motor innervation to the sternomastoid muscle and the upper portion of the trapezius muscle	Observe the infant's head movement from side to side.	Damage to the nerve can result in difficulty in turning the head from side to side.
XII	Hypoglossal Motor innervation to the tongue	Gently pinch the infant's nostrils to produce reflex opening of the mouth and raising of the tongue. Note tongue assymmetry, deviation, or atrophy. Observe the tongue movements during sucking.	Damage to the nerve can result in paresis, paralysis, deviation, or fasciculations.
Child†			
I	Olfactory Sense of smell	Assure that both nasal passages are patent and unobstructed. Ask child to close eyes and identify smells, testing each nostril separately. Use familiar odors, such as peanut butter, oranges, and chocolate.	Unreliable test results are common in toddlers and young children. Damage to this nerve results in perversion or loss of smell. Unilateral loss of smell can indicate a tumor of the anterior fossa. Temporary or permanent loss of smell can also be related to trauma to the olfactory bulbs or tracts or an upper respiratory tract infection.

Table continued on following page

Table 4–5.   **CRANIAL NERVE EVALUATION** (*Continued*)

CRANIAL NERVE	FUNCTIONS	METHODS OF TESTING	COMMENTS
II	Optic Vision	Test visual acuity in the younger child by observing recognition of familiar objects or people at a distance. This nerve can be tested with an eye chart (such as a Snellen chart) when children are about 6 to 7 y of age. Test color acuity through recognition of colored objects. Determine visual fields through the confrontation method: (1) seat the child at your eye level approximately 2 to 3 ft away; (2) ask the child to stare at your nose (using a bright sticker on the end of your nose can help); (3) bring a brightly colored object into his field of vision from the nasal, lateral, superior, and inferior fields; (4) compare the child's visual fields to your own. Inspect the fundus with an ophthalmoscope for optic atrophy or papilledema.	Damage to this nerve can result in ipsilateral visual impairment. Homonymous hemianopsia can result from spastic hemiplegia. Bilateral (bitemporal) hemianopsia can result from a tumor of the optic chiasm or craniopharyngioma. The confrontation method is a rough evaluation of visual fields. Specialized testing is required for an accurate evaluation. Specific fundoscopic findings in the pediatric patient include: (1) the child's retina is lighter than the adult's, (2) the macula is not fully differentiated, and (3) papilledema is rare in children before complete closure of the fontanelles and sutures.
III	Oculomotor Pupillary constriction, elevation of the upper eyelid, and most of the extraocular movements	Check pupillary responses by shining a light directly into each eye from the side and observing the briskness and completeness of the direct pupillary response. Check the consensual response by shining the light into one eye and observing the briskness in response of the other pupil. Record the size of pupil in millimeters. Note the shape and equality of the pupils. Note the opening of the upper eyelids and ptosis (drooping). Check the extraocular movements as described below.	Compression of the parasympathetic nerve fiber on the third cranial nerve allows sympathetic dominance and pupillary dilatation. Since the third nerve is located at the tentorial notch, increases in ICP can result in ipsilateral, contralateral, or bilateral pupillary dilatation. Early signs of increased ICP include a sluggish response to light or incomplete constriction. Other abnormal findings that should be noted include: (1) anisocoria (unequal pupils), (2) bilaterally pinpoint fixed pupils (damage to sympathetic nerves at brain stem), and (3) hippus (rhythmical dilatation and constriction of pupils in response to light).

Table 4–5.   CRANIAL NERVE EVALUATION (*Continued*)

CRANIAL NERVE	FUNCTIONS	METHODS OF TESTING	COMMENTS
IV	Trochlear Downward, inward movement of the eye	Check the six fields of gaze by holding a bright object 18 in from the child and moving it from the midline into each of the six fields of gaze for each eye.	Damage to the fourth nerve can cause diplopia (double vision) and altered downward eye movement.
VI	Abducens Lateral deviation of the eye	Ask the child to follow the object with his or her eyes but to keep the head steady. Note conjugate movements of the eyes and absence of nystagmus except in the extreme lateral position.	Damage to the sixth nerve can produce deviation of the head toward the weak muscle to avoid diplopia. Dysconjugate gaze can indicate blindness, and a conjugate horizontal gaze palsy suggests a lesion of the brain stem or cerebral hemisphere. Vertical gaze paralysis suggests brain stem dysfunction, and upward gaze paralysis suggests hydrocephalus or a tumor of the pineal region.
III	Oculomotor All other extraocular movements	Check for accommodation by bringing an object from 18 in out in toward the nose. As the object is brought toward the nose, check for convergence of the eyes and pupillary constriction.	Damage to the third nerve can result in ptosis, outward and downward displacement of the eye, and a large, sluggish pupil (in addition to the changes noted above).
V	Trigeminal Motor: Innervation to the temporal and masseter muscles; responsible for clenching and lateral movement of the jaw	Motor: While palpating the temporal and then masseter muscles, ask the child to clench his or her teeth or bite on a safe object. Note the muscle strength. Ask the child to move his or her jaw from side to side and observe the symmetry of jaw movement during laughter, crying, or talking.	Damage to the motor component of the nerve can result in impaired mastication. A unilateral paralysis can cause deviation of the jaw to the affected side when the child opens his mouth. Trauma, infections, or tumors can impair facial sensation or produce paroxysmal facial pain.
	Sensory: Innervation to the face with three branches: ophthalmic, maxillary, and mandibular	Sensory: With the child's eyes closed, test the three sensory branches of the nerve by using first a cotton wisp and then a sharp object on the forehead, cheeks, and jaw. Substitute the dull end of the object occasionally to test the child's reliability. If abnormal findings are present, evaluate temperature sensation using test tubes filled with hot and cold water. Test the corneal reflex with a cotton wisp touched lightly to the cornea only. Note the response of blinking and some tearing.	The sensory component of the corneal reflex is the trigeminal nerve, and the motor component is the facial nerve. Use of contact lenses in the older child can diminish or abolish the corneal reflex. If the child in an intensive care setting is being tested frequently for pain sensation, it may be wise to use a sterile needle for testing.

Table continued on following page

Table 4–5. CRANIAL NERVE EVALUATION *(Continued)*

CRANIAL NERVE	FUNCTIONS	METHODS OF TESTING	COMMENTS
VII	Facial Motor: Innervation to the muscles of the face including the forehead, eyes, and mouth	Motor: Inspect the child's face for asymmetry during rest and while talking or crying. Ask the child to raise eyebrows, make a "mad" face, close eyes very tightly, show teeth, smile, puff out cheeks, and make a "funny" face. In the younger child, watch facial expressions during play.	Damage to this nerve can result in facial weakness or paralysis. Central facial damage will result in paralysis from the eye down, while peripheral damage can produce paralysis on the entire side of the face. Damage can also result in the loss of taste sensation on the anterior $2/3$ of the tongue. Younger children may not cooperate or be reliable in responding to taste testing.
	Sensory: Innervation to the anterior $2/3$ of the tongue where sweet, sour, and salty sensors predominate	Sensory: Ask the child to hold out his or her tongue. Using an applicator, apply sweet, salty, or sour substances to the child's tongue.	
VIII	Acoustic Cochlear division: Hearing	Cochlear: Check for fine hearing by holding a tickling watch 1 or 2 in from one ear while occluding the other ear. Repeat on the opposite side. Check for gross hearing by standing one to 2 ft away from the child and whispering something the child will be able to repeat.	Damage to the nerve can result in impaired hearing, tinnitus, vertigo, nystagmus, and unilateral or bilateral deafness. The Rinne and Weber tests can be used for further assessment of this nerve.
	Vestibular division: Balance	Vestibular: Test the vestibular branch with caloric testing. Iced saline (of varying amounts for different ages) is injected into the external ear canal with a syringe. Note the normal response of nystagmus with the eye jerking away from the irrigated ear.	Deviation of the eyes toward the irrigated ear can occur in coma with an intact brain stem. Caloric testing usually results in no response in brain stem lesions.
IX	Glossopharyngeal Sensory: Innervation to the pharynx and taste on the posterior $1/3$ of tongue	Test the two nerves together by asking the child to say "ah" or yawn. During this action, observe the upward motion of the soft palate and uvula and the upward, inward movement of the posterior pharynx.	Damage to these nerves can result in impaired sensation, dysphagia (difficulty swallowing), dysarthria (difficulty talking), dysphonia, excessive drooling, stridor, and autonomic nervous system changes related to the vagus nerve. Adolescent boys can demonstrate hoarseness and voice changes related to normal puberty.

Table 4–5.   CRANIAL NERVE EVALUATION *(Continued)*

CRANIAL NERVE	FUNCTIONS	METHODS OF TESTING	COMMENTS
X	Vagus Sensory: Innervation to the pharynx and larynx Motor: Innervation to the palate and pharynx and parasympathetic functions	Touch the side of the uvula with a tongue blade, and note the upward movement and deviation to the stimulated side. Touch the posterior portion of the tongue with a tongue blade to stimulate a gag reflex. Note any hoarseness, and observe the child's ability to swallow without pain or choking. Note excessive drooling or coughing. Test bitter taste on the posterior ⅓ of the tongue.	
XI	Spinal accessory Motor: Innervation to the sternocleidomastoid muscle and the upper portion of the trapezius muscle	Ask the child to turn his or her head from side to side against the pressure of your hands to test for strength. Note the normal range of motion of approximately 170 degrees. Ask the child to shrug his or her shoulders against the pressure of your hands. You may need to demonstrate this action to younger children.	Damage to this nerve can produce asymmetrical should posture, drooping shoulders, impaired strength in lifting the shoulders, or difficulty in turning the head to either side.
XII	Hypoglossal Motor: Innervation to the tongue	Inspect the younger child's tongue for fasciculations and symmetrical movement. Ask the older child to stick out his or her tongue, and observe for asymetry, deviation, or atrophy.	Damage to this nerve can result in atrophy, weakness, deviation, or fasciculations of the tongue. Fine, irregular, occasional tremors of the tongue are normal when holding out the tongue.

Table 4–6.   COMMON RESPIRATORY PATTERNS IN COMATOSE CLIENTS

PATTERN		LOCATION OF LESION CAUSING COMA
Cheyne-Stokes respiration		Usually bilateral in cerebral hemispheres Cerebellar sometimes Midbrain Upper pons
Central neurogenic hyperventilation		Low midbrain Upper pons
Apneustic breathing		Mid pons Low pons
Cluster breathing		Low pons High medulla
Ataxic breathing		Medulla

From Ignatavicius D et al. *Medical-Surgical Nursing: A Nursing Process Approach,* 2nd ed. Philadelphia: Pa: WB Saunders Co; 1995.

CNS infections (due to the effects of pyrogens on the hypothalamus), and children with status epilepticus (may be due to hypothalamic dysfunction as well as increased total body oxygen consumption) (Tasker and Dean, 1992). Hypothermia may be seen in neonates (same as above) and in brain death because of loss of hypothalamic function.

c. *Pulse and blood pressure:* Changes in pulse and blood pressure are very late and ominous signs of neurologic dysfunction. Cushing's reflex is an increase in systolic pressure greater than diastolic pressure (i.e., widened pulse pressure) and bradycardia. Cardiac dysrhythmias are seen with some traumatic brain injuries (TBIs). Vasodilation with systemic hypotension may be seen with spinal trauma or sympathetic insufficiency (Davis et al, 1992).

C. **BRAIN DEATH DETERMINATION**
1. Most states have adopted guidelines to define death the same way for infants, children, and adults. One of two conditions must exist:
   a. Irreversible cessation of breathing and circulation *or*
   b. Irreversible cessation of whole brain function (i.e., cortical and brain stem)
2. The difference in brain death determination between children and adults is not the legal definition of death but the process of confirming brain death. Several sets of guidelines have been published for the determination of brain death in children. The most widely accepted guidelines are those published by the Ad Hoc Task Force for the Determination of Brain Death in Children (Guidelines, 1987).
   a. *History:* The cause of coma must be known to establish irreversibility. There must be an absence of complicating factors such as hemodynamic instability, use of sedatives and paralyzing agents, severe hypothermia, or hypoxemia.
   b. To determine brain death the *physical examination* should demonstrate coma, normothermia, normal blood pressure, flaccidity, absence of movement (except for spinal cord reflexes), and absence of brain stem function. Loss of brain stem function is determined by nonreactive midposition or fully dilated pupils, absence of oculocephalic (doll's eyes) and oculovestibular (cold calorics) reflexes, absence of movement of bulbar musculature and corneal, gag, cough, sucking, and rooting reflexes, and absence of respiratory effort with standardized apnea testing (Jumah et al, 1992; Outwater and Rockoff, 1984). Following disconnection from the ventilator several conditions must occur: adequate time (5 to 10 minutes) to allow $Paco_2$ to increase to levels sufficient to stimulate respiration, adequate oxygenation, and absence of cardiovascular instability.
   c. Consistent examination techniques are required throughout the observation period. For infants age 7 days to 2 months, two examinations and electroencephalograms (EEGs) are performed 48 hours apart. For infants age 2 months to 1 year, two examinations and EEGs are performed 24 hours apart, or one examination and an initial EEG showing electrocerebral silence (ECS) combined with a radionuclide angiogram showing no CBF is used. In children older than 1 year, two examinations are performed 12 to 24 hours apart. EEG and isotope angiography are optional.
3. **Controversies** (Freeman and Ferry, 1988; Shewmon, 1988): The exact cause of coma is often unknown in the newborn, since many hypoxic-ischemic injuries occur in utero. The accuracy of confirmatory tests in the newborn are unknown.

NEURODIAGNOSTIC MONITORING

A. ASSESSING ANATOMIC INTEGRITY

1. **Radiograph**
   a. *Description:* Roentgenographic films of skull and spine demonstrate structural deficits only. The radiation penetrates all body tissues and is absorbed to varying degrees, resulting in different shadow intensities (Mason, 1992).
   b. *Clinical use: Skull films* are used to determine fractures, widened sutures, tumors, calcification, and bone erosion. *Spinal films* are used to evaluate the integrity of the vertebral structures including the vertebral body, disc interspace, lamina, and pedicles. Spinal films are also used to evaluate fractures, dislocations, and degeneration of bone.
   c. *Nursing implications:* Immobilize fractures with splints, cervical collars, traction devices, or age-appropriate immobilizers. Provide routine safe transport care including use of appropriate monitoring devices, elevation of side rails, good alignment of affected body structure(s), securing standby emergency equipment, and serial monitoring of neurovascular status. Explain the procedure to older children or parents including the length of the procedure, purpose of the procedure, sensations and appearance of the environment, and expectations of the child during the procedure (e.g., to remain quiet without body movement).

2. **Computed tomography (CT) scan**
   a. *Description:* CT scan is based on computer image reconstruction from a series of thin slices of the brain (x-ray film measurements of sections of the brain). CT scan differentiates tissue density relative to water via a computer. Highly dense structures (e.g., bone, fresh blood) appear white, and low-density areas (e.g., air, fat) appear dark (Chesnut, 1994).
   b. *Clinical use:* Because of cost, speed, and availability, CT scan is used for examination of acute neurologic dysfunction. CT scan is superior to magnetic resonance imaging (MRI) in detecting blood (especially subarachnoid hemorrhage) and in evaluating cortical bone structures of skull and spine (Chan et al, 1995). Contrast-enhanced CT (CECT) is used to detect lesions that cause blood-brain barrier breakdown, to visualize blood vessels and well-vascularized lesions, and to rule out cerebral metastases (Curley and Vernon-Levett, 1996). It is difficult to visualize the posterior fossa because of bone obstruction.
   c. *Nursing implications:* Before the procedure the patient and family should be told that the machine surrounds the body and clicking and whirring noises may be heard. The procedure is painless, except for a venipuncture if contrast medium is used. The child is required to remain still throughout the procedure; sedation may be required. If contrast medium is used, the patient may experience an unusual sensation during the procedure (e.g., a burning or warm sensation for about 20 to 30 seconds during injection of the contrast medium). The use of contrast media is contraindicated in patients with acute renal failure.
   d. Postprocedure monitoring includes assessing for an allergic reaction to the contrast medium (e.g., tachycardia, hypotension, fever, chills) and observing contrast injection site (if used) for bleeding, swelling, redness, and pain.

3. **Magnetic resonance imaging (MRI)**
   a. *Description:* MRI differentiates tissues by their response to radiofrequency pulses in a magnetic field; lesions have either a high or low signal (in contrast to x-ray density seen with a CT scan).

b. *Clinical use:* MRI is used to identify small infarcts, infections, inflammatory areas, and demyelinating plaques. MRI provides clear sagittal images; therefore, it is the procedure of choice for suspected lesions of the spinal cord or cervicomedullary junction (Bergman, 1992). MRI can delineate between tissue structure (e.g., white and gray matter).

- The advantages of MRI as compared to CT scan (Chan et al, 1995) include better definition of normal and pathologic lesions (except for those listed above for CT scan), better three-dimensional information and relationships, demonstration of blood and CSF flow, and evaluation of tumors in the posterior fossa that are normally obstructed by bone artifact in CT imaging.

- Disadvantages of MRI as compared to CT scan are the requirement of more time and cooperation from the patient and difficulty in continuously monitoring the patient during the procedure because of the magnetic field; however, newer MRI-compatible monitors are becoming increasingly more available (Kanal and Shellock, 1992). Another disadvantage of MRI is that it is contraindicated in patients with metallic implants (e.g., pacemakers, aneurysm clips).

c. *Nursing implications:* When the patient's condition permits, preprocedural education should include the information that the machine turns around the patient and makes a loud noise much like a washing machine. The procedure is long, and the child must lie still. If a contrast medium is used, an unusual sensation may occur (i.e., a warm rushing sensation for approximately 20 to 30 seconds during injection). The procedure is painless, except for venipuncture when a contrast medium is used. All metallic objects must be removed from the patient, parents, and supportive staff who may accompany the patient. Inquire regarding implantable metallic objects (e.g., pacemakers, electronic implants, surgical clips, ferromagnetic items). Sedation is often required for small children. Postprocedure monitoring is the same as for CT scan.

4. **Cerebral angiogram**

a. *Description:* Intraarterial injection (usually femoral cannulation) of radiopaque dye is followed by sequential skull radiographs or digital subtraction technique. Cerebral angiogram is used to outline the intracranial and extracranial vessels. A series of radiographs are taken once the arterial system is accessed and contrast dye is injected (Mason, 1992).

b. *Clinical use:* Since the advent of CT scan and MRI, angiogram use is more restricted. It is usually reserved for confirmation of lesions and identification of vascular occlusions, recanalization, ulceration and dissection of large arteries, and stenosis of small arteries. It is the procedure of choice for aneurysms and arteriovascular malformations and is used to detect CBF alterations.

c. *Nursing implications*

- Preprocedural education should include describing the purpose of the procedure, the length of the procedure (usually takes several hours), possible sensations the patient may experience during the procedure (e.g., a burning or warm sensation for about 20 to 30 seconds during injection of the contrast medium), and the possible need for sedation and its expected effects. Contrast medium is excreted by the kidneys; patients are encouraged to drink liberally the day before the procedure or intravenous (IV) fluids may be increased as ordered. Nothing by mouth restrictions prior to the test usually apply for 12 hours. All jewelry and hair ornaments must be removed.

- Postprocedure monitoring: Patients should avoid movement of the affected extremity to prevent dislodgment of a clot, bleeding, and hematoma formation. Frequently assess the neurovasculature status and pressure dressing of a cannulated extremity; usually every 15 minutes for an hour, then every 30 minutes for an hour, and then every hour until the patient is stable. Assess for bleeding, hematoma, or infection at the cannulation site. Restrict activity initially; usually 12 to 24 hours. Monitor vital signs for signs of shock (e.g., hypotension, diminished pulses, and tachycardia) at the same intervals as the neurovasculature assessment. Assess for an allergic reaction to contrast medium (e.g., tachycardia, hypotension, fever, chills). Encourage hydration with sips of water or IV fluids. Maintain intake and output record for 24 hours.

5. **Radioisotope scan**
   a. *Description:* A radioisotope is injected into the circulation, and a brain scanning device detects areas of abnormal uptake of the isotope (occurs with altered blood-brain barrier or highly vascularized area).
   b. *Clinical use:* The use of a radioisotope scan has been limited since the development of the CT scan. A radioisotope scan is effective in identifying isodense lesions such as subdural hematoma, blood clots with the same density as adjacent tissue, intracerebral infection, and inflammation. A radioisotope scan is also effective in the evaluation of patients with epilepsy, since it may help to identify epileptic foci prior to excision.
   c. *Nursing implications:* Preprocedural education includes explaining the purpose for and length of the procedure. A small venipuncture is necessary for isotope injection. Time delay may be necessary for adequate uptake of the isotope. There is a small radiation hazard to the patient and staff; however, the half-life of nuclides is extremely short.

B. **ASSESSING PHYSIOLOGIC ALTERATIONS**
   1. **ICP monitoring**
      a. *Description:* ICP monitoring is a technique where a catheter is placed directly within the cranium to measure ICP. Less frequently, a transducer is placed indirectly on the anterior fontanelle to measure ICP.
      b. *Clinical uses* include assessment for the prevention of herniation and the preservation of cerebral perfusion.
      c. *Classification of systems: type of transducer*
         - In *fluid-filled systems,* the compartment that is being monitored is connected to a strain-gauge transducer via a fluid pathway. Fluid column pulsations are converted into millimeters of mercury. Advantages include the low cost, accuracy (with an intraventricular catheter), and ability to zero and recalibrate after insertion. Disadvantages are that the accuracy depends on the catheter location, artifact is present with movement, the procedure requires transducer leveling with position changes, and the system may become obstructed with tissue, blood, air, or bone.
         - *Fiberoptic catheters* have a transducer tip that is non-fluid-filled. A mirrored diaphragm (in the tip of the transducer) moves in response to pressure and is sensed by light fibers. Information is converted into an analog signal and displayed on a pressure monitor (Gambardella et al, 1993). Advantages include the theoretical low risk of infection because of the lack of a fluid column and stopcocks, accurate ICP value, excellent waveform quality with less artifact, placement in brain parenchyma, and the fact that transducer leveling is not required. Disadvantages (McQuillan, 1991) include a greater cost than the fluid-filled system, requirement for dedicated hardware, special handling of the catheter

and cable to avoid breakage, inability to rezero after insertion, and inability to drain CSF as a treatment modality unless a catheter is placed in a lateral ventricle.

- An *external fiberoptic transducer* is applied to the anterior fontanelle and measures ICP indirectly. Fontanelle tonometers are used only rarely in infants. Advantages include its noninvasive nature and lack of complications. Disadvantages include the lack of accurate ICP measurements (amount of external pressure applied to the sensor can alter measurements), the fact that it may underestimate ICP and may not record acute increases in ICP, additional cost, and that compliance testing and CSF drainage are not possible.

d. Classification of systems: *anatomic locations* (fluid-filled or fiberoptic systems)

- The *intraventricular* location is the gold standard of ICP monitoring. Ventricular monitoring is located deeply within the brain and is therefore considered to be more accurate in reflecting whole brain pressure (Schickncer and Young, 1992). The catheter tip is placed in the anterior horn of the lateral ventricle through the nondominant cerebral hemisphere. Waveform quality is excellent. Advantages are that the catheter allows drainage of CSF, is accurate and reliable, permits administration of medications, and permits volume pressure compliance testing. Disadvantages include the high risk of infection and bleeding, the longer insertion time (collapsed or small ventricles make insertion difficult or prohibitive), and the risk of CSF leakage.

- *Subarachnoid bolts* are inserted into the subarachnoid space via a twist drill hole in the nondominant prefrontal cranium behind the hairline just anterior to the coronal suture. Different types of bolts are available (e.g., Philly bolt, Richmond bolt, Leeds screw). Pediatric bolts are usually shorter and lighter compared to adult bolts. Waveform quality is good initially, but may dampen with time with a fluid-filled system. Advantages are that subarachnoid bolts are quick to insert and useful when ventricles are collapsed and access is impossible. Disadvantages are that tissue may occlude the device, CSF leakage may occur, ICP may be underestimated, and the bolt requires the skull to be intact.

- *Subdural catheters* are inserted below the dura mater and above the subarachnoid space in the same manner as the subarachnoid bolt. Used primarily after surgery for evacuation of a clot, the catheter is placed at the operative site (Germon, 1994). Waveform quality is poor and used primarily for trending. Advantages include the low risk of hemorrhage, quick and easy insertion, usefulness when the ventricles are collapsed and access is impossible, and a lower infection risk than with an intraventricular catheter. Disadvantages include the potential underestimation of ICP, the inability to drain CSF, and the requirement of an intact skull.

- *Epidural catheters* are inserted below the skull and above the dura mater. They are considered to be an indirect measure of ICP. Waveform quality is poor and used primarily for trending. Advantages are that epidural catheters have the least invasive placement (dura mater remains intact), there is a low risk of infection, quick and easy insertion, no risk for CSF leakage, and low risk for brain injury. Disadvantages are that epidural catheters provide an indirect measurement that is not as accurate and reliable as measurements made with other catheter systems and that epidural catheters are unable to drain CSF.

- *Intraparenchymal fiberoptic transduced tipped catheters* are placed directly into the brain tissue (via a bolt or screw device) approximately 1 cm below the subarachnoid space. Waveform quality is good. Advantages include the low risk of infection, quick and easy insertion, and the accuracy and reliability. Disadvantages are the same as for all fiberoptic systems (see above).

e. *Nursing implications*

- *Zeroing and calibrating* the fluid-filled systems depends on the manufacturer's recommendation, unit practice, location of the catheter, and the risk of infection. Since fiberoptic transducers are zeroed before insertion and are factory set, no calibration is required. Fiberoptic transducers may be calibrated with the bedside monitor. The fluid-filled transducer (Vos, 1993) should be *level* at the foramen of Monro (e.g., outer canthus of the eye, tragus of the ear). The level should be changed with every position change. Leveling for fiberoptic systems is not required. The transducer is located at the tip of the catheter.

- *Insertion site care* is basically the same for all systems. Maintain a dry and intact occlusive dressing. Maintain aseptic technique with dressing changes. Notify the physician for leakage on and around the dressing. Evaluate the insertion site for CSF leakage, bleeding, hematoma, and infection. The diagnosis of meningitis or ventriculitis is made on the basis of positive results from CSF cultures; fever and leukocytosis are less predictive. Local signs of catheter infection include redness, swelling, and drainage at the insertion site.

- *Maintain infection control* by using aseptic technique when handling the system. In fluid-filled systems, minimize the number of connections and stopcocks. Maintain a closed system by covering all entry ports with dead-ender caps. Minimize the number of times the system is entered. Avoid dislodgment or breakage of the system by avoiding tension on the tubing or fiberoptic cables. Tape the tubing to the dressing, clip or pin the cable to the patient, avoid kinking the cable, and use caution when repositioning or transporting the patient. Notify the physician of any loose connections at the insertion site.

f. **Waveform analysis** (Dean and Moss, 1992; Germon, 1994; McQuillan, 1991; Vos, 1993): The normal ICP waveform (Fig. 4–15) resembles the arterial waveform with three descending peaks:

- P_1 (percussion wave) is the first peak that originates from pulsations of the choroid plexus. It is a sharp peak, consistent in amplitude, and the largest of all waves.

- P_2 (rebound or tidal wave) is more variable in shape and amplitude and smaller than the percussion wave and may become larger than the other two waves with decreased intracranial compliance.

- P_3 (dicrotic wave) follows P_1 and P_2 and is the smallest of the three waves. After the dicrotic wave, pressure usually decreases to diastolic baseline.

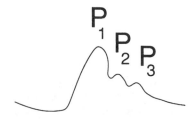

Figure 4–15.   Components of a normal ICP waveform.

g. Abnormal ICP waveforms (Fig. 4–16)
- A waves (plateau) are spontaneous, rapid, irregular increases in ICP to 50 to 100 mm Hg lasting 5 to 20 minutes. A waves are frequently associated with dilated pupil(s), vomiting, abnormal posturing, decreased level of consciousness, widened pulse pressure, dysrhythmias, and decreased respirations. They represent impaired CBF and occur most often with decreases in blood pressure associated with hypovolemia.
- B waves are sharp rhythmic increases in ICP to 50 mm Hg lasting 30 seconds to 2 minutes. B waves are related to respirations. They may precede A waves or seizures or occur during a headache, posturing, or decreased level of consciousness.
- C waves are small waves that occur every 4 to 8 minutes and result from

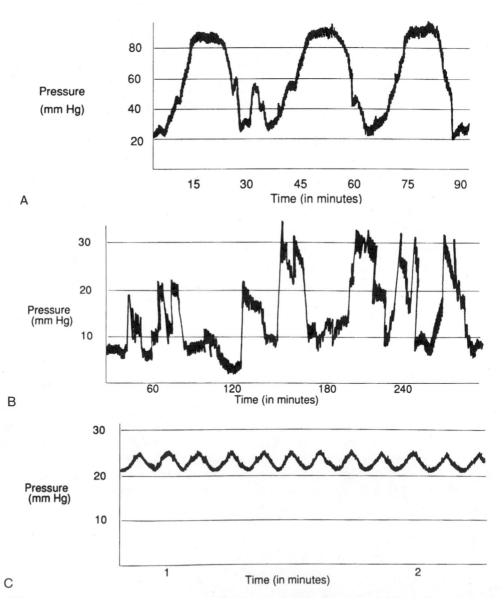

Figure 4–16. Abnormal ICP waveforms. **A,** A or plateau waves. **B,** B waves. **C,** C waves. (Reprinted with permission from McQuillan KA. Intracranial pressure monitoring: technical imperatives. *AACN Clin Issues Crit Care Nurs.* 1991;2[4]:632–633.)

fluctuations in the systemic pulse and respirations. They are clinically insignificant.

2. **Transcranial Doppler ultrasound**
   a. *Description:* Calculation of mean velocity and direction of CBF is achieved by means of a 2-MHz ultrasound probe held to thin areas of the skull. Velocity signals are displayed as pulsatile waveforms that can be recorded. Transcranial Doppler ultrasound does not directly measure blood flow, but the velocity signals are directly proportional to blood flow and therefore can accurately measure any change in flow (Unwin et al, 1991).
   b. *Clinical uses* are for diagnosis of vasospasm, diagnosis of vessel occlusion, monitoring for cerebral emboli, testing of carbon dioxide and blood pressure vasoreactivity, and detection of changes in ICP (an increase in pulsatility).
   c. *Nursing implications:* Ultrasound may be done at the bedside and has no major complications or contraindications. Preprocedural education should include instructing the patient to lie still. Sedation may be required.

3. **Xenon CT scan of CBF**
   a. *Description:* The CT technique uses the high density of stable nonradioactive xenon to measure brain tissue buildup of this atom following inhalation of a xenon gas mixture. It is based on the principle that the rate of uptake or clearance of an inert diffusible gas is proportional to blood flow in the tissue. The brain is scanned before, during, and after the procedure, and end-tidal xenon concentration is measured and computer calculated to estimate CBF.
   b. *Clinical uses* are for diagnosis of stroke, diagnosis of massive cerebral hypertension, confirmatory test for brain death determination (absence of uptake indicates no CBF, which is a definitive diagnosis of brain death), assessment of global hypoxic ischemic injury, and assessment of intracranial trauma.
   c. *Nursing implications:* Preprocedural education includes instructing the patient to lie still and inhale a gas mixture. The CT scanner may frighten patients. There are no known risks with the procedure.

4. **Electroencephalograms (EEGs)**
   a. *Description:* An EEG records spontaneous electrical activity across the surface of the brain. Activity is characterized by the frequency and voltage of electrical signals. Common EEG abnormalities include the following:
      - Diffuse slowing of background rhythms is a common nonspecific finding seen in patients with diffuse encephalopathies and some structural abnormalities.
      - Focal slowing of parenchyma indicates localized dysfunction.
      - Triphasic waves seen in toxic metabolic encephalopathies consist of generalized synchronous waves occurring in brief runs.
      - Epileptic discharges are associated with seizure disorders.
      - Periodic lateralizing epileptiform discharges (PLED) suggest an acute destructive cerebral lesion.
      - Generalized periodic sharp waves are seen most commonly in patients following cerebral anoxia.
   b. *Clinical uses* include the diagnosis of epilepsy, dementia and diffuse encephalopathies, brain lesions, some cerebral infections, and brain death.
   c. *Nursing implications:* Preprocedural teaching should include a description of the sensations and setup of scalp leads. Sleep deprivation may be used to precipitate certain types of seizure discharges. It involves keeping the

patient awake for all or part of the night before the EEG is to be performed. Depending on specific orders, the patient may be awake or asleep during the EEG. Discontinuation of anticonvulsants may be used prior to an EEG as an activation technique for seizure discharges. Describe the testing procedures to the child or family. Hyperventilation is an activation technique (i.e., induces seizure discharges) that requires voluntary hyperventilation. Photic stimulation is an activation technique (flashing a light in the eyes at various frequencies). Routine monitoring during the procedure includes observation of seizure activity, observation of other activity, and monitoring of vital functions as dictated by the patient's condition. Accurate documentation of the patient's behaviors and nursing interventions with continuous EEG recording is essential. Shampoo the patient's hair after the procedure.

5. **Evoked potential (EP)**
   a. *Description:* Evoked potentials measure electrical activity produced by a specific neural structure along a sensory pathway. The measurement is called an evoked response (ER). EP electrical activity is generally much slower than spontaneous cortical electrical activity. EP studies usually characterize neurologic dysfunction as delayed responses (Henneman, 1989). Neural pathways usually studied are visual (VER), brain stem auditory (BAER), somatosensory (SSER), and multimodality (MMER.)
   b. *Clinical uses* are to identify dysfunction in specific sensory pathways. Sometimes, EPs are used as an adjunctive test to confirm brain death or abnormalities with equivocal findings (Garcia-Larrea et al, 1992).
   c. *Nursing implications:* Preprocedural education includes teaching the patient what to expect from stimuli. In visual testing the patient sees a strobe or alternating checkerboard. In auditory testing the patient hears clicks. In somatosensory testing the patient feels electrical current on the skin. The procedure is lengthy. Sedation may be required for agitation or anxiety. After the test, completely remove the gel and glue from the patient's scalp to prevent skin breakdown.

C. ASSESSING METABOLIC ALTERATIONS
   1. **Lumbar puncture and CSF analysis**
      a. *Description:* Lumbar puncture is the most frequently performed neurologic diagnostic test to assess CSF composition. Lumbar puncture is performed by inserting a needle into the spinal subarachnoid space distal to the spinal cord (between L-3 and L-4 or L-4 and L-5 vertebral interspace).
      b. *Clinical use* is to measure CSF pressure, analyze CSF, inject or remove substances, and deliver spinal anesthesia.
      c. *Nursing implications:* Preprocedural education includes a description of the sensations. Local anesthesia is used requiring a small needle insertion at the site of the lumbar puncture. Burning may be felt for a few seconds at the infiltration site. A side-lying position is used most often with the child's knees flexed to the chest. The child is held in place with the back close to the edge of the examining table. The nurse should avoid placing any weight on the child. An alternative position for infants to distend the dural sac slightly, and therefore ease insertion, is the sitting position. The infant's buttocks are placed at the edge of the table, and the infant's neck and hips are flexed and stabilized. Following the procedure, assess the insertion site for bleeding, infection, leak, hematoma, and swelling. Potential complications include brain stem herniation with elevated ICP at the time of the test, hematoma, infection, headache, radiculopathy, and spinal, epidural, or subarachnoid bleeding.

INTRACRANIAL DEVICES

A. **EXTERNAL VENTRICULAR DRAINAGE (EVD)**
   1. **Description:** EVD is a temporary straight, Silastic catheter placed in the lateral ventricle (usually on the right) through a burr hole. The catheter is externalized through the ventriculostomy site or from a secondary incision after being tunneled under the scalp. It may be attached to an ICP monitoring catheter (Fig. 4–17) or may function just as a drainage system. The distal end of the catheter is connected to a simple extraventricular drain.
   2. **Indications** include intermittent drainage of CSF for acute intracranial hypertension, ventricular shunt malfunction, or acute hydrocephalus following intracranial hemorrhage.
   3. **Potential complications** include infection, hemorrhage, collapse of ventricles, leakage of fluid, leakage of air into the ventricular system, and seizures.
   4. **Nursing implications** (Birdsall and Greif, 1990)
      a. Several EVD systems are available but have similar components including a drip chamber, collection bag, and drainage pressure scale.
      b. Specific orders are obtained from the physician for care. With the foramen of Monro or lateral ventricles used as the zero reference point, the drip chamber is moved up or down to adjust the amount of CSF drainage. Anatomic location of the zero reference point is usually the external auditory meatus. The height of the drip chamber is usually 27 cm above the reference point. In this position CSF automatically drains when the ICP is

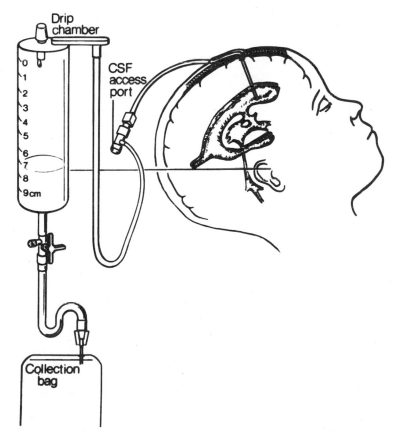

Figure 4–17. Intraventricular ICP monitor with drainage system. (Reprinted with permission from Fuhrman BP, Zimmerman JJ. *Pediatric Critical Care.* St Louis, Mo: Mosby–Year Book Inc; 1992.)

greater than 20 mm Hg (1 mm Hg is equal to 1.36 cm H_2O). Specific times when the tubing should be clamped (e.g., too much CSF drainage, during transport, during vigorous activity) or unclamped (e.g., signs and symptoms of increased ICP) and the level of head elevation are ordered by the physician.

c. Nursing responsibilities include assessing and documenting the amount of CSF drainage. CSF flow is controlled by physician order (i.e., level of the drip chamber), the initial problem, and hydration status. However, normal CSF flow is usually 3 to 5 ml/h in an infant, 5 to 10 ml/h in a toddler or child, and 10 to 15 ml/h in an adolescent. CSF should be clear and colorless. Initially CSF may be blood tinged but it should turn clear in 1 to 2 hours.

- Assess the system for patency by assessing the ICP waveform if a transducer is being used (i.e., the waveform would be dampened). Assess for fluctuation of the CSF fluid in the tubing with each heartbeat and respiration (if the system does not have a one-way valve). When the system is not draining, lower the collection cylinder until you see drainage; if the system has an external valve, compress the valve several times with the clamp open. Refer to the specific manufacturer's recommendations.
- Assess the system for loose connections.
- Notify the physician for significant changes in the patient's neurologic status or abrupt cessation or too much drainage of CSF (i.e., if beyond the initial evacuation period, CSF drainage exceeds the established norms or exceeds the physician's prescribed amount).
- Document the reference level and maintain the drip chamber or drainage bag at the prescribed level.
- Prevent infection of the CSF. Observe the catheter exit site or dressing for drainage. Change the catheter dressing using aseptic technique. Monitor the patient's temperature and other signs of systemic infection (e.g., hypotension, increased WBC count, positive results from blood or CSF cultures).

B. **VENTRICULAR SHUNT**

1. **Description:** A ventricular shunt is an internal catheter system designed to drain the lateral ventricles of CSF by bypassing part of the ventricular system. Many systems are available, but the major components are similar. A ventricular catheter is placed in the anterior horn of the right lateral ventricle. It is inserted through a burr hole usually in the region of the right parietooccipital area; the left side is avoided because of the location of the speech center. The catheter is tunneled under skin to minimize infection. A reservoir and pumping device are placed directly under the scalp on the skull bones. The pump contains a one-way valve that is usually pressure regulated. Distal tubing is attached to the valve and may be placed in one of several body cavities. The peritoneum (Fig. 4–18) is the most common cavity used. The distal catheter is tunneled subcutaneously to the upper quadrant of the abdomen. A small incision is made in the abdomen, and the catheter is guided into the peritoneum, where CSF is absorbed. Extra tubing is coiled in the abdomen to allow for growth. The right atrium is only used if abdominal problems preclude a peritoneal catheter. The distal catheter is inserted into the right atrium via passage through the subclavian vein, or less frequently, inserted directly into the right atrium. The pleural cavity is used infrequently, only when the above locations are contraindicated.

2. **Indicated** for hydrocephalus (acute and chronic).

3. **Complications** of the ventriculoperitoneal (VP) shunt include bowel perforation, ascites, and ileus. Complications of the ventriculoatrial (VA) shunt include

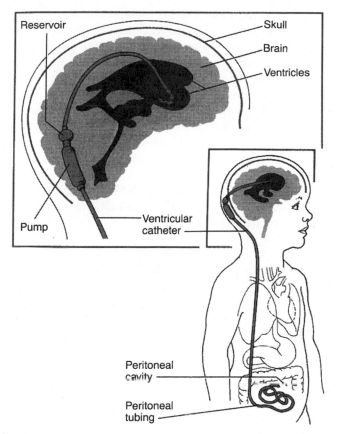

Figure 4–18. Placement of a VP shunt. (Reprinted with permission from Betz CL, Hunsberger MM, Wright S. *Family-Centered Nursing Care of Children.* 2nd ed. Philadelphia, Pa: WB Saunders Co; 1994.)

catheter movement, dysrhythmias, operative risks with more extensive surgery, endocarditis, and congestive heart failure. Complications of the ventriculopleural shunt include pleural effusion, pulmonary infection, and respiratory compromise.

a. All shunting devices and body cavities that are receptacles are at risk for infection including ventriculitis, meningitis, and systemic infection.

b. Mechanical failure, although rare, may occur from valves that stick and reservoirs that become obstructed with debris or disconnected from the distal catheter. The distal catheter may become disconnected and migrate to other areas (e.g., right ventricle or pulmonary artery from a VA shunt, perforated intestine from a VP shunt). Obstruction from tissue, clots, and debris may occur in the ventricular tip, valves, reservoir, internal catheters, and distal catheter tip.

c. Clinical manifestations of shunt obstruction and malfunction are similar and generally relate to increased ICP (e.g., a tense and bulging anterior fontanelle, poor feeding, and increase in head circumference in the infant; headaches, vomiting, or papilledema in the toddler and child).

4. **Nursing interventions**

a. Monitor neurologic status. Rapid evacuation of the ventricles may cause collapse of the ventricles, shearing of small vessels, and intracranial hemorrhage. Obstruction of the system can cause signs and symptoms of increased ICP. Seizures may occur.

    b. Monitor for signs of infection including redness or drainage at shunt site, hypothermia (more often in the neonate) or hyperthermia, redness, swelling, and tenderness along the subcutaneous tract, and nonspecific signs (e.g., lethargy, irritability, poor feeding, weight loss, pallor).

    c. Monitor for signs of excessive CSF drainage including a sunken fontanelle and increased sodium loss.

    d. Prevent skin breakdown by elevating the head of the bed as ordered, positioning the patient on the unaffected side of the skull or using pressure reduction devices to protect skin over the shunt when the patient is lying on the affected side, promoting good nutrition, and turning the patient every 2 hours.

    e. Monitor for signs of ileus including abdominal distention, vomiting, large orogastric residuals (i.e., more than one half of previous hours' intake), and hypoactive or absent bowel sounds.

INTRACRANIAL HYPERTENSION

A. DESCRIPTION

Sustained elevation of ICP above 15 mm Hg. Increased ICP is not a disease state but is a final common pathway for a number of neurologic pathologies.

B. INCIDENCE

Specific occurrence rates are unknown.

C. ETIOLOGY

    1. Neurologic pathologies that produce increased ICP are broadly classified into (specific pathologies are discussed in later sections) those that increase cerebral blood volume, CSF, or brain tissue.

    2. Cerebral edema may increase ICP and results from a number of different pathologies. It is defined as an increase in the fluid content of brain tissue. It is not a single entity and occurs in several different forms (Fishman, 1995).

        a. *Cellular (cytotoxic) edema* is characterized by intracellular swelling. It is caused by hypoxia, producing failure of intracellular active transport systems and an increase in intracellular osmoles as water enters rapidly into the cell or acute hypoosmolality of the plasma that results in water rapidly shifting into cells. This occurs primarily in gray matter.

        b. *Vasogenic edema* is characterized by increased permeability of the capillary endothelium to macromolecules. Large plasma molecules move from the vascular compartment into the extracellular spaces pulling water with them. Vasogenic edema occurs after vascular injury (e.g., abscess, hemorrhage, infarction, contusion), tumors, or disruption of the blood-brain barrier and accumulation of extracellular fluid.

        c. *Interstitial edema* is characterized by transependymal movement of CSF fluid from the ventricles into the extracellular spaces of brain tissue. It results from increased CSF hydrostatic pressure associated with noncommunicating hydrocephalus. This edema is most prominent in the white matter around ventricles.

D. PATHOPHYSIOLOGY

    1. Regardless of the cause, when intracranial volume exceeds the buffering capacity of the brain, ICP increases (see Intracranial Pressure Dynamics discussion).

    2. Increased ICP causes a number of interrelated pathologic processes resulting in distortion and herniation of brain tissue (Fig. 4–19).

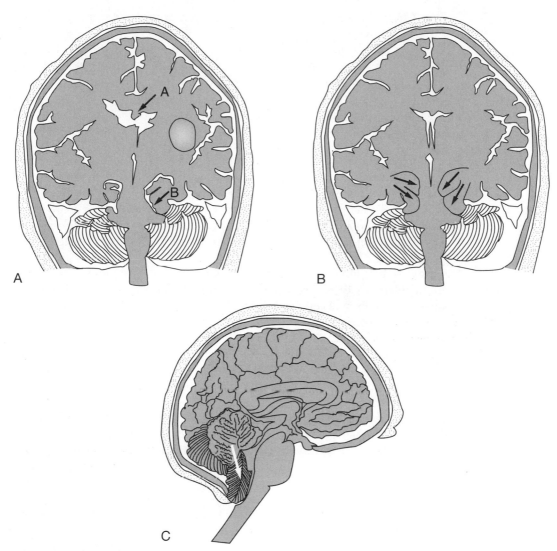

Figure 4–19. Herniation syndromes. **A,** Midline shift indicating cingulate herniation. **B,** Protrusion of uncus through the tentorial notch. Downward displacement of supratentorial region through the tentorial notch as seen in central herniation. **C,** Herniation of cerebellar tonsils into the foramen magnum. (Reprinted with permission from Morrison CAM. Brain herniation syndromes. *Crit Care Nurse.* 1987;7[5]:35–38.)

a. **Supratentorial herniation** occurs with an increase in intracranial volume and ICP in the brain structures above the tentorial membrane.
- *Uncal herniation* is a unilateral displacement of the uncus through the tentorial notch from a large lateral lesion of the middle fossa. Disruption of the parasympathetic fibers to the third cranial nerve causes unilateral pupil dilation on the same side as the lesion and contralateral hemiplegia. Later signs include paralysis of extraocular eye movements, coma, and if left untreated, death.
- *Central herniation* is a symmetric downward displacement of the cerebral hemispheres, basal ganglia, diencephalon, and midbrain through the tentorial notch. Early signs include alteration in the level of consciousness, alteration of the respiratory pattern (e.g., yawning and sighs), small reactive pupils, and bilateral Babinski reflexes. Later signs include

Cheyne-Stokes breathing, decorticate posturing, oculocephalic reflex, and coma.

- *Cingulate herniation* is displacement of the cingulate gyrus under the falx cerebri into the opposite hemisphere, causing compression of the internal cerebral vein. There are few signs specific to cingulate herniation. Changes in the patient's mental status and level of consciousness may be the only clue.

 b. **Infratentorial herniation** occurs with an increase in intracranial volume and ICP in the brain structures below the tentorial membrane. Downward displacement of one or both of the cerebellar tonsils occurs through the foramen magnum, and symptoms occur very rapidly (e.g., cardiorespiratory failure). Upward displacement of the lower brain stem through the tentorial notch can also occur. Clinical signs include developing hydrocephalus and coma. *Midbrain compression* produces downward deviation of the eyes, and *pontine compression* produces small reactive pupils and decerebrate posturing.

3. Increased ICP also results in a reduction in CBF. With loss of cerebral autoregulation, CBF passively follows systemic arterial pressure. Brain ischemia, anoxia, and neuronal cell death occur.

E. **DEFINING CHARACTERISTICS**

Symptoms depend on the age of the child and how rapidly the ICP increases.

1. **Chronic symptoms in infants** are usually nonspecific and include irritability, poor feeding, and lethargy. An abnormal increase in head circumference is noted; patients in the 95th percentile require further evaluation. The normal rate of head growth in the first year of life is 2 cm/mo for 3 months, 1 cm/mo for 3 months, and 0.5 cm/mo for the remaining 6 months (Jacobson, 1989). The setting sun sign is a classic "sunset" appearance of the eyes (i.e., the sclera are visible above the iris, and the infant is unable to look upward with the head facing forward). Vomiting, a large and full anterior fontanelle, the "cracked-pot" sound when the skull is percussed, and separation of cranial sutures also occur.

2. **Chronic symptoms in children** include headache (local or generalized), vomiting in the absence of nausea, especially on rising in the morning, blurred vision and decreased acuity, altered mental status (e.g., confusion, memory loss, fatigue, irritability), papilledema, and gait disturbances.

3. With **acute changes,** age becomes less of a factor in differentiating clinical manifestations. Vital sign changes include a change in the respiratory pattern, progressing from irregular to absent respirations. The systolic pressure increases relative to diastolic pressure (widened pulse pressure), and the pulse decreases. The pupils are dilated and fixed because of cranial nerve III compression. The patient's level of consciousness progresses from restlessness to unresponsiveness. Motor function progresses from hemiparesis, hemiplegia, or decorticate posturing to flaccid paralysis or decerebrate posturing.

F. **NEURODIAGNOSTIC STUDIES**

Selection of specific studies depends on the cause of the increased ICP. CT scan and MRI are used to identify structural causes of increased ICP.

G. **MEDICAL MANAGEMENT**

The cause of increased ICP is identified and corrected (e.g., insert a shunting device for hydrocephalus, excise tumors, and remove extradural hematomas). An ICP catheter is inserted for monitoring ICP, and a ventriculostomy is established for CSF drainage and ICP monitoring. Medications to reduce cerebral swelling (e.g., diuretics and hyperosmolar agents) are administered. Decompressive craniectomy (removal of part of the skull) is used to treat patients with uncontrolled ICP following head trauma (Yamakami and Yamaura, 1993).

H. MULTIDISCIPLINARY MANAGEMENT
  ❖ ALTERATION IN CEREBRAL TISSUE PERFUSION RELATED TO INCREASED ICP
    1. **Expected outcomes**
       a. Maintains a normal ICP range
       b. Maintains a normal MAP for age
    2. **Nursing assessment:** Perform baseline and serial neurologic assessments. Monitor serum medication levels, urine and serum osmolality, electrolytes, arterial blood gases, end-tidal CO_2, and arterial saturation.
    3. **Collaborative interventions to reduce cerebral blood and CSF volumes**
       a. Provide hyperventilation by maintaining the $PaCO_2$ between 28 and 35 torr (individualize). Low $PaCO_2$ causes pH to increase (decreased H^+ concentration) and decreases cerebral tissue acidosis. Precapillary arterioles constrict in response to decreased H^+ concentration. CBF, cerebral blood volume, and ICP decrease. Monitor and trend $PaCO_2$ with end-tidal CO_2 ($ETCO_2$) monitoring. Monitor CPP to prevent ischemia.
       b. Maintain neuromuscular blockade that allows for controlled ventilation to manipulate $PaCO_2$ and prevent increases in the arterial pressure associated with isometric muscle contraction (Mitchell, 1988).
       c. Maintain oxygenation and normal PaO_2. Hypoxemia (PaO_2 below 50 mm Hg) produces vasodilation and an increase in cerebral blood volume. Individualize the endotracheal tube suctioning procedure based on the patient's response. Lidocaine may be given prior to suctioning to blunt increases in ICP during suctioning. Perform serial respiratory assessments and continuously monitor arterial oxygen saturation.
       d. Promote cerebral venous drainage. Elevate the head of the bed 15 to 30 degrees to promote displacement of venous blood volume to extracranial vessels. Prevent increased intraabdominal pressure by using stool softeners, decompressing the stomach, and minimizing gastric residuals. Prevent increased intrathoracic pressure by individualizing the use of positive end-expiratory pressure (PEEP) and avoiding chest physiotherapy during periods of poor cerebral compliance. Maintain body alignment (e.g., flexion of the hips, flexion of the neck) to prevent cerebral venous drainage obstruction.
       e. Minimize environmental stimuli by minimizing noxious procedures, individualizing nursing activities to control ICP, and maintaining effective pain control.
       f. Control cerebral metabolism. An increase causes increased CBF and cerebral blood volume. Treat hyperthermia. Control seizures quickly with anticonvulsants. Barbiturate coma is generally used when all other conventional therapies have been exhausted. An induced barbiturate coma reduces cerebral metabolism and, therefore, decreases CBF and cerebral blood volume. It is associated with significant negative cardiac effects (e.g., decreased contractility, dysrhythmias, vasodilation, and hypotension). Inotropic agents are used concomitantly or are on standby.
       g. Administer hyperosmolar therapy. Mannitol (Osmitrol) is a widely used agent that produces an osmotic gradient between the intravascular and extravascular compartments. The net effect is movement of water from the interstitium into the cerebral vasculature, where it can be removed via the kidneys. A secondary effect of mannitol is a compensatory vasoconstriction due to decreased blood viscosity (with intact autoregulation) (Muizelaar

et al, 1983). Dosing guidelines for mannitol vary, but smaller doses (0.25 mg/kg) given intermittently are as effective as traditional larger doses and have fewer side effects (Dean and Moss, 1992; Dean et al, 1992). Serum osmolality is monitored and maintained in a high normal range (300 to 310 mOsm/L). Potential complications of mannitol when used in high doses and at frequent intervals (i.e., creating hyperosmolality) include acute renal failure, possible rebound intracranial swelling (when mannitol diffuses into the extravascular compartment and reverses the osmotic gradient), electrolyte imbalances from increased diuresis via the kidneys, and fluid shifts.

h. Administer diuretics that can be used alone, or more frequently, in combination with mannitol. The proposed effects are total body fluid reduction and decreased CSF production. Monitor fluid and electrolytes. Fluid restriction must be individualized, since hypovolemia must be avoided. Frequently monitor serum and urine electrolytes and osmolalities.

i. Administer corticosteroids when indicated. The benefit is unclear for cytotoxic and interstitial edema and use is largely empiric. They are effective in reducing vasogenic edema associated with brain tumors, intracerebral hematoma, and abscess. They stabilize endothelial cell function and permeability.

j. Promote CSF drainage by elevating the head of the bed to promote displacement of CSF to the spinal subarachnoid space. Maintain ventricular CSF drainage (see intraventricular devices). Decrease CSF production. Acetazolamide (Diamox) and furosemide (Lasix) have been shown to transiently decrease ICP by reducing CSF. Long-term success of these medications is unproven (Bruce, 1989; Fishman, 1995).

SEIZURES

A. DEFINITIONS
1. A seizure is an uncontrolled, time-limited alteration in behavior that results from abnormal electrical discharge from cortical neurons.
2. *Status epilepticus* is a prolonged seizure (usually defined as 30 minutes or longer) or multiple consecutive seizures without regaining consciousness.
3. *Epilepsy* is a term used to define seizures that are chronic (recurrent seizures).

B. INCIDENCE
Seizures are the most common neurologic disorder seen in children (Holmes, 1992; Pedley et al, 1995). The incidence is highest in the first year of life. New cases of epilepsy occur at a rate of 50 per 100,000 individuals per year. Seventy-five percent of patients who develop epilepsy do so before 20 years of age. Forty million people are affected worldwide. Males are affected more often than females.

C. ETIOLOGY
More than half of the cases are idiopathic (Hauser et al, 1993). Other cases are related to vascular disorders, congenital causes, trauma, neoplastic disease, degenerative disease, infection, and fever (in the young child). Risk factors include age (more common in the young and elderly), family history of previous seizure, neurologic disease, head trauma, and neurodevelopmental abnormalities.

D. CLASSIFICATION OF SEIZURES
Classification of seizures varies among experts, but the most widely used system is from The International Classification of Epileptic Seizures (Dreifuss, 1989). There are two broad categories of classification.
1. **Partial (focal, local) seizures** include simple partial seizures (consciousness not

impaired), complex partial seizures (impairment of consciousness), and partial seizures evolving secondarily to generalized seizures.

2. **Generalized seizures (convulsive or nonconvulsive)** include absence seizures, atypical absence seizures, myoclonic seizures, clonic seizures, tonic seizures, tonic-clonic seizures, and atonic seizures.

E. PATHOPHYSIOLOGY

1. In the absence of a compromised CNS, the brain is usually protected from a seizure by compensatory mechanisms. After approximately 20 to 30 minutes, severe alterations in brain function occur (Hale and Williams, 1989; Littrell and Cantwell, 1991). Seizures increase the metabolic demand and CBF requirements of the parts of the cortex with repeated neuronal discharges. Prolonged seizures cause an uncoupling of CBF and metabolic demand, resulting in regional hypoxia, which leads to cell death.

2. **Systemic effects** may also occur and are most often a result of hypoxia (Hale and Williams, 1989; Orlowski and Rothner, 1992). Cardiovascular effects include alterations in heart rate, cardiac arrest, cardiac failure, hypertension, hypotension, and shock. Respiratory effects include apnea, tachypnea, aspiration, respiratory acidosis, and airway obstruction. Renal effects include oliguria, uremia, and acute tubular necrosis. ANS effects include hyperpyrexia, diaphoresis, vomiting, and hypersecretion. Metabolic or biochemical effects include metabolic acidosis, hypoglycemia, hyperkalemia, and elevated creatine phosphokinase (CPK).

F. DEFINING CHARACTERISTICS

Defining characteristics vary with the type of seizure. The most common type of seizure requiring admission to the ICU is generalized tonic-clonic (GTC) status epilepticus (formerly known as a grand mal seizure).

1. A **prodromal period** may precede a GTC seizure. The prodrome may occur days to hours before the seizure. Symptoms include headache, irritability, loss of appetite, insomnia, and change in mood. The physiologic basis is unknown.

2. An **aura** may precede a GTC seizure by seconds. It represents an abnormal focal electrical discharge from the brain. Clinical manifestations of aura vary considerably among patients and may include focal motor symptoms such as finger movement and clonic movement of an extremity; focal sensory symptoms such as a "needles-and-pins" sensation or numbness; autonomic symptoms such as vomiting, pallor, flushing, sweating, dizziness, erection of body hairs, pupillary dilation, tachycardia, and incontinence; and psychic symptoms such as hallucinations and fear.

3. **Motor symptoms** of a GTC seizure are easily recognized. The tonic phase is characterized by rigid extension of the arms and legs. The clonic phase follows and is characterized by relaxation of the muscles alternating with contractions (rhythmic jerks). Following the clonic phase the bladder sphincter relaxes, and urinary incontinence may occur.

4. The **postictal phase** is characterized by sleep with the extent and duration related to the duration of the GTC seizure (Holmes, 1992).

G. NEURODIAGNOSTIC FINDINGS

Specific studies to identify the underlying cause of the seizure vary depending on the suspected neuropathology (e.g., an MRI or CT scan for a structural lesion). EEG provides adjunctive data for diagnosing a seizure. Most GTC seizures produce abnormal EEG findings. Specific EEG findings vary depending on the type of seizure (Table 4–7).

H. MEDICAL MANAGEMENT

Control of seizures with anticonvulsants is the mainstay of therapy. Identify causes of the seizure and correct underlying pathology.

Table 4–7. CHARACTERISTIC EEG FEATURES IN THE VARIOUS SEIZURE TYPES

SEIZURE TYPE	INTERICTAL EEG ABNORMALITIES
Partial Seizures	
Simple partial	Variable, spikes over involved area of cortex may be normal
Complex partial	Variable, frontal or temporal lobe spikes
Generalized Seizures	
Absence	Generalized spike-wave, often activated by sleep, hyperventilation, or photic stimulation
Generalized tonic-clonic	Variable, frequently normal
Myoclonic	Usually abnormal, generalized spike-wave, multiple spikes
Tonic or atonic	Usually abnormal, generalized abnormalities, spikes, multiple spike-waves

From David RB, ed. *Pediatric Neurology for the Clinician.* Norwalk, Conn: Appleton & Lange; 1992.

I. **MULTIDISCIPLINARY MANAGEMENT FOR STATUS EPILEPTICUS**
   ❖ POTENTIAL FOR INJURY RELATED TO UNCONTROLLED MOVEMENTS OF SEIZURE ACTIVITY
   1. **Expected outcome:** The patient will be free of injury after a seizure.
   2. **Nursing assessment:** Assess the patient's airway for tongue biting. Describe characteristics of seizure activity. Assess the patient's environment for potential hazards.
   3. **Collaborative interventions:** For an unexpected seizure, immediately clear the environment of potentially hazardous materials. In anticipation of seizure activity, maintain seizure precautions (e.g., standby oxygen, padded side rails, suction equipment). The patient should not be restrained during seizures.
   ❖ INEFFECTIVE BREATHING PATTERN FROM SEIZURE OR ANTICONVULSANTS
   1. **Expected outcomes:** The patient will maintain a normal range of $PaCO_2$ and a $PaO_2 > 80$ mm Hg.
   2. **Nursing assessment:** Assess for a patent airway, ventilatory effort, and adequate oxygenation via skin color, arterial blood gases, and pulse oximetry.
   3. **Collaborative interventions:** Maintain an open and unobstructed airway using caution not to inflict oral trauma. Provide supplemental oxygen (FiO_2 1.0). Support ventilations as needed including bag-valve-mask ventilation or tracheal intubation for apnea or prolonged seizure.
   ❖ ALTERATION IN CEREBRAL TISSUE PERFUSION RELATED TO A CEREBRAL METABOLIC RATE IN EXCESS OF SUBSTRATE AND OXYGEN DELIVERY
   1. **Expected outcomes** include control of seizure activity, no significant complications from medication therapy, and resumption of premorbid mental functioning.
   2. **Nursing assessment:** Document seizure activity including information about the prodromal period, aura, duration of the seizure, characteristics of motor behaviors, and characteristics of the postictal phase. Assess mental status following the seizure.
   3. **Collaborative interventions**
      a. Control seizure activity. Secure venous access and administer 25% dextrose (2 to 4 ml/kg) if hypoglycemia is suspected or confirmed by rapid test. Administer anticonvulsants (Table 4–8). Three classifications of anticonvulsants are typically used to control seizures. Benzodiazepines act rapidly and are used as a first-line medication. Lorazepam (Ativan) is frequently used in children because major side effects are infrequent. Phenytoin (Dilantin) is

longer acting and used to maintain seizure control. It is cardiotoxic and must be given slowly (0.5 to 1 mg/min in the child; Hale and Williams, 1989). It is not sedating and is useful for patients with an altered mental status. Phenobarbital is longer acting and used to maintain seizure control.

b. If seizures persist despite conventional anticonvulsant therapy, additional interventions may be required including an increased dosage and frequency of the above medications. Barbiturate coma provides chemically induced ECS. When maintained for approximately 48 to 72 hours, it has been successful in arresting seizure activity following discontinuation of the barbiturate (Orlowski and Rothner, 1992). General anesthesia with inhalation gas (e.g., halothane or isoflurane) is also used to achieve ECS and arrest seizure activity. General anesthesia is not used as often as IV anesthesia (i.e., barbiturates) because it requires gas-scavenging equipment and operating room facilities. Guidelines do not exist regarding depth and duration of inhalation anesthetics. Paraldehyde has been successful in arresting seizure activity; however, the IV form is no longer available and rectal administration is unreliable. The rectal solution can be sterilized and made into a 4% solution for IV use; 0.15 ml/kg is administered over 1 hour. If seizure activity is arrested before the hour is complete, the infusion may be reduced to a level that maintains a seizure-free state (Orlowski and Rothner, 1992).

c. Monitor electrolytes, calcium, glucose, toxic screen, and blood urea nitrogen (BUN). Obtain appropriate neurodiagnostic studies to determine the underlying cause of the seizure.

d. Discuss with the patient and family potential long-term effects of anticonvulsive therapy. Phenytoin (Dilantin) can cause gingival hyperplasia, lymphadenopathy, hirsutism, acromegaloid facies, ataxia, nystagmus, rickets, and folate deficiency. Phenobarbital can cause hyperkinesis, drowsiness, and rash. Carbamazepine (Tegretol) can cause drowsiness and abdominal distress. Valproic acid (Depakene) can cause drowsiness, alopecia, and abdominal discomfort.

Table 4–8. INITIAL ANTICONVULSANTS TO CONTROL STATUS EPILEPTICUS

Drug	Dose	Rate of Administration	Time to Effect	Side Effects
Rapid-Acting Agents				
Diazepam (undiluted)	Begin 0.25 mg/kg IV and titrate to effect	<1 mg/min	1–2 min	Respiratory depression; thrombophlebitis
Lorazepam 2 mg/ml	0.1 mg/kg × 4, 20 min apart, max 4 mg	1 mg/min	2–3 min	Drowsiness, confusion, ataxia
Midazolam	0.075 mg/kg IV			Same as above; respiratory depression
Longer-Acting Agents				
Phenytoin 50 mg/ml; dilute in normal saline 1:10	15 mg/kg, up to 45 mg/kg	20–50 mg/min	~20 min	Heart block; hypotension
Phenobarbital 130 mg/ml	10 mg/kg, up to 30 mg/kg	30 mg/min	10–12 min	Respiratory depression

From Blumer JL. *A Practical Guide to Pediatric Intensive Care.* St Louis, Mo: Mosby–Year Book; 1990.

INTRACRANIAL HEMORRHAGE

A. **ARTERIOVENOUS MALFORMATION (AVM)**

1. **Description:** AVM is an abnormal connection between arteries and veins without an interposed capillary bed. AVMs can occur in any part of the brain and can vary in size from a few millimeters to large formations. Characteristically, they are cone shaped and thin walled and may involve parenchymal or meningeal tissue.

2. **Incidence and etiology:** The exact incidence is unknown, but approximately 2000 new cases are identified annually (McNair, 1988). AVMs are occasionally familial. The majority of cases are parenchymal (85% to 90%). AVMs are present at birth, but the patient may not become symptomatic until 10 to 20 years of age. Eighty-five percent to 90% are supratentorial.

3. **Pathophysiology**

   a. AVMs occur early in fetal development from failure of the capillaries to develop. Supply of blood to adjacent brain tissue is diminished or absent (ischemia) because of the diversion of CBF through the AVM without the benefit of capillaries to allow diffusion of oxygen (i.e., there is a vascular "steal"). Without the inherent resistance to blood flow through a capillary bed, blood flow through the vascular malformation is increased. A pressure gradient develops, and the malformation continues to grow; collateral vessels develop, which add to the mass.

   b. Neurologic dysfunction can occur from compression of surrounding tissue, ischemia of surrounding tissue and gliosis, hemorrhage, and hydrocephalus from obstruction of CSF.

4. **Defining characteristics** (Garcia-Monaco et al, 1991; Johnson, 1994; McNair, 1988; Nevo et al, 1994; Wiggins et al, 1991)

   a. The most common presentation in children is from spontaneous hemorrhage. Increased ICP occurs from mass effect. Meningeal irritation occurs with subarachnoid hemorrhage. Rapid neurologic deterioration ensues with rupture and bleeding into the ventricles. Focal signs may be present and relate to the location of the hemorrhage.

   b. Seizures are the second most common presenting sign.

   c. Congestive heart failure may occur in neonates with a large AVM because of the increased cardiac output necessary to support the AVM blood flow (often seen in vein of Galen aneurysms).

   d. A cranial systolic bruit is heard over the carotid arteries, mastoid bone, or eyes.

   e. Headache occurs from displacement of pain-sensitive arteries and veins. Veins may be enlarged on the scalp or face.

5. **Neurodiagnostic studies**

   a. CT scan may be used as a screening procedure and identifies blood collection and ventricular size. A high-resolution scan may reveal an aneurysm.

   b. Cerebral arteriography is usually obtained if surgery is required. It identifies the size, shape, and location of the aneurysm and vessel anatomy.

   c. MRI may be used as a screening procedure and is superior to the CT scan. It identifies hemorrhage, ventricular size, and vasospasm.

6. **Medical management**

   a. Treatment varies and depends on size and location of the AVM, age of the patient, cerebral dominance, technical support, condition of the patient, and characteristics of feeder vessels.

   b. Surgical options include total surgical excision as the treatment of choice, but some formations are inoperable. Proton beam radiation is directed within the volume of the AVM with the use of stereotactic equipment (skeletal fixation holds the head in place while various x-ray views localize the AVM using three planes of space). The proton beam causes thickening of the vascular channels to reduce the risk of hemorrhage.

 c. Embolization of the AVM is performed by inserting a catheter into the cerebral circulation (e.g., carotid or vertebral arteries) and depositing a substance (e.g., Silastic sphere, Gelfoam, metallic pellet) to block blood vessels within the lesion. The use of transarterial embolization alone rarely obliterates an AVM in its entirety and is most often used as adjunctive therapy (i.e., staged embolizations can reduce the size of an AVM for surgical resection). Laser therapy uses a light beam to photocoagulate vessels of the AVM. Its advantages include the ability to coagulate small, fragile, vessels; provide hemostasis following surgical resection; and clearly define the AVM. However, this therapy is still limited to a few centers, and long-term outcome data are not available.

7. **Multidisciplinary management** (See Intraventricular and Periventricular Hemorrhage.)

B. ANEURYSM

1. **Description:** An aneurysm represents a weakening in the arterial wall. The size may vary from a few millimeters to 2 to 3 cm. Most aneurysms are located at bifurcations in or near the circle of Willis, in the vertebrobasilar arteries, or within the carotid system.

2. **Incidence** (Guertin, 1992; Stewart-Amidei and Hill, 1986): Presentation during childhood is rare. Aneurysms in childhood account for 1.3% of aneurysms for all ages. Aneurysms are usually diagnosed at the time of rupture. The male-to-female ratio is 2 : 1 during childhood. Like adults, 10% to 20% of children have multiple aneurysms.

3. **Etiology:** Aneurysms may be congenital (majority), traumatic, arteriosclerotic, or septic in origin. A high percentage of aneurysms are found in the posterior circulation, and 20% occur at the carotid bifurcation. They may be associated with unrepaired coarctation of the aorta and subacute bacterial endocarditis (SBE; Stewart-Amidei and Hill, 1986). Aneurysms in children are more distal in origin, are more likely giant or mycotic aneurysms, are less likely to be atherosclerotic, and are located more peripherally (e.g., distal branches of the middle cerebral artery) than in adults.

4. **Pathophysiology**

 a. Abnormalities exist in the arterial wall, especially in the elastica and media layers. There are four main types of aneurysms.

  • A *saccular (berry) aneurysm* is rare in childhood. The sac gradually grows over time, usually rupturing between the third to sixth decade of life.

  • A *fusiform (giant) aneurysm* results from diffuse atherosclerotic changes. It is commonly found in basilar arteries or terminal ends of internal carotids.

  • A *mycotic aneurysm* is relatively common in children compared to adults. It results from arteritis due to bacterial emboli.

  • A *traumatic aneurysm* is a weakening of the arterial wall that occurs from a bone fracture or penetrating missile. It is rare in childhood.

 b. An aneurysm is significant when it ruptures and hemorrhages. Patients usually have acute symptoms, with bleeding into the subarachnoid space. A rapid injection of blood into the brain may produce an acute increase in ICP with distortion and compression of tissue. Several complications may occur including vasospasm, rebleeding of the aneurysm, hydrocephalus from obstruction of the absorptive pathways, and hypothalamic disturbances from the proximity of the hemorrhage to the hypothalamus. A clot forms following rupture of an aneurysm. Seven to ten days later the clot dissolves, and the patient is at risk for rebleeding.

5. **Defining characteristics:** Frequently, children are asymptomatic for many years. Nonspecific findings include nausea, back pain, lethargy, and photophobia. Localized periorbital pain and diplopia or ptosis may indicate third cranial nerve compression. A giant aneurysm may present as a mass effect (increased ICP). Symptoms related to hemorrhage (see above), severe headache and seizures may occur.

6. **Neurodiagnostic studies** are the same as for AVM.

7. **Medical management**
   a. The goal of treatment following rupture of an intracranial aneurysm is to prevent rebleeding of the aneurysm and control cerebral vasospasm. Controversy exists as to when an operation is of benefit. Early surgery (i.e., within the first hours or days) carries a high risk because of the critical condition of the patient, and cerebral vasospasm, which may occur between 4 and 12 days after the hemorrhage, may complicate the patient's response to surgery. Postponing surgery until the patient is more stable (e.g., CPP > 60 mm Hg, MAP > 70 mm Hg, ICP < 20 mm Hg, neurologic status unchanged or improved from baseline) and cerebral vasospasm has been relieved carries a risk of a second bleed (the first 48 hours are associated with the highest incidence of rebleeding).
   b. Surgical options include occluding the aneurysm at its neck with clips (most common), occluding the parent vessel on either side of the aneurysm (dependent on collateral circulation), coating the aneurysm with a material after wrapping it in muslin, or embolization of the aneurysm.

8. **Multidisciplinary management** (See Periventricular and Intraventricular Hemorrhage.)

C. **PERIVENTRICULAR AND INTRAVENTRICULAR HEMORRHAGE (PIVH)**
   1. **Description:** PIVH involves bleeding into the subependymal germinal matrix at the level of the foramen of Monro (periventricular) and bleeding into the lateral ventricles spreading throughout the ventricular system (intraventricular).
   2. **Incidence** (Chen et al, 1993; Rozmus, 1992): Thirteen percent of neonates weighing less than 1500 g have PIVH. The incidence increases as the weight and age of the neonate decreases. Ninety percent of PIVH occurs within the first 72 hours of life.
   3. **Etiology** (Ferrari et al, 1992; Gibbs and Weindling, 1994)
      a. Presence of subependymal germinal matrix (periventricular region) is characteristic of prematurity. The matrix is a highly vascular, gelatinous area with vessels that lack supporting structure. Glial and neuronal precursor cells are perfused by numerous fragile capillaries. Neonates have an immature vascular autoregulatory system with increased fibrinolytic activity. Before 32 weeks' gestation, there is increased CBF to this area; after 32 weeks' gestation there is a shift of blood flow to the cerebral cortex and subcortical areas.
      b. Other risk factors include hypoxia, placental abruption, infections that alter the CBF in the periventricular region, respiratory complications such as pneumothorax (or any condition that increases venous pressure and impedes cerebral venous return), and rapid infusion of hyperosmolar infusions.

4. **Pathophysiology**
   a. Bleeding into and around the intracranial ventricles is believed to be related to several developmental factors (Rozmus, 1992): The subependymal germinal matrix is highly vascular and the vessels are thin walled, fragile, and lack supporting structures. Conditions that alter CBF can cause rupture of vessels and bleeding.
   b. Classification of bleeding is used to assess the location and amount of bleeding present:
      • Grade I: Subependymal hemorrhage only
      • Grade II: Intraventricular hemorrhage without ventricular dilation
      • Grade III: Intraventricular hemorrhage with ventricular dilation
      • Grade IV: Intraventricular and parenchymal hemorrhage
   c. Blood clots within the ventricular system may obstruct the flow and absorption of CSF, resulting in progressive hydrocephalus.
5. **Defining characteristics:** Three basic clinical syndromes may be seen (Rozmus, 1992).
   a. A saltatory syndrome is a subtle deterioration that progresses over hours to days. Clinical features include depressed level of consciousness, hypotonia, irritability, drop in hematocrit, abnormal eye movements and position, and alteration in spontaneous movements.
   b. A silent syndrome is clinically undetected and usually diagnosed on routine ultrasound examinations of the head.
   c. A catastrophic syndrome is a rapid deterioration progressing in minutes to hours. Clinical features include coma, apnea, generalized seizures, abnormal posturing, unreactive pupils, drop in hematocrit, and alteration in vital signs (e.g., hypotension, bradycardia) and endocrine function.
6. **Neurodiagnostic**
   a. Real-time cranial sonography is the study of choice. It identifies the degree and location of the hemorrhage. Advantages include its portability, low cost, and noninvasive nature.
   b. CT scan and MRI identify structures as listed above. Disadvantages include transporting the patient to another location, maintaining patient stability during the procedure, and the difficulty of doing serial examinations.
7. **Medical management:** No specific surgical treatment is required for nonprogressive hydrocephalus. Progressive hydrocephalus may require serial lumbar punctures to remove CSF and external ventricular drainage of CSF.
8. **Multidisciplinary Management for Intracranial Hemorrhages**
❖ POTENTIAL FOR ALTERATION IN CEREBRAL TISSUE PERFUSION RELATED TO HEMORRHAGE, INCREASED ICP, VASOSPASM, REBLEEDING, OR HYDROCEPHALUS
   a. *Expected outcomes* include no hemorrhage, rebleeding, or vasospasm, premorbid baseline neurologic status, and no postoperative complications.
   b. *Nursing assessment:* The frequency of serial neurologic assessments is individualized to the patient; however, a general guideline is every 15 minutes if the patient's condition is deteriorating. Once the patient's condition is stable, assessments can be performed every hour. Monitor ICP, analyze waveforms, and calculate CPP at frequent intervals. Monitor cardiovascular status and assess for congestive heart failure. Postoperative monitoring includes temperature, WBC count, ICP monitoring, and wound condition.
   c. **Collaborative interventions**
      • Minimize hemorrhage or rebleeding by maintaining a quiet, dark (if appropriate for the child) environment and enforcing strict bed rest. Administer analgesics for headache. Administer stool softeners and

order soft diet to prevent straining with defecation. Administer sedatives for anxiety and analgesics for pain. Administer anticonvulsants for seizure control.

- Control vasospasm (Armstrong, 1994; Guertin, 1992). Hyperperfusion consists of volume expansion with crystalloids or colloids to increase CPP, and therefore, CBF. Induced arterial hypertension consists of increasing the MAP to a level 20 to 100 mm Hg higher than the pretreatment MAP. Dopamine and dobutamine are usually selected because of the ease of titration. The induced arterial hypertension improves CPP and CBF. Calcium channel blockers are used to inhibit contraction of vascular smooth muscle by blocking the influx of calcium into smooth muscle. The desired effect is reduced vasoconstriction and improved CBF. Nimodipine (Nimotop) is the preferred calcium antagonist because of its affinity for cerebral vessels.
- Provide postoperative craniotomy care (see Space-Occupying Lesions [Tumors] discussion).

❖ POTENTIAL FOR DECREASED CARDIAC OUTPUT AND TISSUE PERFUSION RELATED TO HIGH FLOW AVM (see Congestive Heart Failure in Chapter 3)

❖ POTENTIAL FOR INJURY RELATED TO SEIZURES (see Seizures discussion)

CNS INFECTIONS

A. **DESCRIPTION**
  1. **Meningitis** is an inflammation of the meninges identified by an abnormal number of WBCs in the CSF (Klein et al, 1986). Bacterial (purulent) meningitis is diagnosed with evidence of a bacterial pathogen in the CSF. Viral (aseptic) meningitis is defined as meningitis without evidence of bacterial pathogen in the CSF (by usual laboratory testing).
  2. **Encephalitis** is defined as an acute inflammation of the brain and occasionally the meninges.

B. **INCIDENCE**
  1. Bacterial meningitis (Bijlmer and van Alphen, 1992; Dagan, 1994; Feigin et al, 1992; Fortnum and Davis, 1993) is age specific with the highest incidence in children younger than 1 year of age. Males predominate. Viral meningitis (Beghi et al, 1984; McIntyre and Keen, 1993) is less common than bacterial meningitis. The highest incidence is in infants younger than 1 year. The majority of cases occur in younger children, and males predominate.
  2. Encephalitis (Beghi et al, 1984) occurs most often in children younger than 10 years of age. The incidence decreases after age 10 years and is constant until age 40 years when it decreases further. It is more common in children who are immunosuppressed.

C. **ETIOLOGY**
  1. **Bacterial meningitis** (Feigin et al, 1992; Shattuck and Chonmaitree, 1992) pathogens are age specific. The most common organisms in newborns are group B streptococci, *Listeria monocytogenes, Haemophilus influenzae,* and enterovirus. In children age 2 months to 12 years, *H. influenzae, Neisseria meningitidis,* and *Streptococcus pneumoniae* predominate. In children older than 12 years, *N. meningitidis* and *S. pneumoniae* are the most frequent. There has been a rapid decline in the incidence of *H. influenzae* following widespread use of *H. influenzae* type b (Hib) conjugate vaccines (Adams et al, 1993; Michaels and Ali, 1993). The most common pathogens for **viral meningitis** are enteroviruses, mumps, herpes simplex (type 1), adenoviruses, and California virus.

2. **Encephalitis** pathogens include arthropod-borne viruses and herpes simplex (type 1). It may also occur from systemic viral infections or following vaccination from a live attenuated virus vaccine.

D. PATHOPHYSIOLOGY

1. **Bacterial meningitis** (Ashwal et al, 1992; Quagliarello and Scheld, 1992) pathogens usually arise from a distant site and colonize. They enter the blood stream, producing septicemia, and then invade the meninges. Less frequently, pathogens infect the meninges via a direct route (e.g., depressed skull fracture, penetrating missile). Pathogens proliferate and spread into CSF and then invade parenchyma and blood vessel walls, producing vasculitis or cerebral edema. Purulent exudate may obstruct CSF pathways, producing hydrocephalus. Cell necrosis may also occur. **Viral meningitis** pathogenesis remains unclear. It is believed that the port of entry is the nasal pharynx, where the viral pathogen colonizes and spreads to the CNS via the blood stream. The clinical course is usually self-limiting with improvement seen in 7 to 14 days.

2. **Encephalitis** viral invasion begins in extraneural tissue (e.g., mastoid) and travels to the CNS via the blood stream. Once in the CNS, pathogens may enter the CSF circulation through the choroid plexus or through passive transfer through the blood-brain barrier. Less frequently, pathogens may enter the CNS along peripheral nerves or via the olfactory system (Weil, 1990). Widespread nerve cell degeneration may occur, as well as cerebral edema, cell necrosis, and increased ICP.

E. DEFINING CHARACTERISTICS

1. **Bacterial meningitis** (Akpede, Abiodun, Ambe, and Jacob, 1994; Chotpitaya-sunondh, 1994; Walsh-Kelly et al, 1992) is characterized by nuchal rigidity (stiff neck), Brudzinski's sign (flexion of the hips and knees with passive flexion of the neck), Kernig's sign (back pain and resistance after passive extension of the lower legs), photophobia (abnormal intolerance of light), fever, vomiting, lethargy, headache, and alteration in consciousness. Petechial rash may occur with *N. meningitidis*. Late stages may produce increased ICP and cardiovascular collapse. Symptoms in infants are less specific and include vomiting, lethargy, bulging fontanelle, hypothermia or hyperthermia, diarrhea, and poor feeding. **Viral meningitis** presentation is similar to clinical symptoms seen in bacterial meningitis but usually milder. Most infants younger than 12 months have minimal symptoms (Walsh-Kelly et al, 1992).

2. **Encephalitis'** course of illness varies considerably (mild to elevated ICP and death) and depends somewhat on the infectious agent and the specific CNS structures involved. Clinical manifestations include prodromal symptoms of fever, malaise, myalgia, upper respiratory symptoms, nausea, vomiting, and stiff neck. CNS invasion is indicated by lethargy, drowsiness, stupor that may progress to coma, seizures, and localized symptoms. Severe cases may have signs and symptoms of increased ICP. Meningeal signs may be present and depend on the degree of meningeal involvement (vs. cerebral involvement).

F. NEURODIAGNOSTIC STUDIES

1. **CSF analysis** (Fishman, 1992; Pohl, 1993) is the gold standard for diagnosing bacterial meningitis. Obstructive hydrocephalus must be ruled out before lumbar puncture can be performed.

a. *CSF analysis in bacterial meningitis* demonstrates the following:
   - Elevated WBC count; polymorphonuclear cells predominate
   - Elevated protein content (normal 10 to 30 mg/dl)
   - Decreased glucose content (normal 40 to 80 mg/dl)
   - Positive results from Gram stain
   - Positive results from culture for organism

- Color: Turbid or cloudy
- Results are variable in the neonate (Klein et al, 1986), since the WBC count may be normal, glucose content may be normal (it should be compared to serum), and protein levels are normally higher in neonates (20 to 170 mg/dl).

b. *CSF results in viral meningitis* demonstrate the following:
   - Slightly elevated WBC count; lymphocytes predominate
   - Normal or slightly increased protein content
   - Normal glucose content
   - Negative results from Gram stain or culture for bacteria

c. *CSF results in encephalitis* are variable but may be similar to viral meningitis. Viral antibodies may be found. Large amounts of RBCs may be seen with herpes simplex.

2. **CT scan and MRI** (Heyderman et al, 1992) may demonstrate abnormal findings in children with meningitis but do not predict outcome or the degree of brain swelling. They are not routinely performed unless specific information is being sought (e.g., progressive neurologic focal signs, presence of obstruction of CSF before lumbar puncture).

3. **EEG** is used as adjunctive study in all CNS infections. Abnormal background EEGs are predictive of outcome in neonates with bacterial meningitis. Chequer et al (1992) found infants who had normal or mildly abnormal EEG backgrounds had normal outcomes, and infants with markedly abnormal EEG backgrounds had abnormal outcomes (e.g., death or neurologic sequelae). The abnormal EEG backgrounds are generally nonspecific. The EEG is also helpful in identifying focal abnormalities.

4. **Brain biopsy** is the definitive diagnostic study for encephalitis but is rarely performed because the procedure poses risks to the patient and treatment would remain the same (i.e., supportive).

G. **MEDICAL MANAGEMENT**

Antimicrobial therapy is the mainstay of bacterial meningitis treatment. Chemoprophylaxis is given to close contacts (e.g., family members, day care contacts, and primary caregivers in the hospital) of patients with *H. influenzae* and *N. meningitidis* (Feigin et al, 1992). Supportive care is all that is usually available for encephalitis and viral meningitis. ICP monitoring is not routinely used for CNS infections.

H. **MULTIDISCIPLINARY MANAGEMENT**

❖ DECREASED CEREBRAL TISSUE PERFUSION RELATED TO INCREASED ICP

1. **Expected outcomes** include a normal ICP, premorbid neurologic status, no complications, and normal CSF analysis.

2. **Nursing assessment:** Provide serial neurologic assessment including head circumference in infants; assess for increased ICP; and monitor fluid and electrolyte status.

3. **Collaborative interventions**
   a. Use above interventions to control increased ICP.
   b. Administer antimicrobial therapy for bacterial meningitis. Broad-spectrum antibiotics are used until the pathogen is isolated. Chloramphenicol (Chloromycetin) and ampicillin have been used widely for broad-spectrum coverage; however, some third-generation cephalosporins are effective for resistant organisms (Akpede, Abiodun, Sykes, and Salami, 1994). Administer antimicrobials immediately following culture collections. Appropriate antimicrobial therapy continues for 10 to 14 days. Administration of dexamethasone (Decadron) is recommended in patients with *H. influenzae* to prevent hearing deficits (American Academy of Pediatrics, 1990). Current dosing guidelines are 0.6 mg/kg/d in four divided doses given

intravenously for the first 4 days of antimicrobial therapy. Dexamethasone should be administered at the time of the first antimicrobial dose. It is not used for aseptic meningitis.

   c. Respiratory isolation may be used for 24 hours for patients with bacterial meningitis caused by or suspected to be caused by *H. influenzae* or *N. meningitidis.* Maintain enteric precautions for aseptic meningitis for 7 days from the onset of disease.

   d. Administer acyclovir (Zovirax) 30 mg/kg/d divided every 8 hours for 10 days or longer for herpes simplex encephalitis.

❖ POTENTIAL FOR INEFFECTIVE BREATHING PATTERN RELATED TO INCREASED ICP

  1. **Expected outcomes** include normal arterial blood gases, oxygen saturation >95%, normal respiratory effort and rate, and no supplemental oxygen requirement.

  2. **Nursing assessment:** Monitor respiratory rate, work of breathing, arterial blood gases, and SaO_2.

  3. **Collaborative interventions:** Administer oxygen as needed; support and maintain ventilations as needed (intubation and mechanical ventilation); perform pulmonary toilet for airway secretions; and perform chest physiotherapy as needed (in absence of increased ICP).

❖ POTENTIAL FOR INJURY RELATED TO SEIZURES (see Seizures discussion)

❖ ALTERATION IN COMFORT RELATED TO MENINGEAL IRRITATION, HEADACHE, PHOTO-PHOBIA, FEVER

  1. **Expected outcomes** include no complaints of headache, meningeal signs, or fever and normal light tolerance.

  2. **Nursing assessment:** Monitor pain using pain scales, assess for meningeal signs (e.g., stiff neck, Brudzinski's sign, Kernig's sign), monitor temperature, and assess effectiveness of comfort measures.

  3. **Collaborative interventions**

   a. Maintain body temperature in the normal range using antipyretics and sponging with tepid water.

   b. Maintain a quiet environment by dimming lights and controlling noise.

   c. Alleviate nausea and vomiting by administering oral care and antiemetics.

   d. Eradicate infection (see above).

   e. Control increased ICP (see above).

   f. Administer analgesics for complaints of headache, arthralgia, and neck pain.

❖ POTENTIAL FOR ALTERATION IN FLUID AND ELECTROLYTES RELATED TO SYNDROME OF INAPPROPRIATE ANTIDIURETIC HORMONE (SIADH), DIABETES INSIPIDUS, DIURETICS, FLUID RESTRICTIONS

  1. **Expected outcomes** include normal serum and urine electrolytes and osmolalities, normal range of urine specific gravity, and central venous pressure (CVP) and vital signs within normal limits.

  2. **Nursing assessment:** Monitor urine output, hemodynamic parameters, and serum and urine electrolytes and osmolality.

  3. **Collaborative interventions** (see Chapter 6)

SPACE-OCCUPYING LESIONS (TUMORS)

A. DESCRIPTION

  1. Tumors are an abnormal proliferation of CNS cells producing a space-occupying lesion and increased ICP. Because neurons do not have the capability to reproduce (significantly), most CNS tumors arise from glial cells.

2. Lesions are classified according to histology and location (Lacayo and Farmer, 1991):

a. **Infratentorial** (below the tentorium) tumors include *brain stem gliomas* (malignant), *cerebellar astrocytoma* (malignant tumors that enlarge slowly and worsen over several months), *medulloblastomas* (malignant tumors that enlarge quickly, have symptoms detected within 3 months from onset, and are found almost exclusively in children), and *ependymomas* (benign tumors derived from ependymal cells arising from any part of the ventricular system and frequently located in the fourth ventricle in young children and the lateral ventricles in older children and adolescents).

b. **Supratentorial** (above the tentorium) include *hemispheric tumors* (usually malignant gliomas, low-grade tumors without distinct borders that infiltrate the parenchyma) and *midline tumors* including *optic chiasm tumors* (malignant), *craniopharyngiomas* (malignant), *pineal-region tumors* (usually malignant), and *germ cell tumors* (malignant).

B. INCIDENCE

Brain tumors are the second most common malignancy in children (Donahue, 1992; Duffner and Cohen, 1992; Fitz, 1993; Lacayo and Farmer, 1991). In the United States, 1200 to 1500 new cases of brain tumors are diagnosed annually (Kadato et al, 1989). The posterior fossa is the most frequent site of occurrence. Only 50% of children with any type of brain tumor may be expected to live 5 years. Astrocytomas and teratomas are the most common types of brain tumors seen in infants (Pezzotta et al, 1992).

C. ETIOLOGY

The causes are unknown. Risk factors include neurofibromatosis and von Hippel-Lindau disease (for hemangioblastomas). Past cranial irradiation increases the incidence of developing a secondary cancer; the amount of irradiation varies depending on the initial type of cancer and treatment. However, secondary brain tumors have been documented in children with acute lymphocytic leukemia who were given 18 to 24 Gy cranial irradiation for CNS prophylaxis (DeLaat and Lampkin, 1992).

D. PATHOPHYSIOLOGY

Physiologic changes are based on a space-occupying lesion and the effects of increased ICP. Expanding mass causes distortion and compression of intracranial structures, reduction in CBF, and obstruction of CSF circulation. Left untreated, ischemia and herniation syndromes may occur.

E. DEFINING CHARACTERISTICS

1. Symptoms vary tremendously in children and depend on location, rate of growth, and the age and developmental stage of the child (Barker, 1990).

2. **General symptoms** include increased ICP caused by obstruction of the CSF pathways (most common). Classic signs and symptoms of increased ICP in verbal children include headache (usually on awakening in the morning; diffuse, dull and steady in quality; and less prominent in supratentorial tumors) and nausea.

3. **Localized symptoms of infratentorial tumors:** *Cerebellar tumors* cause impaired coordination and balance, truncal ataxia (irregular muscular coordination of the upper body), and nystagmus. *Brain stem tumors* cause cranial nerve dysfunction, ataxia, and corticospinal tract dysfunction.

4. **Localized symptoms of supratentorial tumors**

a. Tumors located near the cortical surface cause seizures and focal cerebral dysfunction, which depends on the area affected but may include motor dysfunction, irritability, and speech dysfunction.

b. *Deep cerebral hemispheric tumors* cause hemiplegia and visual field defects.

   c. *Frontal lobe tumors* provoke behavioral changes, language dysfunction, motor weakness, and seizures with focal motor onset or tonic-clonic movements.

   d. *Occipital lobe tumors* cause visual field dysfunction (e.g., homonymous hemianopsia, which describes a defect in the right or left halves of the visual fields of the two eyes) and visual hallucinations.

   e. *Temporal lobe tumors* produce auditory and speech dysfunction such as receptive aphasia, olfactory dysfunction such as involuntary smacking or licking of the lips, and psychomotor seizures.

   f. *Sella turcica area tumors* produce eating dysfunction, metabolic dysfunction, and autonomic seizures.

   g. *Parietal lobe tumors* cause reading dysfunction and dysfunction in awareness of contralateral extremities.

5. Infants and toddlers (Albright, 1993) usually present with nonspecific symptoms (e.g., vomiting, lethargy, unsteadiness, and irritability). Weakness and seizures are less common.

F. NEURODIAGNOSTIC STUDIES

1. **CT scan** is performed with and without contrast in approximately 15 minutes. It is useful for urgent diagnostic studies (Albright, 1993).

2. **MRI** (Barkovich, 1992; Yue, 1993) is the preferred diagnostic study and is performed with and without contrast. It provides a better definition of tumor than a CT scan and identifies small tumors not seen on CT scan. MRI demonstrates the tumor in all planes and requires approximately 45 minutes to complete. The child may require sedation. It also avoids irradiation.

3. **Human chorionic gonadotropin (HCG) and alpha-fetoprotein (AFP)** may be elevated in a child with a pineal-region tumor. Elevated levels of HCG and AFP usually indicate nongerminomatous germ cell tumor.

4. **CSF polyamines** may be elevated in several types of brain tumors and hydrocephalus.

5. **Brain biopsy** is required to make a tissue diagnosis for specific treatment protocols and is usually done during surgical tumor debulking.

G. MEDICAL MANAGEMENT

1. The goal is to eradicate the tumor with minimal morbidity (Shiminski-Maher et al, 1991).

2. Therapy usually consists of three elements (Allen, 1992; Friedman and Oakes, 1992).

   a. *Surgery* is used to obtain tissue for histologic examination, reduce tumor size, and create VP shunts for patients with surgically uncorrectable hydrocephalus. Total resection is rarely possible, and postoperative edema may occur; however, debulking improves the effectiveness of radiation and chemotherapy.

   b. *Irradiation* is the frontline therapy for diffuse tumors. It is delayed as long as possible in infants and toddlers to avoid damage to normal developing brain tissue. Stereotactic techniques have improved effectiveness of irradiation and have limited damage to normal tissue (Baron, 1991). Stereotactic procedures consist of a basic frame that attaches to the patient's skull. Side arms (Y axis) and vertical (Z axis) and horizontal (X axis) bars and an arc are attached to the frame. With the use of a CT scan or MRI and the above coordinates, instruments are precisely directed to a specific area of the brain.

   c. Traditional *chemotherapy* (Gajjar et al, 1993; Kramer and Packer, 1992; Packer, 1994) has been limited in part because the blood-brain barrier limits many systemic drugs from entering the CNS. However, chemotherapy's effectiveness has increased over the last decade (Horowitz and Poplack,

1991; Mulligan and Wittman, 1990). It is most effective with treating astrocytomas, medulloblastomas, and chiasmal gliomas. Children younger than 2 years of age are treated with radical surgical resection and chemotherapy to delay irradiation for 1 to 2 years to allow brain tissue development. Lomustine (CCNU) and vincristine are the mainstays of chemotherapy (Albright, 1993; Barker, 1990; Mulligan and Wittman, 1990).

H. MULTIDISCIPLINARY MANAGEMENT OF POSTOPERATIVE CRANIOTOMY
   ❖ ALTERATION IN CEREBRAL TISSUE PERFUSION RELATED TO INCREASED ICP: POSTOPERATIVE CEREBRAL SWELLING, INTRACRANIAL BLEEDING
   1. **Expected outcomes** include normal ICP, premorbid or improved preoperative neurologic status, no intracranial bleeding, no complications, and CPP >50 mm Hg.
   2. **Nursing assessment:** Perform baseline neurologic assessment followed with serial assessments. Calculate the CPP if an ICP monitor is in place. Assess functioning of the ICP monitoring device. Cerebral swelling usually peaks on the third postoperative day. Monitor side effects of chemotherapeutic agents.
   3. **Collaborative interventions** (see Intracranial Hypertension)
   ❖ ALTERATION IN COMFORT RELATED TO INCISIONAL PAIN AND HEADACHE
   ❖ POTENTIAL FOR INJURY RELATED TO SEIZURES (see Seizures discussion)
   ❖ POTENTIAL FOR INFECTION RELATED TO PREOPERATIVE CORTICOSTEROIDS, IMMUNOSUPPRESSION, INVASIVE LINES, SURGICAL WOUND (see CNS Infections)
   ❖ ALTERATION IN FLUID VOLUME STATUS RELATED TO NAUSEA AND VOMITING, SIADH, AND DIABETES INSIPIDUS (see Chapter 6)
   ❖ INEFFECTIVE BREATHING PATTERN RELATED TO ANESTHESIA, INCREASED ICP, DEPRESSED LEVEL OF CONSCIOUSNESS

HYDROCEPHALUS

A. DESCRIPTION
   Hydrocephalus refers to a variety of conditions that result in an excess of CSF in the intracranial compartment.
   1. *Noncommunicating hydrocephalus* is an obstruction within the ventricular system.
   2. *Communicating hydrocephalus* is a blockage to CSF circulation outside of the ventricular system in subarachnoid cisterns or poor CSF absorption at the pacchionian granulations.
   3. *Normal-pressure hydrocephalus* (low-pressure, adult, or occult hydrocephalus) occurs usually in middle age from arachnoid adhesions or communicating hydrocephalus.
   4. *Hydrocephalus ex vacuo* is a ventricular enlargement from loss of brain parenchyma rather than an overproduction of CSF.

B. INCIDENCE
   Congenital hydrocephalus occurs in approximately 4 per 1000 live births. The exact incidence of acquired hydrocephalus is unknown but estimated at 1 per 1000 individuals (Andrews and Mooney, 1990).

C. ETIOLOGY
   Congenital hydrocephalus is present at birth and includes Arnold-Chiari type II deformity, aqueductal stenosis, and congenital arachnoid cysts. *Acquired hydrocephalus* results from obstructive lesions that may include neoplasms, hemorrhage, infection, or trauma.

D. PATHOPHYSIOLOGY
   The cause of hydrocephalus is most often obstruction of the flow of CSF somewhere along its pathway of circulation (usually congenital aqueductal stenosis). Less often

it is due to overproduction or reduced absorption of CSF. Untreated hydrocephalus with increased ICP causes dilation of the ventricles, atrophy of the cerebral cortex, and degeneration of the white matter tracts.

E. **DEFINING CHARACTERISTICS**
   1. Clinical presentation depends on how rapidly the ICP increases. Acute hydrocephalus with increased ICP may present with cerebral hypertension and rapid deterioration.
   2. Slowly progressing hydrocephalus may have more subtle signs. In the infant, these include poor feeding, increased head circumference, setting sun sign (sclera of the eyes are visible above the iris), Macewen's sign or "cracked-pot" sound when the skull is percussed, bulging fontanelles, prominent scalp veins, thin and shiny scalp skin, and high-pitched cry with increased ICP. Older children experience nausea and vomiting, headache, unsteady broad-based gait with history of falling, deterioration in school performance, urinary incontinence, papilledema, diplopia, seizures, and behavioral changes such as irritability, lethargy, and personality changes.

F. **NEURODIAGNOSTIC STUDIES**
   1. Presumptive diagnosis is based on clinical examination and presenting signs.
   2. **CT scan or MRI** demonstrates an enlarged ventricular system and the pathology causing hydrocephalus.
   3. **Ultrasound** is used with open fontanelles and demonstrates enlarged ventricles.
   4. **Skull radiograph** demonstrates separated sutures or widened sutures, a "beaten silver" appearance on x-ray film from thinning of the skull and widened or split sutures, and the size of the cranial vault.
   5. **CSF analysis** may demonstrate the presence of infection or inflammatory process.

G. **MEDICAL MANAGEMENT**
   The cause of obstruction must be corrected (e.g., excision of the tumor compressing the ventricle, antibiotics for inflammation from bacterial meningitis, or third ventriculostomy). Serial lumbar punctures or ventricular taps allow drainage of CSF and are indicated for temporary forms of obstructive hydrocephalus. Surgical insertion of a shunting device may be required. A VP shunt is most commonly used (Choux, 1994).

H. **MULTIDISCIPLINARY MANAGEMENT**
   ❖ DECREASED CEREBRAL TISSUE PERFUSION RELATED TO INCREASED ICP
   ❖ POTENTIAL FOR INFECTION RELATED TO INVASIVE SURGERY
   ❖ ALTERATION IN COMFORT RELATED TO SURGICAL INCISION PAIN, HEADACHE
   ❖ ALTERATION IN SKIN INTEGRITY RELATED TO SUBCUTANEOUS DEVICE WITH EXTERNAL PRESSURE, LARGE HEAD WITH MINIMAL MUSCULAR CONTROL

TRAUMATIC BRAIN INJURY (TBI)

A. **DESCRIPTION**
   A TBI is an insult to the brain caused by an external force and not of a degenerative or congenital nature. It produces a diminished or altered state of consciousness and results in impairment of cognitive abilities or physical functioning, which may be permanent or temporary (National Head Injury Foundation, 1986).

B. **INCIDENCE**
   Beyond the first year of life, multiple trauma is the leading cause of death and disability among children. Sixty to eighty percent of multiple trauma includes a head injury. Approximately 100,000 to 250,000 acute brain-injured children are admitted to hospitals annually. One million children annually are estimated to sustain some

type of head injury. Boys are victims almost twice as often as girls. Nationwide, 1300 individuals die annually from bicycle-related deaths, half of which involve children and adolescents (Altimier, 1992; Henry et al, 1992; Nelson, 1992; Weiss, 1994).

C. Etiology

Many causes are age-related (Coats and Allen, 1991; Graham et al, 1992; Henry et al, 1992; Nelson, 1992; Weiss, 1994). In all age groups, the most common cause of TBI is from a motor vehicle. Children younger than 2 years who have a TBI are usually occupants of motor vehicles, and they often are not restrained or are improperly restrained. Older children with a TBI are more frequently pedestrians or cyclists. Infants sustain TBIs in falls, walker-related injuries, and nonaccidental injuries. Older children and adolescents are injured in bicycle-related or motorcycle-related accidents, with firearms and assaults, and during recreational activities. Risk factors include young age, substance abuse, and lack of protective devices (e.g., helmets). (See discussion on Multiple Trauma in Chapter 9 for a detailed description of incidence, etiology, risk factors, and prevention.)

D. Pathophysiology

1. **Primary injuries** occur at the time or within seconds of traumatic impact.
   a. *Skull fractures* are usually linear in children and occur along a suture line or perpendicular to a suture line. Diastasis (separation of cranial sutures) may occur in infants and small children; the separation may progress to growing fractures (i.e., a gradual erosion and separation of the fracture line) when accompanied by dural tears. Depressed fractures may represent depressed bone fragments or indentation of pliable skull bone without loss of bone integrity ("ping pong" depression in an infant). *Basal fractures* are a break in the basilar portions of the frontal, ethmoid, sphenoid, temporal, or occipital bones.
   b. A *concussion* is a transient loss of awareness immediately following rapid deceleration of brain tissue. It usually involves no structural brain damage. Diagnosis is based on history. Infants do not always lose consciousness. Diffuse axonal injury and damage to neurons may occur from shearing.
2. **Secondary injuries** develop after the traumatic event and are a consequence of the primary injury (Lovasik and Kerr, 1993).
   a. *Cerebral lacerations* are tears in the brain tissue often associated with skull fractures. They are less common in children, since the smoother inner table of the skull offers less resistance between bone and brain tissue.
   b. *Cerebral contusions* are heterogeneous areas of hemorrhage and edema within the brain tissue. They begin as primary injuries, but swelling, hemorrhage, and subsequent increased ICP produce secondary injuries. These are less common in young children compared to adolescents and adults.
   c. *Extradural hematomas:* Subdural hematoma represents bleeding into the dural space, usually venous in origin from bilateral bridging of cerebral veins. They are more common than epidural hematomas in children. Epidural hematoma represents a collection of blood (usually arterial in origin) in the extradural space. The most common location is under the temporal bone from the middle meningeal artery. These are less common in children compared to adults.
   d. *Diffuse generalized cerebral swelling* (Aldrich et al, 1992) is produced by increased blood volume (hyperemia). The basic triggering mechanism is unknown. True cerebral edema (increased water content of brain tissue) may follow with severe injuries.

E. Defining Characteristics

1. Symptoms depend on the type and severity of the injury. Simple linear fractures usually are asymptomatic.

2. **Basilar fractures** present with specific symptoms.
   a. *Battle's sign* represents postauricular hematoma and swelling from damage to the sigmoid sinus temporal bone.
   b. *The raccoon or panda sign* represents a periorbital blood collection from an anterior skull base fracture (there is absence of a subconjunctival hemorrhage).
   c. *Rhinorrhea* represents CSF leakage into the middle ear cavity with drainage through the eustachian tube into the nose. *Anosmia* is the lack of smell from damage to the olfactory nerve. Both are usually related to middle fossa basilar fracture.
   d. *Hemotympanum* represents a blood collection behind the tympanic membrane from a temporal bone fracture. If the dura mater is torn at the same time, CSF may leak out of the ear canal *(otorrhea).*
   e. *Vertigo* may occur with damage to the inner ear.
   f. *Acute deterioration with associated hemorrhage and increased ICP* is most often seen with occipital transverse fractures because of the close proximity to the vital centers of the brain stem.
3. **Cerebral contusion** presentation depends on location of the injury. Most injuries occur on the cortical surface of the temporal and frontal lobes from acceleration-deceleration forces, placing the patient at risk for focal seizures. The size of the injury and the shift in brain structures also affect presentation. Large contusions can produce a significant mass effect with shifting of intracranial structures and increased ICP. Clinical signs of increased ICP and herniation may present. Symptoms also depend on the degree of associated swelling. Swelling occurs around the contusion 3 to 4 days following the injury. Significant swelling can also cause shifting of brain structures and increased ICP.
4. **Concussion** may result in loss of consciousness, retrograde amnesia, headaches, vomiting, fatigue, and posttraumatic seizures. Diaphoresis, pallor, and lethargy may occur in infants.
5. The symptoms of **epidural hematoma** vary. Infants may present with a bulging fontanelle, anemia with significant bleeding, and separation of cranial sutures. Older children demonstrate hemiparesis or hemiplegia and anisocoria. (Anisocoria is an inequality of the pupils usually greater than 1 mm difference; some individuals normally have unequal pupils, usually less than 1 mm difference.) All ages may have symptoms of increased ICP in severe epidural hematoma.
6. The clinical presentation of **subdural hematoma** is usually nonspecific and may include drowsiness, lethargy, and irritability. Retinal hemorrhages and seizures may occur especially in children younger than 3 years of age. Significant bleeding produces tense, bulging, and pulseless fontanelles. Retinal hemorrhages in a child younger than 3 years suggests intentional injury (Buys et al, 1992).
7. **Generalized cerebral swelling** presents with increased ICP.

F. NEURODIAGNOSTIC STUDIES
   1. **CT scan** remains the gold standard for acute evaluation (McMicken, 1986; Scynoll et al, 1993). Mass lesions are identified with and without shifts in brain structures. Bone windows identify basilar fractures. Epidural hematoma demonstrates a double-convex, hyperdense area. Subdural hematoma demonstrates a more diffuse blood collection crossing the suture lines. Cerebral swelling and edema results in changes in density.
   2. The disadvantages of **MRI** (see MRI under Neurodiagnostic Monitoring) limit its use as an initial screening study. It is superior to the CT scan in imaging nonhemorrhagic contusions and posterior fossa and small vas-

cular lesions (Marshall et al, 1990; Snow et al, 1986; Yokota et al, 1991)

3. The **skull radiograph's** routine role in evaluating acute TBI has been supplanted by the CT scan. However, skull radiographs are useful in identifying missile injuries and some depressed skull fractures.

4. **ICP monitoring** is usually recommended for patients with severe injury including those with a Glasgow Coma Score < 8, abnormal CT findings with potential for increased ICP, and comatose patients with or without an abnormal CT scan (O'Sullivan et al, 1994).

G. **MEDICAL MANAGEMENT**

1. Surgical management depends on the type of lesion. In general, children require surgery less often. Extradural hematomas are evacuated. Large intracerebral hemorrhages producing midline shifts are removed. Growing fractures are repaired with cranioplasty.

2. Medical management is supportive and directed toward preventing secondary injury including hypoxia and ischemia, increased ICP, and complications (e.g., seizures, obstructive hydrocephalus).

3. Many traditional therapies for managing increased ICP (e.g., hyperventilation, elevation of the head) require individualization of interventions (Lovasik and Kerr, 1993; Reynolds, 1992; Walleck, 1989).

H. **MULTIDISCIPLINARY MANAGEMENT** (Vernon-Levett, 1991; Walleck, 1989)

❖ ALTERATION IN CARDIOVASCULAR TISSUE PERFUSION RELATED TO CARDIOPULMONARY ARREST

1. **Expected outcomes** include heart rate and rhythm within normal limits; respiratory rate, pattern, and effort within normal limits; and no complications.

2. **Nursing assessment:** Provide baseline and serial cardiovascular, respiratory, and neurologic assessments.

3. **Collaborative interventions:** Maintain ventilation and oxygenation by controlling ventilation (e.g., intubation and manual ventilation) and administering supplemental oxygen. Support the cardiovascular system (e.g., cardiac compressions, inotropic agents, fluids).

❖ ALTERATION IN CEREBRAL TISSUE PERFUSION RELATED TO INCREASED ICP

❖ IMPAIRED GAS EXCHANGE RELATED TO INCREASED PULMONARY INTERSTITIAL WATER CONTENT (NEUROGENIC PULMONARY EDEMA)

1. **Expected outcomes** include normal arterial blood gases, spontaneous respirations, normal respiratory rate and effort, oxygen saturation >90%, and the absence of adventitious breath sounds.

2. **Nursing assessment:** Monitor heart rate and rhythm, respiratory rate and work of breathing, breath sounds, arterial blood gases and pulse oximetry, and intake and output.

3. **Collaborative interventions:** Administer oxygen to maintain SaO_2 >95%. Maintain good pulmonary toilet and PEEP when a patient is receiving manual ventilation. Administer fluids as ordered (may be restricted to approximately three fourths of maintenance) while maintaining adequate perfusion. Administer diuretics as ordered.

❖ POTENTIAL FOR FLUID VOLUME ALTERATIONS RELATED TO SIADH AND DIABETES INSIPIDUS (see Chapter 6)

ENCEPHALOPATHY

A. **DESCRIPTION**

Encephalopathy is a term used to describe any condition that produces a generalized disturbance in brain cellular metabolism resulting in an alteration of consciousness.

In children the list of potential causes is endless; causes may be chronic or acute, static or progressive, and inherited or acquired. The prototypic encephalopathies seen in critically ill children are Reye's syndrome and hypoxic-ischemic encephalopathy.

1. Reye's syndrome is an acute toxic-metabolic encephalopathy associated with hepatic dysfunction. Even though it is rarely seen currently, the principles of its clinical management are used widely.

2. Hypoxic-ischemic encephalopathy is a final common pathway for a number of pathologies that produce brain injury from two physiologic abnormalities. Damage to brain tissue from ischemia results from reduction in blood flow and damage to brain tissue from hypoxia (decreased oxygen) or anoxia (absence of oxygen).

B. **INCIDENCE**

The peak incidence of Reye's syndrome (DeVivo et al, 1976; Keating, 1987) occurred between 1970 and 1980 at 1 to 8 cases per 100,000 individuals. It rarely recurs in survivors. The exact incidence of hypoxic-ischemic encephalopathy is unknown, since the condition is a complication of a number of pathologies.

C. **ETIOLOGY**

The cause of Reye's syndrome (Tasker et al, 1992) is unknown. Possible "triggering" factors include antecedent viral infection (most often influenza B) and concurrent aspirin ingestion (Centers for Disease Control, 1984). Hypoxic-ischemic injury can occur from any disorder that compromises cardiopulmonary functioning (e.g., sudden infant death syndrome [SIDS], drowning and near-drowning, cardiopulmonary arrest, and prolonged seizures).

D. **PATHOPHYSIOLOGY**

1. Reye's syndrome produces acute vomiting and alteration in the level of consciousness during recovery from a viral illness. Microscopic liver changes include fatty infiltration (including other viscera) and swelling and disruption of mitochondria (Trauner, 1992). Hepatic dysfunction occurs, resulting in metabolic and enzymatic alterations such as increased liver enzymes, increased ammonia, coagulation disorders, and alteration in carbohydrate, amino acid, and lipid metabolism. No jaundice is present. Cerebral edema and increased ICP may occur. Multisystem organ failure may develop.

2. Hypoxic-ischemic encephalopathy (Joy, 1989; Rogers and Kirsch, 1989; Traystman et al, 1991) results in damage during the initial hypoxic-ischemic event or during the reperfusion phase. It results from the depletion of vital metabolic substrates and accumulation of toxic by-products. Cellular changes are multifaceted, complex, and interrelated. They include energy depletion and anaerobic metabolism; lactic acidosis contributes to cellular damage, ionic pump failure occurs, and lipid perioxidation develops with free fatty acid accumulation. Another cellular change is loss of ionic homeostasis (resulting in calcium related damage, excitatory amino acid production, and oxygen free radical production). Irreversible cellular damage occurs with cytotoxic edema formation; increased ICP occurs infrequently.

E. **DEFINING CHARACTERISTICS**

1. Reye's syndrome may progress in one of two ways. A mild, self-limiting course lasts several days, or a severe course demonstrates progressive deterioration with loss of neurologic function. The disease process is staged into four or five categories of symptomatology (Chesney, 1992; Owen and Levin, 1991).

   a. Stage I: Lethargic, frightened, confused, but follows commands

   b. Stage II: Stuporous, combative, agitated, and delirious

   c. Stage III: Unresponsive coma, decorticate posturing, and pupils dilated but react to light

      d. Stage IV: Loss of oculocephalic reflex, decerebrate posturing, and dilated pupils

      e. Stage V: Loss of brain stem reflexes (pupillary and oculovestibular), irregular breathing progressing to apnea, and flaccidity

    2. The defining characteristics of hypoxic-ischemic encephalopathy depend on the cause of the hypoxic-ischemic event. Mild cases may demonstrate no apparent neurologic signs. Severe injury may present signs such as coma, increased ICP, vegetative state, or death.

F. NEURODIAGNOSTIC STUDIES

    1. **Reye's syndrome**

      a. *Chemistries* reveal increased transaminases, usually 2 to 3 times normal (normal levels: aspartate aminotransferase [AST] 5 to 55 U/L; alanine aminotransferase [ALT] 5 to 50 U/L), increased prothrombin time (normally 11 to 15 s), increased serum ammonia (normally 29 to 70 µg/dl), hypoglycemia (normally 60 to 100 mg/dl), hyperuricemia (normally 1.7 to 6.6 mg/dl, 1 to 11 y), and hypophosphatemia (normally approximately 130 to 500 U/L, 1 to 11 y).

      b. Findings from *CSF analysis* are normal, except for possible elevated opening pressure.

      c. *EEG* characteristics depend on the stage of the disease process. The typical pattern is a progressive slowing of electrical activity (Owen and Levin, 1991).

      d. *CT scan* is used to rule out structural causes of coma. It may demonstrate cerebral edema.

      e. *Liver biopsy* is used to differentiate other forms of hepatic disease. It demonstrates mitochondrial swelling, membrane changes, and fatty infiltration of the liver.

      f. *ICP monitoring* is used to manage CPP.

    2. **Hypoxic-ischemic encephalopathy**

      a. *Chemistries* vary and depend on the extent of hypoxic-ischemic damage to other organs.

      b. *CSF analysis* reveals normal cell count and routine chemistries. Creatine kinase-BB assay is present (Goe and Massey, 1988).

      c. *EEG* findings depend on the extent of cortical damage (Wauquier et al, 1987). Slight to moderate insults demonstrate changes in peak frequency or asymmetric rhythms from homotopic regions in each hemisphere. Severe insults demonstrate progressive slowing of electrical activity.

      d. *CT scan* is the same as for Reye's syndrome.

      e. *ICP monitoring* is not routinely used for encephalopathy from asphyxial arrest. ICP control does not improve outcome (Kochanek et al, 1992).

G. MEDICAL MANAGEMENT

    1. Reye's syndrome has no specific therapy; supportive care is provided (Owen and Levin, 1991). Maintain fluid and electrolyte balance with supplemental glucose ($D_{10}W$ or $D_{15}W$) to maintain glucose at a high normal level, calcium supplements, and reduction of ammonia with neomycin (Mycifradin). Prevent bleeding by treating elevated prothrombin time and partial thromboplastin time with fresh frozen plasma (FFP), 10 ml/kg, prior to invasive procedures (e.g., liver biopsy, ICP catheter insertion) and vitamim K, 1 mg intravenously, every 2 to 3 days. Increased ICP is the primary cause of mortality; therefore, therapies are directed toward controlling ICP and maintaining CPP (see Intracranial Hypertension discussion).

    2. The mainstay of therapy for hypoxic-ischemic encephalopathy is to resume oxygenated blood flow as soon as possible to prevent secondary brain injury. Even though increased ICP is rare after global cerebral ischemia, ICP-directed

management continues to be used with some exceptions. Hyperventilation is used with caution to prevent further ischemia. Barbiturate coma has not been shown to be beneficial (Brain Resuscitation Clinical Trial I Study Group, 1986; Haun et al, 1992). Several cerebral resuscitation therapies have been proposed, but their efficacy remains to be validated in the clinical setting. Improvement of CBF through induced moderate arterial hypertension has been advocated in the past; however, data do not exist to demonstrate its efficacy (Kirsch et al, 1989; Safar, 1986). Decreased coagulation and viscosity of blood (Safar, 1988; Wauquier et al, 1987), administration of calcium antagonists (Steen et al, 1985), and administration of free radical scavengers (Imaizumi et al, 1990; Liu et al, 1989) have been studied as well.

H. MULTIDISCIPLINARY MANAGEMENT

 ❖ ALTERATION IN CARDIOVASCULAR TISSUE PERFUSION RELATED TO DIFFUSE MYOCARDIAL ISCHEMIA, FATTY INFILTRATION (SEE CHAPTER 3)

 ❖ ALTERATION IN CEREBRAL TISSUE PERFUSION RELATED TO INCREASED ICP, MICROCIRCULATORY CHANGES (SEE INTRACRANIAL HYPERTENSION DISCUSSION)

 ❖ ALTERATION IN FLUID AND ELECTROLYTE STATUS RELATED TO VOMITING AND HYPOGLYCEMIA (REYE'S SYNDROME), SIADH AND DIABETES INSIPIDUS

1. **Expected outcomes** include normal electrolytes, serum glucose, serum and urine osmolalities (or expected values if using hypertonic infusions), and urine output.
2. **Nursing assessment** includes monitoring intake and output, serum and urine chemistries and osmolalities, serum glucose, CVP, and urine specific gravity.
3. **Collaborative interventions:** Administer crystalloids to maintain normal hydration. Reduce fluids for SIADH. With central diabetes insipidus, provide fluid resuscitation for hypovolemia and administer desmopressin (DDAVP). Administer supplemental electrolytes to correct imbalances and glucose for hypoglycemia. Administer neomycin for severely elevated serum ammonia.

 ❖ POTENTIAL FOR INFECTION RELATED TO INVASIVE LINES

 ❖ POTENTIAL FOR INJURY RELATED TO SEIZURE ACTIVITY (SEE SEIZURE DISCUSSION)

SPINAL CORD INJURY (SCI)

A. DESCRIPTION

1. **Complete cord injury** is the complete loss of motor and sensory function due to interruption of nerve pathways below the level of the injury (Nolan, 1994). *Quadriplegia* is the complete loss of leg function and loss or limited use of arms from cervical injury. *Paraplegia* is the loss of leg function alone from high lumbar injury.
2. **Incomplete cord injury** causes some loss of motor and sensory function with some sparing of function below the level of the injury (Hughes, 1990).
    a. *Posterior cord syndrome* is caused by injury to the dorsal columns. There is loss of proprioception but preservation of other sensory and motor function.
    b. *Anterior cord syndrome* from injury to the anterior cord results in loss of motor function below the level of the injury. Sensory function is lost except for proprioception and vibration sense.
    c. *Central cord syndrome* is caused by injury or edema to the central spinal cord in the cervical area. Greater motor deficits occur in the upper extremities compared to the lower extremities. Sensory deficits are variable but are usually greater in the upper extremities. Bowel and bladder dysfunction is common.

d. *Partial spinal cord syndrome* (Brown-Séquard's syndrome) results from injury to one side of the spinal cord, resulting in loss of voluntary motor function on the same side as the injury. Loss of pain, temperature, and touch occurs on the contralateral side.

e. *Conus medullaris* is an injury to the sacral cord and lumbar nerve roots, resulting in an areflexic bladder, bowel, and lower limb.

B. INCIDENCE

1. Nationwide, 5000 to 10,000 SCI injuries occur annually. They are most common in men (80% of victims) 15 to 30 years of age and less common in children. One third die before reaching the hospital. The most frequent sites of injury are the lower cervical region (C-4 through C-7 and T-1) and the thoracolumbar region (T-12, L-1, and L-2) (Hughes, 1990; Nolan, 1994).

2. Cervical injury is rare in children; the upper cervical spine is more commonly injured in small children than in adolescents and adults (Mann and Dodds, 1993). Children have a higher incidence of spinal cord injury without radiographic abnormality (SCIWORA). This condition occurs predominantly in children and is thought to result from severe subluxation and trauma of the vertebral column (Lang and Bernardo, 1993; Mann and Dodds, 1993.) Pang and Wilberger (1982) theorized that SCIWORA is more common in young children because immature spines allow for reduction after momentary subluxation. As a result, the spinal cord is stretched or compressed with subsequent ischemia. Compression fractures are the most common spinal column injuries (Mann and Dodds, 1993).

C. ETIOLOGY

1. The most common cause of SCI is motor vehicle related (Acton et al, 1993; Dincer et al, 1993; Goebert et al, 1991; Mann and Dodds, 1993). Less common causes include bicycle accidents, sports (especially winter sports and diving) accidents, falls, and violence. "Seat belt"–type injuries (flexion-distraction) are almost exclusively seen in children younger than 13 years. Flexion-distraction injuries occur when children are restrained in an automobile with only a lap belt (Mann and Dodds, 1993). Intestinal and lumbar spine injuries occur (Newman et al, 1990) as a result of flexion of the upper body against a fixed lap belt with a high-impact motor vehicle accident.

2. Nontraumatic causes include tumor, disc herniation, infection, spinal stenosis, and congenital abnormalities.

D. PATHOPHYSIOLOGY

1. SCI most often occurs from vertebral injury, usually from acceleration-deceleration or deformation forces (Boss et al, 1990). Hyperextension causes fracture and dislocation of the posterior elements. Hyperflexion causes fracture or dislocation of the vertebral bodies, discs, or ligaments. Vertical compression causes shattering fractures. Rotational forces cause rupture of the supporting ligaments and fractures.

2. **Types of SCIs and consequences**

a. *Concussion of the cord* is caused by stretching and shearing of the spinal cord without tissue trauma. It causes a temporary disruption of cord-mediated functions.

b. *Contusion of the cord* is a bruising and swelling of the cord, causing a temporary or permanent loss of cord-mediated function.

c. *Laceration* is a tearing of neural tissue. The condition is reversible with minimal injury but may result in permanent dysfunction of cord-mediated functions.

d. *Transection of the cord* is severing of the cord, causing permanent loss of cord-mediated function.

      e. *Hemorrhage of the cord* is blood vessel damage with bleeding into neural tissue. There is no major loss of function, depending on the extent of injury.

      f. *Damage to the blood vessels* that supply the cord results in decreased perfusion of the spinal cord with local ischemia. Alteration in function depends on the severity of ischemia.

3. **Intracellular and extracellular changes from SCI** (Nolan, 1994) cause an increase in excitatory amino acids, increase in free oxygen radical formation, alteration in calcium homeostasis, and increase in platelet-activating factor (PAF). Cellular alterations produce edema, damage to cell membranes, ischemia, and cellular death at the level of injury and approximately two segments above and below it. Normal activity is lost at and below the level of the injury.

4. **High cervical injuries** may cause immediate death.

5. **Spinal shock** (complete loss of reflex function) may result from acute SCI. It can occur within 60 minutes of the injury and may last for 7 to 20 days. It results from loss of integrity of the ANS below the level of injury, producing venous pooling, bradycardia, and hypotension.

6. **Autonomic dysreflexia** is a life-threatening complication in SCI. It is rare during the acute phase, but it may occur any time after an SCI. Autonomic dysreflexia results from an uncontrolled, paroxysmal, continuous lower motor neuron reflex arc due to stimulation of the sympathetic nervous system. The response typically occurs from stimulation of sensory receptors (e.g., distended bladder or bowel) below the level of the cord injury. The ANS responds with arteriolar vasospasm resulting in increased blood pressure. Carotid sinus baroreceptors are stimulated and respond with activation of the vasomotor centers in the brain stem via the ninth and tenth cranial nerves. The parasympathetic nervous system (vagus nerve) sends a stimulus to the heart, causing bradycardia and vasodilation. The peripheral vessels and viscera do not respond because the efferent pulse cannot pass through the spinal cord. The vagus nerve is not "turned off," and profound bradycardia may occur (Nolan, 1994).

7. **Temperature regulation** is impaired in patients with injuries above T-1 because of the loss of connection between temperature centers in the hypothalamus and sympathetic outflow of the spinal cord. Body temperature is regulated by the ambient temperature.

E. **DEFINING CHARACTERISTICS**

Sensory and motor dysfunction depends on the type and level of the injury.

1. **Complete transection** results in loss of voluntary movement of body parts, loss of sensation to body parts, and loss of autonomic and spinal reflexes below the level of the injury. Reflex activity may return in 1 to 2 weeks.

2. **Incomplete transection** causes variable levels of vasomotor instability and bowel and bladder dysfunction; and asymmetric flaccid paralysis, asymmetric loss of reflexes, variable sensory function (e.g., pain, temperature, touch, pressure, proprioception), and variable visceral and somatic responses below the level of injury.

3. **Spinal shock in the acute period** results in loss of vasomotor tone with complete transection causing hypotension, poor venous circulation, and bradycardia; loss of perspiration below the level of the injury; and loss of bladder and rectal control.

4. **Autonomic hyperreflexia** is a complication that usually occurs after the acute phase of an SCI. It results from a continuous, uncontrolled, paroxysmal lower motor neuron reflex arc, a massive sympathetic response that causes vasoconstriction with severe hypertension (systolic pressures of more than 200 mm Hg). The vagus nerve responds with bradycardia and vasodilation above the lesion. It occurs primarily in patients with injuries above T-4 through T-6 and is absent

in patients who have injuries that destroy the preganglionic sympathetic fibers. Stimuli that can trigger this response include, bladder dysfunction (e.g., distention, infection, outflow obstruction), surgical procedures, line insertions, tight clothing, pressure sores, and an impacted rectum (Nolan, 1994). Symptoms include paroxysmal hypertension, headache, blurred vision, nausea, bradycardia, nasal congestion, and piloerection.

F. NEURODIAGNOSTIC STUDIES

1. **Radiographic spine films** are examined carefully to determine the integrity of each component of each vertebra and alignment of each segment. Frequently, spinal cord trauma occurs without radiographic findings in children because of their cartilaginous spine.

2. **CT scan** is used when radiographs do not adequately explain the clinical picture. CT scan identifies SCIs and bony lesions.

3. **MRI** is indicated for use the same as a CT scan. It clearly identifies the relationship of the spinal cord and surrounding vertebral elements and readily identifies cord compression. Approximately half of all children with SCI fail to demonstrate radiographic abnormalities on plain films, CT scans, or myelograms. However, MRI can usually identify spinal cord pathology with SCIWORA (Pang and Wilberger, 1982). Clinical assessment should be considered when evaluating SCI. MRI is not routinely used in unstable patients but is an excellent study for follow-up care.

4. **Myelography** is used when pathology is unclear and is helpful in identifying spinal cord abnormalities including cord hematoma, epidural hematoma, swelling, and preexisting disease.

G. MEDICAL MANAGEMENT

Medical management consists of prevention of a secondary injury. .

1. **Immobilization of the spine** until it can be surgically stabilized is imperative. During transport, a semirigid cervical collar and spine backboard (ideally with a head well to keep the head in a neutral position) should be used. Foam blocks or linen rolls and tape help to further stabilize the head and shoulders on a backboard.

2. **Spinal canal decompression** is used to prevent secondary injury to the spinal cord. Cervical traction is used to stabilize fractures or when subluxation has occurred. Muscle relaxants are frequently used with traction. Surgical decompression with posterior laminectomy and debridement may be indicated once the patient has stabilized and bleeding and swelling have stopped (usually after 7 to 10 days).

3. **Stabilization of the spine with surgical fixation** is accomplished by the fusion of two or more vertebrae with the insertion of bone grafts, metal rods, or wires. A halo jacket involves the placement of a halo ring around the skull fixated with screws to the skull. The ring is attached to a padded jacket or cast made into a vest via vertical rods and a horizontal articulation device. Traction is adjusted to stabilize cervical fractures.

4. **Pharmacologic prevention of a secondary injury** with methylprednisolone (Solu-Medrol) has neuroprotective effects (Hall, 1992; Hilton and Frei, 1991) including inhibition of lipid perioxidation, inhibition of arachidonic acid release and eicosanoid formation, maintenance of spinal cord blood flow, improvement of ionic pump function, and decreased intracellular accumulation. The clinical effect is a reduction in spinal cord swelling. Accurate administration is critical to the effectiveness of the drug, and guidelines are followed carefully (McEvoy, 1990). The loading dose is 30 mg/kg IV over 15 minutes, which is followed after 45 minutes by the maintenance dose of 5.4 mg/kg/h IV for 23 hours (continuous). The loading dose is given within 8

hours of the injury, and the maintenance dose is started within 1 hour of the loading dose. Indications are for evidence of an SCI less than 8 hours old. Relative contraindications include pregnancy, uncontrolled diabetes mellitus, medication allergy, and injury more than 8 hours old.

H. MULTIDISCIPLINARY MANAGEMENT

❖ ALTERATION IN RESPIRATORY FUNCTION: BREATHING PATTERN RELATED TO HIGH CERVICAL INJURY (LACK OF INNERVATION OF RESPIRATORY MUSCLES); INEFFECTIVE AIRWAY CLEARANCE RELATED TO ARTIFICIAL AIRWAY AND DIMINISHED RESPIRATORY MUSCLE INNERVATION

1. **Expected outcomes** include normal arterial blood gases, $SaO_2 > 95\%$, adequate ventilation, and no respiratory complications (such as pneumonia, aspiration, edema).
2. **Nursing assessment** is provided to assess for spontaneous or effective ventilations, to monitor oxygenation (e.g., arterial blood gases, SaO_2), assess effectiveness of cough and ability to mobilize secretions, respiratory rate, pattern, and work of breathing (note acute changes), and breath sounds. Decompress the stomach with an indwelling orogastric tube.
3. **Collaborative interventions:** Maintain the artificial airway, assist with ventilatory support, perform chest physiotherapy and postural drainage, administer effective pulmonary toilet, and maintain aseptic technique with invasive procedures.

❖ ALTERATION IN CARDIAC OUTPUT RELATED TO ANS DYSFUNCTION

1. **Expected outcomes** include a normal blood pressure and heart rate and rhythm, capillary refill <3 seconds, and urine output of 1 to 2 ml/kg/h.
2. **Nursing assessment:** Monitor heart rate and rhythm, urine output, and systemic arterial pressure. Perform serial measurements of cardiac output and cardiac index (if available) and assess systemic perfusion (e.g., pulses, color, capillary refill).
3. **Collaborative interventions:** Support circulation as needed using fluids, inotropic and vasopressor agents, and elastic stockings. Maintain functioning of invasive lines. Correct bradycardia with atropine, an anticholinergic drug used to increase the rate of cardiac conduction. Eliminate the precipitating cause (e.g., hypothermia, distended bladder).

❖ POTENTIAL FOR IMPAIRED GAS EXCHANGE RELATED TO PULMONARY EMBOLI FROM IMMOBILITY (DEEP VEIN THROMBOSIS [DVT])

1. **Expected outcomes** include normal arterial blood gases, $SaO_2 > 95\%$, and no swelling, redness, tenderness, or pain in the lower extremities.
2. **Nursing assessment** includes assessment of the respiratory status for acute deterioration, serial measurements of the legs, and assessment for signs of venous thrombosis (pain, swelling, redness, and tenderness in the lower extremities). With vena cava filter use, assess the venous access site for bleeding, swelling, and hematoma.
3. **Collaborative interventions:** Apply antiembolism stockings or mechanical devices designed to improve venous return from the lower extremities. Consult with physical or occupational therapy to plan appropriate range of motion and positioning therapy. Maintain good hydration. Administer subcutaneous heparin or warfarin (Coumadin) as ordered.

❖ POTENTIAL FOR ALTERATION IN SKIN INTEGRITY RELATED TO IMMOBILITY, DECREASED VENOUS BLOOD FLOW, REDUCED SENSORY RECEPTORS; CHILDREN AT RISK FOR OCCIPITAL PRESSURE ULCERS

1. **Expected outcome** is the absence of skin breakdown.
2. **Nursing assessment** includes skin assessment (especially heels, elbows, sacral, and occipital areas) for alterations in integrity (including redness, swelling, and

breakdown), assessment for the degree of mobility, and assessment of the environment for potential sources of skin trauma (including traction, soiled linens, and patient appliances).

3. **Collaborative interventions:** Change the patient's position frequently and use a pressure reduction surface if available; maintain dry and clean bed linens and clothing; provide meticulous skin care; and consult with physical or occupational therapy to plan appropriate range of motion and positioning therapy.

❖ POTENTIAL FOR PULMONARY INFECTION RELATED TO ARTIFICIAL AIRWAY, GENERAL DEBILITATED STATE, AND IMMOBILITY

1. **Expected outcomes** include normal WBC, temperature, and respiratory parameters.
2. **Nursing assessment** includes monitoring oxygenation (e.g., arterial blood gases, SaO_2) and assessing effectiveness of cough and ability to mobilize secretions, respiratory rate, pattern, and work of breathing (note acute changes), and breath sounds. Monitor for infection (e.g., WBC, temperature, tachycardia) and evaluate tracheal cultures.
3. **Collaborative interventions:** Provide pulmonary toilet, maintain hydration, perform chest physiotherapy and postural drainage, and maintain aseptic technique with invasive procedures.

❖ ALTERATION IN TEMPERATURE REGULATION RELATED TO POIKILOTHERMISM (I.E., BODY TEMPERATURE IS CONTROLLED BY THE ENVIRONMENT INSTEAD OF INTERNAL REGULATORY CENTERS)

1. **Expected outcome** is a temperature within normal range.
2. **Nursing assessment** includes monitoring core temperature frequently.
3. **Collaborative interventions** include adjusting the environmental temperature to maintain normal temperature range, adjusting clothing and bed linens, correcting hypothermia (e.g., warming blanket, heating lamps, warm linens), and correcting hyperthermia (e.g., remove excessive clothing, sponge with tepid water).

❖ ALTERATION IN ELIMINATION PATTERNS RELATED TO DIMINISHED INNERVATION OF VISCERA

1. **Expected outcomes** are no constipation, impactions, or urinary retention.
2. **Nursing assessment** includes assessment for bladder or abdominal distention; assessment of intake and output; assessment of stools for frequency, consistency, and color; assessment for presence of bowel sounds; and monitoring of urine cultures.
3. **Collaborative interventions** include maintaining urinary drainage with intermittent or indwelling catheterization, obtaining routine urine cultures and renal studies, maintaining good hydration, and administering stool softeners and bulk-forming agents.

SCOLIOSIS AND SPINAL FUSIONS

A. **DESCRIPTION**

The normal spine has three curves: cervical lordosis, thoracic kyphosis, and lumbar lordosis. Scoliosis is defined as a lateral curvature of the spine greater than 10 degrees. The three major types of scoliosis are congenital, (vertebral abnormalities develop in utero), neuromuscular (resulting from muscle weakness or imbalance), and idiopathic (unknown by definition).

B. **INCIDENCE**

The exact incidence of congenital scoliosis is unknown because some cases go undetected (Weinstein, 1994). The exact incidence of neuromuscular scoliosis is unknown because it is related to the incidence of specific neuromuscular diseases. Two percent of the population have idiopathic scoliosis, and it accounts for 65% to 80% of cases (Marlow & Redding, 1988). Only 15% of the curves progress. Scoliosis can occur at any age. Early onset is defined as birth to 5 years or described as infantile at birth to 3 years. Juvenile onset is onset at 4 to 10 years. Adolescent onset is onset at older than 10 years. The majority of cases are adolescent onset, and 90% of idiopathic adolescent scoliosis cases occur in females.

C. **ETIOLOGY**

Congenital scoliosis is an embryologic malformation during the third to fifth embryonic week (Mason and Wright, 1995). **Neuromuscular scoliosis** occurs secondary to neuropathic or myopathic diseases, resulting in muscle imbalance (Mason and Wright, 1995). **Idiopathic** infantile scoliosis occurs in the first years of life and is associated with intrauterine position. The cause of idiopathic juvenile scoliosis is unknown. Idiopathic adolescent scoliosis most often is caused by X-linked inheritance (Mason and Wright, 1995).

D. **PATHOPHYSIOLOGY**

Initial pathologic changes begin in the soft tissues, which shorten on the concave side of the curve. Vertebral deformity occurs as a result of unequal forces applied to the epiphyseal center of the ossification (growth plates). Curves progress during growth spurts. A large curve can be physically disabling and may compromise respiratory function.

E. **DEFINING CHARACTERISTICS**

The first sign is often uneven hips and shoulders. Physical changes are most noticeable when the child bends forward and may include one more prominent breast or scapula and posterior humping of ribs or hips.

F. **NEURODIAGNOSTIC STUDIES**

1. **Serial radiographs** are used to assess the progression of curve and to document whether it is progressive.
2. **Serial pulmonary function tests** may be used to trend lung capacity.

G. **MEDICAL MANAGEMENT**

Medical management is based on the degree of the curve and the age of the patient (i.e., how much growth remains).

1. Mild curves (in a prepubescent patient) require observation. The young child is evaluated every 3 to 12 months and older children and adolescents are evaluated every 3 to 4 months. (Curves usually progress during growth spurts.)
2. Moderate curves (20 to 40 degrees) commonly require orthotic braces. Electrical stimulation is used less frequently. An electrical stimulator transmits an electrical pulse to muscles on the convex side of the curvature causing the muscles to contract at regular and frequent intervals. Muscle contraction counterbalances the opposing forces, preventing further deformity.
3. Severe curves (greater than 40 degrees in a growing child) require spinal fusion and instrumentation (Krag, 1991; Spivak and Balderston, 1994). Hardware (series of metal rods, hooks, and screws) is used and attached to the vertebrae to stabilize the spine until the bone grafts have time to form a solid bone mass, which usually takes 10 to 12 months (Jacobs-Zacny and Horn, 1988; Partyka, 1991). Posterior fusion with instrumentation is most common. Anterior fusion with and without instrumentation may be used for severe curves, or in children who are lacking the posterior portion of the vertebrae. High anterior fusions disrupt the thoracic cavity and require thoracostomy tube(s) placement.

H. **MULTIDISCIPLINARY MANAGEMENT OF SPINAL FUSION** (Feingold et al, 1991; Jacobs-Zacny and Horn, 1988; Partyka, 1991)

❖ INEFFECTIVE BREATHING PATTERN RELATED TO ANESTHESIA, IMMOBILIZATION, PAIN

1. **Expected outcomes** include normal respiratory rate, pattern, and oxygenation

parameters (e.g., arterial blood gases, SaO_2) and clear breath sounds bilaterally.

2. **Nursing assessment** includes respiratory ventilation (e.g., rate, depth), work of breathing (e.g., use of accessory muscles, retractions), effectiveness of incentive spirometry, and respiratory physiologic parameters.

3. **Collaborative interventions:** Support ventilation as needed by administering supplemental oxygen to maintain SaO_2 >95%, maintaining pain control, assisting with airway clearance (suctioning, position changes, and cough and deep breathing), and administering bronchodilators as needed. Monitor chest tube drainage (for anterior fusions).

❖ DECREASED CARDIAC OUTPUT RELATED TO HEMORRHAGE (LONG PROCEDURE WITH LONG SUTURE LINES)

1. **Expected outcomes** include balanced intake and output, urine output >2 ml/kg/h, CVP within normal range, adequate peripheral pulses, normal vital signs for age, and normal mental status (awake and responsive).

2. **Nursing assessment** includes monitoring of intake and output, vital signs and hemodynamic pressures, thoracostomy tube drainage for amount and color, hemoglobin and hematocrit, surgical drains for amount and color, and surgical dressing for drainage amount and color.

3. **Collaborative interventions** include administering isotonic fluids or blood products as needed to support circulation and maintaining patency of the thoracostomy tubes.

❖ ALTERATION IN COMFORT RELATED TO INCISIONAL PAIN (POSTERIOR, ANTERIOR, OR THORACOTOMY)

1. **Expected outcomes** include pain relief or control, absent physiologic manifestations of pain (e.g., tachycardia, diaphoresis, elevated blood pressure, facial grimacing, restlessness), and decreased need for narcotic analgesics.

2. **Nursing assessment** should include physiologic indicators of pain, asking patient frequently about pain control, using age-appropriate pain scales, and assessing the effectiveness of interventions.

3. **Collaborative interventions:** Use nonpharmacologic measures individualized to age, culture, and past experiences including distractors, imagery, and controlled breathing. Encourage parental involvement. Administer analgesics by continuous infusion or patient-controlled analgesia. Position for comfort.

❖ POTENTIAL FOR INJURY RELATED TO SCI

1. **Expected outcome** is the preoperative neurovascular status.

2. **Nursing assessment** includes monitoring neurovascular status in the lower extremities (e.g., sensation to light touch, movement, pulses, color, and capillary refill).

3. **Collaborative interventions** include positioning as ordered and frequent repositioning. Notify the physician for any neurovascular changes.

❖ POTENTIAL FOR INFECTION RELATED TO SURGICAL TRAUMA, INVASIVE LINES, AND SKIN BREAKDOWN

❖ POTENTIAL IMPAIRED GAS EXCHANGE RELATED TO PULMONARY EMBOLI

❖ ALTERATION IN SKIN INTEGRITY RELATED TO IMMOBILITY

❖ ALTERATION IN ELIMINATION RELATED TO IMMOBILITY

CONGENITAL NEUROLOGIC ABNORMALITIES

A. **DESCRIPTION**

1. **Myelodysplasia, spinal dysraphism,** and **spina bifida** are terms that are used interchangeably to describe a collection of disorders characterized by vertebral arch fusion defects and abnormalities of the spinal cord and coverings. These

defects, as well as all disorders of the neural tube, are collectively referred to as neural tube defects (NTD).

2. **Spina bifida cystica,** incomplete fusion of one or more vertebral laminae, results in external protrusion of the spinal tissue. Two classifications include *myelomeningocele,* a protruding saclike structure containing meninges, spinal fluid, and neural tissue, and *meningocele,* a protruding sac containing only meninges and CSF.

3. **Spina bifida occulta** is incomplete fusion at one level without a protrusion of neural structures. The defect is not apparent to the naked eye.

B. **INCIDENCE**

In the United States, 1 to 2 per 1000 live births have an NTD (Cohen, 1987). In the United Kingdom, 4 to 5 per 1000 live births have an NTD. Irish and Moslems have the highest occurrence of NTDs. Asians and African-Americans have the lowest incidence. Incidence rates may be higher if the defect is related to some stillbirths and spontaneous abortions.

C. **ETIOLOGY**

The cause of congenital neurologic abnormalities is unknown and possibly multi-factorial. The abnormality occurs early in embryonic development.

D. **PATHOPHYSIOLOGY**

The most common part of the spine affected is the lower thoracic lumbar and sacral areas (Reigel, 1989). The anterior aspects of the spinal cord are frequently intact with varying degrees of destruction to the dorsal columns. Sometimes it is associated with brain abnormalities including cellular migration, agenesis of the corpus callosum, arachnoid cysts, and Arnold-Chiari malformations. The degree of func-tional impairment depends on the extent of the defect and associated neural tissue.

E. **DEFINING CHARACTERISTICS**

1. **Spina bifida occulta** often goes undetected (Disabato and Wulf, 1994; Haller, 1992). Possible signs (over the midline of the lumbosacral area) include a palpable mass, dermal sinus, skin discoloration, and a tuft of hair. Spinal cord or nerve involvement may demonstrate asymmetry of the lower extremities, persistent enuresis (late onset), and progressive weakness of one or both legs.

2. **Meningocele** is a visible defect of the cord and covering. It may have minimal to no involvement of the lower extremities.

3. **Myelomeningocele** dysfunction ranges from minimal impairment to total paralysis of the lower extremities. Lumbosacral lesions usually result in some hip, knee, or ankle flexion. Sensory involvement is usually symmetric but patchy. Usually, some degree of bowel and bladder dysfunction exists. Arnold-Chiari type II deformity is present in the majority of cases. It consists of elongation and herniation of the cerebellar vermis through the foramen magnum, displacement and distortion of the medulla (including the fourth ventricle), impeded CSF flow and hydrocephalus, and possibly lower bulbar dysfunction producing apnea, vocal cord paralysis, and stridor.

F. **NEURODIAGNOSTIC STUDIES**

1. **Radiographs** are taken of the entire spine to identify the precise level of deformity and to rule out deformities at other levels.

2. **CT scan or MRI** are done to visualize the ventricular system and brain stem.

3. **Serum AFP** levels are used as a screening tool for open NTDs during the 16th and 18th weeks of gestation. Normal maternal serum AFP at 16 weeks is 38 ng/ml and at 18 weeks is 49 ng/ml. NTD levels vary; therefore, any level above the normal range is further evaluated.

G. **MEDICAL MANAGEMENT**

In recent years, immediate closure of the protruding sac is indicated. The goals of surgery are to preserve all neural tissue, provide a physiologic skin barrier, and control progressive hydrocephalus. Surgical closure involves several steps including dissection of the exposed sac, closure of the dura over preserved neural tissue, and closure of the skin covering the repair. Skin grafting may be necessary. If hydrocephalus is present, a CSF shunting device is inserted, or the foramen magnum is enlarged.

H. MULTIDISCIPLINARY MANAGEMENT

❖ POTENTIAL FOR INFECTION RELATED TO SURGICAL INCISION, FRAGILITY OF COVERING, INVASIVE LINES, URINARY RETENTION

1. **Expected outcomes** include no signs and symptoms of infection and a healed wound incision.

2. **Nursing assessment** includes monitoring vital signs, WBC count, cultures, and urine studies; assessing the sac's protective barrier (before and after the operation) for drainage, odor, and color; assessing neurologic functioning including head circumference and fontanelles and signs of increased ICP; and assessing for bladder distention and monitoring urinary output.

3. **Collaborative interventions** include protecting the sac with a sterile saline moist dressing preoperatively and maintaining the child in a prone or side-lying position before and immediately after the operation to promote wound healing. Provide routine postoperative care, maintain sterile dry wound dressings, administer antibiotics as ordered, and prevent contamination of the wound from feces and urine.

❖ ALTERATION IN CEREBRAL TISSUE PERFUSION RELATED TO INCREASED ICP FROM HYDRO-CEPHALUS

❖ ALTERATION IN ELIMINATION RELATED TO DECREASED INNERVATION OF BLADDER, URINARY SPHINCTER, LOWER INTESTINES

REFERENCES

Abels L, Belcher A, Russo BL. The nervous system. In: Abels L, ed. *Critical Care Nursing: A Physiologic Approach.* St Louis, Mo: The CV Mosby Co; 1986:254–336.

Acton PA, Farley T, Freni LW, Ilegbodu VA, Sniezek JE, Wohlleb JC. Traumatic spinal cord injury in Arkansas, 1980 to 1989. *Arch Phys Med Rehabil.* 1993;74:1035–1040.

Adams WG, Deaver KA, Cochi SL, et al. Decline of childhood *Haemophilus influenzae* type b (Hib) disease in the Hib vaccine era. *JAMA.* 1993;269:264–266.

Akpede GO, Abiodun PO, Ambe JP, Jacob DD. Presenting features of bacterial meningitis in young infants. *Ann Trop Paediatr.* 1994;14:245–252.

Akpede O, Abiodun PO, Sykes M, Salami CE. Childhood bacterial meningitis beyond the neonatal period in southern Nigeria: changes in organisms/antibiotic susceptibility. *East Afr Med J.* 1994;71:14–20.

Albright AL. Pediatric brain tumors. *CA.* 1993;43(5):272–289.

Aldrich EF, Eisenberg HM, Saydjari C, et al. Diffuse brain swelling in severely head-injured children. *J Neurosurg.* 1992;76:450–454.

Allen JC. Complications of chemotherapy in patients with brain and spinal cord tumors. *Pediatr Neurosurg.* 1992;17:218–224.

Altimier LB. Pediatric central neurologic trauma: issues for special patients. *AACN Clin Issues Crit Care.* 1992;3:31–43.

Altman DI, Powers WJ, Perlman JM, Herscovitch P, Volpe SL, Volpe JJ. Cerebral blood flow requirement for brain viability in newborn infants is lower than in adults. *Ann Neurol.* 1988;24:218–226.

American Academy of Pediatrics Committee on Infectious Diseases. Dexamethasone therapy for bacterial meningitis in infants and children. *Pediatrics.* 1990;86:130–133.

Andrews M, Mooney KH. Alterations of neurologic function in children. In: McCance KL, Huether SE, eds. *Pathophysiology: The Biologic Basis for Disease in Adults and Children.* St Louis, Mo: The CV Mosby Co; 1990:531–561.

Anttila M. Clinical criteria for estimating recovery from childhood bacterial meningitis. *Acta Paediatr.* 1994;83:63–67.

Anttila M, Himberg JJ, Peltola H. Precise quantification of fever in childhood bacterial meningitis. *Clin Pediatr.* 1992;31:221–227.

Armstrong SL. Cerebral vasospasm: early detection and intervention. *Crit Care Nurse.* 1994;14:33–37.

Ashwal S, Tomasi L, Schneider S, Perkin R, Thompson J. Bacterial meningitis in children: pathophysiology and treatment. *Neurology*. 1992;42:739–748.

Barker E. Brain tumor. Frightening diagnosis, nursing challenge. *RN*. 1990;53(9):46–55.

Barkovich AJ. Neuroimaging of pediatric brain tumors. *Neurosurg Clin North Am*. 1992;3:739–769.

Baron MC. Advances in the care of children with brain tumors. *J Neurosci Nurs*. 1991;23(1):39–43.

Beghi E, Nicolosi A, Kurland LT, Mulder DW, Hauser WA, Shuster L. Encephalitis and aseptic meningitis, Olmsted County, Minnesota, 1950–1981: I. Epidemiology. *Ann Neurol*. 1984;16:283–294.

Bergman I. Pediatric neurological assessment and monitoring. In: Fuhrman BP, Zimmerman JJ, eds. *Pediatric Critical Care*. St Louis, Mo: Mosby–Year Book Inc; 1992:569–587.

Bijlmer HA, van Alphen L. A prospective, population-based study of *Haemophilus influenzae* type b meningitis in the Gambia and the possible consequences. *J Infect Dis*. 1992;165(suppl):29–32.

Birdsall C, Greif L. How do you manage extraventricular drainage. *Am J Nurs*. 1990;90(11):47–49.

Bishop BS. Pathologic pupillary signs: self-learning module, part 2. *Crit Care Nurse*. 1991;11:58–67.

Boss BJ, Heath J, Sunderland PM. Alterations of neurologic function. In: McCance KL, Huether SE, eds. *Pathophysiology: The Biologic Basis for Disease in Adults and Children*. St Louis, Mo: The CV Mosby Co; 1990;476–530.

Boss BJ, Stowe AC. Neuroanatomy. *J Neurosci Nurs*. 1983;18:214–230.

Brain Resuscitation Clinical Trial I Study Group. Randomized clinical study of thiopental loading in comatose survivors or cardiac arrest. *N Engl J Med*. 1986;314:397–403.

Bruce DA. Treatment of intracranial hypertension. In: Wonsiewicz M, ed. *Pediatric Neurosurgery*. Philadelphia, Pa: WB Saunders Co; 1989:245–254.

Bruno JP. Systematic neonatal assessment and intervention. *MCN*. 1995;20:21–24.

Buys YM, Levin AV, Enzenauer RW, et al. Retinal findings after head trauma in infants and young children. *Ophthalmology*. 1992;99:1718–1723.

Centers for Disease Control. Reye syndrome—United States, *MMWR*. 1984;34:13.

Chan S, Khandji AG, Hilal SK. How to select diagnostic tests. In: Rowland LP, ed. *Merritt's Textbook of Neurology*. 9th ed. Baltimore, Md: Williams & Wilkins; 1995:59–66.

Chen CH, Wang TM, Wu KH, Chi CS. Intraventricular hemorrhage in preterm neonates—a two year experience. *Acta Paediatr Sin*. 1993;34:343–348.

Chequer RS, Tharp BR, Dreimane D, Hahn JS, Clancy RR, Coen RW. Prognostic value of EEG in neonatal meningitis: retrospective study of 29 infants. *Pediatr Neurol*. 1992;8:417–422.

Chesney PJ. Pediatric infectious disease-associated syndromes. In: Fuhrman BP, Zimmerman JJ, eds. *Pediatric Critical Care*. St Louis, Mo: Mosby–Year Book Inc; 1992:1023–1032.

Chestnut RM. Computed tomography of the brain: a guide to understanding and interpreting normal and abnormal images in the critically ill patient. *Crit Care Nurs Q*. 1994;17:33–50.

Chotpitayasunondh T. Bacterial meningitis in children: etiology and clinical features, an 11-year review of 618 cases. *Southeast Asian J Trop Med Public Health*. 1994;25:107–115.

Choux M. Consensus: treatment. *Childs Nerv Syst*. 1994;10:74–75.

Coats TJ, Allen M. Baby walker related injuries—a continuing problem. *Arch Emerg Med*. 1991;8:52–55.

Cohen F. Neural tube defects: epidemiology, detection, and prevention. *J Obstet Gynecol Neonatal Nurs*. 1987;2:105–115.

Crutchfield JS, Narayan RK, Robertson CS, Michael LH. Evaluation of fiberoptic intracranial pressure monitor. *J Neurosurg*. 1990;72:482–487.

Curley MAQ, Vernon-Levett P. Intracranial dynamics. In: Curley MAQ, Smith JB, Moloney-Harmon PA, eds. *Critical Care Nursing of Infants and Children*. Philadelphia, Pa: WB Saunders Co; 1996:336–384.

Dagan R. Epidemiology of pediatric meningitis caused by *Haemophilus influenzae* B, *Streptococcus pneumoniae* and *Neisseria meningitidis* in Israel. *Israel J Med Sci*. 1994;30:351–355.

Davis RJ, Tait VF, Dean JM, Goldberg AL, Rogers MC. Head and spinal cord injury. In: Rogers MC, ed. *Textbook of Pediatric Intensive Care*. Baltimore, Md: Williams & Wilkins; 1992:805–857.

Dean JM, Moss SD. Intracranial hypertension. In: Fuhrman BP, Zimmerman JJ, eds. *Pediatric Critical Care*. St Louis, Mo: Mosby–Year Book Inc; 1992:577–587.

Dean JM, Rogers MC, Traystman RJ. Pathophysiology and clinical management of the intracranial vault. In: Rogers MC, ed. *Textbook of Pediatric Intensive Care*. Baltimore, Md: Williams & Wilkins; 1992:639–666.

DeLaat CA, Lampkin BC. Long-term survivors of childhood cancer: evaluation and identification of sequelae of treatment. *CA*. 1992;42:263–282.

Delgado MR. Status epilepticus. In: Levin DL, Morriss FC, eds. *Essentials of Pediatric Intensive Care*. St Louis, Mo: Quality Medical Publishers; 1990:59–65.

DeVivo DC, Keating JP, Haymond MW. Acute encephalopathy with fatty infiltration of the viscera. *Pediatr Clin North Am*. 1976;23:527–535.

Dincer F, Celiker R, Ozker S, Basgoze O, Ozker R. Etiological and functional evaluation of the pediatric population with spinal cord injuries. *Turkish J Pediatr*. 1993;35:171–175.

Disabato J, Wulf J. Altered neurologic function. In: Betz CL, Hunsberger M, Wright S, eds. *Family-Centered Nursing Care of Children*. 2nd ed. Philadelphia, Pa: WB Saunders Co; 1994;1717–1814.

Donahue B. Short- and long-term complications of radiation therapy for pediatric brain tumors. *Pediatr Neurosurg.* 1992;18:207–217.

Dreifuss FE. Classification of epileptic seizures and the epilepsies. *Pediatr Clin North Am.* 1989;36:265.

Drummond BL. Preventing increased intracranial pressure. *Focus Crit Care.* 1990;17:116–122.

Duffner PK, Cohen ME. Changes in the approach to central nervous system tumors in childhood. *Pediatr Clin North Am.* 1992;39:859–877.

Farley JA. The comatose child: analysis of factors affecting intracranial pressure. *Dimens Crit Care Nurs.* 1990;9:216–222.

Feigin RD, McCracken GH, Klein JO. Diagnosis and management of meningitis. *Pediatr Infect Dis J.* 1992;11:785.

Feingold DJ, Peck SA, Reinsma EJ, Ruda SC. Complications of lumbar spine surgery. *Orthopedic Nurs.* 1991;10(4):39–58.

Ferrari B, Tonni G, Luzietti R, Ciarlini G, Vadora E, Merialdi A. Neonatal complications and risk of intraventricular-periventricular hemorrhage. *Clin Exp Obstet Gynecol.* 1992;19(4):253–258.

Fishman MA. Infectious diseases. In: David RB, ed. *Pediatric Neurology for the Clinician.* Norwalk, Conn: Appleton & Lange; 1992:249–267.

Fishman RA. Brain edema and disorders of intracranial pressure. In: Rowland LP, ed. *Merritt's Textbook of Neurology.* 9th ed. Baltimore, Md: Williams & Wilkins; 1995:302–310.

Fitz C. Magnetic resonance imaging of pediatric brain tumors. *Topics in Magnetic Resonance Imaging.* 1993;1:174–189.

Fortnum HM, Davis AC. Epidemiology of bacterial meningitis. *Arch Dis Child.* 1993;68:763–767.

Foster AH, Salter DR. Cerebral pathophysiologic considerations in patients with coexisting carotid and coronary artery disease. *Adv Cardiac Surg.* 1990;2:203–221.

Freeman JM, Ferry PC. New brain death guidelines in children: further confusion. [Editorial]. *Pediatrics.* 1988;81:301–303.

Friedman HS, Oakes WJ. New therapeutic options in the management of childhood brain tumors. *Oncology.* 1992;6(5):27–36.

Gajjar A, Heideman RL, Kovnar EH, et al. Response of pediatric low grade gliomas to chemotherapy. *Pediatr Neurosurg.* 1993;19:113–120.

Gambardella G, Zaccone C, Cardia E, Tomasello F. Intracranial pressure monitoring in children: comparison of external ventricular device with the fiberoptic system. *Childs Nerv Syst.* 1993;9:470–473.

Garcia-Larrea K, Artru F, Bertrand O, Pernier J, Mauguiere F. The combined monitoring of brain stem auditory evoked potentials and intracranial pressure in coma. A study of 57 patients. *J Neurol Neurosurg Psychiatry.* 1992;55:792–798.

Garcia-Monaco R, Victor DD, Mann C, Hannedouche A, Terbrugge K, Lasjaunias P. Congestive cardiac manifestations from cerebrocranial arteriovenous shunts. *Childs Nerv Syst.* 1991;7:48–52.

Germon K. Intracranial pressure monitoring in the 1990s. *Crit Care Nurs Q.* 1994;17:21–32.

Gibbs JM, Weindling AM. Neonatal intracranial lesions following placental abruption. *Eur J Pediatr.* 1994;153(3):195–197.

Goe MR, Massey TH. Assessment of neurologic damage: creatine kinase-BB assay after cardiac arrest. *Heart Lung.* 1988;17:247–253.

Goebert DA, Ng MY, Varney JM, Sheetz DA. Traumatic spinal cord injury in Hawaii. *Hawaii Med J.* 1991;50(2):44,47–48.

Graham CJ, Kittredge D, Stuemky JH. Injuries associated with child safety seat misuse. *Pediatr Emerg Care.* 1992;8(6):351–353.

Guertin SR. Neurosurgical intensive care: selected aspects. In: Fuhrman BP, Zimmerman JJ, eds. *Pediatric Critical Care.* St Louis, Mo: Mosby–Year Book Inc; 1992:621–635.

Guidelines for the determination of brain death in children. *Pediatrics.* 1987;80:298–300.

Hale BR, Williams TM. Managing tonic-clonic status epilepticus in children. *Indiana Med.* April 1989: 256–260.

Hall ED. The neuroprotective pharmacology of methylprednisolone. *J Neurosurg.* 1992;76:13–21.

Haller JS. Congenital malformations of the central nervous system. In: David RB, ed. *Pediatric Neurology for the Clinician.* Norwalk, Conn: Appleton & Lange; 1992:461–467.

Hamilton MG, Myles ST. Pediatric spinal injury: review of 174 hospital admissions. *J Neurosurg.* 1992;77: 700–704.

Haun SE, Dean JM, Kirsch JR, Ackerman AD, Rogers MC. Theories in brain resuscitation. In: Rogers MC, ed. *Textbook of Pediatric Intensive Care.* Baltimore, Md: Williams & Wilkins; 1992:698–732.

Hauser WA, Annegers JF, Kurland LT. Incidence of epilepsy and unprovoked seizures in Rochester, Minnesota: 1935–1984. *Epilepsia.* 1993;34:453–468.

Hazinski MF. Neurologic disorders. In: Hazinski MF, ed. *Nursing Care of the Critically Ill Child.* St Louis, Mo: Mosby–Year Book Inc; 1992:521–628.

Henneman EA. Clinical assessment and neurodiagnostics. *Crit Care Nurs Clin North Am.* 1989;1:131–142.

Henry PC, Hauber RP, Rice M. Factors associated with closed head injury in a pediatric population. *J Neurosci Nurs.* 1992;24:311–316.

Heyderman RS, Robb SA, Kendall BE, Levin M. Does computed tomography have a role in the evaluation of complicated acute bacterial meningitis in childhood? *Dev Med Child Neurol.* 1992;34:870–875.

Hilton G, Frei J. High-dose methylprednisolone in the treatment of spinal cord injuries. *Heart Lung.* 1991;20:675–680.

Holmes GL. The epilepsies. In: David RB, ed. *Pediatric Neurology for the Clinician.* Norwalk, Conn: Appleton & Lange; 1992:185–228.

Horowitz ME, Poplack DG. Development of chemotherapy treatment for pediatric brain tumors. *Neurol Clin.* 1991;9:363–373.

Hughes MC. Critical care nursing for the patient with a spinal cord injury. *Crit Care Nurs Clin North Am.* 1990;2:33–40.

Imaizumi S, Woolworth V, Fishman RA, Cahn PH. Liposome-entrapped superoxide dismutase reduces cerebral infarction in cerebral ischemia in rats. *Stroke.* 1990;21:1312–1317.

Jacobs-Zacny JM, Horn MJ. Nursing care of adolescents having posterior spinal fusion with Cotrel-Dubousset instrumentation. *Orthopedic Nurs.* 1988;7:17–21.

Jacobson RI. Congenital structural defects. In: Swaiman KF, ed. *Pediatric Neurology: Principles and Practice.* St Louis, Mo: The CV Mosby Co; 1989;1:317–362.

Jensen D. *The Human Nervous System.* New York, NY: Appleton-Century-Crofts; 1980.

Johnson JK. Vascular anomalies in the pediatric age group. *J S C Med Assoc.* 1994;90(1):16–17.

Johnston MV. Development, structure, and function of the brain and neuromuscular systems. In: Fuhrman BP, Zimmerman JJ, eds. *Pediatric Critical Care.* St Louis, Mo: Mosby–Year Book Inc; 1992:559–568.

Joy C. Pediatric cerebral resuscitation. *Crit Care Nurs Clin North Am.* 1989;1:181–187.

Jumah MA, McLean DR, Rajeh SA, Crow N. Bulk diffusion apnea test in the diagnosis of brain death. *Crit Care Med.* 1992;20:1564–1567.

Kadota RP, Allen JB, Hartman GA, Spruce WE. Brain tumors in children. *J Pediatr.* 1989;114:511–519.

Kanal E, Shellock FG. Patient monitoring during clinical MR imaging. *Radiology.* 1992;185:623–629.

Keating JP. Reye syndrome. In: Feigin RD, Cherry JD, eds. *Textbook of Pediatric Infectious Disease.* 2nd ed. Philadelphia, Pa: WB Saunders Co; 1987:1845.

Kirsch JR, Diringer MN, Borel CO, Hart GK, Hanley DF. Brain resuscitation: medical management and innovations. *Crit Care Nurs Clin North Am.* 1989;1:143–154.

Klein JO, Feigin RD, McCracken GH. Report of the task force on diagnosis and management of meningitis. *Pediatrics.* 1986;78(suppl):959–982.

Kochanek PM, Uhl MW, Schoettle RJ. Hypoxic-ischemic encephalopathy: pathobiology and therapy of the postresuscitation syndrome in children. In: Fuhrman BP, Zimmerman JJ, eds. *Pediatric Critical Care.* St Louis, Mo: Mosby–Year Book Inc; 1992:637–657.

Krag MH. Biomechanics of thoracolumbar spinal fixation: a review. *Spine.* 1991;16(suppl):84–99.

Kramer ED, Packer RJ. Chemotherapy of malignant brain tumors in children. *Clin Neuropharmacol.* 1992;15:163–185.

Lacayo A, Farmer PM. Brain tumors in children: a review. *Ann Clin Lab Sci.* 1991;21(1):26–35.

Lang SM, Bernardo LM. SCIWORA syndrome: nursing assessment. *Dimens Crit Care Nurs.* 1993;12:247–254.

Littrell KA, Cantwell GP. Pediatric status epilepticus: managing the complexities. *J Emerg Med Systems.* 1991;Feb:71–79.

Liu TH, Beckman JS, Freeman BA, Hogan EL, Hsu CY. Polyethylene glycol–conjugated superoxide dismutase and catalase reduce ischemic brain injury. *Am J Physiol.* 1989;256:H589–H593.

Lovasik DA, Kerr ME. Controversial treatments of the traumatic brain-injured patient. *Am J Nurs.* 1993;(suppl):28.

Mann DC, Dodds JA. Spinal injuries in 57 patients 17 years or younger. *Orthopedics.* 1993;16:159–164.

Marlow DR, Redding BA. *Textbook of Pediatric Nursing.* 6th ed. Philadelphia, Pa: WB Saunders Co; 1988:1193–1199.

Marshall SB, Marshall LF, Vos HR, Chestnut RM. Head injury and the treatment of increased intracranial pressure. In: *Neuroscience Critical Care: Pathophysiology and Patient Management.* Philadelphia, Pa: WB Saunders Co; 1990:169.

Mason KJ, Wright S. Altered musculoskeletal function. In: Betz A, Hunsberger M, Wright S, eds. *Family-Centered Nursing Care of Children.* 2nd ed. Philadelphia, Pa: WB Saunders Co; 1994:1815–1873.

Mason PJB. Neurodiagnostic testing in critically injured adults. *Crit Care Nurse.* 1992;12(8):64–75.

McEvoy GK. *AHFS Drug Information.* Bethseda, Md: American Society of Hospital Pharmacists; 1990.

McIntyre JP, Keen GA. Laboratory surveillance of viral meningitis by examination of cerebrospinal fluid in Cape Town, 1981–9. *Epidemiol Infect.* 1993;111:357–371.

McMicken DB. Emergency CT head scans in traumatic and atraumatic conditions. *Ann Emerg Med.* 1986;15:274–279.

McNair N. Arteriovenous malformations. *Crit Care Nurse.* 1988;8(4):35–40.

McQuillan KA. Intracranial pressure monitoring: technical imperatives. *AACN Clin Issues Crit Care Nurs.* 1991;2:623–636.

Menkes JH. Introduction: neurologic examination of the child and infant. In: Menkes JH, ed. *Textbook of Child Neurology.* Philadelphia, Pa: Lea & Febiger; 1990:1–26.

Michaels RH, Ali O. A decline in *Haemophilus influenzae* type b meningitis. *J Pediatr.* 1993;122:407–409.

Mitchell PH. Neurologic disorders. In: Kinney MG, Packa DR, Dunbar SB, eds. *AACN's Clinical Reference for Critical-Care Nursing.* New York, NY: McGraw-Hill Book Co; 1988:971–1028.

Moore K. *The Developing Human.* 4th ed. Philadelphia, Pa: WB Saunders Co; 1988.

Muizelaar JP, Wei EP, Kontos HA, Becker DP. Mannitol causes compensatory cerebral vasoconstriction and vasodilation in response to blood viscosity changes. *J Neurosurg.* 1983;59:822–828.

Mulligan CM, Wittman BK. Nursing care of the child with a brain stem glioma. *J Pediatr Nurs.* 1990;5:375–386.

National Head Injury Foundation. *Definition of Traumatic Brain Injury.* Southborough, Mass: National Head Injury Foundation; 1986.

Nelson VS. Pediatric head injury. *Phys Med Rehabil Clin North Am.* 1992;3:461–474.

Nevo Y, Jurgenson U, Harel S. Cranial auscultation in two children with intracranial vascular malformation. *Dev Med Child Neurol.* 1994;36:545–553.

Newman K, Bowman L, Eichelburger M, et al. The lap belt complex: intestinal and lumbar spine injury in children. *J Trauma.* 1990;30:1133–1139.

Noback CR, Strominger NL, Demarest RJ. *The Human Nervous System: Introduction and Review.* 4th ed. Philadelphia, Pa: Lea & Febiger; 1991.

Nolan S. Current trends in the management of acute spinal cord injury. *Crit Care Nurs Q.* 1994;17:64–78.

Orlowski JP, Rothner AD. Diagnosis and treatment of status epilepticus. In: Fuhrman BP, Zimmerman JJ, eds. *Pediatric Critical Care.* St Louis, Mo: Mosby–Year Book Inc; 1992:595–604.

O'Sullivan MG, Statham PF, Jones PA, et al. Role of intracranial pressure monitoring in severely head-injured patients without signs of intracranial hypertension on initial computerized tomography. *J Neurosurg.* 1994;80:46–50.

Outwater KM, Rockoff MA. Apnea testing to confirm brain death in children. *Crit Care Med.* 1984;12:357–358.

Owen DB, Levin DL. Reye's syndrome. In: Levin DL, Morris FC, eds. *The Essentials of Pediatric Intensive Care.* St Louis, Mo: Quality Medical Publishers; 1991:226–231.

Packer RJ. Diagnosis, treatment, and outcome of primary central nervous system tumors of childhood. *Curr Opin Oncol.* 1994;6:240–246.

Pang D, Wilberger JE. Spinal cord injury without radiographic abnormalities in children. *J Neurosurg.* 1982;57:114–129.

Partyka MB. Practical points in the care of the post-lumbar spine surgery patient. *J Post Anesth Nurs.* 1991;6:185–187.

Pedley TA, Scheuer ML, Walczak TS. Epilepsy. In: Rowland LP, ed. *Merritt's Textbook of Neurology.* 9th ed. Baltimore, Md: Williams & Wilkins; 1995:845–870.

Pezzotta S, Locateli D, Arico M. Brain tumours in infants. Preferred treatment options. *Drugs.* 1992;44:368–374.

Plum R, Posner JB. *The Diagnosis of Stupor and Coma.* 3rd ed. Philadelphia, Pa: FA Davis Co; 1982.

Pohl CA. Practical approach to bacterial meningitis in childhood. *Am Fam Physician.* 1993;47:1595–1603.

Quagliarello V, Scheld WM. Bacterial meningitis: pathogenesis, pathophysiology, and progress. *N Engl J Med.* 1992;327:864–872.

Reigel D. Spina bifida. In: McLaurin R, Schut L, Venes J, Epstein F, eds. *Pediatric Neurosurgery.* 2nd ed. Philadelphia, Pa: WB Saunders Co; 1989:35–52.

Renshaw TS. Spinal cord injury and posttraumatic deformities. In: Weinstein SL, ed. *The Pediatric Spine: Principles and Practice.* New York, NY: Raven Press Publishers; 1994:767–780.

Reynolds EA. Controversies in caring for the child with a head injury. *MCN.* 1992;17:246–251.

Rogers MC, Kirsch JR. Current concepts in brain resuscitation. *JAMA.* 1989;261:3143–3147.

Rozmus C. Periventricular-intraventricular hemorrhage in the newborn. *MCN.* 1992;17:74–81.

Safar P. Cerebral resuscitation after cardiac arrest: a review. *Circulation.* 1986;74(suppl IV):138–153.

Safar P. Resuscitation from clinical death: pathophysiologic limits and therapeutic potentials. *Crit Care Med.* 1988;16:923–941.

Schickncer DJ, Young RF. Intracranial pressure monitoring: fiberoptic monitor compared with the ventricular catheter. *Surg Neurol.* 1992;37:251–254.

Schynoll Q, Overton D, Krome R, et al. A prospective study to identify high-yield criteria associated with acute intracranial computed tomography findings in head-injured patients. *Am J Emerg Med.* 1993;11:321–325.

Shattuck KE, Chonmaitree T. The changing spectrum of neonatal meningitis over a fifteen-year period. *Clin Pediatr.* 1992;31:130–136.

Shewmon A. Commentary on guidelines for the determination of brain death in children. *Issues Clin Neurosci.* 1988;24:789–791.

Sieber FE, Traystman RJ. Special issues: glucose and the brain. *Crit Care Med.* 1992;20:104–114.

Shiminski-Maher T, Abbott R, Wisoff JH, Epstein FJ. Current trends in the management of brainstem tumors in childhood. *J Neurosci Nurs.* 1991;23:356–362.

Slota MC. Neurological assessment of the infant and toddler. *Crit Care Nurse.* 1983;3:87–94.

Slota MC. Pediatric neurological assessment. *Crit Care Nurse.* 1983;3:106–12.

Snow RB, Zimmerman RD, Gandy SE, Deck MDF. Comparison of magnetic resonance imaging and computed tomography in the evaluation of head injury. *Neurosurgery.* 1986;18:45–52.

Spivak JM, Balderston RA. Spinal instrumentation. *Curr Opin Rheumatol.* 1994;6:187–194.

Steen PA, Gisvold SE, Milde JH, et al. Nimodipine improves outcome when given after complete cerebral arrest in primates. *Anesthesiology.* 1985;62:406–414.

Stewart-Amidei C, Hill LL. Subarachnoid hemorrhage in children: a nursing perspective. *J Neurosci Nurs.* 1986;18(2):63–70.

Swaiman K. Spinal fluid examination. In: Swaiman L, ed. *Pediatric Neurology.* St Louis, Mo: The CV Mosby Co; 1989.

Tasker RC, Dean JM. Status epilepticus. In: Rogers MC, ed. *Textbook of Pediatric Intensive Care.* Baltimore, Md: Williams & Wilkins; 1992:751–777.

Tasker RC, Dean JM, Rogers MC. Reye syndrome and metabolic encephalopathies. In: Rogers MC, ed. *Textbook of Pediatric Intensive Care.* Baltimore, Md: Williams & Wilkins; 1992:778–804.

Trauner DA. Toxic and metabolic encephalopathies. In: David RB, ed. *Pediatric Neurology for the Clinician.* Norwalk, Conn: Appleton & Lange; 1992;153–168.

Traystman RJ, Kirsch JR, Koehler RC. Oxygen radical mechanisms of brain injury following ischemia and reperfusion. *J Appl Physiol.* 1991;71:1185–1195.

Unwin DH, Giller CA, Lopitnik TA. Central nervous system monitoring: what helps, what does not. *Surg Clin North Am.* 1991;71:733–747.

Vernon-Levett P. Head injuries in children. *Crit Care Nurs Clin North Am.* 1991;3:411–421.

Vernon-Levett P. Neurologic critical care problems. In: Curley MAQ, Smith JB, Moloney-Harmon PA, eds. *Critical Care Nursing of Infants and Children.* Philadelphia, Pa: WB Saunders Co; 1996:656–694.

Vos HR. Making headway with intracranial hypertension. *Am J Nurs.* 1993;93:28–39.

Walleck CA. Controversies in the management of the head-injured patient. *Crit Care Nurs Clin North Am.* 1989;1:67–74.

Walsh-Kelly C, Nelson DB, Smith DS, et al. Clinical predictors of bacterial versus aseptic meningitis in childhood. *Ann Emerg Med.* 1992;21:910–914.

Wauquier A, Edmonds HL, Clincke GHC. Cerebral resuscitation: pathophysiology and therapy. *Neurosci Biobehav Rev.* 1987;11:287–306.

Weil ML. Infections of the central nervous system. In: Menkes JH, ed. *Textbook of Child Neurology.* Philadelphia, Pa: Lea & Febiger; 1990:327–423.

Weinstein SL. Adolescent idiopathic scoliosis: prevalence and natural history. In: Weinstein SL, ed. *The Pediatric Spine Principles and Practice.* New York, NY: Raven Press Publishers; 1994:463–478.

Weiss BD. Bicycle-related head injuries. *Clin Sports Med.* 1994;13:99–112.

Welch K. The intracranial pressure in infants. *J Neurosurg.* 1980;52:693–699.

Wiggins CW, Loisel CW, Budock AM. Intracranial arteriovenous malformation in a neonate: aneurysm of the great vein of Galen. *Neonatal Network.* 1991;9:7–17.

Willis D, Harbit MD. Transcatheter arterial embolization of cerebral arteriovenous malformations. *J Neurosci Nurs.* 1990;22:280–284.

Yamakami I, Yamaura A. Effects of decompressive craniectomy on regional blood flow in severe head trauma patients. *Neurol Med Chir.* 1993;33:616–620.

Yokota H, Kurokawa A, Otsuka T, Kobayashi S, Nakazawa S. Significance of magnetic resonance imaging in acute head injury. *J Trauma.* 1991;31:351–357.

Yue NC. Advances in brain tumor imaging. *Curr Opin Neurol.* 1993;6:831–840.

Zegeer LJ. Oculocephalic and vestibulo-ocular responses: significance for nursing care. *J Neurosci Nurs.* 1989;21(1):46–55.

5 Renal System

CATHERINE L. HEADRICK

ESSENTIAL DEVELOPMENTAL ANATOMY

A. ANATOMIC LOCATION

The kidneys are positioned within the retroperitoneal space. The upper pole is located approximately in the area of the 12th thoracic vertebrae with the lower pole angling toward the abdomen. The right kidney lies slightly lower than the left.

B. ANATOMIC STRUCTURE

1. **Development:** All nephrons are formed by 28 weeks' gestation. Kidney weight doubles in the first month of life. Filtration and absorption capabilities are not developed until the epithelial cells of the nephrons mature. As the loop of Henle matures and elongates, the ability to concentrate urine improves. Infants are more vulnerable to dehydration and fluid overload because of their inability to concentrate or to excrete urine in response to changes in fluid status. Bladder capacity is age dependent: infants, 15 to 20 ml; adult bladder, 600 to 800 ml. The kidneys of infants and children are relatively large for their body size and age, making them more susceptible to trauma.

2. **Gross structures**
   a. The capsule is the thin, fibrous, tough outer covering of the kidney.
   b. The outer portion of the kidney is the cortex. It contains all the glomeruli, the proximal and distal convoluted tubules, the first portions of the loop of Henle, and the collecting ducts.
   c. The inner region contains the medulla and the pelvis. The medulla has a pyramidal shape and contains primarily the collecting ducts and loops of Henle. The pelvis forms the upper end of the ureter. It is formed by the merging of the collecting ducts and tubular structures. It provides the pathway of urine from the kidney to the ureter. The fluid in the pelvis is identical to urine.

3. **Gross renal vasculature:** Approximately 20% of the total cardiac output is delivered to the kidneys. Two renal arteries branch from the descending aorta, and each renal artery branches repeatedly into arterioles.

4. **Microscopic structure**
   a. The nephron is the functional unit of the kidney. Each mature kidney has approximately 1 million nephrons. The nephron wall is composed of a single layer of epithelial cells. The top end (origin) of the nephron is called Bowman's capsule. Bowman's capsules are always found in the cortex. The fluid in Bowman's capsule is a filtrate of blood plasma.
   b. There are two types of nephrons. Cortical nephrons (85% of nephrons)

originate in the outer portion of the cortex and have short loops of Henle that reach only the outer region of the medulla. Juxtaglomerular nephrons originate closer to the medulla, have very long loops of Henle that reach deep into the medulla, and are important for water conservation in the body.

  c. The nephron can be divided into three parts: vascular components, tubular components, and collecting ducts.

  - Vascular components of the nephron: Within Bowman's capsule is a capillary bed, called the glomerulus (Bowman's capsule and the glomerulus may be referred to collectively as the "glomerulus"). Afferent arterioles bring blood to the glomerulus. Efferent arterioles take blood as it exits the glomerulus to the second capillary bed of peritubular capillaries, which supply the proximal and distal tubules in the cortex. Efferent arterioles of juxtaglomerular nephrons send off branches to create the vasa recta, a loop of straight vessels that stretch deep down to supply the medulla, descending alongside the descending limbs of the loop of Henle and back up toward the cortex.

  - Tubular components of the nephron: The proximal tubule is proximal to Bowman's capsule. The tubule begins as coiled and convoluted (proximal convoluted tubule) and then straightens as it extends into the medulla. The descending limb of the loop of Henle is a long, thin tubule that extends deep into the medulla. At its deepest point in the medulla, it turns sharply upward toward the cortex. The ascending limb of the loop of Henle is considerably thicker than the descending limb. It becomes continuous with the distal tubule. The distal tubule is a coiled, convoluted structure responsible for final adjustments of filtrate.

  - Collecting ducts gather fluid from several nephrons and drain into larger ducts, which drain into the minor calices in the renal pelvis.

PHYSICAL ASSESSMENT

A. PAST MEDICAL HISTORY
Past medical history includes significant prenatal history, pain (frequency, intensity, type, and location), unexplained or frequent itching, edema, unusual thirst or dry mouth, change in urinary patterns (for example, increase or decrease in number of wet diapers), change in activity level (lethargy may be secondary to anemia due to the lack of erythropoietin production), and hypertension.

B. ABDOMINAL INSPECTION
Abdominal inspection provides a gross assessment of the gastrointestinal and genitourinary systems. Assessment and findings related to the genitourinary system may include abdominal distention or striae (which may indicate fluid retention) and a sallow complexion (which may be a result of urochrome deposits in the skin).

C. AUSCULTATION
Auscultation of the abdominal region generally does not offer significant information related to renal function.

D. PERCUSSION
Dullness above the symphysis pubis may be indicative of a full bladder.

E. PALPATION
Kidneys are rarely palpable except in neonates. Enlarged kidneys may be indicative of tumor or hydronephrosis. A distended bladder may be palpable under the symphysis pubis.

ESSENTIAL PHYSIOLOGY AND CLINICAL ASSESSMENT OF RENAL FUNCTION

A. **BASIC TRANSPORT MECHANISMS**

1. During **active transport,** substances combine with a carrier and, with the help of adenosine triphosphate (ATP), diffuse against the concentration gradient and through the tubular membrane. Sodium, glucose, amino acids, calcium, potassium, chloride, bicarbonate, and phosphate are reabsorbed from the tubule by active transport.

2. **Passive transport** involves movement of substances in response to changes in the concentration gradient, without the assistance of ATP or a carrier. Diffusion is the spontaneous movement of solutes across a semipermeable membrane from a high concentration to a lesser concentration. As water reabsorbs out of the tubule and urea concentration in the tubule increases, urea diffuses out of the tubule. Osmosis is the spontaneous movement of water across a semipermeable membrane from an area of lesser solute concentration to an area of greater solute concentration. As sodium is reabsorbed from the tubule and concentration increases outside the tubule, water moves out of the tubule to balance the concentration gradient. Serum colloid osmotic pressure is the opposing pressure preventing free water from moving out of the vascular space.

B. **URINE FORMATION**

Urine formation involves the following physiologic processes: filtration, reabsorption, and secretion.

1. **Filtration**

   a. Fluid and various substances, known as the glomerular filtrate, are filtered from the plasma through the porous walls of the glomerular capillaries into Bowman's capsule and on to the renal tubules. Glomerular filtrate is primarily composed of water; it is essentially the same substance as blood plasma except for the larger protein molecules.

   b. The pathway for filtration is through capillary fenestrations across the basement membrane and through slit passages (formed by vacant spaces between the foot processes of podocytes of the epithelial cell layer). The ability and resistance to passing through filtration pathways depends on size, shape, and electrical charge of the molecules. Albumin (protein) molecules are too large to permeate the glomerular membrane, creating a high osmotic pressure that opposes orthostatic filtration from the vascular space.

   c. The "forcing" pressure, or filtration pressure, is the net pressure acting to force substances out of the glomerulus.

   - The primary force is the hydrostatic pressure of the blood inside the capillaries generated by the pumping action of the heart.
   - The secondary forces are the osmotic pressure of the plasma in the glomerular capillaries and the hydrostatic pressure in Bowman's capsule.
   - Filtration pressure can be expressed as the forces favoring filtration minus the forces opposing filtration.

$$\text{Filtration} = \begin{pmatrix} \text{Glomerular} & \text{Capillary} \\ \text{Hydrostatic} + \text{Hydrostatic} \\ \text{Pressure} & \text{Pressure} \end{pmatrix} - \begin{matrix} \text{Glomerular} \\ \text{Osmotic} \\ \text{Pressure} \end{matrix}$$

   d. Regulation of glomerular filtration rate (GFR)

   - Changes in filtration pressure can directly affect GFR. Factors affecting filtration pressure, and thus the GFR, include vasoconstriction or vasodilation of afferent and efferent arterioles, blood flow rate, tubule obstruc-

Table 5–1. FACTORS AFFECTING GLOMERULAR FILTRATION RATE (GFR)

FACTORS	PHYSIOLOGIC RESPONSE	NET EFFECT ON GFR
Afferent arteriole vasoconstriction or efferent arteriole vasodilation or both	Decreased blood flow Decreased glomerular hydration pressure	Decrease
Afferent arteriole vasodilation or efferent arteriole vasoconstriction	Blood backs up in the glomerulus Increased hydrostatic pressure	Increase
Decrease in plasma protein concentration	Decreased plasma osmotic pressure	Increase
Slow blood flow	Larger proportions of the plasma filters out of the glomerulus Plasma osmotic pressure rises	Decrease
Rapid blood flow	Less change in plasma osmotic pressure	Increase
Tubular obstruction	Fluid backs up in the renal tubules Hydrostatic pressure increases in Bowman's capsule	Decrease

tion, and changes in serum osmotic pressure. Renal blood flow is controlled by sympathetic nerve impulses that constrict arterioles. The effect on GFR depends on which arteriole is constricted (Table 5–1).

- Vasodilation and vasoconstriction are autoregulatory responses to changes in systemic arterial pressure. They occur to maintain constant renal blood flow and a stable GFR. A distal tubular feedback mechanism ensures constant delivery of filtrate to the distal tubule (Table 5–2)
- The effect of shock on GFR and renal function is detailed in Table 5–3.

e. Measuring filtration: Clearance is the volume of a specific substance filtered from the plasma over a designated period of time.

$$\text{Clearance (ml/min/1.7 m}^2) = \frac{\text{Concentration of Substance in Urine} \times \text{Volume of Urine Collected}}{\text{Plasma Concentration of that Substance}}$$

- Substances used to assess GFR include creatinine, inulin (nonmetabolizable sugar), and ^{131}I-iothalamate (Glofil; radioactive isotope).
- GFR is approximately equal to creatinine clearance. Creatinine is an endogenous waste product, produced by the muscles and excreted by the kidneys. Creatinine clearance may slightly overestimate GFR.
- GFR as measured by creatinine clearance:
  - First week of life: GFR = 15 to 20 ml/min/1.73 m^2

Table 5–2. AUTOREGULATORY RESPONSE

GFR increases
↓
Solute delivery (primarily chloride) to the juxtaglomerular apparatus increases
↓
Stimulates constriction of arteriole
↓
Decrease in GFR for that nephron

Table 5–3. RENAL RESPONSE TO SHOCK

Glomerular hydrostatic pressure falls
↓
Epithelial cells of the tubules do not receive
sufficient nutrients to support the high metabolic rate
↓
Cells die, tubular necrosis occurs
↓   ↓
Renal function may be lost   Regeneration of renal tubular epithelial cells
↓
Recovery of renal function

- ○ At the second week of life: GFR = 35 to 40 ml/min/1.73 m^2
- ○ At 6 months: GFR = 60 ml/min/m^2
- ○ At 1 year: GFR = 80 to 120 ml/min/m^2 (= Adult Norm)
- • Alteration in GFR occurs with decreased renal perfusion, changes in glomerular perfusion pressures (e.g., shock, glomerulonephritis), and decreases in plasma oncotic pressure (e.g., nephrotic syndrome).
- • The filtration fraction is the percent of fluid filtered into Bowman's capsule by the glomerulus in relationship to the total renal plasma flow (normal = 20%).

2. **Tubular reabsorption:** As fluid flows along the nephron, past the cells of the tubular wall, substances are reabsorbed from the renal tubule and returned to the blood via the peritubular capillaries.
   a. Most of tubular reabsorption occurs in the proximal tubule. By the time the filtrate reaches the end of the proximal tubule, two thirds of the water and virtually all the nutrients have been reabsorbed and returned to the blood. The proximal tubules play a role in acid-base balance and regulation of calcium, magnesium, and phosphorus. The proximal tubules have active transport systems for secretion of organic acids and bases from blood to tubule lumen.
   b. The tubular cells lining the walls of the proximal tubules are surrounded by two different membranes that aid in water and solute reabsorption. The convoluted portion of the proximal tubule has a brushlike border of microvilli that greatly increases surface area exposed to glomerular filtrate and enhances reabsorption. The basolateral membrane has no microvilli but has an abundance of sodium and potassium pumps and other diffusion transport systems for glucose and amino acids.
   c. Segments of the renal tubule use particular modes of transport to reabsorb certain substances. Substances reabsorbed by active transport depend on carriers. If the amount of substance exceeds the number of carriers (renal tubular threshold), the remaining substance will remain in the filtrate and be excreted in urine (e.g., glucosuria).
   d. Fluid reabsorption is determined by the net sodium reabsorption. If the GFR decreases, net sodium reabsorption decreases, and fluid reabsorption decreases. If the GFR increases, net sodium reabsorption increases, and fluid reabsorption increases.
   e. Several factors enhance the rate of fluid reabsorption from the renal tubule. The efferent arteriole is narrower than the peritubular capillary; therefore, blood flowing from the efferent arteriole to the peritubular capillary is under relatively low pressure. The wall of the renal capillary is more permeable than other capillaries.

f. The prime "mover" for most of the proximal tubular transport is the active transport of sodium. Water is reabsorbed by osmosis in response to the reabsorption of sodium ions by active transport. Amino acids and glucose are cotransported (reabsorbed) with sodium into the interstitial fluid and eventually to capillaries. When sodium is reabsorbed from the tubule, it takes chloride with it, changing the osmotic gradient and favoring the reabsorption of water into the interstitium and eventually to the capillaries. When water is absorbed from the tubule, the concentration of the remaining solutes increases, therefore increasing the diffusion of other solutes into the interstitial space and eventually to the capillaries.

g. Measuring reabsorption: The amount of solute reabsorbed is the difference between the amount of solute filtered into the glomerulus and the amount of solute excreted in the urine (assuming the amount filtered is greater than the amount excreted).

3. **Tubular secretion** is the process by which certain substances are removed from the blood or plasma of the peritubular capillary and added to the fluid of the renal tubule through active or passive transport.

a. Certain organic compounds (such as penicillin, creatinine, histamine) are actively secreted into tubular fluid by the epithelium of the proximal convoluted segment.

b. Hydrogen ions are secreted by the distal segment and the collecting ducts. Hydrogen ion secretion plays an important role in acid-base balance.

c. Potassium ions are secreted into tubular fluid because of the electrochemical attraction created by sodium reabsorption.

d. Measuring secretion: The amount of solute secreted is the difference between the amount of solute filtered into the glomerulus and the amount of solute excreted in the urine (assuming the amount filtered is less than the amount excreted). See Table 5–4.

C. WATER AND SODIUM BALANCE

1. **Measuring water balance and regulation of urine concentration:** Normal serum osmolarity is 272 to 290 mOsm/L. It is approximately equal to 2 times the serum sodium concentration. Normal urine osmolarity is approximately 300 mOsm/L. This usually correlates with the urine specific gravity. If renal function is adequate, urine-plasma osmolarity is a 1:1 or higher ratio. The osmolarity of the medullary portion of the kidney sets the limit for maximum urine concentration.

2. **Role of countercurrent mechanism in concentrating and diluting**

a. Filtrate concentration changes as it flows from the proximal tubule to the collecting ducts. Filtrate becomes increasingly concentrated as it moves from the proximal tubule through the descending limb to the loop of Henle. Maximum concentration occurs at the tip of the loop of Henle. Filtrate becomes less concentrated as it moves up the ascending limb of the loop and on to the collecting duct.

b. Juxtamedullary nephrons and the medullary portion of the kidney play a major role in this countercurrent mechanism. Sodium and chloride are actively reabsorbed out of the thick portion of the ascending limb into the interstitial space and peritubular capillaries, creating an osmotic gradient between the interstitium and the tubule. This segment of the tubule is impermeable to water, and water cannot be reabsorbed with sodium. In response to this osmotic gradient, water is passively reabsorbed out of the descending limb into the interstitium and peritubular capillaries. A concentration gradient is created, and filtrate is more dilute as it enters the collecting duct. As this dilute urine enters the distal tubule and collecting

Table 5–4. SUMMARY OF PHYSIOLOGIC FUNCTIONS OF NEPHRON COMPONENTS

COMPONENT	PRIMARY PHYSIOLOGIC FUNCTIONS
Vascular Components	
Glomerulus	Filtration of water and dissolved substances from plasma
Bowman's capsule	Pathway of glomerular filtrate to proximal tubule
Tubular Components	Secretion and reabsorption of solutes (sodium, chloride, glucose, bicarbonate) and water
Proximal convoluted tubule	Reabsorption of proteins, water, chloride ions, glucose, amino acids, creatine, lactic acid, citric acid, uric acid, ascorbic acid, phosphate ions, sulfate ions, calcium ions, potassium ions, sodium ions, bicarbonate (site for 60–70% Na^+ reabsorption from ultrafiltrate)
	Secretion of morphine, aspirin, penicillin, and other drugs; histamine, dopamine, epinephrine; fatty acids; hydrogen ions
	Filtrate leaves this section isotonic
Descending loop of Henle	Reabsorption of water
Ascending loop of Henle	Reabsorption of chloride and sodium ions (20–25% of sodium reabsorbed)
	Filtrate leaves this section hypotonic
Distal convoluted tubule	Final adjustments of filtrate
	Reabsorption of water, sodium ions (5–10% sodium reabsorbed)
	Secretion of hydrogen and potassium ions
	Site for ADH action to reabsorb water
	Site for aldosterone action to reabsorb sodium and water and secrete potassium
	Filtrate leaves this section hypotonic
Collecting Ducts	Gather fluid from several nephrons and transport fluid to calyces
	Similar actions of distal tubule
	Filtrate leaves this section hypotonic

ADH, antidiuretic hormone.

ducts, antidiuretic hormone (ADH) controls the amount of water reabsorption according to the need for dilute or concentrated urine. If dilute urine is needed, ADH is inhibited. If water conservation or concentrated urine is needed, ADH is activated.

3. **Hormonal control of water balance**

   a. Vasopressin, or ADH, plays a role in water balance. The distal convoluted tubule and collecting duct are impermeable to water, so water may be excreted as dilute urine. If ADH is present, the distal tubule and collecting ducts become permeable, water is reabsorbed, and urine is more concentrated. A rise in the solute concentration of the extracellular fluids and blood plasma stimulates cells in the hypothalamus to increase production of ADH and to cause release of ADH from the posterior pituitary. In the kidney, ADH initiates retention of water and decrease in solute concentration. Decreased solute concentration causes decreased ADH, which causes dilute urine. Increased solute concentration causes increased ADH, which causes concentrated urine.

   b. Aldosterone is important in maintaining volume homeostasis and the balance of substances such as sodium, potassium, and hydrogen ions. The adrenal cortex releases aldosterone in response to angiotensin II, hyperkalemia, hyponatremia, decreased pulse pressure, or decreased right atrial distention. Aldosterone stimulates reabsorption of sodium and water in the distal tubule and collecting duct. Aldosterone stimulates the secretion of potassium and hydrogen and decreases potassium reabsorption.

4. **Sodium and water reabsorption**

   a. Sodium concentration is higher in the lumen of the tubule than in the cells lining the tubule, so sodium moves into the tubular cells. Since the proximal tubule's brush border has no sodium pump, the sodium cannot be pumped back into the lumen. Only the basolateral membrane can pump out sodium into the interstitial spaces and then diffuse into the peritubular capillaries. When sodium (positively charged) is reabsorbed, it leaves the tubule and moves into the tubular wall. Negatively charged ions (chloride, phosphate, and bicarbonate) follow.

   b. Every sodium or chloride ion that leaves the tubule means the loss of osmotically active particles from the tubule to the interstitium. The movement of particles creates a change in osmotic gradient favoring water reabsorption, and water follows the sodium and chloride into the interstitium. With less sodium in the tubule, the concentration of solutes in the tubule increases, therefore increasing diffusion of other solutes out of the tubule and into the interstitial space. As water is reabsorbed from the filtrate into the peritubular capillaries, substances remaining in the tubule become more concentrated. As a result, water moves into the tubules. As sodium reabsorption increases, water reabsorption increases and vice versa.

   c. Alteration in the GFR influences the amount of sodium reabsorbed or secreted. When the GFR decreases (e.g., dehydration, sepsis), sodium and water reabsorption increases. Decreased volume decreases venous, atrial, and arterial pressures. Pressoreceptors decrease the number of impulses to the brain stem, which activates sympathetic impulses to stimulate renin release from the juxtaglomerular cells in the afferent arterioles. Renin is converted to angiotensin I, which is converted to angiotensin II, which causes vasoconstriction and secretion of aldosterone. This creates "thirst" in an effort to increase volume. As water volume increases, ADH is secreted to maintain water and solute balance.

D. **ELECTROLYTE BALANCE**

   1. **Potassium ion (K^+)**

      a. Potassium has a normal serum value of 3.5 to 5.5 mEq/L. It is the most abundant solute inside cells (145 mEq/L) with a very small amount present in the serum. Potassium is an important factor in the performance of many enzyme systems, playing a role in the maintenance of cell volume, pH, and cell excitability (membrane potentials).

      b. Decreasing serum potassium depolarizes membranes and raises excitability (e.g., cardiac rhythm deterioration leading to fibrillation). Increasing serum potassium hyperpolarizes membranes and decreases excitability (e.g., skeletal and smooth muscle weakness and decreased reflexes). Potassium shifts frequently occur secondary to acid-base balance changes, hormone imbalance, and pharmacologic agents.

      c. Most potassium is reabsorbed in the proximal tubule and the loop of Henle. The distal tubule and collecting ducts have a high concentration of intracellular potassium due to the action of the sodium-potassium pumps. Changes in renal regulation of potassium are due to changes in potassium secretion in the distal tubule and collecting duct. Increases in intracellular potassium increase secretion and excretion of potassium. Increases in plasma potassium stimulate the adrenal cortex to secrete aldosterone, which promotes secretion and excretion of potassium.

   d. In acidosis, potassium excretion decreases. Distal tubular and collecting duct cells lose potassium to the plasma, leakage and secretion of potassium into tubules decrease, and potassium shifts from the cells into the plasma. In alkalosis, potassium excretion increases. Potassium increases in the distal tubule and collecting duct. Leakage and secretion of potassium increases. Potassium shifts into the cells. With a shift from acidosis to alkalosis, serum potassium decreases because of the shift into the cells.

2. **Sodium**
   a. The normal serum value is approximately 135 to 145 mEq/L. In nonoliguric patients with large sodium losses, hyponatremia may lead to seizure activity. In oliguric patients with minimal sodium losses, hypernatremia leads to edema and hypertension. Dilutional hyponatremia occurs secondary to hypotonic fluid intake and unrecognized oliguric acute renal failure (ARF). The hyponatremia corrects slowly with free water diuresis.
   b. Management may include dialysis or continuous renal replacement therapy for severe or symptomatic hyponatremia (serum Na^+ <125 mEq/L) in the oliguric, hypervolemic patient *or* oliguric, hypernatremic patient (Na^+ >150 mEq/L). Hyponatremic metabolic acidosis may be treated with administration of sodium, partly in the form of sodium bicarbonate. Administer normal saline for fluid loss and dehydration. Administer 3% normal saline for volume overload.

3. **Phosphate (phosphorus, inorganic)**
   a. Normal serum values in the newborn are 4.2 to 9 mg/dl. Normal values in children 1 to 5 years of age are 3.5 to 6.5 mg/dl and in older children range from 2.5 to 4.5 mg/dl. Renal excretion of phosphate is the body's primary mechanism for regulation of phosphate; therefore, patients in renal failure are at high risk for hyperphosphatemia.
   b. Parathyroid hormone (PTH) indirectly affects serum phosphate levels by affecting calcium. Phosphate and calcium are reabsorbed from the bone. Tubular reabsorption of phosphate is decreased as tubular reabsorption of sodium increases. PTH enhances intestinal absorption of calcium and phosphate. Vitamin D is converted to its active form by the liver and kidneys, which regulates phosphate and calcium balance. Active absorption of phosphate (and calcium) by the intestine is stimulated by vitamin D. Reabsorption of phosphate and calcium from bone to extracellular fluid is facilitated by vitamin D. Vitamin D stimulates renal tubular reabsorption of phosphate and calcium.

4. **Calcium**
   a. The normal serum value is 9 to 11 mg/dl (total calcium) and 5.4 to 6.6 mg/dl (ionized calcium). Calcium exists in two forms: ionized and nonionized. Approximately 45% to 50% is ionized, meaning "free" and not bound to albumin. Albumin-bound calcium is not filtered at the glomerulus. Decreased serum albumin levels may affect serum calcium levels.
   b. PTH is the most important regulator of calcium. Hypocalcemia stimulates the release of PTH, which decreases renal excretion of calcium and increases urinary excretion of sodium. Hypercalcemia inhibits the release of PTH.

5. **Magnesium:** The normal serum values are 1.2 to 1.8 mEq/L. Eighty percent of plasma magnesium is filtered at the glomerulus, and only a small amount of this filtrate is excreted. Increased extracellular fluid volume stimulates increased magnesium excretion. Decreased extracellular fluid volume inhibits magnesium excretion.

E. REGULATION OF ACID-BASE BALANCE

1. **Definitions:** An acid is a source of hydrogen ions. A base takes up or absorbs hydrogen ions. A buffer combines with an acid or base to maintain a stable pH.

2. In an effort to achieve an acid-base balance, the lungs regulate carbon dioxide and the kidneys regulate bicarbonate. With normal digestion, metabolic acids (hydrogen ions) are produced. Metabolic hydrogen ions are picked up by serum bicarbonate and form carbon dioxide. An increased level of carbon dioxide and hydrogen ions stimulates increased respiration, which helps eliminate carbon dioxide and reverse acidosis. Respiratory regulation of acid-base balance is generally inadequate in severe metabolic acidosis and alkalosis.

3. The kidney regulates acid-base balance through hydrogen secretion and bicarbonate reabsorption. Hydrogen ions are secreted (removed from the blood and plasma of the peritubular capillary and added to the fluid of the renal tubule) at the distal tubule and the collecting duct.

   a. *Renal response in alkalotic conditions:* Potassium excretion increases. Chloride is reabsorbed with sodium, and bicarbonate is excreted. If an increase in filtrate bicarbonate is secondary to increased serum concentration, bicarbonate excretion increases. If an increase in filtrate bicarbonate is secondary to hypovolemia, hydrogen ion secretion and bicarbonate reabsorption from the tubules increases, preventing excretion of excess bicarbonate. Alkalosis is corrected as volume status is restored.

   b. *Renal response in acidotic conditions:* Potassium excretion decreases. Bicarbonate is reabsorbed with sodium, and chloride is excreted. Bicarbonate diffuses into the extracellular compartment and ultimately into the plasma (via the renal vein), resulting in reabsorption of hydrogen ions. Renal excretion of acid (ammonium excretion) increases.

F. REGULATION OF ARTERIAL BLOOD PRESSURE

1. **Maintenance of circulating blood volume:** Circulating blood volume is maintained by sodium and water balance. A countercurrent mechanism plays a role in concentrating and diluting. Hormonal control of water balance is mediated by ADH and aldosterone.

2. Regulation of peripheral vascular resistance is via the renin-angiotensin-aldosterone system and the CNS. Juxtaglomerular cells release renin in response to a decrease in glomerular pressure (renal perfusion pressure), an increase in sympathetic nervous system stimulation, decreased sodium in the distal tubule, or vasoconstrictive agents. Renin diffuses into the circulatory system and converts angiotensinogen into angiotensin I. As angiotensin I circulates to the lungs, it converts to angiotensin II (and also produces aldosterone). Angiotensin II is a powerful vasoconstrictor of the peripheral vascular system. Angiotensin II stimulates aldosterone secretion, which causes an increase in water and sodium reabsorption. The sympathetic nervous system also regulates peripheral vascular resistance by causing vasoconstriction.

G. REGULATION OF RENAL BLOOD FLOW

Prostaglandins are vasoactive substances that act by either dilating or constricting renal vessels. Their effect is limited to the renal vasculature. Three prostaglandins are produced by cells in the kidney's cortical and medullary structures. Thromboxane A_2 is a vasoconstrictor. Prostacyclin (PGI_2) and prostaglandin E_2 (PGE_2) are vasodilators. **PGI$_2$ and PGE$_2$** produce direct vasodilation of afferent arterioles, which helps to maintain renal blood flow and glomerular perfusion. PGE$_2$ increases urine output by counteracting the actions of ADH. PGE$_2$ increases sodium excretion by inhibiting its reabsorption from the renal tubules.

H. ELIMINATION OF DRUGS, TOXINS, AND METABOLIC WASTES

1. **Urea** is produced in the liver as a by-product of amino acid metabolism. Amino acids and proteins are metabolized in the liver and yield ammonia, which is very toxic unless rapidly detoxified into urea. About 50% of urea is passively reabsorbed, and 50% is excreted in the urine. In the presence of ADH, urea is trapped because the upper portions of the collecting duct are impermeable to urea; as water is reabsorbed, the urea becomes concentrated, thus increasing intracellular fluid solute concentration.

2. **Uric acid** is a by-product of metabolism of certain organic bases in nucleic acids. Ninety percent is reabsorbed in the glomerular filtrate, and 10% is secreted into the renal tubule.

3. **Creatinine** is the end product of protein metabolism. Under normal conditions, creatinine is completely filtered by the kidneys and excreted in the urine. Its complete elimination makes it an excellent marker of renal function. The creatinine level is proportional to the blood urea nitrogen (BUN) level. The normal BUN:creatinine ratio is 10 to 15:1. An increase in both BUN and creatinine signals renal dysfunction. An increase in BUN without an increase in creatinine may be an indication of dehydration, decreased renal perfusion, or catabolism.

I. STIMULATION OF BONE MARROW ERYTHROCYTE PRODUCTION

1. The kidneys play a role in the production of erythropoietin and red blood cells. Erythropoietin is synthesized in the renal cortex. A decrease in oxygen delivery to the kidneys secondary to anemia, hypoxia, or decreased renal blood flow triggers the release of erythropoietin from the kidney. Erythropoietin induces the bone marrow to produce additional red blood cells. If renal function is compromised, the production of erythropoietin and subsequent red blood cell production decrease.

2. Intravenous (IV) recombinant human erythropoietin is available for treatment of anemia secondary to chronic renal failure. Side effects include hypertension, seizures, and vascular access thrombus formation.

ACUTE RENAL FAILURE (ARF)

A. DEFINITIONS

1. ARF is the sudden loss of renal capacity for filtration and tubular reabsorption, resulting in accumulation of wastes, fluid and electrolyte imbalance, and acid-base imbalances.

2. Postrenal failure is usually associated with obstruction of urine flow at any point in the ureters, bladder, or urethral meatus caused by such conditions as Wilms' tumor, renal calculi, blood clots, or edema. ARF secondary to postrenal failure is a relatively small percentage of the cases of ARF.

3. Prerenal failure, the most common cause of ARF, usually is caused by poor perfusion. A decrease in renal perfusion causes decrease in glomerular perfusion and GFR. Impaired renal blood flow may be secondary to impaired cardiac performance, intravascular volume depletion, renal vasoconstriction, or renal artery thrombosis. There is a good prognosis for kidney function if prompt recognition and restoration of adequate renal blood flow is achieved.

4. Intrarenal failure is described below as acute tubular necrosis related to decreased perfusion to the renal parenchyma.

B. **INTRARENAL FAILURE (ACUTE TUBULAR NECROSIS [ATN])**

1. **Definition:** When mean arterial blood pressure drops significantly, renal autoregulatory processes are no longer functional, which often leads to development of ATN and uremic syndrome. Multiple factors (including systemic maldistribution of volume and decrease in blood flow secondary to circulating mediators) affect blood and oxygen delivery to the kidneys.

2. **Etiology**
   a. Nephrotoxic ATN is a toxic insult to the renal tubules secondary to nephrotoxic drugs, radiographic contrast dye, organic solvents, or inappropriate levels of hemoglobin or myoglobin. Tubular epithelium necrosis occurs. The healing process and prognosis are better than that for ischemic ATN because the supporting basement membrane is not affected.
   b. Ischemic ATN (hemodynamically mediated renal failure) is a sudden and sustained decline of GFR and necrosis of the tubule cells secondary to nephrotoxic injury. Compensatory and autoregulatory mechanisms are exhausted. Renal oxygen delivery is critically impaired, causing tubular and cellular damage. The body attempts to compensate and maintain adequate renal blood flow and GFR by sodium and water retention, which results in decreased urine output. Oliguric ATN has a much worse prognosis than nonoliguric ATN.

3. **Pathophysiology**
   a. Vasoactive factors: Arteriolar vasoconstriction is induced.
   b. Tubular factors: As the hydrostatic pressure increases, there is back leak from the tubular lumen to the vasa recta. Cellular sloughing and casts cause tubular obstruction.
   c. Vascular factors: In low blood flow states, nephrotoxins are concentrated in the renal tubular cells. Glomerular capillary permeability increases for proteins and decreases for potassium.
   d. Metabolic factors: Damage to the cell membrane and impaired cellular function occur as the calcium flux is altered and oxygen free radicals are formed.

4. **The clinical course** of ATN can be divided into four phases:
   a. The *onset, or initiating phase,* is the time from the precipitating event until cell injury occurs. The duration is hours to days. It may correspond with prerenal failure. Renal failure is reversible at this point. It may be hours for postischemic ATN vs. days for nephrotoxic ATN.
   b. The *oliguric phase* is the time from cell injury to the development of uremia. Duration is 1 to 2 weeks. Oliguria (urine output <1 ml/kg/h) is more common in postischemic ATN. Nonoliguria is more common in nephrotoxic ATN. Anuria (no urine output) is uncommon in ATN, and more common in postrenal obstruction. The following events characterize development of severe nephron dysfunction and uremia or uremic syndrome during this phase:
      • GFR is significantly decreased.
      • Hypervolemia occurs.
      • BUN and plasma creatinine increase.
      • Electrolyte imbalances occur.
      • Metabolic acidosis is present.
      • Side effects of the accumulation of uremic toxins are evident.
   c. The *diuretic phase* is the beginning of recovery characterized by improved

urine output, increased urea excretion, and solute excretion. Duration is 7 to 14 days. Signs of gradual improvement of overall renal function occur. In the early part of the phase, urine output dramatically increases each day. In the beginning of the diuretic phase, "dumb" urine is excreted; "dumb" urine is similar to filtrate and shows little function of reabsorption or secretion. Throughout the diuretic phase, urea excretion and solute reabsorption and secretion improve. By the end of the this phase, BUN has fallen and stabilized, electrolyte balance and acidosis are improved, and GFR begins to return to normal. Renal replacement therapy may be indicated during this phase until kidney function has returned enough to control fluid and electrolyte balance. Administration of fluid to replace urine output may be necessary if the patient's volume status and assessment indicate.

    d. During the *recovery phase,* renal function slowly reoccurs. It may take years for renal function to return to normal. There may be residual damage, and a certain percentage of unrecoverable renal function.

C. **INVASIVE AND NONINVASIVE DIAGNOSTIC TOOLS**

    1. **Prerenal failure vs. ATN:** Diagnostic laboratory values (urine and serum) are detailed in Table 5–5.

    2. **Other diagnostic tools**

        a. *Radiologic consultation* may be helpful if serum and urine laboratory values are inconclusive. The risk of intravenous pyelography (IVP) outweighs its benefit.

        b. *Ultrasonography* documents the presence and size of one or two kidneys and allows for assessment of the collection system, renal parenchyma, and vessels. Azotemia and small kidneys indicate underlying chronic renal disease. Enlarged kidneys indicate hydronephrosis, renal vein thrombosis, nephrotic syndrome, cystic disease, acute glomerulonephritis, or various infiltrative diseases.

        c. *Radionucleotide scanning* identifies renal perfusion and function (e.g., urinary tract obstruction, renal vein thrombosis, inflammatory conditions of the kidney, renal artery disease).

        d. *Renal biopsy* should be performed only when there is reasonable belief that the test results will alter therapy.

Table 5–5. DIAGNOSTIC LABORATORY VALUES (URINE AND SERUM)

	PRERENAL	**ATN**
Urine output	Decreased	Decreased or normal
Urine sediment	Normal	Red blood cell casts, cellular debris
Specific gravity	High (>1.020)	Low (≤1.010)
Osmolality (urine-to-plasma ratio)	>1.5 (>1.2 in neonates)	<1.2
Urine sodium	Low (<10 mEq/L)	High (>30 mEq/L) (>25 mEq/L in neonates)
Creatinine (urine-to-plasma ratio)	>15:1	<10:1
FE_{Na} (%)*	<1 (<2.5 in neonates)	>2 (>3 in neonates)
Creatinine	Normal or slowly increasing	High and increasing
BUN	High	High and increasing

*Excreted fraction of filtered sodium. Furosemide (Lasix) administration may affect results or measurement of urine sodium.

D. **CLINICAL MANIFESTATIONS OF ARF**

  1. **Hyperkalemia**

  a. Hyperkalemia occurs secondary to decreased renal excretion. Oliguric patients do not excrete sufficient potassium to maintain a normal balance. Hyperkalemia may be exacerbated by metabolic acidosis, which causes a shift of potassium from the intracellular space. Continued acid production occurs from catabolic cellular metabolism, despite loss of renal excretory function. Multiple blood transfusions and red blood cell hemolysis release potassium. The "older" the blood, the greater opportunity for cell breakdown and accumulation of potassium.

  b. *Electrocardiogram (ECG) changes secondary to hyperkalemia* can range from peaked T waves, prolonged PR interval, and complete heart block to ventricular fibrillation as the level of severity of hyperkalemia increases.

  c. *Other clinical manifestations* may include muscle cramps, muscle twitching, abdominal cramps, diarrhea, and ileus.

  d. *Management of hyperkalemia* depends on the severity of electrolyte imbalance. Patients with a serum potassium level greater than 7 mEq/L and evidence of myocardial toxicity are at an extremely high risk for lethal arrhythmias. Prompt and aggressive intervention is critical for survival.

  - Treatment measures include the administration of insulin (0.1 U/kg regular insulin) and hypertonic glucose (0.5 to 1 ml/kg 50% dextrose) to promote cellular uptake of potassium.
  - Movement of the potassium into the cells can be facilitated by hyperventilation and administration of sodium bicarbonate (1 to 3 mEq/kg). (CAUTION: Do not mix calcium and bicarbonate in IV solutions, since precipitation will occur.)
  - Eliminate exogenous sources of potassium (potassium-free hydration).
  - Remove potassium from the patient using resin exchange via the gastrointestinal tract with a Kayexalate enema (1 g/kg). (NOTE: Repeat the enema 2 to 3 times per 24-hour period if necessary.)
  - Stabilize the myocardium with IV calcium (0.2 to 0.3 ml/kg of 10% $CaCl_2$ or 0.5 to 1 ml/kg of 10% calcium gluconate).
  - Renal replacement therapy may be indicated if the K^+ level is life threatening or unresponsive to treatment. Hemodialysis is the most efficient treatment for life-threatening levels. The patient may be transitioned to continuous renal replacement therapy (CRRT) to maintain potassium regulation and homeostasis until renal function returns.

  e. *Desired patient outcomes*

  - Maintain normative K^+ values.
  - Maintain adequate urine output.
  - Absence of acidosis.
  - Absence of dysrhythmia.

  2. **Hyperphosphatemia**

  a. *Pathophysiology* involves decreased phosphate excretion in ARF. An elevation in serum phosphorus occurs when the GFR is less than 30 ml/min. It may be secondary to tumor lysis syndrome or use of sodium phosphate enemas in the presence of gastrointestinal tract abnormalities or renal insufficiency.

  b. *Hyperphosphatemia may not produce signs and symptoms* until levels are very high (above 10 mEq/L); however, a secondary hypocalcemia may develop as an attempt to compensate. See clinical manifestations under Hypocalcemia below.

  c. *Management of hyperphosphatemia* may include IV fluid therapy to increase phosphorus excretion or administration of IV calcium. Management of severe hyperphosphatemia (greater than 10 to 12 mEq/L) may include hemodialysis or renal replacement therapy to decrease phosphate levels.

3. **Hypocalcemia**
   a. *Pathophysiology:* Serum calcium declines reciprocally as phosphorus rises. Alterations in calcium most often occur secondary to hyperphosphatemia. Loop diuretics block tubular reabsorption of calcium and may cause hypocalcemia. Other reasons for hypocalcemia include induced resistance to the action of PTH, crush injury (occurs early), severe muscle damage, and large transfusions of citrate-containing blood products.
   b. *Clinical manifestations of calcium or phosphate imbalance* include central nervous system changes (anxiety, tetany, seizures), muscle cramps, hypotension, and Trousseau's and Chvostek's signs.
   c. *Management of hypocalcemia* includes decreasing the serum phosphate levels and replacing magnesium, if indicated, to increase PTH release. If symptomatic, administer IV 10% calcium gluconate (50 to 100 mg/kg per dose; maximum dose 2 g). If a more rapid response is required, use calcium chloride (10 to 20 mg/kg per dose [infants and children] and 37 to 74 mg/kg per dose [neonates]; maximum dose 1 g). Infuse slowly (do not exceed 1 ml/min) and monitor for bradycardia and asystole with IV calcium infusion. Extravasation with IV administration can cause severe tissue damage.
   d. In ARF, PTH's ability to serve as a regulator of phosphorus and calcium balance is compromised because of the alteration in the renal absorption of calcium and excretion of phosphate. Decreased synthesis of the active form of vitamin D results in hypocalcemia.

4. **Hypermagnesemia**
   a. Mild hypermagnesemia may occur in ARF secondary to decreased renal excretion of magnesium. It may be secondary to the use of magnesium-containing antacids (Maalox) or total parenteral nutrition (TPN).
   b. *Clinical manifestations:* Acute elevations may depress the central nervous system, peripheral neuromuscular junction, and deep tendon reflexes. There is an increased potential for hypotension, hypoventilation, and cardiac arrhythmias.
   c. *Management of hypermagnesemia* usually does not require intervention other than discontinuing magnesium-containing substances (e.g., Maalox). Calcium acts as a direct antagonist to magnesium. In life-threatening situations, IV calcium may be administered. *Dialysis may be used for* removal of magnesium, *since loop diuretics* in particular *enhance magnesium excretion.* PTH stimulates reabsorption of magnesium from the tubules.

5. **Glucose intolerance** may develop secondary to decreased peripheral sensitivity to insulin when renal excretion is decreased. Renal replacement therapy can remove glucose.

6. **Uremia** is related to the accumulation of toxins and waste products normally excreted in the urine and is measured as BUN. *Azotemia* refers to a high serum concentration of nitrogenous wastes.
   a. *Clinical manifestations* are due to toxic effects of substances such as urea and ammonia. Neurologic symptoms include lethargy, confusion, seizures, and coma. Gastrointestinal tract symptoms include anorexia, nausea, vomiting, diarrhea, and gastrointestinal tract bleeding. Cardiovascular symptoms include hypervolemia and hypotension secondary to shifts of fluid into the extracellular space. Hematologic compromise involves anemia, thrombocytopenia, platelet dysfunction, and increased bleeding time. Skin symptoms include pruritus and discoloration. Immunosuppression may result.

Table 5–6.   RENAL RESPONSE TO CHANGES IN ACID-BASE BALANCE

CHANGE IN ACID-BASE BALANCE	RENAL RESPONSE
Respiratory Acidosis	
Retaining of carbon dioxide and bicarbonate	Increase bicarbonate in plasma to take up hydrogen ions
Plasma hydrogen ions rise	Excretion of acid in urine
Respiratory alkalosis	
Increased elimination or blowing off of carbon dioxide	Increase excretion of bicarbonate to conserve hydrogen ions
Decreased plasma hydrogen ion concentration	
Metabolic Acidosis	
Decreased plasma bicarbonate and increased plasma hydrogen ion concentration	Replenish bicarbonate
Metabolic Alkalosis	
Increased plasma bicarbonate	Less intracellular hydrogen ion available for secretion
Decreased plasma and intracellular hydrogen ion concentration	Some bicarbonate escapes into the urine (alkaline urine)
Chronic Acidosis	Increase production of ammonia (NH_3) to bind with hydrogen ions and excrete ammonium (NH_4^+) in urine

    b. *Management* for symptomatic patients may include renal replacement therapy. BUN level is often a marker for indication for therapy, as well as response to treatment.

  7. **Acid-base imbalance**

    a. Metabolic acidosis occurs in ARF because of alterations in renal function including a decrease in GFR, decreased hydrogen ion secretion, decreased bicarbonate reabsorption, and decreased ammonia (NH_3) synthesis and ammonium (NH_4) excretion. Acidosis in ARF results in an increase in the anion gap.

$$\text{Anion Gap} = \text{Sodium} - (\text{Chloride} + \text{Bicarbonate*})$$

$$Na^+ - (Cl^- + HCO_3^-)$$

    b. *Clinical manifestations of acidosis* secondary to ARF include increased minute ventilation, change in mental status as ammonium excretion decreases, and hyperkalemia as potassium excretion decreases, causing an increased potential for lethal dysrhythmias.

    c. *Management* involves correction of metabolic acidosis. Minor adjustments may be made by hyperventilation. IV administration of bicarbonate is necessary for significant correction (Table 5–6).

  8. **Anemia and alteration in red blood cell production and availability** are related to decreased erythrocyte production, changes secondary to volume status (i.e., hemoconcentration or hemodilution), frequent blood sampling, and bleeding. Catabolism develops; as a result, BUN, acidosis, and hyperkalemia increase. Proper nutritional assessment is crucial in correcting catabolism and its complications. A diet high in calories but low in high–biologic value (high

---

* Serum bicarbonate content is represented by the serum carbon dioxide value from laboratory analysis.

amino acids and more liberation of urea nitrogen) protein is ideal. TPN is recommended for the patient who is unable to eat. A TPN calorie-to-nitrogen ratio of 450:1 is recommended. Alterations in potassium, phosphate, and magnesium may be necessary. Insulin infusion may be required to maintain normal serum glucose when using TPN with a large percentage of glucose.

9. Patients are at an increased risk for infection. They have an altered immune response secondary to suppression of macrophages by uremic toxins. Invasive lines increase the risk. Prophylactic antibiotic therapy is generally not indicated.

E. **POTENTIAL PATIENT PROBLEM LIST**
* HYPERVOLEMIA SECONDARY TO FLUID RETENTION DURING THE OLIGURIC OR ANURIC PHASE OF ATN
* HYPOVOLEMIA SECONDARY TO FLUID LOSS DURING THE DIURETIC PHASE OF ATN
* DECREASED CARDIAC OUTPUT RELATED TO DYSRHYTHMIAS AND ALTERATION IN VOLUME STATUS
* ELECTROLYTE IMBALANCE RELATED TO CHANGE IN FILTRATION OR CHANGE IN TUBULAR SECRETION AND EXCRETION
* MULTISYSTEM COMPLICATIONS RELATED TO ELECTROLYTE IMBALANCE
* ALTERATION IN SKIN INTEGRITY SECONDARY TO UREMIC TOXINS (PRURITUS, DRYNESS, FRAGILE CAPILLARIES, EASY BRUISING)
* ALTERATION IN MUCOUS MEMBRANES SECONDARY TO UREMIC TOXINS ON MUCOUS MEMBRANES
* ALTERATION IN CARDIAC FUNCTION (DYSRHYTHMIAS, INCREASED POTENTIAL FOR HYPOTENSION OR HYPERTENSION)
* ALTERATION IN MUSCULOSKELETAL SYSTEM (MUSCLE TWITCHING, MUSCLE WEAKNESS, DEPRESSED DEEP TENDON REFLEXES)
* ALTERATION IN ACID-BASE BALANCE
* INCREASED RISK FOR INFECTION RELATED TO INVASIVE CATHETERS AND ALTERED IMMUNE RESPONSE
* ALTERATION IN COMFORT RELATED TO PAIN, MULTIPLE PROCEDURES, CHANGES IN SKIN INTEGRITY, AND NAUSEA OR VOMITING
* ALTERATION IN NUTRITION RELATED TO DECREASED INTAKE, INTAKE RESTRICTION, AND ALTERED METABOLISM OF NUTRIENTS (see Table 5–7)

F. **RENAL DISEASES OR CONDITIONS THAT MAY LEAD TO ARF**
1. **Hemolytic uremic syndrome (HUS)** is the simultaneous occurrence of hemolytic anemia, thrombocytopenia, and renal failure.

Table 5–7. CLINICAL MANIFESTATIONS OF POTENTIAL MULTISYSTEM COMPLICATIONS SECONDARY TO ACUTE RENAL FAILURE (ARF)

SYSTEM	CLINICAL MANIFESTATIONS
Cardiovascular	ECG changes secondary to hyperkalemia
Respiratory	Pneumonia, pulmonary edema
Gastrointestinal	Hemorrhage, abdominal cramping, nausea and vomiting, diarrhea, malnutrition
Neurologic	Altered mental status
Metabolic	Acidosis, hypocalcemia, hyperkalemia, uremia, hypermagnesemia, hyperphosphatemia, hyperuricemia
Hematologic	Anemia, coagulopathy
Infection	Sepsis, pneumonia

ECG, electrocardiogram.

a. *Pathophysiology* is characterized by microangiopathy with platelet aggregation and fibrin deposition in small vessels in small arterioles in the kidney, gut, and central nervous system. Hemolytic anemia is believed to be a result of the shearing of red cells as they pass through narrowed vessels.

b. *"Typical" HUS* occurs in the summer in the northern hemisphere with diarrhea during the prodromal period. *Escherichia coli* has been found to cause a large number of cases of typical HUS.

c. *"Atypical" HUS* occurs sporadically throughout the year with no diarrheal prodromal period. Atypical HUS has a poorer prognosis. Although a poor prognosis was thought to be age related (children younger than 3 years old have a better outcome), studies show that the prognosis is related to other factors. Factors that potentially indicate an increased risk of developing severe disease include absence of a prodromal diarrhea period, normal urine output, marked proteinuria, hypertension, and occurrences of relapses. Poor prognosis is related to development of neurologic sequelae, including coma.

d. *Clinical symptoms of HUS* include bloody diarrhea (more common in typical HUS), mild to moderate hypertension, fever, lethargy, decreased urine output, and paleness.

e. *Management* is primarily focused on general supportive care and treatment of complications such as ARF, anemia, central nervous system symptoms, and abdominal symptoms.

2. **Acute glomerulonephritis** is initiated by immunologic events within the glomerulus that result in glomerular damage. Antigen-antibody complexes mediate glomerular injury. Hypofiltration occurs as a result of decreased glomerular blood flow. Glomerular blood flow decreases as a result of arteriolar vasoconstriction, capillary obstruction by thrombi, and endothelial cell edema from proliferation of endothelial cells and white blood cell infiltration.

   a. *Clinical signs and symptoms* include salt and water retention secondary to decreased GFR, red blood cell or granular casts in the urine, declining renal function, hypertension, hematuria, oliguria, and other nonspecific symptoms such as fever, malaise, abdominal discomfort, nausea, or vomiting.

   b. *Management* includes the administration of antibiotics to treat the underlying cause, as well as management of declining renal function. (*Note:* Antibiotic doses must be adjusted in patients with decreased renal function.)

3. **Nephrotic syndrome** is defined as proteinuria greater than 3.5 g/d that occurs secondary to glomerular damage.

   a. *Nephrotic syndrome can be induced by drugs or chemicals.* Aminoglycosides (e.g., gentamicin) or amphotericin B (an antifungal agent) can induce renal toxicity because their actions increase the permeability of the distal tubule, cause back leak of hydrogen ions, sodium, and chloride, and incite an ADH-resistant polyuria. The two main effects include renal tubular cell injury (primarily of the distal tubule) and acute afferent arteriolar vasoconstriction.

   b. *Radiocontrast dyes* can also cause nephrotic syndrome. Contrast agents are freely filtered at the glomerulus with the kidneys as the primary mode for excretion. A decrease in GFR is a normal renal response to administration of dye secondary to transient vasodilation followed by vasoconstriction (occurs within minutes of administration and lasts for 10 to 20 minutes) and increased activity of the renin-angiotensin-aldosterone system and local release of a potent vasoconstrictor, adenosine.

   c. *Children with increased risk for nephrotoxicity* include those with preexisting renal dysfunction, diabetes, hypovolemia, proteinuria, and hyperuricemia. Nephrotoxicity is related to proximal tubule toxicity, intratubular cast formation, uric acid crystallization, vasoconstriction, erythrocyte-related changes in renal microcirculation, interstitial edema, and tubular cell necrosis.

d. *Nephrotoxicity generally presents* in the first 24 hours after infusion. Nephrotoxicity may be mild and present with minimal symptoms, or it may be severe and present with oliguria and pathologic changes in the proximal tubule. *Clinical signs of nephrotoxicity* are metabolic acidosis, polyuria, hypokalemia, and salt wasting.

e. Nephrotoxicity is predictable and usually reversible. Maintaining intravascular volume and reducing renal vasoconstriction supports renal function. The severity of the effects on the tubules and filtration is proportional to drug dosage. Protection against nephrotoxicity may be achieved with calcium channel blockers.

4. **Hepatorenal syndrome** is renal failure that develops in the presence of end-stage liver disease. Hepatorenal failure may accompany liver failure related to fulminant hepatic failure, hepatic malignancy, liver resection, or biliary tract obstruction. Primary renal disease is usually not present.

a. *Renal dysfunction* occurs because of decreased renal blood flow and perfusion to the kidneys. Hypoperfusion may be related to a decrease in cardiac output, sympathetic systemic vasoconstriction, or changes in renal prostaglandin levels. Portal hypertension and resultant splanchnic sequestration may occur.

b. *Signs and symptoms* include increased renal vascular resistance, decreased glomerular filtration, increased sodium and water retention (secondary to hyperaldosteronism), decreased urine output, and electrolyte and coagulation abnormalities.

c. *Management* includes treatment of the hepatic failure and support of renal function.

5. **Tumor lysis syndrome** occurs at the initiation of antineoplastic therapy for large, rapidly growing tumors. Metabolic abnormalities occur as a consequence of rapid tumor cell breakdown and release of their intracellular contents into the circulation (most likely to occur in a patient who has Burkitt's lymphoma, T-cell leukemias and lymphomas, a high white blood cell count, or bulky lymphoma).

a. *Potential effects* of tumor lysis include hyperuricemia, hypocalcemia, hyperphosphatemia, hyperkalemia, and hyperxanthinemia. These electrolyte imbalances lead to crystallization, tubular obstruction, decreased urine output, and renal failure. The severity of the condition is proportional to the tumor burden. A previous history of renal impairment increases the likelihood for developing tumor lysis syndrome. *Prevention* of complications from cell breakdown is the optimal goal.

b. *Management* of actual or potential complications includes aggressive IV fluid administration, alkalinization of the urine using IV bicarbonate, administration of allopurinol to reduce uric acid production, and immediate treatment of electrolyte imbalances. Severe electrolyte disturbances may require hemodialysis or continuous renal replacement therapy.

6. **Cardiac failure:** Changes in renal function may be attributed to hypovolemia or hypervolemia, hypotension, and electrolyte imbalance.

G. DESIRED PATIENT OUTCOMES FOR THE CHILD IN ARF

1. Urine output remains adequate.

2. Laboratory values indicate resolving ARF (e.g., stabilized or decreasing BUN and creatinine).
3. Cardiac output remains adequate.
4. Intake and output balance maintained.
5. Fluid and electrolyte balance maintained.
6. Nutritional status is optimized.
7. No signs of infection exist.
8. The child remains comfortable, and anxiety is minimized.

H. MANAGEMENT OF ARF

1. **Response to treatment is related to the extent of nephron damage and ATN**
   a. In prerenal failure, there is no actual nephron damage and the kidneys respond well to treatment for symptoms of decreased urine output or electrolyte abnormalities, or both.
   b. In true intrarenal ATN, actual nephron damage has occurred and response to therapy to treat the underlying problem of renal dysfunction is often futile.

2. **The plan of care to support renal function** includes eliminating the cause of ARF, if known, and discontinuing or altering the dose of potentially nephrotoxic medications. All drugs excreted by the kidneys require an alteration of the dosage based on the level of renal function. Serum concentrations of potentially toxic drugs should be closely monitored. Creatinine clearance and serum creatinine should be monitored when using potentially nephrotoxic agents. Drug dosage alteration is indicated with increased levels of serum creatinine. If a patient is receiving renal replacement therapy, drug supplementation may be necessary to restore the drug that is removed or filtrated.

3. **Maintain adequate intravascular volume and maintain adequate blood pressure.**

4. **Pharmacologic support** includes diuretics and other agents. Common indications for diuretic therapy include pulmonary edema, hypertension, hypercalcemia, hyperkalemia (furosemide), hypercalciuria (thiazides), hypokalemia (spironolactone), generalized edema, hypervolemia, and increased intracranial pressure. Diuretics promote renal excretion of water, either directly or indirectly on different segments of the tubules.
   a. *Loop diuretics* induce water loss secondary to sodium loss. The site of action is the ascending limb of the loop of Henle and the proximal and distal tubules. Furosemide and bumetanide (Bumex) are two of the most potent loop diuretics. Potential complications include hypovolemia, hypokalemia, hyponatremia, metabolic alkalosis, hypercalciuria, hypomagnesemia, hyperglycemia, deafness, renal calculi, and thrombocytopenia.
   b. *Thiazide diuretics* promote water loss secondary to sodium and chloride loss. Hydrochlorothiazide is frequently used as a secondary or adjunct agent in diuretic therapy. Sodium and chloride reabsorption is decreased in the cortical segment of the distal tubule. Potential complications are similar to loop diuretics. Potassium supplemental therapy may be indicated.
   c. *Nonthiazide, sulfonamide diuretics* work at both the proximal and distal tubules. Metolazone is frequently used as a secondary agent in conjunction with loop diuretics (furosemide).
   d. *Potassium-sparing diuretics* inhibit potassium transport in the distal tubule (causing sodium and water excretion) and potassium and hydrogen reabsorption. Spironolactone (aldosterone antagonist) is the most commonly used agent. Potassium-sparing diuretics are used in conjunction with a potassium-depleting diuretic agent to decrease the occurrence

of hypokalemia. They also have minimal side effects or potential complications.

    e. *Osmotic diuretics* are hyperosmolar agents that primarily induce water loss by pulling free water into the filtrate. Mannitol is a sugar that is relatively inert and freely filtered by the glomerulus, however, not greatly reabsorbed by the renal tubule. Mannitol produces diuresis by osmotically inhibiting tubular fluid and sodium reabsorption. The transient pulling of fluid into the intravascular space can increase the intravascular volume significantly; therefore, mannitol should not be used with patients in congestive heart failure and hypervolemia or in renal failure.

    f. *Caffeine* promotes diuresis by inhibiting secretion of ADH from the posterior pituitary gland.

    g. Acetazolamide (Diamox) is a *carbonic anhydrase inhibitor.* Metabolic acidosis may occur secondary to the limitation of secretion of hydrogen ions from the tubule and subsequent decreased reabsorption of bicarbonate and sodium.

    h. Low-dose *dopamine* (1 to 5 μg/kg/min) stimulates dopaminergic receptors located on the afferent arterioles that improve renal blood flow. Afferent arterioles dilate, increasing blood flow to the glomerulus, which increases the GFR, resulting in increased urine output.

5. **Consider renal replacement therapy if unable to support function with above measures.**

6. **Complications of end-stage renal disease (ESRD)** include hypertensive disease, hyperlipidemia, and hyperparathyroidism due to poor control of calcium and phosphate levels.

RENAL REPLACEMENT THERAPIES

    Renal replacement therapies for infants and children include peritoneal dialysis (PD), hemodialysis, and continuous renal replacement therapy.

A. PERITONEAL DIALYSIS (PD)

1. **Indications** for PD include an inability to tolerate anticoagulation, congenital metabolic disease, ATN, renal cortical necrosis, obstructive uropathy, renal agenesis, bilateral renal dysplasia, and other renal dysfunction requiring long-term, nonemergent therapy. PD is often used for infants and children in either ARF or chronic renal failure.

2. **Types** of PD include continuous ambulatory PD (CAPD), manual PD, or continuous cycling PD using a cycler computerized mechanical device. Access is via a soft catheter in the peritoneal space, placed in the operating room or at the bedside.

3. **Process:** The removal of water and solutes (ultrafiltrate) is adjusted by raising the osmolarity of the dialysate by increasing dextrose content or increasing the amount of time the dialysate solution dwells in the peritoneal space. The amount of dialysate placed into the peritoneal space (inflow volume), is determined by gradually increasing volumes from 15 to 50 ml/kg of body weight, as tolerated. Standard dialysate solution contains dextrose, sodium, calcium, magnesium, chloride, and lactate (which is metabolized to produce bicarbonate). Potassium, heparin, antibiotics, or antifungal medications can be added to the peritoneal fluid as needed. CAPD or manual PD may be needed in infants and small children when inflow volumes are less than 50 ml. Excessive inflow volume can be assessed by monitoring for signs of uncomfortable

fullness and pain or discomfort on inflow. The dialysate solution must be warmed to or near body temperature to prevent hypothermia.

    a.   *Manual PD* requires more nursing time than the cycler method because of the need for manual timing of dwell times, exact measurement of inflow and outflow volumes, calculation of net ultrafiltration after each dwell time, and cumulative ultrafiltrate tabulation. Dialysate is infused by gravity into the peritoneal space through the catheter. Clots, kinks, and catheter position can affect the ability to inflow adequately. The catheter is clamped, and a timer is set to mark dwell time completion. Dwell times generally range from 15 to 30 minutes. On completion of the dwell time, the catheter is unclamped, and the outflow drains to a urine collection bag to be measured. Drain times are dependent on catheter patency. The net ultrafiltrate is calculated (outflow volume minus inflow volume). The inflow-dwell-outflow cycle is repeated at ordered time intervals.

    b.   *Computerized PD* using a cycler requires less hands-on nursing time, has a decreased incidence of infection related to a closed system, provides a programmable automated ultrafiltrate calculation, and has a built-in mechanism for dialysate warming.

    c.   Dwell times impact waste removal and fluid removal. Long dwell times may achieve good waste and solute clearance but poor fluid removal. Short dwell times have poor waste and solute clearance but remove a significant amount of fluid.

  4. **Potential complications** of PD include peritonitis, which can be indicated by cloudy dialysate, abdominal pain, tenderness, or sepsis. Mechanical and iatrogenic catheter problems can occur. Such problems include leakage at the insertion site, bowel perforation, retroperitoneal hemorrhage, increased intraabdominal pressure due to obstruction of the catheter, and hernia. Other complications include impaired pulmonary function related to abdominal distention and fluid overload, decreased cardiac output and stroke volume related to fluid volume overload or loss, hypoproteinemia due to loss of protein in the dialysate, and hyperglycemia related to absorption of dextrose. Hyperglycemia may require treatment with insulin.

B. HEMODIALYSIS

  1. **Indications** for hemodialysis may include symptomatic electrolyte imbalance, hypervolemia, pulmonary edema, severe acidosis, anuria that is not responsive to other therapy, severely elevated BUN with elevated creatinine, cardiac failure, tumor lysis syndrome, hepatic failure, and other conditions that require rapid, efficient correction of the abnormality.

  2. **Process:** An extracorporeal circuit carries blood from the child through a filter, an artificial kidney, and back to the child. The artificial kidney has a semipermeable membrane through which water, solutes, and other substances are filtered (ultrafiltrate). Removal of solutes occurs through the filter by diffusion, which is created by the infusion of the dialysate into the filter (the other side of the semipermeable membrane) countercurrent to the flow of blood. Negative pressure is added to the dialysate side of the circuit to increase the fluid and solute removal from the blood. Positive pressure is added to the venous side of the blood circuit, thus increasing resistance to remove excess fluid. Blood access is obtained via a double-lumen central venous catheter, via an arterial catheter and a venous catheter, or via two single-lumen central venous catheters. It is important to consider the extracorporeal circuit volume in relation to the child's circulating blood volume to prevent hypovolemia. If the extracorporeal circuit volume is greater than 10% of the child's circulating blood volume or if

the child weighs less than 10 kg, the circuit may be primed with a colloid substance. Small volume artificial kidneys and circuit sizes have enabled hemodialysis to be an option for small infants.

3. **Potential complications** include hypovolemia, hypervolemia, systemic bleeding, kidney rupture or circuit disconnection, infection, and transfusion reaction.

4. **Nursing implications:** Vital signs, oxygenation, hemodynamics, fluid status, electrolyte balance, and physiologic response to treatment must be closely monitored. Inadequately treated intravascular hypovolemia, rapid electrolyte and pH changes, and hypoxemia will significantly affect cardiac function and lead to severe compromise. Volume expanders such as albumin or colloid products (or both) should be readily available and used as needed. Administration of hyperosmotic agents (mannitol) may increase diuresis. Hemodialysis removes drugs along with the solutes, water, and toxins; therefore, drug dosing must be adjusted for the patient receiving hemodialysis. A hemodynamically unstable child may not tolerate hemodialysis and may require a more gentle therapy such as PD or CRRT.

C. CONTINUOUS RENAL REPLACEMENT THERAPY (CRRT)

1. **Indications** for CRRT include ARF with hemodynamic instability, azotemia, severe electrolyte imbalance, hypervolemia, and symptomatic metabolic abnormalities. CRRT is appropriate for hemodynamically unstable patients who are unable to tolerate hemodialysis and patients who are not candidates for PD.

2. **Process**
   a. *Continuous arteriovenous hemofiltration (CAVH)* uses an arterial catheter and a venous catheter. The circuit is dependent on the arterial blood pressure to propel the blood through the circuit. Therefore, CAVH is limited by the mean arterial pressure of the patient.
   b. *Continuous venovenous hemofiltration (CVVH)* uses a double-lumen venous catheter or two single-lumen venous catheters. This method requires a blood pump to propel the blood through the circuit. So although CVVH does not require arterial access, it requires more mechanical devices. CVVH offers a highly efficient circuit that is driven by a pump, instead of the patient's blood pressure. CVVH is becoming a preferred method of treatment for the hemodynamically unstable patient in many neonatal and pediatric intensive care units.

3. **Methods for measuring filtration capability or performance of the filter and circuit**
   a. Clearance is the removal of solutes from the plasma and is dependent on the device's capability for removing individual molecules, the size of the solute, the solute's protein-binding capacity, and the rate of blood flow through the hemofilter. Negative pull pressure can be added by using an infusion pump to draw ultrafiltrate from the filter. Clearance for a particular molecule can be expressed by the ultrafiltrate-to-plasma ratio, known as the *sieving coefficient.*

$$\text{Sieving Coefficient} = \frac{\text{Concentration of x in Ultrafiltrate } [(x)Uf]}{\text{Concentration of x in Plasma } [(x)Plasma]}$$

(1 = 100% Clearance)

   b. *Another indicator of the efficiency of the system is the filtration fraction (FF).* FF is reflective of the fraction of plasma water that is being removed by ultrafiltration. Optimum FF is a percentage that is high enough to provide adequate solute and fluid removal needs but not so high that blood viscosity and increased oncotic pressure impact filter performance.

$$\text{Filtration Fraction (\%)} = \frac{\text{(Qf) Ultrafiltrate Rate (ml/min)}}{\text{(QP) Plasma Flow Rate at the Inlet (ml/min)}}$$

4. **Methods of solute clearance and water removal: Convection, diffusion, ultra-filtration**

   a. *Convective transport* occurs when water and small particles are carried through membrane pores into ultrafiltrate by a moving stream of fluid containing large protein molecules. The important determinants of convective transport are the direction and rate of the solvent flux across the membrane. Unlike diffusion, it is not influenced by any solute concentration gradient.

   b. *Diffusion* is the removal of a solute from a higher concentration to a lower concentration to establish equilibrium. If adequate clearance is not obtained by convection alone, it may be necessary to influence clearance by diffusion as well. To add the capability of diffusion to CVVH, dialysate is infused into the outer compartment of the hemofilter, countercurrent to the flow of blood through the filter (continuous venovenous hemodialfiltration [CVVHD]). The dialysate, and any solutes that have diffused across the membrane, will pass out of the hemofilter with the ultrafiltrate.

   c. *Ultrafiltration* is the removal of extracellular free water. The rate of removal is determined by the surface area of the filter membrane, the permeability coefficient of the membrane to water, and the transmembrane pressure gradient. With pump-assisted hemofiltration, it is easier to maintain an optimal blood flow rate and in turn maximize the ultrafiltration rate.

5. **Nursing implications for the hemodynamically unstable infant or child during CVVH**

   a. *Limited vascular access sites and catheter diameter* often limit blood pump speed and therefore impact circuit efficiency and solute clearance. *Coagulopathy* presents a challenge for risk of bleeding during catheter placement and prevention of catheter thrombus formation. The additional vascular access adds another potential source of *infection*. If the catheter is placed in the femoral vein, it may be necessary to immobilize the limb, and pharmacologic paralysis or sedation may be required.

   b. *Thermoregulation* is a significant issue with infants and small children. Depending on the extracorporeal volume of the circuit, a significant amount of heat may be lost via the circuit. Fluid and blood warmer infusion systems or external heat sources should be used to maintain normothermia. Small volume, extracorporeal tubing sets are ideal.

   c. *Anticoagulation* is helpful to maintain patency of the circuit. A continuous heparin infusion is generally used. Activated clotting times (ACTs) should be maintained at 1 to 1.5 times normal (approximately 180 to 200 seconds). In the absence of a coagulopathy, a heparin bolus is given to the patient at least 3 minutes prior to initiation of therapy. In the presence of coagulopathy, heparin administration may be contraindicated, and the life span of the circuit may be decreased. The benefit of routine flushes of normal saline, lactated Ringer's, or filter replacement solution to maintain circuit patency and decrease clotting is debatable. The use of PGI_2 or citrate has been discussed in the literature, but little pediatric clinical data exist.

   d. *Hemodynamic stability:* The CVVH circuit volume should be considered in relationship to the child's circulating blood volume. In small infants and children it may be necessary to prime the circuit with albumin, whole blood, or another colloid substance. If the circuit is primed with a blood product preserved with citrate, assess the serum calcium level prior to CVVH initiation and treat if necessary to decrease the risk of hypotension secondary to hypocalcemia. Because of drug clearance by the hemofilter, it may be necessary to titrate the infusion of vasoactive agents just prior to or in the first few minutes after initiation of CVVH. If the preceding precautions are taken, the incidence of hemodynamic instability during initiation of CVVH is rare. Unlike CAVH and pump-assisted hemofiltration, CVVH is able to function independently of the child's mean arterial pressure and can therefore be used in times of low cardiac output.

e. *Fluid balance:* It may be necessary to begin at an ordered zero fluid balance and slowly adjust the balance as tolerated. Strict fluid intake and output are recorded hourly. In a child who is receiving multiple blood products or fluid boluses, it is important to determine what is to be included in the formula as fluid to be "taken off" or removed. The formula for determining the hourly filter replacement fluid (FRF) rate is as follows:

$$FRF = (Total\ Fluid\ Out) - (Total\ Fluid\ In) +/- (Hourly\ Fluid\ Balance)$$

f. *The extracorporeal circuit:* Plasma-free hemoglobin levels may be measured prior to initiation of CVVH and daily to monitor red blood cell destruction. Elevated plasma-free hemoglobin levels indicate the necessity to change the circuit.

RENAL TRANSPLANTATION

A. CRITERIA FOR TRANSPLANTATION
1. All candidates must have end-stage renal disease (ESRD) or rapidly approaching ESRD.
2. **Common causes of ESRD** requiring transplantation include congenital renal disorder, glomerulonephritis, and ESRD secondary to other disease states or treatment.
3. **Pretransplantation evaluation criteria:** Failure to respond to conservative management is no longer a criterion for transplantation. Transplantation may now be considered at the time of diagnosis of ESRD. The child must have a normal or repairable bladder and urinary outflow tract and be free from major multisystem complications (malignancy, advanced cardiopulmonary disease) and active infection. Nutritional status should be adequate and psychiatric and socioeconomic parameters should be viewed as appropriate.
4. **Histocompatibility:** Infection-free successful transplantation is largely dependent on the recipient's immunologic acceptance.
5. **Postoperative management**
   a. *Minimize the risk for infection* by observing strict hand washing and other institutional infection control guidelines and using strict aseptic techniques with all dressing changes.
   b. *Maintain pulmonary toilet.*
   c. *Closely monitor urinary output* and observe for signs and symptoms of infection.
   d. *Maintain adequate nutritional intake.*
   e. *Monitor and maintain metabolic and electrolyte balance* (BUN, creatinine, calcium, phosphorus, urinary protein).
   f. *Maintain comfort for the patient* and administer medications as needed to decrease pain or anxiety.

g. *Administer the daily immunosuppressive medication regimen* as ordered and follow serum levels as appropriate.

h. *Initiate and plan discharge teaching for the patient and family.*

i. *Potential complications* include ATN, rejection, infection, obstruction to urinary flow, hypovolemia, renal artery stenosis, renal vein thrombosis, and ureteral leaks.

RENAL TRAUMA

A. ETIOLOGY AND RISK FACTORS

1. Renal trauma is the most common genitourinary injury (34% to 68% of all genitourinary injuries). Contusion or laceration comprises 80% to 85% of renal injuries.

2. Children have a greater renal vulnerability than adults because of the larger size of a child's kidney in relation to abdomen size, underdevelopment of a child's abdominal wall muscles, and lack of protection from the lower ribs.

3. The most common source of renal trauma is blunt trauma, primarily from motor vehicle accidents. The two types of blunt trauma causing most renal injuries are direct compression from external force or deceleration injury. With deceleration injury, there is a concern about laceration of the renal artery. In addition, acute renal trauma may occur as a result of decreased perfusion. Lumbar scoliosis and fracture of the body or transverse processes of the spine transmit significant injury to the retroperitoneal region of the kidney. Penetrating trauma rarely is a cause of renal injury in children.

B. CLINICAL MANIFESTATIONS

1. **Signs and symptoms** of genitourinary trauma include blood at the urethral meatus, high-riding prostate, gross hematuria, and labial, scrotal, or perianal ecchymosis or hematoma. Hematuria occurs in 90% of cases. If the patient is hypovolemic, hematuria may not manifest until after fluid replacement. There is no correlation between the magnitude of injury and the degree of hematuria. These signs and symptoms are contraindications to bladder catheterization.

2. With **penetrating trauma,** proximity of the wound to the genitourinary area increases suspicion of renal trauma.

3. With **blunt trauma** the child may be asymptomatic or complain of abdominal or flank pain.

C. INTERPRETATIONS FROM DIAGNOSTIC STUDIES

1. **Computed tomography (CT)** is the standard imaging study for acute renal trauma in children. Advantages include more accurate demonstration of renal injury, visualization of nonvascularized regions, and simultaneous visualization of the intraabdominal area. It is less time consuming and easier than arteriography.

2. **Abdominal or kidney, ureter, and bladder (KUB) film** demonstrating obliteration of the renal shadow is suggestive of renal trauma. Up to 85% of plain abdominal films demonstrate normal findings despite proven renal trauma.

3. **Excretory urogram (IVP)** is standard for diagnosis of renal injury.

4. **Ultrasonography** has limited application in evaluation of renal trauma. Doppler-enhanced ultrasound gives information related to renal perfusion and integrity of vascular pedicles of the kidney.

5. **Arteriography** may assist in planning surgical intervention.

6. **Radionucleotide renal scan** demonstrates renal function, perfusion, and urinary extravasation. It is useful if there is a contraindication to contrast dye.

7. Use of **magnetic resonance imaging (MRI)** is limited because of the technique and the amount of information gained.

D. **CLASSIFICATION**

A **minor injury** is a simple contusion or laceration with an intact capsule and stable clinical vital signs. A **major injury** results in more extensive laceration with or without extravasation and stable vital signs. **Critical injuries** involve major vessels, a shattered kidney, uncontrollable hemorrhage, or unstable vital signs.

E. **DESIRED PATIENT OUTCOMES**

1. Absence of hematuria
2. Adequate urine output
3. Absence of hypertension
4. Negative results from radiographic studies

F. **PLAN OF CARE**

Most **penetrating renal injuries** require surgical exploration and potential intervention. **Management of blunt trauma** is dependent on the stability of the child and the extent of injury. Eighty-five percent of blunt trauma cases are minor injuries, requiring only observation and bed rest until gross hematuria resolves. If results from initial radiographic studies are abnormal, continued follow-up for a year or more may be necessary. **Management of major renal trauma** is controversial when considering an operative vs. a nonoperative approach. **Long-term follow-up** (6 months to 1 year) is important because hypertension is subtle yet frequently associated with vascular trauma.

REFERENCES

Allshouse MJ, Betts JM. Genitourinary injury. In: Eichelberger MR, ed. *Pediatric Trauma: Prevention, Acute Care, Rehabilitation*. St Louis, Mo: Mosby–Year Book Inc; 1993:503–520.

Awazu M, Devarajan P, Stewart CL, Kaskel F, Ichikawa I. "Maintenance" therapy and treatment of dehydration and overhydration. In: Ichikawa, ed. *Pediatric Textbook of Fluid and Electrolytes*. Baltimore, Md: Williams & Wilkins; 1989:417–428.

Baer CL, Lancaster LE. Acute renal failure. *Crit Care Nurs Q*. 1992;14:1–21.

Brem AS. An overview of renal structure and function. In: Fuhrman BP, Zimmerman JJ, eds. *Pediatric Critical Care*. St Louis, Mo: Mosby–Year Book Inc; 1992:659–670.

Friedman AL. Acute renal disease. In: Fuhrman BP, Zimmerman JJ, eds. *Pediatric Critical Care*. St Louis, Mo: Mosby–Year Book Inc; 1992:723–737.

Hendix W. Dialysis therapies in critically ill children. *AACN Clin Issues Crit Care*. 1992;3(3):605–613.

Hole JW. *Human Anatomy and Physiology*. Dubuque, Iowa: William C Brown; 1984:747–778.

Kapit W, Macey RI, Meisami E. *The Physiology Coloring Book*. New York, NY: Harper Collins Inc; 1987:54–66.

Kennedy J. Renal disorders. In: Hazinski MF, ed. *Nursing Care of the Critically Ill Child*. St Louis, Mo: Mosby–Year Book Inc; 1992:629–713.

Lancaster LE. Acute renal failure. In: Huddleston VB, ed. *Multisystem Organ Failure: Pathophysiology and Clinical Implications*. St Louis, Mo: Mosby–Year Book Inc; 1992:222–235.

McCormick A, Sterk MB. Acute renal failure of the neonate. *Dimens Crit Care Nurs*. 1986;5:155–161.

Quigley RP, Alexander SR. Acute renal failure. In: Levin DL, Morriss FC, eds. *Essentials of Pediatric Intensive Care*. St Louis, Mo: Quality Medical Publishing Inc; 1990:106–120.

Wood EG, Lynch RE. Fluid and electrolyte balance. In: Fuhrman BP, Zimmerman JJ, eds. *Pediatric Critical Care*. St Louis, Mo: Mosby–Year Book Inc; 1992:671–687.

Endocrine System

6

JANET CRAIG

The **role of the endocrine system** is to maintain the internal environment, including fluid and electrolytes, blood pressure, and maintenance of fat, muscle, and bone. Functions of the endocrine system involve the control and regulation of metabolism and energy stores, growth and development, and reproduction and coordination of the body's response to stress (e.g., trauma, critical illness, major surgery; Guyton, 1986; Toto, 1994a).

The **major glands of the endocrine system** are the hypothalamus, pituitary glands (anterior and posterior), and thyroid/parathyroid glands, adrenal glands (medulla and cortex), pancreas, and gonads (Fig. 6–1).

These glands or organs consist of specialized cells that synthesize and secrete biochemical messengers (hormones) in response to specific signals. **Endocrine glands** secrete hormones directly into the blood stream (e.g., adrenal glands, endocrine pancreas, thyroid gland). **Exocrine glands** secrete biochemical substances that are released into ducts to be delivered to target organs (e.g., salivary glands, sebaceous glands, exocrine pancreas, and sweat glands).

Hormones (Table 6–1) are released directly into the bloodstream from endocrine glands in response to specific stimuli or signals. Hormones facilitate communication between cells, both locally and distally. Negative feedback is the primary mechanism controlling hormonal regulation (Toto, 1994a).

Integrated functions include central nervous system (CNS) input to the endocrine system via the hypothalamic-pituitary complex. The immune system contributes to endocrine regulation via the biologic response modifiers (cytokines, interleukin-1, tumor necrosis factor; Toto, 1994a).

DEVELOPMENTAL ANATOMY AND PHYSIOLOGY

A. PANCREAS
   1. **Location:** The pancreas is shaped like a tadpole with a head, body, and tail and lies across the posterior abdominal wall between the spleen and duodenum.
   2. **Cell types**
       a. *An exocrine system* with acini ducts secretes digestive juices into the duodenum.
       b. The *endocrine system* is a ductless system with direct secretion into the portal circulation. It comprises less than 2% of the total pancreatic volume. The islets of Langerhans (Fig. 6–2) contain beta cells, which secrete insulin and constitute 60% of islet cells; alpha cells, which secrete glucagon and

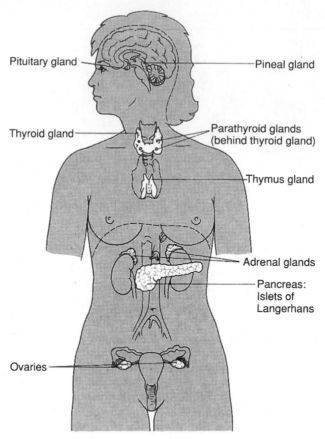

Figure 6–1. Anatomic loci of the principal endocrine glands of the body. (Reprinted with permission from Guyton AC, Hall JE. *Textbook of Medical Physiology.* 9th ed. Philadelphia, Pa: WB Saunders Co; 1996.)

constitute 25% of islet cells; delta cells, which secrete somatostatin and constitute 10% of islet cells; and PP cells, which secrete pancreatic polypeptide and gastrin and constitute 5% of islet cells (Guyton, 1986; Sizonenko, 1993c; Toto, 1994a).

3. **Insulin**

   a. *Biosynthesis:* Insulin is an anabolic hormone, a hormone of fuel storage. Synthesized by the beta cells, proinsulin is stored in secretory granules and converted to insulin when the signal comes for its secretion. Insulin's circulatory half-life is approximately 6 minutes (Guyton, 1986; Sizonenko, 1993c).

   b. *Regulation* (Fig. 6–3): Release of insulin is predominantly stimulated by an increase in the blood glucose level and amino acid levels and occurs in two stages (Table 6–2). Other factors that potentiate release of insulin are gastrointestinal (GI) tract hormones, growth hormone (GH), and glucagon. Insulin release is greater after an oral glucose load than after intravenous (IV) glucose injection, suggesting the presence of anticipatory signals from the GI tract to the pancreas (Guyton, 1986; Sizonenko, 1993c; Toto, 1994a). Inhibition for insulin release is hypoglycemia and the α-adrenergic effects of catecholamines, somatostatin, and some pharmacologic agents. Once blood glucose levels fall to fasting levels, insulin secretion is halted.

   c. *Effects in target cells* are mediated by insulin's binding with specific receptor sites on the cell membrane (Toto, 1994a).

Table 6–1. MAJOR ACTIONS OF ENDOCRINE HORMONES

Pituitary Gland
Anterior Lobe

Growth hormone (GH) or somatotropin (SH)	Stimulates growth of cells, bones, and tissues
	Increases protein synthesis
	Decreases rate of carbohydrate use and resistance to insulin
	Increases mobilization and use of fats for energy
	Necessary for normal growth and development
Thyroid-stimulating hormone (TSH)	Promotes growth and secretory activity of the thyroid gland
	Necessary for normal growth and development
Adrenocorticotropic hormone (ACTH)	Influences the secretory output of the adrenal cortex (cortisol and adrenal androgens)
Follicle-stimulating hormone (FSH)	Stimulates gametogenesis in boys and girls
Lutenizing hormone (LH)	
Prolactin (PRL)	Acts directly on the mammory gland and is responsible for initiation and maintenance of lactation

Posterior Lobe

Antidiuretic hormone (ADH) or vasopressin	Regulates osmolarity and body water volume
	Increases permeability of the collecting ducts in the kidneys, thereby decreasing urine formation by increased water reabsorption
Oxytocin	Stimulates uterine contractions at parturition
	Stimulates release and flow of breast milk

Thyroid Gland

Thyroxine (T_4) Triiodothyronine (T_3)	Regulates the metabolic and oxidative rates in tissue cells
	Stimulates growth and development of various tissues at critical periods, including the central nervous system and skeleton
	Influences rate of metabolism of lipids, proteins, carbohydrates, water, vitamins, and minerals

Thyroxine (T_4) Triiodothyronine (T_3) *Continued*	Maintains cardiac rate, force, and output
	Necessary for muscle tone and function
Calcitonin	Lowers serum calcium by opposing bone-reabsorbing effects of PTH, prostaglandins, and calciferols by inhibiting osteoclastic activity
	Lowers serum phosphate levels

Parathyroid Glands

Parathyroid hormone (PTH)	Maintains normal calcium levels in the blood
	Regulates phosphorous metabolism and increases the rate of calcium reabsorption in the renal tubules
	Enhances the rate of calcium reabsorption from bone
	Influences the rate of calcium absorption from GI tract

Adrenal Glands
Cortex
Mineralocorticoids

Aldosterone*	Influences electrolyte concentrations and fluid volume
	Stimulates renal tubules to reabsorb sodium and excrete potassium
	Necessary for life
Glucocorticoids† Cortisol	Promotes the conversion of protein to carbohydrate (gluconeogenesis) and the storage of carbohydrate as glycogen
	Mobilizes amino acids from proteins in plasma and muscle
	Promotes fat mobilization
	Antagonizes the action of insulin
	Influences the immune system, plasma volume, maintenance of blood pressure, and cardiac output
	Acts as an antiinflammatory
	Necessary for life
Androgens‡	Produce many secondary sexual characteristics in boys and girls (e.g., growth of sexual hair)
	Maintain secondary sexual characteristics

Table continued on following page

Table 6–1.   MAJOR ACTIONS OF ENDOCRINE HORMONES *(Continued)*

Medulla		Pancreas	
Catecholamines		Insulin	Regulates glucose, protein, and lipid metabolism
Norepineph-rine	Acts as an α-adrenergic receptor stimulator whose action is excitatory (vasoconstriction, increased blood pressure, intestinal relaxation)		Promotes the transfer of glucose across the cell membrane
	Regulates basic metabolic processes, including glycogenolysis, lipolysis, inhibition of insulin release, and electrolyte transport		Inhibits the release of glucose from the liver, promoting hepatic glucose storage
			Potentiates the action of GH
Epinephrine	Acts as an α- and β-adrenergic receptor stimulator for which actions are primarily inhibitory and metabolic (increases contractility and excitability of the heart muscle, causing increased cardiac output)	Glucagon	Acts as a counterregulatory hormone to insulin with epinephrine, GH, and the glucocorticoids
			Increases blood glucose
			Promotes amino acid transport from the muscle
	Increases blood flow to muscles, brain, and viscera		Decreases protein synthesis
	Increases the basal metabolic rate		Decreases lipolysis and ketone formation
	Enhances blood glucose		
	Inhibits smooth muscle contractions		

*Aldosterone is the major mineralocorticoid; others include 11-deoxycorticosterone and 18-hydroxy-11-deoxycorticosterone.

†The principal glucocorticoid is cortisol; others include cortisone and corticosterone.

‡The primary androgens secreted during adrenarche are dehydroepiandosterone and androstenedione.

From Recker B. Anatomy and physiology of the endocrine system. In: Jackson DB, Saunders RB, eds. *Child Health Nursing*. Philadelphia, Pa: JB Lippincott Co; 1993:1434.

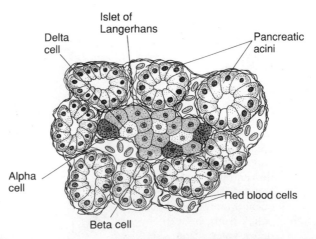

Figure 6–2.   Physiologic anatomy of the pancreas. (Reprinted with permission from Guyton AC, Hall JE. *Textbook of Medical Physiology*. 9th ed. Philadelphia, Pa: WB Saunders Co; 1996.)

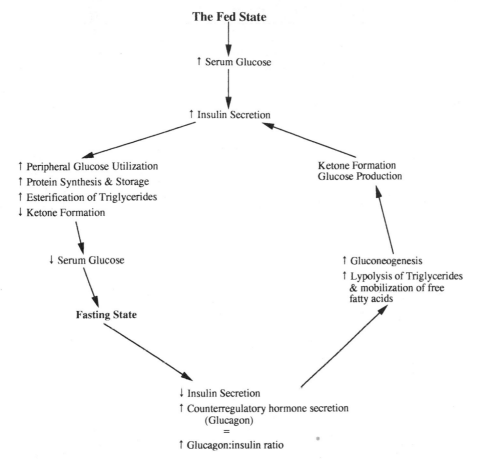

Figure 6–3. Insulin feedback loop. The fasting state normally results in formation of small quantities of ketones. In the patient who does not have diabetes the presences of even small quantities of ketones serves as a stimulus for an increase in insulin secretion. The increase in insulin action suppresses further ketone formation and prevents the progression to ketoacidosis. (Reprinted with permission from Jones TL. Diabetic ketoacidosis to hyperglycemic hyperosmolar nonketotic syndrome. *Crit Care Nurs Clin North Am.* 1994;6(4):705.)

    d. *Effects on carbohydrate metabolism:* Insulin increases glucose uptake by the liver, muscle, and adipose tissue and stimulates glycogen synthesis and storage in the liver and muscle (glycogenesis). Insulin inhibits gluconeogenesis and glycogenolysis (breakdown of glycogen to glucose). Insulin is not necessary for glucose uptake by the brain (Guyton, 1986; Sizonenko, 1993c; Toto, 1994a; Villee and Najjar, 1994).

    e. *Effects on fat metabolism:* Insulin inhibits lipolysis and ketogenesis. Insulin stimulates triglyceride synthesis and transport of fatty acids across the cell membrane. Infants can use ketone bodies for cerebral metabolism during a fast (Sizonenko, 1993a,c; Toto, 1994a).

    f. *Effects on protein metabolism:* Insulin inhibits proteolysis, facilitates transport of amino acids into the cells, works synergistically with GH to promote growth, and stimulates protein synthesis (Guyton, 1986; Toto, 1994a).

    g. *Secondary effects of insulin on other cellular functions* (relatively minor role) involve transport of potassium, magnesium, and phosphate into the cell (Toto, 1994a).

    h. *Effects of lack of insulin:* Lack of insulin markedly reduces the rate of transport of glucose across the cell membrane. Reduced insulin secretion

Table 6–2. STAGES OF INSULIN RELEASE

Stage I
Within 5 min of an acute elevation of serum glucose, there is an immediate release of preformed insulin into the blood; insulin levels increase tenfold. This high level of release is
not maintained, and secretion drops by approximately one half.

Stage 2
Fifteen minutes after an elevation in serum glucose, insulin secretion increases a second time
and reaches a plateau during the next 2–3 h. This is secondary to the synthesis of new insulin, as well as the continued release of preformed insulin by the beta cells.

also increases the amount of stored triglycerides in the liver; increases
serum triglycerides, fatty acids, and cholesterol; and increases serum levels
of acetoacetic acid, acetone, and ketone bodies because of increased
oxidation of fat (lipolysis). Liver and muscle glycogen is converted to
glucose and released into the blood (glycogenolysis). Gluconeogenesis
(formation of glucose from noncarbohydrate sources) includes the breakdown of proteins (proteolysis) to form glucose (Guyton, 1986; Sizonenko,
1993c; Toto, 1994a).

4. **Glucagon**
   a. *Biosynthesis:* Glucagon is a large peptide that is synthesized and secreted by
      the alpha cells of the islet cells.
   b. *Regulation:* Hypoglycemia, amino acids, proteins, and vigorous exercise are
      the most potent stimulants for the release of glucagon. Glucagon release
      may also be stimulated by the rise in α-adrenergic activity that results from
      hypoglycemia (Sizonenko, 1993b). Hyperglycemia and somatostatin sup-
      press release of glucagon.
   c. *Effects:* Glucagon is a catabolic hormone, a hormone of fuel mobilization.
      It is an insulin antagonistic hormone that directs the breakdown of
      liver glycogen (glycogenolysis) and increases gluconeogenesis in the liver
      (Guyton, 1986; Sizonenko, 1993b,c; Toto, 1994a).

5. **Somatostatin**
   a. *Biosynthesis:* Somatostatin is a polypeptide synthesized and secreted by the
      delta cells of the islet cells. It is present in the hypothalamus and GI tract.
   b. *Regulation:* Glucose, amino acids, fatty acids, and GI tract hormones
      stimulate the release of somatostatin. Starvation reduces somatostatin levels
      (Sizonenko, 1993c; Toto, 1994a).
   c. *Effects:* Somatostatin inhibits the secretion of insulin, glucagon, GH, thyroid-
      stimulating hormone (TSH), and gastrin and decreases GI tract motility
      and absorption.

6. **Developmental issues**
   a. Dorsal and ventral pancreatic buds arise from the dorsal section of the
      duodenum. Acini develop from cells around the primitive ducts in the
      pancreatic buds. The islets of Langerhans develop from cell groups that
      separate from the primitive buds and form next to the acini.
   b. Insulin and glucagon secretion begins at approximately 20 weeks' gestation
      (Moore, 1988; Sizonenko, 1993c). The main determinant of fetal glucose
      uptake is maternal blood glucose level.
   c. Maturation of the beta and alpha cells increases progressively after birth,
      and fasting levels of insulin rise progressively during the first 3 months of
      life. Glucagon levels rise sharply after birth, remain stable during the first
      48 hours of life, and then rise progressively throughout the next days
      of life.
   d. Glucose is a poor stimulus for insulin secretion in the premature infant;

however, beta cells become increasingly sensitive to glucose stimulation with age. Glucose and glucagon induce only a moderate increase in insulin secretion in term infants when compared to the older infant. Liver glycogen stores decrease during the first 12 hours of life because of the stress of birth.

e. The high body content of fat in the term newborn is a buffer against hypoglycemia during periods of fast. Premature or small-for-gestational-age infants have less body fat, and therefore, during the first month of life, small-for-gestational-age infants have lower blood glucose levels than term infants. The neonate and young child also exhibit hypoglycemia when fasting for shorter time periods than the older child or adult. Counter-regulatory hormonal responses to hypoglycemia are immature, and the enzymes of the gluconeogenic pathway are not completely functional in the newborn.

f. External sources of glucose are more important in the young child because of limited glycogen stores, which is related to the small muscle mass. Liver glycogen stores are depleted 4 to 8 hours after a meal in the young child (Sizonenko, 1993c).

B. HYPOTHALAMIC-PITUITARY COMPLEX (NEUROENDOCRINE SYSTEM)

1. **Location**
   a. The *hypothalamus* is located at the base of the brain and is connected to the pituitary gland by the pituitary stalk.
   b. The *anterior pituitary (adenohypophysis)* is linked to the hypothalamus by the hypothalamic-hypophysial portal vessels and constitutes 75% of the pituitary gland. The anterior pituitary secretes GH, adrenocorticotropic hormone (ACTH), TSH, prolactin, follicle-stimulating hormone (FSH), and luteinizing hormone (LH).
   c. The *posterior pituitary (neurohypophysis)* (Fig. 6–4) is linked to the hypothalamus via nerve fibers and secretes antidiuretic hormone (ADH) and oxytocin (Gaillard, 1993; Guyton, 1986; Toto, 1994a,b).

2. **Cell types of the hypothalamus, neurohypophysis, and adenohypophysis**
   a. The supraoptic and paraventricular nuclei originate in the hypothalamus.

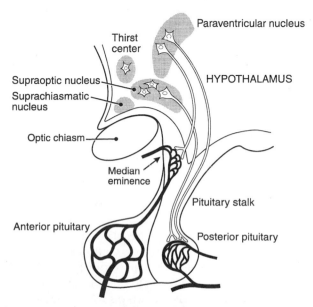

Figure 6–4. Neuroanatomy of the vasopressin pathways. (Reprinted with permission from Toto KH. Regulation of plasma osmolality. *Crit Care Nurs Clin North Am.* 1994;6(4):670.)

Table 6–3.   HORMONES OF THE HYPOTHALAMUS THAT AFFECT THE ANTERIOR PITUITARY

EFFECT	NAME	ACTION
Stimulating	Thyrotropin-releasing hormone (TRH)	Stimulates the release of TSH and prolactin
	Gonadotropin-releasing hormone (Gn-RH)	Stimulates the release of FSH and LH
	Growth hormone–releasing hormone (GH-RH)	Stimulates the release of GH
	Corticotropin-releasing hormone (CRH)	Stimulates the release of ACTH
	Prolactin-releasing factor (PRF)	Stimulates the release of prolactin
	Follicle-stimulating hormone–releasing factor (FSH-RF)	Stimulates the release of FSH
Inhibiting	Prolactin-inhibiting factor (PIF)	Inhibits the release of prolactin
	Growth hormone–inhibiting hormone (GIH; somatostatin)	Inhibits the release of GH

ACTH, adrenocorticotropic hormone; *FSH,* follicle-stimulating hormone; *GH,* growth hormone; *LH,* luteinizing hormone.

Thirst receptors and osmoreceptors are located in the hypothalamus close to the supraoptic nucleus. ADH is primarily formed in the supraoptic nucleus, but small amounts of ADH are produced in the paraventricular nucleus. Therefore, if the supraoptic nucleus is destroyed, the paraventricular nucleus can compensate and produce adequate amounts of ADH (Toto, 1994a,b). Oxytocin is primarily formed in the paraventricular nucleus. Terminal nerve fibers carry the hormones formed in the hypothalamus through the pituitary stalk to the posterior pituitary (Czernichow, 1993b). Terminal nerve endings contain secretory granules that store and secrete ADH and oxytocin into the capillary bed.

  b. The anterior pituitary consists of five different types of secretory cells including the somatotrophs (secrete GH, constitute 30% to 40% of anterior pituitary cells), corticotrophs (secrete ACTH, constitute about 20% of anterior pituitary cells), thyrotrophs (secrete TSH), gonadotrophs (secrete LH and FSH), and lactotrophs (secrete prolactin). Thyrotrophs, gonadotrophs, and lactotrophs each constitute 3% to 5% of anterior pituitary cells (Blevins and Wand, 1992; Gaillard, 1993; Guyton, 1986; Villee and Najjar, 1994).

3. **Role of the hypothalamus**
  a. The hypothalamus functions as a center to integrate incoming stimuli from the CNS and the peripheral nervous system. It modulates neurotransmitter signals and appropriate endocrine response (Gaillard, 1993). Secretion of pituitary hormones is under the control of the hypothalamus, through either hormonal or electrical signals. The anterior pituitary is under the control of hormones secreted by the hypothalamus. The stimulating and inhibiting hormones from the hypothalamus are carried to the anterior lobe of the pituitary gland via the hypothalamic-hypophysial portal vessels (Table 6–3). The posterior pituitary is controlled by the hypothalamus via nerve fibers that terminate in the posterior pituitary. The hypothalamus synthesizes ADH and transports it to the posterior pituitary.

4. **Antidiuretic hormone (ADH;** also referred to as arginine vasopressin)
  a. *Biosynthesis:* ADH is a polypeptide containing nine amino acids (Villee and

Najjar, 1994). The prohormone is carried in vesicles through the axons to the posterior pituitary. Final synthesis of the prohormone to ADH occurs in the vesicles during axonal transport.

b. *Regulation:* Osmoreceptors in the hypothalamus are in close proximity to the supraoptic nucleus. When serum osmolality increases, the cells in this area begin to shrink, stimulating the release of ADH.

c. The most potent *stimulus for ADH release* is a serum osmolality exceeding 280 mOsm/kg (Conley, 1990). Osmotic changes as small as 1% stimulate release of ADH (Czernichow, 1993 a, b). These small changes in osmolality also stimulate the thirst mechanism, a protective mechanism to maintain water balance and prevent dehydration. Infants, small children, patients who are comatose or disoriented, or individuals who have abnormal thirst response are not able to meet these physiologic demands; therefore, they are dependent on others to ensure an adequate intake of water. A 5% to 10% reduction in circulating blood volume also stimulates ADH release. Therefore, hemorrhage, hypotension, and hypoxemia can activate the release of ADH. Catecholamines and angiotensin II can modulate the release of ADH.

d. ADH release is inhibited by a serum osmolality below 280 mOsm/kg (Toto, 1994a). The baroreceptors in the carotid sinus and the volume receptors in the left atrium send signals to the brain stem via the vagus and glossopharyngeal nerves. The stimulus is then carried to the hypothalamus. This pathway is primarily inhibitory; however, a fall in pressure or volume decreases the amount of inhibition, facilitating the release of ADH. This system is less sensitive than the osmoreceptor system. However, in the face of extensive volume loss (hemorrhage), blood levels of ADH exceed those achieved by hyperosmolality (Czernichow, 1993a). Vincristine, cyclosphosphamide, and glucocorticoids inhibit ADH release (Czernichow, 1993b; Toto, 1994a). Atrial natriuretic factor (ANF) inhibits ADH release and its effect on the kidney.

e. *Effects:* There are two target cell receptors responsive to ADH: V_1 and V_2. V_1 receptors are located in blood vessels. When stimulated, they produce vasoconstriction (Toto, 1994b). V_2 receptors are located in the kidney. ADH increases the permeability of the distal renal tubules and the collecting ducts to water. Water is therefore reabsorbed back into the circulation, increasing circulating blood volume. Antidiuresis is the primary action of V_2 stimulation with a resultant increase in urine osmolality. ADH enhances sodium chloride transport out of the ascending limb of the loop of Henle. This serves to maximize the interstitial osmotic gradient in the renal medulla, facilitating water reabsorption and urine concentration (Villee and Najjar, 1994).

5. **Oxytocin**

a. *Biosynthesis:* Oxytocin is a polypeptide consisting of nine amino acids, almost identical to ADH except for the placement of two of the amino acids in the peptide chain. Like ADH, the prohormone for oxytocin is carried in vesicles through axons from the hypothalamus to the posterior pituitary, where the final synthesis of oxytocin occurs during neuronal transport.

b. *Regulation:* The stimulus for oxytocin release is an increase in estrogen, the onset of labor with stretching and stimulation of the cervix and vagina (labor can occur in women with oxytocin deficiency, although the duration is prolonged), suckling stimuli on the nipple, hemorrhage, or psychologic stress. Oxytocin is inhibited by pain, heat, or loud noises (Toto, 1994b).

c. *Effects* include contraction of the uterus in pregnancy (levels are highest during the last stage of labor) and contraction of the myoepithelial cells in the alveoli of the mammary gland, stimulating the release of breast milk.

6. **Growth hormone (GH)**

   a. *Biosynthesis:* GH is a small protein containing 191 amino acids.

   b. *Regulation:* The strongest stimulus for release is growth hormone–releasing hormone (GH-RH) secreted by the ventromedial nucleus in the hypothalamus. GH-RH is transported to the anterior pituitary via the hypothalamic-hypophysial portal vessels. Starvation, hypoglycemia, stress, exercise, and low blood levels of fatty acids can stimulate GH release. Hypoglycemia stimulates the ventromedial nucleus, the same center that causes the sensation of hunger. Catecholamines, dopamine, and serotonin also can stimulate the release of GH. Inhibition of GH release occurs secondary to growth hormone–inhibitory hormone (GHIH), also known as somatostatin, and increased blood sugar. It is secreted by the hypothalamus and the delta cells of the pancreas.

   c. *Effects:* GH is an anabolic hormone that facilitates linear growth in all tissues of the body through increased mitosis and increased cell size. GH increases protein synthesis through increased RNA and DNA replication, increases mobilization of fatty acids, increases blood glucose levels through the diminished use of glucose by the cell, and stimulates bone and cartilage growth.

   d. *Abnormalities of GH secretion:* With growth hormone deficiency (GHD) the anterior pituitary fails to produce enough GH; consequently stature is less than genetic determination would indicate. Most GHD is idiopathic. An excessive level of GH produces gigantism, usually caused by pituitary adenoma. Gigantism is due to excessive GH secretion after the epiphyses of the long bones have closed.

7. **Adrenocorticotropic hormone (ACTH)**

   a. *Biosynthesis:* ACTH is a large polypeptide consisting of 39 amino acids.

   b. *Regulation:* The stimulation for release of ACTH is corticotropin-releasing factor (CRF) secreted by the hypothalamus. Pain and stress also stimulate release. Inhibition to release of ACTH is primarily through negative feedback secondary to increased cortisol levels, that in turn decrease the formation of CRF.

   c. *Effects:* ACTH controls adrenal cortex function, activating adrenocortical cells to produce and secrete cortisol and aldosterone.

   d. *Abnormalities of ACTH secretion:* Long-term ACTH oversecretion stimulates hypertrophy, proliferation, and hyperfunction of the adrenal cortex (Guyton, 1986). Undersecretion of ACTH leads to adrenal insufficiency.

8. **Thyroid-stimulating hormone (TSH)**

   a. *Biosynthesis:* TSH, also known as thyrotropin, is a glycoprotein.

   b. *Regulation:* Stimulation of the hypothalamus causes secretion of thyrotropin-releasing hormone (TRH). TRH stimulates the anterior pituitary to secrete TSH. Exposure to severe cold stimulates release of TSH. Increased blood levels of thyroid hormones provide negative feedback and inhibit TSH release.

   c. *Effects:* TSH stimulates the thyroid gland to release triiodothyronine (T_3) and thyroxine (T_4), which determines the size and shape of the thyroid follicles and epithelial cells (Delange, 1993).

   d. *Abnormalities of TSH secretion:* Hypersecretion of TSH induces a rare form of hyperthyroidism, usually secondary to a pituitary adenoma. Hyposecretion of TSH may be the cause of extrathyroidal abnormalities that induce hypothyroidism (Czernichow, 1993c; Delange, 1993).

9. **Follicle-stimulating hormone (FSH)**
   a. *Biosynthesis:* FSH is a small glycoprotein.
   b. *Regulation:* The stimulus for FSH release is gonadotropin-releasing hormone (Gn-RH) secreted by the hypothalamus. FSH secretion is inhibited through negative feedback secondary to increased levels of estrogen secreted by the ovaries and increased levels of inhibin secreted by the testes.
   c. *Effects:* Following puberty in boys, FSH promotes spermatogenesis. Following puberty in girls, FSH stimulates the growth of the ovarian follicles.

10. **Luteinizing hormone (LH)**
    a. *Biosynthesis:* LH is a small glycoprotein.
    b. *Regulation:* The stimulus for release of LH is Gn-RH secreted by the hypothalamus. Inhibition for release of LH is negative feedback secondary to increased levels of estrogen, progesterone, and testosterone.
    c. *Effects:* LH stimulates production of testosterone and ovulation and maintenance of the corpus luteum.

11. **Prolactin**
    a. *Regulation:* The stimulus for release of prolactin is oxytocin, which is secreted by the posterior pituitary, and TRH and prolactin-releasing factor (PRF) from the hypothalamus. Inhibition for release of prolactin is dopamine, which is secreted by the hypothalamus.
    b. *Effects:* Prolactin stimulates the growth of the ductal system in the breast and production of breast milk.

12. **Developmental issues**
    a. The *hypothalamus* arises from the diencephalon following a proliferation of neuroblasts. The fibers of the supraoptic tract are present by 12 weeks' gestation. ADH and oxytocin production begin at about 12 weeks' gestation. The pituitary concentration of ADH at term is approximately 20% that of the adult.
    b. The *pituitary gland* has a double embryonic origin, contributing to the differentiation of the anterior and posterior lobes. Pituitary development begins between the fourth and fifth week of gestation. The anterior pituitary forms from ectodermal cells from the primitive mouth cavity. The posterior pituitary forms from the neuroectoderm of the diencephalon.
       • The fetal posterior pituitary is capable of maintaining fetal osmolality and blood volume. In the fetus and newborn, increased levels of ADH are found secondary to hypoxia and stress. Serum levels of ADH in the newborn correlate with the length of labor. Data indicate that ADH secretion is fully mature in the newborn; however, renal responsiveness may be decreased.
       • At 5 weeks' gestation the anterior pituitary secretes ACTH. Administration of steroids during pregnancy decreases fetal ACTH and cortisol levels. At birth, ACTH levels are higher than in adults or children, and they remain elevated during the first week of life. GH is present at 60 days' gestation. Fetal GH levels vary widely secondary to maternal nutrition, fetal stress, and sex. GH does not play a major role in fetal growth. Growth promotion secondary to GH is evident soon after birth (Czernichow, 1993b; Gaillard, 1993; Moore, 1988; Sizonenko and Aubert, 1993; Villec and Najjar, 1994).

C. **THYROID GLAND**
   1. **Location:** The thyroid gland consists of two lobes, located on each side of the trachea below the larynx.
   2. **Cell types:** The thyroid gland consists of a large number of follicles filled with colloid. The main constituent of colloid is thyroglobulin, a glycoprotein

containing the thyroid hormones. Follicular cells and a basal membrane constitute the outer boundary of the follicle. Cuboidal epithelioid cells secrete colloid. Between the follicular cells are parafollicular cells that secrete calcitonin. The thyroid gland is highly vascular; follicles are in close contact with blood and lymphatic vessels.

3. **Metabolism of iodine:** Iodine is the major constituent of the thyroid hormones. To form normal amounts of thyroid hormone, iodine must be ingested and absorbed by the GI tract into the blood. The thyroid gland is capable of concentrating iodide to 20 to 40 times the plasma level. This occurs secondary to the thyroid iodide pump that actively transports iodide across the follicular cell membrane. The iodide pump is stimulated by TSH or a low iodine diet (Delange, 1993).

4. **Thyroglobulin:** Thyroglobulin is the thyroid hormone precursor that permits storage of iodide. It is synthesized by thyroid cells and secreted into the thyroid follicle. Following stimulation by TSH, thyroglobulin is ingested by the follicular cell and undergoes enzymatic digestion to cleave T_4 and T_3, which are subsequently released into the thyroid capillary blood (Guyton, 1986).

5. **Thyroxine (T_4)**
   a. *Biosynthesis:* Ninety percent of the thyroid hormone production is T_4. Iodide is converted to an oxidized form of iodine and binds with thyroglobulin. Oxidized iodine in association with the enzyme iodinase within the thyroglobulin molecule promotes the formation of T_4.
   b. *Regulation:* Release of T_4 is stimulated by TSH, low iodide levels, and extreme cold. Release of T_4 is inhibited by excess iodide and negative feedback due to increased levels of thyroid hormones that decrease the anterior pituitary secretion of TSH. Stimulation of the sympathetic nervous system causes a decrease in the secretion of TSH with a subsequent decrease in thyroid hormone secretion.
   c. *Effects:* T_4 is a prohormone necessary for the production of T_3. The effects of T_4 are similar to the effects of T_3, although less potent with a longer duration of action (Delange, 1993; Toto, 1994a).

6. **Triiodothyronine (T_3)**
   a. *Biosynthesis:* T_3 constitutes 10% of the hormones released by the thyroid gland. The formation of T_3 within the molecule of thyroglobulin is similar to that of T_4. In the peripheral cells, T_4 is deiodinated to form T_3.
   b. *Regulation* of T_3 is the same as for T_4.
   c. *Effects:* On release into the blood stream, the thyroid hormones bind with plasma proteins. Due to a high affinity for the plasma binding proteins, the thyroid hormones are released into the peripheral cells very slowly. Once they enter the cell, these hormones bind with intracellular proteins and are stored. Intracellular activity may last days or weeks. T_3 maintains basal metabolic rate and promotes tissue growth through the stimulation of almost all aspects of carbohydrate and fat metabolism. T_3 promotes protein synthesis, regulates body temperature, and stimulates oxygen consumption through an increase in metabolic rate. In addition, T_3 maintains cardiac output, heart rate, and strength of myocardial contraction through increased metabolism and direct effect on the heart; increases rate and depth of respiration secondary to increased metabolism and increased carbon dioxide production; and increases GI tract motility and secretion of digestive enzymes (Guyton, 1986; Toto, 1994a).

7. **Abnormalities of T_3 and T_4 secretion**
   a. *Hypothyroidism* is caused by low levels of thyroid hormones resulting in lowered metabolic rate, subnormal temperature, low heart rate, hypoten-

sion, weight gain, fatigue, and constipation. Infants with untreated congenital hypothyroidism become mentally retarded.

b. *Hyperthyroidism* is caused by high levels of thyroid hormones, and results in a hypermetabolic state with weight loss, tachycardia, hypertension, irritability, increased GI tract motility, and restlessness.

8. **Calcitonin**
   a. *Biosynthesis:* Calcitonin is a large polypeptide with a 32–amino acid chain. It is manufactured by the parafollicular cells of the C cells of the thyroid gland.
   b. *Regulation:* The stimulus for release of calcitonin is an increase in serum calcium and gastrin. Release of calcitonin is inhibited by a low serum calcium level.
   c. *Effects:* Calcitonin plays a minor role in calcium and phosphorus regulation. It inhibits bone resorption of calcium and phosphorus to lower serum calcium and enhances renal excretion of calcium.

9. **Developmental issues:** The thyroid gland is the first fetal endocrine gland to develop. Twenty-four days after fertilization, development of the thyroid gland begins from the endodermal floor of the primitive pharynx. As the embryo grows, the thyroid gland descends into the neck, passing the laryngeal cartilages. This is complete by 7 weeks' gestation. Fetal brain development is dependent on thyroid hormones. The fetal thyroid gland is able to accumulate iodine by 12 weeks' gestation. T_3 and T_4 are present by the end of the first trimester; however, low levels of thyroid hormones and TSH suggest a relative pituitary hypothyroidism during fetal development. Thyroid hormone levels peak at 24 hours of life and slowly decrease over the next few weeks. Newborns and preterm infants are more sensitive than adults to the effects of iodine excess or deficiency. Calcitonin levels are somewhat elevated at birth, possibly contributing to neonatal hypocalcemia (Czernichow, 1993c; Delange, 1993; Moore, 1988).

D. **PARATHYROID GLANDS**
   1. **Location:** There are usually four parathyroid glands. Two pairs are located behind the thyroid gland, on each side of the trachea.
   2. **Cell types:** Chief cells secrete most of the parathyroid hormone (PTH). Oxyphil cells are absent in infants and children. Their function is unknown.
   3. **Parathyroid hormone (PTH)**
      a. *Biosynthesis:* PTH is composed of 84 amino acids. A prohormone is synthesized and cleaved to form PTH. It is stored in the secretory granules in the cytoplasm of the chief cells.
      b. *Regulation:* The stimulus for release of PTH is hypocalcemia and mild hypomagnesemia. Release of PTH is inhibited by increased ionized calcium, hypermagnesemia, and severe hypomagnesemia (Toto, 1994a).
      c. *Effects:* PTH is the major hormone in the regulation of serum calcium, phosphorus, and magnesium levels. In the kidney PTH increases calcium reabsorption and phosphorus excretion. PTH stimulates the conversion of vitamin D, increases GI tract calcium and phosphate absorption, and promotes bone resorption of calcium (movement out of the bone into the extracellular fluid).
   4. **Abnormalities of parathyroid function**
      a. *Hyperparathyroidism* is a rare disorder with elevated levels of PTH causing hypercalcemia.
      b. *Hypoparathyroidism* is the absence of PTH, resulting in hypocalcemia and hyperphosphatemia.
   5. **Developmental issues:** The third and fourth pharyngeal pouches differentiate

into the thymus and parathyroid glands during the fourth to sixth week of gestation. During gestation the mother is the sole source of minerals for the fetus. Following birth the newborn must rapidly adapt to this loss of support. Ionized calcium and PTH levels remain low for 48 hours after birth. Infants develop an appropriate PTH response to hypocalcemia during the first weeks of life (Moore, 1988; Salle et al, 1993).

E. **ADRENAL GLANDS**

1. **Location:** The adrenal glands are small glands that lie atop the kidneys. Each gland has two distinct parts, the cortex, constituting 20% of the gland, and the medulla, constituting 80% of the gland.

2. **Cell types**

   a. The *adrenal cortex* is responsible for the secretion of corticosteroids. The zona glomerulosa is the outer most layer, responsible for the secretion of aldosterone. The zona fasciculata is the middle layer, responsible for the majority of cortisol secretion. The zona reticularis is the deep layer of the cortex, responsible for cortisol and androgen secretion.

   b. The *adrenal medulla* is responsible for the secretion of the catecholamines epinephrine and norepinephrine.

3. **Aldosterone**

   a. *Biosynthesis:* Aldosterone is a steroid compound synthesized from cholesterol absorbed from the blood. Synthesis is catalyzed by a number of specific enzymes. Because of the similar structure of all the steroids, an alteration in one enzyme can produce significant changes in the steroids being formed.

   b. *Regulation:* Volume depletion, decreased renal perfusion, ACTH, and increased levels of angiotensin II increase aldosterone release. An increase in serum potassium of less than 1 mmol/L will triple aldosterone release. Inhibition to aldosterone release is secondary to volume expansion, hypokalemia, and low angiotensin levels (Guyton, 1986; Toto, 1994a).

   c. *Effects:* Aldosterone is responsible for 95% of mineralocorticoid activity. It acts on the distal tubule, collecting tubule, and collecting duct of the kidney to promote sodium reabsorption and potassium excretion. Along with renal reabsorption of sodium, there is a concurrent movement of water into the vascular bed. The net effect is an increase in extracellular sodium, an increase in extracellular volume, and a decrease in extracellular potassium. Aldosterone promotes reabsorption of sodium and excretion of potassium by the sweat and salivary glands and promotes hydrogen ion excretion by the kidney.

4. **Cortisol**

   a. *Biosynthesis:* Cortisol is a steroid compound. Synthesis of cortisol is similar to that of aldosterone.

   b. *Regulation:* The primary stimulus for secretion of cortisol is ACTH. Stress is another strong stimulus. Release of cortisol is inhibited by negative feedback to the anterior pituitary secondary to increased cortisol levels, producing a decrease in ACTH release.

   c. *Effects:* Cortisol increases gluconeogenesis and decreases peripheral use of glucose. The net effect of the above two actions leads to hyperglycemia. Protein synthesis decreases, and catabolism of protein increases. Cortisol promotes mobilization of fatty acids from the tissues. Antiinflammatory effects include stabilization of lysosomal membranes, decrease of capillary permeability, block of allergic reactions, and reduction of the intensity of the inflammatory reaction. Cortisol sensitizes the vascular bed to the alpha effects of norepinephrine to support vascular tone and blood pressure and protects against stress.

5. **Abnormalities of adrenal cortical function**
   a. *Adrenal insufficiency:* Primary adrenal insufficiency (Addison's disease) is due to an absent or damaged adrenal gland. Symptoms are secondary to absent or insufficient glucocorticoids and mineralocorticoids. Chronic deficiency produces weakness, weight loss, anorexia, electrolyte imbalances, and altered metabolism. Adrenal crisis due to an acute depletion of adrenal cortical hormones (secondary to stress or infection) precipitates vomiting, diarrhea, convulsions, coma, hypotension, hyperpyrexia, tachycardia, and cyanosis. Adrenal insufficiency can also result from exogenous suppression with oral or IV steroids. High levels of circulating steroids suppress ACTH release, and abrupt withdrawal of steroids results in symptoms previously described.
   b. *Hyperfunction of the adrenal cortex* (Cushing's syndrome) results in growth retardation; weight gain; moon facies; striae on the hips, abdomen, and thighs; bruises; bone demineralization; emotional lability; and increased blood volume.

6. **Epinephrine**
   a. *Biosynthesis:* Epinephrine is a catecholamine derived from the amino acid tyrosine. Tyrosine is converted to dopamine in the sympathetic nerve endings. Dopamine is transported into vesicles, where it is converted to norepinephrine, which is converted to epinephrine in the adrenal medulla. Eighty percent of the catecholamine secreted by the adrenal medulla is epinephrine (Guyton, 1986).
   b. *Regulation:* Preganglionic sympathetic nerves pass from the spinal cord to the adrenal medulla. These nerve tracts end on secretory cells that secrete epinephrine and norepinephrine directly into the blood. The secretory cells are embryologically derived from nerve cells. Any stress or stimulus that produces a sympathetic (fight-or-flight) response stimulates secretion of epinephrine from the adrenal medulla. ACTH and cortisol also stimulate release of epinephrine. Inhibition of epinephrine is through negative feedback. High levels of circulating catecholamines produce a down regulation of sympathetic receptors.
   c. *Effects* are secondary to the stimulation of β-adrenergic receptors in the end-organs. The greatest effects are due to stimulation of the sympathetic β_1-adrenergic receptors in the heart, resulting in increased cardiac contractility, conduction velocity, and heart rate. The net result is an increase in cardiac output and blood pressure. In isolation, stimulation of the β_2-adrenergic receptors of the vascular bed promotes relaxation; however, during stress the vasoconstricting effects of norepinephrine counteract significant vasodilation. Other effects of stimulation of the β-adrenergic receptors are intestinal, bladder, and uterine relaxation and bronchial dilation. Epinephrine increases metabolic activity to a much greater degree than norepinephrine. It increases glycogenolysis and glucose release, resulting in elevations of blood glucose. Epinephrine accounts for 10% of the sympathetic activity during the stress response (Guyton, 1986; Toto, 1994a).

7. **Norepinephrine**
   a. *Biosynthesis:* Norepinephrine is synthesized in the nerve endings of the sympathetic nervous system. The precursor is dopamine, which is converted in nerve ending vesicles to norepinephrine.
   b. *Regulation* is the same as for epinephrine.
   c. *Effects* are secondary to stimulation of the α-adrenergic receptors in the end-organs. The most significant effect during stress is peripheral vasoconstriction supporting blood pressure. Stimulation of the α-adrenergic recep-

tors also produces dilation of the iris, contraction of the bladder and intestinal sphincters, and pilomotor contraction.

8. The most significant abnormality of adrenal medulla function is hyperfunction. Pheochromocytoma is a catecholamine-secreting tumor arising from the adrenal medulla that produces hypertension, tachycardia, diaphoresis, tremors, and headaches (Agana-Defensor and Proch, 1992).

9. **Developmental issues**
   a. The adrenal glands develop from two different origins: the cortex, arising from the mesoderm, and the medulla, arising from the neural crest cells. Differentiation of the adrenal medulla occurs late in gestation, and the zona reticularis is not developed until the end of the third year of life.
   b. Fetal cortisol is necessary for the enzymatic maturation of the fetal liver. Newborn blood cortisol levels are twice the maternal levels at birth and progressively decrease over the next 2 months of life.
   c. Rates of aldosterone secretion are low in the newborn. The renin-angiotensin-aldosterone system is active in the newborn, with levels of angiotensin II higher in cord blood than in maternal blood.
   d. The sympathetic nervous system is immature in the newborn and infant. α-Adrenergic and β-adrenergic receptors are decreased in number, density, and responsiveness in the infant (Moore, 1988; Sizonenko and Aubert, 1993).

CLINICAL ASSESSMENT OF ENDOCRINE FUNCTION

Many endocrine disorders develop over time so they may not become apparent immediately. Often in hindsight it becomes apparent that a child has had an endocrine disorder for years. Assessment and documentation of past medical conditions, growth patterns, developmental milestones, physical examinations, and family history are critical to the accurate diagnosis of endocrine disorders.

A. **HISTORY**
   1. **Family history** includes the parents' age; height, weight, and body proportions of family members; the parents' age at puberty; familial and genetic diseases; health of parents and siblings; presence of known endocrine disorders in other family members; the child and family's perception of any known endocrine disorders in the family; and the impact of known endocrine disorders on the family's lifestyle.
   2. **Prenatal history** includes complications of pregnancy; prenatal exposure to infections, drugs, radiation, and alcohol; and gestational diabetes.
   3. **Neonatal history** includes gestational age, complications of labor and delivery, method of delivery, Apgar scores, hospitalization as a newborn, congenital anomalies, feeding difficulties, and postnatal complications.
   4. **Growth and development** factors to evaluate include height and weight, recent changes in weight, and developmental milestones and growth patterns.
      a. Diet is assessed including food preferences and aversions, content and time of typical meals, snacking behaviors, changes in appetite, and anorexia. Problems with digestion such as nausea, bloating, food intolerances, abnormal stool patterns, diarrhea, or constipation are noted.
      b. School performance and problems or recent changes in performance are discussed. Assessment of personality and behavioral traits includes recent changes in behavior, irritability, sluggishness, disinterest, lethargy, emotional lability, attention deficits, increased aggressiveness, altered self-esteem, perceptions of body image, family roles, and socialization issues.

    c. Sleep and rest patterns including normal bedtimes, incidence of insomnia, ease of falling asleep, restlessness, snoring, bed-wetting, and nightmares are evaluated. Also, note activity and exercise patterns including the types of exercise normally engaged in, stamina, strength, outside interests, and hobbies.

    d. Sexual maturation including the age of development, any abnormalities, timing and character of menarche, and sexual activity is recorded.

5. **Past medical history** includes known endocrine disorders, neurosurgery, trauma or stress, and previous hospitalizations.

    a. *Medication history* can be significant.

- High-dose steroids can induce hyperglycemia, inhibit normal physiologic release of steroids from the adrenal cortex, suppress ACTH release, and alter serum electrolytes.
- Nonsteroidal antiinflammatory agents enhance renal responsiveness to ADH.
- Sedatives, narcotics, and anesthetics can stimulate the thirst mechanism and alter ADH release.
- Phenytoin inhibits insulin release.
- Chemotherapy alters ADH release.
- Stimulants stimulate the thirst mechanism, alter glucose metabolism, and can modulate release of catecholamines.
- Ethanol stimulates the thirst mechanism, alters serum osmolality and ADH release, and alters glucose metabolism by inhibiting insulin.
- Tricyclic antidepressants stimulate the thirst mechanism and alter ADH release.
- Hypoglycemic agents alter glucose metabolism and serum glucose levels.
- Hormone replacements alter normal feedback mechanisms for hormone release.
- Diuretics stimulate the thirst mechanism, alter serum electrolytes and osmolality, and alter renal response to ADH.

    b. Other diseases can have a relationship with endocrine disorders. Cystic fibrosis can be an underlying cause of diabetes mellitus (DM). Pancreatitis constitutes part of the differential diagnosis for pancreatic disorders. Renal disease can be an underlying cause of diabetes insipidus (DI) and part of the differential diagnosis for ADH abnormalities. Lung disease can be an underlying cause of syndrome of inappropriate antidiuretic hormone (SIADH). Pheochromocytoma is a catecholamine-secreting tumor.

B. PHYSICAL ASSESSMENT (Table 6–4)

1. Height and weight are measured.
2. Body size and proportion, fat distribution, upper and lower body ratios, chest circumference, and arm span are compared to previous measurements if available.
3. Temperature, blood pressure, and heart rate are recorded.
4. Head circumference and percentiles on age- and sex-related growth charts are plotted.
5. Intake and output is monitored.
6. The head, eyes, ears, nose and throat (HEENT) survey includes observation for sunken or protruding eyes, periorbital edema, gaze, pupil symmetry, and visual acuity. The thyroid gland and neck are palpated for masses or thrills, and the neck is auscultated for bruits. The mucous membranes are assessed for moisture and color, and the oral cavity is inspected for abnormalities of the lips and palate, presence of caries, and abnormalities in dentition. Observe for obvious dysmorphic features.

Table 6–4. DEVELOPMENTAL CONSIDERATIONS IN THE PHYSICAL EXAMINATION OF ENDOCRINE FUNCTION

SYSTEM	INFANT	CHILD	ADOLESCENT
Head and neck	Patency and size of fontanelle; symmetry of head, eyes, and ears Dentition appropriate for age Absence of cleft lip or palate Absence of goiter	Symmetry of head, eyes, ears Dentition appropriate for age Absence of goiter	Symmetry of head, eyes, ears Dentition appropriate for age Absence of goiter
Chest	Symmetry, absence of breast development Normally spaced nipples	Breast development (Tanner stage)	Breast development (Tanner stage) Gynecomastia in boys
Abdomen	Absence of umbilical hernia, symmetry	Fat distribution	Fat distribution
Genitourinary	Absence of genital ambiguity, absence of hair, absence of odor and discharge	Absence of hair or pubertal changes Testicular descent in boys Sexual development (Tanner stage) Absence of odor or discharge	Sexual development appropriate for age (Tanner stage) Absence of odor or discharge
Musculoskeletal	Absence of disproportionality, muscle tone (hypotonic vs. normal vs. spastic)	Absence of disproportionality Absence of short metacarpals Absence of muscle weakness	Absence of disproportionality Absence of short metacarpals Absence of muscle weakness
Neurologic	Absence of hypotonia Absence of tremor	Absence of tremor Absence of hyporeflexia or hyperreflexia Absence of gait disturbance Normal stance	Absence of tremor Absence of hyporeflexia or hyperreflexia Absence of gait disturbance Normal stance
Integument	Absence of abnormal texture or coloring (hyperpigmentation or vitiligo) Absence of excessive nevi	Absence of abnormal texture or coloring (hyperpigmentation or vitiligo) Absence of excessive nevi	Absence of abnormal texture or coloring (hyperpigmentation or vitiligo) Absence of excessive nevi

From Parker SH. Nursing assessment and diagnosis of endocrine function. In: Jackson DB, Saunders RB, eds. *Child Health Nursing.* Philadelphia, Pa: JB Lippincott Co; 1993:1450.

7. Integumentary assessment includes turgor and moisture; color including hyperpigmentation, depigmentation, nevi, and café au lait spots; texture of the skin including the presence of excess oil, rough or dry skin, acne, and temperature; hair texture and distribution; and brittle nails.

8. Neurologic assessment includes the level of consciousness (irritability, lethargy,

hyperactivity), cranial nerves, size and shape of the head, palpation of fontanelle and suture lines, pupil responses, fine and gross motor movement, abnormal gait or stance, presence of tremors, reflexes, abnormal deep tendon reflexes, and presence of seizure activity.

9. Cardiovascular evaluation includes rate, rhythm, and character of heart tones; peripheral pulses; perfusion, capillary fill time, warmth, and mottling of skin; palpation for thrills, heaves, and point of maximal impulse (PMI); edema; and blood pressure (hypertension or hypotension, orthostasis).

10. Respiratory assessment includes the rate and depth of respiration, odor of breath (acetone), chest excursion, chest symmetry and deformities, and characteristics of breath sounds (coarse or fine crackles, areas of diminished breath sounds).

11. Abdominal assessment notes the presence of bowel sounds (hypoactive or hyperactive), tenderness and pain, size, and shape (central obesity with thin arms and legs, distribution and character of fat) and includes palpation of the liver, spleen, and masses.

12. Genitourinary survey includes the development of external sexual organs and testicular size, palpation of the kidneys, and the Tanner stage of pubic hair and breast development.

13. Musculoskeletal survey includes disproportionate growth (body habitus, length of extremities), presence of genu valgum or genu varum, short or unusually long metacarpals, and palpation of muscles (Parker, 1993).

C. Diagnostic Studies

1. Laboratory

a. *Blood* (Table 6–5) chemistries are performed for screening and include electrolytes (magnesium, phosphorus, calcium), glucose, pH, osmolality, blood urea nitrogen (BUN) and creatinine, and cortisol levels to assess the pituitary-adrenal axis (plasma levels vary with age and time of day). Screening is done for inborn errors of metabolism (part of the differential diagnosis of endocrine dysfunction); inborn errors of metabolism alter fat and glucose metabolism, and normal growth. Screening is done for enzyme deficiencies; various enzyme deficiencies may be the underlying cause of alterations in metabolism and growth. Glycosylated hemoglobin is measured to assess blood glucose control. Vasopressin levels determine the type of DI.

b. *Urine* is tested for electrolytes, fractional excretion of sodium, specific gravity, osmolality, glucose, ketones, and pH.

c. *Dynamic tests of function*
   - The water deprivation test is described later under DI.
   - With a glucose tolerance test (rarely obtained), an oral or IV glucose load is administered following an overnight fast, and serial blood glucose determinations are made (Table 6–6). It can help in the diagnosis of DM type I.
   - An insulin tolerance test is used to assess the hypothalamic-pituitary-adrenal axis. Following an overnight fast, regular insulin is administered intravenously to produce hypoglycemia, and serial blood sampling is performed to determine cortisol, blood glucose, and GH levels. This test requires continuous patient monitoring, and is hazardous to those with panhypopituitarism.
   - TRH stimulation is used to assess the hypothalamic-pituitary-thyroid axis. TRH is administered intravenously, and serial blood determinations of T_3, T_4, and TSH are obtained to diagnose thyroid dysfunction.
   - An ACTH stimulation test is used to assess the hypothalamic-pituitary-

Table 6–5. BLOOD INDEXES OF ENDOCRINE FUNCTION

TEST	APPROPRIATE RANGE*	DEVIATIONS	CLINICAL IMPLICATIONS
Growth hormone (GH) Somatomedin C or insulin-like growth factor (IGF-1)	>10 ng/ml after pharmacologic stimulation Normal ranges specific for laboratory and child age	<10 ng/ml Low	Growth hormone deficiency Growth hormone deficiency Malnutrition
17-hydroxyprogesterone	Less than 200 ng/dl	Elevated	Adrenal hyperplasia, in poor control
Karyotype	46 xy (male) 46 xx (female)	Abnormal karyotype associated with many syndromes	45 xo Turner's syndrome, 47 xxy Klinefelter's syndrome, 15 q Prader-Willi syndrome
Luteinizing hormone (LH) and follicle- stimulating hormone (FSH)	Prepubertal: <10 mIU/ml After puberty: 10–25 mIU/ml	Elevated with precocious puberty Low Very high	Primary gonadal failure, pre- cocious puberty Hypogonadotrophic Hypogonadism Primary gonadal failure
Total thyroxine (T$_4$)	4.5–12.5 µg/dl	Elevated Low	Hyperthyroidism Increased thyroid-binding globulin (TBG) Hypothyroidism Decreased TBG
Triidothyronine (T$_3$) resin uptake	33–50%	Elevated Low	Hyperthyroidism Decreased TBG Hypothyroidism Increased TBG

Test	Normal value*		Clinical significance
Thyroid-stimulating hormone (TSH)	0.3–5 mIU/ml	Elevated	Primary hypothyroidism
		Low	Hyperthyroidism
			TSH deficiency
		Normal	
Calcium	Premature: 6–10 mg/dl	Low	Hypocalcemia due to rickets,
	Full term <1 wk: 7–12 mg/dl		hypoparathyroidism
	Child: 8–10.5 mg/dl	Elevated	Hyperparathyroidism
	Adult: 8.5–10.5 mg/dl		
Phosphorus	<1 y: 4.2–9 mg/dl	Low	Rickets, renal phosphate loss
	1 y: 3.8–6.2 mg/dl		(X-linked rickets), hyper-
	2–5 y: 3.5–6.8 mg/dl		parathyroid
	Adult: 3–4.5 mg/dl	Elevated	Renal disease, hyperpara-
			thyroid, neonatal tetany
Alkaline phosphatase	<2 y: 150–400 U/L	Low	Hypoparathyroid
	2–10 y: 100–300 U/L		Hypophosphatasia
	11–18 y	Elevated	Rickets, hyperparathyroid,
	Male: 50–375 U/L		familial
	Female: 30–300 U/L		
	Adult: 30–100 U/L		

*Normal ranges vary between laboratories. Compare patient values to normals for the laboratory performing the tests.

From Parker SH. Nursing assessment and diagnosis of endocrine function. In: Jackson DB, Saunders RE, eds. *Child Health Nursing.* Philadelphia, Pa: JB Lippincott Co; 1993:1453.

Table 6–6. BLOOD LEVELS OF GLUCOSE FOLLOWING AN ORAL GLUCOSE TOLERANCE TEST

	NORMAL		IDDM	
	WHOLE BLOOD	PLASMA	WHOLE BLOOD	PLASMA
Fasting	<100 mg/dl	<115 mg/dl	>120 mg/dl	>140 mg/dl
30, 60, and 90 minutes	<180 mg/dl	<200 mg/dl	>180 mg/dl	>200 mg/dl

IDDM, insulin-dependent diabetes mellitus.

adrenal axis. Following an IV dose of ACTH, serial cortisol levels are obtained to diagnose adrenal insufficiency.
- GH stimulation is used to diagnose GHD. Insulin, clonidine, arginine, or glucagon may be administered to stimulate the release of GH (Bertrand et al, 1993; Parker, 1993).

2. **Pitfalls in the interpretation of endocrine function tests** (Toto, 1994a): Many hormones are secreted according to a specific rhythm. Plasma hormone levels are dependent on the time and circumstances of measurement. A single measurement of blood levels may not accurately reflect mean levels. Factors that interfere with endocrine tests include drug therapy, nutritional status, stress, and pathology.

3. **Radiologic tests:**
   a. Chest radiographs are used to evaluate for pleural effusions or congestive heart failure (CHF).
   b. Computed tomography (CT) scan of the head and neck determines the presence of cerebral edema, tumors, or midline defects. CT scan of the abdomen is used to determine the presence of pancreatic or renal tumors.
   c. Magnetic resonance imaging (MRI) of the head is used to determine the presence of tumors.
   d. Ultrasound of the neck and abdomen is used to determine renal and pancreatic function, to evaluate for pancreatic tumors, and to determine thyroid function.
   e. Bone age evaluates normal growth patterns.

4. An **electrocardiogram (ECG)** is used to evaluate myocardial function and the presence of dysrhythmias.

DIABETES MELLITUS (DM)

A. DEFINITIONS
   1. **Type I: Insulin-dependent diabetes mellitus (IDDM):** IDDM (10% of the DM population) is an autoimmune disease, resulting in the destruction of beta pancreatic cells. The process may be slow, since some children maintain a limited ability to secrete insulin for up to 5 years (Palmer, 1994; Villee and Najjar, 1994). IDDM (DM type I) occurs in genetically susceptible children usually in response to an environmental agent that triggers the autoimmune process (Millward, 1993). Eighty percent to 90% of the beta cells must be destroyed prior to clinically detectable hyperglycemia (Plotnick, 1994). IDDM is the most common form of diabetes in infants and children and requires insulin replacement therapy. IDDM is associated with ketoacidosis and abrupt onset of diabetes.
   2. **Type II: Non-insulin-dependent diabetes mellitus (NIDDM):** NIDDM (90% of

the DM population) was previously referred to as adult-onset diabetes. It can often be treated with oral hypoglycemic agents, diet, or exercise. NIDDM is associated with obesity, a strong family history, and older age. It is not an autoimmune process but, instead, is due to insulin resistance (Villee and Najjar, 1994). Enough insulin is produced to prevent ketoacidosis, so onset is slow.

B. **DIABETIC KETOACIDOSIS (DKA)**
1. **Pathophysiology**
   a. DKA is a relative or absolute insulin deficiency (Fig. 6–5). In the absence of insulin, stored substrates are mobilized, and cellular uptake of glucose is inhibited (Jones, 1994; Miller, 1994; Plotnick, 1994). Glycogenolysis, proteolysis, and lipolysis occur.
   b. An increase in counterregulatory hormones contributes to hyperglycemia. Hyperglycemia results from increased glucose production and decreased glucose utilization. Glycosuria occurs when the renal threshold for glucose is exceeded, and polyuria results from an osmotic diuresis due to glycosuria. Passive electrolyte losses occur secondary to the diuresis. Hyperosmolality is secondary to hyperglycemia and free water loss with diuresis. Nausea and vomiting occur secondary to ketoacidosis, electrolyte imbalances, and

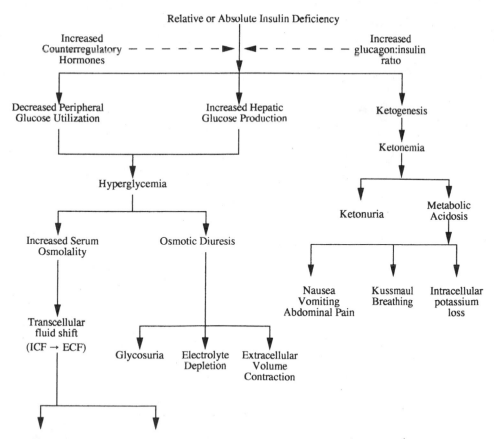

Figure 6–5. The physiologic alterations responsible for the clinical presentation of DKA begin with a relative or absolute insulin deficiency and an increase in counterregulatory hormones, most notably glucagon. The resulting increased glucagon-to-insulin ratio leads to hyperglycemia and ketogenesis, which ultimately leads to disturbances in fluid and electrolyte and acid-base balance. (Reprinted with permission from Jones TL. Diabetic ketoacidosis to hyperglycemic hyperosmolar nonketotic syndrome. *Crit Care Nurs Clin North Am.* 1994;6(4):706.)

possible viral illness. Dehydration occurs secondary to osmotic diuresis and vomiting (Rosenbloom and Schatz, 1994; Villee and Najjar, 1994).

   c. Lack of insulin results in mobilization and incomplete oxidization of fatty acids. There is a resulting increase in ketone bodies (acetoacetic acid, β-hydroxybutyric acid, and acetone) that contributes to the development of metabolic acidosis (Jones, 1994; Laron and Karp, 1993; Miller, 1994). Metabolic acidosis contributes to the extracellular movement of potassium with a resultant depletion of total body potassium, although serum levels may be normal (Ellis, 1990).

2. **Etiology** is related to inadequate endogenous insulin secretion (DM initially presents as DKA in 40% of children newly diagnosed with diabetes [Larson and Karp, 1993]), deliberate or inadvertent omission of insulin, or to acute stress or infection in patients with IDDM.

3. **Risk factors** include a previous history of IDDM with poor metabolic control; initial presentation of IDDM is precipitated by stress, acute infection, or trauma (Laron and Karp, 1993); adolescents with diabetes who do not comply with their treatment plan (Millward, 1993); stress or acute illness in patients with diabetes; cystic fibrosis; and high-dose steroids.

4. **Signs and symptoms** (Table 6–7) include polyuria, polydipsia, and polyphagia. Generally a serum glucose greater than 200 mg/dl. However, DKA can occur with normoglycemia or hypoglycemia if severe vomiting is present. pH is less than 7.3 (Miller, 1994; Plotnick, 1994), and serum bicarbonate is less than 18 mmol/L (Villee and Najjar, 1994). Hyperosmolality is noted. Serum sodium may be high, low, or normal with total body sodium depletion; and serum potassium may be high, low, or normal with total body potassium depletion.

Table 6–7. SIGNS AND SYMPTOMS OF DIABETIC KETOACIDOSIS (DKA)

CLINICAL PRESENTATION	UNDERLYING MECHANISMS
Shock	Osmotic diuresis secondary to hyperglycemia
Acidosis	Build up of ketones, ketoacids and lacic acid in serum from oxygenation of fatty acids
Sodium alterations	Total body sodium depletion due to passive loss of sodium as a result of osmotic diuresis; serum sodium may be high due to hemoconcentration
Potassium alterations	Intracellular to extracellular potassium shifts due to acidosis, potassium may be normal or inceased then decrease as a result of osmotic diuresis
Cardiac arrhythmia	Hypokalemia, hyperkalemia
Ketonuria	Ketones rise above the renal threshold and are spilled into the urine
Hyperpnea	A compensatory mechanism in effort to blow off carbon dioxide and normalize pH
Mental status changes and cerebral edema	Possibly related to rate of correction, hyperosmolar state, or fluid shifts
Nausea, vomiting, abdominal pain	Electrolyte disturbances, acidosis, and underlying factors
Glucosuria	Glucose spilled into the urine when blood glucose exceeds the renal threshold, creating an osmotic diuresis
Weight loss	Due to ketogenesis and fat metabolism (lipolysis) when cells are deprived of glucose and dehydration
Hyperosmolality	Hyperglycemia Hypernatremia secondary to hemoconcentration

Elevated serum triglycerides are present. The white blood cell (WBC) count is elevated with a shift to the left (Miller, 1994). Other symptoms include weight loss, weakness and lethargy, nausea and vomiting, abdominal pain, dehydration, tachycardia, hypovolemia, poor perfusion, shock, glycosuria, ketonuria, rapid deep respiration (Kussmaul's breathing) and lethargy, stupor, or coma.

5. **Interpretation of diagnostic studies**
   a. Hyperglycemia is due to insulin deficiency, decreased glucose uptake, gluconeogenesis, and an increase in the counterregulatory hormones.
   b. Glycosuria is secondary to hyperglycemia.
   c. pH less than 7.30 and bicarbonate less than 18 mmol/L are due to acetoacetic acid and β-hydroxybutyrate dehydrogenase (ketones) production.
   d. Ketonuria is due to the high levels of serum ketones.
   e. Serum osmolality is greater than 300 mOsm/kg because of hyperglycemia and diuresis (dehydration).
   f. Electrolyte disturbances are related to electrolyte loss with osmotic diuresis and metabolic acidosis.
   g. Islet cell antibodies and insulin autoantibodies may offer a screening tool for detecting patients with pre–type I IDDM in the future, but they are not diagnostic for DKA (Boulware and Tamborlane, 1992; Chase et al, 1991; Palmer, 1994).
   h. A glucose tolerance test can be used to diagnose glucose intolerance but is not necessary to make the diagnosis of DKA (Laron and Karp, 1993; Villee and Najjar, 1994; Table 6–6).
   i. Glycosylated hemoglobin reflects blood glucose control over the last 2 to 3 months. Elevated levels are correlated with high serum glucose concentrations.
   j. CT scan is used to diagnose cerebral edema, an uncommon manifestation associated with rapid correction of hyperosmolar states.

6. **Diagnoses**
   a. *Differential diagnoses* include adrenocortical dysfunction, high-dose steroids, pheochromocytoma, pancreatitis, cystic fibrosis, exogenous catecholamines, stress response, DI, alcoholic ketoacidosis, starvation, and inborn errors of metabolism.
   b. *Collaborative diagnoses*
      ❖ FLUID VOLUME DEFICIT RELATED TO OSMOTIC DIURESIS SECONDARY TO HYPERGLYCEMIA
      ❖ POTENTIAL FOR LOW CARDIAC OUTPUT RELATED TO FLUID VOLUME DEFICIT
      ❖ POTENTIAL FOR CEREBRAL EDEMA RELATED TO TREATMENT
      ❖ ARRYTHMIAS RELATED TO ELECTROLYTE IMBALANCES
      ❖ ACID-BASE IMBALANCE RELATED TO KETOACIDOSIS
      ❖ ELECTROLYTE IMBALANCES RELATED TO OSMOTIC DIURESIS OR TREATMENT, OR BOTH
      ❖ POTENTIAL FOR HYPOGLYCEMIA RELATED TO TREATMENT
      ❖ POTENTIAL FOR SELF-CARE DEFICITS RELATED TO LIFELONG TREATMENT AND MONITORING, WITH POSSIBLE NONCOMPLIANCE
      ❖ ALTERATION IN BODY IMAGE RELATED TO CHRONIC ILLNESS AND FUTURE COMPLICATIONS
      ❖ ALTERATION IN NUTRITION RELATED TO POOR METABOLIC CONTROL
      ❖ POTENTIAL FOR INFECTION RELATED TO SECONDARY COMPLICATIONS
      ❖ POTENTIAL FOR KNOWLEDGE DEFICIT REGARDING HOME MANAGEMENT

7. **Treatment goals**
   a. Correct fluid and electrolyte imbalances.

    b. Correct metabolic acidosis.

    c. Provide insulin to treat and prevent ketosis and to lower serum glucose.

    d. Prevent neurologic complications.

    e. Maintain good metabolic control (long term).

    f. Treat underlying disorders.

8. **Management**

    a. *Fluid and electrolyte therapy:* Assume that the child is 10% dehydrated (Rosenbloom and Schatz, 1994). Administer 20 ml/kg normal saline (NS) during the first 1 to 2 hours as volume expansion. Reassess and administer another fluid bolus if needed to treat poor perfusion (Jones, 1994). Calculate the fluid deficit and replace over the next 48 hours, including ongoing losses (urine, vomiting), with 0.5 NS. Do not exceed 4 $L/m^2/d$ to prevent the development of cerebral edema (Table 6–8). Replace potassium when the serum potassium level is less than 6 mEq/L as a combination of 20 mEq/L KCl and 20 mEq/L KPO_4 (Jones, 1994; Rosenbloom and Schatz, 1994). Bicarbonate replacement is very controversial in children and it should only be instituted if pH is less than 7.10 or the bicarbonate level is less than 5 mmol/L, or shock, cardiac insufficiency, or renal failure is present. If given, sodium bicarbonate should be given *slowly* in the replacement fluids and discontinued when the pH reaches 7.20 (Miller, 1994; Villee and Najjar, 1994); sodium bicarbonate should not be given as a bolus. Phosphate replacement is necessary, usually given as KPO_4 in the replacement fluids.

    b. The initial bolus of regular insulin (Table 6–9) 0.1 U/kg IV or subcutaneously (SC) is followed by continuous infusion of regular insulin 0.1 U/kg/h (Rosenbloom and Schatz, 1994). Blood glucose should drop 50 to 150 mg/dl/h; if this does not occur, the insulin dose can be increased to 0.2 U/kg/h. When the blood glucose falls to 250 mg/dl, IV fluids should have 5% dextrose added (Ellis, 1990; Miller, 1994). If blood glucose falls to less than 150 mg/dl, 10% dextrose should be added to the IV fluids. Do not stop insulin if the blood glucose falls in the face of persistent acidosis. Decrease the insulin dose if the blood glucose falls to less than 100 mg/dl (Plotnick, 1994). Give SC insulin 30 to 60 minutes prior to discontinuing the continuous infusion. IV insulin should continue until the pH is greater than

Table 6–8. GUIDELINES FOR FLUID THERAPY REQUIREMENTS

ESTIMATION OF FLUID VOLUME DEFICIT	
% WEIGHT LOSS	FLUID DEFICIT
4–5	40–50 ml/kg
6–9	60–90 ml/kg
>10	100–110 ml/kg

DAILY IV MAINTENANCE FLUIDS*	
100 ml/kg	First 10 kg body weight
50 ml/kg	Next 10–20 kg body weight
20 ml/kg	Each additional kg over 20 kg

*Maintenance requirements may be altered by renal function, insensible losses, mechanical ventilation, and the administration of humidified gases.

Data from Paschall JA, Melvin T. Fluid and electrolyte therapy. In: Holbrook PR, ed. *Textbook of Pediatric Critical Care.* Philadelphia, Pa: WB Saunders Co; 1993.

Table 6–9. INSULIN PREPARATIONS

TYPE	ONSET	PEAK EFFECT	DURATION
Regular	0.5–1 h	2–3 h	5–7 h
Semilente	0.5–1 h	4–7 h	12–16 h
NPH	1–2 h	4–12 h	18–24 h
Lente	1–2 h	8–12 h	18–24 h
Ultralente	4–8 h	16–18 h	36 h

From Taketomo CK, Hodding JH, Kraus DM. *Pediatric Dosage Handbook 1997–98*. 4th ed. Cleveland, Ohio: Lexi-Comp; 1997:395.

7.25, bicarbonate is greater than 15 mmol/L, and the child is tolerating oral intake.

c. *Monitoring:* Vital signs, blood pressure, and neurologic checks are done every 30 minutes. Hourly glucometer determination of blood glucose is done at the bedside. Initial laboratory tests should include complete blood count (CBC), electrolytes, BUN, creatinine, glucose, and pH. Electrolytes and pH are monitored every 2 hours until stable. Sodium deficits range from 4 to 11 mEq/kg and potassium deficits range from 1 to 10 mEq/kg in children, although serum levels may not reflect total body depletion (Ellis, 1990). A gradual rise in serum sodium as the glucose levels fall can help prevent rapid changes in serum osmolality, therefore maintaining normal serum osmolality (Plotnick, 1994). BUN and creatinine are assessed every 12 hours. Intake and output, daily weights, and urine ketones (every void) are monitored.

9. **Complications**
   a. *Acute*
      - Hypoglycemia is due to infrequent blood glucose monitoring and delayed glucose replacement.
      - Persistent acidosis can be related to inadequate insulin dose or method of delivery. Lactic acidosis is secondary to inadequate volume resuscitation (Rosenbloom and Schatz, 1994).
      - Hypokalemia can occur because of inadequate potassium replacement.
      - Cerebral edema is possibly due to a precipitous fall in blood glucose, excessive fluid resuscitation (>4 L/m^2), excessive use of bicarbonate, or failure to elevate serum sodium levels with treatment. Cerebral edema is often unpredictable and is frequently fatal, particularly in children younger than 5 years (Ellis, 1990; Plotnick, 1994).
      - Mucormycosis infection is an opportunistic fungal infection that is a complication of frequent episodes of DKA. Mucormycosis can present as pneumonia, pulmonary infarction, ulceration and necrosis of the nasal cavities or sinuses, orbital cellulitis, or inflammation and infarction of the GI tract. It is often fatal (Rosenbloom and Schatz, 1994).
      - Fluid overload and CHF can occur because of treatment.
      - Aspiration is possible if the level of consciousness is depressed.
   b. *Chronic complications* of DM include poor metabolic control with episodes of hypoglycemia and hyperglycemia, poor growth, insulin resistance, hypertrophy and lipoatrophy (lipoatrophy is rare with purified insulins) of injection sites, limited joint mobility, vaginitis and candidiasis, retinopathy, nephropathy, neuropathy (rare in childhood), and macrovascular disease.

HYPERGLYCEMIC, HYPEROSMOLAR, NONKETOTIC SYNDROME (HHNS)

A. **PATHOPHYSIOLOGY**

The occurrence of HHNS is rare in children, and the pathogenesis is controversial. Insulin secretion is present but inadequate, or insulin actions are diminished. This produces hyperglycemia without ketogenesis and ketoacidosis. The absence of ketosis in the presence of profound hyperglycemia is the most puzzling component of HHNS. Postulated mechanisms for this phenomenon include (1) insulin secretion is enough to prevent ketosis but not hyperglycemia; (2) counterregulatory hormone levels are lower, therefore lipolysis and ketogenesis may be suppressed; and (3) dehydration with hyperosmolality may suppress ketogenesis (Ellis, 1990; Jones, 1994). There is marked hyperosmolality with significant dehydration. Polyuria is secondary to osmotic diuresis due to hyperglycemia. Electrolyte losses occur secondary to osmotic diuresis. The degree of hyperglycemia, hyperosmolality, and dehydration is much greater in HHNS than in DKA. Because of the absence of ketoacidosis and the associated physical symptoms (Kussmaul's breathing, anorexia, nausea and vomiting), there may be a delay in treatment; therefore these patients often present with profound cardiovascular collapse and neurologic sequela (coma) (Ellis, 1990). Shock and neurologic deficits are secondary to progressive and profound dehydration.

B. **ETIOLOGY**

HHNS may be on the continuum of uncompensated diabetes ultimately resulting in DKA. Phenytoin has been associated with HHNS because of its inhibition of insulin release. Corticosteroids, β-blockers, and thiazide diuretics have been associated with HHNS. Preexisting cardiovascular and renal disease have been associated with HHNS. Infections, trauma, burns, pancreatitis, thyrotoxicosis, heat stroke, dialysis (peritoneal dialysis and hemodialysis), and IV hyperalimentation may precipitate HHNS.

C. **RISK FACTORS**

Risk factors include stress or infection, infants or children who are dependent on others for fluid intake (such as debilitated, mentally incompetent children or children with altered thirst mechanisms who are unable to meet the fluid demands of osmotic diuresis and dehydration), previously undiagnosed NIDDM, and patients receiving IV fluids with high levels of dextrose.

D. **SIGNS AND SYMPTOMS** (Table 6–10)

Signs and symptoms include polyuria, polydipsia, serum glucose greater than 600 mg/dl, serum osmolality greater than 330 mOsm/kg, normal pH or mild metabolic acidosis, and serum bicarbonate of 18 to 24 mmol/L. Serum sodium levels may be high, low, or normal with total body sodium depletion; deficits range from 2 to 8 mmol/L (Ellis, 1990). Serum potassium levels may be high, low, or normal with total body depletion; deficits range from 0.5 to 3 mmol/L (Ellis, 1990). Serum phosphate levels are normal. Tachycardia, hypotension, low central venous pressure (CVP), shock, and glycosuria without ketonuria may occur. Lethargy, stupor, or coma may occur. Neurologic impairment is significantly higher in children with HHNS than DKA because of the severity of hyperosmolality and dehydration.

E. **INTERPRETATION OF DIAGNOSTIC STUDIES**

1. Hyperglycemia is due to decreased release or action of insulin. Insulin levels are adequate to prevent ketosis.
2. Glycosuria is secondary to hyperglycemia.
3. Hyperosmolality is secondary to hyperglycemia and loss of free water with osmotic diuresis.

Table 6–10. DIFFERENTIATION BETWEEN DIABETIC KETOACIDOSIS (DKA) AND HYPERGLYCEMIC, HYPEROSMOLAR, NONKETOTIC SYNDROME (HHNS)

	DKA	HHNS
Nausea and vomiting	Present	Absent
Neurologic changes	Present	Present
Polyuria	Present	Present
Respiratory rate	Kussmaul's breathing	Normal
Blood glucose	Usually >200 mg/dl	>600 mg/dl
Blood ketones	Elevated	Normal
Urine ketones	Present	Absent
Blood HCO_3^-	<18 mmol/L	>18 mmol/L
Blood pH	<7.30	>7.30
Serum osmolality	>300 mOsm/kg	>330 mOsm/kg
Sodium deficits	4–11 mEq/kg	2–8 mEq/kg
Potassium deficits	1–10 mEq/kg	0.5–3 mEq/kg
Water deficits	50–100 ml/kg	60–170 ml/kg

    4. Mild metabolic acidosis is secondary to dehydration, low cardiac output, renal insufficiency, and lactic acidosis.

    5. Electrolyte disturbances are due to urinary losses.

F. DIAGNOSES

    1. **Differential diagnoses** include DM, pancreatitis, renal insufficiency, and adrenocortical dysfunction.

    2. **Collaborative diagnoses**

       ❖ FLUID VOLUME DEFICIT RELATED TO OSMOTIC DIURESIS

       ❖ LOW CARDIAC OUTPUT RELATED TO FLUID VOLUME DEFICIT

       ❖ POTENTIAL FOR ARRHYTHMIAS RELATED TO ELECTROLYTE DISTURBANCES

       ❖ ACID-BASE IMBALANCE RELATED TO LOW CARDIAC OUTPUT AND LACTIC ACIDOSIS

       ❖ ELECTROLYTE IMBALANCES RELATED TO OSMOTIC DIURESIS AND TREATMENT

       ❖ POTENTIAL FOR CEREBRAL EDEMA RELATED TO TREATMENT

       ❖ POTENTIAL FOR HYPOGLYCEMIA RELATED TO TREATMENT

G. TREATMENT GOALS

    1. Treat underlying disorder.

    2. Correct hyperglycemia and hyperosmolality.

    3. Correct fluid and electrolyte deficits.

    4. Prevent neurologic complications.

H. MANAGEMENT

    1. **Fluid and electrolyte therapy** involves volume resuscitation of hypotensive patients with 20 ml/kg NS. Once blood pressure is normalized, IV fluids can be changed. Calculate the fluid volume deficit (Table 6–8); replace half during the first 12 hours and the remainder during the next 36 hours. Fluid and sodium replacement should be accomplished over 48 hours. Initial IV replacement fluid should be at least 0.5 NS. Because of the frequency of renal insufficiency with HHNS, potassium is not added until renal function is known, urine output is adequate, and serum potassium levels are less than 4.5 mmol/L. Potassium replacement can be added to the IV fluids as a combination of KCl and KPO_4 or as KCl alone dependent on laboratory values (Ellis, 1990; Jones, 1994). Once serum glucose reaches 300 mg/dl, dextrose should be added to the IV fluids.

    2. **Insulin therapy:** Often hyperglycemia is corrected with fluid therapy alone. Insulin therapy should be used with caution in HHNS. Low-dose insulin therapy can be used to achieve a gradual decline in hyperglycemia and osmolality, often after the institution of fluid therapy. Continuous infusion of

0.5 U/kg is usually adequate to decrease blood glucose levels. It should be discontinued once blood levels fall below 300 mg/dl to prevent hypoglycemia.

3. **Monitoring:** Vital signs, blood pressure, and neurologic checks are done every 30 to 60 minutes. Hourly determination of blood glucose is performed at the bedside. Initial laboratory studies include CBC, electrolytes, BUN, creatinine, glucose, and pH. Electrolytes and pH are monitored every 2 hours until stable, and BUN and creatinine are done every 12 hours until stable. Intake and output and daily weights are monitored.

I. **COMPLICATIONS** include hypoglycemia (from treatment), neurologic deficits (due to hyperosmolality), and cerebral edema and death due to rapid correction of the hyperosmolar state. Mortality averages 15% to 20% (Ellis, 1990).

ACUTE HYPOGLYCEMIA

A. **PATHOPHYSIOLOGY**

Hypoglycemia is defined as serum glucose less than 60 mg/dl. Energy failure may contribute to cell death, particularly in the brain (Sizonenko, 1993b). Nonketotic hypoglycemia is associated with hyperinsulinism (Miller, 1994). Ketotic hypoglycemia is secondary to metabolic derangements associated with lack of glucose for metabolism, with resulting fat metabolism.

B. **ETIOLOGY**

1. **Neonatal hypoglycemia** (Sizonenko, 1993b) is related to hyperplasia of beta cells and hyperinsulinism (infants of diabetic mothers), lack of exogenous supply (Schwartz, 1991), depletion of glycogen stores, defective gluconeogenesis, adrenocortical deficiency, infections, cerebral hemorrhage, or inborn errors of metabolism.

2. **Childhood hypoglycemia** can be caused by inborn errors of metabolism, growth hormone deficiency, cortisol deficiency, stress, hepatic dysfunction, excessive insulin in IDDM, severe malnutrition, infections, or drugs.

C. **RISK FACTORS**

1. Infants of diabetic mothers
2. Small-for-gestational-age infants
3. Stress or acute illness
4. Insulin infusion
5. Infants or children with compromised IV access and nothing-by-mouth (NPO) status
6. Increased metabolism
7. Poor nutrition

D. **SIGN AND SYMPTOMS**

1. **Neonates** (Miller, 1994; Sizonenko, 1993b) demonstrate symptoms of temperature instability, irritability, tremor, lethargy, hypotonia, feeding or sucking difficulties, cyanosis, and bradycardia.

2. **Toddlers and children** (Miller, 1994; Schatz, 1994) experience sweating, tremor or irritability, hunger, confusion, weakness, slurred speech, headache, tachycardia, and changes in the level of consciousness or coma.

E. **INTERPRETATION OF DIAGNOSTIC STUDIES**

1. Blood glucose is less than 60 mg/dl with serum sample confirmation of glucometer result. Glucose tolerance test is of little value.
2. Low plasma carnitine levels can indicate medium-chain acyl-CoA deficiency (very rare).
3. Low plasma levels of growth hormone indicate growth hormone deficiency.
4. Low cortisol levels are due to cortisol deficiency.

5. Elevated blood insulin levels indicate hyperinsulinemia.
6. Urine-reducing substances indicate fructose intolerance or galactosemia.
7. Urinary ketones can differentiate between ketotic and nonketotic hypoglycemia.
8. Abdominal CT scan is used to determine the presence of a pancreatic tumor.
9. Abdominal ultrasound can identify insulinoma.

F. **DIAGNOSES**
   1. **Differential diagnoses** include hepatic failure, pancreatic tumors, cardiovascular disease, neurologic disease, endocrine deficiencies, tumors, and sepsis.
   2. **Collaborative diagnoses**
      ❖ POTENTIAL FOR ALTERATIONS IN NUTRITION DUE TO LOW BLOOD GLUCOSE, DECREASED SUBSTRATE FOR METABOLISM, OR ALTERED METABOLIC PATHWAYS
      ❖ POTENTIAL FOR NEUROLOGIC ALTERATIONS DUE TO DECREASED AMOUNTS OF THE PRIMARY METABOLIC SUBSTRATE OF THE BRAIN (GLUCOSE)

G. **TREATMENT GOALS**
   1. Normalize blood glucose.
   2. Support cellular metabolic requirements.

H. **MANAGEMENT**
   1. **Neonatal treatment** includes early feedings (Schwartz, 1991), IV boluses of 10% or 20% glucose (0.5 to 1 g/kg over 1 to 3 minutes), 10% dextrose (4 to 8 mg/kg/min) continuous infusion (Miller, 1994), identification and treatment of underlying cause, maintenance of normothermia, and decrease in environmental stress.
   2. **Infant and childhood treatment** includes feedings (if possible), IV boluses of 25% dextrose (2 to 4 ml/kg) (Miller, 1994), continuous infusion of 5% or 10% dextrose, initiation of nutritional support (hyperalimentation or parental feedings), or subtotal pancreatectomy for treatment of pancreatic adenomas. Add dextrose or decrease insulin infusion in patients with DKA who develop hypoglycemia. Treat underlying metabolic disorders.

I. **COMPLICATIONS**
Complications include neuronal death, coma, seizures, neurologic deficits, and death.

SYNDROME OF INAPPROPRIATE ANTIDIURETIC HORMONE (SIADH)

A. **PATHOPHYSIOLOGY**
SIADH is characterized by inappropriate, excessive secretion of ADH in the absence of normal physiologic stimuli. SIADH occurs in the face of low serum sodium and low serum osmolality that would normally serve to inhibit ADH secretion through negative feedback (Batcheller, 1994). This results in water retention and expansion of extracellular volume. Hyponatremia is secondary to hemodilution. Renal function is normal. Clinical signs and symptoms are secondary to increased blood volume and hyponatremia (Berry and Belsha, 1990).

B. **ETIOLOGY AND RISK FACTORS**
   1. **Conditions associated with SIADH**
      a. Meningitis (Brown and Feigin, 1994; Padilla et al, 1991).
      b. Head trauma.
      c. Cerebral tumors: Germ cell tumors, craniopharyngiomas, pituitary tumors, hypothalamic gliomas, and third ventricle tumors. Often children who have tumors fluctuate between SIADH and DI (Shiminski-Maher, 1991).
      d. Cerebral hemorrhage.

   e. Pulmonary disease: Tuberculosis, pneumonia, abscesses.
   f. Chronically ill or malnourished children may develop chronic increased ADH secretion due to a downward resetting of the osmotic receptors. Hyponatremia is chronic, and ADH secretion occurs at a lower serum osmolality (Berry and Belsha, 1990).
   2. **Medications associated with SIADH** (Batcheller, 1994) include analgesics, vincristine, cytoxan, carbamazepine, chlorpropamide, and barbiturates.
   3. **Other precipitating conditions** include severe pain, temperature changes, and positive pressure ventilation.
C. SIGNS AND SYMPTOMS (Table 6–11)
   Clinical manifestations: The severity of the clinical presentation depends on the degree and rapidity with which hyponatremia occurs (Batcheller, 1994; Berry and Belsha, 1990). Symptoms include altered level of consciousness, headache, confusion, lethargy, coma, or seizures. Nausea and vomiting may occur. Children gain weight but have no peripheral edema and normal skin turgor. Normal or increased filling pressures are present. Urine output is low in the absence of hypovolemia. Hypertension and tachycardia are late signs.
D. LABORATORY DATA
   1. Serum osmolality is less than 280 mOsm/kg. Urine osmolality is elevated inappropriately relative to serum osmolality (Batcheller, 1994; Gildea, 1993).
   2. Serum sodium is less than 135 mEq/L. Continued renal excretion of sodium occurs with urine sodium greater than 30 mEq/L.
   3. Urine specific gravity (SG) is greater than 1.020.
E. INTERPRETATION OF LABORATORY RESULTS
   1. Hyponatremia and hypoosmolality occur secondary to water retention and hemodilution.
   2. Excessive concentration of urine occurs with high specific gravity and increased osmolality because of ADH's effect on the renal tubules, resulting in increased water reabsorption by the kidney. Increased fractional excretion of sodium is noted.
   3. Renal, thyroid, and adrenal function tests are normal (Brown and Feigin, 1994).
F. DIAGNOSES
   1. **Differential diagnoses** (Berry and Belsha, 1990) include congestive heart failure, water intoxication, glucocorticoid deficiency, hypothyroidism, renal failure, nephrotic syndrome, third space losses, heat exhaustion (increased sweating), GI tract losses, laboratory error, and cerebral salt wasting (a syndrome of hyponatremia, natriuresis, and hypovolemia without elevated ADH levels that requires fluid replacement [Sivakumar et al, 1994]).

Table 6–11. DIFFERENTIATION BETWEEN DIABETES INSIPIDUS (DI) AND SYNDROME OF INAPPROPRIATE ANTIDIURETIC HORMONE (SIADH)

	DI	SIADH
Serum Na^+	>145 mEq/L	<135 mEq/L
Urine Na^+	<30 mEq/L	>30 mEq/L
Serum osmolality	>300 mOsm/kg	<280 mOsm/kg
Urine specific gravity	<1.005	>1.020
Urine output	High	Low
Central venous pressure	Low	High
Weight	Decreased	Increased

2. **Collaborative diagnoses**
   ❖ FLUID AND VOLUME EXCESS RELATED TO EXCESSIVE ADH SECRETION AND WATER RETENTION
   ❖ ALTERATION IN MENTAL STATE RELATED TO UNDERLYING CONDITIONS (E.G., MENINGITIS, BRAIN TUMORS), RAPID DEVELOPMENT OF HYPONATREMIA, OR ACUTE INCREASES IN SERUM OSMOLALITY
   ❖ POTENTIAL FOR SEIZURES RELATED TO SERUM SODIUM LESS THAN 120 MMOL/L
   ❖ POTENTIAL FOR CEREBRAL HEMORRHAGE DUE TO RAPID CORRECTION OF HYPO-OSMOLAR STATE

G. **TREATMENT GOALS**
   1. Normalize serum sodium.
   2. Normalize serum osmolality.
   3. Decrease extravascular fluid volume.
   4. Prevent neurologic sequela.

H. **MANAGEMENT**
   1. Serum sodium should be normalized over 24 to 48 hours to prevent neurologic sequela. Acute increases in serum sodium and osmolality can cause the brain cells to shrink, precipitating cerebral hemorrhage and brain injury (Berry and Belsha, 1990). Treatment is based on the degree of hyponatremia and hypoosmolality. Usually fluid restriction to insensible losses (or 800 to 1000 $L/m^2/d$) is sufficient to decrease blood volume and increase serum sodium (Brown and Feigin, 1994). If serum sodium is less than 120 mEq/L and the child is symptomatic (seizures), 3% NaCl 3 to 5 ml/kg is administered slow IV push, and furosemide (Lasix) 1 mg/kg should be given until the serum sodium reaches 125 mEq/L (Gildea, 1993). Once serum sodium is greater than 135 mmol/L, fluid restriction may be liberalized to a maintenance fluid rate.
   2. **Monitoring** includes intake and output, SG with every void, serum electrolytes and osmolality (every 4 to 6 hours until normal), and daily weights. Urine electrolytes and osmolality may be obtained to help make the initial diagnosis; however, frequent monitoring may not be necessary. CVP is obtained if possible, and heart rate and blood pressure are monitored.

I. **COMPLICATIONS** (Berry and Belsha, 1990)
   Complications include seizures (if serum sodium is less than 120 mEq/L), cerebral edema (if serum sodium falls too rapidly), cerebral dehydration and hemorrhage (if corrected too quickly), muscle cramps or weakness (secondary to hyponatremia), and pulmonary edema or hypertension (secondary to fluid overload).

DIABETES INSIPIDUS (DI)

A. **PATHOPHYSIOLOGY**
   1. DI is a clinical condition that is characterized by a decrease in both urine concentrating ability and water conservation, resulting in excessive diuresis and low urine osmolality. There are two types: central (or neurogenic) and nephrogenic (Fig. 6–6). DI can be transient, as it occurs in many neurosurgical patients, or permanent (Bell, 1994; Blevins and Wand, 1992).
   2. Central DI is the most common form found in children and in the critical care environment. Deficiency of ADH is due to failed synthesis or secretion by the posterior pituitary, or both.
   3. Nephrogenic DI is characterized by normal secretion of ADH by the posterior pituitary. The distal tubule and the collecting duct in the kidney, however, are resistant to the effects of ADH. Nephrogenic DI is the most difficult form of DI to treat.

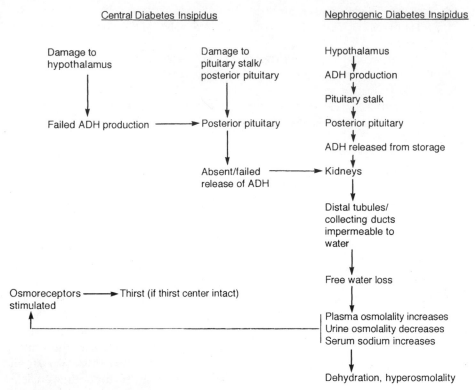

Figure 6–6. Pathophysiology of DI. (Reprinted with permission from Bell TN. Diabetes insipidus. *Crit Care Nurs Clin North Am.* 1994;6(4):678.)

B. **Etiologies and Risk Factors**
1. **Central DI** results from pituitary and suprasellar surgery, midline defects (septooptic dysplasia and agenesis of the corpus callosum), head trauma (usually an ominous sign), CNS infections, cerebral edema, cerebral hemorrhage or infarct, or sickle cell crisis. About 25% of adolescent cases are idiopathic, but there is a familial, autosomal dominant trait (Blevins and Wand, 1992; Masera et al, 1994; Seckl et al, 1990; Shiminski-Maher, 1991).
2. **Nephrogenic DI** is related to chronic renal disease, polycystic kidney disease, familial tendency, pregnancy, chronic hypokalemia, chronic hypercalcemia, starvation, and medications such as lithium, amphotericin B, loop diuretics, and gentamicin. Sickle cell nephropathy can also cause DI (Bell, 1994; Blevins and Wand, 1992).

C. **Signs and Symptoms** (Table 6–11)
Signs and symptoms of DI include polyuria, dilute urine with SG less than 1.005, urine osmolality less than 200 mOsm/kg, polydipsia, dehydration, low CVP, hypernatremia (serum sodium greater than 145 mmol/L), serum hyperosmolality (greater than 300 mOsm/kg), tachycardia, hypotension, poor skin turgor, dry mucous membranes, weight loss, lethargy, confusion, and coma.

D. **Interpretation of Tests**
1. Hypernatremia and hyperosmolality are due to water loss and hemoconcentration.
2. Low SG and urine osmolality are due to the kidney's inability to reabsorb water and concentrate urine.
3. Vasopressin levels are low or unmeasurable in central DI. Vasopressin levels are normal or high in nephrogenic DI.

4. MRI or CT scan is used for the diagnosis of cerebral edema or underlying conditions such as cerebral tumors, calcifications, hypopituitarism, or midline defects.

5. Pituitary function tests determine GH or ACTH defects.

6. A water deprivation test can be used to further define the type of DI (Leung et al, 1991). This requires careful supervision and monitoring. All medications that can interfere with the secretion or action of ADH should be discontinued prior to the test (including alcohol and tobacco). Unrestricted access to fluids should be allowed until the test starts. At the beginning of the study a baseline weight, serum sodium and osmolality, urine osmolality, and volume are recorded. Over the next 6 to 8 hours all fluids and foods are withheld. The child is weighed every hour, and urine volume and osmolality are measured with every void. At the end of the study serum laboratory specimens are redrawn. The test is terminated if body weight falls 3% to 5%. If serum osmolality remains high and hypotonic polyuria continues in spite of water deprivation, the diagnosis of DI is made. To differentiate between central and nephrogenic DI, the patient is given a dose of vasopressin or desmopressin (DDAVP). If urine volume falls and becomes more concentrated, the patient has central DI; if there is no response to vasopressin, the patient has nephrogenic DI (Blevins and Wand, 1992).

E. DIAGNOSES

1. **Differential diagnoses** include DM, sodium excess (improperly mixed formula or iatrogenic sodium administration), overuse of diuretics, adipsia, increased insensible water loss, and primary polydipsia (Conley, 1990).

2. **Collaborative diagnoses**
   * POTENTIAL FOR LOW CARDIAC OUTPUT RELATED TO DIURESIS AND INTRAVASCULAR VOLUME LOSS
   * POTENTIAL FOR NEUROLOGIC INSULT RELATED TO UNDERLYING CAUSES (E.G., MIDLINE DEFECTS, HEAD TRAUMA) OR RAPID RISE IN SERUM OSMOLALITY
   * POTENTIAL FOR THE DEVELOPMENT OF CEREBRAL EDEMA RELATED TO RAPID CORRECTION OF HYPEROSMOLAR STATE
   * FLUID AND ELECTROLYTE IMBALANCE RELATED TO EXCESSIVE DIURESIS

F. TREATMENT GOALS

1. Correct dehydration and fluid deficits.
2. Correct hypernatremia.
3. Control free water loss by the kidney.
4. Prevent neurologic sequela.

G. MANAGEMENT

1. Identify and treat underlying cause.
2. In **central DI,** the decision to use fluid or ADH replacement therapy or both is often based on the severity of the illness, patient condition, and the underlying cause. Children with an intact thirst mechanism are allowed unlimited access to fluids. Once serum osmolality rises and stimulates the thirst center, these children can meet the fluid needs precipitated by polyuria. Infants, comatose patients, or children with an abnormal thirst response require fluid therapy. If dehydration is severe and shock is present, resuscitate with isotonic fluids (NS or lactated Ringer's solution) 10 to 20 ml/kg, reassess, and inject another bolus if necessary until perfusion improves (Conley, 1990). In patients who are dehydrated, replace fluid volume deficits with hypotonic fluids for a period of 48 hours. In acute, sudden-onset DI, urine replacement milliliter per milliliter with hypotonic fluids in addition to maintenance fluids normalizes serum electrolytes and blood volume, or ADH replacement therapy is titrated to keep SG greater than 1.010 and urine output at 2 ml/kg/h with normal serum sodium.

Table 6–12.   ANTIDIURETIC HORMONE (ADH) REPLACEMENT THERAPIES

NAME	DOSE	DURATION
Aqueous vasopressin, IM	2.5–10 U 2–4 times a day	2–6 h
Aqueous vasopressin, IV	0.5 mU/kg/h–maximum of 10 mU/kg/h	2–6 h after discontinued
Desmopressin (DDAVP) Intranasal IV bolus	5 µg/d in 1–2 divided doses, range 5–30 µg/d 1/10 of maintenance intra- nasal dose	5–21 h

Data from Taketomo CK, Hodding JH, Kraus DM. *Pediatric Dosage Handbook 1997–98.* 4th ed. Cleveland, Ohio: Lexi-Comp; 1997.

ADH replacement may be intranasal, IV, IM, SC, or continuous infusion (Table 6–12). Normal fluid intake or maintenance fluids are continued.

3. **Nephrogenic DI** is difficult to treat. A sodium-restricted diet may help. Hydrochlorothiazide (diuretic) 2 mg/kg/d in two divides doses paradoxically reduces polyuria by causing excessive sodium reabsorption in the proximal portion of the nephron, with resultant reduction of volume delivered to the distal tubule and less urine formed. This mechanism is not well understood. Nonsteroidal antiinflammatory agents inhibit renal production of prostaglandin, enhancing renal responsiveness to ADH (Blevins and Wand, 1992; Bonioli, 1991). ADH replacement therapy is of no value.

4. **Monitoring** (Bell, 1994) includes intake and output, daily or twice daily weights, frequent hemodynamic and neurologic assessments, urine SG every void, and urine osmolality and serum sodium and osmolality every 4 to 6 hours until normal.

H. COMPLICATIONS

Complications include cardiac collapse and shock from rapid diuresis; neurologic sequela from rapid rise in serum osmolality; cerebral edema, herniation, and possible death due to rapid correction of hyperosmolar state; electrolyte imbalances secondary to inadequate monitoring of serum electrolytes during therapy; and water intoxication and fluid overload related to overtreatment with ADH replacement therapy.

REFERENCES

Agana-Defensor R, Proch M. Pheochromocytoma: a clinical review. *AACN Clin Issues Crit Care Nurs.* 1992;3(2):309–318.

Batcheller J. Syndrome of inappropriate antidiuretic hormone secretion. *Crit Care Clin North Am.* 1994;6(4):687–692.

Bell TN. Diabetes insipidus. *Crit Care Clin North Am.* 1994;6(4):675–685.

Berry PL, Belsha CW. Hyponatremia. *Pediatr Clin North Am.* 1990;37(2):351–363.

Bertrand J, Rappaport R, Sizonenko PC. Assessment of endocrine functions. In: Bertand J, Rappaport R, Sizonenko PC, eds. *Pediatric Endocrinology: Physiology, Pathophysiology and Clinical Aspects.* Baltimore, Md: Williams & Wilkins; 1993.

Blevins LS, Wand GS. Diabetes insipidus. *Crit Care Med.* 1992;20(1):69–79.

Bonioli E. Therapy for hereditary nephrogenic diabetes insipidus. *J Pediatr.* 1991;119(2):331.

Boulware SD, Tamborlane WV. Not all severe hyperglycemia is diabetes. *Pediatrics.* 1992;89(2):330–332.

Brown LW, Feigin RD. Bacterial meningitis: fluid balance and therapy. *Pediatr Ann.* 1994;23(2):93–98.

Chase HP, Garg SK, Butler-Simon N, et al. Prediction of the course of pre-type 1 diabetes. *J Pediatr.* 1991;118:838–841.

Conley SB. Hypernatremia. *Pediatr Clin North Am.* 1990;37(2):365–372.

Czernichow P. Hormonal regulation of water metabolism. In: Bertand J, Rappaport R, Sizonenko PC, eds. *Pediatric Endocrinology: Physiology, Pathophysiology and Clinical Aspects.* Baltimore, Md: Williams & Wilkins; 1993a.

Czernichow P. Posterior pituitary hormones. In: Bertand J, Rappaport R, Sizonenko PC, eds. *Pediatric Endocrinology: Physiology, Pathophysiology and Clinical Aspects.* Baltimore, Md: Williams & Wilkins; 1993b.

Czernichow P. Thyrotropin and thyroid hormones. In: Bertand J, Rappaport R, Sizonenko PC, eds. *Pediatric Endocrinology: Physiology, Pathophysiology and Clinical Aspects.* Baltimore, Md: Williams & Wilkins; 1993c.

Delange F. Thyroid hormones: biochemistry and physiology. In: Bertand J, Rappaport R, Sizonenko PC, eds. *Pediatric Endocrinology: Physiology, Pathophysiology and Clinical Aspects.* Baltimore, Md: Williams & Wilkins; 1993.

Ellis EN. Concepts of fluid therapy in diabetic ketoacidosis and hyperosmolar hyperglycemic nonketotic coma. *Pediatr Clin North Am.* 1990;37(2):313–321.

Gaillard RC. Neuroendocrine regulation. In: Bertrand J, Rappaport R, Sizonenko PC, eds. *Pediatric Endocrinology: Physiology, Pathophysiology and Clinical Aspects.* Baltimore, Md: Williams & Wilkins; 1993.

Gildea JH. High and dry—low and wet: the key to DI and SIADH. *Pediatr Nurs.* 1993;19(5):478–481.

Guyton AC. *Textbook of Medical Physiology.* Philadelphia, Pa: WB Saunders Co; 1986.

Herskowitz-Dumont R, Wolfsdorf JI, Jackson RA, Eisenbarth GS. Distinction between transient hyperglycemia and early insulin-dependent diabetes mellitus in childhood: a prospective study of incidence and prognostic factors. *J Pediatr.* 1993;123:347–354.

Jones TL. From diabetic ketoacidosis to hyperglycemic hyperosmolar nonketotic syndrome. *Crit Care Nurs Clin North Am.* 1994;6(4):703–720.

Laron Z, Karp M. Diabetes mellitus in children and adolescents. In: Bertand J, Rappaport R, Sizonenko PC, eds. *Pediatric Endocrinology: Physiology, Pathophysiology and Clinical Aspects.* Baltimore, Md: Williams & Wilkins; 1993.

Leung AKC, Robson WLM, Halperin ML. Polyuria in childhood. *Clin Pediatr.* 1991;30(11):634–640.

Masera N, Grant DB, Stanhope R, Preece MA. Diabetes insipidus with impaired osmotic regulation in septo-optic dysplasia and agenesis of the corpus callosum. *Arch Dis Child.* 1994;70:51–53.

Miller KL. Endocrine disorders in critically ill children. *Crit Care Nurs Clin North Am.* 1994;6(4):785–803.

Millward A. Childhood diabetes. *Practitioner.* 1993;237:730–733.

Moore KL. *The Developing Human.* Philadelphia, Pa: WB Saunders Co; 1988.

Padilla G, Ervin MG, Ross MG, Leake RD. Vasopressin levels in infants during the course of aseptic and bacterial meningitis. *Am J Dis Child.* 1991;145:991–993.

Palmer JP. What is the best way to predict IDDM? *Lancet.* 1994;343:1377–1378.

Parker SH. Nursing assessment and diagnosis of endocrine dysfunction. In: Jackson DB, Saunders BR, eds. *Child Health Nursing.* Philadelphia, Pa: JB Lippincott Co; 1993.

Plotnick L. Insulin-dependent diabetes mellitus. *Pediatr Rev.* 1994;15(4):137–148.

Rosenbloom AL, Schatz DA. Diabetic ketoacidosis in childhood. *Pediatr Ann.* 1994;23(6):284–288.

Salle BL, Delvin EE, Glorieux FH. Calcium, parathormone and vitamin D. In: Bertrand J, Rappaport R, Sizonenko PC, eds. *Pediatric Endocrinology: Physiology, Pathophysiology and Clinical Aspects.* Baltimore, Md: Williams & Wilkins; 1993.

Schatz DA. Hypoglycemia in childhood diabetes. *Pediatr Ann.* 1994;23(6):289–291.

Schwartz R. Neonatal hypoglycemia: back to basics in diagnosis and treatment. *Diabetes.* 1991;40(2):71–73.

Seckl JR, Dunger DB, Bevan JS, et al. Vasopressin antagonist in early postoperative diabetes insipidus. *Lancet.* 1990;335:1353–1356.

Shiminski-Maher T. Diabetes insipidus and syndrome of inappropriate secretion of antidiuretic hormone in children with midline suprasellar brain tumors. *J Pediatr Oncol Nurs.* 1991;8(3):106–111.

Sivakumar V, Rajshekhar V, Chandy MJ. Management of neurosurgical patients with hyponatremia and natriuresis. *Neurosurgery.* 1994;34(2):269–274.

Sizonenko PC. Biochemistry and physiology. In: Bertrand J, Rappaport R, Sizonenko PC, eds. *Pediatric Endocrinology: Physiology, Pathophysiology and Clinical Aspects.* Baltimore, Md: Williams & Wilkins; 1993a.

Sizonenko PC. Hypoglycemia. In: Bertrand J, Rappaport R, Sizonenko PC, eds. *Pediatric Endocrinology: Physiology, Pathophysiology and Clinical Aspects.* Baltimore, Md: Williams & Wilkins; 1993b.

Sizonenko PC. Pancreatic hormones: insulin and glucagon. In: Bertrand J, Rappaport R, Sizonenko PC, eds. *Pediatric Endocrinology: Physiology, Pathophysiology and Clinical Aspects.* Baltimore, Md: Williams & Wilkins; 1993c.

Sizonenko PC, Aubert ML. Hypothalamopituitary axis and adrenal cortex: fetoplacental unit. In: Bertrand J, Rappaport R, Sizonenko PC, eds. *Pediatric Endocrinology: Physiology, Pathophysiology and Clinical Aspects.* Baltimore, Md: Williams & Wilkins; 1993.

Taketomo CK, Hodding JH, Kraus DM. *Pediatric Dosage Handbook 1993–1994.* Cleveland, Ohio: Lexi-Comp; 1993.

Toto KH. Endocrine physiology: a comprehensive review. *Crit Care Nurs Clin North Am.* 1994a;6(4):637–653.

Toto KH. Regulation of plasma osmolality. *Crit Care Nurs Clin North Am.* 1994b;6(4):661–674.

Villee D, Najjar S. Endocrinology. In: Avery ME, First LR, eds. *Pediatric Medicine.* Baltimore, Md: Williams & Wilkins; 1994.

Yagi H, Nagashima K, Miyake H, et al. Familial congenital hypopituitarism with central diabetes insipidus. *J Clin Endocrinol Metab.* 1994;78(4):884–889.

7

Gastrointestinal System

SARAH MARTIN and SHARI DERENGOWSKI

ANATOMY AND PHYSIOLOGY

A. **STRUCTURE AND FUNCTION** (Fig. 7–1)
1. **Oral cavity:** The oral cavity serves as a reservoir for chewing and mixing food with saliva. *Salivary glands* include the submandibular, sublingual, and parotid glands. Saliva is composed of water, small amounts of mucus, sodium bicarbonate, chloride, potassium, and amylase. Amylase begins carbohydrate digestion.
2. The **esophagus** propels swallowed food to the stomach. The upper esophageal sphincter prevents air from entering the esophagus during respiration. The lower esophageal sphincter prevents reflux of gastric contents into the esophagus.
3. **Stomach**
   a. The stomach is a hollow, muscular organ that acts as a reservoir for ingested food. It secretes digestive juices that mix with digested food (chyme). *Parietal cells* (oxyntic) secrete hydrochloric acid and intrinsic factor. The secretion is regulated by stimuli (e.g., H_2-histamine receptors). *Chief cells* secrete pepsinogen, which combines with hydrochloric acid to break down protein.
   b. *Gastric emptying* is affected by the volume of food, osmotic pressure, and chemical composition of the contents. Emptying is controlled by the pyloric sphincter. Delayed emptying is caused by foods with high fat content, solid foods, sedatives, sleep, secretin, and cholecystokinin hormones. Accelerated emptying is caused by foods with high carbohydrate content, liquids, increased volume, and aggression.
4. The **small intestine** is the primary site for digestion and absorption of fats, amino acids, sugars, and vitamins.
   a. The *duodenum* is the primary site for the absorption of iron, trace metals, and water-soluble vitamins.
   b. The *jejunum* is the principal absorption site for proteins and sugars, since the epithelial cells contain villi. Ninety percent of nutrients and 50% of water and electrolytes are absorbed here.
   c. The *ileum* is responsible for absorption of bile salts and vitamin B_{12}. The ileocecal valve controls the entry of digested material from the ileum into the large intestine and prevents reflux into the small intestine. There is continued digestion in the ileum by the action of pancreatic enzymes, intestinal enzymes, and bile salts. Carbohydrates are broken down into monosaccharides and disaccharides and absorbed by villus capillaries.

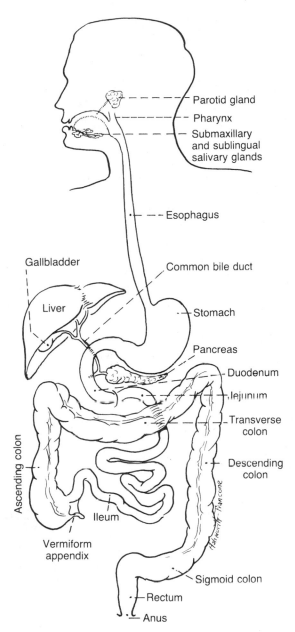

Figure 7–1.   The GI tract and associated structures. (Reprinted with permission from Jacob SW, Francone CA. *Elements of Anatomy and Physiology*. 2nd ed. Philadelphia, Pa: WB Saunders Co; 1989.)

Proteins are degraded to amino acids and peptides and absorbed by villus capillaries. Fats are emulsified and reduced to fatty acids and monoglycerides.

5. **Colon:** The anatomic segments of the colon include the cecum, ascending colon, transverse colon, descending colon, sigmoid colon, and rectum. Water and electrolytes are reabsorbed. Feces are stored in the rectum. The greatest growth of anaerobic and gram-negative aerobic bacteria is in the colon. *Bacteroides fragilis* (anaerobic) and *Escherichia coli* (aerobic) play a role in metabolizing bile salts and synthesizing vitamins.

6. **Pancreas:** The pancreas's exocrine function is to secrete bicarbonate and enzymes for digestion and absorption of fats, carbohydrates, and proteins. The

pancreas's endocrine function involves islet cells, which function in glucose homeostasis by synthesizing and secreting insulin.

7. **Liver**
   a. Liver functions include the following:
      - Formation of clotting (coagulation) factors I, II, V, VII, IX, X, and XI
      - Synthesis of plasma proteins (albumin, fibrinogen, and 60% to 80% of globulins)
      - Synthesis and transportation of bile (bile salts, pigment, and cholesterol)
      - Storage of glycogen, fat, and fat-soluble vitamins
      - Metabolism of fats, carbohydrates, and proteins
      - Metabolism and deactivation of bilirubin and many toxins by oxidation or conjugation reactions
   b. Three fourths of the blood supply to the liver is supplied by the portal venous system (blood rich in nutrients) and one fourth by the hepatic artery (blood rich in oxygen).

8. **Biliary tree and gallbladder:** The biliary tree serves as the conduit for bile flow from the liver to the duodenum. The gallbladder provides a storage and concentration site for bile.

9. **Splanchnic circulation:** The splanchnic circulation supplies blood to the stomach, small intestine, and colon. It receives one fourth of cardiac output. The major arterial branches are the celiac, superior mesenteric, and inferior mesenteric. Venous drainage from the stomach, pancreas, small intestine, and colon flows to the portal vein to the liver and then to the heart through the hepatic vein and inferior vena cava.

B. **REGULATION OF FLUID AND ELECTROLYTE MOVEMENT**

Large volumes of water, electrolytes, proteins, and bile salts are secreted and reabsorbed throughout the gastrointestinal (GI) tract, resulting in massive fluid and electrolyte shifts. Fluid and electrolyte movement occurs concurrently with digestion and absorption of nutrients.

DEVELOPMENTAL ANATOMY AND PHYSIOLOGY

A. **GI TRACT DEVELOPMENT** (Motil, 1993)

Formation of the GI system is dependent on embryologic folding by the fourth week of gestation. Development of the gut is nearly complete by the 20th week of gestation. Functional maturity occurs by the 33rd to 34th week of gestation, providing nutrition to support fetal growth.

B. **GASTRIC ACTIVITY**
   1. Gastric motility is decreased and somewhat irregular in comparison to the adult. Gastric emptying is increased.
   2. Gastroesophageal reflux is common during the first 6 months because of a complex set of factors (hormonal changes, anatomic relationships) causing inappropriate relaxation of the lower esophageal sphincter (Kocoshis, 1992).

C. **IMMATURE NEONATAL LIVER**

The liver matures in function during the first year of life. Toxic substances are inefficiently detoxified. Synthesis of liver enzymes and degradation is impaired. Adjust therapeutic drug dosing for hepatoxicity as necessary.

D. **METABOLIC RATE IN CHILDREN**
   1. Caloric requirements per kilogram of weight are higher in children than in adults. The basal metabolic rate (BMR) is highest during the first 2 years of life and increases during growth spurts.
   2. Children require baseline calories, regardless of their activity level, to promote

Table 7–1. **CALORIC REQUIREMENTS IN CRITICALLY ILL CHILDREN**

AGE	kcal/kg/d
High-risk neonate	120–150
0–6 mo	120
6–12 mo	100
1–2 y	90–100
2–6 y	80–90
7–9 y	70–80
10–12 y	50–60
>12 y	40

growth and development and require additional calories during acute illness (e.g., disease, surgery, fever, and pain) (Table 7–1). The BMR increases 12% with each centigrade degree of temperature increase above 37° C. Children on bed rest have decreased caloric needs. Caloric needs can be supplied by parenteral or enteral feedings.

E. **GENERAL ANATOMIC CONSIDERATIONS**
1. The abdominal wall is less muscular in the infant and toddler, making the abdominal organs easier to palpate. In the infant, the liver can be palpated 1 to 2 cm below the right costal margin (RCM).
2. In younger children the contour of the abdomen is protuberant because of immature abdominal musculature. After 4 years of age, the abdomen is no longer protuberant when the child is in a supine position; but because of lumbar lordosis, the abdomen remains protuberant when the child stands.

CLINICAL ASSESSMENT

A. **GENERAL PRINCIPLES OF ABDOMINAL ASSESSMENT**
Examination of the abdomen is difficult in a healthy child. A frightened child will not cooperate with the examination. A child suffering from multisystem trauma will be unable to localize pain. The preferred order of assessment is inspection, auscultation, palpation, and percussion.

B. **ABDOMINAL EXAMINATION ASSESSMENT TECHNIQUES**
1. **Inspection:** Evaluate for size, contour, symmetry, integrity, visible peristalsis, umbilicus, masses, and wounds. Underdeveloped abdominal musculature in children allows easier visualization of masses and fluid waves. Abdominal distention (abdomen is normally rounded in infants and toddlers) is the hallmark sign of obstruction.
2. **Auscultation**
   a. Determine the absence, presence, and character of peristalsis or bowel sounds. Bowel sounds are absent in paralytic ileus and peritonitis. A venous hum heard over the upper area of the abdomen suggests portal obstruction. A bruit (caused by turbulent blood flow through a partially occluded artery) suggests an arteriovenous malformation.
   b. Bowel sounds should be heard every 5 to 30 seconds. Listen to all four quadrants for 2 to 5 minutes to confirm absent bowel sounds.
3. **Palpation:** Palpation should be performed before percussion, since palpation is a less threatening technique to a child. Begin with light palpation and assess for guarding and tenderness. With deep palpation, assess for abdominal tone, masses, pulsations, fluid, and organ enlargement. The liver is normally pal-

pated at the right costal margin (RCM) or is nonpalpable. The spleen is not normally palpable.

4. **Percussion:** Percussion is used to estimate the size of organs and aids in the diagnosis of ascites, obstruction, and peritonitis. *Assess* for abdominal distention, fluid, masses, or organ enlargement. The normal liver and spleen are dull. Dullness over the liver may be decreased or absent in the presence of free air in the abdomen from perforation. The stomach is tympanic when empty. The intestines are hyperresonant to tympanic in tone, depending on contents.

PHARMACOLOGY

A. **ANTIBLEEDING AGENTS**
1. **Vasopressin (Pitressin)** (Goff, 1993)
   a. *Action:* Nonselective, short-acting vasoconstrictor.
   b. *Uses:* Decreases splanchnic blood flow and portal hypertension.
   c. *Dose:* Continuous intravenous (IV) infusion: 0.1–0.3 U/min; titrate dose as needed.
   d. *Side effects* include hypertension, bradycardia, arrhythmias, abdominal cramping, vomiting, decreased urine output, and hyponatremia.
2. **Somatostatin** (Goff, 1993)
   a. *Action and uses:* Selective for splanchnic circulation with decreased incidence of hypertension. Use of somatostatin in children has not been studied; somatostatin is used when conservative treatment fails.
   b. *Dose:* 0.5–1 µg/kg IV bolus; infusion rate 7.5 µg/min.
   c. *Side effects* are minimal in adults.
3. **Propranolol (Inderal)**
   a. *Action:* β-adrenergic blocker causing vasoconstriction resulting in decreased splanchnic arterial blood flow and decreased portal hypertension.
   b. *Uses:* Used to prevent variceal rebleeding.
   c. *Dose:* 0.5–4 mg/kg/d PO in divided doses q6h or 0.01–0.1 mg/kg slow IV push over 10 minutes in children. Maximum dose is 1 mg.
   d. *Side effects* include hypotension, hypoglycemia, GI tract upset, bradycardia, arrhythmias, and mental depression. The efficacy and safety of long-term administration in children is unknown.
4. **Vitamin K_1, Phytonadione (AquaMEPHYTON, Mephyton)**
   a. *Action:* Provides vitamin K activity.
   b. *Uses:* Prevents and treats hypoprothrombinemia caused by drug- or anticoagulant-induced vitamin K deficiency.
   c. *Dose:* 1–2 mg per single dose IV, intramuscular (IM), or subcutaneous (SC). Dosages up to 10 mg/d have been used. Dilute in 5–10 ml of IV fluid for IV infusion over 15 to 30 minutes. The maximum rate of IV administration should not exceed 1 mg/min at a maximum concentration of 10 mg/ml.
   d. *Side effects* include a transient flushing reaction, rarely hypotension, rarely dizziness, rash, and urticaria. Vitamin K_1 may cause anaphylaxis or hypersensitivity (rare).
B. **ANTIULCER AGENTS**
1. **Cimetidine (Tagamet)**
   a. *Action:* Histamine antagonist.
   b. *Uses:* Short-term treatment of active duodenal ulcers and benign gastric ulcers or for long-term prophylaxis and prevention of upper GI tract bleeding.
   c. *Dose:* 20–40 mg/kg/d IV, IM, or PO in divided doses q6h. Continuous IV

infusion is used with GI tract bleeding. The IV dose should be titrated to maintain pH greater than 5.0. Adjust dosage for renal failure.

    d. *Side effects* include bradycardia, tachycardia, hypotension, diarrhea, nausea, vomiting, dizziness, headache, agitation, elevated serum creatinine, elevated aspartate aminotransferase (AST) and alanine aminotransferase (ALT), and neutropenia.

2. **Ranitidine (Zantac)**

    a. *Action:* Histamine antagonist.

    b. *Uses:* Short-term treatment of active and benign ulcers or long-term prophylaxis and prevention of hypersecretory states and bleeding.

    c. *Dose:* Neonate: 1.5 mg/kg/d IV divided q12h. Child: 2–4 mg/kg/d IV divided q6–8h. 0.1–0.15 mg/kg/h continuous IV infusion.

    d. *Side effects* include headache, nausea, vomiting, bradycardia, tachycardia, elevated serum creatinine, hepatitis, and arthralgia.

3. **Famotidine (Pepcid)**

    a. *Action:* Histamine antagonist.

    b. *Uses:* Therapy and treatment of ulcers and control of gastric pH and hypersecretory states.

    c. *Dose:* 0.6–0.8 mg/kg/d IV in divided doses q8–12h to a maximum of 40 mg/d; 1–1.2 mg/kg/d PO in divided doses q8–12h up to a maximum of 40 mg/d.

    d. *Side effects* include headache, dizziness, constipation, and diarrhea.

4. **Omeprazole (Prilosec)**

    a. *Action:* Protein pump inhibitor; direct inhibitor of hydrochloric acid secretions at the cellular level.

    b. *Uses:* Treatment of severe erosive esophagitis and short-term treatment of severe gastroesophageal reflux disease.

    c. *Dose:* 0.75–3.3 mg/kg/d PO q12h. This is a sustained release capsule. The capsule can be opened, and the beads can be mixed with water for delivery through a nasogastric tube. The beads of medication should *not* be crushed.

    d. *Side effects* include nausea, diarrhea, abdominal cramps, headache, dizziness, skin rash, leukopenia, and increased levels in liver function tests (LFTs).

5. **Sucralfate (Carafate)**

    a. *Action:* Gastric protectant; paste formation and ulcer adhesion occurs within 1 to 2 hours and can persist up to 6 hours.

    b. *Uses:* Short-term management of duodenal ulcers and gastritis.

    c. *Dose:* 40–80 mg/kg/d PO in divided doses q6h. Administer before meals or on an empty stomach.

    d. *Side effects* include constipation, diarrhea, nausea, dry mouth, rash, and pruritus. Safety and efficacy in children have not been established.

6. **Magnesium hydroxide and aluminum hydroxide (Maalox), aluminum hydroxide (Amphojel), and calcium carbonate (Titralac)**

    a. *Action:* Antacid.

    b. *Uses:* Prophylaxis against GI tract bleeding or in the treatment of peptic ulcer disease.

    c. *Dose:* Infant: 0.5 ml/kg per dose PO q2h; titrate to gastric pH greater than 5.0. Child: 2.5–5 ml per dose up to 4 times per day or 5–15 ml/d PO q1–2h; titrate to gastric pH greater than 5.0. In peptic ulcer disease: 5–15 ml per dose PO q3–6h; 5–15 ml per dose PO 1 to 3 hours after meals and at bedtime.

    d. *Side effects:* Magnesium can cause diarrhea, aluminum can cause constipation, and sodium can cause fluid retention.

7. **Glycopyrrolate (Robinul)**
   a. *Action:* Antimuscarinic and antispasmodic.
   b. *Uses:* Adjunct in the treatment of peptic ulcer disease; inhibits secretions.
   c. *Dose:* 2.5–5 µg/kg per dose IV q4–8h. Maximum dose is 0.2 mg per dose or 0.8 mg/24 h.
   d. *Side effects* include dry mouth, tachycardia, headache, nausea, and vomiting.
8. **Atropine**
   a. *Action:* Antimuscarinic and antispasmodic.
   b. *Uses:* Adjunct in the treatment of peptic ulcer disease; inhibits secretions.
   c. *Dose:* 0.01 mg/kg per dose to a maximum of 1 mg IV q4–6h. Minimum dose is 0.1 mg.
   d. *Side effects* include tachycardia, blurred vision, decreased GI tract motility, constipation, and headache.

C. OTHER AGENTS
   1. **Lactulose (Cephulac)**
      a. *Action:* Hyperosmotic laxative; ammonia detoxicant.
      b. *Uses:* Used to prevent and treat portal-systemic encephalopathy.
      c. *Dose:* Infant: 2.5–10 ml/d PO. Child: 40–90 ml/d PO in divided doses 3 to 4 times per day. Adjust dosage to produce three to four stools per day.
      d. *Side effects* include abdominal discomfort, diarrhea, nausea, and vomiting.
   2. **Magnesium citrate (Citroma) and magnesium hydroxide (Milk of Magnesia)**
      a. *Action:* Cathartic and laxative.
      b. *Uses:* Bowel evacuation and treatment of hyperacidity. Contraindicated with appendicitis, intestinal obstruction, colostomy, or ileostomy.
      c. *Dose*
         • Citroma: In children younger than 6 years: 2–4 ml/kg given as a single daily dose or divided. Ages 6 to 12 years: ⅓–½ bottle. Older than 12 years: ½–full bottle.
         • Magnesium hydroxide: As a laxative in children younger than 2 years: 0.5 ml/kg per dose. Ages 2 to 5 years: 5–15 ml/d or in divided doses. Ages 6 to 12 years: 15–30 ml/d or in divided doses. As an antacid, 2.5–5 ml as needed.
      d. *Side effects* include respiratory depression, diarrhea, hypermagnesemia, and hypotension.

D. IMMUNOSUPPRESSIVE THERAPY
   1. **Basic principles:** Combination therapy is used to maximize therapeutic benefit of agents while minimizing associated toxicities. Institution of specific protocols and organ-specific therapies exist. Generally, when the patient exhibits toxicities of the therapy, the patient is receiving excessive amounts of the drugs. Drug doses are decreased in the posttransplantation period as tolerated.
   2. **Tacrolimus (Prograf)**
      a. *Action:* Blocks the production of interleukin-2 and other lymphokines that promote T-cell proliferation.
      b. *Dose:* 0.05–0.1 mg/kg/d via a continuous IV infusion; 0.3 mg/kg/d PO in divided doses twice a day. Dosing is variable.
      c. *Side effects:* With IV use greater toxicity is observed including hypertension, renal impairment, central nervous system (CNS) effects (insomnia, headache, tremor, seizure, paresthesia), hyperkalemia, hypomagnesemia, hyperglycemia, GI tract symptoms, and lymphoproliferative disease.
   3. **Cyclosporine (Sandimmune)** (Marsh et al, 1992)
      a. *Action:* Inhibits T-cell proliferation through inhibition of interleukin-2 synthesis.

b. *Dose:* 5 to 6 mg/kg/d IV in divided doses q12–24h after transplantation; 15 mg/kg/d PO for first 2 weeks after transplantation. Maintenance: 5–10 mg/kg/d based on serum levels.

c. *Side effects* include hypertension, renal impairment, CNS toxicity (headache, tremor, seizure, paresthesia), hypomagnesemia, GI tract symptoms, gum hyperplasia, hirsutism, and lymphoproliferative disease.

4. **Corticosteroids: Methylprednisolone (Solu-Medrol) and prednisone**

a. *Action:* Depress the immune system by decreasing lymphocytes, macrophage motility, and leukocyte chemotaxis.

b. *Dose*
- Methylprednisolone: 0.1–1.6 mg/kg/d in divided doses q6–12h PO, IM, or IV.
- Prednisone: 0.05–2 mg/kg/d in divided doses 1 to 4 times.

c. *Side effects* include hyperglycemia, ulcers, weight gain, hypertension, sodium and water retention, infection, and acne.

5. **Azathioprine (Imuran)** (Marsh et al, 1992)

a. *Action:* Inhibits DNA synthesis.

b. *Dose:* Initial dose is 3–5 mg/kg/d IV or PO. Maintenance: 1–3 mg/kg/d.

c. *Side effects* include bone marrow suppression (anemia, leukopenia), pancreatitis, nausea and vomiting, and mucosal ulceration.

6. **Muromonab-CD3 (Orthoclone OKT3)** (Marsh et al, 1992)

a. *Action:* Monoclonal antibody that complexes with CD3 receptor of the T cell and blocks cell function.

b. *Uses:* Generally used in the treatment of intractable rejection.

c. *Dose:* Children weighing less than 30 kg: 2.5 mg/d once daily or 0.1 mg/kg/d for 10 to 14 days. Adults: 5 mg/d once daily for 10 to 14 days.

d. *Side effects:* The first dose should be administered in an intensive care unit (ICU) because of the potential adverse reactions. Administration of methylprednisolone sodium succinate prior to the first dose and hydrocortisone sodium succinate 30 minutes after the first dose are recommended to decrease the incidence of reactions. A first-dose effect (flulike symptoms, anaphylactic-type reaction) may occur in 30 minutes to 6 hours or up to 24 hours after the first dose. Administration may result in infection, pulmonary edema with fluid overload, hypotension, anaphylaxis, and the need for cardiopulmonary resuscitation.

ACUTE ABDOMINAL TRAUMA

A. PATHOPHYSIOLOGY AND ETIOLOGY AND RISK FACTORS

1. **General principles:** Acute abdominal trauma is the most common potentially lethal injury (Schafermeyer, 1993) and is often associated with other traumatic injuries. Anatomic differences in children as compared to adults include a body size that allows for greater distribution of injury, a larger body surface area that allows for greater heat loss, abdominal organs that are more anterior with less subcutaneous fat protection, and a smaller blood volume resulting in hypovolemia with relatively smaller volume losses.

2. **Mechanism of injury** (Schafermeyer, 1993)

a. *Blunt* injuries are caused by compression of solid or hollow viscous organs against the spine, rapid acceleration and deceleration with subsequent tearing of structures, or increased abdominal pressure resulting in contusion, laceration, or bursting of organs with subsequent hemorrhage. Solid organs are injured more commonly than hollow organs, and the most commonly injured organ is the spleen. Blunt trauma can result in lethal injury without visible signs of trauma.

   b. *Penetrating* injuries are most often caused by gunshot or stab wounds. The most common injury is to the hollow viscera. Major vascular injuries are common. The onset of peritonitis may be immediate.

B. Signs and Symptoms of Acute Abdominal Trauma

1. Significant injuries to the head and extremities may overshadow abdominal injuries.
2. Signs of injury are often subtle and include rebound tenderness, pain, rigidity, pallor, grunting respirations, hypotension, failure to respond to fluid resuscitation, and increasing abdominal girth. Acute abdominal distention occurs even with minor trauma, especially in infants and often in children as a result of crying and swallowing air. Distention may lead to vomiting and aspiration.
3. Signs of retroperitoneal bleeding include Cullen's sign (discoloration around the umbilicus) and Turner's sign (discoloration on the flank).

C. Diagnostic Studies

1. **Computed tomography (CT) scan** may be indicated if there is bleeding or for further diagnosis related to the mechanism of injury.
2. **Diagnostic peritoneal lavage (DPL)** may be performed using 10 ml/kg of normal saline (NS) or lactated Ringer's solution (LR) (Foltin and Cooper, 1992) (Table 7–2).
3. **Complete blood count (CBC) and coagulation studies** are used to evaluate bleeding.
4. **Chest and abdominal x-ray examinations** determine gastric dilation (which is common in children related to crying), ground glass appearance (suggests intraperitoneal blood or urine), associated lower rib fractures (indicates severe force), and signs of ileus (Foltin and Cooper, 1992).
5. **Urinalysis** evaluates the presence of blood.
6. **Nuclear scan** is a gold standard used for follow-up of hepatic and splenic injuries.
7. **Ultrasound** is used to evaluate pancreatic injuries.

D. Nursing and Collaborative Diagnoses

  ❖ Potential fluid volume deficit related to bleeding due to blunt or penetrating trauma

  ❖ Potential for infection related to impaired viscera integrity

  ❖ Potential alteration in nutrition, less than body requirements related to inadequate nutritional intake

  ❖ Pain related to abdominal injury

E. Desired Patient Outcomes

1. Child will maintain adequate intravascular volume. Treat hypovolemic shock with adequate volume resuscitation. Prevent or control bleeding.
2. Child will demonstrate no signs of infection. Monitor vital signs and CBC for

Table 7–2.   CRITERIA FOR POSITIVE DIAGNOSTIC PERITONEAL LAVAGE (DPL)

Hemorrhage	Perforation*
1. >100,000 RBCs/mm^3 in effluent	1. >500 WBC/mm^3 in effluent
2. Free blood aspirated	2. Amylase >175 mg/dl
	3. Stool aspirated

*Data from Foltin GL, Cooper A. Abdominal trauma. In: Barkin RM, Asch SM, Caputo GL, et al, eds. *Pediatric Emergency Medicine*. St Louis, Mo: The CV Mosby Co; 1992:276–292.

Table 7–3.   CALCULATION OF CIRCULATING BLOOD VOLUME (CBV) IN CHILDREN

AGE OF CHILD	BLOOD VOLUME (ml/kg)
Neonates	85–90
Infants	75–80
Children	70–75
Adults	65–70

Modified from Hazinski MF. *Nursing Care of the Critically Ill Child.* 2nd ed. St Louis, Mo: The CV Mosby Co; 1992.

evidence of leukocytosis (elevated white blood cell [WBC] count). Administer antibiotic therapy as ordered. Observe for signs of peritonitis: abdominal distention, diffuse pain, tenderness, fever, and tachycardia.

3. Child will maintain adequate nutrition and positive nitrogen balance. Calculate daily caloric requirements and notify the physician if the child's caloric intake is inadequate. Monitor serum glucose as appropriate while the child is NPO. Administer peripheral or central parenteral nutrition while the child is NPO. Maintain a warm environment to prevent cold stress in infants.

4. The child's pain will be controlled. Assess for signs and symptoms of pain. Give narcotic analgesics as needed. Position the child to maximize comfort. Use techniques appropriate for the child's developmental age.

F. **GENERAL PATIENT CARE MANAGEMENT**

1. Early management of airway, breathing, and circulation (ABCs) has the most direct impact on survival. Inadequate airway and fluid resuscitation is the leading cause of preventable death.

2. Serial monitoring of vital signs and abdominal girth is the key to appreciating the progression of findings associated with abdominal injury. Avoid deep palpation as it may cause further injury.

3. Insertion of nasogastric (NG) or orogastric (OG) tube allows for gastric decompression and maximizes respiratory effort.

4. Serial hematocrits are imperative to assess bleeding.

5. Military antishock trousers (MAST) are useful to stabilize pelvic, hip, and long bone fractures (Moloney-Harmon, 1991). They are beneficial if systolic blood pressure is less than 60 mm Hg and the patient is not responding to fluid resuscitation. Usually only the leg compartments are inflated. Abdominal compartments are inflated only if abdominal bleeding is present or there is a pelvic fracture. If the abdominal compartment is inflated, observe for respiratory compromise.

6. Most abdominal trauma can be managed medically. Indications for surgery include massive bleeding (40 to 60 ml/kg or 50% of blood volume) (Table 7–3), penetrating trauma, and certain blunt injuries.

G. **SPECIFIC INJURIES**

1. The **spleen** is the most commonly injured abdominal organ.

   a. *Signs and symptoms* include left upper quadrant (LUQ) tenderness, bruising, or abrasion, positive Kehr's sign (LUQ pain radiating to the left shoulder), signs of decreased perfusion (pallor, tachycardia, delayed capillary refill, and hypotension), and nausea and vomiting.

   b. *Diagnostic studies:* Abdominal x-ray examinations are rarely helpful but may demonstrate a medially displaced lateral stomach border suggesting splenic laceration. The hematocrit may be decreased related to bleeding, or an increased WBC count may be noted. Definitive diagnosis is made by CT scan. DPL is not indicated.

   c. *Management* involves supportive care to maintain stable vital signs if transfusion requirements are less than half of the child's estimated total blood volume. *Splenectomy* is rarely performed but is indicated for a spleen completely separated from the blood supply or a hemodynamically unstable patient with multiple severe injuries. *Splenorrhaphy* is an alternative to splenectomy. Indications include complete severation of the spleen from the blood supply, hemodynamic instability, and associated injuries including head trauma. Splenorrhaphy involves inspection, control of bleeding, and repair of lacerations. The majority of injuries heal spontaneously on a regimen of limited activity beginning with 7 to 10 days of strict bed rest (Foltin and Cooper, 1992).

    d. *Complications* include rebleeding or splenic laceration 3 to 5 days after the initial injury. Splenectomized children are at risk for infection, require immunization with pneumococcal vaccine (Pneumovax), and should receive prophylactic antibiotics with dental care and elective surgeries.

2. The **liver** is second only to the spleen as a major source of hemorrhage and is the most common source of lethal hemorrhage. Bleeding stops spontaneously with the majority of injuries.

    a. *Injuries are graded* according to increasing severity. Grading varies based on the scale used (Buntain, 1995; Moore et al, 1989):
- Grade I: Subscapular hematoma, capsular tears
- Grade II: Minor lacerations of the parenchyma (right lobe injured most frequently)
- Grade III: Deep parenchymal lacerations
- Grade IV: Burst liver injuries with or without associated major vascular injury

    b. *Signs and symptoms* include right upper quadrant (RUQ) tenderness, ecchymosis, abrasion, enlarging abdominal girth, signs of shock, lower rib fractures, elevated AST greater than 200 IU/L, and ALT greater than 100 IU/L (Torres and Garcia, 1993).

    c. *Diagnostic studies:* Definitive diagnosis is made with CT scan. The hematocrit decreases with major laceration. Serial CT scans are performed to assess healing or continued bleeding.

    d. *Management* is supportive. Surgery is indicated if the child is hemodynamically unstable, signs of peritoneal irritation are evident, or transfusion requirements exceed 50% of the estimated blood volume during the first 24 hours (Foltin and Cooper, 1992; Torres and Garcia, 1993).

3. Infrequently injured, the **pancreas** is located deep in the upper abdomen and is well protected unless a significant, sustained force compresses it against the spine. Associated injuries occur in 90% of all children (Buntain, 1995). The classic injury is bicycle handlebar injury.

    a. *Signs and symptoms* include diffuse abdominal tenderness and deep epigastric pain radiating to the back, bilious vomiting, elevated amylase (extent of increase does not usually correlate with the severity of injury), and elevated lipase (which usually follows elevated amylase).

    b. *Diagnostic studies*
- DPL demonstrates a high amylase concentration (rarely performed in children).
- Amylase is elevated (normal 0 to 88 IU/L). The extent of increase does not correlate with the severity of injury. Three times normal suggests injury. A trend of increasing amylase is indicative of significant injury. Amylase begins to rise 2 to 12 hours following the onset of symptoms, peaks by 12 to 24 hours, and gradually returns to normal by the fourth or fifth day after injury (Mader and McHugh, 1992).

- Lipase (normal 20 to 180 U/L) rises after injury and remains elevated longer than amylase.
- Diagnosis is definitive with abdominal CT scan with contrast.
- Ultrasound is useful for diagnosis of pseudocyst.
- Endoscophic retrograde cholangiopancreatography (ERCP) may be necessary to visualize pancreatic ductal disruption or post-traumatic stricture.

    c. *Management* is supportive and nonoperative if there is no ductal disruption. An NG tube is used for gastric decompression. Children are monitored for signs of infection. If pancreatic pseudocyst develops, patients require 6 to 8 weeks of bowel rest with total parenteral nutrition (TPN) (Foltin and Cooper, 1992). Surgery is indicated if pain, fever, ileus, and elevated amylase persist or develop. Surgery involves drainage, partial resection, or repair of lacerated ducts.

    d. *Complications* involve development of pancreatic fistulas and pseudocyst formation resulting in chronic intermittent attacks of abdominal pain, nausea, and vomiting.

4. **Stomach**

    a. *Signs and symptoms* of injury include abrasion or contusion in the upper abdomen and bloody gastric drainage. A boardlike abdomen with severe pain is indicative of perforation.

    b. *Diagnostic studies:* Abdominal x-ray examination detects free air or demonstrates that the NG tube is in an abnormal position. An upper GI tract series locates the exact area of injury.

    c. *Management* includes surgical repair as appropriate.

5. **Small and large intestine:** The **colon and rectum** are rarely injured in children. Such an injury occurs most often in the presence of abuse.

    a. *Signs and symptoms* include bloody gastric drainage, absent bowel sounds, tympanic sounds on percussion, and pain that increases as peritonitis develops.

    b. *Diagnostic studies:* Abdominal x-ray examination detects intraperitoneal air or retroperitoneal emphysema. An upper GI tract series is diagnostic.

    c. *Management* includes supportive care and surgical repair as indicated.

ACUTE GI TRACT HEMORRHAGE

A. **PATHOPHYSIOLOGY**

The child presenting with sudden massive blood loss is at risk for hemodynamic instability. The first priority is to determine the extent of the blood loss and establish if perfusion is compromised. Greater than 15% circulating blood volume (CBV) loss results in stimulation of autonomic cardiovascular responses to maintain blood pressure and perfusion. Greater than 20% CBV loss results in decreased systolic blood pressure and metabolic acidosis. Rapid fluid resuscitation is required, or cardiovascular collapse and death may occur.

B. **ETIOLOGY**

Etiology is based on age (Table 7–4) (Vinton, 1994).

C. **SIGNS AND SYMPTOMS** (TABLE 7–5)

1. The location of bleeding can be identified by the color and source of the bleeding. **Hematemesis** is the result of acute blood loss from the upper GI tract (esophageal or gastric). **Hematochezia** is the result of frank bleeding from the rectum. **Melena** is caused by the digestion of blood in the GI tract. **Occult bleeding** is the result of chronic blood loss.

Table 7–4. COMMON CAUSES OF GI TRACT BLEEDING IN INFANTS AND CHILDREN

AGE	CAUSES
Neonates	Congenital intestinal malrotation
	Intestinal duplication
	Meckel's diverticulum
	Vascular malformations
	Neonatal necrotizing enterocolitis
Infancy	Hirschsprung's disease
	Cow's milk protein intolerance
	Gastroesophageal reflux disease
	Intussusception
	Infectious colitis
	Portal hypertension and esophageal varices
Preschool	Schönlein-Henoch purpura
	Hemolytic-uremic syndrome
	End-stage liver disease
	Juvenile polyps
School-age and adolescence	Peptic ulcer disease
	Inflammatory bowel disease
	Stress ulcer
	Esophagitis
	Schönlein-Henoch purpura

    2. Signs and symptoms of hypovolemic shock occur with acute bleeding: tachycardia, weak peripheral pulses, pallor and mottled color, and cool and clammy skin. Blood pressure may be normal despite significant blood loss; hypotension is a late sign of shock.

D. NURSING AND COLLABORATIVE DIAGNOSES
   ❖ FLUID VOLUME DEFICIT RELATED TO BLEEDING
   ❖ POTENTIAL INEFFECTIVE BREATHING PATTERNS RELATED TO ELEVATION OF THE DIAPHRAGM FROM INTRAABDOMINAL BLEEDING
   ❖ POTENTIAL ALTERATION IN NUTRITION, LESS THAN BODY REQUIREMENTS RELATED TO NPO STATUS
   ❖ ALTERATION IN COMFORT RELATED TO MULTIPLE INVASIVE PROCEDURES

E. DESIRED PATIENT OUTCOMES
    1. Child will maintain adequate intravascular volume as evidenced by effective

Table 7–5. PRESENTATIONS OF GI TRACT BLEEDING

PRESENTATION	DEFINITIONS
Acute Bleeding	
Hematemesis	Bloody vomitus; either fresh, bright red blood or dark, grainy digested blood with "coffee ground" appearance
Melena	Black, sticky, tarry, foul-smelling stools caused by digestion of blood in the GI tract (seen in both upper GI and lower GI tract bleeding)
Hematochezia	Fresh, bright red blood passed from the rectum
Chronic Bleeding	
Occult	Trace amounts of blood in normal-appearing stools or gastric secretions; detectable only with a guaiac test

Modified from Huether SE, McCance KL, Tarmina MS. Alterations of digestive function. In: McCance KL, Huether SE, eds. *Pathophysiology: The Biological Basis for Diseases in Adults and Children.* 2nd ed. St Louis, Mo: Mosby–Year Book Inc; 1994.

peripheral perfusion. Treat hypovolemic shock with volume resuscitation. Prevent or stop bleeding.

2. Child will maintain effective breathing patterns and rate. Maintain airway patency; monitor respiratory status and effort; and maintain the position of comfort to maximize diaphragm excursion. Optimize oxygenation by providing oxygen as needed, and prepare for intubation as needed.

3. Child will maintain adequate nutrition and positive nitrogen balance. Monitor serum glucose as appropriate while the child is NPO. Administer peripheral or central parenteral nutrition while the child is NPO. Calculate daily caloric requirements and notify the physician if the child's caloric intake is inadequate.

4. Child will achieve a maximal level of comfort. Allow the child's parents to be present as much as possible. Use pain control measures appropriate for the child's developmental age.

F. DIAGNOSTIC STUDIES

1. **Laboratory studies** are used to monitor for metabolic acidosis (ABGs), monitor decreased hematocrit, hemoglobin, and thrombocytopenia (CBC), evaluate for coagulopathies, serum fibrinogen and fibrin split products if disseminated intravascular coagulation (DIC) is suspected (prothrombin time [PT], partial thromboplastin time [PTT]), detect occult blood in stool or gastric fluid, and to screen for liver disease (LFTs).

2. The **upper and lower GI tract study** involves a fluoroscopic x-ray examination by which the location and cause of bleeding is identified in 85% to 95% of patients (Hyams et al, 1985). Complete volume resuscitation must be achieved prior to the procedure. The upper GI tract study is therapeutic for esophageal varices (sclerotherapy).

3. **Abdominal x-ray examination** involves a supine and lateral decubitus view to rule out bowel obstruction and free intraabdominal air.

4. **Endoscopy** provides direct visualization of the GI tract (upper or lower) to determine injury, structural defects, or source of bleeding.

5. **Radionuclide studies** are indicated for midintestinal bleeding (Berry and Perrault, 1996). The studies are an effective method for locating subacute or intermittent bleeding. Two types are used: technetium-labeled sulfur colloid (more sensitive) and technetium-pertechnetate-labeled red blood cells.

6. **Angiography** is used infrequently because of endoscopy and safer, improved noninvasive methods. Angiography may be effective in determining arteriovenous malformations, hemangiomas, and telangiectasias.

G. GENERAL PATIENT CARE MANAGEMENT

1. Assess for signs of respiratory distress.

2. Secure two large-bore IVs for fluid resuscitation. Administer fluid (20 ml/kg of NS or LR) or blood (10 ml/kg) as needed until peripheral circulation is adequate. Whole blood should be administered with massive bleeding. Monitor central venous pressure (CVP) and blood pressure for response to fluid resuscitation and the need for continued therapy. The initial hematocrit may be misleading with acute bleeding.

3. Monitor PT, PTT, and fibrinogen for coagulopathies. Administer vitamin K (AquaMephyton), platelets, or fresh frozen plasma (FFP) as necessary.

4. Monitor electrolytes, blood urea nitrogen (BUN), and creatinine for potential renal dysfunction. Monitor urine output via a Foley catheter.

5. Monitor serum ionized calcium following transfusion.

6. Monitor for signs of further bleeding: poor perfusion, abdominal pain, increased abdominal girth, decreased bowel sounds, hematemesis, and hematochezia.

7. Assess for signs and symptoms of abdominal perforation: fever, severe or persistent abdominal pain, and abdominal rigidity.

8. Administer room temperature gastric saline lavage (10 ml/kg) until bleeding stops. Therapeutic effectiveness of room temperature lavage is not established. Prevent hypothermia if iced lavage is used.

9. Monitor gastric pH. Administer antacid if pH is less than 4. Bleeding usually stops when gastric pH is greater than 5 with acute hemorrhage secondary to peptic disease. H_2-histamine receptor antagonists are effective for chronic suppression.

10. Prevent stress ulcers and increase gastric cytoprotection by administering sucralfate (Carafate).

H. ESOPHAGEAL VARICES

1. **Acute treatment** involves the administration of vasopressin (Pitressin) or somatostatin (Berry and Perrault, 1996). Insertion of a Sengstaken-Blakemore tube (Fig. 7–2) is helpful. Three separate lumens are used for gastric suction, inflation of the gastric balloon, and inflation of the esophageal balloon. Balloons must be deflated every 12 to 24 hours. Ensure patency of the gastric suction lumen by irrigating frequently. Assess for complications including perforation or erosion of the esophagus or stomach (due to hyperinflation or prolonged inflation of the balloons).

2. **Endoscopic variceal sclerosis** is the current treatment of choice. The sclerosing

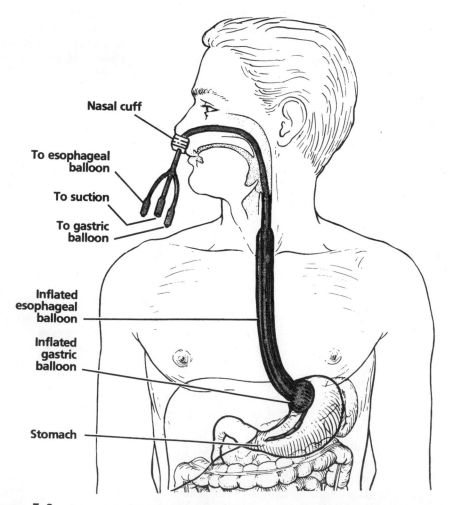

Nasal cuff

To esophageal balloon

To suction

To gastric balloon

Inflated esophageal balloon

Inflated gastric balloon

Stomach

Figure 7–2. Sengstaken-Blakemore tube. (Reprinted with permission from Quinless FW. Severe liver dysfunction: client problems and nursing actions. *Focus Crit Care.* 1985;12:24–32.)

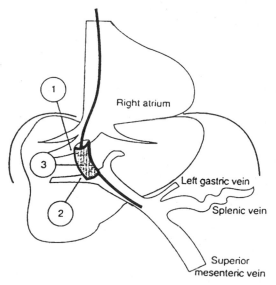

Figure 7–3. Technique of transjugular intrahepatic portal-systemic shunt (TIPS). Following transjugular catheterization of a hepatic vein *(1)* and puncture of a main branch of the portal vein *(2)*, the shunt is established by implanting a stent spanning the hepatic parenchyma between sites *1* and *2*. (Reprinted by permission of *The New England Journal of Medicine* from Rossle M, Haag K, Ochs A, et al: The Transjugular Intrahepatic Portosystemic Stent-Shunt Procedure for Variceal Bleeding. *N Engl J Med.* 1994;330:165. Copyright 1994, Massachusetts Medical Society.)

agent is injected directly into or alongside varices. Assess for complications including ulceration with rebleeding, perforation, and stricture formation.

3. **Preventive therapy** includes a transjugular intrahepatic portosystemic shunt (TIPS) (Fig. 7–3). This is a nonsurgical approach to palliate portal hypertension. It is effective but associated with a high rate of shunt thrombosis. Propranolol (Inderal) is a long-term treatment modality that decreases portal blood flow and prevents bleeding of esophageal varices. Bleeding must be stopped before administration of propranolol. TIPS is contraindicated in the presence of heart disease. Repeated injection sclerotherapy may also be used.

4. **Development of new therapies** includes laser surgery, ligation of varices with endoscopically placed elastic bands, and electrocoagulation (Berry and Perrault, 1996).

5. **Complications** include rebleeding, sepsis, and hepatic encephalopathy.

CONGENITAL GI TRACT ABNORMALITIES

See Table 7–6.

BOWEL INFARCTION, OBSTRUCTION, AND PERFORATION

A. ETIOLOGY AND RISK FACTORS

1. **Acute abdomen** refers to sudden onset of abdominal pain and tenderness that warrants evaluation for surgical intervention.

2. **Etiology:** Causes in neonates include necrotizing enterocolitis (NEC), intussusception, volvulus, birth trauma, and Hirschsprung's disease. Causes in children and adolescents include appendicitis (common cause of peritonitis), Meckel's

Text continued on page 446

Table 7–6. CONGENITAL GI TRACT ABNORMALITIES

Diagnosis	Etiology and Risk Factors	Pathophysiology	Signs and Symptoms	Nursing Diagnoses	Patient Care Management	Complications

Omphalocele	Cause unknown; may be caused by incomplete closure of the anterior abdominal wall or incomplete return of the bowel into the abdomen by 10–11 wk gestation	Herniation of abdominal viscera into the umbilical cord usually covered by a peritoneal sac with the umbilical arteries and veins inserting into the apex of the defect
		
		Associated anomalies include cardiac defects; neurologic, genitourinary, skeletal, and chromosomal abnormalities; malrotation of the intestine; Beckwith–Wiedemann syndrome
			Size of the defect is variable
			Signs and symptoms of dehydration, hypothermia, hypoglycemia, respiratory distress (dependent on lesion size)
				Potential for alteration in breathing patterns: ineffective r/t abdominal hernia
				Potential for fluid volume deficit: actual r/t increased insensible water loss and third spacing
				Potential for alteration in nutrition: actual r/t NPO status
				Impairment of skin integrity: actual r/t abdominal hernia
				Alteration in comfort r/t postoperative pain
					1. Cover exposed abdominal hernia with warm, moist dressing; cover dressing with plastic
					2. Maintain NPO status
					3. Place OG/NG tube
					4. Maintain neutral thermal environment
					5. Monitor I & O
					6. Monitor electrolyte status
					7. Provide IV hydration
					8. Provide IV antibiotic therapy
					9. Surgical repair of defect
					10. Postoperative care
					  a. TPN
					  b. Management of fluid and electrolyte status
					  c. Monitor for infection
					  d. Encourage pulmonary toilet
					  e. Pain management
						Intestinal obstruction
						Respiratory distress
						Sepsis
						Wound infection
						Feeding intolerance

| Gastroschisis | Cause unknown; theories include a failure of closure of the lateral fold of the abdominal wall or intrauterine vascular accident involving the omphalomesenteric artery with subsequent disruption of the abdominal ring | Herniation of the abdominal wall usually includes the small and large intestine; no protective sac Associated anomalies include intestinal stricture and atresia | Size of defect usually smaller than an omphalocele, usually includes the small and large intestine, no sac covering the defect Intestine may be edematous and inflamed due to exposure to amniotic fluid | Potential for alteration in breathing patterns: ineffective r/t abdominal hernia Potential for fluid volume deficit: actual r/t increased insensible water losses and third spacing Alteration in nutritional status: actual r/t NPO status Impairment of skin integrity: actual r/t abdominal hernia Alteration in comfort r/t surgical procedure | 1. Cover exposed abdominal hernia with warm, moist dressing; cover dressing with plastic 2. Maintain NPO status 3. Place OG/NG tube 4. Maintain neutral thermal environment 5. Monitor I & O 6. Monitor electrolyte status 7. Provide IV hydration 8. Provide IV antibiotic therapy 9. Surgical repair of defect 10. Postoperative care a. TPN b. Management of fluid and electrolyte status c. Monitor for infection d. Encourage pulmonary toilet e. Pain management | Intestinal obstruction Respiratory distress Sepsis Wound infection Feeding intolerance |

Table continued on following page

Table 7-6. CONGENITAL GI TRACT ABNORMALITIES (*Continued*)

DIAGNOSIS	ETIOLOGY AND RISK FACTORS	PATHOPHYSIOLOGY	SIGNS AND SYMPTOMS	NURSING DIAGNOSES	PATIENT CARE MANAGEMENT	COMPLICATIONS
Volvulus (malrotation)	Abnormal rotation and fixation of the intestine; most commonly occurs in infancy; however, may occur at any age	The intestine returns from the umbilical cord at about the 10th wk gestation, undergoes a counterclockwise rotation about the axis of the superior mesenteric artery, followed by fixation to the posterior abdominal wall; this twisting causes gangrene as the superior mesenteric artery is strangulated	Bilious vomiting Melena or currant-jelly stools Abdominal distention X-ray examination shows evidence of duodenal obstruction and poor air distribution throughout the remaining intestine	Alteration in nutrition: actual r/t NPO status Alteration in comfort: actual r/t pain associated with vascular compromise and associated postoperative pain	1. Maintain NPO status 2. Provide IV hydration 3. Provide IV antibiotics 4. Prepare child for emergency surgery 5. Postsurgical care a. TPN b. Management of fluid and electrolyte status c. Monitor for infection d. Encourage pulmonary toilet e. Pain management	Sepsis Complete bowel infarction with resultant short-gut syndrome
Intestinal atresia	Etiology thought to be related to in utero vascular accident (e.g., volvulus, intussusception) due	Four types: Type 1: Intact mucosal membrane obstructs the intestinal lumen Type 2: Gaps in bowel continu-	Signs of bowel obstruction: bilious vomiting, abdominal distention	Alteration in nutritional status: actual r/t NPO status Alteration in comfort r/t associated postoperative pain	1. Provide IV hydration 2. Provide IV antibiotics 3. Maintain NPO status 4. Prepare for palliative/corrective surgery 5. Postoperative care a. TPN	Intestinal perforation Ileus

	to constriction of the superior mesenteric artery Obliteration of the intestinal lumen due to occlusion or total absence	ity, short fibrotic bands connect proximal and distal segments Type 3: No connective tissue between gaps on the intestine Type 4: Atretic segments that are numerous and continuous		b. Management of fluid and electrolyte status c. Monitor for signs and symptoms of infection d. Encourage pulmonary toilet e. Pain management	

Intussusception	Frequently preceded by gastroenteritis, 5% of the cases have a specific anatomic instigator (e.g., polyp, enlarged lymph node, tumor); most commonly occur in children aged 6 mo to 18 y	One segment of the intestine invaginates into another (usually the ileum into the cecum); the entrapped bowel initially develops venous obstruction with eventual arterial obstruction and gangrene	Recurrent and severe abdominal pain
			Bloody stool
			Signs of bowel obstruction: bilious vomiting, abdominal distention
			RUQ may have sausage-shaped mass
				Alteration in nutrition: actual r/t NPO status
				Alteration in comfort: pain associated with lesion
					1. Provide IV fluids
					2. Maintain NPO status
					3. Nonsurgical repair with barium enema
					4. Surgical repair of defect if nonsurgical repair fails
					5. Postsurgical care
					  a. Provide IV hydration
					  b. Provide IV antibiotics
					  c. Monitor for infection
					  d. Encourage pulmonary toilet
					  e. Pain management
						Intestinal perforation
						Intestinal infarction
						Shock

Table continued on following page

Table 7–6. CONGENITAL GI TRACT ABNORMALITIES (*Continued*)

DIAGNOSIS	ETIOLOGY AND RISK FACTORS	PATHOPHYSIOLOGY	SIGNS AND SYMPTOMS	NURSING DIAGNOSES	PATIENT CARE MANAGEMENT	COMPLICATIONS

Tracheoesophageal fistula (TEF) (see Chapter 2 for pulmonary implications)	History of maternal polyhydramnios
	
	Abnormal separation of the esophagus in relation to the trachea
		Five types of the anomaly can occur:
		
		Type 1: Blind proximal esophageal pouch with distal esophagus originating at the transbronchial junction (80%)
		
		Type 2: Blind proximal esophageal pouch with blind distal esophageal pouch (8%)
		
		Type 3: An H-type TEF (4%)
		
		Type 4: Fistulization of proximal esophagus into trachea with blind distal esophageal pouch (2%)
			Dependent on type of anomaly
			
			Dysphagia
			
			Inability to pass OG/NG tube
			
			Choking/cyanosis with feeding
			
			Recurrent pneumonia
				Potential for ineffective airway clearance r/t dysphagia
				
				Potential for fluid volume deficit r/t continuous suctioning of oral/gastric secretions
				
				Alteration in nutritional status: actual r/t feeding difficulties, NPO status
					1. Maintain NPO status
					2. Provide IV hydration
					3. Maintain the head of the bed elevated
					4. Provide constant suctioning of upper airway to clear oral secretions
					5. Surgical repair/palliation of defect
					6. Postoperative care
					  a. Management of fluid and electrolyte status
					  b. Monitor for infection
					  c. Wound care
					  d. Encourage pulmonary toilet
					  e. Pain management
						Respiratory distress
						Aspiration

Disorder	Etiology	Pathophysiology	Clinical manifestations	Nursing diagnoses	Nursing management	Complications
Type 5: Interrupted esophagus with both proximal and distal esophagus communicating with trachea (<1%; Kocoshis, 1992)						
Diaphragmatic hernia (see Chapter 2 for pulmonary implications)	Failure of diaphragm closure or return of the intestine prior to diaphragmatic closure	Herniation of the abdominal organs into the thoracic cavity. Herniation of the intestine into the thorax results in hypoplasia of the lung (usually left, right may be affected if there is displacement of the mediastinum)	Respiratory distress Heart tones shifted to the right Scaphoid abdomen	Alteration in breathing patterns: ineffective r/t pulmonary hypoplasia Alteration in nutritional status: actual r/t NPO status	1. Maintain NPO status 2. Place NG tube for gastric decompression 3. Place right-side down, to augment pulmonary perfusion 4. Pulmonary management: mechanical ventilation, ECMO may be indicated 5. Prepare for emergent surgical repair	Respiratory failure Pneumothorax Sepsis Survival dependent on severity of presenting symptoms

ECMO, extracorporeal membrane oxygenation; *I & O*, intake and output; *IV*, intravenous; *NG*, nasogastric; *NPO*, nothing by mouth; *OG*, orogastric; *r/t*, related to; *RUQ*, right upper quadrant; *TPN*, total parenteral nutrition.

diverticulum, inflammatory bowel disease, and trauma. Blunt trauma from motor vehicle accidents, falls, and abuse and penetrating trauma from gunshot wounds and stab wounds are also risk factors.

B. **PATHOPHYSIOLOGY** (Barnard and Hazinski, 1992)

1. Inflammation or trauma may result in perforation with resultant leakage of GI tract contents into the peritoneum. An abscess forms if peritoneal defenses are successful in localizing the insult. If peritoneal defenses are unsuccessful in localizing the insult, peritonitis can occur. Peritonitis is associated with increased blood flow and capillary permeability, causing transudation of fluid into the peritoneal cavity with resultant third spacing and hypovolemia.

2. Upper GI tract perforations result in leakage of hydrochloric acid, digestive enzymes, or bile causing chemical peritonitis.

3. Lower GI tract perforation results in the leakage of fecal material, which releases aerobic and anaerobic bacteria into the peritoneum. Endotoxins may be released. The release of bacteria and endotoxins may cause bacterial peritonitis and sepsis.

4. Injury to the peritoneum causes decreased bowel motility and may result in an ileus.

C. **SIGNS AND SYMPTOMS**

1. Obstruction results in abdominal distention, vomiting, fever, and absence of bowel sounds.

2. Perforation causes signs of respiratory distress including tachypnea, retractions, flaring, grunting, cyanosis, hypoxemia, and acidosis.

3. Signs of third spacing include increased abdominal girth and hypovolemia (tachycardia, decreased peripheral perfusion, decreased urine output, and hypotension [late sign]).

4. Symptoms of peritonitis include fever, nausea, abdominal distention and rigidity, absent or hypoactive bowel sounds, diffuse abdominal pain, guarding of the abdomen, and rebound tenderness.

D. **DIAGNOSTIC STUDIES**

1. **Abdominal x-ray examination** determines the presence of free air in the abdomen and indicates bowel wall edema and distribution of intraluminal air.

2. **Abdominal CT scan** provides definitive imaging of abdominal solid organs.

3. **DPL** is diagnostic for perforation if the effluent contains stool, greater than 500 WBC/mm^3, amylase greater than 175 µg/dl, and an ALT greater than 6 IU/L (Foltin and Cooper, 1992).

4. **Radionuclide studies** determine rupture or laceration of the liver or spleen and determine the size, position, and shape of abdominal organs.

E. **NURSING AND COLLABORATIVE DIAGNOSES**

❖ POTENTIAL FOR INFECTION RELATED TO IMPAIRED BOWEL INTEGRITY

❖ ALTERATION IN NUTRITION, LESS THAN BODY REQUIREMENTS RELATED TO INADEQUATE NUTRITIONAL INTAKE

❖ ALTERATION IN FLUID VOLUME DEFICIT RELATED TO THIRD SPACING

❖ POTENTIAL ALTERATION IN ELECTROLYTE STATUS RELATED TO FLUID LOSSES FROM THE GI TRACT AND THIRD SPACING

❖ ALTERATION IN COMFORT RELATED TO MULTIPLE INVASIVE PROCEDURES OR INJURY

F. **DESIRED PATIENT OUTCOMES**

1. Child will demonstrate no signs of infection. Monitor vital signs. Monitor CBC for leukocytosis (elevated WBC count). Observe for signs of peritonitis including abdominal distention, diffuse pain and tenderness, fever, and tachycardia. Observe for signs of an abscess including localized pain, fever, or leukocytosis. Administer antibiotics as ordered.

2. Child will maintain adequate nutrition and positive nitrogen balance. Monitor

serum glucose as appropriate while the child is NPO. Administer TPN while the child is NPO. Calculate daily caloric requirements and notify the physician if the child's caloric intake is inadequate.

3. Child will maintain adequate intravascular volume. Provide volume resuscitation for hypovolemic shock.

4. Child will maintain normal electrolyte balance. Monitor serum electrolytes per physician order. Provide electrolyte replacement as needed.

5. Child will achieve a maximal level of comfort. Allow the parents to remain with the child. Provide pharmacologic intervention as appropriate. Use age-appropriate techniques for coping with pain.

G. Patient Care Management

1. Provide frequent vital sign monitoring with assessment for respiratory distress. Elevate the head of the bed 30 to 45 degrees to enhance respiratory effort. Prepare for intubation and ventilation if respiratory failure is evident.

2. Place an NG tube for gastric decompression and drainage.

3. Surgical intervention may be indicated for persistent abdominal pain, evidence of localized peritonitis (erythema over a portion of the abdomen) and presence of free air on abdominal x-ray examination.

H. Complications

Complications include decompensated shock, perforation, infarction, or death.

NECROTIZING ENTEROCOLITIS (NEC)

A. Etiology and Risk Factors (Roberts, 1991)

1. NEC is a disease of the newborn characterized by abdominal distention, bloody stools, and presence of gas in the wall of the intestine. NEC is primarily seen in premature infants following a hypoxic or hypoperfusion insult.

2. Prenatal risk factors include maternal infection, hypotension, and placental or cord problems. Perinatal risk factors include prematurity, meconium aspiration, and asphyxia. Postnatal risk factors include catheterization of the umbilical vessels, early feedings, hyperosmolar feedings, hypotension, shock, sepsis, and cold stress.

B. Pathophysiology

1. There appears to be three essential precipitating factors that act either individually or together to produce NEC (Israel, 1991): ischemic damage to the intestine, bacterial colonization of the intestine, and enteral feeding.

2. Bowel ischemia leads to injury and disruption of the intestinal mucosal epithelium. Bowel wall injury allows bacterial colonization and can lead to extensive tissue damage, including necrosis and ulceration.

3. The introduction of feeding produces hydrogen gas. Hydrogen gas penetrates the perforated intestinal wall, resulting in the diagnosis of free air on abdominal x-ray films. The entry of hydrogen gas into the submucosal tissue is called pneumatosis cystoides intestinalis.

C. Signs and Symptoms

1. Initially, symptoms of NEC are nonspecific and include unexplained apnea and bradycardia, hypoglycemia, electrolyte imbalance, lethargy, temperature instability, and poor feeding. The **classic triad** is abdominal distention, bilious vomiting, and blood in the stools with gastric residuals.

2. Signs of progressive NEC include discoloration of the abdominal wall, respiratory distress, hypotension, neutropenia, thrombocytopenia, and a WBC count reflecting a shift to the left.

3. Staging criteria are detailed in Table 7–7.

Table 7–7. STAGING CRITERIA FOR NECROTIZING ENTEROCOLITIS (NEC)

Stage 1 (Suspect)

a. History of perinatal stress

b. Systemic manifestations: Temperature instability, lethargy, apnea, bradycardia

c. GI tract manifestations: Poor feeding, increasing gastric residuals, emesis (may be bilious or have positive results for occult blood), mild abdominal distention, occult blood in stool

Stage 2 (Definite)

a. Above history and signs and symptoms plus persistent occult or gross GI tract bleeding

b. Marked abdominal distention

c. Abdominal radiographs show significant intestinal distention with ileus, small bowel separation, pneumatosis cystoides intestinalis

Stage 3 (Advanced)

a. Same signs and symptoms as in stage 2 plus deterioration in vital signs

b. Evidence of septic shock or marked GI tract hemorrhage

c. Abdominal radiographs show pneumoperitoneum

Modified from Bell MJ, Ternberg JL, Reign RD, et al. Neonatal necrotizing enterocolitis: therapeutic decisions based upon clinical staging. *Ann Surg.* 1978; 1:187.

D. **DIAGNOSTIC STUDIES**

Abdominal x-ray examination with a lateral view determines pneumatosis cystoides intestinalis, intestinal distention with multiple dilated loops of small bowel, and pneumoperitoneum if perforation has occurred.

E. **PATIENT CARE MANAGEMENT**

1. Infants are kept NPO with an NG tube to low intermittent suction for gastric decompression. Fluids and electrolytes are monitored, and TPN is provided. Umbilical artery or vein catheters are discontinued. Broad-spectrum antibiotic therapy is prescribed.

2. Respiratory and cardiac status is closely monitored with frequent monitoring of vital signs and abdominal girth.

3. Guaiac stool testing is used to detect occult bleeding. Serial platelet counts and serial abdominal x-ray examinations are used to monitor progression.

4. Surgery is indicated if signs of perforation, peritonitis, or clinical deterioration are evident.

F. **COMPLICATIONS**

Complications include short-gut syndrome, neurologic impairment, shock, or death.

HYPERBILIRUBINEMIA

A. **ETIOLOGY AND RISK FACTORS**

1. Bilirubin is the by-product of the heme portion of the breakdown of the hemoglobin molecule.

2. Hyperbilirubinemia is an elevated level of serum bilirubin. Indirect-prehepatic-unconjugated bilirubin elevations may be physiologic vs. pathologic. Direct-posthepatic-conjugated bilirubin elevations are always pathologic.

3. Premature neonates and infants with traumatic births and increased hemolysis are at higher risk for developing hyperbilirubinemia.

B. **PATHOPHYSIOLOGY**

1. Fat-soluble bilirubin binds to albumin as indirect (prehepatic-unconjugated) bilirubin for transport to the liver. In the liver, fat-soluble bilirubin is detached

from albumin and conjugated with glucuronic acid, rendering the bilirubin water soluble. Increases in indirect bilirubin result when the liver is not able to conjugate the bilirubin with impaired synthetic function.

2. Direct (posthepatic-conjugated) bilirubin is excreted into the hepatic ducts and eventually into the intestine. Impaired excretion of direct bilirubin into the bile ducts leads to increased levels of conjugated bilirubin as increased amounts are reabsorbed into the blood.

3. Impaired synthetic function and obstruction increase total bilirubin.

4. Three types of jaundice (prehepatic, hepatocellular, cholestatic) can occur. **Prehepatic** is usually caused by hemolysis. The total bilirubin is increased with the majority of the bilirubin in the indirect form. **Hepatocellular** jaundice results from liver dysfunction characterized by hepatic inflammation (infection, hepatitis, drug induced). The total bilirubin is increased. **Cholestatic** jaundice results from failure of biliary excretion. An increase in direct bilirubin is present.

C. SIGNS AND SYMPTOMS

Indirect, direct, and total bilirubin levels (Table 7–8) are elevated. Jaundice is an accumulation of yellow pigment in the skin and other tissues and is evident when total bilirubin is greater than 3 mg/dl. Kernicterus is the presence of yellow pigment in the basal ganglia of the brain. Dark-colored urine and pale-colored stool may occur.

D. NURSING AND COLLABORATIVE DIAGNOSIS
   ❖ POTENTIAL FOR ALTERED NEUROLOGIC STATUS RELATED TO KERNICTERUS

E. DESIRED PATIENT OUTCOME

Child's hyperbilirubinemia will resolve without long-term sequelae.

F. PATIENT CARE MANAGEMENT

1. Management of indirect hyperbilirubinemia includes phototherapy. As much skin surface as possible should be exposed. Cover eyes to protect from light and provide eye care every 4 hours. Fluid requirements are increased up to 20% because of increased insensible water losses. With excessive hyperbilirubinemia, exchange transfusion and pharmacologic interventions are required.

2. Management of direct hyperbilirubinemia depends on the etiology. (See the discussion under Hepatic Failure.)

G. COMPLICATIONS

Indirect hyperbilirubinemia can result in brain damage.

HEPATIC FAILURE

A. ETIOLOGY AND RISK FACTORS OF ACUTE HEPATIC FAILURE

1. **Hepatitis (inflammation of the liver)** is the most frequent cause of hepatic failure. Infectious causes include the following:
   a. Hepatitis A virus (HAV)
      • The incubation period is approximately 30 days.
      • Serologic markers for HAV include hepatitis A antibodies of the IgM class (anti-HAV IgM), whose presence reflects active HAV infection, and hepatitis A antibodies of the IgG class (anti-HAV IgG), whose presence reflects immunity.
      • Disease transmission is via the oral-fecal route. (Food, water, and shellfish contaminated by the virus are the usual sources.)
      • HAV is the most common form of viral hepatitis (Balisteri, 1988). One third of affected persons are children.

Table 7–8.   LIVER FUNCTION TESTS (LFTs)

LFT	FUNCTION	PEDIATRIC REFERENCE VALUE	CHANGES WITH HEPATIC FAILURE
Alanine ami-notransferase (ALT)	ALT catalyzes the reversible transfer of an amino group between the amino acid alanine and α-glutamic acid (Cella and Watson, 1989).	<37 IU/L	ALT initially increases with cell destruction. Following cell necrosis, enzyme level peaks and then decreases. It may be an ominous sign if the enzyme level peaks and falls rapidly. ALT is more hepatic specific as compared to AST. Isolated increases are characteristic of hepatitis.
Aspartate ami-notransferase (AST)	AST catalyzes the reversible transfer of the amino group between the amino acid aspartate and α-ketoglutamic acid (Cella and Watson, 1989).	<34 IU/L	AST initially increases with cell destruction. Following cell necrosis, enzyme level peaks and then decreases. It is an ominous sign if the enzyme level peaks and falls rapidly. Isolated increases are characteristic of hepatitis.
Alkaline phosphatase (ALP)	ALP cleaves phosphates from compounds with a single phosphate group. The hepatic isoenzymes are believed to be largely derived from the epithelium of the intrahepatic bile ducts, rather than from hepatocytes.	Newborn: <310 IU/L 1 mo–1 yr: <360 IU/L 1–10 y: <290 IU/L 10–15 y: <400 IU/L >15 y: <110 IU/L	ALP levels increase with inflammation or obstruction of the hepatobiliary tract.
γ-Glutamyl transpeptidase (GGTP)	GGTP is an isoenzyme of ALP. GGTP catalyzes the transfer of glutamyl groups among peptidase and amino acids (Johnson and McFarlane, 1989).	<120 IU/L	Hepatobiliary causes should be considered with increased levels. Significantly increased levels reflect hepatobiliary obstruction, whereas moderately elevated levels may suggest hepatocellular destruction.
Bilirubin	Bilirubin is a by-product of the heme portion of the breakdown of the hemoglobin molecule. Fat-soluble bilirubin binds to albumin as indirect bilirubin for transport to the liver.	Total bilirubin Newborn: 1–12 mg/dl Child: 0.2–1.3 mg/dl Direct: 0.1–1.3 mg/dl Indirect: 0.1–0.3 mg/dl	Increased indirect bilirubin levels occur as the liver is unable to conjugate the bilirubin with impaired synthetic function or in the presence of an excessive load of biliru-

Table 7–8.   LIVER FUNCTION TESTS (LFTs) *(Continued)*

LFT	FUNCTION	PEDIATRIC REFERENCE VALUE	CHANGES WITH HEPATIC FAILURE
	In the liver, fat-soluble bilirubin is detached from the albumin and conjugated with glucuronic acid, rendering it water soluble. Direct bilirubin is excreted into the hepatic ducts and eventually into the intestinal tract.		bin in cases of hemolysis. Impaired excretion of direct bilirubin into the bile ducts or biliary tract results in increased levels of direct bilirubin with increased amounts absorbed into the blood. Impaired synthetic function and obstruction increase total bilirubin levels.
Prothrombin time (PT)	PT is the laboratory measure of the time for a fibrin clot to form after tissue thromboplastin (factor III) and calcium are added to the sample. PT allows for clinical evaluation of the extrinsic clotting cascade.	10.5–13.5 s	A prolonged PT reflects poor utilization of vitamin K due to parenchymal disease or low levels of vitamin K due to obstructive jaundice. With clinical hepatic failure, the failure of the PT to respond after the administration of IV vitamin K reflects significant parenchymal injury.
Albumin	Albumin is the major circulating plasma protein responsible for maintaining plasma oncotic pressure. Albumin levels reflect a component of liver synthetic function.	3.8–5.4 g/d	The half-life of albumin is 21 d; therefore, hypoalbuminemia is present with chronic hepatic failure. Interpret with caution, as protein intake and albumin administration may alter the albumin level.
Ammonia	Ammonia is formed from the deamination of amino acids during protein metabolism and is a by-product of the breakdown of colonic bacteria proteins.	Newborn: 50–84 μg/dl Child: 12–38 μg/dl	Increased ammonia levels reflect decreased synthetic function. Elevated ammonia levels can occur in the presence of acute or chronic hepatic failure. Elevated ammonia levels may alter neurologic status.

Adapted from Martin SA, The ABCs of pediatric LFTs. *J Pediatr Nurs.* 1992;18(5):445–449.

    b. Hepatitis B virus (HBV)

- The incubation period is 4 weeks to 6 months with an average of 60 days (Gurevich, 1993).
- Synthetic hepatitis B vaccine is available and is part of the American Academy of Pediatrics recommended immunization schedule.
- Serologic markers of HBV include hepatitis B surface antigen (HbsAg), whose presence reflects acute or chronic infection; hepatitis B e antigen (HbeAg), whose presence reflects active HBV infection with active viral replication and high infectivity; and antibody to hepatitis B surface antigen (anti-HBs), whose presence reflects clinical recovery and immunity.
- Disease transmission occurs through the exchange of blood or body fluids. Neonates can acquire the virus via maternal transmission.
- Disease presentation varies. Fifty percent of cases are subclinical (Gurevich, 1993). Five to ten percent of patients develop chronic liver disease. Ninety percent of affected infants develop chronic hepatitis and a chronic carrier state (Balisteri, 1988). Eighty-five to ninety-five percent of affected persons recover (Gurevich, 1993). A small percentage (5% to 10%) of infected individuals develop fulminant hepatic failure (FHF).

    c. Hepatitis D virus (HDV)

- HDV is caused by an incomplete virus and requires the helper function of the HBV HbsAg for replication; therefore, only individuals infected with HBV can be HDV positive. HDV is directly cytopathic to the liver cells and tends to cause more severe hepatitis as compared to HBV.
- Serologic markers for HDV include antibody to HDV (anti-HDV), whose presence reflects exposure to the delta virus, and RNA of HDV (HDV RNA), whose presence reflects active transmission of HDV. Coinfection can be identified by simultaneous detection of antibody of the IgM class to the hepatitis B core antigen (anti-HBc IgM) plus HbsAg, which establishes acute HBV infection.

    d. Hepatitis C virus (HCV)

- HCV is one of approximately four non-A, non-B viruses. HCV is the cause of 20% of posttransfusion hepatitis (Gurevich, 1993). Twenty-five percent of those infected manifest symptoms of hepatitis (Gurevich, 1993).
- Serologic markers for HCV include HCV antibody testing (IgG, IgM, polymerase chain reaction [PCR] whose presence reflects the presence of antibodies of HCV).

    e. *Clinical presentation of hepatitis* involves three stages (Barnard and Hazinski, 1992).

- *Preicteric stage* has a duration of approximately 1 week. Signs and symptoms include fever, chills, anorexia, malaise, abdominal pain, nausea, vomiting, joint pain, hepatomegaly, and lymphadenopathy. HAV is characterized by nonspecific features of viral illness including fever, headache, anorexia, and nausea. HBV is characterized by urticaria, arthralgia, and arthritis preceding the full-blown illness (Balisteri, 1988).
- *Icteric stage* has a duration of 2 to 6 weeks. Signs and symptoms include weakness, fatigue, pallor, jaundice, dark urine, pale-colored stool, pruritus, and palmar erythema.
- During the *posticteric stage,* there is resolution of the jaundice, darkening of the stools, and normalization of LFT values. Complete recovery occurs in most cases.

    f. *Other viral causes* include herpes simplex virus, Epstein-Barr virus, adenovirus, and cytomegalovirus (which may be congenitally acquired). Infants are at risk if the mother is infected with a primary infection and active infection is present at birth.

2. **Neonatal "giant cell" hepatitis** represents a histologic descriptive term. The disease is characterized by large cells with many nuclei. The cause is unknown.

3. **Drug-induced acute hepatic failure**
   a. The liver is the most common site for drug metabolism. Children receiving drugs known to be hepatotoxic should have serial LFT monitoring while receiving therapy. The risk of developing FHF increases with continued use of the drug in the presence of developing hepatitis.
   b. The most common toxic drugs are acetaminophen (Tylenol), anticonvulsants (phenytoin [Dilantin] and valproate [Depakene]), halothane, and isoniazid (INH).

4. **Reye's syndrome** is a multisystem disease characterized by severe encephalopathy, with fatty changes to the viscera (particularly the liver). The disorder is associated with viral illnesses treated with aspirin.

B. **ETIOLOGY OF CHRONIC HEPATIC FAILURE**

1. The difference between acute and chronic disease presentation relates to the rate of parenchymal (organ-specific tissue) injury. Fibrosis leads to cirrhosis with development of portal hypertension evidenced by the presence of hepatosplenomegaly, varices, and ascites.

2. The majority of children have a chronic presentation of hepatic failure vs. an acute presentation. (See the chronic disease categories in the Liver Transplantation discussion.)

C. **PATHOPHYSIOLOGY OF ACUTE HEPATIC FAILURE**

1. **Pathophysiology** of acute hepatic failure is presumed to be multifactorial. Portal-systemic shunting (caused by progressive liver destruction) allows blood flow from the intestine to be shunted around the liver, bypassing any remaining viable hepatocytes. The liver is unable to remove toxic metabolites normally formed by intestinal bacteria's degradation of proteins, amino acids, and blood (e.g., ammonia). Altered blood-brain permeability is hypothesized to be related to toxin(s) of intestinal origin bypassing the portal filtration, resulting in a disruption of the blood-brain barrier.

2. **Fulminant hepatic failure (FHF)** is diagnosed in children who develop signs of encephalopathy within 8 weeks of the onset of liver disease and in whom there is no evidence of previous liver dysfunction. Multiple organ or system failure occurs.

3. **Neurologic pathophysiology:** Four hypotheses (Treem, 1991) exist to attempt to explain the encephalopathy that occurs.
   a. *Ammonia accumulation hypothesis:* Encephalopathy caused by ammonia accumulation from intestinal bacteria, dietary protein, and GI tract bleeding)
   b. *Synergistic neurotoxin hypothesis:* Excessive production of serotonin and dopamine (neurotransmitters that mediate the postsynaptic action of neurons) and a deficient synthesis of norepinephrine and dopamine
   c. *False neurotransmitter hypothesis:* Excessive production of brain inhibitory neurotransmitter (serotonin) and false neurotransmitter (octopamine) and deficiency of norepinephrine and dopamine
   d. *γ-Aminobutyric acid (GABA-ergic) inhibitor neurotransmitter hypothesis:* Increased GABA-ergic and glycinergic transmission, which are principal inhibitory neurotransmittors

4. **Renal pathophysiology**
   a. More than one type of renal failure may be present. Careful differentiation of the type of renal failure must be made before appropriate therapy can be initiated.

       b. Prerenal azotemia occurs when prerenal blood flow and renal perfusion are compromised. Treatment includes addressing the cause of decreased renal perfusion (e.g., fluid resuscitation).

       c. Acute tubular necrosis is related to parenchymal damage to the kidney related to a chronic prerenal condition or postrenal condition (e.g., toxic chemical exposure or glomerulonephritis). It may occur with concomitant sepsis, hemorrhage, and ischemia.

       d. Hepatorenal syndrome (functional renal failure of liver disease) is likely to be related to an unidentified substance causing oliguric renal failure in the presence of hepatic failure. Renal failure resolves with improvement of the hepatic dysfunction; however, the associated mortality is high.

  5. **Hematologic pathophysiology**

       a. Coagulopathy is related to an abnormal production of prothrombin and other clotting factors produced by the liver and ineffective removal of activated clotting factors.

       b. Hypersplenism results from increased portal venous pressure's delaying the blood flow through the splanchnic bed with resultant congestion and enlargement of the spleen. Splenic overactivity increases destruction of red blood cells (RBCs), platelets, and WBCs. The sequelae of splenomegaly include anemia, thrombocytopenia, leukopenia, and DIC.

D. Signs and Symptoms of Acute Hepatic Failure

  1. **Staging of hepatic encephalopathy**

       a. Stage I: Normal level of consciousness, periods of lethargy and euphoria

       b. Stage II: Disorientation, increased drowsiness, and agitation with mood swings

       c. Stage III: Marked confusion, sleeping most of the time

       d. Stage IV: Coma

  2. **Jaundice:** Yellow discoloration of the skin, mucous membranes, and sclera is caused by excessive bilirubin levels.

  3. **Renal failure** symptoms are dependent on the type of renal failure the child is experiencing. Azotemia should be evaluated carefully in the presence of hepatic failure, as nitrogenous wastes cannot be metabolized appropriately. Increased serum creatinine levels and oliguria are present.

  4. **Coagulopathy** is recognized by an elevated PT. A PT that is uncorrectable despite IV vitamin K (AquaMephyton) administration reflects significant parenchymal disease. Other signs include bruising and bleeding from mucosal surfaces.

E. Signs and Symptoms of Chronic Hepatic Failure

  1. **Hepatosplenomegaly:** The liver becomes firm and enlarged with regeneration, and the spleen becomes enlarged due to vascular engorgement. An enlarged spleen and liver, bruising, and petechiae are noted.

  2. **Varices:** With intrahepatic fibrosis there is obstruction of blood flow with formation of collaterals in the esophagus and rectum. These veins are thin walled and prone to the development of varicosities (e.g., rectal, esophageal) and GI tract bleeding.

  3. **Ascites** is related to the accumulation of fluid in the abdomen related to altered plasma oncotic pressure (decreased albumin production) and increased portal venous pressure. Increased abdominal girth, positive fluid wave, and respiratory distress are noted.

  4. **Malnutrition** is evident because of inadequate bile salts and the child's inability to absorb fat-soluble vitamins (A, D, E, and K). Poor weight gain and deficiencies of vitamin A (causing atrophy of the epithelial tissue and night blindness when severe), vitamin D (causing rickets), vitamin E (causing muscle degen-

eration, megaloblastic anemia, hemolytic anemia, creatinuria, target cell anemia, spur cell anemia, and peripheral neuropathology), and vitamin K (causing hypoprothrombinemia resulting in coagulopathy) are noted. Adequate glucose is necessary to maintain normal blood glucose levels.

5. **Pruritus** is related to bile salt deposition on the epidermis. Constant itching can be accompanied with skin breakdown.
6. **Asterixis:** "Liver flap" is a flapping tremor of the hand noted when both arms are raised with forearms fixed and the hands dorsiflexed.
7. **Fetor hepaticus** is a fecal breath that is intestinal in origin.
8. **Rickets** are caused by an abnormal bone formation related to a deficiency of vitamin D, calcium, and phosphorus. Pathologic fractures and bone malformations result.
9. **Telangiectasis** (vascular spiders, spider angiomas, spider nevi) are skin lesions consisting of a central arteriole from which smaller vessels radiate. Spontaneous bleeding from lesions can occur.
10. **Xanthomas** are fatty nodules that develop in the subcutaneous skin layer due to the accumulation of cholesterol.

F. INVASIVE AND NONINVASIVE DIAGNOSTIC STUDIES
Comprehensive blood chemistries, hematology and coagulation studies, ultrasound, CT scan, liver biopsy, endoscopy, and LFTs (see Table 7–8) may be useful in the determination of pathology as described above.

G. NURSING AND COLLABORATIVE DIAGNOSES
❖ POTENTIAL FOR ALTERED THOUGHT PROCESSES AND CEREBRAL PERFUSION RELATED TO HEPATIC ENCEPHALOPATHY WITH RESULTANT INCREASED INTRACRANIAL PRESSURE (ICP)
❖ POTENTIAL FOR ALTERATION IN FLUID AND ELECTROLYTE STATUS RELATED TO ACUTE TUBULAR NECROSIS, PRERENAL AZOTEMIA, AND HEPATORENAL SYNDROME
❖ POTENTIAL FOR BLEEDING AND GI TRACT BLEEDING RELATED TO COAGULOPATHY, PORTAL HYPERTENSION, AND THE PRESENCE OF VARICES
❖ POTENTIAL FOR ALTERED NUTRITIONAL STATUS, LESS THAN BODY REQUIREMENTS RELATED TO ALTERED FAT, PROTEIN, AND CARBOHYDRATE METABOLISM

H. PATIENT CARE MANAGEMENT
1. **Management of encephalopathy**
   a. Monitor for signs of increased ICP or neurologic dysfunction. Placement of an ICP monitoring device may be contraindicated in the presence of coagulopathy. Provide intubation when appropriate for airway control and hyperventilation.
   b. Intervene to decrease serum ammonia with administration of neomycin to decrease GI tract ammonia formation and lactulose (Cephulac) to acidify colonic flora and promote ammonia elimination. Restrict dietary protein.
2. **Management of hepatorenal syndrome:** Monitor fluid and electrolyte status and correct electrolyte imbalances. Dialysis may be indicated (hemodialysis or continuous venovenous hemofiltration).
3. **Management of coagulopathy:** Administration of blood products (FFP by bolus or continuous infusion, platelets, packed RBCs), IV vitamin K (AquaMephyton) therapy, and plasmapheresis may be required.
4. **Management of portal hypertension**
   a. Variceal bleeding is treated with pharmaceutic agents (e.g., vasopressin [Pitressin], somatostatin, and propranolol [Inderal]), injection of a sclerosing agent into or around varices, the Sengstaken-Blakemore tube (see Fig. 7–2 and Acute GI Tract Hemorrhage section), a portal-systemic shunt (see Fig. 7–3), or any combination of the above.
   b. Central shunts (portacaval shunt) are created by anastomosis of the portal vein to the inferior vena cava. Distal splenorenal shunts are created by

anastomosis of the splenic vein to the left renal vein. (For a description of the TIPS procedure, see the Acute GI Tract Hemorrhage section.) Complications of shunting procedures include thrombosis of the anastomotic vessel, elevated ammonia levels, peptic ulcers, aggravated hepatic failure, and ascites.

5. **Management of hepatosplenomegaly:** A spleen guard is a custom-fitted plastic device to cover and protect the liver. Children must avoid contact sports.

6. **Management of ascites:** Sodium restriction and diuretic therapy (IV furosemide [Lasix] or bumetanide [Bumex]) can help to control fluids. Paracentesis may be used when respiratory compromise occurs. It may precipitate fluid shifts. Complications include infection and hemorrhage.

I. COMPLICATIONS

Complications of acute hepatic failure include encephalopathy, cerebral edema (major cause of mortality for children with FHF), hepatorenal syndrome, and coagulopathies resulting in GI tract, cerebral, and pulmonary hemorrhage. Associated mortality for children is as high as 70% to 90% (Psacharopoulos et al, 1980; Vickers et al, 1988).

LIVER TRANSPLANTATION

A. ETIOLOGIES AND RISK FACTORS

1. **Biliary atresia** is the most common indication for pediatric liver transplantation. The incidence is 1 per 10,000 to 20,000 births (MacDonald, 1991). Biliary atresia is a congenital defect of unknown cause that involves the absence or obstruction of the intrahepatic and extrahepatic ducts of the biliary system. With the development of fibrosis, bile flow is obstructed. Progressive disease with resultant fibrosis and eventual cirrhosis occurs.

2. **Metabolic diseases**

   a. Alpha-1 antitrypsin (α_1AT) deficiency is transmitted via an autosomal codominant trait. Only 5% to 20% of α_1AT–deficient children develop liver disease. The disorder involves a deficiency of α_1AT, which is a polymorphic glycoprotein synthesized by the liver. The enzyme is the principal inhibitor of destructive enzymes such as leukocyte elastase, which cleaves connective tissue (Balisteri, 1990). The enzyme is trapped within hepatocytes causing liver damage. Liver dysfunction is usually evident as cholestasis during the neonatal period and cirrhosis develops in later childhood. Children with α_1AT deficiency have an increased risk for developing hepatocellular carcinoma (Whitington, 1990).

   b. Tyrosinemia is an autosomal recessive trait that results in the deficiency of fumarylacetoacetate hydrolase (FAH) activity. Children with tyrosinemia have an increased risk for developing hepatocellular carcinoma (Whitington, 1990).

   c. Wilson's disease is an autosomal recessive disorder that results in excessive accumulation of copper in the organs. The biochemical defect is not known (Pleskow and Grand, 1991). Liver dysfunction manifestations are variable and the child may present with FHF. Medical therapy includes administration of D-penicillamine and dietary restrictions of copper. Liver transplantation is indicated in the presence of FHF or cirrhosis with decompensation or progression of liver disease.

3. **Intrahepatic cholestasis**

   a. Progressive familial intrahepatic cholestasis (PFIC) is of probable autosomal recessive inheritance. It is characterized by paucity (few) of bile duct development. Symptoms usually develop before 6 months of age with severe pruritus and moderate jaundice (Whitington et al, 1994). Effective treatment includes surgical biliary diversion and liver transplantation.

   b. Alagille syndrome (arteriohepatic dysplasia) is an autosomal dominant trait (Alagille et al, 1987). The syndrome's characteristics include a broad forehead, indented chin, vertebral defects, pulmonary artery stenosis, and congenital heart disease. Cholestasis may resolve in infancy with recurrence in childhood.

4. **Metastatic disease**
   a. Hepatoblastoma usually occurs as a single-mass lesion composed of epithelial cells or a mixture of epithelial and mesenchymal components. Seventy-five percent occur before age 3 years. The abdomen enlarges with the presence of an abdominal mass.
   b. Hepatocellular carcinoma is a highly malignant tumor, characterized by anaplastic hepatocytes. It has a peak incidence in infancy, with another peak between the ages of 10 and 15 years. Signs and symptoms include abdominal swelling with associated pain and discomfort, fever, nausea, vomiting, weight loss, lethargy, and jaundice.

B. CONTRAINDICATIONS TO TRANSPLANTATION
There are no absolute contraindications to liver transplantation. The presence of metastatic disease or sepsis are relative contraindications.

C. PRETRANSPLANT CONSIDERATIONS
Pretransplant considerations involve a medical workup including a thorough history and examination, laboratory tests, assessment for evidence of portal hypertension, and assessment of portal vein patency. Family preparation and education are extensive.

D. NURSING AND COLLABORATIVE DIAGNOSES
   ❖ AIRWAY CLEARANCE: INEFFECTIVE RELATED TO THE LENGTHY ABDOMINAL PROCEDURE, LARGE TRANSVERSE ABDOMINAL INCISION, AND POSTOPERATIVE PAIN
   ❖ IMPAIRED GAS EXCHANGE: POTENTIAL RELATED TO POSTSURGICAL ATELECTASIS (FORTY PERCENT OF CHILDREN EXPERIENCE COLLAPSE OF THE RIGHT UPPER AND MIDDLE LOBES [SHAW ET AL, 1988].)
   ❖ ALTERED BREATHING PATTERNS: RELATED TO ASCITES, LARGE DONOR ORGAN, BLEEDING, AND PHRENIC NERVE PARESIS
   ❖ POTENTIAL FOR HEMODYNAMIC INSTABILITY RELATED TO HYPERTENSION ASSOCIATED WITH THE USE OF IMMUNOSUPPRESSIVE AGENTS OR HYPOTENSION ASSOCIATED WITH GRAFT DYSFUNCTION OR SURGICAL BLEEDING
   ❖ POTENTIAL FOR VESSEL THROMBOSIS RELATED TO SMALL VESSEL SIZE

E. DESIRED PATIENT OUTCOMES
   1. Child will be extubated after recovering from anesthesia.
   2. The child will not experience hemodynamic instability (hypertension or hypotension).
   3. All existing coagulopathies will resolve in the immediate postoperative period.
   4. All vascular anastomoses (portal vein, hepatic artery, and caval anastomoses) will remain patent.

F. PATIENT CARE MANAGEMENT
   1. Promote pulmonary toilet. After resolution of the existing coagulopathies, initiate chest physiotherapy. Evaluate diaphragm function with an ultrasound if the child fails extubation twice.
   2. Treat hypertension with antihypertensives. The first-line drug in the immediate postoperative period is sodium nitroprusside. The second line of treatment is often sublingual nifedipine (Procardia) when necessary.
   3. Monitor Jackson-Pratt drainage. Bloody drainage greater than 30 ml/kg/h may indicate surgical bleeding.
   4. Avoid rapid correction of coagulopathies. Hematocrit is maintained at approxi-

mately 30%. Subclinical anticoagulation is used for vessel thrombosis prophylaxis and is initiated when the PT is less than 17 seconds. Aspirin decreases platelet aggregation. Dipyridamole (Persantine) is a platelet adhesion inhibitor. Dextran decreases blood viscosity and platelet adhesiveness. Heparin is used as a prophylactic anticoagulant.

5. Other commonly used medications include immunosuppressive therapy (see Pharmacology section) and drugs for infection prophylaxis. Broad-spectrum IV antibiotics are given for the first 48 hours. If the patient is afebrile, the antibiotics are then discontinued. Co-trimoxazole (Bactrim) is prescribed indefinitely for *Pneumocystis carinii* prophylaxis. Nystatin (Mycostatin) is an antifungal agent used for thrush prophylaxis while steroids are prescribed. Ganciclovir (Cytovene) is administered intravenously for 14 days for cytomegalovirus and Epstein-Barr virus prophylaxis.

G. **COMPLICATIONS**

1. **Rejection**
   a. Signs and symptoms include fever, RUQ tenderness, lethargy, light-colored stools, dark-colored urine, and elevated LFT values (see Table 7–8).
   b. Liver biopsy is used for definitive diagnosis. Before the biopsy, check platelet count and PT. Ultrasound marking is used when necessary (e.g., may be done in the presence of abnormal anatomic findings, as in the presence of a reduced-size graft following liver transplantation). Monitoring for complications of the biopsy includes frequent vital signs for the assessment of hemorrhage, chest x-ray examination to rule out pneumothorax, and serial hematocrit measurements.
   c. Treatment is augmentation of the child's immunosuppression.

2. **Infection** is the leading cause of morbidity and mortality following transplantation. Causes include bacterial, viral, and fungal infections (Green and Michaels, 1996).
   a. Bacterial infections occur most often within the first 30 days. Common causes include preexisting disease conditions, central lines, surgical intervention, and posttransplantation factors including transfusion requirements and dosing of immunosuppressive agents. Treatment is antibiotic therapy.
   b. Viral infections usually occur from 31 to 180 days following transplantation. Primary infections occur when the patient becomes infected with a virus with no previous exposure. Secondary infection involves the reactivation of a latent virus. Recovery from a secondary infection is usually easier than recovery from a primary infection. Common organisms include cytomegalovirus and Epstein-Barr virus. Treatment is antiviral therapy. Acyclovir (Zovirax) inhibits viral DNA synthesis of the herpesviruses. Dosing is 500 mg/m^2 per dose q8h. Side effects include impaired renal function. Ganciclovir (Cytovene) inhibits DNA polymerase. Dosing is 5 mg/kg per dose q12h. Side effects include impaired renal function, neutropenia, thrombocytopenia, confusion, and nausea.

3. **Lymphoproliferative disease (LPD) and Epstein-Barr infection:** LPD is characterized by the development of continually proliferating B lymphocytes, presumably stimulated under the influence of the Epstein-Barr virus. LPD is diagnosed by clinical, laboratory, and pathologic examination. Tissue biopsy with histologic evidence is necessary to confirm the diagnosis. Treatment involves reducing or discontinuing the child's immunosuppression and initiating antiviral therapy.

REFERENCES

Alagille D, Estrada A, Hadchouel M, Gautier M, Odièvre M, Dommergues JP. Syndromic paucity of interlobular bile ducts (Alagille syndrome or arteriohepatic dysplasia): review of 80 cases. *J Pediatr.* 1987;110:195–200.

Balisteri WF. Liver disease associated with alpha-1 antitrypsin deficiency. In: Balisteri WF, Stocker JT, eds. *Pediatric Hepatology.* New York, NY: Hemisphere Publishing Co; 1990:159–181.

Balisteri WF. Viral hepatitis. *Pediatr Clin North Am.* 1988;35(2):375–405.

Barnard JA, Hazinski MF. Pediatric gastrointestinal disorders. In: Hazinski MF, ed. *Nursing Care of the Critically Ill Child.* St Louis, Mo: The CV Mosby Co; 1992:715–801.

Bell MJ, Ternberg JL, Feign RD, et al. Neonatal necrotizing enterocolitis: therapeutic decisions based upon clinical staging. *Ann Surg.* 1978;1:187.

Berry R, Perrault J. Gastrointestinal bleeding. In: Walker AW, Durie PR, Hamilton JR, Walker-Smith JA, Watkins JB, eds. *Pediatric Gastrointestinal Disease: Pathophysiology, Diagnosis, Management.* Philadelphia, Pa: BC Decker Inc; 1996:323–342.

Buntain WL. *Management of Pediatric Trauma.* Philadelphia, Pa: WB Saunders Co; 1995.

Cella JH, Watson J. Blood chemistry. In: *Nurses' Manual of Laboratory Tests.* Philadelphia, Pa: FA Davis Co; 1989:130–288.

Foltin GL, Cooper A. Abdominal trauma. In: Barkin RM, Asch SM, Caputo GL, et al, eds. *Pediatric Emergency Medicine.* St Louis, Mo: The CV Mosby Co; 1992:276–292.

Goff JS. Gastroesophageal varices: pathogenesis and therapy of acute bleeding. *Gastroenterol Clin North Am.* 1993;22(4):779–799.

Green M, Michaels MG. Infections in solid-organ transplant recipients. In: Long SS, Pickering LK, Prober CG, eds. *Principles and Practices of Pediatric Infectious Diseases.* New York, NY: Churchill Livingstone, Inc; 1996:626–633.

Gurevich I. Hepatitis part II: viral hepatitis, B, C, and D. *Heart Lung.* 1993;22(5):450–458.

Hazinski MF. Children are different. In: Hazinski MF, ed. *Nursing Care of the Critically Ill Child.* St Louis, Mo: The CV Mosby Co; 1992:1–17.

Huether SE. Structure and function of the digestive system. In: McCance KL, Huether SE, eds. *Pathophysiology: The Biological Basis for Disease in Adults and Children.* 2nd ed. St Louis, Mo: The CV Mosby Co; 1994.

Hyams JS, Leichtner AM, Schwartz AN. Recent advances in diagnosis and treatment of gastrointestinal hemorrhage in infants and children. *J Pediatr.* 1985;106(1):1–7.

Israel EJ. NEC. In: Walker WA, Durie PR, Hamilton JR, Walker-Smith JA, Watkins JB, eds. *Pediatric Gastrointestinal Disease: Pathophysiology, Diagnosis, Management.* Philadelphia, Pa: BC Decker Inc; 1991;1: 639–649.

Johnson PJ, McFarlane IG. The standard of liver function tests. In: *The Laboratory Investigation of Liver Disease.* Philadelphia, Pa: WB Saunders Co; 1989:11–47.

Kocoshis SA. Disorders and diseases of the gastrointestinal tract and liver. In: Furman BF, Zimmerman JJ, eds. *Pediatric Critical Care.* St Louis, Mo: Mosby–Year Book Inc; 1992:867–879.

Kucharski SA. Fulminant hepatic failure. *Crit Care Nurs Clin North Am.* 1993;5(1):141–151.

MacDonald CA. Biliary atresia. *J Pediatr Nurs.* 1991;6:374–383.

Mader TJ, McHugh TP. Acute pancreatitis in children. *Pediatr Emerg Care.* 1992;8(3):157–161.

Marsh JW, Vehe KL, White HM. Immunosuppressants. *Gastroenterol Clin North Am.* 1992;21(3):679–692.

Martin SA. The ABCs of pediatric LFTs. *J Pediatr Nurs.* 1992; 18(5):445–449.

Moloney-Harmon PA. Initial assessment and stabilization of the critically injured child. *Crit Care Nurse Clin North Am.* 1991;3(3):399–409.

Moore EE, Shackford SR, Pachter HL, et al. Organ injury scaling: spleen, liver, and kidney. *J Trauma.* 1989;29(12):1664–1666.

Motil KJ. Development of the gastrointestinal tract. In: Wyllie R, Hymans JS, eds. *Pediatric Gastrointestinal Disease: Pathophysiology, Diagnosis and Management.* Philadelphia, Pa: WB Saunders Co; 1993:3–16.

Pleskow RG, Grand RJ. Wilson's disease. In: Walker WA, Durie PR, Hamilton JR, Walker-Smith JA, Watkins JB, eds. *Pediatric Gastrointestinal Disease: Pathophysiology, Diagnosis, Management.* Philadelphia, Pa: BC Decker Inc; 1991;2:1014–1024.

Psacharopoulos HT, Mowat AP, Davies M, Portmann B, Silk DBA, Williams R. Fulminant hepatic failure in childhood: an analysis of 31 cases. *Arch Dis Child.* 1980;55:252–258.

Roberts P. Neonatal necrotizing enterocolitis: etiology, treatment, prevention, and nursing care. *Crit Care Nurs* 1991;10(4):38–53.

Schafermeyer R. Pediatric trauma. *Emerg Med Clin North Am.* 1993;11(1):187–205.

Shaw BW, Wood RP, Kaufman SS, et al. Liver transplantation therapy in children: part II. *J Pediatr Gastroenterol Nutr.* 1988;7:797–815.

Torres AM, Garcia VF. Hepatobiliary trauma. In: Eichelberger MR. *Pediatric Trauma: Prevention, Acute Care, Rehabilitation.* St Louis, Mo: The CV Mosby Co; 1993.

Treem WR. Hepatic failure. In: Walker WA, Durie PR, Hamilton JR, Walker-Smith JA, Watkins JB, eds. *Pediatric Gastrointestinal Disease: Pathophysiology, Diagnosis, Management.* Philadelphia, Pa: BC Decker Inc; 1991;1: 141–161.

Vickers C, Neuberger J, Buckels J, McMaster P, Elias E. Transplantation of the liver in adults and children with fulminant hepatic failure. *J Hepatol.* 1988;7:143–150.

Vinton NE. Gastrointestinal bleeding in infancy and childhood. *Gastroenterol Clin North Am.* 1994:93–122.

Whitington PF. Advances in pediatric transplantation. In: Barnes LA, ed. *Advances in Pediatrics.* St Louis, Mo: The CV Mosby Co; 1990:357–389.

Whitington PF, Freese DK, Alonso EM, Schwarzenberg SJ, Sharp HL. Clinical and biochemical findings in progressive familial intrahepatic cholestasis. *J Pediatr Gastroenterol Nutr.* 1994;18(2):134–141.

Hematology and Immunology

LINDA L. OAKES and CATHY ROSENTHAL-DICHTER

8

DEVELOPMENTAL ANATOMY AND PHYSIOLOGY

A. HEMATOPOIESIS

Hematopoiesis is the process by which blood cells are formed.

1. Sites for the hematopoietic process vary with age.
   a. During embryonic and fetal life, there are several sites for blood cell production including the yolk sac, liver, spleen, thymus, lymph nodes, and bone marrow (Tortora and Grabowski, 1993).
   b. After birth, hematopoiesis takes place in the red bone marrow of all bones. During the first 5 years of life, many bones containing red marrow are employed including the proximal epiphyses of long bones (e.g., humerus, tibia, femur), fat bones (e.g., sternum, ribs, cranium), and the vertebrae and pelvis. After 5 years of age, involvement of the shafts of long bones is reduced, since these sites become progressively fatty while other sites predominate (Leonard, 1989).
2. Pluripotential hematopoietic stem cells give rise to many differentiated blood cells but also replenish themselves (Tortora and Grabowski, 1993). Stem cells, also called colony-forming units, predominantly reside in the bone marrow and reproduce throughout life but decrease in numbers with age (Guyton, 1986). Stem cells are not committed to a specific cell line and therefore are referred to as pluripotential stem cells. They eventually develop a commitment to a specific cell line (referred to as unipotential stem cells) with the capability of forming only a particular type of cell, such as red blood cell (RBC) or white blood cell (WBC; Guyton, 1986).
3. Five types of cells arise from the stem cell. Each of these cells end with "-blast," which refers to a nucleated precursor cell (Tortora and Grabowski, 1993). Proerythroblasts form the mature erythrocyte (RBCs). Myeloblasts form the mature neutrophils, eosinophils, and basophils (a type of WBC). Monoblasts form the mature monocytes (a type of WBC). Lymphoblasts form the mature lymphocytes (a type of WBC). Megakaryoblasts form the mature thrombocytes (platelets) (Fig. 8–1).
4. Development of the pluripotential stem cell into a mature hematopoietic cell (RBC, WBC, or platelet) occurs in approximately 1 to 2 weeks.
5. Differentiation and proliferation of committed cells is stimulated by various hematopoietic growth factors. Erythropoietin (EPO) stimulates the production of erythrocyte precursors. Thrombopoietin stimulates the production of thrombocytes (platelets). Cytokines, such as colony-stimulating factors

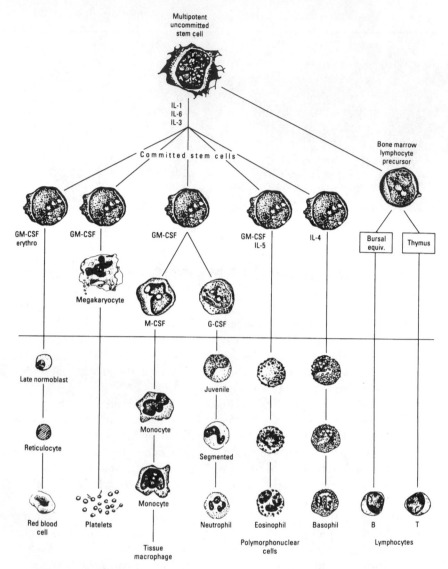

Multipotent
uncommitted
stem cell

IL-1
IL-6
IL-3

Committed stem cells

Bone marrow
lymphocyte
precursor

GM-CSF
erythro

GM-CSF

GM-CSF

GM-CSF
IL-5

IL-4

Bursal
equiv.

Thymus

Megakaryocyte

M-CSF

G-CSF

Late normoblast

Monocyte

Juvenile

Reticulocyte

Segmented

Monocyte

Red blood
cell

Platelets

Neutrophil

Eosinophil

Basophil

B

T

Tissue
macrophage

Polymorphonuclear
cells

Lymphocytes

Figure 8–1. Cell differentiation from stem cells. The process of hematopoiesis in which the most primitive cells differentiate and ultimately give rise to erythrocytes, granulocytes, thrombocytes, and macrophages. Colony-stimulating factors (CSFs) act on blood precursors to stimulate production of specific cell lineages, and the principal sites of action of these CSFs are indicated. Cells below the horizontal line are found in normal peripheral blood. *G,* granulocyte; *M,* macrophage; *IL,* interleukin. (From Ganong WF. Circulating body fluids. In: Ganong WF, ed. *Review of Medical Physiology.* 16th ed. Norwalk, Conn: Appleton & Lange; 1993:471.)

([CSFs]; e.g., granulocyte colony-stimulating factor [G-CSF]) and interleukins, stimulate the production of several different blood cell types.

6. Alterations in the development of blood cell lines include aplasia, where the bone marrow completely fails to develop stem cells, and hypoplasia, where the bone marrow develops an abnormally low number of stem cells.

7. Tissues or organs of the body involved in development of blood cells are classified according to the primary or secondary roles they play in the development of blood cells, particularly WBCs.

a. Primary lymphoid tissue or organs are those that participate in the development and maturation of lymphocytes.

• Bone marrow is the primary site of hematopoiesis and thought to be the site of maturation and differentiation of B lymphocytes. The storage site contains approximately 1 week's worth of developing RBCs and WBCs.

- The thymus is an encapsulated structure located in the anterior mediastinum directly behind the sternum. It is very large relative to body size at birth, reaches peak mass at prepuberty, and then shrinks throughout life. Its primary function is thought to be the maturation and differentiation of T lymphocytes. The thymus produces and secretes thymosin and other thymic hormones, influencing the formation of lymphocytes and the development and maturation of T lymphocytes.

b. Secondary lymphoid tissue or organs are sites for storage, division, and activation of mature lymphocytes.

- The spleen is a large vascular organ beneath the diaphragm, behind and to the left of the stomach, and is occasionally palpable in young healthy children. It is not essential for life, but performs many important functions. Hematopoiesis is active during fetal life and, later in life, may be recruited for severe anemia or skeletal marrow failure. The spleen is a temporary reservoir for platelets and to a lesser extent for WBCs. Immunologically it functions as an active site for defense mechanisms. The white pulp consists of lymphoid tissue that is primarily concerned with humoral immunity and B-lymphocyte function. Macrophages that line the sinuses filter the blood of foreign materials. B and T lymphocytes reside in splenic tissue. The red pulp consists of venous sinuses with reticuloendothelial cells that destroy and remove old and damaged erythrocytes. Target cells undergo antibody-mediated hemolysis or phagocytosis, as seen in some autoimmune hemolytic anemias.

  ○ The spleen modulates the course of numerous illnesses by being a mechanical filter and a site for early antibody production. After a splenectomy, patients are at increased risk of infection with encapsulated microorganisms and need prompt recognition and treatment of any fever to prevent the development of septic shock.

- The lymphatic system consists of fluid called lymph, which flows through a series of vessels (lymphatics), and several organs and structures that contain lymphatic tissue (Tortora and Grabowski, 1993). The functions of the lymphatic system are to drain excess interstitial fluid, transport dietary fats such as lipids and lipid-soluble vitamins, and protect against invasion by concentrating foreign substances in lymphatic organs and circulating lymphocytes through lymphatic organs.

  ○ Lymph is a pale yellow fluid that passes from the interstitial space to the lymphatic vessels (also called interstitial fluid if located in the interstitium). Lymph (in comparison with blood) (Jennings, 1991) contains WBCs, including lymphocytes, granulocytes, and humoral substances (antibodies) but is deficient in RBCs, platelets, and fibrinogen and therefore coagulates at a slow rate (Jennings, 1991). Lymph travels from lymphatic capillaries into lymphatic vessels and through lymph nodes. After passage through the most proximal lymph nodes, lymph is eventually carried either to the right lymphatic duct or to the thoracic duct. The thoracic duct is the main collecting duct of the lymphatic system, receiving lymph from the left side of the head, neck, and chest, the upper left extremity, and the entire body below the ribs. The right lymphatic duct drains lymph from the upper right side of the body, and the ducts drain lymph into the subclavian vein and into the systemic circulation.

  ○ Lymph nodes are oval or bean-shaped structures located along the length of the lymphatic vessels (Fig. 8–2). Distribution is scattered throughout the body and clustered in groups, both superficial and deep. Superficial nodes may be palpated, whereas deep nodes may be visualized on radiographic examination (Jennings, 1991). The parenchyma is specialized into two regions. The cortex is the outer region that contains densely packed lymphocytes arranged in masses, called follicles. The medulla is the inner region where macrophages, lymphocytes, and plasma cells are arranged into strands, referred to as medullary cords (Tortora and Grabowski, 1993). Functions are to filter bacteria and other foreign substances carried by lymph and to act as sites of lymphocyte distribution, production, and activation.

- Mucosa-associated lymphoid tissue (MALT) is a dispersed aggregate of lymphoid tissue located in areas to protect the body from microorganism invasion. MALT is located within or close to potential sites of invasion. Three types exist:
  - Skin: Skin-associated lymphoid tissue (SALT)
  - Respiratory: Bronchus-associated lymphoid tissue (BALT)

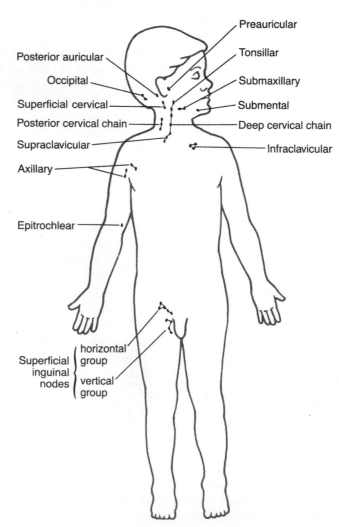

Figure 8–2.   Lymph nodes of the body. (From Betz CL, Hunsberger, MM, Wright S, eds. *Family-Centered Nursing Care of Children.* 2nd ed. Philadelphia, Pa: WB Saunders Co; 1994:474.)

        ○ Gastrointestinal (GI): Gut-associated lymphoid tissue (GALT; e.g., tonsils, Peyer's patches)

- The liver is a large organ located in the right upper quadrant of the abdomen. Liver reticuloendothelial functions are similar to the spleen but are performed by Kupffer's cells (stellate reticuloendothelial cells). The liver filters old and misshapen cells; however, it does so much less effectively than the spleen. The liver synthesizes amino acids, albumin, globulins, and most of the plasma clotting factors (Jennings, 1991) and clears RBC breakdown products.

B. RED BLOOD CELLS (ERYTHROCYTES)

1. The **proerythroblast,** the earliest identifiable precursor of the RBC, develops from a pluripotential stem cell.

2. **Reticulocytes,** precursors to RBCs (normally 1% to 2% in the peripheral blood), mature into erythrocytes (RBCs) within 24 to 48 hours of release into the blood stream. Reticulocytosis (increased numbers of reticulocytes in the blood), which occurs with increased bone marrow activity, usually indicates increased blood loss or hemolysis.

3. **Erythrocytes** are mature reticulocytes released into the circulation with a normal life span of 120 days; transfused RBCs have a shorter life span. The life span of RBCs is determined by their ability to get through narrow splenic passages. The innermost lining (stroma) of erythrocytes has a spongelike substance to which hemoglobin, an iron-containing protein, attaches. The outer membrane contains antigenic material that defines blood type: A or B. Absence of antigenic material results in blood group O.

4. **Hemoglobin synthesis**
   a. HbA is the normal hemoglobin.
   b. HbF, the major hemoglobin in the fetus, gradually decreases over the first year of life. HbF is able to transport oxygen when smaller amounts of oxygen are available because of its increased oxygen affinity. HbF is present in only minimal amounts in the child and adult; levels higher than 3% in a child older than 3 years of age are abnormal.
   c. HbS is the type of hemoglobin associated with sickle cell anemia.
   d. Thalassemias are associated with decreased production of globin chains (α or β).
   e. HbSC and HbSD are examples of HbS (a heterozygous condition with another abnormal hemoglobin).

5. **Production of RBCs:** Erythropoiesis
   a. Production is controlled by EPO, a hormone produced primarily in the kidney and also in the liver in small amounts. Production of RBCs also requires folic acid, iron, and vitamin B_{12}.
   b. Increased RBC production occurs with hypoxemia secondary to EPO release.
   c. Decreased RBC production occurs with chronic illnesses (such as infections or renal failure secondary to decreased EPO production), endocrine disorders, nutritional deficiencies, diseases of the bone marrow (e.g., cancer), and chemotherapy or radiation therapy.
   d. Anemia is a decrease in red cell mass or hemoglobin content below normal levels for age due to an increased loss or decreased production of RBCs. Anemia is not a disease but an indication of the presence of a disorder related to bleeding, lack of red cell production, or excessive red cell destruction (hemolysis). Anemia is measured as a decrease in hematocrit and hemoglobin; it is usually defined as a hemoglobin level below 11 g/dl (age related). Gradual losses can be compensated with few clinical signs and

symptoms until the hemoglobin falls to 8 g/dl. Aplastic anemia is associated with decreased RBCs, platelets, and WBCs. Peripheral blood also indicates a low reticulocyte count. Bone marrow tests reveal a markedly decreased hematopoietic activity, although the bone marrow architecture is normal and no other cells (such as leukemic cells) have replaced the normal marrow components.

6. **Hemolysis** involves the removal of normal and abnormal RBCs (misshapen, nonfunctional cells) either intravascularly or extravascularly.

   a. *Intravascular hemolysis* is relatively rare and occurs with acute blood transfusion reactions, prosthetic heart valve dysfunction, and heat stroke. Hemoglobin is released from the injured cells into the plasma. If the free hemoglobin cannot be cleared from the circulation by complexing to haptoglobin, hemoglobin is eliminated in the urine (hemoglobinuria). Accumulation of RBCs stroma in the renal vessels can lead to acute renal failure.

   b. *Extravascular hemolysis* is more common and represents removal of RBCs sequestered by the fixed phagocytes of the spleen and liver. The heme iron is recycled for further RBC production with only a small amount of the removed hemoglobin being released into the plasma. The level of unconjugated (indirect) bilirubin indicates the net effect of the rate of the hemolysis and the ability of the liver to process the bilirubin.

   c. *Anemia* occurs if the rate of hemolysis exceeds the production of RBCs. Hemolytic anemia is the term used for anemia that results from an increased rate of RBC destruction due to abnormalities of the red cell membrane, enzymes, or hemoglobin; antibody interactions with the red cell membrane; toxins or antibiotics; heat; or mechanical trauma. If the hemolytic anemia is chronic, hepatomegaly or splenomegaly may occur, as the liver and spleen hypertrophy to eliminate the increased numbers of damaged RBCs from the circulation.

C. WHITE BLOOD CELLS (LEUKOCYTES)

WBCs comprise a heterogeneous group of cells that mediate the inflammatory or immune response; WBCs are the mobile units of the immune system. Classification of leukocytes was first based on morphologic criteria and divided into granulocytes, mononuclear phagocytes, and lymphocytes.

1. **Granulocytes** (myeloid series) are referred to as polymorphonuclear neutrophil leukocytes (PMNs) because of the multilobular nucleus and abundant granules in their cytoplasm. Granulocytes (neutrophils, eosinophils, and basophils) are nonspecific in nature and have a critical role in engulfing and phagocytosing microorganisms.

   a. *Neutrophils* account for the largest component of total circulating WBCs, usually 60% to 70% (age related). Neutrophils are the most active in phagocytosis.

      • Neutrophils originate and mature in the bone marrow and can be found in the following locations:
         ○ Marginal pool: Neutrophils are temporarily sequestered in small vessels or adhered to the walls of large blood vessels.
         ○ Intravascular space: Neutrophils in the circulation and in the marginal pool are included in this category.
         ○ Tissues: Nearly twice as many neutrophils are found in the tissues as in the intravascular space.
         ○ Bone marrow: The adult bone marrow reserve is approximately 10 times the quantity of the neutrophils in the circulation and tissue and body cavities (Jennings, 1991). The infant and young child have

smaller bone marrow reserves of neutrophils and are less able to rapidly replenish these cells (Rosenthal, 1989).

- The mature form of the neutrophil is polymorphonucleated (PMNs or "poly") and segmented ("seg") reflecting the appearance of the nucleus. PMNs normally constitute the majority of the circulating neutrophils and are phagocytic and active in inflammation and tissue damage. PMNs are the first WBCs to respond to infection and the most numerous WBCs at the site of infection.
- The immature form of the neutrophil has an unsegmented appearing nucleus and is referred to as a "band." The immature form lacks complete phagocytic ability and normally constitutes less than 10% of the circulating neutrophils.
- Neutrophilia is an increased number of circulating neutrophils often accompanied by an increase in the number of immature neutrophils (bands). Neutrophilia is associated with situations that increase cardiac output (stress response associated with surgery, hemorrhage or emotional distress such as intense crying) or increase release of epinephrine, adrenocorticotropic hormone (ACTH), or adrenal corticosteroids. Neutrophilia is also associated with administration of CSFs (e.g., G-CSF).
- Neutropenia is a decreased number of circulating neutrophils ($<1500/$ mm^3); it is often associated with pathologic or malignant conditions.
- WBCs mature in the bone marrow for approximately 10 days. WBCs then are released into the circulation to be distributed to the marginal pool or the tissues. WBCs circulate in the blood for 4 to 8 hours and then circulate another 4 to 5 days in the tissues. The life span of WBCs is shortened in the presence of an infection.

b. Eosinophils normally account for 2% to 5% of the circulating WBC and have weak phagocytic activity. Eosinophils may have a role in "turning off" the immune response, since the eosinophil is the last to arrive at the site of infection. Cytoplasmic granules contain chemical substances that destroy parasitic worms and act on immune complexes involved in allergic responses.

- Eosinophilia is an increased number of eosinophils, greater than normally present. The eosinophil count may increase as high as 50% of the circulating WBC with parasitic infection and less often with allergic conditions (Jett and Lancaster, 1983). Eosinopenia is a decreased number of eosinophils, which is not clinically significant.
- From the bone marrow, eosinophils are released into the circulation and migrate to tissues. Unlike other granulocytes, eosinophils may recirculate back and forth between the circulation and the tissues.

c. Basophils represent the smallest proportion of granulocytes, accounting for less than 1% of circulating WBCs. Cytoplasmic granules contain chemical substances (e.g., histamine, heparin, and probably serotonin) that are released and participate in inflammation and allergic responses.

- Production and life span of the basophil is not thoroughly understood. Basophilia is an increased number of circulating basophils. Basopenia is a decreased number of circulating basophils, not clinically significant.

2. **Mononuclear phagocytes** (monocytes and macrophages)

a. Monocytes normally comprise 3% to 8% of circulating WBCs. Produced in the bone marrow and spending only a brief time in the circulation, most monocytes migrate into the tissues and differentiate into macrophages.

- Monocytosis, an increase in the number of circulating monocytes, is observed in patients with viral, parasitic, or rickettsial infections.

- Monocytopenia, a decrease in the number of circulating monocytes, is not clinically significant. It is sometimes seen with human immuno-deficiency virus (HIV) infection or in patients receiving prednisone therapy.

b. Macrophages usually are located in various body tissues. These cells are not quantified in the serum and have a long life span; some live for years. Macrophages commonly reside in a specific tissue, although a small percentage may wander. Examples of fixed macrophages include alveolar macrophage, Kupffer's cells in the liver, microglial cells of the brain, and spleen sinus macrophages. Macrophages play a primary role in *nonspecific* defenses through the ability to phagocytose. They are capable of phagocy-tosing larger and greater numbers of particles than the neutrophil or the monocyte. Macrophages also play a primary role in *specific* defense through processing and presentation of the antigen to the helper T cell.

3. **Lymphocytes** (lymphoid lineage) are the primary immune cells associated with humoral and cell-mediated immunity (CMI), although a small portion of lymphocytes (natural killer cells) are nonspecific in nature.

a. *Lymphocytes* account for 10% to 40% of the circulating WBCs. They are produced in the bone marrow and then migrate to other parts of the body to differentiate and mature into several distinct subsets. Cells that migrate to the thymus differentiate into T lymphocytes (T cells) and mediate CMI. Cells that migrate to the bursa equivalent in the human (thought to be the bone marrow) differentiate into B lymphocytes (B cells) and mediate humoral immunity (involving antibody production). A subset of lympho-cytes that is nonspecific in nature are the NK cells.

- Lymphocytosis, an increase in the number of circulating lymphocytes, is often noted in patients with viral infections (such as infectious mono-nucleosis or infectious hepatitis) or lymphocytic leukemia or lymphoma.
- Lymphopenia, a decrease in the number of circulating lymphocytes, is often noted in patients with congenital immunodeficiency, acquired immunodeficiency syndrome (AIDS), uremia, or following administra-tion of corticosteroids or ACTH.

b. *T lymphocytes, or T cells,* normally comprise 65% to 85% of all lymphocytes. T cells mediate CMI, which comprises a component of specific, acquired immunity and protects from infections with intracellular organisms, such as viruses, fungi, protozoa, and helminthic parasites. T cells are involved in the elimination of mutated or tumor cells and the immune response triggered during tissue graft or organ transplantation.

- Subsets of T lymphocytes have been identified through the identifica-tion of specialized molecules of the cell membrane surfaces, referred to as clusters of differentiation (CD). **Helper T cells** (CD4) send chemical signals (via lymphokines) to the cytotoxic T cells, macrophages, and NK cells. They have an important role in the activation of B cells. **Suppressor T cells** (CD8) send a signal to inhibit actions of B cells, helper T cells, and killer T cells. **Cytotoxic or killer T cells** (CD8) eliminate targets *directly* by chemical destruction and play a role in the rejection of tissue transplantation.

c. *B lymphocytes, or B cells,* normally comprise up to 35% of circulating lymphocytes. B cells mediate humoral immunity (HI) through transfor-mation into a plasma cell, which then secretes immunoglobulin. HI comprises a component of specific, acquired immunity and protects the host from bacterial infection and viral invasion.

d. *Natural killer (NK) cells* normally comprise 5% to 10% of the total lympho-cyte count. NK cells have neither B- nor T-cell markers and are referred to by many other names (non-B non-T cells, null cells). The target for the NK cell is the tumor cell or virally infected cell. The NK cells' cytotoxic abilities are nonspecific in nature, since they can destroy the target without prior sensitization.

e. *Memory cells* have cluster differentiation (CD) according to the various distinct cell types (helper, suppressor, or cytotoxic T cell or B cell). They are programmed to recognize the original invading microorganism on subsequent invasions. Memory cells initiate a secondary response and may result in elimination prior to any signs or symptoms of infection.

D. PLATELETS (THROMBOCYTES)

1. Megakaryoblasts mature into megakaryocytes.

   a. Megakaryocytes break into pieces (budding) forming platelets, which are released into the blood stream. It is unclear if EPO increases the production rate. Granulocyte-macrophage colony-stimulating factor (GM-CSF), stem cell factor, and interleukin-3 (IL-3) have been shown to stimulate the growth of megakaryocytes but are ineffective clinically. Thrombopoietin may be effective but is unavailable for clinical use in humans at this time.

   b. Two thirds of mature platelets circulate in the blood stream, and one third are stored in the spleen but released if needed to maintain hemostasis. The life span of platelets produced in vivo is 7 to 10 days; transfused platelets have a shorter life span, usually 3 to 4 days. Thrombocytes usually are removed by the spleen or incorporated into a clot.

2. **Characteristics:** Thrombocytes are minute, round or oval discs. Platelet performance depends on the quantity of platelets (platelet count: 150,000 to 400,000/mm^3) and the quality of function. Adhesiveness is stickiness, the ability to attach to blood vessel walls and surfaces. Aggregation is the process in which first platelets release substances, which further recruit platelets so that a platelet plug is formed. Aggregation is increased with secretion of epinephrine and serotonin, substances found on the surface of platelets. Functions are decreased in the presence of antiprostaglandins such as aspirin (see Relevant Pharmacology section). Newly produced platelets are more effective than those that have been in the circulation for a few days.

E. PLASMA FACTORS

More than 40 substances or protein molecules in blood and tissues are involved in the clotting cascade.

1. **Procoagulants,** also known as plasma clotting factors (Table 8–1), promote coagulation. Clotting factors lead to the formation of a fibrin clot. They are referred to by Roman numerals and the name of the substance. Anticoagulants are produced in the liver except for factor VIII (formation site unknown). Vitamin K is required for production of factors II, VII, IX, and X. Factors are circulated in inactive form until stimulated to initiate clotting (see Plasma Factors discussion). All factors act in concert in vivo to respond to tissue or blood-cell injury. Consumption of the substances results in their destruction.

2. **Anticoagulants** inhibit coagulation.

   a. Circulating anticoagulants are antithrombin III, protein C, and protein S. Antithrombin III inactivates thrombin and inhibits factor X. Protein C inactivates factors V and VIII, stimulates fibrinolysis, and elevates levels of tissue plasminogen activator (tPA). Protein activates protein C.

   b. The fibrinolytic system's major component is plasminogen. Plasminogen is produced in the liver and circulated in the plasma. Concentrations increase in response to inflammatory states. Plasminogen is converted to plasmin, which has the ability to digest fibrinogen and fibrin. A by-product is D-dimer, an indicator of the breakdown of cross-linked fibrin. tPA further stimulates the conversion of plasminogen to plasmin. It is synthesized

Table 8–1. NOMENCLATURE FOR COAGULATION FACTORS

FACTOR	SYNONYM
I	Fibrinogen
II	Prothrombin
III	Tissue thromboplastin
IV	Calcium
V	Proaccelerin
VI	Not assigned
VII	Proconvertin
VIII	Antihemophilic factor (AHF)
IX	Plasma thromboplastin component (Christmas factor)
X	Stuart factor (Stuart-Prower factor)
XI	Plasma thromboplastin antecedent (PTA)
XII	Hageman factor
XIII	Fibrin-stabilizing factor (FSF)

Modified from Gordon JB, Bernstein ML, Rogers MC. Hematologic disorders in the pediatric intensive care unit. In: Rogers M, ed. *Textbook of Pediatric Intensive Care.* 2nd ed. Baltimore, Md: Williams & Wilkins; 1992:1380.

    by endothelial cells of the vessels and stimulated by tissue anoxia or damage to the endothelial lining of vessels. tPA will not activate plasminogen in the absence of fibrin.

    c. The antithrombin system involves a plasma protein that inactivates thrombin and active clotting factors not used in the clotting process.

  3. **Coagulation** depends on a balance between the procoagulants and the anticoagulants. A balance is needed to maintain blood as a fluid when the vasculature is intact and uninjured. Anticoagulants usually predominate until a blood vessel or tissue is injured.

FUNCTION AND PHYSIOLOGIC MECHANISMS

A. **RBCs**

RBC function is to transport oxygen from the lungs to the tissues. Oxygen-carrying capacity is determined by the amount of hemoglobin available to combine with the oxygen.

B. **WBCs**

  1. **Functions** (Bellanti, 1985; Mudge-Grout, 1992)

    a. Defense: WBCs protect the body's internal environment from "nonself" antigens or microorganism invasion by inactivating, destroying, or eliminating "nonself" antigens.

      • A DNA code at the molecular level assists the immune system in discriminating "self" from "nonself" or "altered self." "Nonself" is composed of foreign or alien molecular structures and is referred to as antigenic or as an antigen. Antigens are identified by characteristic shapes on their cell surfaces, referred to as epitopes. Antigens carry numerous epitopes, sometimes hundreds, on their cell surface (Mudge-Grout, 1992).

      • Major histocompatibility complex (MHC) molecules serve as the genetic blueprint and are different for each mammalian species. The MHC molecules specific to the human species are human leukocyte antigens (HLA) and are located on chromosome 6. HLA antigens are located on the surfaces of most nucleated cells in the body, as well as on platelets. HLA antigens are inherited according to Mendelian laws, with an individual's genotype determined by one paternal and one maternal haplotype. Close relatives share some of these antigens, whereas identical twins share all these antigens.

- HLA antigens of the MHC are divided into three classes (I, II, and III) based on function, types of cell antigens expressed on the cell membrane surfaces, and structure.
  - Class I includes HLA-A, -B, and -C antigens and are found on all nucleated cell surfaces and platelets. Class I antigens serve as identification markers of self, assist in the elimination of cells infected with intracellular microorganisms and of mutated or malignant cells, and are involved in the rejection of tissue grafts. Class I antigens are the target antigens recognized by the cytotoxic T cells.
  - Class II includes HLA-D and HLA-DR antigens and are located nearly exclusively on the surfaces of certain immune cells (macrophages and B lymphocytes). Class II antigens serve as identification markers of exogenous antigens and assist in the elimination of extracellular microorganisms.
  - Class III antigens are located between class I and class II antigens on chromosome 6 and are involved in the alternative and classical pathways of complement (Mudge-Grout, 1992).
  b. Homeostasis: WBCs remove old or damaged debris from the circulation.
  c. Surveillance: WBCs recognize and guard against the development, growth, and dissemination of abnormal cells.
2. Physiologic mechanisms of WBCs are usually categorized by three lines of defense, each representing increasingly more complex and sophisticated means of protection and methods of elimination.
  a. The *first line of defense* involves the child's natural, innate barriers with unique physical, chemical, and mechanical capabilities. This provides a nonspecific or generic defense with immediate onset.
  - Physical and mechanical barriers prevent or minimize entry and attachment of antigen. These include the phenomenon of colonization and bacterial interference, mucus traps in the respiratory and GI tract, hair and cilia traps, saliva, tears, and urine (dilution and washing away of antigens), defecation and vomiting (expulsion of invading organisms), and an intact GI lining. Many factors associated with critical illnesses are thought to threaten the barrier role of the gut mucosa and increase the risk of translocation of gram-negative bacteria or endotoxin (see Septic Shock discussion in Chapter 9).
  - Chemical barriers deter attachment, survival, and replication of antigen. These include the acid pH of the skin; lysozymes present in saliva, tears, and nasal secretions; gastric secretions; and unsaturated fatty acids in sweat and sebaceous glands.
  - The first line of defense has distinct developmental implications.
    - Skin: The newborn's skin is about 1 mm thick at birth and increases to approximately twice that thickness at maturity. The newborn has scant amounts of stratum corneum, the barrier component of the skin, resulting in increased skin permeability (Malloy and Perez-Woods, 1991). The stratum corneum develops quickly and is considered an adequate barrier at 2 weeks of age (Harpin and Eutter, 1983). After the neonatal period, the sebaceous glands involute and produce only small amounts of sebum until puberty. The differences noted in sweating may be related to the immaturity of autonomic (sympathetic) control of sweating rather than to the structural immaturity of the glands.

Complete neural control of sweat glands is noted between 2 and 3 years of age. Diminished sweat production may result in lower quantities of bactericidal and fungicidal substances and, in some, alteration in the physical barrier of the infant or young child's skin.

○ Respiratory: The small airways of the infant and young child make a significantly greater contribution to airway resistance compared to the adult (Bellanti and Kadlec, 1990). This increased resistance to flow places the child at greater risk for airway occlusion secondary to edema or inflammatory exudate. Normal defense mechanisms of the respiratory tract may be disrupted by such narrowing or obstruction.

○ GI tract: Newborn saliva contains no secretory IgA. At birth the gastric pH is approximately 6 but normally reaches a pH of 2 to 3 within the first 24 hours of life (Ebers et al, 1956; Grand et al, 1976). Acidity of the stomach gradually increases through childhood and then plateaus to adult levels at 10 years of age. The newborn's intestinal epithelium allows certain molecules to pass into the systemic circulation. The maturation of the intestinal epithelium is thought to occur in response to hormones and a variety of growth factors, but the specifics are unknown (Bousvaros and Walker, 1990).

○ Ophthalmologic: Tearing is present by approximately 6 weeks of age, and lysozyme levels in the infant and the normal adult are comparable.

b. The *second line of defense* involves the inflammatory response, phagocytosis, and complement activation. It is nonspecific or generic in nature with immediate onset once triggered if the first line of defense is ineffective.

• The local inflammatory response is a sequential reaction to injury hallmarked by the release of numerous chemical mediators such as histamine, bradykinin (and other kinins), serotonin, and prostaglandins. The goals of inflammation include localization, dilution, and destruction of the offending antigen, maintenance of vascular integrity and minimization of tissue damage, and transportation of cells and substances to the area.

○ Vascular response is characterized by immediate vasoconstriction, which facilitates fibrin plug formation and WBC, RBC, and platelet margination. Vasodilation facilitates cell and cell products to move close to the area of injury. Capillary permeability assists in cell and cell product movement from the vascular space into the tissues. Local increases in hydrostatic pressure and increased oncotic pressure of proteins in the interstitium leads to edema (Jennings, 1991).

○ Cellular response involves **margination** or pavementing the lining of cells along the capillary endothelium to prepare for movement from the intravascular space to the tissue. Margination is facilitated by the vascular response, since fluid leakage into the interstitium results in an increased blood viscosity and a decreased blood flow. **Diapedesis** is an ameboid type movement of WBCs through the junctions between the endothelial lining from the intravascular space to the site of injury (Jennings, 1991). The sequence of cell movement is neutrophils first, followed by monocytes, and much later lymphocytes. **Chemotaxis** involves chemical signals to attract cells to the site of injury. Substances that serve as chemotactic chemicals include microbial products, components of damaged WBCs and tissue, activated complement proteins, and others. Once WBCs are in the area of injury, phagocytosis may begin.

○ Other components of the inflammatory response, biochemical mediators and plasma enzyme cascades, facilitate the inflammatory response through diverse, but complementary actions. Numerous biochemical mediators have been identified, such as prostaglandins, leukotrienes, endorphins, and histamine. The primary nonspecific plasma enzyme cascades include complement, coagulation (involved in the vascular response via hemostasis; see Coagulation Cascade), fibrinolysis (primary activity is the degradation of fibrin clot; see Fibrinolytic System), and kallikrein or kinin (bradykinin; enhances inflammatory response by promoting vasodilation, increased capillary permeability, neutrophil chemotaxis, and other actions).

- Phagocytosis: Phagocytes include granulocytes (especially neutrophils) and monocytes or macrophages. The purpose of phagocytosis is to capture, engulf, and destroy the antigen. Additionally, phagocytosis may eventually present the antigen to the helper T lymphocyte. The process of phagocytosis is complex and involves several mechanisms:
  ○ Recognition of the antigen as nonself.
  ○ Adherence or attachment of the phagocyte to the antigen or invader.
  ○ Ingestion or engulfment is performed through the use of pseudopods. Eventually the antigen is taken into the phagocyte's cytoplasm where it is enveloped in a sac (phagosome).
  ○ Killing and degradation: The antigen-containing sac is subjected to lysozyme and the process known as the respiratory (oxidative) burst, containing hydrogen peroxide, superoxide anion, and hydrochlorite anion. Some microorganisms are ingested but not necessarily killed. For instance, the toxins from staphylococci may in turn kill the phagocyte. Others, such as tubercle bacilli, may multiply within the phagosome and eventually destroy the phagocyte.

- The complement system is a complex group of more than 20 enzymes and proteins that, like the coagulation system, react sequentially in a cascading manner. There are 11 principal proteins labeled C1 through C9 (Jennings, 1991). Complement system activation can occur through two separate, but interrelated, pathways. However, both pathways lead to the generation of C3 and C3b and a final common pathway. The classical pathway activation is stimulated by antigen-antibody interaction. The alternate pathway activation is stimulated without antigen-antibody interaction, but with more generic activators; it is a slower process than classical pathway activation (Jennings, 1991). The final common pathway of complement activation is various events that limit the damage posed by the antigen including enhancement of inflammation, chemotaxis, opsonization (the process of coating an organism with antibodies or proteins to increase its palatability to phagocytes), and target cell membrane lysis.

- Developmental distinctions in the second line of defense
  ○ Local inflammatory response: Infants and young children are less able to localize infection, perhaps because of the following: The newborn's neutrophil chemotaxis is altered (Anderson et al, 1983; Masuda et al, 1989); this chemotactic activity remains unchanged for the first 24 months of life and may not reach adult activity until approximately 16 years of age (Klein et al, 1977). The infant's neutrophils have less ability to aggregate and are less deformable than the adult's (Miller, 1983). It appears that the neutrophil surface is more rigid, which may

impair the cell's movements though capillary walls and bone marrow sinusoids. This may partially explain impaired chemotaxis and thus the inability to localize infection.

○ Systemic response to infection: The infant has considerably smaller numbers of stored neutrophils per kilogram of body weight than the adult (Abramson et al, 1989). Due to the smaller neutrophil storage pool, there is less ability to repeatedly replace the number of circulating neutrophils. Infants and young children may display neutropenia rather than neutrophilia in the presence of infection, and increased release of immature neutrophils in the presence of infection may be exaggerated in the infant and young child (Christensen and Rothstein, 1980).

○ Phagocytosis: Some evidence indicates that phagocytosis in the newborn is deficient (Goldman et al, 1985), whereas others report that phagocytic activity is normal (Abramson et al, 1989; Miller, 1980).

○ Complement proteins gradually increase to 60% to 80% of normal adult levels at birth for the classical pathway and lower percentages for the alternative pathway (Berger and Frank, 1989; Goldman et al, 1985), but it is not until about 3 to 6 months of age that serum complement levels are within normal adult range (Goldman et al, 1985). Low levels may lead to relative and subtle deficiencies in complement system function and at birth may contribute to the newborn's afebrile and absent leukocytic response to infection (Berger and Frank, 1989).

c. The *third line of defense* involves specific, acquired immunity and is triggered if the first and second lines of defense are ineffective in eliminating or containing the antigen. The immune response is a highly complex sequence of events that are triggered by an antigen and integrally associated with other physiologic events including, but not limited to, complement activation and the clotting and fibrocytic systems (Mudge-Grout, 1992). Hallmarks of the third line of defense include specificity, the ability of a lymphocyte to respond to a single antigen for which it was designed, and memory, the ability of a lymphocyte to recall prior exposure to an antigen and respond in an accelerated, potentiated manner. Specific, acquired immunity may be obtained either passively or actively and naturally or artificially (Table 8–2).

• Specific acquired immunity occurs in phases. Recognition and processing of the antigen is the primary responsibility of the macrophage, although the B lymphocyte may participate. Once identified as nonself or foreign, the macrophage ingests the antigen and through an enzyme-mediated reaction begins "antigen processing." When "antigen processing" is complete, the macrophage re-expresses the processed antigen on its membrane surface in conjunction with HLA antigen. "Antigen presentation" to the B or T lymphocyte occurs (Mudge-Grout, 1992). Processing and presentation of the antigen triggers the immune response to facilitate elimination.

• Acquired immunity is comprised of two different, but closely interrelated, antigen-specific immune responses (Fig. 8–3): (1) Humoral immunity (HI), which is mediated by B lymphocytes, results in the synthesis and secretion of immunoglobulins and *indirectly* eliminates or impedes the antigen. HI provides protection primarily from encapsulated pyogenic bacterial infections. (2) Cell-mediated immunity (CMI), which is mediated by T lymphocytes, *directly* eliminates the antigen. CMI protects from viral, fungal, protozoal, and mycobacterial infections, plays a role in

Table 8–2. ACQUIRED, SPECIFIC IMMUNITY: DEFINITION, ACQUISITION, AND CHARACTERISTICS

TYPES OF ACQUIRED, SPECIFIC IMMUNITY	DEFINITION AND ACQUISITION	CHARACTERISTICS
Passive Immunity		
Natural	Acquired through natural contact with *antibody* transplacentally or through colostrum and breast milk (e.g., IgG and IgA from mother to fetus or neonate)	No participation of the host; a transfer of preformed substances or sensitized cells from an immunized host to a nonimmunized host
Artificial	Acquired through the administration of *antibody* or antitoxin (e.g., γ-globulin, tetanus)	Onset is immediate, but duration is temporary
Active Immunity		
Natural	Acquired through natural infection; the body is exposed to an *antigen* and mounts an immune response to that antigen (e.g., chickenpox)	Active participation of the host following exposure to an antigen either naturally (subclinical or clinical disease) or artificially through immunization
Artifical	Acquired through inoculation with a variant *antigen,* but usually not the entire antigen (e.g., immunization, attenuated virus)	Provides slow antigen-specific development of antibody, but provides permanent or long-lived immunity to that antigen

Adapted from Mudge-Grout CL. *Immunologic Disorders.* St Louis, Mo: Mosby–Year Book Inc, 1992.17.

the response to malignancies, and participates in the rejection of transplanted tissues and in hypersensitivity reactions (Mudge-Grout, 1992).

- HI: B lymphocytes can be activated without the help of the T lymphocyte, as in T-cell-independent antigen response but most commonly are activated with the assistance of the T lymphocyte, as in the T-cell-dependent antigen response. B cells transform into plasma cells, which synthesize and secrete immunoglobulins and subsequently interact with the antigen for which it was made. Immunoglobulins (antibodies) are glycoproteins produced by plasma cells in response to an antigen. The nature of the antibody response varies with the chemical and physical nature of the antigen, the antigen's route of entry, and the immunization history of the child (Mudge-Grout, 1992). There are five major classes of immunoglobulins (Table 8–3).
  - Outcomes of antigen-antibody interaction include neutralization (antibody binds the antigen, causing the antigen to be ineffective or promoting removal by phagocytes), agglutination (antibody combines with the antigen to form clumps), precipitation (antibody combines with the antigen to make an insoluble lattice formation that precipitates), opsonization (antibody coats the antigen, enhancing phagocytosis), complement (antibodies activate complement, thus causing target cell lysis), and antibody-dependent cytotoxicity (antibody facilitates lysis of the antigen by another immune cell).
  - Primary response: Antibody production occurs within 2 to 10 days after the first exposure, and the response peaks in 1 to 3 weeks. IgM is followed by an IgG response.

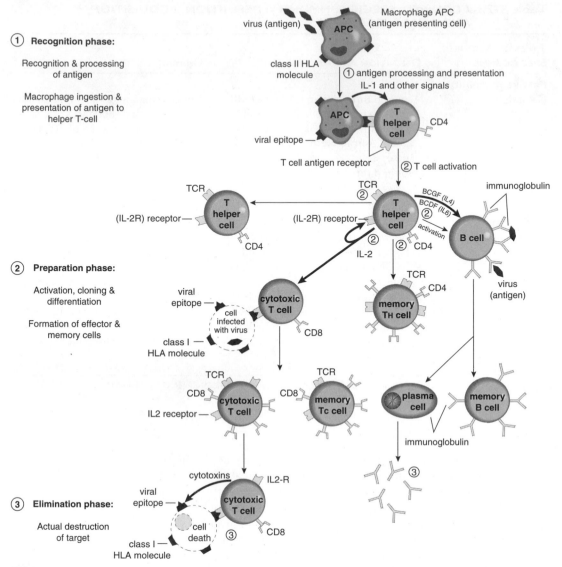

Figure 8–3. Overview of specific acquired immunity. The grand scheme of specific acquired immunity is comprised of humoral (immunoglobulin) immunity (HI) orchestrated by the B cell and cell-mediated immunity (CMI), orchestrated by the T cell. Note the interdependence between the B and T cells. The three phases of the specific immune response are indicated by numbers in the figure: *1,* recognition phase, *2,* preparation phase, and *3,* elimination phase. (Adapted from Goodman JW. The immune response. In: Stites DP, Terr AI, Parslow TG, eds. *Basic and Clinical Immunology.* 9th ed. Norwalk, Conn: Appleton & Lange; 1997.)

- Secondary response is the response that occurs with exposure to a previously encountered antigen. Memory cells are responsible for the rapid (1 to 2 days), prolific, sustained response to the familiar antigen. Antibody response is primarily IgG at much higher titers for a shorter period of time as compared to the primary response (Mudge-Grout, 1992).
- CMI involves T-lymphocyte recognition and activation. T lymphocyte binds to the antigen *and* to a class I or class II protein on the surface of an antigen presenting cell (usually the macrophage). Class I HLA antigens are required for cytotoxic T-lymphocyte activation. Class II HLA antigens are required for helper T-lymphocyte activation.

- Communication among all the cells participating in the immune response is facilitated through the secretion of cytokines. Cytokines are hormonelike substances that function to up regulate and down regulate immunologic, inflammatory, and reparative host responses. Cytokines secreted by lymphocytes are referred to as lymphokines. Cytokines secreted by monocytes or macrophages are referred to as monokines. Cytokines are distinct from endocrine hormones, since they are produced by a number of cells rather than a specialized gland, do not usually present in the serum, and act in paracrine (locally near the producing cell) or autocrine (directly on the producing cell) fashion rather than on distant target cells. Selected cytokines are described in Table 8–4.
- Developmental distinctions in the third line of defense: The infant's B cells are deficient in producing comparable adult levels and subclasses of immunoglobulins. Serum immunoglobulin levels, the degree of synthesis at birth, and the age in which the levels are comparable to the adult are

Table 8–3. HUMAN IMMUNOGLOBULINS

Ig	PERCENTAGE IN SERUM	LOCATION	ACTIVITY AND FUNCTION
IgG	75%	Most abundant intravascularly Also in extravascular spaces (e.g., lymph, colony-stimulating factor)	Only immunoglobulin to cross placenta Primary antibody class Activates complement Takes 10–14 d after antigen stimulation to develop sufficient IgG titer in primary response; only 4 d in secondary response Appears 1 wk after IgM and peaks in 1–3 wk or longer after IgM peaks Promotes phagocytosis via opsonization
IgA	15%	Found in mucous membrane secretions Intravascular	Two types: Serum and secretory Primary defense against local invasion of body surfaces and orifices
IgM	10%	Intravascular only	Promotes phagocytosis Can activate complement Participates in blood transfusion reactions; makes antibodies for "nonself" ABO blood groups Made in utero and may indicate the presence of an intrauterine infection or ABO incompatibility First made in response to an antigen Predominant in a primary infection Peaks 1–2 wk after infection Increases in chronic infections
IgE	0.1%	Found in serum bound to mast cells and basophils	Triggers release of histamine and other mediators from mast cells and basophils Involved in type I immediate hypersensitivity or anaphylactic reactions Defense against parasite infections
IgD	<1%	Found in serum located on surface of B cells	Function not yet defined May participate in B-cell differentiation Increases in chronic infection

Data from Grady C. Host defense mechanisms: an overview. *Sem Oncol Nurs.* 1988:4(2):92; Mudge-Grout C. *Immunologic Disorders.* St Louis, Mo: Mosby–Year Book Inc; 1992:19; and Selekman J. Pediatric problems related to the immunologic system. In: Feeg VD, Harbin RE, eds. *Pediatric Nursing: Core Curriculum and Resource Manual.* Pitman, NJ: Anthony Jannetti, Inc; 1991:202.

Table 8–4. SELECTED CYTOKINES: SOURCE AND FUNCTIONS

TYPE	SOURCE	FUNCTIONS
Interleukins (ILs)		
IL-1 (endogenous pyrogen)	T cell, B cell, macrophage, endothelium, tissue cell	Enhances T-cell growth and function; stimulates macrophages; immuno-augmentation
IL-2 (T-cell growth factor)	T cells	Promotes T-cell and B-cell growth; activates T cell; enhances NK activity
IL-3 (multi-CSF)	T cells, mast cells	Stimulates growth of immature hematopoietic precursor cells (e.g., granulocytes, macrophages, RBCs, platelets, and mast cells)
BCGF (IL-4)	T cells	Enhances B-cell growth and function
BCDF (IL-6)	T cells	Enhances B-cell growth and function
Interferons		
Interferon alfa	Lymphocytes, NK cells, macrophages, fibroblasts, epithelial cells	Enhances NK activity; provides antiviral protection; induces HLA-I expression; induces fever; generates cytotoxic T lymphocytes; induces macrophage killing of tumor cells
Interferon beta	Fibroblasts, macrophages, epithelial cells	Provides antiviral protection
Interferon gamma	T cells, NK cells	Activates macrophages; induces macrophage killing of microorganism and tumor cells; regulates action of certain cytokines; increases NK cell activity; increases expression of Fc receptor and HLA-I antigens
Tumor Necrosis Factor	Macrophages, T cells, and others	Enhances destruction of tumor cells
Colony-Stimulating Factors (CSFs)		
G-CSF	Monocytes, macrophages, endothelial cells, and fibroblasts	Stimulates growth and activation of neutrophils
M-CSF	Monocytes, macrophages, endothelial cells, and fibroblasts	Stimulates growth and activation of monocytes
GM-CSF	T cells, endothelial cells, and fibroblasts	Stimulates growth and activation of neutrophils, eosinophils, and macrophages

HLA, human leukocyte antigen; *NK,* natural killer; *RBCs,* red blood cells.
Data from Mudge-Grout CL. *Immunologic Disorders.* St Louis, Mo: Mosby–Year Book Inc; 1992:23; and Plaeger SF. Principal human cytokines. In: Stiehm ER, ed. *Immunologic Disorders in Infants and Children.* 4th ed. Philadelphia, Pa: WB Saunders Co; 1996:1063–1064.

reflected in Table 8–5. The IgG level seems comparable between the newborn and the adult, but this level reflects the transplacental acquisition of maternal antibody during primarily the third trimester of gestation. The infant is lowest in immunoglobulin concentrations at about 4 to 5 months of age, when maternal IgG begins to decrease through natural catabolism and when infant synthesis of immunoglobulin is low. This period of time is referred to as physiologic hypogammaglobulinemia. During this time, the infant is most susceptible to infections caused by viruses, candida, and acute inflammatory bacteria (*Staphylococcus aureus, Streptococcus pyogenes, Streptococcus pneumoniae, Haemophilus influenzae* type B, *Neisseria meningitidis*). This state can be prolonged to such an extent that the young child suffers from recurrent and severe infections.

Table 8–5.   SERUM IMMUNOGLOBULINS: DEVELOPMENTAL PERSPECTIVES

Ig	SYNTHESIS BY FETUS (GESTATION-WK)	PERCENTAGE OF ADULT LEVELS AT BIRTH	AGE AT WHICH ADULT LEVELS ARE ACHIEVED
IgM	10.5	10%	1–2 y
IgD	14	Small amount	1 y
IgG*	12	110%†	4–10 y
IgA	30	Small amount or none	6–15 y
IgE	10.5	Small amount	6–15 y

*Crosses placenta.

†Greater than or equal to maternal level.

From Rosenthal CH. Immunosuppression in the pediatric critical care patient. *Crit Care Nurs Clin North Am.* 1989;1(4):779.

C. PLATELETS

The function of platelets is to maintain normal hemostasis and vascular integrity when a blood vessel wall is injured.

1. **Hemostasis** is a complex interaction among three responding systems:
   a. Blood vessel walls have a "nonstick" lining that normally repels platelets and keeps blood cells flowing smoothly.
   b. Injury to a vessel wall leads to constriction of the injured vessel within seconds. The sympathetic nervous system responds with a catecholamine surge. The vessel immediately constricts, cutting off the blood supply.
   c. Hemostatic response of platelets: Circulating platelets rush to the injured area to form a protective plug. Platelets change to become "sticky" with hairlike projections and adhere to the injured area. As platelets aggregate, they release substances (prostaglandin, serotonin, thromboxane A_2) that attract additional platelets to the area (Fig. 8–4). Formation of a platelet plug or clot occurs within 1 to 3 minutes. Further activation of platelets is influenced by plasma clotting proteins, particularly thrombin. This process is referred to as primary hemostasis and is completed in minutes to about an hour. Secondary hemostasis involves the plasma clotting factors (see section on Plasma Factors).
2. **Physiologic conditions** influencing platelet response can be quantitative (increase or decrease in number) or qualitative (abnormal function).
   a. An increase in the number of circulating platelets (platelet count) usually occurs after acute blood loss to enhance hemostasis.

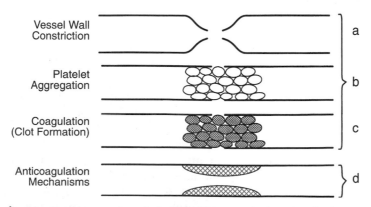

Figure 8–4.   Hemostatic response of platelets. Major mechanisms involved in primary hemostasis (*a* through *c*). Injury results in vessel wall constriction, platelet aggregation, and clot formation. Anticoagulation mechanisms (*d*) reestablish blood flow by lysing the clot. (From Harvey M. *Study Guide to Core Curriculum for Critical Care Nursing.* Philadelphia, Pa: WB Saunders Co; 1986:162.)

b. *Thrombocytopenia,* defined as a platelet count lower than $150,000/mm^3$, can result from decreased production, increased destruction, or increased trapping in the spleen (splenic sequestration). Causes of thrombocytopenia include medications (see Relevant Pharmacology discussion), renal or liver disease, cardiopulmonary bypass or hemodialysis, aplastic anemia, auto-immune or idiopathic thrombocytopenic purpura (ITP), viral diseases, disseminated intravascular coagulation (DIC), radiation to the bones, and malignancies involving the bone marrow (displacement of normal stem cells with malignant cells). Thrombocytopenia may also result from congenital disorders, such as thrombocytopenic absent radii (TAR), Wiskott-Aldrich syndrome, and May-Hegglin anomaly.

c. Platelet function can be impaired by medications (e.g., aspirin, nonsteroi-dal antiinflammatory drugs [NSAIDs]); see Relevant Pharmacology discus-sion) and renal disease. Uremia causes reversible impairment of qualitative platelet function. Impaired platelet function results in bleeding in areas abundant in capillaries such as the mucous membranes in the GI tract, vagina, bladder, and nasopharynx, producing petechiae or ecchymosis or both.

d. Most platelet problems in critical care are due to thrombocytopenia rather than a decreased function of the platelets. Hemostasis begins to be affected when the platelet count is below 80,000 to $100,000/mm^3$, but bleeding is unlikely until the platelet count is less than $25,000/mm^3$. If the plate-let count is less than $50,000/mm^3$, easy bruising may occur. If the platelet count is less than 10,000 to $20,000/mm^3$, spontaneous bleeding may occur especially if the child is anemic or febrile. If the platelet count is $10,000/mm^3$, severe spontaneous or intracranial bleeding may occur.

D. PLASMA FACTORS

1. **Procoagulants** contribute to the process of secondary hemostasis, which is represented by the formation of a fibrin clot and trapping of RBCs at the site of the initiating primary hemostatic plug.

2. Different substances **(enzymes and proteins)** amplify initial activation of a soft clot to an appropriately sized, fully developed clot (Fig. 8–5).

3. **Factors** play a role in initiating primary nonspecific plasma enzyme cascades.

4. **Coagulation cascade** starts within the blood stream itself (intrinsic) or outside the blood stream (extrinsic). The process results in blood changing from a liquid to a gel state by the ultimate conversion of fibrinogen to insoluble fibrin polymers. Contraction of the fibrin network follows, causing the plug to retract, pull the walls of the damaged vessel together, and seal shut the injured vessel wall.

a. The *intrinsic pathway* is activated when platelets contact collagen or dam-aged endothelium. Its function is screened by partial thromboplastin time (PTT).

b. The *extrinsic pathway* is activated when a tissue factor (nature of which is not well understood) is released from injured tissues, such as when tissues have been cut in surgery. Its function is screened by prothrombin time (PT).

c. The *common pathway* is the part of the coagulation cascade that is activated by the intrinsic or extrinsic pathway. The final step is a fibrin mesh within the platelet plug. Thrombin stimulates the platelets to further aggregate. Fibrin is an essential portion of a clot, soluble until polymerized by factor XIII, which converts it to a stable (insoluble) clot. The function of the common pathway is screened by both the PT and PTT.

5. **Anticoagulant mechanisms** function to maintain blood as a fluid to maintain

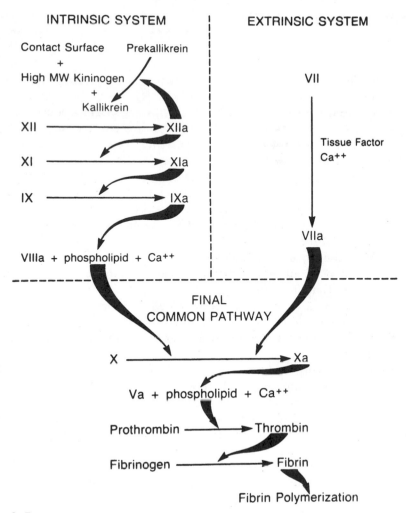

INTRINSIC SYSTEM

EXTRINSIC SYSTEM

Contact Surface   Prekallikrein
+
High MW Kininogen
+
Kallikrein

XII ————————→ XIIa

XI ————————→ XIa

IX ————————→ IXa

VIIIa + phospholipid + Ca++

VII

Tissue Factor
Ca++

VIIa

FINAL
COMMON PATHWAY

X ————————→ Xa

Va + phospholipid + Ca++

Prothrombin ———→ Thrombin

Fibrinogen ———→ Fibrin

Fibrin Polymerization

Figure 8–5.   Platelet clotting factors. Secondary hemostasis. The coagulation cascade starts within (intrinsic) or outside (extrinsic) the blood stream, both leading to a common pathway. Inactive components and factors become active indicated by the *"a."* (From Farmer JC, Parker RI. Coagulation disorders. In: Civetta JM, Taylor RW, Kirby RR, eds. *Critical Care.* 2nd ed. Philadelphia, Pa: JB Lippincott Co; 1992:1701.)

vascular patency. The system must turn off the various coagulation pathways to reestablish blood flow through an injured vessel, maintain vascular patency, and modulate the balance between the clotting and lysing systems.

a. The *fibrinolytic system* involves the process of lysing a clot. Plasminogen is the precursor to the active part, which is plasmin. It is produced in the liver and circulated in the plasma. The conversion to plasmin is increased in states such as inflammation and coagulation or in the presence of tPA. Plasmin lyses fibrin clots by digesting fibrin or fibrinogen. Plasmin splits fibrin into smaller elements called fibrin split products (FSPs) or fibrin degradation products (FDPs). FSPs impair platelet aggregation, reduce prothrombin, and interfere with polymerization of fibrin.

b. The *antithrombin system* defends against excessive clotting and maintains blood as a fluid. The blood vessel wall has sites that allow thrombin to be inactivated by antithrombin III. Disorders of antithrombin mechanism include congenital thrombotic disorder and hepatic failure.

CLINICAL ASSESSMENT

A. Nursing History

1. The **chief complaint** is noted in the patient's or the primary caretaker's own words.

    ❖ Potential for decrease in RBCs related to activity intolerance, fatigue, and weakness; shortness of breath and dyspnea; and "racing heart"

    ❖ Potential increase or decrease in WBCs related to fever or chills, chronic or recurrent infection, lymphadenopathy, skin rash, and joint pain

    ❖ Potential for decrease in platelets related to petechiae, bruising or abnormal bleeding (either prolonged after a minor injury or spontaneous)

2. A **family history** of RBC, WBC, and platelet abnormalities is noted.

    a. RBC abnormalities include jaundice, anemia, and RBC dyscrasia, such as sickle cell anemia.

    b. WBC abnormalities include malignancies; frequent, recurrent, or chronic infections; congenital immunodeficiencies; acquired immunodeficiencies; and autoimmune disorders.

    c. Platelet abnormalities include any bleeding disorders or predisposition to bleeding or clotting.

    d. Any symptoms of blood disorders similar to the patient's symptoms are noted.

3. **Patient health history**

    a. Record immunizations and previous immunologic testing.

    b. The patient's diet and nutrition history is described including recent weight gain or loss, dietary restrictions and food dislikes and intolerance, and routine dietary intake, including cultural adherence. All blood cell lines are dependent to some extent on adequate nutritional intake. In particular, iron, vitamin B_{12}, and folic acid are needed for RBC development.

    c. Allergies and hypersensitivities are noted, including allergies to inhalants (e.g., animal dander, pollens), contactants (e.g., fibers, chemicals), injectables (e.g., drugs, blood transfusions), or ingestants (e.g., foods, food additives, drugs) and the symptoms accompanying the allergic or hypersensitivity reaction.

    d. *Previous surgeries* that may impair hematologic or immunologic status are noted, including organ or tissue transplantation, thymectomy, splenectomy, or any surgery that imposed trauma to lymph nodes.

    e. Inquire about *medical conditions* that may impair hematologic or immunologic status. RBCs are affected by anemia or malabsorption syndrome or problems. WBCs are affected by liver or spleen disorders (functional splenectomy), chronic or recurrent infections, mononucleosis, or problems with wound healing. Platelets may be abnormal with prolonged or excessive bleeding or menorrhagia. Plasma factors may be implicated in hemarthrosis.

    f. *General symptoms* include fatigue, change in level of activity, weakness, headache, chills, fever, weight loss, failure to thrive, night sweats, poor wound healing, malaise, pain, prolonged or excessive bleeding, excessive bleeding related to dental extractions, and menorrhagia.

    g. *Specific symptoms*
      - Mental status: Note confusion, restlessness, syncope, irritability, impaired consciousness, or somnolence.
      - Skin: Note prolonged bleeding, bruising easily, petechiae, jaundice, pallor, lesions, ulcers, rhinitis, dermatitis, urticaria, or eczema.

- Eyes: Note visual disturbances and retinal hemorrhages and examine conjunctivae for erythema or pallor.
- Nose and mouth: Note epistaxis, gingival bleeding, sore or ulcerated tongue, mucositis, candidiasis, or vesicular crusting lesions (herpes simplex).
- Lymph nodes: Note enlargement (adenopathy) or tenderness.
- Chest: Note tachypnea, respiratory tract infections, respiratory distress, dyspnea, orthopnea, cough, hemoptysis, sputum, or chest pain.
- Abdomen: Note anorexia, altered bowel sounds, diarrhea, constipation, melena, vomiting, hematemesis, protuberant abdomen (not age related), abdominal pain, masses, or hepatosplenomegaly.
- Genitourinary: Note hematuria, menorrhagia, and urinary tract infections.
- Motor and sensory function: Note ataxia and paresthesias.
- Back and extremities: Note pain in joints, back, shoulders, or bone and hemarthrosis (joint bleeding).

    h. *Psychosocial history* should include recent stresses or life-changing events, response to stress, and coping methods.

4. **Medication history**

    a. *Prescription agents* used to treat existing hematologic or immunologic conditions may include multivitamins, iron preparations (oral or parenteral), vitamin B_{12}, folic acid, or EPO for RBC deficiencies. A wide variety of agents used to treat infection, autoimmune disorders, and malignancies affect WBC number and function and the ability of the body to mount an inflammatory response. Examples of such agents include antineoplastic agents, antibiotics, antivirals or antiretrovirals, antifungals, NSAIDs, and CSFs. Antiplatelet agents such as aspirin may compromise clotting functions. Anticoagulants affect plasma factors. Evaluate agents used to treat nonhematologic or immunologic conditions that adversely affect hemopoietic function (see Relevant Pharmacology discussion).

    b. *Nonprescription* drugs include common agents such as aspirin but also recreational use of substances.

5. **Social-cultural history**

    a. Environmental exposures may include radiation, either inadvertent exposure or radiation therapies (total or localized), or inadvertent exposure to chemicals such as benzene, lead, and insecticides.

    b. Discuss recent travel, especially outside the United States.

    c. Determine whether the child is sexually active (including nonconsensual sex). Evaluate sexual preference, safer sex practices, and multiple partners.

    d. Determine tobacco and alcohol use. Alcohol consumption reduces the intake of essential nutrients and vitamins and may affect RBC production, platelet function, and clotting mechanisms.

    e. Evaluate folk practices and interventions for sickness.

B. **PHYSICAL EXAMINATION OF THE PATIENT**

1. **Inspection** (see Nursing History, specific symptoms)

2. **Palpation**

    a. Palpate superficial lymph nodes for location, size, tenderness, fixation, and texture (see Fig. 8–2*B*).

    b. Examine for sternal or rib tenderness, joint mobility and tenderness, and bone or abdominal tenderness.

    c. Evaluate liver and spleen size and tenderness. Tenderness may be indicative of an inflammatory process or an enlarged organ with the stretching of the capsule secondary to bleeding or malignancy. Check for hepatomegaly or splenomegaly (may be a complication of portal hypertension). Hepato-splenomegaly is noted in patients with numerous immune disorders (e.g., hemolytic anemia, immunodeficiency disorders, and ITP).

3. **Auscultate** heart sounds including gallop, rhythm, and pericardial rubs (may indicate an inflammatory process) and lung sounds including rales, rhonchi, and pleural rubs.

NONINVASIVE AND INVASIVE DIAGNOSTIC TESTS

A. **COMPLETE BLOOD CELL COUNT (CBC)**
  1. **RBC count**
     a. Normal: approximately 4.5 to 6×10^6 million/mm^3 (varies with age) (see Table 8–6).
     b. RBCs are reduced in anemia, hemorrhage, and fluid overload.
     c. RBCs are increased in chronic hypoxemia, high altitude, and polycythemia.
  2. **Hemoglobin (Hb)** measures the oxygen-carrying capacity of the RBC and gives it the red color.
     a. Normal: See Table 8–6.
     b. Hb × 3 is an approximation of the patient's hematocrit.
     c. Hb is reduced in sickle cell disease, hemorrhage, anemia, fluid overload, and iron deficiencies.
     d. Hb is increased in dehydration and polycythemia.
  3. **Hematocrit (Hct)** compares the volume of RBCs with the volume of plasma; it is measured as percent of total RBC volume.
     a. Normal: See Table 8–6.
     b. Hct is reduced in hemorrhage, anemia, fluid overload, and iron deficiencies.
     c. Hct is increased in dehydration and polycythemia.
  4. **Peripheral smear** enables a more exact evaluation of blood cell size, shape, and composition and is especially useful in evaluating anemia and confirmation of thrombocytopenia.
  5. **Reticulocyte count** is the number of young RBCs. It indicates the proportion of immature RBCs in the circulation and is helpful in determining the cause of anemia in some children. The reticulocyte count measures the responsiveness and potential of the bone marrow to respond to bleeding or hemolysis.
     a. Normal: 0.5% to 1%.
     b. The reticulocyte count is reduced after a blood transfusion, in aplastic conditions, or in nutritional anemias.
     c. The reticulocyte count is increased in anemia, blood loss, and bone marrow recovery as a compensatory mechanism.
  6. **Total WBC count**
     a. Normal is approximately 5000 to 10,000/mm^3 (age specific) (see Table 8–6).
     b. Variations in the total WBC count include leukocytosis, an elevation in WBC count above normal range, and leukopenia, a reduction in WBC count below normal range.
     c. Total WBC count reflects *only* those WBCs in the intravascular space (excluding the marginal pool). WBCs are also located in the following:
        • Marginal pool: Cells are temporarily sequestered in small vessels or adhere to the walls of large blood vessels.
        • Tissues: Nearly twice as many neutrophils are found in the tissues as intravascularly.

Table 8–6. HEMATOLOGIC VALUES DURING INFANCY AND CHILDHOOD

AGE	HEMOGLOBIN (g/dl)		HEMATOCRIT (%)		RETICU-LOCYTES (%)	MCV (fl)	LEUKOCYTES (WBC/mm³)		NEUTROPHILS (%)		LYMPHO-CYTES (%)	EOSINO-PHILS (%)	MONO-CYTES (%)
	MEAN	RANGE	MEAN	RANGE	MEAN	LOWEST	MEAN	RANGE	MEAN	RANGE	MEAN*	MEAN	MEAN
Cord blood	16.8	13.7–20.1	55	45–65	5	110	18,000	(9,000–30,000)	61	(40–80)	31	2	6
2 wk	16.5	13–20	50	42–66	1		12,000	(5,000–21,000)	40		63	3	9
3 mo	12.0	9.5–14.5	36	31–41	1		12,000	(6,000–18,000)	30		48	2	5
6 mo–6 y	12.0	10.5–14	37	33–42	1	70–74	10,000	(6,000–15,000)	45		48	2	5
7–12 y	13.0	11–16	38	34–40	1	76–80	8,000	(4,500–13,500)	55		38	2	5
Adult													
Female	14	12–16	42	37–47	1.6	80	7,500	(5,000–10,000)	55	(35–70)	35	3	7
Male	16	14–18	47	42–52		80							

*Relatively wide range.

fl, femtoliters; *MCV*, mean corpuscular volume; *WBC*, white blood cells.
From Christensen RD, Ohs RK. Development of the hematopoietic system. In: Behrman RE, Kliegman RM, Arvin AM, eds. *Nelson Textbook of Pediatrics*. 15th ed. Philadelphia, Pa: WB Saunders Co; 1996:1379.

- Bone marrow: The adult bone marrow reserve is approximately 10 times the quantity of the neutrophils in the circulation and tissue and body cavities (Jennings, 1991). The infant and young child have smaller bone marrow reserves of neutrophils and are less able to repeatedly replenish these cells (Rosenthal, 1989).

7. **Differential WBC count** measures the five subcategories of circulating WBCs and is reported as a percentage. It evaluates the bone marrow's ability to produce those particular cells (see Table 8–6). Neutrophil shifts are the number of "segs," "polys," or "bands" as reported in the differential WBC count, which may be interpreted in two ways:

    a. As an indication of the cell's maturity, a "shift to the left" indicates predominantly immature neutrophils (bands), as seen in overwhelming infection or use of colony stimulating factors. A "shift to the right" indicates an increased number of mature neutrophils (polys or segs), which can be observed in patients experiencing pernicious anemia (vitamin B_{12} deficiency), folate deficiency, and morphine addiction.

    b. The differential count also is an indication of the type of cell that is excessively prominent.

8. **Absolute cell counts** are more important than the total count or differential percentage. The absolute count specifically quantifies that particular cell line. Absolute counts may be derived for any cell line.

    a. Following is an example calculation of an absolute neutrophil count:

        - Obtain patient's total WBC count (i.e., WBC = 5 k/mm^3).
        - Translate the total WBC count into an absolute number ("k" means 1000 cells; therefore, $5 \times 1000 = 5000$ or an absolute WBC count of 5000/mm^3).
        - Obtain WBC differential and add the percentages of "polys" plus "bands" (polys = 60% plus bands = 10%; therefore, 60% + 10% = 70%).
        - Translate the percentage of "polys" plus "bands" into an absolute number by dividing by 100 (70% ÷ 100 = 0.7).
        - Multiply the absolute WBC count by the absolute "polys" plus "band" count ($5000 \times 0.7 = 3500$; therefore, absolute neutrophil count = 3500/mm^3).

    b. *Absolute granulocyte or neutrophil counts* (AGC or ANC)

        - Normal: 1800 to 7200/mm^3.
        - Interpretation:
            - ANC <1000: Moderate risk for infection.
            - ANC <500: High risk for infection.

    c. *Absolute lymphocyte counts* were once thought to be comparable across ages. Although total lymphocyte count and subsets of lymphocytes are equivalent percentages of the WBC count in all ages, the young child's higher WBC count yields greater absolute numbers of lymphocytes and subsets of lymphocytes.

        - A lymphocyte count of less than 15% to 20% of the differential WBC count is considered abnormal.
        - Lymphocyte subset determinations are capable through monoclonal antibody technology. Quantifying lymphocyte subsets is useful in monitoring a patient's response to immunosuppressive therapy during the organ transplant process, an infectious process or an immune disorder, and the effect of medications on the patient's immune system.
            - CD4 count (helper T lymphocyte): Cytomegalovirus (CMV) and Epstein-Barr virus (EBV) may result in a transient decrease in CD4 helper cells (Mudge-Grout, 1992).

- ○ CD8 count (suppressor or cytotoxic T lymphocyte): Viral illnesses may result in a marked increase in CD8 suppressor or cytotoxic cells (Mudge-Grout, 1992).
- ○ CD4:CD8 (helper-to-suppressor or cytotoxic) lymphocyte ratio: Normally there are more helper than suppressor or cytotoxic T lymphocytes. The normal ratio is considered 0.8:2.9 (Mudge-Grout, 1992). Patients initially diagnosed with AIDS commonly demonstrate an elevation of CD8 suppressor or cytotoxic cells and a decrease of CD4 helper cells, resulting in a low CD4:CD8 ratio (Mudge-Grout, 1992).

B. OTHER IMMUNE-RELATED DIAGNOSTIC TESTING

1. **Erythrocyte sedimentation rate (ESR)** is a nonspecific indicator of systemic inflammation. In many cases, the ESR is so nonspecific that it has little clinical utility as a single value, but following trends is helpful to assess the effectiveness of therapies. In the immunocompromised child, it may be one of the few objective measurements of response to therapy or relapse.
   a. ESR measures the amount of RBCs that settle in 1 hour: Normal values for the modified Westergren technique range from 0 to 10 mm/h for a child, 0 to 15 mm/h for adult males, and 0 to 20 mm/h for adult females (Harkins et al, 1989).
   b. Elevated rates occur in many conditions including acute and chronic inflammatory conditions, such as Kawasaki syndrome, juvenile arthritis, and rheumatic fever; hypersensitivity conditions, such as Stevens-Johnson syndrome; and malignancy (Harkins et al, 1989).
   c. Decreased rates occur in hypofibrinogenemia, sickle cell anemia, and congestive heart failure (Mudge-Grout, 1992).

2. **C-reactive protein** is a nonspecific indicator of active inflammation.
   a. C-reactive protein, produced by the liver during periods of inflammation, enhances phagocytic activity of phagocytes, particularly of the neutrophil.
   b. Normal value is less than 6 μg/ml.

3. **Histocompatibility testing** identifies the HLA antigens, the child's genetic blueprint. Although HLA antigens are present on all nucleated cells, lymphocytes are commonly used (Mudge-Grout, 1992).
   a. Histocompatibility testing is used for tissue typing for transplantation, paternity testing, and the diagnosis of various autoimmune diseases (Jennings, 1991).
   b. Two methods are used for histocompatibility testing: tissue typing and crossmatching.
      - Tissue typing is the determination of an individual's HLA class I and II specificities. This is routinely performed for organ and tissue transplantation using complement-dependent cytotoxic assay (Mudge-Grout, 1992).
      - Crossmatching is performed prior to organ transplantation to prevent (*or* minimize) risk of rejection after surgery (Mudge-Grout, 1992). Crossmatching detects the presence of antibodies in the recipient's serum that are directed against the HLA antigens of the potential donor (Mudge-Grout, 1992). Various methods are used to complete HLA testing with most patient's awaiting transplantation undergoing four initial crossmatching tests including lymphocytes, T or B lymphocyte–enriched preparations, preformed antibodies, and autocrossmatch (Mudge-Grout, 1992).
   c. Molecular typing (only available in some centers) can be performed to further define DNA sequencing and assist in the selection of a more

complete or precise match between the donor and recipient bone marrow cells.

4. **Complement assays** evaluate the primary complement components of the classical pathway and some of the components of the alternate pathway (Mudge-Grout, 1992). Total complement hemolytic 50 (CH50) is used to test the integrity of the entire complement system, since the entire cascade must be intact to reflect a normal level. The individual complement components (both from a total and functional perspective) also are measured.

5. **Total immunoglobulin level** and levels for the various classes and subclasses are measured. Normal Ig levels vary with age; therefore, it is imperative that age-adjusted values be used for all comparisons. Ig levels can be diagnostic of congenital or primary immunodeficiencies (quantitative testing). If Ig levels are normal, in spite of suspected immunodeficiency, evaluation of the function and effectiveness of the immunoglobulin responding to an antigen may be indicated (qualitative testing).

6. **Coombs test or antiglobulin test** will detect any immunoglobulin (antibody) that is bound to antigen (RBC) or circulating in the plasma by using a solution of antiimmunoglobulins (Mudge-Grout, 1992). Agglutination or clumping occurs if the RBCs are coated with antibodies or complement. The greater the quantity of antibodies against the RBCs, the more clumping will occur. Any clumping is read as a positive result using a scale of trace to +4. Coombs test differentiates types of hemolytic anemia and detects immune antibodies (Jennings, 1991).

   a. Direct Coombs test is an antiglobulin test that determines that serum antibodies (IgG) have attached to RBCs but do not result in agglutination (Mudge-Grout, 1992). It is used to detect newborn hemolytic disease, autoimmune processes in newborns and children, or hemolytic transfusion reactions. After transfusion a positive result may indicate an antibody-mediated hemolytic reaction, but a negative result does not rule out such a condition because the transfused RBCs may have been completely destroyed in the recipient's blood stream by the time the sample was drawn. A normal response is negative.

   b. Indirect Coombs test is a type of antibody screening that detects specific serum antibodies (IgG) to RBC antigens that are in the serum but not attached to the RBCs (Mudge-Grout, 1992). It is used to detect IgG positive antibodies in maternal blood and the newborn and is performed prior to RBC transfusions to detect any incompatibilities other than major ABO groups. A normal response is negative.

7. **Detection of antibody and antigens** is accomplished through a variety of in vitro techniques such as immunodiffusion, agglutination, enzyme-linked immunosorbent assay (ELISA), monoclonal antibodies, radioimmunoassay (RIA), and others.

   a. *ELISA:* See use of ELISA in the diagnosis of HIV infection.

   b. *Monoclonal antibodies* are laboratory-produced antibodies for a single "destiny" antigen that are used for prevention, diagnosis, and treatment of graft rejection and graft-vs.-host disease (GvHD).

      • Anti-T-lymphocyte monoclonal antibodies, such as muromoab-CD3 (Orthoclone OKT3), are often given in rejection episodes unresponsive to steroid therapy. Muromonab-CD3 blocks T-lymphocyte function and clears T-lymphocyte infiltrates from graft sites of rejection (Miller, 1995). Muromonab-CD3 may be administered to prevent the child's mature T lymphocytes from rejecting the grafted or transplanted organ. To prevent GvHD in bone marrow transplant patients, the donor marrow

may be incubated with anti-T-lymphocyte monoclonal antibodies before the marrow is infused into the recipient to purge the donor marrow of immunocompetent T cells.

- Monoclonal antibodies can also be used to monitor subsets of T lymphocytes at the site of organ graft to assist in the diagnosis or monitoring of graft rejection (Mahon, 1991; Shaefer and Williams, 1991).
- Monoclonal antibodies are used on serum, urine, sputum, and stool samples (among others) to diagnose infections with microorganisms such as herpes simplex virus, streptococci, *Chlamydia,* and *Pneumocystis carinii.*
- Monoclonal antibodies assist in the identification of cells and tissues (e.g., B- and T-lymphocyte differentiation, or HLA or blood typing) and are used in the diagnosis of various diseases (e.g., cancer, autoimmune disease). Monoclonal antibodies to various tumor antigens or tumor products can be used in vitro to confirm the diagnosis of certain types of cancers. A radioactive tracer can be attached to monoclonal antibodies so that after the monoclonal antibodies are administered, a body scan may reveal where the cancer is located.

C. COAGULATION

1. **Platelet count**
   a. Normal: 150,000 to 400,000/mm^3.
   b. In adults 50,000/mm^3 is adequate for hemostasis.
2. **Bleeding time** is the time needed for a standard skin wound to spontaneously stop bleeding. It is an indicator of platelet function if platelet number is adequate, and it measures primary hemostasis. Bleeding time is sensitive to qualitative defects in platelet function but is nonspecific as to type of defect. A standardized incision is made on a relatively vascular area of the forearm, and the time required for bleeding to stop is measured.
   a. Normal: less than 10 minutes.
   b. Bleeding time is prolonged in thrombocytopenia or abnormal platelet function. It is difficult to interpret in the presence of a low platelet count.
3. **PT:** Assesses the extrinsic coagulation system by measuring factor VII and the common pathway or factors X, V, II (prothrombin), and I (fibrinogen).
   a. Normal: Control is usually 12 to 15 seconds (normal controls are established by the individual laboratory).
   b. PT is prolonged with oral anticoagulants, DIC, liver disease, long-term use of antibiotics, vitamin K deficiency, and phenytoin.
4. **Activated partial thromboplastin time (aPTT)** assesses the intrinsic coagulation system by measuring the kinins; factors VIII, IX, XI, and XII; and the common pathway (II, V, X). aPTT measures the time needed for a fibrin clot to form after an activating agent (calcium) and phospholipid have been added to a blood sample and measures factor X related to the intrinsic system. It is used frequently to monitor heparin therapy used during procedures such as continuous renal replacement therapies.
   a. Normal: Usually 25 to 40 seconds (normal controls are established by the individual laboratory).
   b. aPTT is prolonged with heparin therapy, DIC, severe vitamin K deficiency, liver disease, hemophilia A, and von Willebrand's disease.
   c. Any sample with heparin contamination falsely elevates the PTT, thrombin time (TT), and FSPs. Research has questioned the accuracy of using heparinized indwelling catheters for obtaining samples for PTT measurement (Almadrones et al, 1987; Harper, 1988; Kajs, 1986; Laxon and Titler, 1994; Molyneaux, 1987; Pinto, 1994). Venipuncture is a more reliable method

for obtaining accurate values, although accurate samples can be obtained from arterial catheters as follows (not studied for pediatric, systemically heparinized, pulmonary artery, central venous, or Hickman catheters):

- Withdraw a quantity of blood that is a minimum of 6 times the dead space of the catheter or tubing the blood is passing through before collection of 20 ml (Laxon and Titler, 1994). Then draw the sample for coagulation tests.
- Any results in contradiction of the patient's clinical status should result in repeated coagulation tests from a nonheparinized site.

5. **TT** reflects the time for thrombin to convert fibrinogen to fibrin.
   a. Normal: 10 to 15 seconds.
   b. Results are normal in factor VIII deficiencies.
   c. Results are prolonged when coagulation is inadequate owing to decreased thrombin activity, DIC, antithrombin activity such as heparin therapy, insufficient or abnormal fibrinogen, or uremia.

6. **Fibrinogen**
   a. Normal: 200 to 400 mg/dl; only 70 to 100 mg/dl is needed for hemostasis to occur.
   b. Decreased values reflect a risk of bleeding.
   c. Increased values may reflect a hypercoagulable state or inflammatory conditions secondary to activation of plasma enzyme cascades.

7. **FSP** (also called fibrin degradation products [FDP]) is a measure of the fibrinolytic system. FSPs act as anticoagulants that further increase bleeding.
   a. Normal: None; but 1 to 10 μg/ml may be present without impairing coagulation.
   b. Elevated levels indicate activation of fibrinolysis.
   c. Assay for D-dimer (fibrin that has actually crosslinked as part of the clot formation) is a more specific test for DIC in which increased amounts of D-dimer are found in the assay, and an indication of thrombin generation followed by active fibrinolysis is found. It is not detected by assay when primary fibrinolysis is the process, since the fibrinogen has not crosslinked forming the D-dimer.

8. **Specific factor assays** measure amounts of each of the various plasma proteins such as II, V, VII, VIII, and IX.

9. **Activated clotting time (ACT)** is the time it takes a patient's whole blood to clot using a bedside ACT instrument. ACT provides a rapid measurement useful in titrating heparin infusions safely because the ACT responds linearly to changes in heparin levels.
   a. Normal: 90 to 150 seconds.
   b. The goal of heparinization is to have ACT twice the preheparinization measurement. ACTs correlate directly with a patient's aPTT. Blood sample must be fresh, therefore requiring the test to be done at the bedside with fresh whole blood.

D. **BLOOD TYPING**

Over 300 different antigens have been identified against human blood cells, each of which can cause antigen-antibody reactions.

1. **ABO** is one system for typing the antigens for individuals.
   a. There are four blood groups (phenotype). An individual inherits a specific type of blood; each type of blood has a specific antigen makeup with the antibodies described.
      - Group A: Natural anti-B antibodies are present in the plasma.
      - Group B: Natural anti-A antibodies are present in the plasma.

- Group AB: No natural anti-A or anti-B antibodies are present in the plasma.
- Group O: Both natural anti-A and anti-B antibodies are present in the plasma.

b. ABO compatibility is essential for blood transfusion.

2. **Rh system** is a second important blood antigen grouping system involving several other antigens found on RBCs.

   a. The most potent and easy to detect is the Rh D antigen. The absence of the D antigen is termed *Rh negative.* If the Rh D antigen is detected, the blood is termed *Rh positive.*

   b. A person must be first exposed to Rh antigen before a significant reaction will occur. IgG antibodies can develop to the Rh antigens after sensitization by prior transfusion or pregnancy. A transfusion of Rh positive blood to a sensitized Rh negative person can provoke acute hemolysis.

   c. Coombs test is used to determine the presence of IgG antibodies (Rh factor antibodies in an Rh negative person).

3. **Cold agglutinins:** IgM antibodies present in the plasma of some persons can cause RBCs to clump when blood plasma temperature is below normal body temperature. Antibodies react to RBCs regardless of the blood type of donor blood and may lead to circulatory impairment and RBC hemolysis. Screening is done by indirect agglutination tests and actual measurement by the antiglobulin test. Prognosis is good; the reaction is not significant because optimal activation of these antibodies is at 4° C. Reduce reactions by administering blood through a warming system.

E. **RADIOLOGIC EXAMINATION**

1. The **chest x-ray examination** is commonly valuable in detecting and tracking various inflammatory or malignant processes. However, just as other signs and symptoms of infection are masked during neutropenia, the chest x-ray examination also *may* be unreliable in revealing pneumonia in some immunocompromised children. The immune response in the neutropenic child may be so diminished that even in the presence of a fulminant pneumonia the chest x-ray examination may inadequately reflect this process. It has been observed in some neutropenic patients that once the neutrophil count begins to increase to a near-normal level, the chest x-ray results may worsen, revealing the existing pneumonia.

2. **Diagnostic imaging studies** of other areas of the body are indicated by the child's history and physical examination.

F. **BIOPSIES**

1. **Bone marrow:** Aspiration of the fluid bone marrow and needle core biopsy of the bone.

   a. *Purpose:* Histologic and hematologic examination of cellular components of the blood (Mudge-Grout, 1992).

   b. *Technique:* The patient is usually deeply sedated. The preferred site is the posterior iliac crest. If the patient is less than 1 month of age, the preferred site is the tibia.

   c. A *contraindication* is respiratory compromise such that positioning the patient for the procedure would exacerbate the compromise.

   d. *Complications* include bleeding and infection at the site.

   e. Transfusions given just prior to biopsy will not affect bone marrow results.

2. **Lymph node biopsy or excision**

   a. *Purpose:* To evaluate the architectural structure and histologic characteristics.

      b. *Techniques:* The patient is usually under general anesthesia. Areas other than the inguinal area are preferred as less risk for infection. Use the inguinal site only if other sites do not demonstrate enlargement.

      c. *Contraindication:* Bleeding.

      d. *Complications* include bleeding and infection at the site.

G. SKIN TESTING

  1. **Delayed hypersensitivity (DH) skin testing**

      a. *Purpose:* It evaluates CMI function (T-cell responsiveness). DH skin testing is not antibody related. DH skin testing involves the intradermal administration of antigens; if T cells sensitized to that antigen are present, the injection will cause the body to mount an inflammatory response. Since DH response depends on the T lymphocyte's prior exposure to the specific antigen and normal cellular chemotaxis, it is imperative to remember developmental differences in the infant and young child. The child may lack previous exposure to antigens and thus may not recognize the antigen as foreign and may not mount an immune response (Miller, 1977).

      b. *Technique:* DH skin testing is performed with the use of a wide variety of accepted antigens. One or more antigens are injected intradermally with the dermal reaction evaluated at 24, 36, 48, or 72 hours after application. A positive reaction is manifested by induration (hardened swelling), not erythema, and indicates intact CMI. Different diseases yield lesser and greater degrees of induration. The lack of dermal response generally indicates anergy, a lack of CMI, to the antigen. Anergy is associated with immunodeficiency disorders such as AIDS and severe combined immunodeficiency (SCID).

  2. **Immediate hypersensitivity testing:** In contrast to DH skin testing, immediate hypersensitivity testing determines a patient's sensitivity to allergens such as dust, animals, and hair. DH and immediate hypersensitivity skin testing differ in purpose, immune cells involved, antigens used, the technique of administration, and the time in which the tests are read.

RELEVANT PHARMACOLOGY

Numerous medications affect the hematologic and immunologic systems of the body. Mechanisms by which pharmacologic agents *intentionally* affect the hematologic and immunologic systems include those that increase production of cell lines (e.g., CSFs or growth factors) or decrease production or increase destruction of cell lines or entire bone marrow production (e.g., chemotherapeutic agents). Side effects of pharmacologic agents on the hematologic and immunologic systems vary in intensity and range of cells affected (one cell line vs. entire bone marrow function) and can be categorized as expected (e.g., cancer chemotherapy), dose related (e.g., acyclovir), idiosyncratic (e.g., neutropenia resulting from vancomycin), or toxic (e.g., anemia resulting from chloramphenicol).

A. THERAPEUTIC MODALITIES, INCLUDING CSFs (PRODUCED IN RECOMBINANT FORM), THAT ENHANCE THE FUNCTIONS OF THE HEMATOLOGIC AND IMMUNOLOGIC SYSTEMS

  1. **EPO**

      a. *Indications* include physiologic anemia, anemia of prematurity, zidovudine (AZT)-induced anemia, anemia associated with chronic renal failure, or anemia from bone marrow suppression following chemotherapy or medication administration and bone marrow transplant. EPO is useful in other conditions for which transfusions are to be avoided such as those not consenting to transfusions for religious reasons.

b. *Mechanisms of action:* EPO promotes RBC production by stimulating erythroid progenitors, but proliferation of immature progenitors into mature RBCs also requires the presence of IL-3 and GM-CSF. EPO increases hematocrit but requires adequate iron sites.

c. *Side effects* are generally well tolerated.
   - Uncommon and self-limiting side effects include nausea, vomiting, and flulike syndrome.
   - In adult patients who have had long-term hemodialysis therapy, hypertension and seizures have been reported to be associated with EPO.

2. **Myeloid growth factors:** G-CSF, GM-CSF, and IL-3 (see Table 8–4 and Fig. 8–1)
   a. *Indications* include treatment of neutropenia related to bone marrow transplantation or standard-dose chemotherapy. These growth factors are also currently being evaluated for use in primary neutropenia such as in congenital neutropenia (Kostmann's syndrome) or neutropenia secondary to bone marrow failure such as in aplastic anemia, lymphoproliferative disease, bone marrow infiltration, or AIDS (Blackwell and Crawford, 1992).
   b. *Mechanism of action:* Growth factors stimulate maturation of myeloid precursors.
      - G-CSF effects are more specific than those of GM-CSF and IL-3, as G-CSF produces an increase in the neutrophil count without affecting monocytes or eosinophils. Other activities of G-CSF include the increase of neutrophil phagocytosis and the enhancement of EPO activity.
      - GM-CSF is multipotent or has the potential to differentiate several cell lineages including granulocytes, monocytes, and eosinophils. Other biologic activities include the induction of mature neutrophils and monocytes to increase phagocytosis, antibody-dependent cytotoxicity, and enhanced monocyte tumor necrosis factor.
      - IL-3 is multipotent or has the potential to differentiate several cell lineages including granulocytes, monocytes, and erythroid and megakaryocyte precursors. IL-3 also supports mast cell growth.
   c. The most common *side effect* is a flulike syndrome including low-grade fever, bone pain, chills and rigor, myalgias, and headache. The severity of symptoms is variable and is influenced by the dose, route of administration, and schedule. Symptoms are reversible once the agent is discontinued and recovery time is variable ranging from days to several weeks (Woolery-Antill and Colter, 1993).

3. Megakaryocyte colony-stimulating factor, also called thrombopoietin, presently is not available for clinical use. It appears to increase the precursors for platelets in vitro.

B. **THERAPEUTIC MODALITIES THAT DEPRESS THE FUNCTIONS OF THE HEMATOLOGIC AND IMMUNOLOGIC SYSTEMS**
   1. Marrow suppressive agents given for another purpose that suppress RBC and WBC production and activity.
      a. *Chemotherapeutic agents*
         - Indications include cancer and immunologically mediated diseases such as rheumatoid arthritis.
         - Mechanisms of action: Chemotherapeutic agents interfere with the normal cycle of the cell replication, especially affecting cells with short life spans or in a constant state of reproduction such as blood cells, hair cells, and cells lining the GI tract.
         - Hematologic side effects involve failure of the bone marrow to develop the cell line. Such aplasia is dose dependent and usually reversible.

b. *Antibiotics, antivirals, and antiretrovirals*
- Chloramphenicol (Chloromycetin)
  - Indications include infection from a wide variety of bacteria including gram-positive, gram-negative, aerobic, and anaerobic organisms; and from spirochetes, rickettsiae, *Chlamydia,* and mycoplasmas. Chloramphenicol crosses the blood-brain barrier and is particularly effective in central nervous system (CNS) infections caused by susceptible organisms. Newer cephalosporins, however, have largely replaced chloramphenicol for *H. influenzae* meningitis.
  - Mechanism of action is through inhibition of bacterial protein synthesis. It is usually bacteriostatic but can be bacteriocidal against common meningeal pathogens *(H. influenzae, N. meningitidis, S. pneumoniae).*
  - Hematologic side effects are dose related and idiosyncratic (e.g., aplastic anemia) (Steele and Kearns, 1989). Reversible suppression, which primarily is characterized by anemia (with or without thrombocytopenia and leukopenia), is *dose related.* It is more likely to occur in patients receiving large doses, prolonged therapy, or serum concentrations ≥ 25 µg/ml. It is more common than aplastic anemia and is reversible within 1 to 3 weeks after the drug is discontinued. *Bone marrow aplasia* is rare, *idiosyncratic* and frequently fatal. It is not dose related and occurs weeks to months after the drug is discontinued. The mechanism of action is unknown.
- Trimethoprim-sulfamethoxazole (TMP-SMZ, Bactrim, Septra)
  - Indications include *P. carinii* pneumonia (PCP) prophylaxis and treatment.
  - Mechanisms of action: TMP-SMZ interrupts thymidine synthesis by inhibiting sequential enzymatic processes. These two folate antagonists are combined for synergism. Most bacteria are more susceptible to the combination of agents than to either agent used alone. Individual agents at therapeutic levels are bacteriostatic, but the combination is usually bacteriocidal.
  - Side effects: Most common are rash (secondary to a hypersensitivity to the sulfonamide component), fever, nausea and vomiting, and neutropenia. Less common are thrombocytopenia, hepatitis, azotemia, bone marrow aplasia, and hemolytic anemia (secondary to hypersensitivity and G6PD deficiency). Discontinuation of medication is associated with complete resolution of neutropenia.
- Zidovudine (previously known as azidothymidine, AZT) (see HIV/AIDS section) was the first licensed antiretroviral drug for HIV infection.
  - Mechanisms of action: Zidovudine, a reverse transcriptase inhibitor, belongs to a family of compounds called dideoxynucleosides and acts by terminating the growth of the DNA chain produced by the viral RNA template. Other dideoxynucleosides have been tested in clinical trials with children (e.g., didanosine or ddI, zalcitabine or ddC, stavudine, lamivudine) and have less hematologic toxicity than zidovudine.
  - Hematologic side effects involve anemia, neutropenia, and thrombocytopenia.
- Ganciclovir
  - Indications include CMV in the immunosuppressed patient.
  - Mechanisms of action: Ganciclovir is a derivative of acyclovir that belongs to a class of agents called purine nucleosides. This purine analog acts by incorporation into nucleic acids of DNA or RNA. This leads to abnormal transcription and translation and the loss of viral infectivity.

      ○ Hematologic side effects: Neutropenia is common and appears to be related to the dose and duration of therapy. Thrombocytopenia is less common.

2. Marrow suppressive agents given to suppress one or more types of WBCs (therapeutic immunosuppression) that have dose-related effects leading to an increased risk of infection.

    a. *Corticosteroids*

       • Indications include malignancies, treatment of acute or chronic GvHD, and prevention of rejection of transplanted tissue. As an antiinflammatory agent, its use in HIV-infected children with PCP or in children with lymphocytic interstitial pneumonitis (LIP) is under investigation. In adult patients a tapering course of prednisone decreases the risk of pulmonary deterioration (e.g., hypoxemia, ventilatory failure; National Institutes of Health and University of California, 1990). In bacterial meningitis, dexamethasone administered prior to and up to several hours after the initial antibiotic dose may decrease neurologic sequelae. Corticosteroids do not reduce hemolysis in transfusion reactions, but ameliorate drug-induced hemolysis. In ITP corticosteroids are thought to act by inhibiting the phagocytosis of antibody-associated coated platelets, thus increasing platelet life span.

       • Mechanisms of action: Corticosteroids alleviate temporary lymphocytopenia and reduce the migration of neutrophils and monocytes to sites of inflammation. Other actions include decreasing the number of cells available to participate in the inflammatory response, stabilizing the vascular beds, thus inhibiting the movement of cells from the vascular space to the tissues, and reducing the functional capabilities of immunologically active cells. Corticosteroids increase neutrophil count secondary to mature neutrophil release from the bone marrow and a decrease of movement of the neutrophils from the blood to the tissues.

       • Side effects include hyperglycemia, hypertension, sodium and water retention, depression and sleep disturbances, and delayed wound healing.

    b. *Cyclosporine A (CSA)*

       • Indications include the prevention and treatment of GvHD and the prevention of rejection of transplanted tissue.

       • Mechanisms of action: CSA depresses the body's natural response to "non-self" tissue. The exact mechanism is not fully known, but it inhibits the production and activation of the cytotoxic T lymphocytes. Once T cells are activated, however, CSA cannot suppress T-cell proliferation. Thus, CSA works well at preventing but not treating rejection of transplanted tissues. CSA inhibits macrophage release but has little effect on function of B lymphocytes or T suppressor cells and antibody production.

       • Administration: CSA is given intravenously or orally. Absorption of oral preparations is unpredictable and incomplete. Continuous infusion is less toxic than short infusions. It is often given in combination with steroids.

       • Side effects include nephrotoxicity, hypertension, hepatotoxicity, neurologic disturbances (seizures), hirsutism, and gingival hypertrophy.

    c. *Azathioprine (AZA) (Imuran)*

       • Indications include prevention of acute rejection of transplanted tissues and treatment of rejection (less effective than as a preventive agent).

       • Mechanisms of action: AZA blocks RNA and DNA synthesis, thus preventing cytotoxic T-cell proliferation and antibody production. It inhibits promyelocyte proliferation within the bone marrow.

       • Side effects include GI tract disturbances (nausea, vomiting, anorexia, diarrhea), fever, hepatotoxicity, increased risk of other cancers, and thrombocytopenia.

- Special considerations: Serious drug interactions can occur with allopurinol (Zyloprim); therefore, a reduced dose of AZA is recommended.

d. *Antilymphocyte preparations*

- Production: Purified polyclonal immune globulins derived from horses are injected with human thymus or lymphoid cells. Antibodies are formed against these cells and accumulate in the animal's serum. Extraction of the antibodies from the animal's serum is done followed by purification to yield the immune globulin.
- Indications include prevention or treatment of acute rejection of transplanted tissue, prevention and treatment of GvHD following bone marrow transplantation, and aplastic anemia.
- Mechanisms of action: A purified, concentrated, and sterile γ-globulin (primarily IgG) reduces the number of circulating lymphocytes, making them susceptible to phagocytosis by macrophages.
- Currently two preparations are approved for use in the United States:
  - Antilymphocyte globulin (mALG), a lymphocyte-selective immunosuppressant, is available only for investigational use.
  - Antithymocyte globulin (ATGAM), also known as lymphocyte immune globulin, is produced from the serum of horses immunized with human thymus lymphocytes. Theoretically it is more specific than mALG because it is directed toward thymocytes only. It reduces the number of circulating, thymus-dependent lymphocytes.
- Side effects of ATGAM and mALG include fever, chills, anemia, thrombocytopenia, skin reactions (rash, pruritus, urticaria, wheal), and serum sickness–like symptoms (dyspnea; arthralgia; chest, back, and flank pain; diarrhea; nausea and vomiting). Anaphylaxis is uncommon but may occur at any time during therapy. Observe the child continuously for possible allergic reactions throughout the infusion. Consider preinfusion treatment with an antipyretic, antihistamine, or steroid. An intradermal skin test before administration to rule out serious allergic reactions is recommended. The patient may require ATGAM desensitization if the patient has positive results from a skin test. Other effects may include reactivation of CMV, herpes simplex virus, or EBV or antigen- or antibody-induced glomerulonephritis.

e. *Monoclonal antibodies: Muromonab-CD3 (Orthoclone OKT3)*

- Production: Monoclonal antibodies are made from mouse cells and are derived from a single antibody-producing clone (vs. mALG or ATGAM, which are polyclonal in origin), which provides less variability between lots of drug. They are more selective in action than immune globulins.
- Indications include rejection of transplanted tissues unresponsive to steroids and prevention of rejection of transplanted tissues.
- Mechanisms of action: Monoclonal antibodies bind to mature T lymphocytes, leading to T-cell depletion, and have no direct effect on B lymphocytes or antibody production.
- Side effects include influenza-like symptoms (fever, chills, tremors, headache, nausea, vomiting, diarrhea), dyspnea, pulmonary edema, or anaphylaxis. Consider preinfusion treatment with an antihistamine or steroid. They may reactivate CMV and herpes simplex infections 2 to 3 weeks after therapy.

3. **Platelet suppressive agents** given for another purpose that result in the suppression of platelet activity

a. *Aspirin*
  - Indications include the desire for antipyretic, antiinflammatory, and analgesic actions.
  - Mechanisms of action: ASA inhibits platelet aggregation. It inhibits thromboxane A_2 for the life of an exposed platelet (7 to 10 days). Effects do not disappear with drug clearance. ASA also inhibits prostacyclin.
  - Hematologic side effects include the prolongation of bleeding time to 1 to 3 times the normal. If aspirin is given to those with liver disease or to those receiving anticoagulant therapy, the effects are greatly amplified.

b. *NSAIDs* (such as *ibuprofen and naproxen)*
  - Indications include the desire for antiinflammatory, analgesic, and antipyretic actions.
  - Mechanism of action involves a decrease in function of platelets, which is reversible on the affected platelet when the NSAID is eliminated from the blood.
  - Hematologic side effects include prolonged bleeding time.

4. **Agents affecting plasma clotting factors**
  a. *Heparin* is an anticoagulant made from porcine intestinal mucosa or bovine lung.
    - Indications include deep vein thrombosis, pulmonary embolism, mural thrombosis, and minimization of clotting during cardiopulmonary bypass surgery, hemodialysis or hemofiltration, cardiac catheterization, or hemodynamic monitoring. Heparin may also be used for selected causes of DIC such as acute promyelocytic leukemia and to maintain patency of vascular access devices such as Hickman lines.
    - Mechanisms of action: Heparin inhibits clot formation but has no effect on formed clots. It dramatically accelerates the body's own anticoagulant mechanism, particularly that which is provided by antithrombin III (enhances the inactivation of thrombin II, inhibits X). Heparin promotes the destruction of factor X and has a direct inhibitory effect on factors IX and X and thrombin. It also interferes with in vitro platelet aggregation, increases plasminogen activation levels (thereby promoting fibrinolysis), and inhibits thrombin.
    - For acute thrombosis, continuous IV infusion is preferred. Titrate to maintain the PTT or ACT 1.5 to 2 times the normal. After acute anticoagulation is achieved, initiate oral therapy with warfarin (Coumadin); however, continue the heparin for the first 3 to 5 days of warfarin therapy.
    - Side effects are reversed with protamine sulfate, which binds heparin to a complex that lacks anticoagulant activity. Bleeding occurs, especially with those children who have deficiencies of coagulation factors such as hemophilia or those with liver disease, platelet dysfunction syndromes (such as with aspirin therapy), peptic ulcer disease, and severe hypertension. Heparin-induced thrombocytopenia is a process not fully understood. It usually occurs after 1 or more weeks of heparin therapy. Occurrence is not dose dependent or related to the method of administration (can be seen with IV bolus or low-dose subcutaneous methods or with small amounts given to flush IV lines). It is more common with bovine-origin heparin. Serious bleeding is not common but may be life threatening.
  b. *Warfarin (Coumadin)* is an anticoagulant.
    - Indications include chronic anticoagulant therapy such as long-term treatment of deep venous thrombosis and prevention of intracardiac clot

formations associated with decreased wall motion such as chronic atrial fibrillation.

- Mechanisms of action: Warfarin inhibits the liver's activation of factor VII, followed by depression of factors II, IX, and X. It also increases plasma antithrombin III levels. Effectiveness is dependent on absorption from the GI tract, vitamin K status of the patient, and rate of hepatic metabolism of warfarin.
- Administration: The oral route is used. Titrate to maintain the PT at 1.5 to 2 times the normal (control). Some centers use the international normalized ratio (INR) to provide a more consistent relationship between the patient's PT and the control between institutions. Titrate the INR to the 1 to 3 range. Warfarin must be given for 5 to 7 days, overlapping with heparin when necessary, before adequate anticoagulation is assumed.
- Side effects: Minor to life-threatening GI tract bleeding may occur. Side effects are reversed with vitamin K. Many drug interactions are possible, resulting in excessive anticoagulation; therefore, the nurse should consult with the pharmacist about any possible drug interactions before administration of warfarin.

c. *Fibrinolytic agents:* Drugs that break up clots (fibrin)
- Indications include great vein, atrial, arterial, and renal vein thromboses; occlusion of grafts; superior vena cava syndrome; and obstruction of vascular access devices such as central lines.
- Mechanisms of action: Fibrinolytic agents promote conversion of plasminogen into plasmin and induce systemic fibrinolysis. Plasmin is a proteolytic enzyme that reacts with proteins other than fibrin being lysed.
- Specific agents
  - Streptokinase, a biologic product of certain strains of streptococci, is antigenic in nature. Over time, antibodies will neutralize it, necessitating larger doses.
  - Urokinase, initially isolated from urine and fetal kidney cells, is now produced using recombinant DNA technology and is not antigenic. This enzyme directly activates plasminogen. It has a lower incidence of allergic reactions than streptokinase.
  - tPA will not activate plasminogen in the absence of fibrin. Concurrent heparin or antiplatelet therapy is sometimes given. It has the advantage of relatively selectively activating only the plasminogen bound to fibrin.
- Administration: Monitor fibrinogen levels.
- Side effects: Bleeding from lysing other existing clots increases the risk of use in children who have had major surgery within the preceding 10 days, a biopsy in an inaccessible site, intracranial bleeding, or active bleeding, especially from the GI tract. As with heparin, risks of bleeding must be weighed against the risks of the thrombosis. Effects can be reversed with the administration of fresh frozen plasma (FFP).

BLOOD COMPONENT THERAPY

A. RED BLOOD CELLS
1. **Whole blood**
   a. *Volume:* About 500 ml/U
   b. *Contents:* RBCs and plasma components; however, the WBCs, platelets, and

labile coagulation factors (V and VIII) are only viable if given without any refrigeration time.

c. *Indications:* Whole blood replaces whole blood losses such as in patients with hemorrhagic shock who require volume expansion and oxygen-carrying capacity. Whole blood is rarely administered except for exchange transfusions and priming tubing for cardiovascular bypass or continuous renal replacement therapies (CRRT). It is physiologically reasonable and more cost effective to separate each unit of donated blood into components that can be used to treat as many as five different recipients.

d. *Considerations:* The blood must be ABO and Rh compatible (Table 8–7). Whole blood, 6 ml/kg of body weight, increases the hemoglobin by 1 g/dl. In adolescents given whole units of blood (500 ml), 1 U increases the hemoglobin by 1 g/dl and the hematocrit by 3% to 5%. Begin the infusion slowly (no more than 2 ml/min) and stay with the patient for the first 15 minutes. Infuse the transfusion over 2 to 4 hours for slow replacement; infuse as rapidly as possible in shock states.

e. *Advantages:* Whole blood replaces RBCs and plasma and provides a source of proteins with oncotic properties.

f. *Limitations:* The volume required to raise hemoglobin and hematocrit may not be well tolerated in infants and young children. Infusion time can be long. There is a potential for transmission of disease (CMV, hepatitis B and C, HIV, and other blood-borne infections). Usually component therapy for specific indications is better than whole blood.

2. **Packed RBCs**

   a. *Volume:* 200 to 350 ml/U (120 to 180 ml of RBCs and 70 to 100 ml of plasma)

   b. *Contents:* RBCs and a small amount of plasma

   c. *Indications:* RBCs improve oxygen-carrying capacity and are useful as a volume expander after acute blood loss when it is difficult to assess the rate of volume depletion. RBCs are used in symptomatic anemia, slow blood loss when hemoglobin is less than 8 g/dl, and congestive heart failure because the volume of whole blood would not be well tolerated.

   d. *Considerations:* RBCs must be ABO and Rh compatible; O negative unmatched blood may be used for infants up to 4 months of age. Packed RBCs, 3 ml/kg of body weight, increase the hemoglobin by 1 g/dl, and 10 ml/kg of body weight increases the hematocrit by 10%. In adolescents given whole units of packed RBCs, 1 U increases the hemoglobin by 1 g/dl and the hematocrit by 3% to 5%. A usual transfusion is calculated to give 10 ml/kg; volume should not exceed 15 ml/kg; for hemorrhagic shock, rates and volumes must be higher.

Table 8–7. RED CELL COMPATIBILITY

RECIPIENT	DONOR
A	A, O
B	B, O
AB	AB, A, B, O
O	O
Rh+	Rh+ or −
Rh−	Rh−
Undetermined	O−

Adapted from Pavel JD, Lowe CR. Transfusion therapy guidelines for nurses. Monrovia, Md: Department of Transfusion Medicine, Clinical Center, National Institutes of Health. 1990.

- The rate of transfusion is usually 5 ml/kg/h (2 ml/kg/h if the child has cardiac dysfunction or severe anemia). If the transfusion will take longer than 4 hours, the unit should be divided into smaller aliquots and administered serially.
- In situations requiring transfusion before crossmatching can be complete, transfuse with type O Rh negative blood or group type specific blood (if time to determine the blood type of the patient) to greatly minimize the risk of a significant transfusion reaction.
- Leukocyte (WBC)-poor RBCs are produced by filtration of the blood with a special leukocyte-reduction filter in the blood bank or at the bedside. It reduces the number of WBCs in a unit from 5×10^9 to less than 5×10^6 and will decrease the likelihood of febrile reactions, the development of anti-WBC antibodies, and the transmission of CMV. However, they require more preparation time, add cost to the product, and result in some RBC loss; and if WBC-poor RBCs are filtered at the bedside, the infusion rate cannot be rapid through the special filter.

   e. *Advantages:* RBCs increase hemoglobin and hematocrit faster than whole blood and with less risk of hypervolemia.

   f. *Limitations:* RBCs are viscous; therefore, the rate of the infusion may be limited by the size of the IV catheter.

B. WHITE BLOOD CELLS

1. **Granulocyte transfusion**

   a. *Volume:* 200 to 500 ml/U.

   b. *Contents:* WBCs are obtained through leukopheresis and separated from other blood constituents. For infants, enough WBCs may be obtained from a unit of whole blood. A minimum of 1×10^{10} granulocytes, less than 10% of lymphocytes, and a variable amount of RBCs, platelets, and plasma are required.

   c. *Indications:* WBCs are used only as an adjunct to other measures for the containment of infections in high-risk patients or for sepsis in neonates. General pediatric indications include the presence of severe acquired neutropenia or congenital white cell dysfunction, proven bacterial infection in a neutropenic patient, *and* failure to respond to appropriate antibiotic treatment.

   d. *Considerations:* Premedication 1 hour prior to transfusion is commonly used to lessen or prevent side effects or reactions and may include antihistamines, acetaminophen, steroids, or meperidine. Infuse WBCs as soon as the transfusion is available. Granulocytes have a short survival time. (Optimal time period is to give within 10 hours; maximum storage period is 24 hours.)

- Dose and administration: The average pediatric dose is 10 to 15 ml/kg, usually given daily for at least 4 days (Foley, 1993). Infuse slowly over 2 to 4 hours. Use with a routine 170 μm blood filter; never use a microaggregate (Foley, 1993) or leukocyte-depleting filter. Precede and follow the transfusion with *only* 0.9% sodium chloride.
- Observe the child closely for granulocyte transfusion reactions. Febrile reaction is common and includes chills and a rise in temperature, usually less than 40° C. Premedications may need to be supplemented with additional doses. Severe pulmonary reactions may be seen and are thought to be due to the accumulation of granulocytes in the pulmonary capillaries and the activation of complement. Reactions may be minimized with slow infusion rates, premedication and supplementation of premedications, and serologically compatible donors.

- No increase to a minimal increase in the circulating WBC count is observed following granulocyte transfusion.
- **Do not administer amphotericin B and granulocyte transfusion at the same time.** Concurrent administration of amphotericin B and granulocytes has been associated with an acute onset of severe pulmonary insufficiency. Although there is no national standard, it is recommended that there be 4 to 12 hours between amphotericin B and granulocyte transfusions.

   e. *Advantages:* Neutropenia is an important predisposing factor to infection, especially in the child who has received a transplant or has cancer. Granulocyte transfusions are *thought* to decrease this risk by providing additional granulocytes, although this remains unproven. If the patient is also thrombocytopenic, platelets found in the average granulocyte transfusion may also be therapeutic. Successful granulocyte transfusions may lead to a more localized pyogenic reaction than was previously possible. This may be accompanied by radiologic evidence of pulmonary consolidation, if the etiology of the patient's infection was pulmonary.

   f. *Limitations:* The incidence of febrile, nonhemolytic reactions is increased. Improvement in clinical condition or the resolution of infection is the only measure of granulocyte transfusion effectiveness. Long-term therapeutic benefit of granulocyte transfusions in patients with congenital white cell dysfunction remains questionable and continues to be evaluated.

2. **Intravenous immunoglobulin (IVIG)**

   a. *Volume:* Varies with preparation and prescribed dose.

   b. *Contents:* Made from pools of plasma from at least 1000 donors, but usually between 3000 to 10,000 donors. Ninety to ninety-five percent of content is IgG. Small quantities of IgA, IgM, IgD, IgE, and other proteins are also present. Nine preparations are currently available in the United States. Each preparation varies in mode of preparation, use of additives, IgA content, and pH level:
      - Preparations with the lowest IgA content are Iveegam (Immuno) with 2 µg/ml of IgA and Gammagard (Hyland) with less than 10 µg/ml of IgA content.
      - Preparations with highest IgA content include Gamimune N (Cutter Biologicals) with 270 µg/ml of IgA and Sandoglobulin (Sandoz) with 720 µg/ml of IgA.

   c. *Indications:* IVIG primarily is indicated in antibody deficiency disorders, both congenital and acquired. Generally it serves as replacement therapy, enhances humoral immunity, and has a half-life of approximately 21 days.
      - In severe bacterial infections in premature and newborn infants, the rationale for use of IVIG is based on the child's increased risk of infection, incomplete acquisition of maternal antibodies, immature phagocyte and complement systems, and physiologic hypogammaglobulinemia (Suez, 1995). Some studies indicate the therapeutic value in high-risk, low-birth-weight infants; however, this has not been proven in all infants or all studies (Baker et al, 1992; Clapp et al, 1989; Fanaroff et al, 1992).
      - In some patients following transplantation, the use of IVIG has been found to decrease the incidence of bacterial, viral, and fungal infections (Suez, 1995). In particular, studies indicate that IVIG is effective in the prevention of CMV infections in bone marrow transplant recipients (Gale and Winston, 1991; Kubanek et al, 1985; Winston et al, 1987).
      - Children with HIV infection display an increase in immunoglobulins

with a concomitant depressed production of antibody to specific antigens, increasing the risk of recurrent bacterial infections. IVIG has been shown to decrease the frequency of infections and to improve various immune functions and survival in infants with AIDS (Calvelli and Rubenstein, 1986; Oleske et al, 1986).

- The efficacy of IVIG varies greatly in immunoregulatory disorders such as ITP and Kawasaki syndrome. The mechanism of action of IVIG in these instances is not fully understood.
- IVIG is used as respiratory syncytial virus (RSV) *prophylaxis* for certain high-risk groups of children (e.g., infants younger than 24 months old with bronchopulmonary dysplasia and infants born at less than 35 weeks' gestation) (Groothuis, 1994; Groothuis et al, 1995).

    d. *Considerations:* The usual transfusion varies with the indication for administration. IVIG is considered a blood product; therefore, administration guidelines and vital sign monitoring should be performed similarly as with traditional blood products. Obtain vital signs every 15 minutes twice after beginning the infusion.

- Rate of administration: Infusion rate guidelines vary among the manufacturers because of the differences in concentrations of IVIG. The most common recommendation is to infuse slowly for the first 15 to 30 minutes and then gradually increase to a maximum rate, as patient tolerates.
- Untoward reactions occur in approximately 10% to 15% of IVIG infusions. Most frequently side effects are caused by an interaction between antibodies in the IVIG preparations with antigens present in the patient at the time of the IVIG infusion resulting in the formation of immune complexes and the activation of complement (Suez, 1995). Reactions are *usually* mild, self-limiting, and are not considered anaphylactic. Symptoms include tachycardia, elevated blood pressure, flushing, fever, chills, dizziness, headache, nausea, abdominal pain, and muscle aches. Reactions are usually related to the rate of administration with symptoms managed by either slowing the rate or stopping the infusion for a brief period of time or by pretreatment such as steroids (Suez, 1995). Febrile reactions are attributed to impurities in the IVIG preparation (Camp-Sorrell and Wujcik, 1994).
- Anaphylactic reactions occur in patients with anti-IgA antibodies with reactions mediated by IgE antibodies to IgA. Anaphylactic reactions occur in patients with no detectable serum IgA (IgA < 5 mg/dl) (Suez, 1995). For these patients, screen for the presence of IgE anti-IgA antibodies and administer preparations with lower concentrations of IgA. For symptoms of anaphylaxis, IVIG therapy should be discontinued and treatment for anaphylaxis given.

    e. *Advantages:* Donors are screened for hepatitis A, B, and C and antibodies to HIV to reduce disease transmission, although the risk is never completely eliminated.

    f. *Limitations:* Some preparations and prescribed doses require a large volume of fluid administration. Note signs and symptoms of fluid overload.

C. COAGULATION COMPONENTS

  1. **Platelet concentrate**

    a. *Volume:* 50 to 75 ml for random donor units and 200 to 300 ml for pheresed units. If volume overload is a concern, the volume can be reduced, but it also decreases the quantity of the platelets in the unit.

    b. *Contents:* Random-donor platelets (also called pooled platelets) are obtained from multiple individual units (4 to 10) of whole blood. Platelets are separated from other components by centrifugation and suspended in a small amount of plasma. Single-donor platelets are obtained by platelet-pheresis from one donor. Whole blood is removed from a donor; platelets are separated from the other components; and the rest of the blood except the platelets and some plasma is reinfused into the donor. Platelets have a short (5 days) shelf-life. Pheresed single-donor platelets (HLA matched) may be given to improve transfusion effectiveness for those patients whose platelet count does not rise after they have been given pooled platelets.

c. *Indications:* Clinical judgment must be used; transfusions are usually limited to patients with an absolute platelet count of less than 10,000 to 20,000/mm^3 or patients who have a platelet count of less than 50,000/mm^3 when bleeding is present or major surgery is anticipated

- Patients with abnormal platelet function or production are more likely to be transfused if their platelet count is less than 50,000/mm^3. However, if the platelet count is 20,000 to 30,000/mm^3, transfusions may be held if the bone marrow biopsy indicates it is recovering with the presence of young, large, sticky platelets. Also, patients with CNS bleeding, brain tumor, liver disease, or uremia and patients taking medications that affect platelet function are more likely to be transfused. Generally, prophylactic transfusions for platelet counts higher than 20,000/mm^3 is not advocated; however, preprocedure platelet transfusion may be considered for patients about to have an invasive procedure with risk of significant bleeding.

d. *Considerations:* ABO and Rh compatibility are preferred; Rh sensitivity is especially important in an Rh-negative female because Rh antigen sensitization could affect an Rh positive fetus in a future pregnancy.

- The posttransfusion platelet count depends on the size of the patient, number of platelets per bag, and clinical factors. In general, 1 U of random donor platelets for every 7 to 10 kg body weight or 1 U of pheresed platelets for every 90 kg should increase the platelet count by 50,000/mm^3. However, if the patient is bleeding or having a process in which platelets are consumed, the increase can be less than predicted.
- Use a standard 170-µm filter for administration. Give by direct push or infusion as fast as the patient can tolerate (usually over 20 to 30 minutes) to provide the optimal level of circulating platelets. Premedicate with acetaminophen or diphenhydramine (Benadryl) to reduce symptoms of febrile reactions and allergic reactions.
- There is a less effective response or increase in platelet count if the patient is febrile; has ongoing oozing or bleeding; has an infection, splenomegaly, or DIC; or is receiving antibiotics or other drugs that may reduce platelet function. More platelet transfusions will be needed to raise the platelet count in the presence of peripheral destruction of platelets.
- ABO antigens are present on platelets; conflicting data exist concerning the survival and effects of transfusing ABO-incompatible platelets. Although processing of platelets involves separating the platelets from the other blood components, RBCs are present in platelet concentrates. Transfusion of platelets from Rh-positive donors can lead to Rh sensitization in Rh-negative recipients. If Rh-positive platelets are administered to Rh-negative females, Rh immunoglobulin (RhoGAM) should be administered to prevent sensitization and future hemolytic reactions. If ABO-incompatible platelets are to be transfused, the volume may be reduced to 100 ml or less; however, the product must be transfused as soon as possible following plasma reduction as platelet viability deterio-

rates after storage of units with high platelet counts. Transfusion of ABO-identical platelets improves the transfusion response.

e. *Advantages:* Platelet concentrate raises the platelet count without adding other components. Other blood products do not have sufficient viable platelets to obtain the needed increase in platelet count.

f. *Limitations:* For patients with conditions in which antibodies attach to the platelets such as ITP, transfusions of platelets will not increase the platelet count because they are coated with antibody and are rapidly removed from the circulation by the spleen, sometimes within minutes of the transfusion. Transfusions are thus limited to only the most life-threatening conditions (Table 8–8).

2. **Fresh frozen plasma (FFP)**

a. *Volume:* 200 to 250 ml/U

b. *Contents:* FFP contains all clotting factors except platelets and is frozen to preserve factors V and VIII.

c. *Indications:* FFP is used for known deficiencies of plasma clotting factors when no specific concentrated product is available and for control of bleeding for patients who require replacement of plasma coagulation factors when simultaneous blood volume expansion is required.

d. *Considerations:* Donor's plasma should be ABO compatible with the recipient's RBCs; Rh type need not be considered (Table 8–9). Blood banks usually require confirmation of a clotting factor deficit that cannot be corrected with another product to reduce the patient's exposure to potential blood-borne diseases. Administer 10 to 15 ml/kg for a period of 2 to 3 hours (within 24 hours of thawing the product). Monitor results with PT and aPTT levels.

e. *Advantages:* FFP provides most of the clotting factors not contained in sufficient quantity in whole blood.

f. *Limitations:* Other alternatives such as crystalloids or colloids (i.e., Plasmanate and albumin) are available for volume expansion. For invasive surgical procedures, the volume required to give the clotting factors will be excessive. Studies do not indicate the efficacy of FFP if it is used prophylactically. FFP is not a treatment for deficiencies of factor V and VIII because of low levels in this product. Transmission of hepatitis B and C and HIV infection is possible.

3. **Cryoprecipitate**

a. *Volume:* 10 to 40 ml per bag (usually 25 ml per bag)

b. *Contents:* Factor VIII (70 to 100 U), von Willebrand's factor, and fibrinogen; obtained from FFP after slow thawing

c. *Indications:* Cryoprecipitate is used to control bleeding associated with

Table 8–8. INDICATIONS FOR SPECIFIC PLATELET PRODUCTS

PLATELET PRODUCT	INDICATION
Leukocyte poor	Repeated febrile nonhemolytic transfusion reactions
Washed	Repeated major allergic transfusion reactions or respiratory compromise
Cytomegalovirus (CMV) negative	CMV seronegative allogeneic bone marrow transplant patients
Irradiated	Neonates and severely immunocompromised oncology patients
HLA-matched	Patients who have developed antibodies to tranfused platelets (alloimmunization)

Adapted from Fuller AK. Platelet transfusion therapy for thrombocytopenia. *Semin Oncol Nurs.* 1990;6(2):124.

Table 8–9. PLASMA COMPATIBILITY

RECIPIENT	DONOR
A	A, AB
B	B, AB
AB	AB
O	O, AB, A, B
Undetermined	AB

Adapted from Pavel JD, Lowe CR. Transfusion therapy guidelines for nurses. Monrovia, Md: Department of Transfusion Medicine, Clinical Center, National Institutes of Health. 1990.

congenital or acquired quantitative or qualitative deficiencies of fibrinogen (DIC, significant liver disease), complex coagulation factor deficiencies, hemophilia A (when other noninfectious factor VIII concentrates are not available), and von Willebrand's disease.

d. *Considerations:* ABO compatibility is not required because of the extremely small volume of plasma being transfused. Cryoprecipitate is stored as a frozen product; once it is thawed, administer the product within 4 hours or as rapidly as tolerated. For DIC, usually 1 to 2 bags per 10 kg of body weight are given with additional doses at 8- to 12-hour intervals, based on the measurement of factor VIII levels and the clinical status of the patient. Repeat coagulation measurements are necessary to avoid inappropriate infusions.

e. *Advantage:* Cryoprecipitate can replace these factors without the hypervolemia risked by FFP.

f. *Limitations:* Development of antibodies to factor VIII will result in less effectiveness of the transfused product. Transmission of infections such as HIV and hepatitis B and C can occur. Large doses of cryoprecipitate in a patient with normal fibrinogen may produce elevations of fibrinogen leading to acute thrombosis and DIC.

4. **Factor VIII concentrates** (also known as antihemophilic factor [AHF])

a. *Volume* varies as this is reconstituted prior to administration, as well as differences per lot from the manufacturer.

b. *Contents:* Made from large pools of normal plasma

c. *Indications:* Hemophilia A

d. *Considerations:* The usual dosage is 10 to 50 U/kg; administer 20 U/kg for mild hemorrhage and 40 U/kg for more severe hemorrhage. One unit of factor VIII will raise the level about 2%. No typing or crossmatching is required. The development of anti–factor VIII antibodies or inhibitors may result even with one dose.

e. *Advantages:* Factor VIII provides needed factor using less fluid volume than required by FFP or cryoprecipitate and allows for accurate dose calculations. It is convenient for home use for hemophilia A patients, since it is stable refrigerated for weeks to months and can be rapidly prepared for self-administration.

f. *Limitations:* In the past, transmission of blood-borne infections was significant, as this product is pooled from multiple donors, and no method was known to reduce or inactivate viruses such as HIV or hepatitis B. Currently, the risk of transmission is reduced by the use of virus-inactivation methods such as solvent-detergent and heat treatments and by testing of donor blood to determine that it is hepatitis and HIV-negative. Therefore, factor VIII products are considered safer than FFP or cryoprecipitate. Factor VIII is costly.

D. OTHER

1. **Albumin** is supplied as 5% and 25% solutions.
   a. *Volume:* Various size bottles available
   b. *Contents:* Blood proteins
   c. *Indications:* The 5% solution is used for volume expansion and hypoproteinemia. The 25% solution is used for severe burns and cerebral edema.
   d. *Considerations:* No typing or crossmatching is necessary.
      • Dosage and administration
         ○ 5% solution: 1 g/kg = 20 ml/kg given 1 to 2 ml/min
         ○ 25% solution: 1 g/kg = 4 ml/kg given 0.2 to 0.4 ml/min
      • Use the filter and administration set provided in the package.
      • Preparation of this product eliminates the risk of transmission of infection.

2. **Plasma protein fraction** (Plasmanate)
   a. *Volume:* 250-ml bottles
   b. *Contents:* Albumin plus some globulins
   c. *Indications:* Volume expansion and hypoproteinemia
   d. *Considerations:* No typing or crossmatching is necessary. Dosage is 10 to 15 ml/kg per dose at a rate of 5 to 10 ml/min. Use the filter and administration set provided in the package. Preparation of this product eliminates the risk of transmission of infection.

E. COMPLICATIONS

Be alert for transfusion complications by staying with the patient and infusing slowly during the first 15 minutes of any infusion; begin ordered rate after 15 minutes.

1. **Hemolytic transfusion reactions** occur when donor RBCs and recipient plasma are incompatible (or donor plasma is incompatible with the recipient's RBCs). They are most commonly associated with an ABO mismatch. Antibodies formed by the recipient's plasma attach to antigens on transfused RBCs, causing RBC destruction. Vasoactive chemical mediators are generated and released in response to the immunologic challenge of transfused antigens with subsequent activation of the coagulation system and organ ischemia. Severity of the reaction depends on the antibody titer and the volume of the mismatched blood infused. Acute onset usually occurs when as little as 10 to 15 ml has been transfused. Symptoms may start with subtle signs such as a vague uneasiness.
   a. *Clinical manifestations* of hemolysis include immediate symptoms of fever, chills, headache, severe flank and back pain, substernal tightness and dyspnea, tachypnea, hypotension, and shock, possibly leading to cardiac arrest and death. Early symptoms may be followed by DIC; bleeding from previous sites of trauma, surgery, or venipuncture; oliguria and hemoglobinuria leading to anuria and acute renal failure; hemoglobinemia; and jaundice (which may develop within minutes or hours).
   b. *Management*
      • Recognize the signs of reaction and terminate the transfusion immediately, since severe consequences are less likely if a minimal volume has been given. Maintain venous access with fluids and notify the physician of the incident. Send the blood unit and a sample of the patient's blood to the blood bank for testing and complete a transfusion reaction report. A complete workup requires that a sample taken from the transfused unit confirms that the blood has been mismatched to the recipient.
      • Assess the severity of the reaction. Administer antihistamine for signs of allergic reaction (itching, wheezing, laryngeal edema, rash) to prevent the release of histamine associated with the body's recognition of a foreign protein. Promote urine output with fluids, diuretics, and manni-

tol. Insert a Foley catheter if it is necessary to monitor urine output carefully. Send a urine specimen to the laboratory. Dialysis may be necessary for severe oliguria and anuria. Treat hypotension and shock with fluids and medications. Treat any hemorrhage and continue additional transfusion therapy after approval of the blood bank.

- Delayed hemolytic reactions can occur weeks after a transfusion resulting from past transfusions or pregnancies and patient sensitization to RBC antigens not in the ABO system. Symptoms (many incidences are asymptomatic) include malaise and fever. Shock and renal failure are rare. These antibodies do not activate complement at a rapid rate and tend not to produce acute hemolysis; instead they cause shortened RBC life span and produce extravascular hemolysis. A decreased hematocrit and an increased bilirubin and jaundice may be present.

   c. *Prevention:* Meticulous verification of the patient's identification and specific unit crossmatching via bracelet identification and crosschecking of discrete number identification are essential. When a blood product requiring crossmatching is ordered, assure that the sample of blood for the crossmatch is less than 3 days old.

2. **Febrile reactions** are much more common than hemolytic reactions. However, it is hard to separate symptoms from other causes of fever in critically ill children. They are usually associated with antibodies that agglutinate WBCs or by-products from RBC metabolism or destruction and are most common with previous sensitization by transfusions.

   a. *Clinical manifestations* include fever and chills shortly after the transfusion (which may last up to 12 hours) and tachycardia, hypotension, and tachypnea.

   b. *Management* is supportive. Terminate the transfusion and retest the donor blood to rule out hemolytic transfusion reaction. Send unit and tubing to the blood bank so that bacteriologic cultures of the transfused unit can be prepared. Acetaminophen may be helpful in preventing future reactions. Decrease the incidence by using leukocyte-poor products, washed RBCs and pheresed platelets with the premise that this reaction is due to the presence of WBCs. Prognosis is good, since severe reactions are rare.

3. **Allergic reactions** are reactions by the recipient to substances or plasma proteins in the donor blood. They may occur with only 1 to 2 ml of transfused blood.

   a. *Clinical manifestations* range from mild to severe; however, hemolysis does not occur. Symptoms include urticaria, pruritus, vomiting, hypotension, laryngeal edema, and anaphylaxis.

   b. *Management:* Discontinue the transfusion temporarily. Administer an antihistamine such as diphenhydramine (Benadryl). If the antihistamine was effective and the reaction was mild, the blood product may be restarted after 20 to 30 minutes. For recurrences, give antihistamines 30 minutes prior to each transfusion prophylactically. If bronchospasm or other life-threatening symptoms occur, discontinue the unit and treat with epinephrine and antihistamines. Future transfusions may require administration of steroids.

4. **Bacterial contamination** is a rare complication since modern blood banking practices use closed blood collecting systems that guard effectively against bacterial contamination and donors are screened for a recent history of fever, dental work, or other signs of infection. It is more likely for products that require thawing in a water bath or those stored at room temperature such as platelets.

   a. *Clinical manifestations* occur within 30 minutes of initiation of the transfusion. This diagnosis is suspected when the patient develops shaking chills, fever, vomiting, diffuse erythema, hypotension, and shock shortly after transfusion begins, followed by hemoglobinuria, renal failure, and DIC. Contamination is confirmed by prompt Gram staining of the residual blood in the blood bag. Also, culturing the blood bag and filter may provide further evidence of the specific organism.

   b. *Management:* Stop infusion immediately and send samples of patient's blood and the blood product to the laboratory for bacterial culture. Provide supportive therapy such as broad-spectrum antibiotics, fluids, and vaso-pressors.

5. **Transmission of infections** is greatest with paid donors, multiple transfusions, and pooled plasma fractions. Mandatory screening of donor blood for hepatitis (B and C), HIV, and CMV before it is transfused decreases the risk.

   a. *Risk of hepatitis (B and C) infection:*
   - Hepatitis B: $1:200,000/U$ of transfused product
   - Hepatitis C: $1:2000$ to $1:6000/U$ of transfused product
   - Cases of hepatitis vary in severity and may be fatal or result in chronic liver disease.

   b. *Risk of HIV infection:* $1:225,000/U$ of transfused product (Statistic was obtained before implementation of HIV screening tests of significantly increased sensitivity became the standard; therefore, this infection rate may be too high.)
   - All blood banks screen products for HIV antibody and antigen; however, the virus (antigen) may be present in the donor's blood for 25 days before antibodies are detectable. Risk of infection is also decreased by screening the donors for lifestyles associated with HIV infection.

   c. *Risk of CMV infection* is decreased if patients are given products not containing WBCs.
   - Approximately 50% of donors are CMV antibody–positive, indicating a prior or current CMV infection (ranges from 10% to 90% depending on the region of the country). The virus may persist in the WBCs, leading to a carrier state despite the presence of antibody; for this reason blood from antibody-negative donors is less likely to transmit CMV.
   - Clinical symptoms range from mild febrile illness to extensive disseminated disease resulting in death, particularly in immunocompromised patients.
   - If possible, transfuse very high risk CMV-negative patients (i.e., after bone marrow transplant) with CMV antibody–negative blood. If the patient is CMV antibody–positive, no additional benefit will occur by transfusing CMV antibody–negative blood. Irradiation does not prevent CMV transmission from the donor to the recipient.

6. **Alloimmunization** occurs when the recipient develops antibodies to transfused RBCs, WBCs, plasma, and platelets (especially from multiple donors).

   a. Antibodies against foreign antigens found on the cell membrane of transfused blood can result in rapid destruction of transfused cells that have these antigens. It is usually not life threatening, and it does not cause immediate symptoms on initial exposure. To lessen the reaction, further screening for specific antigens must be done to provide donor blood that is free from the antigens.

   b. The cause of alloimmunization of platelets is not fully understood; however, HLA-incompatibility is related in 75% of the cases. Subsequent transfusions of platelets lead to a less than expected increase in the platelet count. This is managed by giving single-donor pheresed platelets, preferably by a family member, which improves the platelet count somewhat.

7. **GvHD** occurs when transfused, viable T lymphocytes present in donated blood (engrafted cells) proliferate and react against donor (host) tissues. It most often occurs in patients with underdeveloped or impaired immune systems or bone marrow transplants. GvHD is prevented by the irradiation of blood obtained from donors to render the T lymphocytes incapable of proliferation

8. **Metabolic complications** are associated with large amounts of transfused blood (equal to or greater than the patient's blood volume in a few hours) or when the patient has severe liver or kidney disease.

   a. *Hypothermia:* The degree is directly proportional to the rate and volume of blood infusion. It leads to cardiac dysrhythmias and decrease in the release of the oxygen from the hemoglobin. To manage, monitor temperature frequently. Use an approved blood warming device for frequent transfusions or exchange transfusion for an infant or small child and for patients with potential for cold agglutinins (those identified by pretransfusion agglutination tests).

   b. *Hypocalcemia:* The citrate in the donated blood binds to the recipient's Ca^{++}, leading to a decrease in the serum ionized calcium. It leads to a range of symptoms from muscle tremors to cardiac arrhythmias. Use IV replacement of calcium and slow the infusion if possible.

9. **Iron overload** occurs with chronic infusions over an extended period of time (such as years) in patients with severe chronic anemia not due to blood loss, such as sickle cell disease. It is due to the quantity of iron administered by transfusion being greater than that which can be excreted. Overload results in deposits of iron in the cells of the myocardial, endocrine, and liver cells, leading to organ damage. It is managed by giving an iron-chelating agent (deferoxamine mesylate).

IMPLICATIONS OF SYSTEM DYSFUNCTION

A. **RED BLOOD CELLS**

   ❖ DECREASED GAS EXCHANGE DUE TO DECREASED HEMOGLOBIN

   1. **Assessment:** Signs and symptoms of anemia vary with the rapidity of its onset and with the underlying disease. If anemia develops rapidly, signs and symptoms may be more pronounced. If anemia develops more slowly, compensatory mechanisms such as expanding plasma volume decrease the cardiovascular symptoms. The patient may have only slight dyspnea on exertion despite significant anemia. Young children will prevent dyspnea by decreasing their activity level.

      a. *Clinical signs and symptoms* include tachycardia, tachypnea, diminished level of consciousness, light-headedness, postural hypotension, and pallor of skin and mucous membranes.

      b. *Laboratory data:* Hemoglobin less than 8 g/dl (threshold considered to be 10 g/dl for children with chronic illnesses such as pulmonary disease that require a higher level).

   2. **Interventions**

      a. Administer blood products as ordered.

      b. Improve oxygenation. Reduce fear and anxiety to minimize oxygen demand. Assist in activities to reduce physiologic oxygen demand. Administer supplemental oxygen as ordered (only effective if adequate hemoglobin is present to carry the oxygen). Use semi-Fowler's position for maximum ventilation-perfusion match.

      c. Administer EPO to promote endogenous RBC production.

3. Prevent **iatrogenic anemia** caused by large quantities of blood required for diagnostic procedures. Use smaller blood collection tubes; modern blood chemistry analyzers can perform a number of tests on a few drops of serum. Keep a cumulative total of the volume of blood drawn. Use fingerstick techniques to obtain capillary blood for testing whenever practical.

B. WHITE BLOOD CELLS: HYPOACTIVITY

❖ ACTUAL OR POTENTIAL FOR INFECTION DUE TO UNINTENTIONAL STRESSORS (e.g., immunodeficiency, malnutrition, iatrogenic interventions such as placement of multiple invasive devices, immobility, or environmental pathogens) OR INTENTIONAL STRESSORS (e.g., bone marrow suppression in preparation for transplantation or therapeutic regimens including chemotherapy or radiation)

1. **Assessment**

   a. *Local signs and symptoms of inflammation* include edema (tumor); redness (rubor); pain (dolor); heat (color); and decreased function of an affected area. Also note the presence and characteristics of exudate: Serous (clear) or suppurative/purulent (a creamy colored pus indicating an accumulation of dead WBCs and necrotic debris) (Selekman, 1991)

   b. *Systemic clinical signs and symptoms of infection* include body temperature below 36° or above 38° C, tachycardia, tachypnea, cloudy mentation, confusion, irritability, diaphoresis, rigors or chills, and generalized symptoms such as change in activity level, fatigue, or malaise.

   c. *Laboratory data*
      • Alterations in WBC count: Leukocytosis, leukopenia, increased number of bands
      • Positive blood or body fluid cultures
      • Significant findings in site-specific diagnostic tests (e.g., pneumonia demonstrated on a chest radiograph)

2. **Interventions**

   a. Assess and monitor skin integrity, body orifices, IV sites, and pressure areas for evidence of inflammation, infection, or skin breakdown.

   b. Maintain skin integrity (Jennings, 1991). Turn the patient at least every 2 hours during the day and every 4 hours during the night. Use protective or pressure reduction devices, as needed. Keep skin clean and dry. Progressively mobilize and ambulate the patient. Minimize tissue injury (Jennings, 1991). Ensure gentle removal of tape and other adhesive devices. Avoid intramuscular and subcutaneous injections. Reduce the number of venipunctures and initiate IV therapy judiciously. Reduce the frequency of blood pressure readings using a cuff sphygmomanometer; alternate extremities used for readings. Pad side rails if the patient is combative or at risk for seizure activity.

   c. Assess for and differentiate between inflammation and infection, which are not synonymous terms. Although all infections occur in the presence of inflammation, not all inflammation indicates infection. Infection is the presence of an organism in the body tissue or fluid *with* a local or systemic effect (Ackerman, 1992). Special attention must be paid to patients in whom the cardinal signs of the local inflammatory response may be diminished or absent (e.g., immunocompromised patients, patients receiving medications suppressing the inflammatory response, newborns with a delayed or limited ability to localize infection). In these patients, the most reliable signs of the local inflammatory response are often pain and fever.

   d. Assess and monitor specific sites for infectious processes.
      • Pulmonary or lower respiratory tract infection: Note tachypnea, change

in level of consciousness, feeding, behavior or activity level, presence of cough, signs of respiratory distress, and abnormal breath sounds (see Chapter 2).
- Bacteremia, both primary and catheter related: Note systemic signs and symptoms of infection.

e. Assess for and differentiate between systemic infection and a systemic inflammatory response syndrome (SIRS). SIRS is the acute development of two or more of the following (American College of Chest Physicians [ACCP] and Society of Critical Care Medicine [SCCM], 1992):
- Fever (>38° C) or hypothermia (<36° C)
- Tachycardia (outside age appropriate range)
- Tachypnea (outside age appropriate range)
- Alteration in WBC count, either leukocytosis (WBC >12,000/mm^3; use age-appropriate range [see Table 8–6]), leukopenia (WBC <4000/mm^3), or greater than 10% bands.

f. Administer prescribed antimicrobial agents and monitor response. Dilute medication to diminish venous irritation and ensure complete administration by following antibiotic with an adequate flush. Establish a schedule to maximize pharmacologic effects and minimize late administration. Assess for superinfections that may occur with long-term antibiotic use. Accurately obtain drug levels (serum drug concentrations, SDC), as ordered.

g. Administer granulocytes or biologic response modifiers, as ordered.

h. Institute measures to decrease the patient's risk of infection with endogenous organisms. Assist in personal hygiene measures (oral care, etc.) as indicated by the extent of mucositis (see section below on mucositis). In collaboration with the physician, explore alternatives to use the patient's GI tract for feeding to minimize the risk of bacterial translocation.

3. **Prevention:** Institute good hand washing and universal precautions for all individuals who may have contact with the patient. Use proper technique for initiating and maintaining all intravascular lines and during all invasive procedures. Promote optimal fluid and nutritional intake. Ensure a clean environment and restrict the patient's contact with individuals who may have infectious processes. Use a health screening tool for siblings wishing to visit the patient. Prevent the spread of infectious processes through the use of appropriate isolation procedures.

❖ HYPERTHERMIA OR CHILLS DUE TO INFECTIOUS PROCESSES

1. **Assessment**
    a. Hyperthermia is an elevation in body temperature above normal temperature. Patients may also experience chills (quivering or shaking as if cold).
    b. Clinical signs and symptoms include elevated temperature of 38° to 41° C. Young infants may respond with hypothermia in the presence of infection. Other symptoms include tachycardia; tachypnea; cloudy or altered mentation, confusion, or irritability; warm and dry skin with flushed cheeks; and diaphoresis.
    c. Positive implications of increased temperature include enhanced activity of cells of the immune system and nonconductive environment for the growth and activity of invading microorganisms (antigens). Negative implications of increased temperature include increased metabolic demand, increased insensible water loss and potential dehydration, and fatigue.

2. **Interventions** (Clark et al, 1987)
    a. Monitor, document, and report each temperature elevation. In collaboration with the physician determine the cause of fever. **Fever may be the *only***

sign of infection in the immunocompromised patient, and the patient is presumed to have an infection until proven otherwise. Drug reactions may also cause fever.

b. Monitor for dehydration. Estimate insensible water loss. In collaboration with the physician, evaluate the need for adjustment of fluid requirements.

c. Institute measures to decrease the temperature when the patient is febrile. Remove excess clothing or bed linens. Give a tepid water bath. Alcohol is *not* recommended. Apply cool moist compresses, especially to the forehead and axilla (Selekman, 1991). Use a cooling blanket but discontinue use if shivering ensues. Prevent chills or shivering because the associated peripheral vasoconstriction may actually further increase body temperature. Shivering raises basal metabolic rate and increases heat production and body temperature (Selekman, 1991). Shivering may increase intracranial pressure and predisposes to intracranial bleeding in thrombocytopenic patients (Jennings, 1991).

d. Institute measures to increase comfort when the patient is febrile. Change wet bed linens in the presence of diaphoresis or with the use of the cooling blanket. Cool the patient's room if possible. Provide rest periods. Provide cool fluids, ice, popsicles, or Jello (Selekman, 1991) unless contraindicated.

e. In collaboration with the physician, consider the administration of antipyretics (only after the fever is evaluated) and broad-spectrum antibiotic therapy (until the specific cause of the infection is determined).

f. Identification of the source of infection is a primary concern in a febrile patient (Pizzo, 1989). Indwelling catheters should be sampled for culture. If possible, two peripheral blood samples should be obtained from separate venipuncture sites. Other cultures that may be obtained include sputum, routine urinalysis and culture, and a stool examination and culture (especially if diarrhea is present).

g. If possible, discontinue medications that may cause fever as an adverse reaction.

❖ ALTERED INTEGRITY OF MUCOUS MEMBRANES DUE TO ORAL INFECTION OR THE SIDE EFFECTS OF CHEMOTHERAPY OR RADIATION

1. **Assessment**

a. *Definitions* (Clark et al, 1987)
   - Mucositis: Generalized inflammation of the mucous membranes
   - Stomatitis: Inflammation of the mucous membranes of the oral cavity
   - Esophagitis: Inflammation of the mucous membranes of the esophagus

b. *Clinical signs and symptoms* are often graded systematically (from grade 0 to grade III), such as in the St. Jude Children's Hospital Oral Care Guidelines noted in Table 8–10. Differentiate between stomatitis and candidiasis (Jennings, 1991). Candidiasis (moniliasis or thrush) can be distinguished by its severity. Subacute candidiasis is demonstrated by soft white patches on mucosa. Chronic candidiasis is demonstrated by dry, red buccal mucosa. A specimen should be cultured and the regimen supplemented with an antifungal agent.

c. Implications of altered oral mucous membranes include impaired integrity and increased risk to infection, inadequate nutritional intake or absorption, pain, and difficulty swallowing or speaking (if not intubated).

2. **Interventions** (see Table 8–10): Assess and monitor the condition of the oral mucosa. Institute measures to prevent inflammation (mucositis) or prevent further injury to existing inflammation. Avoid exposure to chemical or physical irritants and provide adequate fluid intake. Provide oral hygiene measures at

Table 8–10.   AN EXAMPLE OF ORAL CARE GUIDELINES

ASSESSMENT	TREATMENT
Normal Mucosa and Gingivae: Grade 0 (No Mucositis)	
Oral mucosa is pink, moist; no lesions, crusts, or debris; gingivae are pink, firm, and stippled	Aid and encourage brushing, flossing, and rinsing after meals, particularly in evenings. Use soft bristle brush, fluoride toothpaste, and ½-strenth Cepacol.
Mucositis and Gingivitis: Grade I (Early, Mild Form)	
Oral mucosa or gingivae are red, shiny, with possible white patches; gingivae may appear swollen; patient may complain of a burning sensation or general discomfort in the mouth; tongue may appear coated, red, dry, or swollen	1. Rinse with alkaline-saline solution q2–4h while awake. 2. Debride teeth and gingivae b.i.d. using an Ultra-Suave toothbrush dipped in ½-strength Peroxyl. Rinse with water. 3. Swish and hold 5–10 ml of ½-strenth S.T. 37 for 30 s; then spit. Use q.i.d. 4. If white patches are present, candidiasis should be considered and cultures done. Add Nilstat to the regimen.
Mucositis with Ulceration: Grade II (Moderate Form)	
Mucositis and gingivitis as previously described, but with the addition of focal ulceration; patient hesitates to eat because of pain from chewing or swallowing	On a t.i.d. schedule: 1. Debride teeth and gingivae using an Ultra-Suave toothbrush dipped in ½-strength Peroxyl. Rinse copiously with alkaline-saline solution. For pain relief: 1. For isolated, small ulcers, apply Kank A solution with provided applicator directly to the ulcer. 2. For more extensive and numerous ulcers, swish and hold 5–10 ml of Ulcer-Ease solution in the mouth for 30 s; then spit out.
Mucositis with Severe Ulceration: Grade III (Severe Form)	
Severe erythema and ulceration or white patches present; patient complains of severe pain and cannot eat, drink, or swallow; saliva may appear thick and viscid with much "drooling"	1. Rinse for 30 s with Ulcer-Ease to anesthetize mucosa. 2. Debride teeth and gingivae using an Ultra-Suave toothbrush dipped in alkaline-saline solution. Rinse copiously with alkaline-saline solution. *Do not use Peroxyl in grade III mucositis.* 3. For pain relief: Use Ulcer-Ease solution or ½-strength Dyclone (1%). Use systemic analgesia if not effective.
Mouth Dryness (Xerostomia)	
Thick "ropy" saliva (early sign) or an obviously dry mouth	1. Mucositis mouth care (see "Mucositis" above). 2. Rinse mouth with saline, ad lib. 3. Swab mouth with Moi-Stir oral swabsticks several times daily. 4. Administer artifical saliva (Xero-Lube) p.r.n. 5. Lip care (see "Lip care") p.r.n.
Lip Care	
Lips dry, chapped, rough, but free of crusts and debris	Treatment varies based on assessment: Moisten lips with lanolin q2–4h
Lips cracked, ulcerated, or crusted	Clean q2–4h with gauze saturated with saline. Pat dry and apply Lanoline or K-Y jelly.
Fissuring or cracking at the corners of the mouth (usually indicates candidiasis)	Apply Mycolog ointment q.i.d.

Table continued on following page

Table 8–10. AN EXAMPLE OF ORAL CARE GUIDELINES *(Continued)*

ASSESSMENT	TREATMENT
Debris on Teeth	
Platelet count >20,000 and no or minimal pain on brushing	Gentle brushing of teeth and gingivae with a *soft* bristle brush. Hold brush under hot water to further soften brush bristles.
Platelet count <20,000; patient unable to tolerate brushing or spontaneous bleeding noted from gingivae	1. Rinse mouth with alkaline-saline solution. 2. An Ultra-Suave toothbrush dipped in very dilute Peroxyl or alkaline-saline solution can be used. Rinse copiously with either water or more alkaline-saline solution. 3. A moistened gauze wrapped over a finger may also be used to debride teeth and gums. Toothettes are *not* effective.

Modified from Hopkins K. *Oral Care Guidelines for Patients Receiving Chemotherapy and Radiation Therapy.* Memphis, Tenn: St Jude Children's Research Hospital; 1993.

least 3 times a day. Provide treatment based on assessment findings and institute measures to increase comfort.

C. **WHITE BLOOD CELLS: HYPERACTIVITY**

Hypersensitivity reactions are classified according to the source of the antigen that stimulates the immune response (Table 8–11).

❖ INCREASED INFLAMMATORY RESPONSE RELATED TO INCREASED IMMUNE SYSTEM ACTIVITY

1. **Type I immediate hypersensitivity reaction or anaphylaxis:** Hyperactivity of the surveillance function of the immune system

    a. *Assessment:* Clinical signs and symptoms are the result of the action of inflammatory mediators on surrounding tissues and blood vessels (Mudge-Grout, 1992). Increased capillary permeability can lead to profound hypotension, circulatory collapse, and facial edema. Constriction of smooth muscle can result in wheezing, crackles, and progressive difficulty in breathing and stridor. An influx of eosinophils can produce erythema and pruritus.

    b. *Intervention:* Diagnosis of anaphylaxis is based on clinical manifestations.
    - Maintain airway and breathing with oxygen administration. This may require intubation and mechanical ventilation. If there is tracheal and laryngeal edema, intubation may be difficult and there is a possibility that the patient may require a tracheostomy. Epinephrine is administered for bronchoconstriction.
    - Support circulation with fluid administration and epinephrine administration to counteract vasodilation. Other vasoactive medications (e.g., dopamine and norepinephrine) may be required.
    - Administer prescribed medications. Antihistamines serve as antagonists to most of the effects of histamine. Bronchodilators relax bronchial smooth muscle. Corticosteroids are antiinflammatory agents and serve to enhance the effects of bronchodilators.
    - Identify the antigen and avoid future exposures.

2. **Autoimmune disease** represents the hyperactivity of the homeostasis function of the immune system

    a. The homeostasis function of the immune system removes old and damaged "self" components from the body.

    b. The immune system mistakenly identifies itself as "nonself" and begins to form antibodies (autoantibodies) against its own healthy cells (autoanti-

Table 8–11. HYPERSENSITIVITY REACTIONS

TYPE	DESCRIPTION	EXAMPLE
Type I (anaphylactic reaction)	Triggered in response to an exposure to an environmental antigen. Mediated by IgE antibodies that bind to specific receptors on the surface of mast cells and basophils. Results in the release of a host of mediators to produce a classic anaphylactic response.	Anaphylaxis Asthma Allergic rhinitis, hay fever
Type II (tissue specific hypersensitivity)	Triggered by the presence of an antigen found only on a cell or tissue. Mediated by antibody (usually IgM, but also IgG) through two different mechanisms (complement and Fc receptors on phagocytes). Results in the destruction of the antibody-coated cell with consequences dependent on the cell that is destroyed (e.g., RBC, WBC, or platelet).	ABO incompatibility Rh incompatibility Drug-induced thrombocytopenia
Type III (immune complex reaction)	Triggered by the formation of antigen-antibody complexes that activate the complement cascade. Immune complexes are formed in the circulation and are later deposited in blood vessels or healthy tissue. Multiple forms of the response exist depending on the type and location of the antigen. Results in local edema and neutrophil attraction and thus degradative lysosomal enzymes resulting in tissue injury.	Serum sickness Glomerulonephritis
Type IV (delayed hypersensitivity)	Triggered by the recognition of an antigen. Mediated by activated T lymphocytes and release of lymphokines, which then stimulate the macrophage to phagocytize foreign invaders and some normal tissue. Results in a delayed onset. Does not have an antibody component; this response is strictly a cellular reaction.	Contact sensitivities such as poison ivy and dermatitis Tuberculin reactions Graft rejection

RBC, red blood cell; *WBC,* white blood cell.

gens). This results in the development of immune complexes that are deposited in tissues (e.g., skin, joints, kidneys) and in tissue damage.

   c. Examples of autoimmune disease in children are juvenile onset diabetes mellitus and systemic lupus erythematosus.

3. **Malignancy**

   a. The surveillance function of the immune system identifies and destroys cells that are "nonself" or "self" cells that have undergone mutation.

   b. Although malignancy is not the primary reason for the patient's admission into the critical care area, complications of malignancy or its treatment are not uncommon reasons for admission. The most common complications include the following:

     • Sepsis and septic shock (See Septic Shock discussion in Chapter 9.)

     • Tumor lysis syndrome is a group of metabolic effects associated with rapidly growing tumors such as leukemia cells that are very sensitive to being destroyed by chemotherapy. Tumor lysis syndrome leads to hyperkalemia, hyperphosphatemia, hyperuricemia, and hypocalcemia. It can be life threatening, requiring dialysis (see Treatment of Hyperkalemia). Effects are managed with vigorous hydration (to promote a rapid renal tubular flow rate and thus less accumulation of uric acid and phosphates in the kidneys), allopurinol (to lower serum uric acid), and sodium bicarbonate (to promote urine alkalinity, which promotes uric acid excretion).

- Superior mediastinal syndrome is associated with a mass leading to a narrowing of the tracheal diameter and obstruction of blood flow returning by the superior vena cava. The syndrome is more frequently associated with lymphomas and acute lymphocytic leukemia. The syndrome may be associated with respiratory distress on admission, sometimes necessitating intubation. Sedation for any procedures may be risky without prior intubation, as these medications will likely lead to airway collapse. Emergent radiation treatments or chemotherapy may be needed to provide relief of the respiratory distress by decreasing the size of the mediastinal mass.

- For patients diagnosed with cancer, tumor invasion of the epidural space may result in compression of the spinal cord. Common symptoms include bowel or bladder dysfunction. Less frequently hypoventilation occurs because of compromise of diaphragmatic and intercostal muscle function. Motor dysfunction precedes sensory losses. Early intervention is critical in preventing permanent damage. If paraplegia occurs, treatment must begin within a few hours or full neurologic function may be lost. Management involves radiation, the treatment of choice. Surgical decompression is indicated if radiation is not effective and clinical deterioration continues.

D. PLATELETS AND PLASMA FACTORS
  ❖ HYPOVOLEMIA RELATED TO BLEEDING
  1. **Assessment** should include vital signs (tachycardia and hypotension), fluid and electrolyte status (decreased urine output, emesis, diarrhea), characteristics of fluid losses (assess for gross or occult blood), perfusion status, capillary refill, mental status, and urine output. Use urine and stool tests to detect the presence of blood.
  2. **Interventions**
     a. *Volume replacement:* Administer fluids, blood products, and vasoactive infusions as ordered.
     b. *Control of bleeding:* Apply direct pressure or cold compresses and elevate the extremity. Apply topical hemostatic agents such as an absorbable gelatin sponge (Gelfoam).
  3. **Prevention**
     a. Avoid intramuscular and subcutaneous injections; if necessary, apply pressure for 10 minutes. If intravascular access is needed, peripheral IV access vs. central access poses less risk for trauma and bleeding to the patient.
     b. Provide a safe environment such as padding the side rails and other firm surfaces especially if the child is combative or at risk for seizure activity.
     c. Do not administer aspirin or NSAIDs because of the effects on platelets. Parents should be taught to read nonprescription medication labels to avoid giving the child aspirin.
     d. Prevent intracranial bleeding from increased intracranial pressure. Teach the patient to avoid the Valsalva maneuver and to cough, sneeze, and blow nose gently. Administer stool softeners.

   e. Provide mouth care with foam swabs and a mild saline or bicarbonate and peroxide solution.
   f. Administer vitamin K (normally obtained from diet and enteric bacterial synthesis). Vitamin K deficiency is the most common cause of prolonged PT in the ICU. Vitamin K is needed for factors II, VII, IX, and X to be effective. Deficiencies are seen with malnutrition, obstructive biliary disease, liver disease, and with use of certain cephalosporins such as cefamandol. With first sign of PT prolongation, administer vitamin K IV or SC or add to TPN. PT should correct within 24 hours. Anaphylactoid reactions are rare but more often are seen with the IV route.

RED BLOOD CELL DISORDERS: SICKLE CELL DISEASE (SCD)

A. **PATHOPHYSIOLOGY**
   SCD affects all organ systems. RBCs have hemoglobin HbSS (an abnormal form of hemoglobin associated with sickle cell disease) not HbA (normal hemoglobin).
   1. When the oxygen level falls, RBCs with HbSS become crescent shaped (sickle shaped), and sickled RBCs are trapped in small vessels, leading to erythrostasis. Deoxygenation and decreased pH leads to further sickling and increased viscosity of the blood; a vicious cycle results, leading to more sickling.
   2. Masses of sickled RBCs occlude blood vessels, leading to thrombosis, ischemia, and infarction. Specific organs involved will present with signs of hypoperfusion, vascular occlusion, and tissue ischemia. The body recognizes and hemolizes the abnormal RBC structure. Sickled RBCs may return to normal shape when the blood is more oxygenated (such as in the pulmonary vein). However, after repeated occasions, a portion of RBCs released into free circulation will be more sensitive to mechanical trauma, even normal trauma experienced during circulation, or will not return to their nonsickled shape even if the blood is well oxygenated.
B. **ETIOLOGY AND RISK FACTORS**
   1. **SCD** is a serious, chronic, hereditary (autosomal recessive), hemolytic disease. It presents in a variety of forms that result in a child inheriting from both parents a copy of a defective gene that encodes for an abnormal Hb protein (HbS).
      a. HbSS is the hemoglobin type associated with sickle cell anemia, the most severe form of SCD, and the result of inheriting a sickle cell gene (SS) from each parent.
      b. HbSC is the hemoglobin type associated with HbSC disease, a more moderate form of the disease with lower mortality, and the result of inheriting a gene of HbSS that combines with an HbC gene.
      c. Hb-β-thal is the hemoglobin type associated with sickle cell–β-thalassemia, a more moderate form of the disease with lower mortality, and the result of inheriting an HbS gene in the presence of the thalassemia trait.
      d. HbAS (sickle cell trait) is the hemoglobin type associated with asymptomatic SCD except in extreme hypoxic states. It results from inheriting one HbS gene and a normal HbA gene, producing both types of Hb. Children with this hemoglobin type are carriers of the disease.
   2. SCD occurs almost exclusively in individuals of African descent and manifests after 6 months of age when fetal hemoglobin (HbF) is replaced with HbSS or HbSC. Increased sickling is associated with dehydration, hypoxemia, and acidosis.

C. **SIGNS AND SYMPTOMS**

Signs and symptoms result from anemia and organ dysfunction due to vascular occlusion by sickled cells' clumping together. SCD is not associated with bleeding. Impaired growth and development, failure to thrive, and increased tendency to develop serious infections are due to decreased splenic function. Specific symptoms include aching joints, especially hands and feet, sudden severe abdominal pain, chest pain, cardiomegaly, and splenomegaly (if spleen is not enlarged, it may be fibrosed and is not functional).

D. **INTERPRETATION OF DIAGNOSTIC STUDIES**

1. Peripheral blood smear will show sickle cells (normal if only the trait). Hemoglobin chromatography or electrophoresis indicates the precise type of hemoglobinopathy.
2. CBC reflects hemolytic anemia with reduced hemoglobin, hematocrit, and RBC count because the spleen has destroyed sickled cells. Platelets and reticulocyte count may be elevated as a compensatory response to anemia.
3. Serum iron and bilirubin may be elevated because of the hemolysis of the sickled cells.
4. Radiologic findings
   a. Bone x-rays show increased density or aseptic necrosis secondary to infarction.
   b. Chest x-rays may show pulmonary infiltrate.
   c. Computed tomography (CT) scan may be performed after stabilization if a cerebral vascular accident (CVA) is suspected.

E. **NURSING AND COLLABORATIVE DIAGNOSIS**

   ❖ ACTIVITY INTOLERANCE
   ❖ POTENTIAL FOR IMPAIRED GAS EXCHANGE
   ❖ PAIN

F. **GOALS AND DESIRED PATIENT OUTCOMES: PREVENTION OF COMPLICATIONS**

1. Promote early diagnosis through newborn screening.
2. Encourage follow-up in a comprehensive sickle cell clinic.
   a. Educate the family regarding the importance of mandatory prophylactic penicillin starting at age 3 months until age 5 years.
   b. Teach parents that fever (temperature >38.5° C) must be promptly evaluated to determine the source of the fever and the need for treatment.
   c. Teach parents to palpate the spleen for possible enlargement.
3. Prevent crises through prevention of dehydration, hypoxemia, and acidosis.
4. Prevent infection with vaccines such as for pneumococcal organisms and *H. influenzae.* However, vaccines do not fully protect against all pathogenic strains of pneumococcus. Children younger than 2 years old will have poor immunologic response to the vaccine and may need future revaccination.

G. **PATIENT CARE MANAGEMENT**

1. Pain management: Supportive interventions
   a. Prevent pain by treating dehydration, hypoxemia, and acidosis to prevent sickling.
   b. Use analgesics ranging from acetaminophen to IV narcotics, as indicated and ordered; monitor effectiveness to decrease pain.
   c. RBC transfusion or exchange transfusion is given to "dilute out" HbSS-containing RBCs. Goal is usually a hematocrit of 25% to 30% with 50% of Hb as non-HbSS. Avoid raising the hematocrit more than 35%, since this increase in viscosity will contribute to the increase in viscosity of the blood from the sickled cells.
2. Bed rest decreases oxygen demand and consumption.
3. Cytotoxic agents (such as hydroxyurea) increase the level of RBCs with HbF,

which will decrease the ability of the RBCs with HbSS to sickle. Cytotoxic agents force hematopoiesis to produce more RBCs with HbF, thereby reducing the sickling process. The response is quite variable from patient to patient. Use is considered experimental and is limited to only those most severely effected by SCD because of the associated toxicity including mutagenesis and possible carcinogenesis.

4. Bone marrow transplant and gene transfer to correct the molecular defect in the hemoglobin are options being considered as future treatments.

H. COMPLICATIONS

1. **Infections** are a major cause of morbidity and mortality for children.
   a. Compromised function of the spleen leads to an increased susceptibility to encapsulated bacteria. There is an increased risk of *S. pneumoniae* (pneumococcus) and *H. influenzae* type b infections. *S. pneumoniae* is a leading cause of death in the first 3 years of life; it can progress from onset of fever to death in less than 12 hours. *H. influenzae* infections have an insidious onset. Any clinical pneumonia decreases the effectiveness of oxygenation, thereby increasing sickling of RBCs.
   b. *Assess* for infections requiring immediate attention and admission to the hospital. Note significant pain, fever, and chills. Patients with SCD typically have a slightly elevated WBC count; but with infection the WBC count further increases to greater than $30,000/mm^3$. Chest x-ray examination demonstrates significant pulmonary infiltrates if infection involves the pulmonary system.
   c. *Management:* Obtain blood cultures and immediately begin antibiotics including coverage for pneumococcus and *H. influenzae* if the child is younger than 5 years of age. Transfuse with RBCs; give sufficient volume to alleviate signs or symptoms of inadequate tissue oxygenation.

2. **Splenic sequestration crisis** is the second most common cause of morbidity and mortality in the first decade of life. The exact cause is unknown but often is associated with viral illnesses and prior sequestration crises. Blood pools in the spleen, further leading to acute splenic enlargement, increased anemia, and, if severe, signs of hypovolemia leading to shock and death.
   a. *Assessment:* Clinically, pallor of the mucosal surfaces, tachycardia, abdominal fullness, splenomegaly, left upper quadrant pain, and weakness are noted. Laboratory results demonstrate a rapid fall in hematocrit.
   b. *Management*
      - A mild crisis (moderate increase in spleen size, a decrease in hemoglobin of less than 3 g/dl) may resolve spontaneously without treatment; continue to observe closely for further deterioration of status.
      - For a severe crisis (massive splenomegaly, a decrease in hemoglobin of more than 3 g/dl, signs of hypovolemia), administer oxygen and infuse normal saline followed by RBC transfusion as soon as possible. Recheck the hemoglobin 4 hours after the transfusion. Usually when hypovolemia is corrected, sequestered RBCs are released from the spleen. If the child is younger than 2 years of age, initiate a long-term transfusion program to maintain HbSS at less than 30%. If the child is older than age 2 years, splenectomy is performed. With splenectomy or if the spleen fibroses, the child will need preventive strategies for infection. Adults are not susceptible to these crises, as their spleens are atrophied (called "autosplenectomy") because of repeated infarctions.

3. **Aplastic crisis** is a transient episode of failure of RBC production that can be life threatening. It is associated with human parvovirus B19, leading to bone marrow failure of erythropoiesis

   a. *Assessment:* Clinically, fever, anorexia, lethargy, tachypnea, tachycardia, nausea, vomiting, abdominal pain, and headache are noted (**not** splenomegaly). Laboratory results show a rapid decrease in hemoglobin, low reticulocyte count (<1%) in peripheral blood, and low RBC precursors in the bone marrow aspirate.

   b. *Management:* Transfuse with RBCs slowly to alleviate signs or symptoms of inadequate tissue oxygenation. Place hospitalized patients in isolation. Pregnant caretakers should not be exposed, since human parvovirus can lead to second and third trimester abortions. Repeat transfusions to maintain the hemoglobin at higher than 8 g/dl until bone marrow function resumes, usually within a few days to 2 weeks.

4. **Acute chest syndrome**

   a. The usual cause is probably in situ vasoocclusion, resulting in a painful crisis; associated with infections (bacteria, *Mycoplasma,* and viral agents), thromboembolism, and sickling of RBCs in the pulmonary vasculature. The major concern is that a vicious cycle may be initiated of pulmonary vasoocclusion, poor oxygenation of blood, increased RBC sickling, and more vasoocclusion. Vascular occlusion of branches of the pulmonary artery leads to infarction of the lung. The syndrome may be self-limited, particularly when it involves a small area of pulmonary parenchyma, but it can rapidly progress and become massive and fatal. A chronic pattern of this syndrome will lead to chronic scarring of the lung seen on x-ray examination. Repeated episodes lead to restrictions of vital capacity, pulmonary hypertension, and cor pulmonale.

   b. *Assessment:* Clinical course is variable, ranging from mild pneumonia to a rapidly progressing and fatal respiratory failure.

- Clinical appearance: Fever accompanied by pleuritic chest pain, cough, dyspnea
- X-ray: Pulmonary infiltrate that may not be present for the first 2 to 3 days, especially if the patient is dehydrated; may progress to a complete "white out"
- Laboratory results: Blood and sputum cultures may be positive for organisms. Arterial blood gases: Because the patient with SCD may have a low PaO_2 during stable periods, it is not until the PaO_2 is lower than 70 mm Hg that symptoms of hypoxia occur.

   c. *Management:* Because this condition can deteriorate rapidly, the child should be hospitalized and carefully monitored.

- Pneumonia must be ruled out; however, it is usually impossible to distinguish between pulmonary infarction and pneumonia, and the processes are likely to coexist. In patients younger than 5 years of age, pneumonia is more likely to be the cause of symptoms. In patients older than 5 years, pulmonary infarction is the more common cause.
- Initiate broad-spectrum antibiotics for *S. pneumoniae, H. influenzae, Mycoplasma pneumoniae* immediately if new pulmonary infiltrates are seen on x-ray examination.
- Administer oxygen to maintain an oxygen saturation of greater than 95%. Administer RBCs if the patient is hypoxic or has respiratory distress or a decrease in hemoglobin of more than 2 g/dl. Consider a partial exchange transfusion if signs of respiratory failure (PaO_2 <75 mm Hg) are present, if multiple lobes are affected, or if the patient's condition continues to deteriorate.

5. **Vasoocclusive crisis (pain crisis)** is one of the most debilitating problems for SCD patients. It is caused by obstruction of small arterioles by sickled RBCs,

resulting in ischemia of tissues; frequency, intensity, duration, and severity are variable. Onset is unpredictable with varied frequency and severity; may be precipitated by infection, fever, dehydration, trauma, or exposure to cold. It is self-limited and may last only minutes to 2 to 3 weeks (usually 4 to 5 days).

  a. *Assessment:* Diagnosis is by history, not by laboratory test or x-ray examination. Clinical appearance demonstrates severe deep pain at any site, commonly musculoskeletal, extremities, back, chest, or abdomen; fever greater than 40° C, respiratory distress, lethargy and joint swelling. Chest x-ray examination is used if chest pain is present to rule out acute chest syndrome. During infancy the syndrome is characterized by a "hand-foot" syndrome with soft tissue swelling, heat, and pain of the dorsum of the hands, feet, fingers, and toes.

  b. *Management*
  - Initially, rule out other causes of pain such as osteomyelitis, bone infarction, and other causes for chest or abdominal pain.
  - Hydration: Give D_5NS at 1 to 2 times normal maintenance rate.
  - Provide oxygen if PaO_2 is less than 75 mm Hg, but it will not be effective in reducing pain in diseased segments of lungs.
  - Pain control measures: It is important not to withhold analgesics because of excessive concern about possible addiction. Determine degree of pain. For mild pain, give acetaminophen with codeine; for severe pain, give morphine or meperidine (Demerol). Avoid PRN schedule, as this will promote cycles of recurring pain. Reevaluate the pain control plan every 24 hours; taper and switch to oral analgesics after pain control has been achieved.
  - Long-term transfusions are used if analgesics are not effective during the acute crisis.
  - If fever is higher than 38.5° C, blood cultures should be obtained and IV antibiotics begun.

6. **Cerebrovascular accident (CVA)** usually is caused by in situ vasoocclusion; fat embolism is a rare cause. The exact cause is age related. In younger children CVA is usually from cerebral thrombosis, and in older children CVA is usually from intracranial bleeding. No reliable predictive factors are known to identify patients at risk.

  a. *Assessment:* Clinical appearance demonstrates hemiparesis, severe unilateral headache, dizziness, lethargy, aphasia, seizures, or change in school performance as signs of increased intracranial pressure.
  - X-ray examination: For CT scan and arteriogram, hyperosmolar contrast requires preparation with hydration and transfusion to lower HbSS to less than 30% before the scan is done. Contrast material may increase sickling; low-ionic strength contrast medium is preferable. Use of MRI is ideal, since no contrast is needed. Results may be normal initially, since several days of evolution is necessary to detect an edematous infarcted area.

  b. *Management:* Goal is to prevent progression of the CVA. Partial exchange transfusion is used to decrease HbSS level to less than 40%; replacement of approximately 35 to 40 ml/kg of the patient's blood with RBCs. Reduce increased intracranial pressure and administer anticonvulsants if seizures occur. Patients are at risk for recurrence of CVAs; therefore, a chronic RBC transfusion program may be initiated to maintain HbSS levels at less than 30%. Patients may need iron chelation therapy for iron overload.

7. **Bone marrow necrosis and fat embolism** is caused by microinfarctions of bone or marrow. Secondary embolization of fat or marrow particles leads to pulmo-

nary infarction or fat globules in the coronary, cerebral, and renal microvasculature, resulting in renal, neurologic, or respiratory failure, which frequently is fatal.

    a. *Assessment:* Clinically, severe bone pain, fever, neurologic abnormalities, or respiratory distress is noted. Lipid or fat may be present in sputum specimens.

    b. *Management* includes exchange transfusion and oxygen and respiratory support.

8. **Acute multiorgan dysfunction syndrome** is an unusual clinical condition for patients with SCD resulting from several of the above complications. Episodes of pain complicated by the acute failure of at least two of three organs (lung, liver, or kidney) results in a severe, life-threatening complication of pain episodes in patients with otherwise mild SCD. It is associated with an unusually severe vasoocclusive crisis for the child and a high baseline hemoglobin level, which may or may not be associated with an infection. The cause is undefined but is assumed to be from the diffuse microvascular occlusion and tissue ischemia simultaneously in multiple organs and the sequestration and destruction of RBCs, leading to further tissue ischemia from the decreased oxygen-carrying capacity.

    a. *Assessment:* Clinically the child has fever, rapid fall in hemoglobin and platelet count, nonfocal encephalopathy (confusion, lethargy), and rhabdomyolysis. Laboratory results show hypoxia and elevation of liver enzymes, bilirubin, PT, and creatinine. X-ray findings include pulmonary infiltrates.

    b. *Management:* Transfusion, if aggressive and prompt, will reverse the syndrome. Exchange transfusion is used for young children. Provide hydration and IV analgesia.

9. **Priapism,** a painful, involuntary erection of the penis, occurs as sickled cells are trapped in the penis. Although it may resolve spontaneously and need only analgesics, management may involve hydration, exchange transfusion (if condition does not resolve in 4 to 6 hours), and surgery to evacuate the stagnant blood.

WHITE BLOOD CELL DISORDERS

Despite the type of stressor (e.g., congenital, acquired, intentional, or unintentional), the final common pathway or outcome of immunodeficiency or immunosuppression is impaired immune function or immunocompromise.

A. Definition of Terms

1. **Immunodeficiency:** A permanent state of impaired immune function that is usually genetic or congenital

2. **Immunosuppression:** A state of impaired immune function that can be intentional or unintentional and is usually temporary

B. Congenital Immunodeficiency Diseases

1. Disorders are characterized by an **inadequate number or inadequate function** of one or more of the components of the immune system (Mudge-Grout, 1992) resulting from a genetic or congenital condition. Disorders are divided by involvement of B lymphocytes, T lymphocytes, phagocytes, complement, or a combination of these components

2. **B-lymphocyte disorders** are characterized by a diminished ability to form immunoglobulins, thus resulting in an inability to generate effective antibody-antigen interactions (Heinzel, 1989)

    a. These are a diverse group of immunodeficiencies and may be manifested as a deficiency in all classes of immunoglobulins (panhypogammaglobulinemia), or as a deficiency in only one class of immunoglobulin (hypogamma-globulinemia), or as a combination of deficiencies in some classes with overproduction of immunoglobulin in another class.

b. IgA deficiency is the most common B-lymphocyte disorder and results in increased incidence of allergy and autoimmune conditions. Another example of a B-lymphocyte disorder includes X-linked agammaglobulinemia.

c. B-lymphocyte deficiencies are frequently interrelated with T-lymphocyte dysfunction.

d. *Etiology and pattern of infections* are often pyogenic bacteria, such as pneumococci, meningococci, streptococci, staphylococci, and *H. influenzae,* and enteroviruses. Less frequent causes are gram-negative organisms (Heinzel, 1989). Because of the inability of antibodies to form from mature plasma cells, reinfection from the same organism is common, even following normal childhood immunization.

3. **T-lymphocyte disorders** are characterized by an inadequate number or function of T lymphocytes. These patients have a limited ability to produce mature T lymphocytes, resulting in the inability to assist in the activation of the immune response.

a. T-lymphocyte disorders are associated with the survival and replication of intracellular organisms inside host immune cells. There is an increased incidence of certain malignancies (such as leukemia or lymphoma), since patients with T-cell disorders may have uncontrolled T-lymphocyte regulation of B-lymphocyte growth (Wood and Sampson, 1989). These disorders are usually associated concomitantly with antibody deficiencies.

b. Examples of T-lymphocyte disorders include DiGeorge syndrome and chronic mucocutaneous candidiasis.

c. *Etiology and pattern of infections* most often are viruses, fungi, protozoa, and intracellular bacteria (Wood and Sampson, 1989; Young, 1989). Opportunistic infection with organisms such as *Candida albicans* and *P. carinii* pose a risk to these patients (Mudge-Grout, 1992). The patient is more susceptible to the development of GvHD after transplantation or the transfusion of lymphocytes (Mudge-Grout, 1992).

4. **Phagocyte dysfunction disorders** (e.g., chronic granulomatous disease [CGD]) are disorders resulting from diverse extrinsic or intrinsic factors.

a. *Extrinsic factors*
   - Deficiency in opsonization related to decrease in either antibody or complement
   - Suppression of neutrophils or altered chemotaxis of neutrophils related to deficiency or alteration in complement
   - Decreased circulating lymphokines
   - Medications with immunosuppressive effect on phagocyte function or number

b. *Intrinsic factors:* Defects in the metabolic pathway of phagocytes.

c. *Etiology and pattern of infection* demonstrate an increased incidence of staphylococcal infections. Patients with phagocytic disorders are considered at risk for infection with gram-negative bacterial and fungal infections despite a "normal" WBC count.

d. Patients with *inadequate numbers* of phagocytes are referred to as neutropenic (total WBC number is decreased) or granulocytopenic (number of PMNs and bands decreased). These are clinical states rather than immunodeficiency disorders.

5. **Complement disorders** are characterized by the absence of an inhibitor or a deficiency in one or more of the specific complement components.

a. *Deficiencies* for each of the key components of complement have been described; however, an increase in the susceptibility to infection is commonly noted for deficiencies in C2, C3, C5, C6, C7, and C8 (Cooper and Buckley, 1982).

b. *Pattern of infection* varies with the complement component that is deficient and can range from recurrent infection to autoimmune disorders (Mudge-Grout, 1992).

6. **Combined B- and T-lymphocyte disorders** (e.g., SCID, Wiskott-Aldrich syndrome)

a. This is the most severe of all the immunodeficiencies because the patient is unable to form antibody (B lymphocyte), orchestrate the immune response (T lymphocyte), and destroy virally infected cells and cells infected with intracellular microorganisms (T lymphocyte).

b. *Etiology and pattern of infection* include infection from all types of microorganisms (bacterial, fungal, viral, and protozoal). Infections are often severe and recurrent

C. **SEVERE COMBINED IMMUNODEFICIENCY (SCID)**

SCID is a rare (1 in 1 million live births in the United States) combined B- and T-lymphocyte disorder.

1. **Etiology and risk factors:** Most cases (70%) are inherited in an autosomal or X-linked recessive pattern (Ackerman, 1992; Mudge-Grout, 1992). Many variants of the disorder exist and range from partial to almost complete loss of T-lymphocyte function. Approximately 50% of the autosomal recessive inherited cases involve a deficiency of the enzyme adenosine deaminase (ADA; Ackerman, 1992).

2. **Pathophysiology**

a. SCID can occur as a consequence to autosomal recessive inheritance: The responsible gene codes for a cytokine receptor.

b. SCID can occur as a consequence of ADA deficiency. B and T lymphocytes produce chemicals that can accumulate to toxic levels within these cells. Normally, these cells produce an enzyme (ADA) that destroys the excess amount of the toxins. When this key "detoxifying enzyme" is missing, these toxins accumulate, poisoning the B and T lymphocytes.

3. **Signs and symptoms**

a. SCID is characterized by recurrent and life-threatening infection of bacterial, fungal, protozoal, or viral origin, with onset within the first year of life (Ammann, 1991; Mudge-Grout, 1992); infants are particularly susceptible to *Candida, P. carinii,* and CMV.

b. Infection is not present at birth, since the infant is protected from bacterial infections by transplacental delivery of maternal IgG antibody; but signs and symptoms of infection develop soon after birth.

c. Infections are characteristic (Mudge-Grout, 1992) in terms of severity, recurrence (persistent in nature), type of organism, and location (common sites include the respiratory tract, mucous membranes, liver, GI tract, and blood). Oral candidiasis is resistant to therapy. Chronic diarrhea responds poorly to alterations in diet and may become life threatening.

4. **Interpretation of findings** from invasive and noninvasive diagnostic studies

a. *WBC count and differential* (Mudge-Grout, 1992)
   - Total lymphocyte count: Decreased, but variable
   - Absolute lymphocyte count: Decreased, usually less than 1500/mm^3; in newborns, less than 2500 is abnormal.

b. *HI:* Immunoglobulins are low to undetectable with minimal to no antibody response to immunizations. The number of B cells is variable.

c. *CMI*
- Lymphocyte subsets
  - Helper T lymphocytes (CD4): Low to absent
  - Suppressor or cytotoxic T lymphocytes (CD8): Low to absent
- Lymphocyte function: There is diminished or absent lymphocyte response to antigens. Delayed hypersensitivity skin testing is usually not helpful since these patients are so young that normal exposure and sensitization has not usually occurred (Ammann, 1991).

d. *Erythrocyte and leukocyte enzymes,* such as ADA and nucleoside phosphorylase, are assessed to determine the cause of SCID. ADA is not detectable in ADA deficiency SCID and will be normal in X-linked SCID.

e. *Chest x-ray examination:* Thymus shadow is absent.

f. *Lymph node biopsy* demonstrates severe depletion of lymphocytes without corticomedullary differentiation and follicle formation (Ammann, 1991)

5. **Nursing and collaborative diagnoses**
   - ALTERED PROTECTION RELATED TO PRIMARY IMMUNODEFICIENCY
   - POTENTIAL FOR INFECTION RELATED TO PRIMARY IMMUNODEFICIENCY, EFFECTS OF PRESCRIBED MEDICATIONS, AND MALNUTRITION
   - POTENTIAL FOR HYPERTHERMIA DUE TO INFECTIOUS PROCESSES
   - POTENTIAL FOR IMPAIRED GAS EXCHANGE RELATED TO PULMONARY INFECTIONS (E.G., PCP OR OTHER OPPORTUNISTIC INFECTIONS)
   - POTENTIAL FOR FLUID VOLUME DEFICIT DUE TO INFECTIOUS PROCESSES, CHRONIC AND UNRESPONSIVE DIARRHEA, AND FEVER
   - POTENTIAL FOR ALTERED NUTRITION, LESS THAN BODY REQUIREMENTS, RELATED TO FREQUENT OR CHRONIC INFECTIOUS PROCESSES AND CHRONIC AND UNRESPONSIVE DIARRHEA
   - POTENTIAL ALTERED GROWTH AND DEVELOPMENT RELATED TO PROLONGED OR REPEATED ILLNESS OR HOSPITALIZATION

6. **Goals and desired patient outcomes**
   a. Augment or improve the child's immune system.
   b. Protect from acquisition of infection (avoid live virus immunizations).
   c. Detect, identify, and eradicate infections or neoplastic disease.

7. **Patient care management**
   a. *Management* is often targeted at alleviating symptoms and eradicating the identified organism.
   b. Prevent or minimize the risk of infection. Provide prophylaxis with TMP-SMZ to minimize the risk of PCP for patients with SCID, undergoing organ transplantation, or receiving intensive immunosuppressive therapy. Provide varicella zoster immunoglobulin within 72 hours of exposure to varicella.
   c. *Immune reconstitution* involves palliative enhancement of immune function. IVIG administration (see IVIG section) is used in severely ill children: 100 to 400 mg/kg IV every 1 to 4 weeks.
   d. Enzyme replacement therapy remains controversial. Replacement therapy with polyethylene glycol–modified bovine ADA (PEG-ADA) administered subcutaneously once weekly results in clinical and immunologic improvement for *some* children with SCID associated with ADA deficiency.
   e. *Innovative treatment modalities* involve bone marrow transplantation (see Bone Marrow Transplantation section) and gene therapy. Gene therapy is a revolutionary means of replacing defective genes within the body (Carr, 1992). An experimental procedure was first used in children with SCID related to ADA deficiency (Blaese, 1992). Multistep treatment requires the removal of mature T lymphocytes or bone marrow from the patient, the

modification of these cells in the laboratory, and the return of the modified cells to the patient (Antoine, 1990; Garnett, 1990). Therapy results show potential in the cure of other diseases that are the result of a defective gene.

8. **Complications**
   a. Infection can progress to sepsis, septic shock, and death (see Septic Shock discussion in Chapter 9).
   b. Failure to thrive and malnutrition may require the use of parenteral nutrition.
   c. These patients are at risk for the development of GvHD through the following (Ammann, 1991; Mudge-Grout, 1992):
      • Immunocompetent lymphocytes are transfused from the mother to the fetus or infant during gestation or delivery.
      • Nonradiated blood is administered.
      • In the event of BMT the donor should be matched for HLA-A, HLA-B, HLA-C, and HLA-D with the mixed leukocyte reaction (MLR) (Ammann, 1991) (see Bone Marrow Transplantation section).
   d. Progressive poliomyelitis may occur if diagnosis is not made early and the child receives the live attenuated poliovirus immunization (Ammann, 1991). No live attenuated vaccines should be given.

D. **ACQUIRED IMMUNODEFICIENCY SYNDROME (AIDS)**
   1. **Definition** of terms (Jones et al, 1996)
      a. HIV infection is the disease spectrum from exposure to the virus to patient death.
      b. AIDS is the portion of the HIV disease when the immune system fails and clinical illness appears, usually an opportunistic infection.
      c. The incubation period is the period of time from the HIV infection to clinical manifestations of the disease; shorter incubation periods in children with perinatally acquired HIV have been noted than for children or adults with other modes of transmission (Berkowitz et al, 1992).
   2. **Pathophysiology**
      a. AIDS is caused by HIV, an RNA retrovirus. When a retrovirus infects a cell, the viral RNA is transcribed backward ("retro-") into the host DNA. The virus then uses the host cell's enzymes to direct the synthesis of new viral RNA and proteins to assemble new virus particles. The HIV interrupts normal cellular activity and function and ultimately causes the host cell to die, thereby releasing new virus into the circulation and infection of more host cells.
      b. The principal, but not exclusive, target of the HIV is the helper T lymphocyte, which orchestrates both CMI and HI. HIV causes the number and function of the helper T lymphocytes to decline, creating a decline in immune function and response and an imbalance in the ratio of helper T lymphocytes to suppressor or cytotoxic T lymphocytes (CD4 to CD8). As the number of CD4 (helper T lymphocytes) declines, the patient becomes increasingly immunocompromised and at risk for opportunistic infection or malignancy.
   3. **Etiology and risk factors**
      a. AIDS in children was first described in 1982, but retrospective evaluation of previously existing medical records revealed undiagnosed cases as early as 1979 (Lott and Kenner, 1994).
      b. *Incidence:* 9117 children have been reported to the Centers for Disease Control and Prevention (CDC) through October 1995. This represents approximately 2% of the cases of AIDS in the United States (Berkowitz et al, 1992).

- Incidence according to age (CDC, 1995)
  - Infants and children less than 4 years of age: 5432 cases reported
  - Children 5 to 12 years: 1385 cases reported
  - Children between 13 and 19 years: 2300 cases reported
- AIDS represents the ninth leading cause of death in children 1 to 4 years old and the twelfth leading cause of death in children 5 to 14 years old (Berkowitz et al, 1992).
  c. *Mode of transmission:* Children are most commonly infected by HIV through one of the following means:
  - Prenatal exposure is thought to be the most prevalent mode of transmission via the placenta during fetal development, but the transmission may also occur intrapartally (e.g., secretions) or postnatally (e.g., with exposure to maternal secretions such as breast milk contaminated with maternal blood). Of infants born to an HIV-positive mother, 25% to 35% will be HIV infected (presence of the HIV virus in the blood).
  - More rarely, children are infected through parenteral exposure to infected blood or blood products or sexual contact with an infected individual (accounts for <5% of cases). The latter is primarily applicable to sexually active adolescents, although younger children may be at risk if they are victims of child abuse (Landor and Rubinstein, 1993).
4. **Classification system** for HIV in children (Table 8–12): Children are classified into mutually exclusive categories. Once classified, the child may not be reclassified in a less severe category despite improvement in the child's immunologic or clinical condition.
5. **Signs and symptoms**
  a. *Clinical course and manifestations* are very different from those manifested in adult patients. The course of the disease is more accelerated, with most children symptomatic before 2 years compared to 8 to 10 years for adults. The pattern of disease also varies with the age of the patient, with children experiencing a higher incidence of bacterial infections compared to adult patients, neurodevelopmental alterations (including developmental delay), failure to thrive, and different types of cancers rather than Kaposi's sarcoma (e.g., lymphoma).
  b. *Clinical signs and symptoms* are nonspecific (Grossman, 1988; Lott and

Table 8–12. CENTERS FOR DISEASE CONTROL AND PREVENTION (CDC) 1994 REVISED CLASSIFICATION SYSTEM FOR HUMAN IMMUNODEFICIENCY VIRUS IN CHILDREN*

	CLINICAL CATEGORIES			
IMMUNOLOGIC CATEGORIES	N: NO SIGNS AND SYMPTOMS	A: MILD SIGNS AND SYMPTOMS	B†: MODERATE SIGNS AND SYMPTOMS	C†: SEVERE SIGNS AND SYMPTOMS
1: No evidence of suppression	N1	A1	B1	C1
2: Evidence of moderate suppression	N2	A2	B2	C2
3: Severe suppression	N3	A3	B3	C3

*Children whose HIV infection status is not confirmed are classified by using the above grid with a letter E (for perinatally exposed) placed before the appropriate classification code (e.g., EN2).

†Both category C and lymphoid interstitial pneumonitis in category B are reportable to state and local health departments as acquired immunodeficiency syndrome.

From Centers for Disease Control and Prevention. 1994 revised classification system for human immunodeficiency virus in children less than 13 years of age. *MMWR.* 1994;43(RR-12):1–10.

Kenner, 1994). The child who is HIV positive (antibodies for HIV) may remain asymptomatic before clinical signs develop, although the child may still transmit the virus. Symptoms include oral candidiasis, recurrent bacterial infections, chronic diarrhea, lymphadenopathy, hepatospleno-megaly, failure to thrive, eczematous rash, neurologic abnormalities (e.g., microcephaly, encephalopathy, dementia, developmental delay, or loss of attained milestones), fever, and salivary gland (parotid) enlargement.

6. **Interpretation of findings** from invasive and noninvasive diagnostic studies
   a. *Diagnostic considerations*
      - Serum antibodies that are produced in response to the HIV serve as the basis for HIV testing (Lott and Kenner, 1994). A confirmed positive test result indicates that antibodies have developed secondary to exposure to the virus, but it does *not* mean the child has AIDS. The following tests are most commonly used:
         ○ ELISA is highly sensitive and specific to the HIV antibody but cannot differentiate between maternal and infant antibody in the infant. A positive ELISA is always repeated, since other antibodies may produce a false-positive result.
         ○ Western blot is highly sensitive and specific to the HIV antibody but cannot differentiate between maternal and infant antibody in the infant. It is usually performed to confirm the result of ELISA.
      - More ideal methods involve testing for the virus itself.
         ○ p24 Antigen is the base antigen of HIV. The test is specific but not always sensitive. Therefore some HIV-positive individuals may have a negative p24 antigen result. If p24 is positive, the child is considered HIV positive, even in the presence of a negative ELISA result (Lott and Kenner, 1994). Lymphocyte p24-FCA test is a test similar to the p24 test but is based on the presence of p24 antigen on the surface of the lymphocyte. This test may be useful in the future (Lott and Kenner, 1994).
         ○ HIV culture indicates reverse transcriptase activity of the HIV in T cells. It requires a long incubation time (60 days).
      - There are challenges with the diagnosis of HIV in infancy, since maternal antibody is present in all infants born to HIV-positive mothers. Therefore, these infants have positive results from ELISA and Western blot tests, but approximately 75% of these are false-positive results, since these tests reflect the presence of maternal rather than infant antibody. It may take up to 18 months for the maternal antibody to clear. A viral specific test is required (viral culture or PCR) for accurate diagnosis in this age group.
   b. *Immune response to HIV:* HIV, especially vertically transmitted HIV, not only destroys mature and immature immune cells, but also interferes with the normal development and maturation of the immune system (Landor and Rubinstein, 1993).
      - Children may or may not have a profound lymphopenia (Grossman, 1988; Lott and Kenner, 1994); lymphopenia is uncommon in early infancy.
      - HI is decreased. Especially with vertical (prenatal) transmission, B-cell dysfunction may be evident. During fetal life the B-cell system matures after the T-cell system and is thought to be more vulnerable to damage by the HIV infection (Landor and Rubinstein, 1993). Congenital HIV infection presents with profound defects in HI and *initially* spares CMI (Landor and Rubinstein, 1993). Markedly elevated serum immuno-globulins is the most frequent pattern in pediatric HIV infection; it

may denote a relatively mild disease course (Landor and Rubinstein, 1993). Hypogammaglobulinemia, when present, is associated with progressive disease (Landor and Rubinstein, 1993; Rubinstein, 1986). Antibody synthesis is impaired after immunization. Secondary antibody response is more profoundly compromised than the primary response is (Landor and Rubinstein, 1993), thereby leading to repeated infections with the same organism. Dysregulation of HI is manifested by the formation of autoantibodies directed against platelets, neutrophils, lymphocytes, and RBCs (Landor and Rubinstein, 1993).

- CMI is affected. Suppressor or cytotoxic T lymphocytes (CD8) are increased. Helper T lymphocytes (CD4) are decreased. The helper–to–suppressor or cytotoxic T lymphocyte ratio (T4/T8 ratio) is decreased, first reflecting an increase in suppressor T lymphocytes and then later a helper T lymphocyte depletion (Landor and Rubinstein, 1993). Lymphocyte function is decreased. In skin testing there is a defective or complete failure of delayed hypersensitivity (DH) reactions because of a decreased lymphocyte response to antigens. IL-2 receptor expression is abnormal, and IL-2 secretion is diminished (Landor and Rubinstein, 1993), as is nonspecific cytotoxicity (decreased NK cell function) (Landor and Rubinstein, 1993).

c. *CBC* reveals anemia and thrombocytopenia.

d. *Coombs test* is positive (Grossman, 1988).

e. *Lymph node biopsies* often reveal marked follicular hyperplasia with an abundance of B cells

7. **Nursing and collaborative diagnoses**

❖ POTENTIAL FOR INFECTION RELATED TO THE HIV/AIDS DISEASE PROCESS, IMMUNODEFICIENCY, EFFECTS OF PRESCRIBED MEDICATIONS, AND MALNUTRITION

❖ POTENTIAL FOR IMPAIRED GAS EXCHANGE RELATED TO PULMONARY INFECTIONS (E.G., PCP OR OTHER OPPORTUNISTIC INFECTIONS)

❖ POTENTIAL FOR FLUID VOLUME DEFICIT DUE TO CHRONIC DIARRHEA AND FEVER

❖ POTENTIAL FOR ALTERED NUTRITION, LESS THAN BODY REQUIREMENTS, RELATED TO THE HIV/AIDS DISEASE PROCESS, NAUSEA, VOMITING, DIARRHEA, AND EFFECTS OF PRESCRIBED MEDICATIONS

❖ POTENTIAL NEUROLOGIC STATUS CHANGES RELATED TO HIV/AIDS DISEASE PROCESS

❖ POTENTIAL ALTERED PARENTING RELATED TO CHRONICITY OF DIAGNOSIS AND CRITICAL ILLNESS

❖ POTENTIAL FOR INEFFECTIVE COPING (PARENT, CHILD, SIBLING) RELATED TO THE CHRONICITY OF THE DISEASE, REPEATED HOSPITALIZATIONS, CRITICAL ILLNESS, DEATH OF A FAMILY MEMBER, OR ANXIETY AND FEAR OF INFECTION OR STIGMA

❖ POTENTIAL FOR TRANSMISSION OF THE DISEASE RELATED TO HIGH-RISK-TAKING BEHAVIOR AND LACK OF KNOWLEDGE REGARDING MODE OF TRANSMISSION

8. **Goals and desired patient outcomes**

a. Suppress retroviral replication.

b. Augment or improve the child's immune system.

c. Detect, identify, and eradicate infections or neoplastic disease.

9. **Patient care management**

a. Suppress or inhibit viral replication and prevent the development or progression of immunodeficiency. Most antiretroviral medications work by interfering with reverse transcription:

- Zidovudine (previously known as azidothymidine or AZT): Studies of IV and oral therapy indicate beneficial effects in children with HIV/AIDS (improved neurodevelopment) with minimal side effects (Landor and

Rubinstein, 1993). Zidovudine does not decrease the incidence of serious bacterial infections (Landor and Rubinstein, 1993) and has a hematopoietic suppressive effect commonly leading to anemia (Landor and Rubinstein, 1993).

- Dideoxycytidine (ddc) is characterized by little hematologic toxicity (Landor and Rubinstein, 1993).
- Dideoxyinosine (ddI) is associated with the incidence of pancreatitis.

b. Augment the child's immune system with CSFs (see Table 8–4) and IV gamma globulin.

c. Management of children with HIV/AIDS in the ICU varies with the reason for their admission.

- Respiratory failure secondary to PCP
  - ○ PCP with respiratory failure is the most common serious opportunistic infection in children with AIDS (Mudge-Grout, 1992), constituting two thirds of all opportunistic infections (Rubinstein, 1986). It is expected that approximately 50% of children with AIDS will have PCP (Hughes, 1994). *P. carinii*, a one-celled protozoa, is ubiquitous and benign to the healthy individual. In the immunocompromised host the organism is an aggressive pathogen with a corresponding high risk of respiratory failure and death (Mudge-Grout, 1992). Infection with *P. carinii* is thought to spread by the respiratory route from person to person. The organism targets the pulmonary tissue and once in the alveolus adheres to the epithelial cell surface. The immunocompetent individual is thought to undergo an asymptomatic infection, and the organism may persist indefinitely (Hughes, 1994). If immunocompromised, pneumonitis is characterized by diffuse, bilateral, interstitial and alveolar infiltrates (Hughes, 1994; Mudge-Grout, 1992). The incidence of PCP in adults with AIDS is closely correlated with the number of absolute helper T lymphocytes (CD4), but this relationship is less so in infants and young children (Hughes, 1994).
  - ○ Signs and symptoms: PCP is characterized by a tetrad of symptoms in all ages of patients and in all immunocompromised patients (with or without AIDS), but vary in intensity: cough (unproductive), tachypnea, dyspnea (or change in the young child's level of activity), and fever (with or without chills). Breath sounds are often clear. Child may demonstrate an acute onset with respiratory distress (without wheezing) and progressive respiratory failure. Blood gases are helpful in evaluating the severity of the pneumonitis (Hughes, 1994). Blood gases often reveal hypoxemia, respiratory alkalosis, and decreased diffusing capacity.
  - ○ Diagnostic findings: Definitive diagnosis is made when clinical symptoms are accompanied by evidence of the organism. Chest x-ray findings initially may be normal or reveal only mild interstitial infiltrates. Early findings typically begin in the perihilar region, progress peripherally, and finally to the apical portions of the lung (Hughes, 1994). Bilateral diffuse alveolar disease appears as pulmonary involvement worsens (Hughes, 1994). A late finding is diffuse and extensive bilateral pulmonary consolidation ("whiteout"). Diagnosis is made by obtaining evidence of the organism (Hughes, 1994). Lower respiratory tract secretions are obtained by bronchoscopy with bronchoalveolar lavage (BAL) or by sputum induction, which is less sensitive but also less invasive than BAL but may obviate the need for bronchoscopy. If an adequate specimen can be obtained and properly evaluated, diagnosis

may be confirmed by sputum induction even in very young children (Ognibene et al, 1989). Pulmonary parenchyma is obtained via transbronchial lung biopsy or open lung biopsy. Results are most sensitive and specific (Hughes, 1994), but this test rarely is needed to confirm the diagnosis (Landor and Rubinstein, 1993).

o Treatment: Definitive treatment is aimed at eradicating the organism. Two major drugs are available to treat *P. carinii*. Both are equally effective but differ in their adverse effects (Hughes, 1994). Trimethoprim-sulfamethoxazole (TMP-SMZ, Bactrim, Septra) is preferred over pentamidine because it has fewer adverse effects. It is recommended for initial treatment of PCP. TMP-SMZ initially is administered intravenously in all but the mildest of cases but may progress to oral doses once the infection is resolving (Hughes, 1994). The IV dose is trimethoprim 15 to 20 mg and sulfamethoxazole 75 to 100 mg/kg/d divided in three to four equal doses and infused over 1 hour. PO dose (tablets or suspension) is trimethoprim 20 mg and sulfamethoxazole 100 mg/kg/d divided in three to four equal doses. The course of treatment is 2 to 3 weeks. At the completion of treatment, doses are reduced to prophylactic range but are continued indefinitely (Hughes, 1994). Adverse effects occur with both IV and PO route of administration. The most common adverse effect is a transient erythematous maculopapular rash that resolves following withdrawal of the drug. Less common adverse effects include nausea and vomiting, neutropenia, diarrhea, anemia, and methemoglobinemia. Indications for discontinuing TMP-SMZ and considering another medication are side effects in the absence of clinical improvement after 3 to 5 days, no clinical improvement after 5 to 7 days, and urticarial rash or Stevens-Johnson syndrome.

o Pentamidine isethionate is the next drug of choice (Hughes, 1994). It is given IM or IV; IV is the preferred route since it is associated with fewer adverse effects. IM use is uncommon and very painful. The IV dose is 4 mg/kg/d. The course of treatment is 2 to 3 weeks. Adverse effects are frequent and include hypotension, hypoglycemia or hyperglycemia, hepatic and renal toxicity, rash, thrombocytopenia, anemia (Hughes, 1994).

o Use of steroids may prevent or suppress the inflammatory response and reduce pulmonary edema secondary to PCP (Mudge-Grout, 1992).

o Supportive treatment is provided. Most patients require oxygen administration. Mechanical ventilation is indicated with respiratory failure if PaO_2 cannot be maintained at 60 mm Hg or greater with inspired O_2 fraction of 50% or greater. A poor response to anti-*Pneumocystis* drugs may indicate the presence of another infection. Superinfections with *Pseudomonas*, *Klebsiella*, *Candida*, and CMV are very common (Landor and Rubinstein, 1993).

o Prognosis (Mudge-Grout, 1992): During early days of treatment the best indicator of clinical response is blood gases (Hughes, 1994). Patients with an alveolar-arterial oxygen gradient less than 30 mm Hg at the time of therapy have a better prognosis than those with ≥30 mm Hg gradient (Hughes, 1994). Chest x-ray examination is less helpful in revealing clinical improvement or deterioration. Subsequent episodes of *P. carinii* infection greatly diminish the child's chances of survival; therefore, lifelong prophylaxis is instituted regardless of clinical status or CD4 counts (Centers for Disease Control and Prevention [CDC], 1995b). Prophylaxis regimens include *one* of the following (Hughes, 1994): TMP-SMZ (Bactrim, Septra) twice daily taken 3 days per week, *or* aerosolized pentamidine once a month, *or* Dapsone daily.

- ○ Despite previous guidelines for prophylaxis of *P. carinii* infection among HIV infected infants and children, no substantial decrease had been noted in *P. carinii* infection incidence. Therefore prophylaxis is initiated in infants born to HIV-infected women. Prophylaxis should begin at 4 to 6 weeks of age, regardless of CD4 counts. All HIV-infected infants and infants whose infection status has not yet been determined should remain on prophylaxis until 12 months of age (CDC, 1995b). HIV-infected children older than 12 months of age should have regular CD4 monitoring to determine the need for *P. carinii* prophylaxis (CDC, 1995b): HIV-infected 1- to 5-year-old children require prophylaxis if the CD4 count is less than 500 cells/µL or CD4 percentage is less than 15%. HIV-infected 6- to 12-year-old children require prophylaxis if the CD4 count is less than 200 cells/µL or CD4 percentage is less than 15%.

- • Respiratory failure secondary to lymphocytic interstitial pneumonitis (LIP) or pulmonary lymphoid hyperplasia (PLH)
  - ○ LIP/PLH is defined as diffuse infiltration of alveolar walls by mature lymphocytes, plasma cells, and reticuloendothelial cells. Although associated with other immunodeficiencies and autoimmune diseases, it affects up to 51% of children with HIV infection (Mudge-Grout, 1992; Rubinstein, 1986; Rubinstein et al, 1988). In the child with AIDS, LIP is characterized by atypical, rather than mature, lymphocytes invading the bronchioles and creating the pulmonary infiltrate (Mudge-Grout, 1992). The cause of LIP is unknown. It is unclear whether LIP and PLH are two extremes of the same disease or two unrelated entities (Landor and Rubinstein, 1993). EBV DNA has been isolated in the lung tissue of children with LIP/PLH, suggesting persistent EBV infection as a cause (Landor and Rubinstein, 1993).
  - ○ Signs and symptoms present as chronic and progressive. Respiratory symptoms are nonproductive cough, tachypnea, dyspnea, and normal to decreased breath sounds; basilar rales are possible. Other symptoms are generalized lymphadenopathy and parotid gland enlargement.
  - ○ Diagnostic findings: Chest x-ray examination discloses diffuse miliary pattern similar to that seen in tuberculosis (Mudge-Grout, 1992) and diffuse reticulonodular infiltrates, at times with hilar and mediastinal adenopathy. Nodular densities are distributed throughout the lung (Landor and Rubinstein, 1993). Pulmonary physiology resembles that of PCP and includes hypoxemia, respiratory alkalosis, decreased diffusing capacity, and restrictive lung volumes. The lack of fever, acute respiratory distress, and significant auscultatory findings assist in the distinction between LIP/PLH and PCP (Landor and Rubinstein, 1993). Diagnosis is often made using clinical findings but may be confirmed with an open lung biopsy.
  - ○ Treatment: LIP/PLH responds well to corticosteroid administration, although it is recommended only when the PaO_2 is less than 70 mm Hg (Landor and Rubinstein, 1993). Prednisone is given daily for 4 weeks, followed by an alternate-day therapy regimen at lower doses (duration of alternate-day therapy ranges from months to years; Landor and

Rubinstein, 1993). Administration of steroids does not seem to affect the acceleration of viral replication (Landor and Rubinstein, 1993). Treatment is largely supportive.

- Prognosis: The child with AIDS experiencing LIP has a better prognosis than a child with a documented opportunistic infection (Mudge-Grout, 1992).

10. **Transmission precautions**

a. Although HIV is detected in many body fluids, the single most infectious medium for HIV is blood (Berkowitz et al, 1992). Universal blood and body fluid precautions should be used for *all* patients, including those children experiencing HIV/AIDS. Use gloves when handling any body secretions including blood, stool, vomitus, or nasogastric (NG) drainage or performing invasive procedures. Use barrier precautions or protective wear (gown and protective eyewear) to prevent skin and mucus membrane contamination. Hands should be washed following glove removal.

b. Parenteral exposure to infected blood by accidental needle stick injury is the overwhelming cause of HIV in health care workers (Berkowitz et al, 1992). There is decreased risk with the use of needleless systems, placement of needles and other "sharps" in puncture-resistant containers for disposal, and avoidance of recapping, bending, or removing needles from disposable syringes (Berkowitz et al, 1992).

11. **Impact of HIV on other organ systems**

a. *Respiratory system:* Respiratory dysfunction occurs in almost 70% of HIV-infected children and is the most frequent cause of death (Berkowitz et al, 1992). Acute respiratory failure (the most common reason for admission into an ICU) often occurs.

b. *Cardiovascular system:* The most common cardiovascular derangement is septic shock. The most frequently isolated pathogens (Wilkinson and Greenwald, 1988) are *S. pneumoniae, Salmonella* species, and *H. influenzae.* Common pediatric bacterial infections include otitis media, sinusitis, bacteremia, recurrent pneumonia, and enterocolitis. Common viral infections are caused by CMV, hepatitis B, and EBV. Severe congestive heart failure occurs secondary to AIDS-associated cardiomyopathy (Wilkinson and Greenwald, 1988). Cardiomyopathy is manifested by tachycardia, arrhythmias, conduction abnormalities, cardiomegaly, or congestive heart failure.

c. *CNS* (Wilkinson and Greenwald, 1988): The most common CNS derangement is secondary infection by usual or opportunistic pathogens such as *H. influenzae, S. pneumoniae,* and *N. meningitidis.* Primary HIV infection of the brain results in encephalopathy.

d. *Hematologic system* (Wilkinson and Greenwald, 1988): The most common disorders are autoimmune thrombocytopenia and drug-induced (therapy) granulocytopenia.

E. SECONDARY IMMUNODEFICIENCY

A large percentage of children admitted to the ICU are immunocompromised as a result of an acquired defects in immune function.

1. Secondary immunodeficiency is caused by a variety of stressors including, but not limited to, anesthesia, tissue injury (e.g., surgery, trauma, thermal injuries), medications (see Relevant Pharmacology section), and malnutrition (acute and chronic).

2. Although the pathophysiology of the defects in immune function differs slightly with each of the aforementioned stressors, the implications of these are the same as found in the section on White Blood Cells: Hypoactivity.

COAGULOPATHIES AND PLATELET DISORDERS

A. **DISSEMINATED INTRAVASCULAR COAGULATION (DIC)**

DIC is a serious bleeding disorder resulting from accelerated normal clotting with a subsequent decrease in clotting factors and platelets, leading to uncontrolled bleeding.

1. **Pathophysiology:** Coagulation mechanisms are abnormally stimulated.

   a. *Clotting component:* Widespread and rapid formation of fibrin thrombi in the microcirculation results in the consumption of certain clotting factors and platelets. The presence of fibrin thrombi in the microcirculation (microclots) leads to ischemic tissue injury. If significant microinfarction occurs, organ function is impaired leading to brain, kidney, liver, or lung injury.

   b. *Hemorrhagic component:* As the clots are lysed and clotting factors (factors V and VIII), fibrinogen, and platelets are consumed, blood loses its ability to clot (consumptive coagulopathy). A stable clot, therefore, cannot be formed at injury sites, thus predisposing to hemorrhage. Clotting factors and platelets cannot be made by the body as fast as they are used.

2. **Etiology and risk factors:** DIC is not a primary disease or primary bleeding disorder. DIC is always a result of another disease or condition. It is often associated with shock, infections, hemolytic processes (such as transfusion of mismatched blood), and severe tissue damage (such as extensive burns or trauma, rejection of transplants, and postoperative damage, especially following extracorporeal circulation). Possible additional causes are neoplastic disorders (especially acute promyelocytic leukemia), fat and pulmonary embolisms, snake bites, acute anoxia, hepatic insufficiency or splenectomy, obstetric emergencies and complications, fresh water near drowning, and heat stroke.

3. **Signs and symptoms:** Two categories of symptoms occur; however, many patients may have laboratory evidence of DIC without clinical signs.

   a. *Clotting* is related to the microvascular thromboses. Symptoms include spontaneous, easy, or disproportionately severe bruising; intramuscular hematoma (spontaneous or trauma related); cool, mottled skin; pallor; and circulatory failure. Thrombosis of peripheral or central veins leads to absent popliteal, posterior tibial, or pedal pulses; cyanosis of fingers, toes, earlobes, or tip of the nose; and tissue necrosis and gangrene.

   b. *Bleeding* in a patient with no previous bleeding history or out of proportion to the degree of thrombocytopenia is noted as a range from prolonged oozing from venipuncture sites and bleeding around intranasal, endotracheal, and urethral catheters to profuse hemorrhage from all orifices. Subtle to occult bleeding occurs. Systemic signs include the following:

      • Skin: Petechiae, ecchymosis, purpura, and hematoma
      • Head: Gingival bleeding and epistaxis
      • Genitourinary: Hematuria
      • GI tract: Hematemesis and melena
      • Neurologic: Headache and altered level of consciousness
      • Cardiovascular: Symptoms of shock

4. **Interpretation of findings** from invasive and noninvasive diagnostic studies: No single laboratory test confirms the diagnosis of DIC.

   a. *Platelet count* is decreased.

   b. *Coagulation tests*
      • PT is prolonged.
      • PTT is prolonged.

- Thromboplastin time is increased.
- Fibrinogen level is decreased.
- FSP is elevated (>40 µg/ml), with increased amounts of D-dimer in the assay.

5. **Nursing and collaborative diagnoses**
   ❖ POTENTIAL FOR BLEEDING AND HEMORRHAGE
   a. Maintain mucous membrane and skin integrity.
   b. Monitor internal bleeding and control overt bleeding.
   ❖ IMPAIRED CARDIAC OUTPUT DUE TO BLOOD LOSS
   ❖ POTENTIAL FOR IMPAIRED GAS EXCHANGE RELATED TO BLOOD LOSS
   a. Maintain hemoglobin above 10 g/dl.
   b. Treat hypoxemia.

6. **Goals and desired patient outcomes**
   a. Correct primary problem.
   b. Perfuse vital organs until primary problem and DIC are controlled.

7. **Patient care management:** Early detection and prompt management can prevent complications and death. Primary disorders associated with DIC must be treated.
   a. *Supportive treatment:* If the symptoms of thrombosis or bleeding are mild, no specific therapy is needed. Begin specific treatments only when significant bleeding or organ dysfunction related to DIC occurs.
      - Administer blood products, replacing coagulation factors. Provide platelet transfusion if platelet count is less than 20,000/mm^3. FFP provides clotting factors; give with packed RBCs if the platelet count is greater than 50,000/mm^3 and the patient is still bleeding. Cryoprecipitate provides needed fibrinogen and factor VIII. Use if FFP or whole blood is not available. Give if fibrinogen is below 75 g/dl. Fresh whole blood is used if bleeding is profuse to supply all clotting factors and platelets. This will also serve as a volume expander and increase oxygen-carrying capacity by increasing the hemoglobin. If after 6 to 8 hours of aggressive treatment and the patient is still in shock and bleeding, consider double-volume exchange transfusion with heparinized fresh blood, reconstituted FFP, and packed RBCs.
      - Heparin by continuous infusion is a controversial treatment. The goal is to tip the balance within the microcirculation toward physiologic fibrinolysis and allow reperfusion of the vital organs. Although it may stop the clotting, it may initially worsen the bleeding. Administer 10 to 20 U/kg/h as a continuous infusion after an initial loading dose of 50 U/kg while continuing supportive treatment with blood products. Titrate the infusion to decrease bleeding and increase the fibrinogen with a decrease in the D-dimer. Oral anticoagulants are of no benefit or substitute for heparin.
      - Provide normal perfusion by fluid replacement.
   b. Improvement is reflected by increased fibrinogen concentrations and platelet count. Any increase in fibrinogen or platelet count is an encouraging indication that the consumption process has been interrupted and bleeding will be under control.

8. **Complications** are related to end-organ hypoxic or ischemia changes. Multifocal neurologic defects are due to multiple small brain infarcts. Thrombosis of blood vessels supplying the kidney cortex may result in renal failure. Pulmonary embolism and adult respiratory distress syndrome (ARDS) may occur. Acute ulceration and GI bleeding, intraabdominal bleeding, intrahepatic hemorrhage, and mesenteric thrombosis may occur.

B. IDIOPATHIC THROMBOCYTOPENIC PURPURA (ITP)

1. **Pathophysiology:** "Idiopathic" means the exact cause of the disease is not known; purpura means bruises caused by bleeding into the skin. ITP is also called autoimmune thrombocytopenic purpura.

   a. Exact cause is often not known; other possible causes of the thrombocytopenia must be ruled out such as toxin or drug exposure. Viral illnesses precede the onset of symptoms in half the cases.

   b. The body develops antibodies against its own platelets. These antibodies coat the surface of the platelets and cause the immune system to see the platelet as "foreign" or "nonself" and destroy it. IgG antibodies directed against specific platelet antigens lead to platelet destruction. Immunoglobulin coating of the platelets may interfere with platelet function, and bleeding may occur when platelets are less than $50,000/mm^3$. The spleen is the site of antibody production and of destruction of sensitized platelets. Bone marrow produces platelets as rapidly as possible, but the platelets are quickly destroyed (in a few hours). Increased sequestration of platelets in the spleen further limits the availability of platelets to the circulation.

2. **Etiology and risk factors:** Children usually have had a viral-induced upper respiratory tract infection, measles, mumps, or chickenpox a few weeks prior to the onset of ITP. Clinical course is generally a severe but self-limited thrombocytopenia in children under age 12 years. Most cases resolve within 6 weeks to 6 months; 10% go on to develop chronic ITP.

3. **Signs and symptoms:** Patients present with bleeding and thrombocytopenia, particularly into their skin and mucous membranes. The bleeding may be seen in all body parts and may be severe enough to result in shock. Splenomegaly is rare.

4. **Diagnosis**

   a. Exclude other causes of accelerated platelet destruction or decreased production of platelets by the bone marrow. Rule out leukemia, meningococcal meningitis, sepsis, systemic lupus erythematosus, and DIC.

   b. The history of the child indicates previous good health; some report a recent viral illness.

   c. Examination reveals bruises and petechiae appearing almost overnight, with no apparent cause.

5. **Interpretation of findings** from invasive and noninvasive diagnostic studies

   a. *CBC*
      - Platelet count is decreased.
      - Platelet function may be normal or show diminished aggregation.

   b. *PT and PTT* are usually normal.

   c. *FSP levels* are normal.

   d. *Bone marrow aspirate* is obtained to see if the bone marrow is producing enough platelets. It may reveal increased megakaryocytes.

6. **Nursing and collaborative diagnoses**
   - ❖ POTENTIAL FOR IMPAIRED SKIN AND MUCOUS MEMBRANE INTEGRITY
   - ❖ POTENTIAL FOR HEMORRHAGE

7. **Goals and desired patient outcomes:** Individualization of the treatment plan

   a. Protection from sources of trauma. Parents should be taught to make the environment as safe as possible (bumper pads on the crib, avoid toys with sharp or hard surfaces). Older children should not play contact sports; restrict bicycles.

   b. Avoid other platelet-damaging drugs such as aspirin.

c. Control bleeding.

d. Maintain normal platelet count and function.

8. **Patient care management:** Acute ITP is usually self-limited with most patients recovering without treatment. Life-threatening bleeding occurs only rarely.

   a. *Steroids* produce prolonged remission in most cases. They have been shown to decrease the removal of the sensitized platelets from the circulation and to increase production and mobilize platelets from the platelet pool. Steroids prevent bleeding by decreasing the rate of platelet destruction in the spleen and will result in a platelet increase within 5 to 21 days.

   b. The *IVIG mechanism of action* is the same as that of steroids in that it increases the platelet count by blocking the antibodies that destroy the sensitized platelets in the spleen. High doses (1 g/kg) have been shown to elevate the platelet count to higher than $30,000/mm^3$ within 3 days. Some patients may not require further doses of IVIG with a permanent increase of their platelet counts. Other patients may require repeated doses of IVIG because of transient increases in their platelet counts.

   c. *Splenectomy* may be used if ITP does not respond to medical treatment and bleeding continues. It is generally avoided in the young child because of the association with a risk of sepsis after splenectomy.

   d. *Platelets* are transfused only if life-threatening bleeding such as CNS or GI tract bleeding occurs. Platelets will be destroyed by antiplatelet antibodies. When platelets are transfused, they are complexed with antibody and rapidly removed from the circulation by the spleen, sometimes within minutes of the transfusion.

   e. Vincristine and cyclophosphamide may be given to suppress the immune system, producing the platelet antibody with variable success.

9. **Complications**

   a. Intracranial bleeding: Most serious complication; occurs in less than 1% of patients with ITP

   b. Bleeding from nose or gums, not as severe, more frequent

   c. GI tract and kidney bleeding

10. Differentiation from hemolytic-uremic syndrome (HUS)

   a. HUS is a triad of hemolytic anemia, thrombocytopenia, and renal failure, all of which involve diffuse endothelial cell damage, activation of platelets, and widespread involvement of multiple organ systems.

   b. HUS is similar to ITP in that HUS is usually associated with infection or viral illness and that many children have bruising and petechiae.

   c. HUS is different from ITP in that HUS is associated with oliguria or anuria with elevated BUN and with neurologic symptoms such as seizures or coma.

   d. Average course of illness for HUS is 4 to 6 weeks.

PLASMA CLOTTING FACTOR DISORDER: HEMOPHILIA

A. **PATHOPHYSIOLOGY**

   Hemophilia is a disorder of hemostasis of one or more clotting factors.

   1. **Types:**

      a. Hemophilia A: Deficient in factor VIII; also called classic hemophilia

      b. Hemophilia B: Deficient in factor IX; also called Christmas disease

   2. Formation of a normal clot at sites of bleeding is prevented. The degree of

bleeding is related to the degree of factor deficiency. Hemophiliacs are susceptible to persistent bleeding or severe hematoma formation following relatively minor trauma. Severe hemophilia is more likely to be associated with spontaneous bleeding.

B. **ETIOLOGY AND RISK FACTORS**

1. Sex-linked recessive traits occur almost exclusively in males, but female carriers transmit the disease. In hemophilia A, inheritance of an abnormal gene produces a defective factor VIII protein with little or no clotting activity. Hemophilia B is caused by a defective factor IX gene and protein.

2. Because the gene easily mutates, one third of affected individuals do not have a family history.

3. Diagnosis can be done during pregnancy for those parents identified as at risk for transmitting the disease.

C. **SIGNS AND SYMPTOMS**

1. Presentation of bleeding varies. Bleeding can occur anywhere in the body following trauma or normal activity or spontaneously.

2. Specific signs and symptoms include the following:

   a. Slow, persistent, prolonged bleeding from minor injuries and small cuts

   b. Uncontrollable hemorrhage subsequent to dental extraction or irritation of the gums

   c. Epistaxis, especially after a facial injury

   d. Hematuria from genitourinary trauma

   e. Ecchymosis and subcutaneous hematomas (petechiae are rare)

   f. Neurologic manifestations ranging from bleeding near peripheral nerve leading to compression of the nerves

   g. Bleeding into joints (hemarthrosis) that may lead to severe joint deformity, especially knees, ankles, and elbows; causes permanent crippling

D. **INTERPRETATION OF FINDINGS FROM INVASIVE AND NONINVASIVE DIAGNOSTIC STUDIES**

1. **Hemophilia A**

   a. *Factor VIII assay:* Decreased levels

      • Less than 1% of normal level represents severe hemophilia. Child is at risk for spontaneous and trauma-induced hemorrhage from infancy.

      • 2% to 5% of normal level: Child will have a moderate clinical course except with trauma or surgery, when supportive treatment will be necessary.

      • Greater than 5% of normal level: A mild clinical course; supportive treatment is not often needed.

   b. *PTT* is significantly prolonged and is used to assess effectiveness of correction by blood products

   c. *CBC:* Normal results including platelet count

2. **Hemophilia B**

   a. *Factor IX assay:* Decreased levels

      • Less than 1% of normal level represents a severe bleeding tendency.

      • 1% to 3% of normal level represents a moderate degree of bleeding tendency.

      • 5% to 25% of normal level represents normal clotting time and no spontaneous bleeding.

      • Greater than 25% of normal level represents significant bleeding only if trauma or surgery.

   b. *PT* is normal, and PTT is prolonged (usually at least 60 seconds in children with severe deficiencies).

   c. *CBC* results are normal, including platelet count.

3. **X-ray findings:** Major joint destruction following repeated hemorrhages

E. **NURSING AND COLLABORATIVE DIAGNOSIS**

   ❖ POTENTIAL FOR HEMORRHAGE RELATED TO DEFICIENCY OF FACTOR VIII OR IX

   1. Local control of hemarthrosis includes elastic wraps and ice packs to the affected limb to reduce swelling, bleeding, and pain. Elevation of the extremity, restriction of normal activity for 48 hours to prevent rebleeding, and pain control are important.

   2. Administer factor VIII or IX or cryoprecipitate, depending on the diagnosis.

   ❖ POTENTIAL FOR IMPAIRED SKIN AND MUCOUS MEMBRANE INTEGRITY

   1. Prevent injury. Venipunctures should be only antecubital, external jugular, or other superficial veins. Counseling should include the appropriate level of activity for the child including contact sports.

   2. Avoid NSAIDs and aspirin.

   ❖ TEACHING NEEDS OF PARENTS

   1. Provide genetic counseling.

   2. Teach how to recognize a bleeding episode, which measures should be done first, and how to differentiate between episodes that can be controlled at home vs. ones that require hospital care.

F. **GOALS AND DESIRED PATIENT OUTCOMES**

   1. Restore normal clotting activity.

      a. *Hemophilia A:* For mild hemorrhages, at least 30% of normal level is needed to control bleeding. For major bleeding, correction to at least 70% of normal level and perhaps to 100% activity is recommended.

      b. *Hemophilia B:* At least 10% to 25% of the normal level of factor is needed; for major bleeding, at least a 40% level is needed.

   2. Minimal tissue and joint damage

   3. Preparation for the child in need of surgery is 80% to 100% of normal factor level. Keep level above 30% to 50% during the postoperative course.

G. **PATIENT CARE MANAGEMENT**

   1. Blood products for children with hemophilia A

      a. For severe bleeding, give factor VIII (AHF) concentrate. Half-life is 10 to 12 hours; subsequent transfusions are needed depending on response and severity of bleeding. One to several days of maintenance therapy are needed for advanced lesions to resolve; must give subsequent infusions every 24 hours (75% of the original dose). The initial dose should not be delayed, and all subsequent doses should be administered on time to assure hemostasis is achieved quickly and maintained.

      b. FFP requires more quantity than factor VIII concentrates to control bleeding and is rarely used.

      c. For less severe bleeding in mild hemophilia (factor VIII > 5% to 10%), use desmopressin (DDAVP), which causes release of factor VIII from endothelial cells.

      d. Platelets may correct thrombocytopenia but will not correct the coagulopathy

   2. Blood products for children with hemophilia B

      a. Factor IX concentrate of monoclonal factor IX or recombinant factor IX (when available) is used.

      b. FFP may be used as a source of factor IX for mild bleeding.

      c. Prothrombin complex concentrates are a major treatment source for children with severe deficiencies of factor IX.

H. **COMPLICATIONS**

   1. Hematoma formation, which can be large in size, results in compression of vital structures. Hematomas may produce fever, leukocytosis, severe pain, and hyperbilirubinemia due to RBC degradation.

2. Progressive arthropathy: Inflammatory and hypertrophic changes occur in the synovial tissue. Over time this results in erosion of cartilage and bone.

3. Intracranial bleeding associated with trauma may be associated with subdural, epidural, intracerebral, subarachnoid, or rarely intraspinal sites.

4. Inhibitor to factor VIII may develop.

BONE MARROW TRANSPLANTATION (BMT)

A. **DEFINITION**

A BMT is the transplantation of pluripotential hematopoietic stem cells capable of self-renewal and terminal differentiation, giving rise to an entirely new hematopoietic system for the patient.

1. BMT is primary therapy in patients whose endogenous marrow function is defective and is also for rescue following treatment of malignancies with very high doses of chemotherapy and radiotherapy.

  a. Leukemia: Acute lymphocytic, acute myelogenous, chronic myelogenous

  b. Solid tumors: Lymphoma, neuroblastoma, Wilms' tumor, brain tumors, other tumors

  c. Hematopoietic stem cell defect: Aplastic anemia, congenital severe immunodeficiencies, osteopetrosis, thalassemia, sickle cell anemia

2. Success of this treatment is related to prevention of rejection or GvHD and appropriate control over the potential multiorgan complications that occur in the weeks after transplant while waiting for the return of the transplanted bone marrow function.

3. Purposes of conditioning regimens: Chemotherapy with or without radiation is used to eliminate the tumor from the recipient, to ablate the recipient's marrow in preparation for the donated marrow, and to suppress the recipient's immunity to prevent rejection of the graft (donated marrow).

B. **TYPES**

1. **Autologous transplant** uses bone marrow from the patient's own marrow. The marrow is harvested (removed) during a known period of time in which the marrow is in remission or the malignancy does not involve the bone marrow. The marrow is then treated and frozen to preserve viability of the cells. After very high doses of chemotherapy and radiation to remove cancer cells from the patient's marrow or other organs, the marrow is thawed and reinfused into the patient as a hematopoietic "rescue" from the marrow ablation secondary to high doses of chemotherapy.

2. A **syngeneic transplant** is bone marrow taken from an identical twin and reinfused into the ill twin. Usually there are few complications because of identical gene makeup. It does not require as aggressive a conditioning regimen because only removal of the tumor is needed, not ablation of the marrow to prevent graft rejection. Marrow is reinfused as a "rescue" as an autologous transplant.

3. **Allogeneic transplant**

  a. There are several types of donors who undergo a bone marrow harvest.

    • Genotypic match (sibling): A family member who has demonstrated histocompatibility (similar HLA antigens)

    • Related mismatched (parent): A family member who has demonstrated partial HLA matching

    • Unrelated phenotypic match: Marrow from a nonrelative that is HLA matched at the major loci. Donor found through bone marrow donor registries. At some centers, removal of the T lymphocytes from the

marrow before reinfusing the marrow into the donor may minimize the incidence of GvHD
   - Unrelated mismatched: Partially HLA matched and from a different gene pool. A donor is found through bone marrow donor registries. Donor marrow preparation involves removal of the T lymphocytes as per unrelated phenotypic matches.
   b. The donated marrow is infused into the patient who has undergone intense chemotherapy or irradiation as part of the treatment of the disease and ablation of the marrow in preparation for transplanted marrow cells (also known as the conditioning regimen).
   c. Engraftment typically occurs in 2 to 4 weeks in an HLA-matched allogeneic BMT. RBC and platelet function return when normal laboratory values return. Normal WBC count may return in a few weeks; however, effective function of the WBCs may take up to a year. If the transplanted marrow cells are of a different RBC type, close collaboration with the Blood Bank is needed to administer the appropriate product as outlined in Table 8–13.

C. MANAGEMENT

1. Reconstitution of a near-normal immunologic status takes place progressively over a period that may last several months to more than a year following the BMT.
   a. To prevent GvHD, patients are given immunosuppressive drugs (see section on Relevant Pharmacology).
   b. Supportive care is needed to manage electrolyte imbalances and nutritional deficits, deficient blood components, and infections. Total parenteral nutrition and fluid replacements may be needed. RBCs should be used to

Table 8–13. BLOOD PRODUCT TRANSFUSION GUIDELINES FOR BONE MARROW TRANSPLANTATION (BMT)

DONOR	RECIPIENT	PACKED RBCs	WBCs	PLATELETS AND PLASMA
ABO Compatible				
O	O	O	O	O
A	A	A	A	A, AB
B	B	B	B	B, AB
AB	AB	AB	AB	AB
Major ABO Incompatibility				
A	B	O	O	AB
A	O	O	O	A, AB
B	A	O	O	AB
B	O	O	O	B, AB
AB	A	A	A	AB
AB	B	B	B	AB
AB	O	O	O	AB
Minor ABO Incompatibility				
O	A	O	O	A, AB
O	B	O	O	B, AB
O	AB	O	O	AB
A	AB	A	A	AB
B	AB	B	B	AB

Modified from Quinones RR. Bone marrow transplantation. In: Fuhrman BP, Zimmerman JJ. *Pediatric Critical Care.* St Louis, Mo: The CV Mosby Co; 1992:846.

keep the hematocrit higher than 25%. Platelet transfusions should be used to keep the platelet count higher than $20,000/mm^3$ unless the patient is actively bleeding or an invasive procedure is planned; then the platelet count should be in the 50,000 to $100,000/mm^3$ range. Clotting factors should be replaced with appropriate blood products such as FFP when the PT or PTT is greater than 1.5 times the control value, if the fibrinogen level is less than 100 mg/dl, or if there is active bleeding. Antibiotics may be required.

c. Pain related to severe mucositis and liver enlargement usually is effectively managed through the use of continuous narcotic infusions.

D. ACUTE COMPLICATIONS

1. **Infection** is the leading cause of morbidity and mortality in the posttransplantation patient

   a. For weeks after the transplant the patient remains profoundly immunosuppressed and highly susceptible to bacterial, viral, and fungal infections despite aggressive antibiotic and antifungal therapy and protective environments. The most common strategy for prevention of infection is high-efficiency particle air (HEPA), filtered air and positive pressure rooms to decrease risk of fungal infections. Some centers use reverse isolation particularly for transplants for children with congenital immunodeficiency diseases. Other requirements include strict hand washing techniques, meticulous central venous catheter care, prophylactic antibiotics, and daily mouth care. CMV-negative blood products are used if both the donor and recipient of the marrow are CMV-negative.

   b. Identification of the *signs and symptoms* of infection must be immediately followed by prompt and aggressive treatment to avoid septic shock and death.

   c. *Management* includes antibiotics and antiviral agents.

2. **Hepatic dysfunction:** Venoocclusive disease (VOD) is seen in the first few days up to 2 to 3 weeks after a BMT.

   a. VOD is caused by obliteration of small hepatic venules, resulting from hepatotoxicity of intensive chemotherapy and radiation. Deposits of fibrous material plug the small venules in the liver. Pressure and fluids back up into the sinusoids of the liver, leading to liver engorgement as venous outflow becomes more and more occluded. Anoxia leads to further injury and necrosis of hepatic tissue with the result that hepatic blood flow and function is even more impaired.

   b. *Diagnosis:* VOD must be differentiated from GvHD, drug-induced liver injury, and hepatitis. Liver biopsy assists in definitive diagnosis; however, this is a high-risk procedure in the critically ill post-BMT patient because of a high risk of bleeding. Signs and symptoms range from moderate liver dysfunction to hepatic coma. Clinical symptoms include jaundice or hyperbilirubinemia, right upper quadrant pain or hepatomegaly, and ascites or unexplained weight gain.

   c. *Management:* Presently no treatment to prevent or reverse VOD is available. Clinical efforts are directed toward supportive and symptomatic care until VOD runs its course and the regenerative capabilities of the liver have a chance to repair the damage. Correct fluid and electrolyte imbalances. Minimize adverse effects of ascites. Adjust drugs to reflect impaired hepatic clearance. Attend to coagulopathies.

3. **GI tract dysfunction**

   a. GI tract dysfunction is caused by direct toxicity of chemotherapy and

radiation, which provides a portal of entry for infection from the denuding of the epithelial lining of the entire GI tract mucosa.
  b. *Diagnosis*
    • Signs and symptoms include mucositis (inflammation of all mucous membranes, which is quite painful); nausea, vomiting, and diarrhea (hypovolemia and significant electrolyte imbalances); and hemorrhage from a site in the GI tract.
    • Endoscopic procedures
  c. *Management*
    • Mucositis: Use appropriate antibiotics, meticulous oral hygiene, and pain control.
    • Nausea and vomiting: Aggressive use of antiemetics, especially in combinations individualized to patient response, is indicated.
    • Diarrhea: Control fluid and electrolyte imbalances; provide symptomatic relief; and protect the skin in the rectal area from severe excoriation and breakdown.
    • Hemorrhage: Maintain hemodynamic stability and find and treat the source; angiography and surgery may or may not be performed, depending on the determination of the risks vs. the benefits.
4. **Renal dysfunction**
  a. Renal dysfunction is caused by toxicities of chemotherapy, antibiotics, antifungals, and CSA and is aggravated by any prerenal problems such as decreased renal perfusion from hypovolemia.
  b. Diagnosis, signs and symptoms, and laboratory results are detailed in Chapter 5.
  c. Specific differences regarding renal dysfunction in the BMT patient include the following:
    • Hyperkalemia may not occur, since in patients receiving CSA or amphotericin B, potassium continues to be wasted in the urine unless the patient becomes anuric.
    • Hypokalemia frequently occurs, often requiring IV potassium replacement.
    • Increased BUN is difficult to interpret, as it is influenced by processes other than decreased glomerular filtration rate. Steroids and the presence of blood in the GI tract can significantly increase BUN without any alteration in renal function.
  d. Rarely, dialysis is required to eliminate waste products, restore fluid balance, and correct life-threatening electrolyte imbalances.
5. **Pulmonary complications** are the most common cause of death in patients receiving allogenic BMT, with interstitial pneumonitis being a major cause. It is associated with a high mortality despite aggressive management.
  a. *Interstitial pneumonitis* is a general term referring to an inflammatory process involving the interalveolar lining of the lung. Risk factors include immunocompromise of the host from pretransplant and posttransplant immunosuppressive therapy, lung damage from conditioning regimens such as radiation or chemotherapy or interaction of both radiation and chemotherapy, and the presence of an infection, many of which are opportunistic microorganisms (often CMV). It can be confirmed by lung biopsy, but this is a high-risk procedure for the post-BMT patient and is not done often. Interstitial pneumonitis often is described as idiopathic, a pulmonary process that does not yield a positive culture, similar to ARDS.
  b. *Diagnosis:* Although distinguishing radiation-induced pneumonitis from

other causes of the symptoms would be helpful, this process is difficult by diagnostic imaging or other studies. Signs and symptoms include dry cough, rales, dyspnea, nasal flaring, fever, and restricted ventilatory capacity due to decreased pulmonary compliance.

- Laboratory results: Arterial blood gases indicate hypoxia.
- X-ray findings: Diffuse interstitial infiltrates are noted on the chest x-ray film.

  c. *Management:* Prompt recognition of the condition is followed by treatment. If interstitial pneumonitis is radiation induced, steroids are used. If it is infection induced (with or without a positive culture), broad-spectrum antibiotics are used; therapy can be more specific if a pathogen is identified by bronchoalveolar lavage or transbronchial biopsy during bronchoscopy, thoracentesis, or open lung biopsy (rarely done because of the high risk for the BMT patient). If the child's condition deteriorates, intubation and mechanical ventilation may be required. Recovery is slow, and aggressive supportive care is required. Toxicity to the lungs is exacerbated by high oxygen and airway pressure settings.

6. **Cardiac complications** are a greater risk with autologous transplants.
   a. *Cardiac complications* are caused by cancer therapy, especially anthracyclines or cyclophosphamide or radiation to the chest, as part of the conditioning regimen or given prior to BMT. Heart failure often leads to pulmonary edema. This results from a loss of myocardial fibrils, mitochondrial changes, and cellular degeneration; chronic changes such as fibrosis are common. Cardiac complications may occur early in post-BMT period.
   b. *Diagnosis*
      - Signs and symptoms include weight gain, peripheral edema, tachycardia, dyspnea on exertion, orthopnea, rales, and rhonchi.
      - Echocardiogram is used to measure shortening or ejection fractions.
   c. *Management:* Patients may continue to deteriorate, as chronic and cumulative damage is usually irreversible. Treatment is limited to supportive measures, including precise fluid management, judicious use of diuretics and inotropic agents, and decreasing stress of the heart (such as bed rest).

7. **Hemorrhagic cystitis** causes significant morbidity for the BMT patient.
   a. Cystitis is caused by bladder toxicity from chemotherapy, most often associated with cyclophosphamide. A metabolite produces ulceration of the bladder mucosal tissue. Small vessels in the underlying tissue hemorrhage into the bladder. Viruses of the bladder mucosa may also cause hematuria.
   b. *Diagnosis*
      - Signs and symptoms include red-tinged urine with clots, dysuria or frequency of urination, and symptoms of urethral obstruction from clots such as pain. This can lead to postrenal failure if not corrected.
      - Bladder ultrasound indicates the presence of clots or thickened bladder wall.
   c. *Management*
      - Mild cases respond to aggressive hydration with resolution in 1 to 2 days.
      - Severe cases may require continuous bladder irrigation with a three-way Foley catheter at 500 ml to 3 L/h to clear developing clots and prevent obstruction. Platelets are used to maintain platelet counts at higher than $20,000/mm^3$ for a child who is not bleeding or higher than $50,000/mm^3$ for a child who is bleeding. Cystoscopy is used to cauterize the bleeding ulcerative areas; it is usually not a long-term solution because of the diffuse widespread area affected. Instillation of chemicals can be used to further stop the bleeding. Continued irrigation is critical as further

damage to the bladder may occur if the chemicals are not rinsed from the bladder.

8. **GvHD** (also see Chapter 7)

a. GvHD represents engraftment of donor T lymphocytes in the recipient that reject the tissue of the recipient. It predominantly involves the skin, GI tract, and the liver. It is rare for GvHD to occur in syngeneic or autologous transplants. There is increased risk with partially matched allogenic transplants.

b. GvHD results from histocompatibility differences between the donor cells (graft) and the recipient (host). Donor cells can contain viable immunocompetent T lymphocytes that can recognize the foreign antigens of the host and, therefore, mount an immunologic response against the host. Recipient with profound cellular immunodeficiency, either congenital or acquired, cannot respond against and reject the donor marrow.

c. GvHD occurs in two forms, acute and chronic, despite HLA-identical donor and recipient transplants and prophylactic immunosuppressive therapy.

d. Acute GvHD occurs within the first 100 days after transplantation with a range in severity from mild and transitory to severe, prolonged, and lethal.

- Signs and symptoms are not always immediately recognized, since symptoms may mimic other problems such as infection, VOD, hepatitis, and toxic effects of chemotherapy.
  - Skin GvHD: Onset of a maculopapular skin rash initially involving the palms and soles and later progressing centrally may cause intense pruritus and progress to bullous lesions and ulceration.
  - GI GvHD: There is nausea, vomiting, abdominal pain, anorexia, paralytic ileus, green and watery, heme-negative diarrhea. Later heme-positive diarrhea occurs as more of the intestinal mucosa begins to slough. Hypoalbuminemia is noted.
  - Liver GvHD: Right upper quadrant pain, hepatomegaly, jaundice, ascites (rare), and elevated liver enzymes and bilirubin occur.
- The degree of organ system involvement is graded from I to IV, describing the severity of illness, prognosis, and response to therapy (Table 8–14).
- Diagnosis is made by biopsy of the skin or rectal or liver tissue.
- Prophylaxis: Morbidity and mortality is lessened by prevention rather than treatment of established GvHD. Interventions include selection of histocompatible donors, immunosuppressive therapy, and removal of T cells from the donor marrow prior to transplant (associated with a risk of engraftment failure). Irradiation of all blood products before transfusion results in the inactivation of T lymphocytes while adequate platelet and

Table 8–14. CLINICAL STAGES OF ACUTE GRAFT-VS.-HOST DISEASE (GvHD)

STAGE	SKIN	LIVER: BILIRUBIN LEVEL	GUT: DIARRHEA VOLUME
1	Maculopapular rash, <25% of body surface area	2–3 mg/ml	7–13 ml/kg/d
2	Maculopapular rash, 25–50% of body surface area	3–6 mg/dl	14–20 ml/kg/d
3	Generalized erythroderma	6–15 mg/dl	21–27 ml/kg/d
4	Desquamation and bullae	>15 mg/dl	>27 ml/kg/d

Data from Cassano WF, Gross S, Graham-Pole J, Rudder S. Graft versus host disease. In: Blumer JL. *A Practical Guide to Pediatric Intensive Care.* St Louis, Mo: The CV Mosby Co; 1990:510; and *Research Protocols for Bone Marrow Transplant.* Memphis, Tenn: St Jude Children's Research Hospital; 1995.

RBC function is maintained. Irradiation should be maintained for 1 year for uncomplicated BMT (return of T cell immunity).

- Treatment of acute GvHD includes corticosteroids, CSA, azathioprine, and antilymphocyte preparations (see Relevant Pharmacology section). Various combinations have not shown consistent impact on reducing GvHD and improving long-term survival as patients continue to die from infections. Mild (grade I) GvHD does not warrant therapy. Treatment of grades II to IV is recommended.
  - Assess early clinical manifestations of GvHD. Distinguish GvHD from other complications such as antibiotic or chemotherapy reactions, irritated bowel, infections, and radiation toxicity.
  - Appropriate skin care will provide comfort and reduce the risk of infection. Oil in the bath water decreases skin dryness and soothes pruritus; if bullae occur, prevent infection and bleeding. Low air-loss beds decrease discomfort of pressure points and facilitate exudate absorption. Other skin care products such as hydrogel absorb wound exudate, provide a physiologically moist environment, and promote wound healing and tissue granulation. Provide pain control measures for the pain associated with skin desquamation.
  - Provide measures to resolve the GI tract effects of GvHD. Watch for hypovolemia and shock through strict monitoring of intake and output, daily weights, and assessment of electrolytes. The patient may need to be NPO to further reduce gut activation of the GvHD. Clean the perineal area and soothe irritated skin. Assess for rectal lesions. Hemoccult test all emesis and stool to determine presence of GI tract bleeding.

  e. Chronic GvHD occurs beyond 100 days up to 2 years often following acute GvHD. Often it is fatal and disabling and is more likely if the child had the acute form of GvHD.

  - Signs and symptoms affect the same target organs as affected in acute GvHD but different symptoms occur including skin lesions, sclerosis, hair loss, dystrophic nails, dysphagia, heartburn, chronic diarrhea, and malabsorption.
  - Management involves steroids, CSA, azathioprine, and artificial tears to prevent ocular damage from the associated keratoconjunctivitis.

REFERENCES

Abramson JS, Wheeler JG, Quie PG. The polymorphonuclear phagocytic system. In: Stiehm ER, ed. *Immunologic Disorders in Infants and Children*. 3rd ed. Philadelphia, Pa: WB Saunders Co; 1989:68–80.

Ackerman AD. Primary and secondary immunodeficiencies. In: Rogers MC, ed. *Textbook of Pediatric Intensive Care*. 2nd ed. Baltimore, Md: Williams & Wilkins; 1992:921–952.

Almadrones L, Godbold J, Raff J, Ennis J. Accuracy of activated partial thromboplastin time drawn through central venous catheters. *Oncol Nurs Forum*. 1987;14(2):15–18.

American Association of Blood Banks, American Red Cross, Council of Community Blood Centers. *Circulation of Information for the Use of Human Blood and Blood Components, 1994*. Washington, DC: The Red Cross, 1994.

American College of Chest Physicians, Society of Critical Care Medicine Consensus Conference. Definitions for sepsis and organ failure and guidelines for the use of innovative therapies in sepsis. *Crit Care Med*. 1992;20(6):864–873.

Ammann AJ. Combined antibody (B cell) and cellular (T cell) immunodeficiency disorders. In: Stites DP, Terr AI, eds. *Basic and Clinical Immunology*. 7th ed. Norwalk, Conn: Appleton & Lange; 1991:341–355.

Anderson DC, Hughes BJ, Edwards MS, Buffone GJ, Baker CJ. Impaired chemotaxigenesis by type III group B streptococci in neonatal sera: relationship to specific anticapsular antibody and abnormalities of serum complement. *Pediatr Res*. 1983;17(6):496–502.

Andreoli TE, Bennett JC, Carpenter CC, Plum F, Smith LH Jr. *Cecil Essentials of Medicine*. 3rd ed. Philadelphia, Pa: WB Saunders; 1993.

Antoine FS. *Landmark Gene Therapy Trial Progresses.* NIH Record, XLII (18), September 4. Bethesda, Md: The National Institutes of Health; 1990.

Baker CJ, Melish ME, Hall RT, et al. Intravenous immunoglobulin for the prevention of nosocomial infection in low-birth-weight neonates. *N Engl J Med.* 1992;327:213–219.

Ballard B. Renal and hepatic complications. In: Whedon MB, ed. *Bone Marrow Transplantation: Principles, Practice and Nursing Insights.* Boston, Mass: Jones and Bartlett Publishers; 1991:240–261.

Bellanti J. *Immunology III.* Philadelphia, Pa: WB Saunders Co; 1985.

Bellanti JA, Kadlec JV. Host defense mechanisms. In: Chernick V, Kernig EL, eds. *Kernig's Disorders of the Respiratory Tract in Children.* 5th ed. Philadelphia, Pa: WB Saunders; 1990:182–201.

Berger M, Frank MM. The serum complement system. In: Stiehm ER, ed. *Immunologic Disorders in Infants and Children.* 3rd ed. Philadelphia, Pa: WB Saunders Co; 1989: 97–115.

Berkowitz ID, Berkowitz FE, Johnson JP. The critically ill child and human immunodeficiency virus infection. In: Rogers MC, ed. *Textbook of Pediatric Intensive Care.* 2nd ed. Baltimore, Md: Williams & Wilkins; 1992:953–975.

Blackwell S, Crawford J. Colony-stimulating factors: clinical applications. *Pharmacotherapy.* 1992;12(suppl 2):20S–31S.

Blaese RM. Development of gene therapy for immunodeficiency: adenosine deaminase deficiency. *Pediatr Res.* 1992; 33(suppl 1):S49–S53.

Blatt J. Structure and function of hematopoietic organs. In: Fuhrman BP, Zimmerman JJ. *Pediatric Critical Care.* St Louis, Mo: The CV Mosby Co; 1992:805–813.

Bontempo FA. Coagulation abnormalities: bleeding and thrombosis. In: Pinsky MR, Dhainaut JA. *Pathophysiologic Foundations of Critical Care.* Baltimore, Md: Williams & Wilkins; 1993a:805–814.

Bontempo FA. General hematology and transfusion. In: Pinsky MR, Dhainaut JA. *Pathophysiologic Foundations of Critical Care.* Baltimore, Md: Williams & Wilkins; 1993b:815–822.

Bousvaros A, Walker WA. Development and function of the intestinal mucosal barrier. In: MacDonald T, ed. *Ontogeny of the Immune System of the Gut.* Boca Raton, Fla: CRC Press; 1990:2–16.

Calvelli TA, Rubenstein A. Intravenous gamma-globulin in infant acquired immunodeficiency syndrome. *Pediatr Infect Dis J.* 1986;5:207–210.

Camp-Sorrell D, Wujcik D. Intravenous immunoglobulin administration: an evaluation of vital sign monitoring. *Oncol Nurs Forum.* 1994;21(3):531–535.

Carabasi M. Bone marrow failure. In: Groeger JS. *Critical Care of the Cancer Patient.* St Louis, Mo: The CV Mosby Co; 1991:86–102.

Carr E. Commentary on genes in a bottle. *ONS Nurs Scan Oncol.* 1992;1(1):16.

Cassano WF, Gross S, Graham-Pole J, Rudder S. Graft versus host disease. In: Blumer JL. *A Practical Guide to Pediatric Intensive Care.* St Louis, Mo: The CV Mosby Co; 1990:509–513.

Caudell KA. Graft-versus-host disease. In: Whedon MB, ed. *Bone Marrow Transplantation: Principles, Practice and Nursing Insights.* Boston, Mass: Jones and Bartlett Publishers; 1991:160–179.

Centers for Disease Control and Prevention. First 500,000 AIDS cases—United States, 1995. *MMWR.* 1995a;44(46):849–853.

Centers for Disease Control and Prevention. 1995 revised guidelines for prophylaxis against *Pneumocystis carinii* pneumonia for children infected with or prenatally exposed to human immunodeficiency virus. *MMWR.* 1995b;44(RR-4):1–10.

Centers for Disease Control and Prevention. 1994 revised classification system for human immunodeficiency virus in children less than 13 years of age. *MMWR.* 1994;143(RR-12):1–10.

Christensen RD, Rothstein G. Efficiency of neutrophil migration in the neonate. *Pediatr Res.* 1980;14:1147–1149.

Clapp DW, Kleigman RM, Baley JE, et al. Use of intravenously administered immune globulin to prevent nosocomial sepsis in low birth weight infants: report of pilot study. *J Pediatr.* 1989;115:973–978.

Clark J, Landis L, McGee R. Nursing management of outcomes of disease, psychological response, treatment, and complications. In: Ziegfeld CR, ed. *Core Curriculum for Oncology Nursing.* Philadelphia, Pa: WB Saunders Co; 1987:271–319.

College of American Pathologists. Practice parameters for the use of fresh frozen plasma, cryoprecipitate, and platelets. *JAMA.* 1994;271:777–781.

Cooper MD, Buckley RH. Developmental immunology and the immunodeficiency diseases. *JAMA.* 1982; 248(20):2658–2669.

Dodd RY. Infectious complications of blood transfusions. *Hematol Oncol Ann.* 1994;2(4):280–286.

Driscoll V. Life threatening coagulopathy. *Am J Nurs.* November 1994;(suppl):57–63.

Ebers DW, Smith DI, Gibbs GE. Gastric acid in the first day of life. *Pediatrics.* 1956;18(5):800.

Esparaz B, Green D. Disseminated intravascular coagulation. *Crit Care Q.* 1990;13(2):7–12.

Fanaroff A, Wright E, Korones S, et al. Controlled trial of prophylactic IVIG to reduce nosocomial infection in low-birth-weight infants. *Pediatr Res.* 1992;31:202.

Farmer JC, Parker RI. Coagulation: essential physiologic concerns. In: Civetta JM, Taylor RW, Kirby RR, eds. *Critical Care.* Philadelphia, Pa: JB Lippincott Co; 1988: 1461–1468.

Farmer JC, Parker RI. Coagulation disorders. In: Civetta JM, Taylor RW, Kirby RR, eds. *Critical Care.* Philadelphia, Pa: JB Lippincott Co; 1988:1469–1480.

Foley MK. Nursing management of the child or adolescent with blood component deficiencies. In: Foley GV, Fochtman D, Mooney KH, eds. *Nursing Care of the Child with Cancer.* Philadelphia, Pa: WB Saunders Co; 1993:385–395.

Gale RP, Winston D. Intravenous immunoglobulin in bone marrow transplantation. *Cancer.* 1991;68:1415–1453.

Garnett C. *First Human Gene Therapy Trial Debuts at NIH.* NIH Record, XLII (20), October 2. Bethesda, Md: The National Institutes of Health; 1990.

Gloe D. Common reactions to transfusions. *Heart Lung.* 1991;20(5):506–513.

Goldman AS, Ham-Pong AJ, Goldblum RM. Host defenses: development and maternal contributions. *Adv Pediatr.* 1985;32:71–100.

Gordan JB, Berstein ML, Rogers MC. Hematologic disorders in the pediatric intensive care unit. In: Rogers M, ed. *Textbook of Pediatric Intensive Care.* 2nd ed. Baltimore, Md: Williams & Wilkins; 1992:1357–1402.

Gordan JB, Yeager AM. Management of the child with malignant disease in the pediatric intensive care unit. In: Rogers M, ed. *Textbook of Pediatric Intensive Care.* 2nd ed. Baltimore, Md: Williams & Wilkins; 1992:1403–1440.

Grand RW, Watkins JB, Torti FM. Development of the human gastrointestinal tract: a review. *Gastroenterology.* 1976;70(5):790–810.

Griffin J. *Hematology and Immunology: Concepts for Nursing.* Norwalk, Conn: Appleton-Century-Crofts, 1986.

Groothuis JR. Role of antibody and use of respiratory syncytial virus (RSV) immune globulin to prevent severe RSV disease in high risk children. *J Pediatr.* 1994;124(5, part 2):S28–S34.

Groothuis JR, Simones EAF, Hemming VG, et al. Respiratory syncytial virus (RSV) infection in preterm infants and the protective effects of RSV immune globulin (RSVIG). *Pediatrics.* 1995;95(4):463–467.

Grossman M. Children with AIDS. In: Sande MA, Volberding PA, eds. *The Medical Management of AIDS.* Philadelphia, Pa: WB Saunders Co; 1988:319–329.

Gunderson LP, Gumm B. Neonatal acquired immunodeficiency syndrome: human immunodeficiency virus infection and acquired immunodeficiency syndrome in the infant. In: Kenner C, Brueggemeyer A, Gunderson LP, eds. *Comprehensive Neonatal Nursing Care: A Physiologic Perspective.* Philadelphia, Pa: WB Saunders Co; 1993:940–967.

Guyton A. *Textbook of Medical Physiology.* 6th ed. Philadelphia, Pa: WB Saunders Co; 1986.

Happ M. Life threatening hemorrhage in children with cancer. *J Assoc Pediatr Oncol Nurses.* 1987;4(3):36–40.

Hardaway RM, Adams WH. Blood problems in critical care, I. *Probl Crit Care.* 1989a;3(1):40–49, 72–77, 108–116, 121–131, 157–160, 165–170.

Hardaway RM, Adams WH. Blood problems in critical care, II. *Probl Crit Care.* 1989b;3(2):249–268.

Harkins A, Crandall M, Foster R. Nursing strategies: altered immune function. In: Foster RLR, Hunsberger MM, Anderson JJT, eds. *Family-Centered Nursing Care of Children.* Philadelphia, Pa: WB Saunders Co; 1989:1524–1611.

Harpin VA, Eutter N. Barrier properties of the newborn infant's skin. *J Pediatr.* 1983;102(3):419–425.

Harper J. Use of heparinized intraarterial lines to obtain coagulation studies. *Focus Crit Care.* 1988;15(5):51–55.

Harvey M. *Study Guide to Core Curriculum for Critical Care Nursing.* Philadelphia, Pa: WB Saunders Co; 1986:162.

Hassell KL, Eckman JR, Lane PA. Acute multiorgan failure syndrome: a potentially catastrophic complication of severe sickle cell pain episodes. *Am J Med.* 1994;96:155–162.

Heinzel FP. Infections in patients with humoral immunodeficiency. *Hosp Pract.* 1989;24(9):99–130.

Hoekelman RA. The physical examination of infants and children. In: Bates B. *A Guide to Physical Examination.* 3rd ed. Philadelphia, Pa: JB Lippincott Co; 1983:447–512.

Hopkins K. *Oral Care Guidelines for Patients Receiving Chemotherapy and Radiation Therapy.* Memphis, Tenn: St Jude's Children's Research Hospital; 1993.

Hughes WT. *Pneumocystis carinii* pneumonia. In: Pizzo PA, Wilfert CM, eds. *Pediatric AIDS: The Challenge of HIV Infection in Infants, Children and Adolescents.* Baltimore, Md: Williams & Wilkins; 1994:405–418.

Imbach P. Intravenous immunoglobulin therapy for idiopathic thrombocytopenic purpura and other immune related disorders. *Pediatr Infect Dis J.* 1988;7:S120–S124.

Jennings BM. The hematologic system. In: Alspach JG, ed. *Curriculum for Critical Care Nursing.* 4th ed. Philadelphia, Pa: WB Saunders Co; 1991:675–747.

Jett MR, Lancaster LA. The inflammatory-immune response. The body's defense against invasion. *Crit Care Nurse.* 1983;3(5):64–86.

Jones K, LeBoeuf F, Dillman P. HIV in the critically ill child. In: Curley MAQ, Smith JB, Moloney-Harmon PA, eds. *Critical Care Nursing of Infants and Children.* Philadelphia, Pa: WB Saunders Co; 1996.

Kajs M. Comparison of coagulation values obtained by traditional venipuncture and intraarterial line methods. *Heart Lung.* 1986;15(6):622–627.

Kedar A, Gross S. Disseminated intravascular coagulation. In: Blumer JL. *A Practical Guide to Pediatric Intensive Care.* St Louis, Mo: The CV Mosby Co; 1990:517–519.

Kempin S. Disorders of hemostasis. In: Groeger JS. *Critical Care of the Cancer Patient.* St Louis, Mo: The CV Mosby Co; 1991:103–139.

Klein RB, Fischer TJ, Gard SE, Biberstein BS, Rich KC, Stiehm ER. Decreased mononuclear and polymorphonuclear chemotaxis in human newborns, infants, and young children. *Pediatrics.* 1977;60(4):467–472.

Kubanek B, Ernst B, Ostendorf P, et al. Preliminary data of controlled trial of intravenous hyperimmune globulin in the prevention of cytomegalovirus infection in bone marrow transplant recipients. *Transplant Proc.* 1985;17:468–469.

Landier WC, Barrell ML, Styffe EJ. How to administer blood components to children. *Matern Child Nurse J.* 1987;60(4):12,178–184.

Landor M, Rubinstein A. Human immunodeficiency virus infection in children. In: Spirer Z, Roifman CM, Branski D, eds. *Pediatric Immunology: Pediatric and Adolescent Medicine.* New York, NY: Karger; 1993:102–130.

Laxon CJ, Titler MG. Drawing coagulation studies from arterial lines: an integrative literature review. *Am J Crit Care.* 1994;3(1):16–22.

Leonard MS. Nursing strategies: altered hematologic function. In: Foster RL, Hunsberger MM, Anderson JJT, eds. *Family-Centered Nursing Care of Children.* Philadelphia, Pa: WB Saunders Co; 1989:1339–1374.

Lewis KD, Thomson HB. Infants, children, and adolescents. In: Flaskerud JH, ed. *AIDS/HIV Infection: A Reference Guide for Nursing Professionals.* Philadelphia, Pa: WB Saunders Co; 1989:111–127.

Lott JW, Kenner C. Keeping up with neonatal infection: designer bugs, part II. *MCN.* 1994;19(5):264–271.

Luban N. Basics of transfusion medicine. In: Fuhrman BP, Zimmerman JJ. *Pediatric Critical Care.* St Louis, Mo: The CV Mosby Co; 1992:829–840.

Mahon PM. Orthoclone OKT3 and cardiac transplantation: an overview. *Crit Care Nurs.* 1991;11(8):42–50.

Malloy MB, Perez-Woods RC. Neonatal skin care: prevention of skin breakdown. *Pediatr Nurs.* 1991;17(1):41–48.

Masuda K, Kinoshita Y, Kobayashi Y. Heterogeneity of Fc receptor expression in chemotaxis and adherence of neonatal neutrophils. *Pediatr Res.* 1989;25(1):6–10.

Mehta P, Gross S, Kao K. Platelet transfusions. In: Blumer JL. *A Practical Guide to Pediatric Intensive Care.* St Louis, Mo: The CV Mosby Co; 1990a:1008–1009.

Mehta P, Gross S, Kao K. Transfusions with packed red blood cells. In: Blumer JL. *A Practical Guide to Pediatric Intensive Care.* St Louis, Mo: The CV Mosby Co; 1990b:1001–1007.

Miller D. Immunosuppression in pediatric transplant patients. *Pediatr Nurs.* 1995;21(1):21–29.

Miller ME. Host defenses of the human neonate. *Pediatr Clin North Am.* 1977;24(2):413–423.

Miller ME. Immunocompetence of the newborn. In: Chandra RK, ed. Primary and secondary immunodeficiency disorders. New York, NY: Churchill Livingstone Inc; 1983:157–164.

Miller ME. The inflammatory and natural defense systems. In: Stiehm ER, ed. *Immunologic Disorders in Infants and Children.* 2nd ed. Philadelphia, Pa: WB Saunders Co; 1980:165–180.

Molyneaux RD, Papciak B, Rorem DA. Coagulation studies and the indwelling heparinized catheter. *Heart Lung.* 1987;16(1):2–23.

Morrison RA, Vedro DA. Pain management in the child with sickle cell disease. *Pediatr Nurs.* 1989;15(6):595–597.

Mudge-Grout CL. *Immunologic Disorders.* St Louis, Mo: Mosby–Year Book Inc; 1992.

National Blood Resource Education Program's Nursing Education Working Group. Preventing and managing transfusion reactions. *Am J Nurs.* June 1991a:48–50.

National Blood Resource Education Program's Nursing Education Working Group. Transfusion nursing: trends and practices for the '90's. Choosing blood components and equipment. *Am J Nurs.* June 1991b:42–46.

National Institutes of Health, University of California Expert Panel for Corticosteroids as Adjunctive Therapy for *Pneumocystis* Pneumonia. Consensus statement on the use of corticosteroids as adjunctive therapy for *Pneumocystis* pneumonia in acquired immunodeficiency syndrome. *N Engl J Med.* 1990;323(21):1500–1504.

Nugent DJ, Tarantino MD. Hematology-oncology problems in the intensive care unit. In: Fuhrman BP, Zimmerman JJ. *Pediatric Critical Care.* St Louis, Mo: The CV Mosby Co; 1992:815–827.

Oakes L. Oncologic disorders. In: Moloney-Harmon PA, Czerwinski SJ, eds. *Review of Pediatric Critical Care.* Philadelphia, Pa: WB Saunders Co; 1997.

Ognibene FP, Gill VJ, Pizzo PA. Induced sputum to diagnose *Pneumocystis carinii* pneumonia in immunosuppressed pediatric patients. *J Pediatr.* 1989;115:430–433.

Oleske JM, Connor EM, Boblia R, et al. The use of intravenous gammaglobulin (IVGG) in children with acquired immunodeficiency syndrome (AIDS). 1986;20:318.

Panzarella C, Duncan J. Nursing management of the physical care needs. In: Foley GV, Fochtman D, Mooney KH, eds. *Nursing Care of the Child With Cancer.* 2nd ed. Philadelphia, Pa: WB Saunders Co; 1993:335–352.

Peterson K. Iatrogenic immune suppression. *Pediatr Nurs.* 1995;21(1):11–15.

Pinto K. Accuracy of coagulation values obtained from a heparinized central venous catheter. *Oncol Nurs Forum.* 1994;21(3):573–575.

Pitel P, Gross S. Sickle cell crisis. In: Blumer JL. *A Practical Guide to Pediatric Intensive Care.* St Louis, Mo: The CV Mosby Co; 1990:501–515.

Pizzo PA. Combating infections in neutropenic patients. *Hosp Pract.* 1989;24(7):93–110.

Querin JJ, Stahl LD. 12 simple, sensible steps for successful blood transfusions. *Nursing '83.* 1983:35–45.

Quinones RR. Bone marrow transplantation. In: Fuhrman BP, Zimmerman JJ. *Pediatric Critical Care*. St Louis, Mo: The CV Mosby Co; 1992:841–851.

Rosenthal CH. Immunosuppression in pediatric critical care patients. *Crit Care Nurs Clin North Am*. 1989;1(4):775–785.

Rosenthal-Dichter CH, Allen M. Host defenses. In: Curley MAQ, Smith JB, Moloney-Harmon PA, eds. *Critical Care Nursing of Infants and Children*. Philadelphia, Pa: WB Saunders Co; 1996.

Rubinstein A. Pediatric AIDS. *Curr Probl Pediatr.* 1986;16:361–409.

Rubinstein A, Morecki R, Goldman H. Pulmonary effects of AIDS: pulmonary disease in infants and children. *Clin Chest Med*. 1988;9:507–517.

Rudder S. Bone marrow transplant. In: Blumer JL. *A Practical Guide to Pediatric Intensive Care*. St Louis, Mo: The CV Mosby Co; 1990:505–508.

Saunders-Laufer D, DeBruin W, Edelson PJ. *Pneumocystis carinii* infections in HIV-infected children. *Pediatr Clin North Am*. 1991;38(1):69–88.

Sears DA. Hematologic disease requiring critical care. In: Civetta JM, Taylor RW, Kirby RR, eds. *Critical Care*. Philadelphia, Pa: JB Lippincott Co; 1988:1503–1516.

Selekman J. Pediatric problems related to the immunologic system. In: Feeg VD, Harbin RE, eds. *Pediatric Nursing: Core Curriculum and Resource Manual*. Pitman, NJ: Anthony J Janietti Inc; 1991:199–207.

Shaefer M, Williams L. Nursing implications of immunosuppression in transplantation. *Nurs Clin North Am*. 1991;26(2):291–307.

Steele RW, Kearns GL. Antimicrobial therapy for pediatric patients. *Pediatr Clin North Am*. 1989;36(5):1321–1349.

Suez D. Intravenous immunoglobulin therapy: indications, potential side effects, and treatment guidelines. *J Intravenous Nurs*. 1995;18(4):178–190.

Thomason T, et al. Clinical safety and cost of heparin titration using bedside activated clotting time. *Am J Crit Care*. 1993;2(1):81–87.

Tortora GJ, Grabowski SR. *Principles of Anatomy and Physiology*. 7th ed. New York, NY: Harper Collins College Publishers; 1993.

US Public Health Service: Guidelines for testing and counseling blood and plasma donors for human immunodeficiency virus type I antigen. Atlanta, Ga: Public Health Service: Centers for Disease Control and Prevention; 1996:5.

Vanacek KS. Gastrointestinal complications of bone marrow transplant. In: Whedon MB, ed. *Bone Marrow Transplantation: Principles, Practice and Nursing Insights*. Boston, Mass: Jones and Bartlett Publishers; 1991:182–205.

Wahrenberger A. Pharmacologic immunosuppression: cure or curse? *Crit Care Q*. 1995;17(4):27–36.

Wang W, et al. Medical management and prevention guidelines for children with sickle cell disease. *J Tenn Med Assoc*. 1992;85(5):209–214.

Whitlock D, Whitlock J, Coates TD. Hematologic and oncologic emergencies requiring critical care. In: Hazinski MF. *Nursing Care of the Critically Ill Child*. 4th ed. St Louis, Mo: Mosby–Year Book Inc; 1992:803–827.

Wilke TJ. Pulmonary and cardiac complications of bone marrow transplant. In: Whedon MB, ed. *Bone Marrow Transplantation: Principles, Practice and Nursing Insights*. Boston, Mass: Jones and Bartlett Publishers; 1991:182–205.

Wilkinson JD, Greenwald BM. The acquired immunodeficiency syndrome: impact on the pediatric intensive care unit. *Crit Care Clin*. 1988;4(4):831–844.

Wingard JR. Historical perspectives and future directions. In: Whedon MB, ed. *Bone Marrow Transplantation: Principles, Practice and Nursing Insights*. Boston, Mass: Jones and Bartlett Publishers; 1991:3–17.

Winston DJ, Ho WG, Lin C, et al. Intravenous immune globulin for prevention of cytomegalovirus infection and interstitial pneumonia after bone marrow transplantation. *Ann Intern Med*. 1987;106:12–28.

Wood RA, Sampson HA. The child with frequent infections. *Curr Probl Pediatr.* 1989;19(5):234–281.

Woolery-Antill M, Colter C. Biologic response modifiers. In: Foley GV, Fochtman D, Mooney KH, eds. Nursing care of the child with cancer. Philadelphia, Pa: WB Saunders Co; 1993:179–207.

Yeston NS, Niehoff JM, Dennis RC. Transfusion therapy. In: Civetta JM, et al, eds. *Critical Care*. Philadelphia, Pa: JB Lippincott Co; 1988:1481–1493.

Young LS. Infections in patients with cellular immunodeficiency. *Hosp Pract.* 1989;24(8):191–212.

9 Multisystem Issues

LISA MARIE BERNARDO, ROSE ANN GOULD SOLOWAY,
CATHY ROSENTHAL-DICHTER, PAULA DICKERSON,
MARY GORDON, and PAM WALTER

MULTIPLE TRAUMA   LISA MARIE BERNARDO

Critically injured children and their families require the expertise of pediatric nurses, intensivists, and other health care professionals for trauma care. Their admission to an intensive care unit (ICU) is unplanned and unexpected, causing stress and anxiety. The pediatric intensive care (PICU) nurse must have knowledge of injury, treatment, and prevention to effectively care for the injured child and family.

EPIDEMIOLOGY AND INCIDENCE

Injuries are the leading cause of childhood mortality and disability in the United States. Injuries were responsible for 37,529 deaths among children and adolescents in 1991 (Ray and Yuwiler, 1994). This number is increased from the 21,210 children who died from trauma in 1985 (Guyer and Ellers, 1990). Motor vehicle crashes continue to be responsible for the highest number of pediatric deaths, and head injury is the primary cause of death in this population (Division of Injury Control, 1990; Table 9–1).

Table 9–1.   1991 FIVE LEADING CAUSES OF INJURY DEATH

0–4 y	5–9 y	10–14 y	15–19 y
Homicide	Motor vehicle occupant	Motor vehicle occupant	Motor vehicle occupant
Fires and burns	Motor vehicle pedestrian	Homicide	Homicide
Drownings	Fires and burns	Suicide	Suicide
Motor vehicle occupant	Drownings	Motor vehicle pedestrian	Motor vehicle other
Motor vehicle pedestrian	Homicide	Drownings	Drownings

Data from Ray L, Yuwiler J. *Child and Adolescent Fatal Injury Databook.* San Diego, Calif: Children's Safety Network; 1994.

Trauma-related deaths result in 2,232,939 years of potential life lost and over $40 billion dollars in lifetime productivity losses annually (Ray and Yuwiler, 1994). An estimated 600,000 children are hospitalized annually for injuries and 80,000 more sustain permanent disabling conditions (Horowitz and Andrassy, 1994).

Childhood injuries cause more hospitalization days than any other disease, cause the highest proportion of admissions to rehabilitation facilities, and result in the highest proportion of children who require home health care after hospital discharge (Division of Injury Control, 1990). The costs of injuries to children are estimated to exceed $7.5 billion each year (Division of Injury Control, 1990).

CAUSES OF INJURY RELATED TO PSYCHOSOCIAL AND PHYSICAL DEVELOPMENT

A. **INFANTS**
1. Infants explore their world through motion, touching, mouthing, and feeling. They are learning to chew, roll, sit, crawl, cruise, and walk, which can lead them into dangerous situations.
2. Falls are the most frequent mechanism of injury in this age group. Infants frequently fall while rolling from high surfaces or from an adult's arms. Walker-related injuries are frequent, especially falls down stairs, and the most frequent injuries are to the head and neck (Chiaviello et al, 1994).
3. Suffocation, choking, aspiration, and poisoning are possible injuries to infants who put objects into their mouths.
4. Nationwide, almost half the burn- and fire-related deaths were in children 4 years of age or younger and were concentrated in the Midwest and South (Ray and Yuwiler, 1994). Severe burns are sustained in house fires and from scalding liquids. As infants push themselves to a standing position, they can burn their hands on an open, hot oven door. Contact burns from hot irons or curling irons can also occur.
5. Injuries are sustained in motor vehicle crashes when the parent does not have a car seat secured properly in the vehicle, the seat harness is not connected correctly, or an infant carrier not manufactured for vehicular travel is in use (Graham et al, 1992). Injuries also occur when the passenger is holding the child. Resulting injuries include head injuries, skull and femoral fractures, and brain hemorrhage (Graham et al, 1992).
6. Homicide (child maltreatment) was the leading cause of death among children aged 4 years and younger (Ray and Yuwiler, 1994).

B. **TODDLERS**
1. Toddlers become increasingly mobile and are eager to discover and explore their selves, bodies, and world. They have no concept of danger or right and wrong. Toddlers have to repeat their mistakes many times through trial and error before they can grasp the cause-and-effect relationship between their action and their injury.
2. Falls are the most common mechanism of injury, as locomotion is the toddler's chief means of gaining independence. When compared with infants, toddlers tend to fall from greater heights such as open windows, porches, and some playground equipment.
3. Burns occur from toddlers' grabbing pot handles on the stove or faucet handles or pulling on electrical cords attached to appliances, resulting in hot liquid scalds. Electrical burns occur from biting plugged-in electrical cords or contact with electrical outlets. Chemical burns occur from ingesting or playing with caustic substances such as cleaning products.

4. Drownings occur most often in the home setting in bathtubs, buckets, toilets, and backyard pools. In the out-of-home setting, drownings occur in ponds, lakes, rivers, and other bodies of water.
5. Injuries also occur during motor vehicle crashes when the toddler is unrestrained or improperly restrained. Unrestrained toddlers become projectiles within the vehicle, striking into the vehicle's interior and other passengers, and are more likely to be ejected from the vehicle. Toddlers restrained with lap belts can experience a multitude of injuries, including spinal column injury, intestinal rupture or tear, solid abdominal organ injury, and lumbar (Chance) fracture, all from rapid acceleration-deceleration forces. Parents or family members may permit toddlers to sit unrestrained on their laps while driving a riding lawn mower or tractor. This dangerous practice can lead to serious injury, as the child can fall off the mower and be run over, sustaining severe injuries to the head and chest or death.

C. PRESCHOOLERS

1. Preschoolers like to imitate adults. Playing with real tools and kitchen equipment can be dangerous. Preschoolers are egocentric; they believe that if they do not want something to happen, it will not happen. They have a rich fantasy life; the boundaries between fantasy and reality are easily blurred with their active imaginations. This age group has increasing motor skills and has increased independence. Less adult supervision may be provided when preschoolers participate in group activities.
2. Preschoolers have a poor sense of direction and underdeveloped peripheral vision, which can be dangerous when they attempt to cross a busy street. Most common injuries associated with pedestrian motor vehicle crashes include head, chest, and extremity injuries (Waddell's triad).
3. Tricycle-related injuries can occur when the child rides in unsafe areas. Children have been run over by vehicles while riding in their own driveway, since drivers may not see the tricycle so low to the ground. Preschoolers are often permitted to ride as passengers on lawn mowers, all-terrain vehicles, tractors, and in the back of pickup trucks.
4. Burns occur from hot liquid spills; flame burns are not common. Children 4 years of age and younger who experience flame burns do so in house fires where they suffer extensive burns and smoke inhalation.

D. SCHOOL-AGE CHILDREN

1. School-age children are very independent and enjoy pleasing others. While their motor skills are well developed, they may lack the cognitive skills to analyze and judge situations accurately. Competition in sports and other recreational activities develops. Parents may have unrealistic expectations for their preschoolers and school-age children. They may erroneously assume that their children can recognize dangers and therefore do not teach them ways to be safe.
2. Restrained and unrestrained child passengers sustain injuries in motor vehicle crashes. They also are involved in pedestrian motor vehicle crashes as well, where they dart out from between parked cars or at intersections. Riding bicycles requires coordination of cognitive and motor functioning, as well as the ability to judge time, space, and distance. Bicycle-related injuries include head injuries, long bone fractures, and chest and abdominal injuries. Using farm and lawn equipment and motorized vehicles (all-terrain vehicles, snow mobiles, speed boats) can also lead to serious injuries.
3. Falls from heights include trees, buildings, playground equipment, and rope swings. Burns occur from playing with matches, working with chemicals, and scalds.

E. **ADOLESCENTS**

1. Adolescents are risk takers, who easily succumb to peer pressure. They engage in activities that they know may cause injury; however, they believe that injury will not happen to them. Their motor skills and cognitive skills are well developed, but their judgment may not be well defined.

2. Motor vehicle crash injuries occur now that adolescents are drivers, and drugs and alcohol may play a role. Driving without restraints at high speeds and riding motor cycles without helmets also lead to serious injuries and death.

3. Homicide and suicide are on the rise in this age group. Suicide is the second leading cause of death for white youth younger than 25 years of age and is one of the leading causes of death in this group in the West and Pacific Northwest (Ray and Yuwiler, 1994). Homicide is the leading cause of death (56%) among black youth (Ray and Yuwiler, 1994).

4. Sports injuries include spinal cord injuries, head injuries, and long bone fractures. Work-related injuries include burns, sprains and strains, and fractures. Drowning while playing with friends in lakes and streams is common.

F. **ALL AGE GROUPS**

In all age groups, prevention of injury is paramount to being safe and healthy. Table 9–2 outlines injury prevention strategies for the pediatric population.

MECHANISMS OF INJURY

There are seven mechanisms of injury responsible for pediatric trauma.

A. **KINETIC FORCES**

Kinetic energy (the energy of motion) is responsible for most traumatic injuries. Kinetic forces cause blunt, crush, shear, acceleration-deceleration, and penetrating injuries.

1. Most pediatric injuries are due to **blunt force trauma,** which results in injuries to the solid and hollow organs, as well as the long bones.

   a. *Falls* are the most common cause of nonfatal head injury and the most common cause for hospitalization following injury. Falls from a window are the most common mechanism of injury for children younger than 13 years of age (Mosenthal et al, 1995). Injuries sustained during falls most often involve the head, chest, abdomen, and extremities. Deaths in young children have resulted from falling 120 cm (4 ft) or less. When such fatalities occur unwitnessed or are witnessed by only one person, child abuse must be suspected and investigated (Chadwick et al, 1991).

   b. Children account for about 10% of all *traffic-related fatalities* (Pautler et al, 1995). Motor vehicle crashes serve as the leading cause of death among children 5 through 18 years of age (Ray and Yuwiler, 1994). The distribution of these fatalities is relatively equal among boys and girls until 14 years of age, when young men are two to three times more likely to succumb to motor vehicle–related trauma (Ray and Yuwiler, 1994).

      • Injury occurs during a motor vehicle crash (Pautler et al, 1995) when the vehicle strikes another moving vehicle or a stationary object, causing a sudden change in the vehicle's velocity and direction. This energy change causes the vehicle occupants to continue their velocity, until they are stopped by the steering wheel, dashboard, air bag, or other object. The body's organs continue to move until they strike their confining spaces. For example, the brain strikes the cranium, leading to a concussion, or the descending aorta pulls forward, separating from the ligamentum arteriosum. The nature and extent of injury in a motor vehicle crash

Text continued on page 561

Table 9–2. INJURY PREVENTION STRATEGIES FOR INFANTS, CHILDREN, AND ADOLESCENTS

	INFANTS	TODDLERS	PRESCHOOLERS	SCHOOL-AGE CHILDREN	ADOLESCENTS
Burns	Do not drink hot liquids while holding infants. Test food and formula temperature before feeding the infant. Test water temperature before bathing the infant. Do not smoke cigarette while holding infant. Only use flame-retardant infant night wear.	Do not drink hot liquids while holding toddlers. Test water temperature before bathing toddlers. Use electrical outlet covers. Keep pot handles turned inward. Keep small appliances unplugged and electrical cords out of toddlers' reach. Avoid using tablecloths to avoid toddlers' spilling hot foods by grabbing at the cloth.	Keep pot handles turned inward. Keep small appliances unplugged and electrical cords out of preschoolers' reach. Teach preschoolers to stop, drop, and roll. Keep matches and lighters out of reach.	Keep matches and lighters out of children's reach. Teach children two routes of escape from the home. Teach children fire safety (how to extinguish a small flame). Keep chemicals out of children's reach. Supervise school-age children while they are cooking, baking, or using chemistry sets or household cleaners.	Teach adolescents to avoid high-voltage areas. Teach on-the-job safety to avoid burns.
Falls	When placing infants in a high chair or safety seat, secure the infant with the safety strap. Keep doors closed to stairways and laundry chutes.	Keep doors closed to stairways and laundry chutes. Secure window screens; windows should only be opened from the top or 10–12.5 cm (4–5 in) from the bottom and secured at the desired height with a "burglar lock" or window lock.	Keep doors closed to stairways and laundry chutes. Secure window screens. Avoid placing furniture near open windows. Ensure that the preschooler uses the lower bunk of a bunk bed.	Teach use of protective equipment for spelunking or rock climbing and for riding bicycles or using skateboards. All children and adolescents who ride skateboards should wear protective gear (helmet, knee, and elbow pads) and skate in safe, nontraffic areas.	Teach the use of protective equipment for riding bicycles or using skateboards and for spelunking or rock climbing.

Data from Mofenson H, Greensher J. Accident prevention. In: Hoekelman R, ed. *Primary Pediatric Care*. 2nd ed. St Louis, Mo: Mosby–Year Book Inc; 1994:260–284; Bernardo L, Trunzo R. Pediatric trauma. In: Kitt S, Selfridge-Thomas J, Proehl J, Kaiser J, eds. *Emergency Nursing: A Physiologic and Clinical Perspective*. 2nd ed. Philadelphia, Pa: WB Saunders Co; 1995:431–432.

Table continued on following page

Table 9–2. INJURY PREVENTION STRATEGIES FOR INFANTS, CHILDREN, AND ADOLESCENTS *(Continued)*

	Infants	Toddlers	Preschoolers	School-Age Children	Adolescents
Falls *Continued*	Keep crib side rails up when the infant is in the crib; as soon as the infant is able to sit unsupported, lower the crib mattress. Keep out of the crib any toys that the infant can stand on to climb out of the crib. The crib should not be used once the height of the side rail is less than three fourths of the infant's height or when the infant is 87.5 cm (35 in) tall. Keep one hand on the infant while the infant is on the dressing table.	Avoid placing furniture near open windows. The crib should not be used once the height of the side rail is less than three fourths of the toddler's height or when the toddler is 87.5 cm (35 in) tall. Supervise play in playground areas.	Supervise play in playground areas. Teach preschoolers to avoid rough play on playground equipment. Follow the manufacturer's instructions for proper equipment set up and maintenance.	Place bunk beds in the corner of the room so that walls are on two of the four sides; keep the guard rails in place; assure that the ladder is secure; keep a nightlight on to visualize the ladder.	

| Choking, strangulation, aspiration | Keep cribs away from window blind drawstrings. Do not use necklaces on the infant. Avoid using accordion-style gates to prevent head entrapment and strangulation. Avoid covering crib mattress or box springs with plastic materials. Cribs should have at least 12 slats to a side no more than 5.9 cm (2⅜ in) apart to meet federal safety standards. Avoid inflated or uninflated latex balloons with infants and toddlers. | Toy parts for toddlers younger than 3 y should be a minimum size of 3.2 cm (1¼ in) in diameter and should not fit into a truncated circular cylinder 5.6 cm (2¼ in) long. Teach toddlers not to run or walk with objects in the mouth. Avoid giving foods that require a grinding motion (i.e., hot dogs, peanuts, chewable tablets) until the age of 4 y. Cut food into bite-sized pieces; teach toddlers not to talk, laugh, or engage in horseplay while eating. | | | |
| Motor vehicles, bicycles, skate boards | Children 4 years of age and younger should be restrained in an approved seat. Infants weighing less than 9 kg (20 lb) who cannot sit upright must be secured in their child | Use an approved child safety seat; the child safety seat should be secured in the rear seat, when possible, especially with a passenger-side air bag. | Preschoolers 4 to 5 y of age or who weigh more than 18 kg (40 lb) may, if necessary, use a standard lap belt or a lap belt or shoulder harness in combination with a booster seat. | Lap and shoulder belts (three-point restraints) are optimal restraints for children 5 to 14 years of age. Purchase the proper size bicycle for the child's size. | Use safety restraints during vehicular travel. Teach adolescents not to drink and drive. Encourage adolescents to take driver safety courses. |

Table continued on following page

Table 9–2. INJURY PREVENTION STRATEGIES FOR INFANTS, CHILDREN, AND ADOLESCENTS (*Continued*)

	INFANTS	TODDLERS	PRESCHOOLERS	SCHOOL-AGE CHILDREN	ADOLESCENTS
Motor vehicles, bicycles, skate boards *Continued*	safety seat at a semireclined angle in a rear-facing position in the rear seat.			When the child straddles the center bar, both feet should be flat on the ground with a 2.5 cm (1-in) space between the crotch and bar. Assure that children wear properly fitting bicycle helmets. Younger children should have coaster brakes, as hand brakes require too much strength and coordination. For skateboarding and in-line skating, encourage the use of helmets, knee and elbow pads, and properly fitting skates.	Encourage adolescents to use helmets with motorcycles, snowmobiles, mopeds, and other vehicles.
Drowning	Do not leave an infant unattended near water.	Never leave a toddler unattended near water. Keep toilet seat lids down and keep buckets out of a toddler's play area. Use buckets smaller than the toddler's head so that the toddler cannot accidentally fall head first into the bucket.	Never leave a preschooler unattended near water; use life preservers or water wings but do not rely on these devices as life preservers. Teach preschoolers how to swim and how to be safe in the water.	Teach children to swim with a buddy. Teach children not to dive into unknown water ("feet first, first time"). Encourage the use of life preservers and other safety equipment. Encourage attendance at swimming classes.	Encourage safe swimming, including the avoidance of alcohol and substances. Encourage safe swimming and safe boating practices.

Overall Safety

Burn Safety

Teach all children fire safety. Know the flammability potential of clothes, furniture, fabrics, and floors in the home.

Safely store gasoline and other flammable liquids.

Use space and water heaters safely.

Keep water heater temperature between 48.9° and 54.4° C (120° and 130° F).

Inspect electric equipment for safe wiring.

Avoid smoking cigarettes in bed; dispose of ashes properly.

Avoid the use of hot steam vaporizers.

Never leave children younger than 10 years of age home alone.

Assure an adequate fire escape plan.

Stay with young children while they are in the bathtub.

Assure that smoke detectors are located on every floor of the house and that they are in working order.

Children of all ages should use sunscreen to avoid sunburn; an SPF of 15 or higher should be used.

Encourage children to drink plenty of salt-containing fluids on hot, humid days to avoid dehydration and heat emergencies; limit the intensity of outdoor play in school-age children and adolescents.

Animal Safety

Teach children how to approach pets and how to respect them; set a good example for them.

Teach children to avoid unfamiliar pets or animals and what to do if a strange pet (i.e., dog) approaches them.

Vehicular Safety

Keep children indoors during lawn mower use.

Do not let children ride as passengers on riding lawn mowers, all-terrain vehicles, or other off-road vehicles.

Always use safety restraints.

Do not allow children and adolescents to ride in the back of pickup trucks or to lean out of open hatchbacks.

Before putting the car in motion, assure that everyone's safety belt is secured, all doors are locked, all groceries and other objects are secured in the trunk, and the rear window is free of obstructions.

Children should be taught proper behavior for riding in the car; distractions, such as toys or games, should be used to occupy the children.

Arms, legs, and heads should not be placed out of the window.

Assure that driveways are clear of toys and pedestrians prior to putting the car in motion.

Pedestrian Safety

Teach children how to cross the street safely.

Encourage children to wear reflective clothing.

Table continued on following page

Table 9–2.   INJURY PREVENTION STRATEGIES FOR INFANTS, CHILDREN, AND ADOLESCENTS (*Continued*)

Water Safety

Never leave children unattended near water, including backyard wading pools.

A fence or barrier at least 120 cm (4 ft) high should surround the home pool, not counting the house as a barrier.

The pool gate should be self-closing and self-latching, with the latch out of a young child's reach.

Have children swim with a buddy or with adult supervision.

Keep first aid and life preservers nearby.

Keep bicycles and other riding toys away from the pool area; do not allow rough-housing, running, or pushing near the pool area.

Teach children of all ages safe swimming practices, such as no dunking, no diving head first, and staying out of the pool during a thunderstorm.

Bicycle Safety

Use bicycle paths when possible.

Walk the bicycle through intersections.

Try to avoid riding in inclement weather.

Wear properly fitting shoes and avoid riding barefoot.

Children older than 9 months should be placed in carrier seats equipped with foot guards, foot rests, foot straps, and seat belts.

Firearm Safety

Keep all firearms unloaded under lock and key; keep a trigger lock in place.

Store ammunition in a separate, locked area.

Horseplay with firearms is strictly prohibited.

Fireworks Safety

Keep fireworks away from children.

Sledding Safety

Assure that the sled is in good working condition.

Encourage sledding in approved areas clear of rocks and holes.

Encourage sledding during daylight hours.

Avoid sledding in high traffic areas.

Teach children how to start and stop the sled.

Dress children warmly with hats, gloves, socks, and boots during inclement weather.

Allow young children limited time in the snow and ice to avoid hypo-thermia.

560

is a function of the mass of the occupant, the speed of travel, the tolerance of the impacted tissues to mechanical energy, and the degree of energy absorbed by the impacting surfaces, their configuration, and the area and length of contact (Robertson, 1985). Projectiles within the vehicle, such as passengers, groceries, or other objects, strike the vehicle occupants, causing additional injuries.

- Injuries are incurred from *restraining devices*. The young child's center of gravity is higher (near T-11 to T-12 in the infant), allowing the child to jackknife forward on impact (Pautler et al, 1995). Resulting injuries include flexion-distraction injuries to the lumbar spine, small bowel contusion and perforation, pancreatic fracture, and cutaneous contusions. Cervical hyperflexion and hyperextension can lead to high spinal cord injuries in young children. In children who are improperly secured with loose-fitting restraints, submarining under the belt can occur and lead to injury. Thus, lap belts, two-point restraints, and three-point restraints should not be used in children younger than 4 years of age. Among 10,098 children aged 15 years and younger who were passengers in motor vehicle crashes, 40% were optimally restrained, 29% were suboptimally restrained, and 31% were unrestrained (Johnston et al, 1994). Car seat usage was very high for infants and toddlers; however, 10- to 14-year-olds had the highest noncompliance for restraints.
- The leading cause of death in unrestrained children in motor vehicle crashes is head injury. Chest injuries sustained after ejection from the vehicle are the second leading cause of death (Templeton, 1993). *Air bags* have been implicated in the deaths of infants and young children. Unrestrained or improperly restrained front seat passengers can strike the dashboard near the point of air bag deployment. The inflating air bag can propel the child against other passengers and interior vehicle structures, causing injury or death (Centers for Disease Control and Prevention [CDC], 1995). To prevent such injury, the National Highway Traffic Safety Administration (NHTSA) proposes that infants riding in rear-facing car safety seats should be secured in the rear seat, and children should ride restrained in a car's rear seat. If a car does not have a rear seat, the child should be secured as far back as possible from the air bag (CDC, 1995).

c. Each year in the United States, 50,000 children are injured as *pedestrians*. Pedestrian injuries are the second leading cause of death among children 5 to 9 years of age and the fourth leading cause of death in children 10 to 14 years of age (Ray and Yuwiler, 1994). *Pedestrian–motor vehicle collisions* differ from other types of motor vehicle–related trauma in that very few victims escape multiple injuries. Although only 1% of pedestrians struck by cars are uninjured, 94% of all motor vehicle collisions involve no personal injuries (Rivara, 1990). Most pedestrian injuries occur in the afternoon and early evening, when school is over and traffic is increasing. Injury occurs when the child is hit by the vehicle and then is thrown onto the car hood. Waddell's triad of chest, extremity, and head trauma can be observed in this population (Halpern, 1989). The long bone injury results from contact with the car fender, the abdominal and chest injuries are due to the blunt forces from the car radiator, and the head injury results from the child being propelled upward onto the hood and hitting the windshield and then landing on the ground head first. If the child's shoes were stricken from the body, the vehicle was probably traveling at greater than 40 mph (Templeton, 1993). Left-sided injuries are most common in the

United States, as motorists drive on the right side of the road (Templeton, 1993).

d. The Consumer Product Safety Commission's National Electronic Injury Surveillance System (NEISS) rates the *bicycle* as the leading hazardous product in the United States (Mofensen and Greensher, 1992). Bicycle-related injuries result in significant short- and long-term disabilities (Nakayama, Gardner, and Rogers, 1990). Bicycles are 17 times more dangerous than cars on a miles-driven basis. Head injuries account for more than 60% of bicycle-related deaths (Li et al, 1995). Wearing properly fitting bicycle helmets reduces the incidence of head injury. National Pediatric Trauma Registry data shows 2333 pediatric patients having bicycle-related trauma, with 54% sustaining head injuries (usually concussions and skull fractures). Only 26 patients (1%) were wearing a helmet at the time of injury. Those patients with head injuries were more likely to receive ICU treatment as compared to those who did not have a head injury. Other bicycle-related injuries included neck fractures, facial fractures, and upper extremity fractures. Nonfatal injuries occur more frequently in boys (Li et al, 1995; McKenna et al, 1991) most often during unsafe riding practices (McKenna et al, 1991).

e. *Skateboard-related injuries* also occur in children, with extremity injuries most often occurring in older children. Children younger than 13 years of age may not have the muscle coordination to maintain balance and sufficient experience and maturity to judge the safety of skateboard maneuvers (Mofenson and Greensher, 1992).

2. A **crush injury** occurs when compressive strain (energy) is concentrated in one body area. Crush injuries include animal bites or being caught in machinery or equipment (i.e., finger caught in a car door). Animal bites can lead to a localized infection, cellulitis, and in some instances, surgical intervention. Bites vary from a small puncture wound or laceration to crushing of major arteries, veins, and nerves. Pets are most likely to be involved in animal bites and include cats, dogs, ferrets, and other small animals. One study of factors associated with dog bites showed that German shepherds and chow chows are most frequently involved. Unneutered male dogs living in a home with one or more children are prone to biting. These animals are usually chained in their yard at the time of the attack (Gershman et al, 1994). Rabies, which is always fatal when untreated, is a concern for any child bitten by a household or stray pet, domestic animal (i.e., horse, cow), or wild animal (i.e., squirrel, bat, raccoon).

3. A **shear injury** occurs when forces are applied in opposite directions. A subdural hematoma from a motor vehicle crash is an example, where due to inertial forces the brain is moving in relation to the surrounding dura, shearing the bridging veins connecting to the sinus (Pautler et al, 1995). Young children's brains appear to be more susceptible to shearing, especially at the base.

4. **Acceleration-deceleration forces** occur when a body stops suddenly and the internal organs keep moving inside the body. The internal organs and vessels rupture or tear, such as the spinal cord, hepatic artery and vein, and descending thoracic aorta.

5. **Penetrating forces** occur from firearms, knives, or other objects.

a. Injuries from low-velocity weapons are generally less destructive than from high-velocity weapons, such as semiautomatic weapons, because high-velocity weapons include hydrostatic pressure (Creel, 1988). Injuries from firearms are related to the type of weapon, type and caliber of bullet, muzzle velocity of the projectile, number of bullets penetrating the body, and distance from which the firearm was discharged. Dense organs, such as the liver and muscle, sustain greater damage than less dense organs, such as the lungs (Creel, 1988). The damage to body tissues from a bullet or missile is related to shock waves, cavitation, and pulsation of the cavity (Creel, 1988), as well as the type of jacket in the projectile. Bullets may become lodged in the body or exit through a separate wound. The severity of knife wounds is related to the anatomic area inflicted with the knife, the length of the blade, and the angle of penetration (Creel, 1988). An exit wound may or may not be present, and the blade may be impaled. Objects and toys can become missiles that can penetrate a child's body. For example, the young child running with a toy in his or her mouth who subsequently falls can sustain a penetrating injury to the oropharynx. Penetrating forces produce entrance and, most often, exit wounds. Damage to the internal organs results from kinetic force along the path of the penetrating object.

    b. *Penetrating injuries* accounted for 25% of admissions to one urban pediatric trauma center, with gunshot wounds being the most frequent injury in the 12- to 15-year-old age group (Hall et al, 1995). Boys 15 to 19 years old living in urban areas accounted for the highest risk group for homicide. Hand-guns were involved in the vast majority (72%) of these firearm injuries. It is estimated that half of American homes contain firearms; this means that there are approximately 200 million firearms, with 60 million being hand-guns (Committee on Injury and Poison Prevention, 1992). Societal factors have been implicated in the preponderance of firearm use; violence in the media, violence in the school and home, and the "glamour" of gun play all contribute to the appeal of firearms in children and adolescents.

B. THERMAL INJURY

Thermal injury occurs when the rate of heat absorption is greater than the rate of heat dissipation and results in scalds and flame burns (see Burns).

C. ELECTRICAL INJURY

When electricity, either through current or lightning, comes into contact with the body, its electrical energy is converted to heat, causing injury. Most electrical injuries are due to low-voltage alternating current in the home setting (see Burns).

D. CHEMICAL INJURY

When a chemical is applied to the body, it causes injury by either producing heat or denaturing protein (see Burns and Toxicology).

E. RADIANT BURNS

Exposure to the sun, nuclear, or therapeutic radiation can cause radiant burns (see Burns).

F. LACK OF OXYGENATION

Lack of oxygenation occurs with near-drowning or near-hanging episodes. Neuro-logic damage and death occur after a near-hanging episode from one of three mechanisms (Digeronimo and Mayes, 1994): (1) direct injury to the brain stem and spinal cord, (2) mechanical constriction of the neck, and (3) cardiac arrest, which may be secondary to a massive vagal response from bilateral carotid body stimulation. Children are at risk from airway edema following a near-hanging episode; however, laryngeal and vertebral fractures are rare to nonexistent (Digeronimo and Mayes, 1994).

G. LACK OF THERMOREGULATION

    1. Prolonged environmental exposure during extreme cold results in frostbite and hypothermia. Hypothermia begins when a child's temperature is ≤35° C. In trauma, hypothermia is related to prolonged environmental exposure, blood loss, alcohol use, and the injuries themselves. Children are at risk for hypother-mia because of their large body surface area (BSA)–to-mass ratio and less sub-cutaneous fat for heat production. Children whose core temperatures are lower than 32° C should be admitted to the ICU (Barkin and Rosen, 1994). Extracor-poreal circulating bypass may be required for severe cases of hypothermia.

2. Frostbite occurs when ice crystallizes in the body's cells. It is usually found in the fingers, hands, feet, toes, ears, and nose (Barkin and Rosen, 1994). The severity (degree) of frostbite depends on the environmental temperature and humidity, duration of exposure, windchill factor, immobility, and tightness of clothing (Barkin and Rosen, 1994). For frostbite, initial treatment includes careful touching of the frostbitten areas. Rewarming is initiated only if there is no chance for a second freezing during transport to the hospital (Barkin and Rosen, 1994). Tables 9–3 and 9–4 outline cold-related emergencies.

Table 9–3. COLD-RELATED EMERGENCIES: HYPOTHERMIA MANAGEMENT

CORE TEMPERATURE	COMMON SIGNS AND SYMPTOMS	MANAGEMENT
		Temperatures ≥32° C (Mild or Moderate)
35° C (95° F)	Slurred speech, lapse of memory, shivering	1. Initiate passive external rewarming (apply blankets, warm the room).
32° C (89° F)	Diminished mental status: Drowsy, amnesic, confused, disoriented	2. Attempt to raise the temperature 0.5°–2° C/h.
	Muscle rigidity, poor muscle coordination	3. If there is no increase in temperature in 2 h, evaluate for underlying disease and initiate active rewarming.
		Temperatures <32° C (Moderate or Severe)
30° C (86° F)	Skin cyanotic, edematous	1. Begin active rewarming at 0.5° C/h. Active external rewarming is used for the *stable* patient. Active core rewarming is used for the *unstable* patient (humidified and heated oxygen 40.5°–42° C; warmed IVF (36°–40° C) D$_5$W/ 0.9% NS without K; peritoneal dialysis without K heated to 40.5°– 42.5° C; warmed gastric, bladder, or pleural lavage; hemodialysis and ECMO are controversial).
	Stuporous, irritable	
	Progressive decline in basal metabolic rate	
	Shivering stops	
	Myocardial irritability, bradycardia, J (or Osborne) waves on electrocardiogram (ECG), decreased cardiac output, and hypotension	
	Decreased minute ventilation	
28° C (82° F)	Dysrhythmias common; bradycardia refractory to atropine with progression to ventricular fibrillation and asystole	2. Observe for rewarming shock during treatment (vasodilation may cause transient fall in blood pressure); handle patient carefully.
	Ventricular fibrillation can be induced by stimulation	3. Avoid inserting intracardiac monitors and administering adrenergic drugs until the temperature is about 28° C if possible. If necessary, preoxygenate patient before performing invasive procedures.
26° C (79° F)	Loss of consciousness, areflexive	
25° C (77° F)	Respirations cease, dead appearance	4. Discontinue active rewarming when the core temperature reaches 32°–34° C to prevent overheating.

D$_5$W, 5% dextrose and water; *ECMO,* extracorporeal membrane oxygenation; *IVF,* intravenous fluid; *NS,* normal saline. From Barkin R, Rosen P. Environmental emergencies. In: Barkin R, Rosen P, eds. *Emergency Pediatrics.* 4th ed. St Louis, Mo: Mosby–Year Book Inc; 1994:314–316.

Table 9–4.   COLD-RELATED EMERGENCIES: FROSTBITE

DEGREE (FROSTBITE)	CLINICAL PRESENTATION	MANAGEMENT
First	Skin mottled, edematous, hyperemic, with burning and tingling Peaks in 24–48 h and may persist for 1–2 wk	Warm affected fingers by holding them in the armpits or blowing warm air on them. When warmed, cover with a clean, dry cloth.
Second	Blister formation with paresthesia and anesthesia	
Third (deep)	Necrosis of skin with ulceration and edema Involves subcutaneous tissue	Immerse area in tepid water (40.5°–43.3° C) for 20 min after core rewarming is initiated. After warming, apply sterile gauze and elevate for 40 min.
Fourth (deep)	Necrosis with gangrene; vesicle followed by eschar and ulceration; progression for 24–36 h Demarcation may take several weeks	Consider administration of tetanus prophylaxis and analgesics; handle the affected areas gently.

From Barkin R, Rosen P. Environmental emergencies. In: Barkin R, Rosen P, eds. *Emergency Pediatrics*. 4th ed. St Louis, Mo: Mosby–Year Book Inc; 1994:314–316.

3. Prolonged environmental exposure to heat may result in heat cramps, heat exhaustion, and heat stroke. Children are at risk for heat-related emergencies because they acclimatize more slowly to exercise in the heat as compared to adults (Barkin and Rosen, 1994). Children's larger BSA-to-weight ratio allows them to produce more metabolic heat per mass unit when walking or running; furthermore, children's sweating capacity is not as great as adults' nor is their ability to convey heat through the circulation from the core to the periphery (Barkin and Rosen, 1994). Table 9–5 differentiates the characteristics of and treatment for each heat-related emergency.

HISTORY

A. **TRAUMA RESUSCITATION**

Trauma resuscitation begins immediately after the injury, with first aid initiated by family or bystanders, and continues with the prehospital care providers and emergency department staff. The first 20 minutes of management is crucial in determining the outcome for the multiply injured child. The initial assessment and treatment must be organized and methodical to decrease trauma-related morbidity and mortality.

B. **INJURY HISTORY**

1. The history surrounding the injury is obtained from family, bystanders, prehospital providers, and the patient (if possible). Pertinent historical information is obtained and relates to three important areas: mechanism of injury, patient history, and plausibility of mechanism of injury and patient history. Pertinent information related to the mechanism of injury is as follows:

   a. *Motor vehicle occupant:* Scene fatalities, use of restraining devices (car seat, three-point restraints, lap belt), front or back seat passenger, ejection from the vehicle; site of impact (side, rear-end, head-on), motor vehicle speed,

Table 9–5. HEAT-RELATED EMERGENCIES

CONDITION	CAUSE	SYMPTOMS	RECTAL TEMPERATURE	TREATMENT
Heat cramps	Sodium depletion from prolonged exercise; drinking salt-poor fluids	Alert, oriented, severe muscle cramps	<40° C	Mild: 1 tsp salt/500 ml water PO. Severe: 0.9% NS at 20 ml/kg/h over 1–2 h; observe for low serum sodium level.
Heat exhaustion	Exposure to high temperature environment; may be water or salt depleted; gradual onset	Sweating, irritable, headache, thirst; may have muscle cramps, nausea, and vomiting	<40° C	Mild: oral fluids; sprinkle water over body to increase evaporative heat loss. Severe: 0.9% NS at 20 ml/kg over 30 min; treat for dehydration; observe for shock, seizures, and coma; monitor serum sodium.
Heat stroke	Nonexertional: Develops over a few days' time, usually during a heat wave; infants and ill children are most often affected. Exertional: Rapid onset, usually in young children who have not acclimated to a hot environment	Headache, listlessness, confusion, seizures, psychosis, coma, hot dry skin (no sweating), tachycardia, hypotension	>40° C	Airway, breathing, and circulation stabilization; observe for cardiac dysrhythmias; monitor rectal temperature; give an ice bath or sprinkle cold water on patient; use fans to increase evaporative heat loss; use a cooling blanket; avoid shivering; 0.9% NS at 20 ml/kg over 45–60 min; place an indwelling bladder catheter and nasogastric tube.

NS, normal saline; *PO*, orally.
From Barkin R, Rosen P. Environmental emergencies. In: Barkin R, Rosen P, eds. *Emergency Pediatrics*. 4th ed. St Louis, Mo: Mosby–Year Book Inc; 1994:309–312.

object of collision (oncoming vehicle, stationary vehicle or object), passenger compartment intrusion, entrapment

b. *Pedestrian–motor vehicle crash:* Speed of vehicle, travel of patient after the impact, run over by or pinned under the vehicle, type of surface on which the patient landed, the point of impact on the patient's body

c. *Bicycle–motor vehicle crash:* Speed of bicycle, speed of vehicle (if moving), use of bicycle helmet

     d. *Fall:* Height from which the patient fell, surface onto which the patient landed, area of body that hit the ground first

     e. *Penetrating injury:* Type of weapon used, number of bullets fired, caliber of bullets, firing range, number and location of stab wounds

  2. Pertinent information related to the patient's history is as follows:

     a. *Airway:* Did the child have a choking or vomiting episode? Was assistance needed to maintain the child's airway?

     b. *Breathing:* Did the child stop breathing or have difficulty breathing? For what length of time did this occur? Was rescue breathing initiated?

     c. *Circulation:* Was blood lost? About how much? Was cardiopulmonary resuscitation (CPR) initiated? How long was it in progress?

     d. *Disability:* Did the child sustain a loss of consciousness? For how long? Was the child easily arousable? Does the child have antegrade (loss of memory after the injury) or retrograde (loss of memory before the injury) amnesia? Does the child recognize family members and familiar objects? Was the child able to wiggle his or her fingers and toes? Did the child appear flaccid? Did the child appear frightened, apprehensive, anxious?

     e. *Other:* Was any first aid administered? Were any splints or bandages applied? Did the child get up and walk around after the injury, or was the child found in the same position as immediately following the injury?

  3. Pertinent information related to the mechanism of injury and the patient's history is as follows:

     a. *Developmental plausibility:* Does the mechanism of injury match the patient's history? That is, if the mechanism of injury in an infant was a fall from a couch (approximately 1 ft) onto a carpeted floor, and the infant is in cardiopulmonary arrest, intentional injury must be suspected.

     b. *Credibility of witnesses:* Are family members or bystanders changing their stories to match the child's injuries? Or, are witnesses reluctant to divulge information? For example, the mechanism of injury in a 13-year-old is a gunshot wound to the chest due to a drive-by shooting. It is a warm evening, all the neighbors are outside, yet no one sees the car or driver. Such witnesses may be afraid to come forward for fear of gang retaliation.

     c. *Patient's overall appearance:* How does the child appear overall? Does the child appear well-nourished and clean? Does the child appear to be developmentally appropriate? Does the child appear to be the correct size and weight appropriate for age? Does the child have any bruises, scars, or other signs of child maltreatment? How is the parent-child relationship? Does the parent or caregiver comfort the child or scold the child for the injury? Does the parent label the child as "clumsy" or "accident prone"? Does the child go willingly to strangers or does the child shrink from human touch?

C. PATIENT PAST HEALTH HISTORY

Parents may have been involved in the injury and may be receiving treatment elsewhere. Family members called to the hospital may not be able to provide information on the patient's past health history. Parents or legal guardians must be notified when an injury occurs; however, emergency treatment is not withheld until parental consent is obtained. A basic history to obtain is AMPLE:

  1. *A*llergies to medications

  2. *M*edications the patient regularly receives (over-the-counter and prescription)

  3. *P*ast medical history or illness, as well as special needs (hearing impairment, use of special devices)

  4. *L*ast meal eaten

  5. *E*vents or environment leading up to the injury (obtained in injury history).

INITIAL ASSESSMENT

The initial assessment of the multiply injured child includes the primary and secondary assessments. Children have unique anatomic and physiologic features that make them different from adults; these features should be taken into consideration when conducting the primary and secondary assessments.

A. Primary Assessment

1. In the primary assessment, life-threatening injuries are detected and treated. Life-threatening injuries include airway obstruction; open, tension, and bilateral hemopneumothoraces; traumatic arrest; flail chest; cardiac tamponade; and hemorrhagic shock.

2. Life-saving interventions are initiated simultaneously with the detection of these injuries and include airway stabilization and restoration of breathing and circulation.

3. **Airway and cervical spine assessment**

   a. *Developmental considerations*

      • Because the young child's airway has a narrow diameter, airway obstruction occurs very easily. The tongue is relatively large in comparison to the oral cavity and can easily obstruct the airway. The larynx is more cephalad and anterior, with the vocal cords being short and concave (Chameides and Hazinski, 1994). The epiglottis is U-shaped and protrudes into the pharynx. The cricoid cartilage is the narrowest area of the airway in children younger than 10 years of age. If the neck is hyperflexed or hyperextended, airway obstruction results from the laxity of the airway structures. The lower airways are small in diameter, with less supporting cartilage in infants and young children; thus, airway obstruction from mucus and edema easily occurs. (See also Chapter 2.)

      • Children younger than 8 years of age are susceptible to cervical spine injury because of their larger head size, weak neck musculature, and horizontal facets (Schafermeyer, 1993). Furthermore, these young children have lax intraspinal ligaments and capsules, thus increasing their susceptibility to pseudosubluxation of the cervical spine (Scully and Luerssen, 1995). Their fulcrum of cervical mobility is high (C2-3) as compared to C5-6 and C6-7 in the adult (Ludwig and Loiselle, 1993), thus accounting for the fact that C1-3 fractures are the most common cervical fracture in pediatric patients. Therefore, cervical spine injuries should always be suspected until proven otherwise.

   b. *Assessment and interventions*

      • The airway is assessed for patency. The presence of loose teeth, vomit, and blood is determined. The cervical spine is maintained in neutral alignment, usually by securing the child on a pediatric long board with a cervical immobilization device and a cervical collar. Flexion of the cervical spine must be avoided to prevent airway compromise or aggravation of an existing spinal cord injury. The front of the cervical collar is opened to inspect the neck for jugular vein distention and tracheal deviation and to palpate the carotid pulse; the collar is then closed. The cervical collar must fit properly to prevent flexion and extension of the cervical spine. A properly fitting collar has these features: the chin rests securely in the chin holder; the ears are not covered by the collar; and the bottom of the collar rests on the upper sternum (Bernardo and Waggoner, 1992).

      • Signs and symptoms of spinal cord injury are quickly ascertained, such as numbness, tingling, and inability to wiggle the toes and fingers. Full spinal immobilization is maintained throughout the initial treatment.

4. **Respiratory assessment**
   a. *Developmental considerations*
      - The chest wall in younger children is cartilaginous, allowing blunt and penetrating energy forces to be easily transmitted to underlying lung and cardiac tissues. Therefore, when rib fractures are present, a tremendous amount of blunt force was applied to the chest wall. An increasing number of fractures correlate with increasing mortality. Similarly, flail segments indicate severe parenchymal injury (Reynolds, 1995). The mediastinum is mobile, allowing for more of a problem with pneumothoraces.
      - Breathing is primarily diaphragmatic until the age of 7 to 8 years. Chest retractions can be observed during respiratory distress. The crying child swallows air, resulting in gastric distention. This distention impedes diaphragmatic movement and respiratory excursion.
      - Children have fewer alveoli and therefore less respiratory reserve as compared to adults. The work of breathing must be continuously assessed. Breath sounds may be easily transmitted because of the thin chest wall, allowing for a false assumption that breath sounds are equal. Standing at the foot of the bed and observing for equal bilateral chest rise is one way to determine symmetry of breathing (Bernardo and Trunzo, 1995).
      - Oxygen consumption is higher in infants (6 to 8 ml/kg/min) as compared to adults (3 to 4 ml/kg/min), allowing hypoxemia to occur rapidly (Chameides and Hazinski, 1994). This higher consumption results in more rapid respiratory rates.
   b. *Assessment and interventions*
      - Respirations are assessed by observation and inspection. The quality of respirations are determined by assessing the presence of breath sounds high in the axillae and anterior chest. Unequal bilateral breath sounds may indicate a pneumothorax on the diminished side. Signs of respiratory distress include retractions of the intercostal muscles, nasal flaring, grunting (in infants), adventitious breath sounds, or diminished or absent breath sounds. Rescue breathing with 100% oxygen by bag-valve-mask is initiated in the apneic or bradypneic child.
      - The chest is exposed and inspected for any surface trauma, penetrating wounds, paradoxical movements, and flail segments. The rib cage is gently palpated for tenderness, crepitus, and flail segments. The sternum is palpated for tenderness as well.

5. **Circulatory assessment**
   a. *Developmental considerations*
      - Children have a higher oxygen requirement and faster metabolic rate, requiring a higher cardiac output per kilogram of body weight (Soud et al, 1992). Although the child's circulating blood volume of 80 ml/kg is small, it is larger on a milliliter per kilogram basis as compared to an adult's. Even small amounts of blood loss can decrease circulating blood volume and compromise perfusion. Hypotension does not develop until a 20% to 25% blood loss occurs (Nakayama, 1991); therefore, hypotension is a *late* sign of circulatory compromise in the child. Adequate tissue perfusion is reflected by a capillary refill time of less than 2 seconds. (See Chapter 3.)
      - Tachycardia is the initial response to hypovolemia and occurs with decreased oxygen delivery. This increased heart rate increases blood pressure; when this compensatory mechanism fails, tissue hypoxia and

hypercapnia occur, leading to bradycardia (Chameides and Hazinski, 1994) and hypotension. Bradycardia and hypotension, therefore, are *late* signs of cardiac failure. Bradycardia and hypotension are both ominous signs of impending respiratory and circulatory collapse.

b. *Assessment and interventions*

- Circulation is assessed by auscultating heart sounds for their rate, rhythm, and quality. If the pulse is absent, or if peripheral pulses or blood pressure are nonpalpable in the presence of an electrical rhythm (PEA), chest compressions are immediately initiated. Muffled heart tones, distended veins, and shock (Beck's triad) may indicate cardiac tamponade, which may necessitate pericardiocentesis or open pericardiotomy (Nakayama, 1991). Major external hemorrhage is controlled by application of direct pressure.

- Peripheral circulation is assessed by palpating a radial or brachial pulse, measuring capillary refill (should be less than 2 seconds), and assessing skin color (pink) and temperature (warm). Deviations in peripheral circulation may indicate decreased blood flow to the periphery, which can result in decreased oxygen and substrate delivery to the tissues.

6. **Neurologic assessment**

a. *Developmental considerations*

- Infants and children are susceptible to brain injury for a number of reasons. They have a larger head-to-body ratio. The skull is malleable due to its thin cranial bones, so less protection is afforded to the brain tissues. Nerve myelinization is not complete at birth, and this unmyelinated brain tissue is particularly vulnerable to injury, especially shearing forces. Continued development of fiber tracts and myelinization may aid recovery from localized injuries.

- Fontanelles and sutures may remain open until approximately 18 to 24 months. Following head injury, the open fontanelles and sutures may help to equalize increased intracranial pressure (ICP), thus hiding the signs of intracranial injury. (See Chapter 4.)

b. *Assessment and interventions*

- A brief neurologic evaluation establishes the patient's level of consciousness and pupillary size and reactivity. Responsiveness may be more difficult to evaluate in the preverbal child. Alterations in developmentally-expected behaviors, such as lack of stranger anxiety in an 8-month-old infant, decreased muscle tone in a 2-month-old infant, or inability to focus and follow objects in a 6-month-old infant may indicate changes in neurologic functioning. Changes in the child's level of consciousness may indicate decreased oxygenation (pulmonary exchange) or perfusion (hypovolemia) and not necessarily brain injury.

- Throughout the primary assessment, the nurse talks to the child to determine his or her level of consciousness and to provide emotional support. The *AVPU* method of evaluation determines the child's response to stimulation (Committee on Trauma, 1989):
  *A*wake
  Responsive to *v*erbal stimuli
  Responsive to *p*ainful stimuli
  *U*nresponsive

- The infant should respond by looking around and being wary of strangers. The verbal child should be able to state his or her name and perhaps other information. The child who changes from awake to sleepy to disoriented should be watched closely. The pediatric Glasgow Coma

Scale (GCS) score (Table 9–6) should be obtained to record the best eye, motor, and verbal responses.

7. **Exposure**

a. *Developmental considerations:* Children have a larger BSA-to-weight ratio as compared to adults. This ratio renders them susceptible to convective and conductive heat loss. Infants younger than 6 months of age do not have the neuromuscular maturity to shiver to maintain body heat. Nonshivering thermogenesis then occurs, where brown fat is broken down to provide warmth; unfortunately, oxygen consumption increases, and decompensation ensues (Soud et al, 1992).

b. *Assessment and interventions:* The child is completely undressed to allow for visualization of all injuries. Overhead warming lights and warm ambient temperature should help maintain body temperature within a normal range. Warm blankets are applied to respect modesty, prevent convective heat loss, and promote comfort.

B. **SECONDARY ASSESSMENT**

A complete head-to-toe assessment is conducted to detect and treat all non-life-threatening injuries.

1. The **head** is examined for depressions, lacerations, hematomas, and impaled objects. The anterior and posterior fontanelles in infants are palpated; a tense and bulging fontanelle may indicate increased ICP. The scalp is palpated for lacerations and observed for dirt, glass, and other debris.

2. The **face** is inspected for deformities, lacerations, foreign bodies, and impaled objects. The orbits, facial bones, and mandible are palpated for pain and

Table 9–6. PEDIATRIC COMA SCALE*

	SCORE	Age Older than 1 y	Younger than 1 y	
Eye opening	4	Spontaneously	Spontaneously	
	3	To verbal command	To shout	
	2	To pain	To pain	
	1	No response	No response	
Best motor response	6	Obeys		
	5	Localizes pain	Localizes pain	
	4	Flexion withdrawal	Flexion withdrawal	
	3	Flexion—abnormal (decorticate rigidity)	Flexion—abnormal (decorticate ridigity)	
	2	Extension (decerebrate rigidity)	Extension (decerebrate rigidity)	
	1	No response	No response	
		Older than 5 y	**2–5 y**	**23 Mo or Younger**
Best verbal response	5	Oriented and converses	Appropriate words and phrases	Smiles, coos
	4	Disoriented and converses	Inappropriate words and phrases	Cries appropriately
	3	Inappropriate words	Cries or screams	Cries, screams
	2	Incomprehensible sounds	Grunts	Grunts
	1	No response	No response	No response
Total	3–15			

*Modification of Glasgow Coma Scale.
From Wong DL. *Whaley and Wong's Essentials of Pediatric Nursing* (ed. 5). St Louis, Mo: Mosby; 1997.

crepitance. Asymmetric facial movement is observed, which may indicate facial nerve paralysis. Le Fort (facial) fractures should be suspected in any blunt force or penetrating facial trauma. Malocclusion is indicative of a fractured mandible.

3. The **eyes** are assessed for pupillary reactivity and symmetry and extraocular movements. Blood in the anterior chamber of the eye (hyphema) should be reported immediately, as this indicates a serious injury. Foreign bodies should be noted, and penetrating objects are stabilized in place with gauze and tape. A ruptured globe is possible if the eye is swollen shut and bruised and a penetrating or direct blunt force was applied during the injury. The presence of tearing should be noted as well. Visual acuity may be easily assessed by asking the young child to point to an object or by having an older child verbalize his or her ability to see. The presence of contact lenses should be ascertained, and the contact lenses should be removed. Periorbital bruising or "raccoon's sign" is indicative of a basilar skull fracture. Scleral hemorrhage may be observed if compression forces were applied at the time of injury.

4. The **ears** are examined for cerebrospinal fluid or bloody drainage. Such drainage can be collected onto a gauze pad; however, the ear is never packed with gauze. Hematotympanum should be noted. Ecchymosis over the mastoid process, or Battle's sign, is indicative of a basilar skull fracture; when noted, the skull fracture is more than 12 hours old. Ear lacerations should be covered with gauze soaked in normal saline (NS) until definitive repair is scheduled.

5. The **nose** is examined for cerebrospinal fluid or bloody drainage, deformities, lacerations, or bruising. Drainage can be collected onto a gauze pad, but the nares are not packed with the gauze.

6. The **oral cavity** including the tongue, mucous membranes, and teeth are examined for injury. Displaced permanent teeth can be placed in milk or NS and dated; the debris should not be removed from the tooth, as this material aids in reimplantation. Dental apparatus, such as braces, may have been damaged during the injury and should be assessed by a pediatric dentist or orthodontist.

7. The **neck** examination involves opening the front piece of the cervical collar for visualization of the anterior neck. The neck is assessed for lacerations, swelling, deformities, jugular vein distention, and impaled objects. The neck is palpated for pain, tenderness and subcutaneous emphysema. Tracheal positioning is noted, with the normal position being midline. Tracheal deviation is noted above the sternal notch in young children. The larynx is palpated for integrity, as a fractured larynx is easier palpated than visualized. The awake child's voice is assessed for hoarseness or changes. A hoarse or "gravelly" voice may also indicate tracheal trauma and the possible need for airway intervention. After the neck is assessed, the collar is secured.

8. The **chest** is reinspected for symmetry, flail segments, open wounds, and impaled objects. The anterior chest is examined for cutaneous lesions that may indicate underlying pulmonary or cardiac injury. The chest is auscultated for the presence of normal and adventitious breath sounds. The anterior rib cage and both clavicles are palpated for pain and tenderness. Pain with inspiration should be noted. The heart sounds are auscultated and should be clear and distinct. The point of maximal impulse (PMI) should be noted.

9. The **abdomen** is observed for distention, bruising, penetrating wounds, and impaled objects. Next, bowel sounds should be auscultated. The abdomen is then palpated for pain, rigidity, and tenderness. The lower abdomen is palpated for bladder tenderness and distention.

10. The **pelvis** is palpated for tenderness and intactness. Any pain or displacement on palpation is indicative of a pelvic fracture. Femoral pulses are assessed for equality and strength. The bladder is palpated for distention. The genitalia, urinary meatus, perineum, and rectum are inspected for signs of trauma, bleeding, and impaled objects. Blood at the urinary meatus may indicate a urethral tear. A rectal examination is performed to assess for the presence of blood or pelvic fractures, rectal wall integrity, and sphincter tone quality (Committee on Trauma, 1989). The prostate gland is difficult to palpate in the preadolescent boy. A flaccid rectal sphincter is indicative of spinal cord injury. The rectal examination may be deferred in cases of severe rectal trauma when an examination under anesthesia (EUA) or surgical intervention is needed or when a foreign body is lodged in the rectal vault. Priapism is noted.

11. The **extremities** are inspected for any deformities, open wounds or fractures, contusions, and impaled objects. Each extremity is palpated for pain, and the peripheral pulses are assessed for equality and amplitude. Skin color and temperature are reassessed, as well as capillary refill time. Asking the child to wiggle his or her toes and fingers and asking if he or she can feel the nurse touching the toes and fingers indicate neurovascular and neuromotor integrity. Hand grasps and foot flexion and extension determine strength and motor nerve functioning.

12. The **back** examination involves carefully logrolling the child to inspect the back. To logroll the child, one person (usually the surgeon) is assigned to keep the child's head midline and execute the move. An additional one or two staff members are needed to roll the child onto his or her side at the surgeon's command. Another person examines the back for any deformities, lacerations, hematomas, impaled objects, or abrasions on the posterior surface and flank. Each vertebra is palpated for stability and the presence of pain. After this examination, the surgeon gives the command to roll the child to the supine position, maintaining in-line cervical stabilization the entire time. The child's motor and neurovascular status are assessed immediately before and after the logrolling to assess the presence of spinal cord injury.

13. **Vital signs and pulse oximetry** readings are measured continuously and recorded every 5 minutes until the child is stable and then every 15 minutes for the first hour of treatment. Temperature is measured frequently to evaluate the effectiveness of warming measures and to detect and treat hypothermia. The child's vital signs should be compared with the age-appropriate norms for heart and respiratory rates and blood pressure ranges. Immediately after the injury, however, the child's physiologic requirements may not fall within age-appropriate ranges. Therefore, these parameters should serve as a guide only.

C. TRAUMA SCORING

1. After the primary and secondary assessments are completed, a trauma score and pediatric GCS score are assigned. A trauma score is an adjunct to, not a substitute for, full and ongoing clinical assessments (Reynolds, 1995).

2. Three trauma scores are used in pediatric trauma. The Pediatric Trauma Score (PTS) assesses six parameters important in the outcome of pediatric trauma: size, airway, blood pressure, CNS, fractures, and wounds. The Trauma Score (TS) assesses respiratory rate and effort, blood pressure, and capillary refill; it also includes the GCS score. The Revised Trauma Score (RTS) is comprised of the GCS score, blood pressure, and respiratory rate. The TS and RTS are adult scores, but they are used in children. One recent study demonstrated that the TS was more useful in predicting the outcome of pediatric trauma patients in

the emergency department and after hospitalization as compared to the PTS (Nayduch et al, 1991). Ideally, trauma scores are calculated in the prehospital setting, on arrival to the emergency department, and 1 hour later.

INITIAL TREATMENT

A. AIRWAY AND CERVICAL SPINE

1. In the unconscious child, the **airway initially is opened** and maintained using the jaw thrust maneuver. This maneuver is the safest technique for opening the airway in the child with a suspected cervical spine injury (Chameides and Hazinski, 1994). The head-tilt/chin-lift method is not used in pediatric trauma patients, as this method may convert a cervical spine fracture without neurologic injury into a cervical spine fracture with neurologic injury. Because the child's oral cavity is relatively small, the upper airway is easily obstructed by the lax oropharyngeal musculature in the unconscious child.

2. **Foreign material,** such as teeth, vomit, or blood, is cleared from the oral cavity with a tonsillar tip (Yankauer) suction tube. Stimulation of the gag reflex must be avoided in the child with an intact gag reflex, as gagging, vomiting, and aspiration may result. Blind finger sweeps are not recommended for foreign body removal in infants and young children, since foreign material may be displaced distally and injury to the friable oral mucosa may result.

3. An **oropharyngeal airway** may be placed in unconscious children to maintain airway patency. Oral airway size must be appropriate, since an airway that is too small may push the tongue backward and one that is too large may damage the delicate, soft intraoral tissues, causing bleeding and swelling and further complicating airway management (Nakayama, Venkataraman, et al, 1992). The oropharyngeal airway is measured from the corner of the mouth to the angle of the jaw (Chameides and Hazinski, 1994). This type of airway is inserted directly using a tongue blade to pull the tongue forward. This airway is *not* rotated 90 degrees as in the adult because damage may occur to the oral tissues. Furthermore, the tongue may be displaced posteriorly into the pharynx, causing an airway obstruction.

4. **Nasopharyngeal airways** are not recommended in pediatric trauma patients. In the child with a head injury, a basilar or cribriform plate fracture may be present. During insertion of a nasopharyngeal airway, entry into the cranial vault may occur.

5. These **basic airway maneuvers** are acceptable for short-term airway control. Endotracheal intubation is preferred for extended periods. The equipment is prepared, and cardiorespiratory and pulse oximetry monitors are used. The child's vital signs are closely monitored for cardiac dysrhythmias, lower oxygen saturations, or bradycardia. During endotracheal intubation, neutral cervical spine alignment is maintained by the surgeon or another skilled practitioner to avoid hyperextension. Endotracheal intubation is best accomplished by rapid-sequence technique by a skilled practitioner. Medications administered for rapid-sequence intubation may include thiopental (Pentothal), fentanyl and diazepam (Valium) or midazolam, lidocaine, and vecuronium. This combination of medications should be used to prevent increased ICP and to produce adequate states of sedation, analgesia, and paralysis (Nakayama, Waggoner, et al, 1992). An uncuffed endotracheal tube is used in children 8 years of age and younger because the cricoid cartilage serves as an effective seal. The orotracheal route is preferred. The endotracheal tube is secured with tape and benzoin or with commercially prepared devices. After intubation, a nasogastric

(if a basilar skull fracture is not present) or orogastric tube is inserted and connected to low continuous suction. Young children are aerophagic, and aggressive ventilation may lead to gastric distention (Semonin-Holleran, 1992). The gastric tube is measured from the corner of the mouth, over the ear to the xiphoid process, and marked with tape. Once the tube is properly placed, it is secured with tape. A chest radiograph is taken to confirm the endotracheal tube placement. Other indicators of correct tube placement include symmetric chest movement, equal bilateral breath sounds auscultated in all fields, a color change in the end-tidal carbon dioxide detector, and condensation in the endotracheal tube. Endotracheal suctioning may be required if copious secretions or oral trauma is present.

6. The **most common complication of endotracheal intubation** is inadvertent intubation of the right main stem bronchus or dislodgment of the endotracheal tube into the right main stem bronchus if the patient is positioned for procedures or transported within the facility. When this situation arises, chest expansion may not be equal, and breath sounds are absent or diminished in the left side of the chest. Pulse oximetry readings may be low, and ventilation may be difficult. Prompt recognition of this complication is essential; it is corrected by withdrawing the endotracheal tube until equal breath sounds and equal chest movement are observed.

7. In children where airway patency and control is not possible because of extensive craniofacial injuries, an **emergency tracheostomy or cricothyrotomy** may be performed by a surgeon skilled in the technique.

8. **Spinal precautions** are maintained during emergency treatment. Spinal precautions include the application of a rigid cervical collar, cervical immobilization device (CID), and an immobilization board. If the child should vomit, the child is logrolled as a unit with the equipment remaining intact, and then suctioning is performed. Anteroposterior, lateral, oblique, and odontoid cervical spine radiographs from C-1 through T-1 are obtained to determine the presence of spinal fractures. When obtaining the lateral views, the child's arms are pulled downward by a surgeon or nurse to allow for radiographic visualization of T-1. The radiographs are assessed for vertebral symmetry, alignment, and spacing. If the child does not have radiographic evidence of bony spinal abnormalities *and* the child has normal neurologic findings, the spinal immobilization devices may be removed.

B. BREATHING

1. High-flow oxygen through a non-rebreather face mask at a flow rate of 10 to 15 L is administered. The face mask fits properly if it is snug and covers the nose and mouth. If the child will not tolerate a face mask and oxygen saturation levels are maintained at 96% to 98%, the oxygen can be administered in a blow-by fashion.

2. If apnea or shallow, ineffective respirations are present, artificial ventilation is initiated with a bag-valve-mask and 100% high-flow oxygen. If spontaneous, effective respirations are not achieved, endotracheal intubation is performed. The chest should rise and fall symmetrically when the bag is squeezed. If the chest does not rise, the face mask and head should be carefully repositioned while maintaining spinal precautions (Nakayama, Venkataraman, et al, 1992). The bag-valve-mask device should have a bag capacity of at least 450 ml, be self-refilling, and come in pediatric and adult sizes. The pop-off valve should be occluded to allow for the need for higher ventilation pressures (Guidelines for Cardiopulmonary Resuscitation and Emergency Cardiac Care, 1992).

3. A **pulse oximeter** detects the percent of oxygen saturation in the blood and is a useful adjunct for determining adequacy of oxygenation.

4. **Mechanical ventilation** is initiated once proper endotracheal placement and adequate ventilation are achieved. The initial settings include an age-appropriate rate, 100% oxygen, and a low positive end-expiratory pressure (PEEP). The ventilator settings are adjusted according to the child's response to treatment.

5. **Life-threatening thoracic injuries** include tension hemothoraces, pneumothoraces, and pericardial tamponade. All these conditions are rare but must be anticipated. Pneumothoraces are initially treated with rapid needle (14- or 18-gauge) decompression in the fourth or fifth intercostal space, midaxillary line, or anterior axillary line, followed by chest tube placement. Pericardial tamponade is treated with a pericardiocentesis or pericardial window in the operating room.

C. CIRCULATION

1. A cardiorespiratory and blood pressure monitor are employed immediately after the child's arrival at the hospital. The appropriate cuff size should be two thirds the size of the child's upper arm or thigh. Intravenous (IV) cannulation with the largest catheter diameter possible is attempted in the upper, preferably uninjured extremity. If IV access is not obtained after three attempts or 90 seconds, intraosseous access is considered in the tibial plate. If intraosseous access is unsuccessful, central venous cannulation is attempted by an experienced physician or surgeon by cutdown in the antecubital space or via the saphenous system.

2. During IV cannulation, blood is obtained and sent for the following tests: hemoglobin, hematocrit, and platelet count; electrolytes and glucose; blood urea nitrogen (BUN) and creatinine; amylase, lipase, aspartate aminotransferase (AST; previously serum glutamic-oxaloacetic transaminase [SGOT]) and alanine aminotransferase (ALT; previously serum glutamic-pyruvic transaminase [SGPT]) in suspected abdominal trauma; creatine phosphokinase (CPK; in suspected cardiac trauma); type and crossmatch or type and screen (if operative management is anticipated or blood will be administered); and blood toxicology screening (in suspected drug or alcohol use).

3. IV crystalloid fluid of choice is lactated Ringer's solution (LR), which is administered at a maintenance rate in the absence of hypovolemic shock. The fluid is warmed if rapid infusion is administered. A stopcock can be connected to the tubing if fluid boluses are anticipated. Overhydration is avoided in children with significant head injury to prevent cerebral edema.

4. In the hypotensive child, a 20-ml/kg fluid bolus of crystalloids is administered. If no improvement in heart rate or blood pressure is observed, a second bolus is administered. If no improvement is observed, a third bolus is administered. If no response is apparent, a 10-ml/kg bolus of warm, O-negative blood is administered rapidly.

5. External hemorrhaging is controlled with direct pressure to the wound. Elevation of a bleeding extremity, in conjunction with direct pressure, may help to slow the bleeding process. Tourniquet and hemostat application are controversial and are not used.

6. The application of a pneumatic antishock garment (PASG) has limited value in the pediatric population. Their use in children is generally limited to inflation of a leg compartment for splinting of a femur fracture.

7. Traumatic arrest (empty heart syndrome) is treated with cardiopulmonary resuscitation and rapid infusion of warmed crystalloid and blood products. Thoracotomy and open cardiac massage are rarely performed for blunt trauma and are usually a last-chance effort to resuscitate the child. Prognosis is poor. In one study of 12 critically injured children who received closed cardiac massage

and 15 critically injured children who received open cardiac massage, none of the children regained consciousness or survived, indicating that open cardiac massage does not improve survival in those children who receive prehospital CPR for more than 20 minutes (Sheikh and Brogan, 1994).

D. DISABILITY AND NEUROLOGIC CHECKS

1. Frequent neurologic checks are performed to observe for changes in level of consciousness, motor, and sensory function. The pediatric GCS score is helpful to document serial neurologic assessments. Changes in the child's level of consciousness may indicate hypovolemia or increased ICP. Vomiting and irritability are early signs of increased ICP. In infants, a bulging fontanelle is a *late* sign of increased ICP.

2. Normoventilation with 100% oxygen is initiated in the child with a severe head injury to keep the $PaCO_2$ at approximately 35 mm Hg. Hyperventilation is initiated to achieve a $PaCO_2$ of approximately 30 mm Hg if signs of a lesion (i.e., epidural) or rapid decompensation are present. A $PaCO_2$ of ≤28 mm Hg may contribute to brain ischemia.

3. Procedures and treatments are explained to the child at a level he or she can understand. Words of praise and comfort go far to help reassure the frightened, injured child.

E. EXPOSE

1. Passive and active warming measures are initiated to prevent conductive and convective heat loss. Passive warming measures include warm blankets and increased ambient room temperature. Active warming measures include the administration of normothermic IV fluids and blood products to help with core warming.

2. Temperature measurements are obtained via the oral, rectal, or tympanic routes. Temperature probes on endotracheal tubes, esophageal probes, or urinary bladder thermistors are other options for temperature measurement.

F. GASTROINTESTINAL (GI) AND GENITOURINARY (GU) TRACTS

1. An orogastric or nasogastric tube should be inserted to prevent gastric distention, vomiting, and aspiration. Initial drainage can be tested for the presence of blood. Gastric contrast can be administered through the gastric tube prior to computed tomography (CT) testing.

2. In the absence of trauma or blood at the urinary meatus or suspected urethral trauma, an indwelling bladder catheter may be inserted and connected to a urinary drainage bag. If urethral trauma is suspected, a retrograde urethrogram must be performed prior to indwelling bladder catheter insertion. Urine should be sent for a urinalysis; urine toxicology testing is indicated when drug or alcohol use is suspected. In postmenarchal females, urinary chorionic gonadotropin (UCG) testing should be done.

3. A stool smear should be tested for occult blood.

G. MUSCULOSKELETAL

1. All long bone fractures are immobilized. The child's neurovascular status is assessed immediately before and after splinting to assure that an injury has not occurred or been aggravated. Open fractures, lacerations, or wounds require careful evaluation and cleaning. Amputated body parts are wrapped in dry or moistened gauze, sealed in a plastic bag, and then placed in an ice water bath. At no time must the amputated part touch the ice directly, as tissue necrosis may occur. The child's amputated parts are evaluated by subspecialists (i.e., plastic surgery, reimplantation specialists) to determine if reattachment is possible. Whether the child and family view the amputated part or injured limb is decided on an individual basis. Younger children may become frightened of the wound, whereas older children may be curious, as their imagined injury may be

worse than the reality. Tetanus prophylaxis, antibiotics, and analgesic administration are necessary.

ADDITIONAL INTERVENTIONS

A. DIAGNOSTIC TESTING
   1. During any intrahospital transport, the child is attended to by an experienced nurse and physician. Appropriate resuscitation equipment is taken during the transport should the child's condition deteriorate.
   2. Chest radiographs are obtained to determine the placement of endotracheal, gastric, and chest tubes. These films also confirm the presence of pneumothoraces or hemopneumothoraces, rib and clavicle fractures, and diaphragm integrity. Abdominal radiographs confirm the placement of gastric tubes and bladder catheters; stomach and intestine intactness can be observed as well. Free air is noted, and the pelvis is examined for fracture. Skeletal radiographs are obtained according to the suspected injury. Radiographs are obtained in the trauma room with portable x-ray equipment or in the radiology suite. The child's primary nurse should remain with the child during these studies to explain procedures and monitor the child's condition.
   3. CT scanning is undertaken in children with significant head, face, chest, or abdominal trauma. Xenon testing may be indicated in children with severe head injury. Xenon testing allows for the determination of cerebral oxygenation. Angiography may be obtained for suspected severe vessel injury from blunt or penetrating trauma.
   4. Peritoneal lavage is rarely performed to diagnose hemorrhage or visceral perforation in the pediatric population, as CT scanning is the procedure of choice (Donnellan, 1990). Peritoneal lavage may be indicated when a multiply injured child requires immediate operative intervention (e.g., head injury), when CT scan is unavailable, or when CT scan findings are normal but a hollow viscus (bowel) injury is presumed (Nichols et al, 1991).

B. PAIN MANAGEMENT
   1. The child's pain is assessed through age-appropriate pain assessment scales and verbal communication. The conscious, verbal child may be asked if he or she hurts or has pain. For the preverbal or nonverbal child, observations of the child's behavior may indicate the presence of pain. Behaviors associated with pain include facial grimacing, guarding, lying still, or resisting movement. Physiologic responses to pain include increased heart rate, increased respiratory rate, increased blood pressure, and increased perspiration. These measures are not specific for pain and may vary among children (Acute Pain Management Guideline Panel, 1992); therefore, they should be used in combination with pain assessment scales and behavioral observations.
   2. Pharmacologic management of pain is not usually initiated in the child with a head injury or severe injuries leading to shock. When invasive procedures, such as chest tube insertion, are undertaken, local anesthesia should be administered. Pharmacologic management of pain includes the use of narcotic and nonnarcotic analgesics.
   3. There are a variety of nonpharmacologic techniques for pain and anxiety ablation and control. Distraction techniques, progressive relaxation, positive self-talk, holding a nurse's hand, holding a stuffed animal or blanket, and storytelling are possibilities.

C. EMOTIONAL SUPPORT
   1. The injured child experiences many painful and frightening events before, during, and after the injury's occurrence. Children have fears of parental

separation, pain, disfigurement, and mutilation. It is a nursing responsibility to provide comfort and emotional support to the child during this time of crisis.

2. The assignment of a primary nurse to the patient helps the child focus on one person. Speaking in a calm, reassuring voice may help the child to gain composure. For the child who receives spinal immobilization, standing at the child's side near the chest level allows the child to see the nurse without attempting to move the head sideways; standing over the child's head may be frightening and intimidating. Holding the child's hand, stroking the hair, and talking calmly and confidently help the child to gain trust.

3. The awake or unconscious child should receive age-appropriate explanations for procedures. The truth is told about any pain or discomfort that may occur. Coping measures for painful procedures include deep breathing, guided imagery, counting, singing, or other activities. Allowing the child to wiggle a hand or foot gives the child some sense of control. Child life specialists may be able to enhance the child's repertoire of coping skills during procedures.

4. The parents or family members should be permitted to see the child as soon as possible. The nurse can explain to the family what they will see, hear, and smell on entering the child's room. Explain the present plans for the child's treatment to the family in language they can understand. Encourage the family to touch the child and to ask questions. Having a social worker, religious counselor, or other support person may be welcomed by the family. Parental presence during resuscitation is advocated, along with the proper support and understanding that goes with this type of intervention (Emergency Nurses Association, 1994).

SPECIFIC INJURIES

The specific body system injuries are briefly addressed in this section. Detailed discussions are found in previous chapters of this book.

A. HEAD INJURIES

1. Head injury usually results from blunt force inflicted during motor vehicle crashes, bicycle crashes, falls, or child maltreatment. Mild (GCS 13 to 15) to moderate (GCS 9 to 12) head injuries are more common than severe (GCS ≤8) head injuries and account for 90% of hospital admissions, whereas severe head injuries account for approximately 5% of admissions (Goldstein and Powers, 1994). Children with severe head injuries typically require admission to the ICU for management of increased ICP (see Chapter 4).

2. Signs of a **mild-to-moderate head injury** include persistent vomiting, posttraumatic seizure, and loss of consciousness. Most often, children with mild-to-moderate head injuries are hospitalized if they have any neurologic deficits, seizures or vomiting, a severe headache, fever, prolonged loss of consciousness, skull fracture, altered level of consciousness, or suspected child maltreatment (Ward, 1995). The evaluation of children with mild-to-moderate head injuries include serial neurologic evaluations with measurement of level of consciousness, pupillary response, motor and sensory response, and vital signs. Changes in the child's level of consciousness indicate increasing ICP, and treatment must be initiated to prevent subsequent deterioration and possible brain stem herniation. A CT scan without contrast may be performed to identify specific drainable blood collection, intraparenchymal injuries, and signs of increased ICP evidenced by compressed ventricles.

3. Signs of a **severe head injury** include a decreased level of consciousness, posturing, combative behavior, and abnormal neurologic findings. Children with severe head injuries require airway and ventilatory control, with a rapid

neurologic assessment performed prior to the administration of paralytic and sedative agents. The child's $Paco_2$ is kept at approximately 35 mm Hg for adequate cerebral blood flow. A $Paco_2$ of 28 or less may result in cerebral ischemia. The Sao_2 is kept at ≥95%, with the mean arterial pressure (MAP) at slightly higher than age-appropriate norms. IV crystalloid fluids are administered at maintenance rate. IV administration of mannitol (1 g/kg) removes fluid from the interstitial spaces. Mannitol is administered for signs of acute increases in ICP or for increased pressure with ICP at various infusion rates ranging from 0.25 to 1 g/kg. Phenobarbital or phenytoin may be administered to prevent seizures. A CT scan without contrast is performed to determine the extent of the injury, followed by operative management as indicated.

B. MAXILLOFACIAL INJURIES

1. Children sustain maxillofacial injuries from blunt forces, such as pedestrian, motor vehicle crash, or bicycle injuries. Maxillofacial injuries include trauma to the dentition, mandible, and midface. Maxillofacial injuries are suspected in children who sustain blunt or penetrating forces to the face. The face is observed for bruising, lacerations, open wounds, and impaled objects. The awake child is asked to open and close the mouth; if the child is unable to do so or malocclusion is present, mandibular fracture is suspected. The face is observed for symmetry, and the cranial nerves are assessed for intactness. The nose is palpated for tenderness and observed for bruising, and the nares are observed for bleeding or blood clots. The face is palpated for "step-offs," tenderness, and pain. The maxilla is palpated between two gloved fingers for continuity. Loose and missing teeth are noted, as well as the presence of orthodontic appliances or false teeth. Anteroposterior, open mouth, panorex radiographs, and CT scanning may be obtained in the stable child to determine the extent and location of facial injuries.

2. Dental injuries occur from direct forces to the face. In very young children, only the temporary (primary) teeth may be involved; however, if the injury displaces or avulses the temporary dentition, the underlying follicles (location of the developing permanent teeth) may be involved (Chase, 1995). The most serious damage to teeth occurs in the permanent teeth that have a partially developed root (Chase, 1995).

3. There are four methods for preserving an avulsed permanent tooth (Chase, 1995). The tooth should be replaced immediately into its socket provided the child is awake, alert, and old enough to understand what is required. If the tooth is not able to be replaced into its socket, it can be placed under the child's tongue, again provided the child is conscious, alert, and old enough to understand what to do. The next option is to place the tooth in a small container with milk; if milk is not available, a cup of water is sufficient. The container is labeled with the child's name, date, and time. The tooth is not cleaned or debrided and is held by its crown; it should be reimplanted within 1 hour. The socket is not cleaned but is left intact. Treatment involves splinting of the teeth.

4. Mandibular fractures are classified according to their location: condylar, angle, symphysis, dentoalveolar, and body fracture. Intermaxillary fixation is an option for fractures of the mandibular condyles, whereas open reduction and internal fixation of angle and body fractures are conducted (Chase, 1995). Antibiotics are administered to prevent infection. Scrupulous attention to airway management and oral hygiene are imperative. Children may have concerns about their inability to talk, and alternative methods for communication are required. The older child and adolescent may have concerns about his or her appearance and should be reassured that any bruising and edema will subside over time.

5. Midfacial fractures are classified using the Le Fort categories. A Le Fort I fracture is horizontal across the maxilla above the alveolar process and horizontal plate of the palatine and palatal process of the maxilla. The Le Fort II fracture involves the orbital floors, lamina papyracea of the ethmoid bone, and separation of the frontal nasal suture. A Le Fort III fracture involves craniofacial disarticulation where the facial bones are separated from the cranial buttress systems (Chase, 1995). Le Fort fractures are treated with internal fixation.

6. Nasal fractures occur in the bony pyramid, cartilaginous nasal vault, the septum, or all three. A pediatric speculum is inserted into the naris to observe for a septal hematoma; if not detected early, such a hematoma may lead to an abscess and destruction of the nasal cartilage. Treatment may be immediate or delayed, depending on the child's condition. Treatment includes a closed reduction while the young child receives general anesthesia, whereas a topical cocaine application and local anesthetic with IV sedation may be adequate for older children (Gussack and Simpson, 1995).

C. SPINAL CORD INJURIES

1. Spinal cord injuries are relatively uncommon in young children. When they do occur, the outcomes are permanent and devastating. The laxity of the juvenile spine allows spinal cord injury without bony abnormalities to occur, a phenomenon known as *spinal cord injury without radiographic abnormalities* (SCIWORA; Pang and Pollack, 1989; Pang and Wilberger, 1982). It is estimated that there is a 35% incidence of SCIWORA in children with traumatic myelopathy (Pollack and Pang, 1995). In SCIWORA, transient displacement of the cerebral column during flexion-extension or acceleration-deceleration forces occurs (Pollack and Pang, 1995). During a hyperflexion or hyperextension episode, the spinal cord stretches, leading to injury or transection. The spinal cord and vertebrae then return to their normal length and alignment, respectively. The child displays signs of spinal cord injury, but radiographs show no evidence of bony abnormality. SCIWORA injuries occur most often at the cervical level, but thoracic SCIWORA is also possible. Younger children (<8 years of age) tend to have high cervical cord SCIWORA with a subsequent higher severity of injury as compared to older children (Pollack and Pang, 1995). Among seven children diagnosed with SCIWORA who received magnetic resonance imaging (MRI) testing, ligamental and disc injuries and cord disruption were found. These findings demonstrate that self-reducing transient subluxation or distraction is the cause of the neurologic injury (Grabb and Pang, 1994). These MRI findings of abnormalities such as major cord hemorrhage, were consistent with permanent, complete cord injuries; likewise, normal MRI spinal cord findings were associated with complete neurologic recovery (Grabb and Pang, 1994). (See Chapter 4.)

2. Spinal injuries are always suspected in multiply injured children. Complete spinal immobilization is maintained until it is clinically determined that a spinal cord injury is not present. Children with high spinal cord injuries must receive airway control and mechanical ventilation, and children with lower cervical injuries are closely observed for worsening of their respiratory status. Children with high spinal cord lesions may require more IV fluid than children with lower spinal cord lesions, as spinal shock causes peripheral vasodilation (warm shock) and relative hypovolemia. Therefore, at minimum, normal maintenance infusion rates are required. The infusion of vasopressors, such as dopamine or phenylephrine (Neo-Synephrine), may also be indicated. High-dose methylprednisolone (30 mg/kg) is administered early in treatment (within 6 to 8 hours of the injury) to be effective. Lateral, anteroposterior, and odontoid radiographs of the cervical spine are obtained, and anteroposterior and lateral

views of the thoracic and lumbar spine are obtained as indicated. Flexion-extension radiographs to determine for stability of the bony canal are not performed until it is determined that spinal cord injury is not present. Such flexion-extension tests may be performed in SCIWORA injury once additional diagnostic testing is completed. Serial neurologic assessments are performed to determine if the injury is worsening.

3. Unconscious, multiply injured children remain in complete spinal immobilization until they are awake and able to complete a neurologic examination. Additional diagnostic tests, such as somatosensory evoked potentials (SSEPs), may be indicated to determine the presence or extent of the spinal cord injury. Operative management for bony spinal stabilization or other vertebral repair may be indicated in children with vertebral fractures or dislocations.

D. THORACIC INJURIES

1. Thoracic injuries in infants and young children usually result from blunt force trauma due to falls. Older children usually sustain thoracic injuries in motor vehicle crashes as pedestrians or passengers (Reynolds, 1995). Penetrating chest trauma occurs more often in adolescents from violence.

2. Common thoracic injuries and their symptoms and treatments are outlined in Table 9–7. (See Chapter 2.)

E. ABDOMINAL INJURIES

1. Blunt forces are the most common cause of abdominal trauma in children, with subsequent hemorrhaging a cause for traumatic death. The compactness of the abdominal contents allows kinetic forces to be transmitted to multiple organs. The most commonly injured organ is the spleen, followed by the liver (Schafermeyer, 1993). Injuries also occur to the pancreas and intestinal tract (see Chapter 7).

2. Signs of abdominal trauma include tenderness on palpation and abdominal distention, abrasions, or contusions. Hypovolemic shock may be observed if internal hemorrhaging is present. The absence of bowel sounds does not confirm an abdominal injury, as an ileus can occur as a result of the child crying, swallowing air, or being frightened (Tepas, 1987). Although elevations in liver function test (LFT) results may be noted with liver injuries, such elevations are not specific to the liver trauma. Tenderness in the left upper quadrant may be associated with a splenic injury. Pain in the left shoulder may be elicited on abdominal palpation or deep breathing (Kehr's sign). Elevation of serum amylase and lipase levels indicate a possible pancreatic injury, and a tender mass in the epigastric region may also be palpated (Tepas, 1987). Free air may be noted on radiographs when injuries occur to the GI tract, whereas CT scan identifies specific injuries to each solid abdominal organ.

3. Most, if not all, gunshot wounds to the abdomen require surgical exploration, whereas many stab wounds to the abdomen may be selectively (i.e., observed) managed if the surgeon determines the knife has not penetrated into the abdominal cavity. CT scanning with contrast is indicated in the stable child sustaining blunt abdominal trauma. This diagnostic method is preferred over peritoneal lavage because of its accuracy in detecting the location and extent of abdominal injuries. Such children receive serial hemoglobin and hematocrit testing to determine if internal bleeding is present. Nursing care involves maintaining IV infusions, an NPO status, and close evaluation of level of consciousness, circulatory status, and abdominal findings (abdominal girth, presence of pain, tenderness, bruising). Although conservative, nonoperative management is usually indicated for most blunt injuries, a surgical approach is indicated if hemorrhaging or peritonitis are suspected.

Table 9–7. CLINICAL MANIFESTATIONS AND TREATMENT OF THORACIC INJURIES

CONDITION	CLINICAL MANIFESTATIONS	TREATMENT
Rib fractures	Pain Crepitus Bruising	Medicate for pain; splinting
Closed pneumothorax	Dyspnea Tachypnea Decreased or absent breath sounds on the affected side Pain Dullness with percussion	Needle thoracostomy; insertion of chest tube
Open pneumothorax	Sucking noise on inspiration Bubbling noise on expiration Dyspnea Tachypnea	Application of an occlusive dressing, taped on three sides
Tension pneumothorax	Dyspnea Jugular vein distention Decreased or absent breath sounds on the affected side Tracheal deviation away from the affected side Decreased or absent chest wall movement Hyperresonance with percussion Possible mediastinal shift away from the affected side	Needle thoracostomy; insertion of a chest tube
Hemothorax	Dyspnea Tachypnea Tachycardia Pallor Restlessness Hypotension Dullness with percussion Decreased or absent breath sounds	Insertion of a chest tube Fluid resuscitation
Pulmonary contusion	Dyspnea	Oxygenation Ventilation
Cardiac contusion	Tachycardia Dysrhythmias Chest pain	Oxygenation Fluid administration Cardiac monitoring
Tracheobronchial rupture	Crepitus Subcutaneous emphysema Pneumomediastinum Pneumopericardium	Intubation Ventilation
Pericardial tamponade	Beck's triad (muffled heart tones, decreased arterial pressure, elevated venous pressure) Agitation Decreased peripheral perfusion Pulsus paradoxus Jugular vein distention	Ventilation Pericardiocentesis Fluid resuscitation Cardiac monitoring Thoracotomy

From Bernardo LM, Trunzo R. Pediatric trauma. In: Kitt S, Selfridge-Thomas J, Proehl J, Kaiser J, eds. *Emergency Nursing: A Physiologic and Clinical Perspective.* 2nd ed. Philadelphia, Pa: WB Saunders Co; 1995:428–454.

4. The unstable child who does not respond to fluid resuscitation is prepared for transfer to the operating room for operative management.

F. **GENITOURINARY (GU) TRACT INJURIES**

1. GU tract injuries usually result from blunt force trauma (Hoover and Belinger, 1987); however, the incidence of penetrating trauma is on the rise. (See Chapter 5.)

2. Injuries to the female genitalia occur from falls, straddle injuries, and sexual abuse or assault. Since these injuries are not easily observed in the emergency department, they require EUA in the operating room (Lynch et al, 1995). Testicular trauma results from straddle-type injuries. The majority of testicular injuries occur in adolescents who are struck in the scrotum while playing sports or during an altercation (Corriere, 1994). Testicular fractures can be diagnosed with ultrasound and are then repaired. Direct forces are the most common causes of penile injuries (i.e., zipper injuries and toilet seat trauma).

3. The child's GU tract system is more vulnerable to certain injuries as compared to the adult's. Children's kidneys are larger and have less perinephric fat. The rib cage affords less protection to the kidneys. Preexisting abnormalities (i.e., Wilms' tumor, ectopic kidneys, and hydronephrosis) can predispose a kidney to injury. Ureteral elasticity and torso mobility allow for ureteral injuries to occur. The bladder is an abdominal organ in the younger child and less protected when full. A full bladder can rupture between the seat belt and vertebral column as a result of a deceleration injury (Corriere, 1994). The bladder neck, especially in girls, is less protected. Boys are more vulnerable to urethral injuries as a result of the length and position of the urethra (Hoover and Belinger, 1987). The tissues of prepubescent girls are smaller and considerably more rigid than those of the adolescent or adult, thus increasing the risk of tearing with either blunt or penetrating trauma. Prepubescent girls also have a thin vesicovaginal septal wall.

4. Symptoms of renal trauma include abdominal, back, or flank tenderness, while physical signs include localized abrasions, bruises, lacerations, and hematuria. The degree of hematuria does not correlate with the degree of injury, as minor or no hematuria may occur in serious injuries such as a renal pedicle or parenchymal injury, and gross hematuria may result from a minor renal injury (Corriere, 1994). Renal injury should be suspected when the lower ribs are fractured. Severe GU tract hemorrhaging can lead to hypovolemic shock.

5. Urinalysis evaluation is performed to determine the presence of hematuria. The awake, stable child may be able to void spontaneously. The unstable child may require an indwelling bladder catheter for evaluation and output measurement, unless catheterization is contraindicated. Urinary catheterization in boys younger than 5 years of age may be harmful and should be avoided if at all possible (Lobe et al, 1995). A retrograde urethral contrast study should be performed prior to catheterization in suspected urethral injuries (Hoover and Belinger, 1987).

6. Treatment is specific for the location and extent of injury, ranging from observation and bed rest to surgical exploration.

G. **MUSCULOSKELETAL INJURIES**

1. Musculoskeletal injuries commonly occur in children and include open and closed fractures, dislocations, nerve injuries, tendon injuries, and amputations. Growing bones are porous, and the periosteum is strong and thick. These features lead to partial fracturing of the bone, such as greenstick fractures, as compared to complete fractures. Although the thicker periosteum allows for quicker fracture healing, it may impede fracture reduction (Olney and Toby, 1995). The ligaments are strong, allowing for the higher occurrence of

fractures vs. ligamentous injury. Children have an epiphyseal growth plate (physis) located at the articulating ends of the bones between the epiphysis and metaphysis (Phelan, 1994). The physis is responsible for longitudinal bone growth, and injury to the growth plate may result in growth disturbance or arrest. Growth generally is completed in boys by 16 years of age and in girls by 14 years of age. Children sustaining injuries near the physis require follow-up to detect limb length discrepancies and angular deformities (Olney and Toby, 1995). Nerve and tendon injuries occur from crushing forces, such as wringers, lawn mowers, or farm equipment. Amputations occur from knives, bicycle spokes, and crushing injuries from lawn mowers, farm equipment, motor vehicles, and power boats.

2. **Musculoskeletal trauma** is suspected in the child with point tenderness, soft tissue swelling, discoloration, limitations in range of motion, loss of function, altered sensory perception, and changes in pulses, temperature, or capillary refill distal to the injury (Phelan, 1994). Musculoskeletal trauma is rarely life threatening, so the priorities of airway, breathing, and circulation are addressed prior to treating any fractures. Neurovascular status is assessed before and after any intervention such as splinting, swathing, or dressing. Analgesics should be administered. Radiographs include the joint above and below the injury and comparative views (radiographs of the injured and uninjured extremities).

3. Most fractures are simple and nondisplaced, only requiring the application of a cast. A schematic representation of fractures is found in Figure 9–1. The casted extremity is assessed for swelling of the toes or fingers, odor from the cast, and changes in skin color and temperature. Should the child complain of sharp pain or numbness, compartment syndrome should be suspected.

   a. *Nondisplaced fractures* may be too edematous to allow for casting. In such cases a splint is applied, and the cast is applied later when the swelling has resolved. *Displaced fractures* may require a closed reduction, where the orthopedic specialist and nurse apply manual traction-countertraction to realign the fractured bone. Conscious sedation is administered, using intravenous analgesics and sedatives such as midazolam, fentanyl, or ketamine. Once the fracture is reduced, the medications are stopped, the cast is applied, and postreduction radiographs are obtained. If the closed reduction was not successful, an open reduction and internal fixation is required.

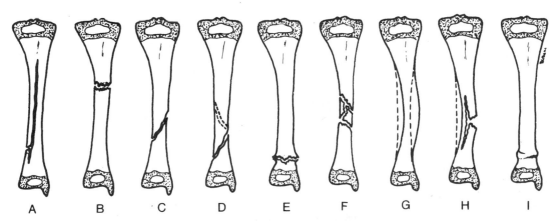

Figure 9–1. Schematic of tibia of a 3-year-old child showing types of fractures. **A,** Longitudinal. **B,** Transverse. **C,** Oblique. **D,** Spiral. **E,** Impacted. **F,** Comminuted. **G,** Bending, bowing. **H,** Greenstick. **I,** Cortical, torus. (Reprinted with permission from Ogden JA. *Skeletal Injury in the Child.* 2nd ed. Philadelphia, Pa: WB Saunders Co; 1990:7.)

b. Open fractures are divided into three types. *Type I open fractures* are less than 1 cm in length, are usually a clean puncture with little soft tissue involvement (Olney and Toby, 1995), and can be treated with casting, provided a window is cut into the cast to allow for wound visualization and dressing changes. *Type II open fractures* have a laceration greater than 1 cm with slight or moderate crushing and no extensive soft tissue damage (Olney and Toby, 1995). *Type III injuries* have extensive damage to soft tissues, muscle, skin, and neurovascular structures; contamination is present (Olney and Toby, 1995). Antibiotics are administered intravenously; they are also irrigated into the wound. Sterile dressings are applied to open fractures, and tetanus prophylaxis is administered. Debridement is continued every 24 to 48 hours until the wound is clean (Olney and Toby, 1995). Type II and III injuries may be treated with external fixation.

c. *Physeal fractures* are described using the Salter-Harris classification and are outlined in Table 9–8. Open fractures that involve the growth plate may be treated with smooth K-wires in addition to external fixation (Olney and Toby, 1995).

d. *Elbow fractures* occur in children, with the supracondylar fractures being the most common. If not assessed rapidly and treated properly, complications can result. A complete neurovascular assessment is performed, along with Doppler examination of the arterial blood supply. Unfortunately, Volkmann's ischemia and compartment syndrome can occur with supra-

Table 9–8. SALTER-HARRIS CLASSIFICATION, FRACTURE DESCRIPTIONS, AND OUTCOME

	DESCRIPTION OF FRACTURES	TREATMENT AND OUTCOME
Type I	Horizontal separation of epiphysis and metaphysis; point tenderness; radiographs may be normal; mild soft tissue swelling produced by shearing forces	No disturbance in growth if properly diagnosed; favorable prognosis; treated with closed reduction and casting
Type II	Separation of epiphysis and metaphysis with some avulsion of the metaphysis produced by shearing forces	No disturbance in growth if properly diagnosed; favorable prognosis; treated with closed reduction and casting
Type III	Produced by intraarticular shearing forces; intra-articular fracture; fracture extends through the epiphyseal plate into the metaphysis	Angular deformities may occur; requires good reduction; variable or poor prognosis
Type IV	Fracture starts at the articular surface and extends through the epiphysis, epiphyseal plate, and metaphysis; intraarticular fracture produced by shearing forces	Open reduction and external fixation is needed; variable poor prognosis; angular deformity may result
Type V	Epiphyseal plate is crushed without physeal fracture or displacement; radiographic diagnosis virtually impossible, produced by crushing forces	Poor prognosis, even when correctly identified and treated

Bernardo LM, Trunzo R. Pediatric trauma. In: Kitt S, Selfridge-Thomas J, Proehl J, Kaiser J, eds. *Emergency Nursing: A Physiologic and Clinical Perspective.* 2nd ed. Philadelphia, Pa: WB Saunders Co; 1995:428–454.

condylar fractures. Operative management for a closed reduction is undertaken. Skeletal or skin traction can be implemented, and closed reduction and percutaneous pinning are options as well (Olney and Toby, 1995). Careful ongoing evaluation of the child's neurovascular status is imperative. If the injured arm is the child's dominant one, the child must learn to use the nondominant arm. This learning requires patience, as the child may become frustrated. The prolonged immobilization also plays havoc on the child's development and temperament, and opportunities for creative release of energy are necessary.

e. *Femoral fractures* are common, with approximately 70% occurring in the midshaft area (Olney and Toby, 1995). The injured thigh is swollen, firm, and shortened in length and may be bruised. The child is unable to move the leg and complains of pain. An anteroposterior radiograph is obtained. Treatment varies according to the child's age. Hip spica casts are applied in infants and toddlers, an intervention that may be performed in the ICU. Most children aged 2 years through 10 years also benefit from the hip spica (Olney and Toby, 1995). Spica casting is contraindicated in these children if the shortening is 2 to 3 cm and if there are multiple injuries (Olney and Toby, 1995). In cases of shortening, skeletal or skin traction is indicated until early callus formation is observed on radiographs; in multiple injuries, open reduction and external fixation is the treatment of choice (Olney and Toby, 1995). Children older than 11 years of age may receive internal fixation or intermedullary fixation. When skeletal traction is used, pin care is performed on a routine schedule to avoid infection. Signs of pin infection include tenting of the insertion site, redness, and drainage.

f. Children with *pelvic fractures* require bed rest. Unstable pelvic fractures may require the application of an external fixation device, or in rare cases, internal fixation may be required. Again, the psychologic effects of immobility must be addressed, and options for movement must be given.

4. **Nerve injury** is suspected in any crushing trauma. Open wounds near the anatomic location for peripheral nerves should be an indication for nerve involvement (Olney and Toby, 1995). Sensory loss is difficult to ascertain in young children; however, there are two tests that can be administered to determine nerve damage. The first test is to observe for a lack of sweating in the affected area using an iodine starch test or a Ninhydrin print test. The second test is the wrinkle test, where the extremity is placed in warm water; if the skin wrinkles, the nerve is intact (Olney and Toby, 1995). Nerve injuries are graded from I to V, with grades I through II having the best chances for full recovery. Peripheral nerve injuries tend to heal better in children than in adults; it is believed that the child's brain plasticity assists in nerve regeneration. Children seem to need less formal sensory reeducation following peripheral nerve repair than adults, which may be due to their natural curiosity. The shorter distances required by axons to regenerate before reaching their end-organ may also enhance nerve recovery (Olney and Toby, 1995).

5. **Amputated digits or extremities** require reimplantation. Such microsurgical techniques are highly specialized and may only be available at level I trauma centers. Prior to reimplantation, the child's health condition and the condition of the digit or limb must be carefully evaluated. For example, severe crushing injuries and excessive warm ischemia for more than 6 hours are contraindications for reimplantation (Olney and Toby, 1995). Amputated digits and limbs are carefully wrapped in sterile gauze moistened with NS and placed in a cup or container. The cup or container is then placed in an ice water bath. The cup is labeled with the child's name, date, and time. An amputated digit cooled

according to the aforementioned method can be replanted up to 24 hours after the injury (Olney and Toby, 1995). The attached body area is assessed for bleeding and neurovascular integrity. The amputated area is carefully wrapped in sterile dressings, and care should be taken to shield the young child's view from the injury. The success of the reimplantation is related to the child's health condition and the viability of the tissues. If the reimplantation is not viable, the child may require prosthesis and subsequent rehabilitation. Even with viable repairs, rehabilitation may still be required. The child and family should be prepared for the possibility of permanent loss and counseled accordingly.

6. **Tendon injuries** also occur with crush or open injuries, usually in the forearm and hand. The child may not be able to move or wiggle the fingers or may refuse to do so because of pain and discomfort. Operative management is necessary to repair tendons. Following tendon repair, the area is assessed for function and neurovascular status; passive flexion exercises are performed with the parents or therapist (Olney and Toby, 1995).

7. **Compartment syndrome** occurs when external (e.g., tight ace wrap, tight cast) or internal (e.g., blood, edema) pressure is applied to a muscle. As this pressure increases, the vasculature is impaired; ischemia to the extremity occurs and leads to nerve and circulatory damage. Assessment of the five *P*s (*p*ain, *p*allor, *p*ulselessness, *p*aralysis, and *p*aresthesia) is ongoing and essential. Compartmental pressures can be measured, but obtaining such pressures should not delay operative management. Treatment of compartment syndrome includes a fasciotomy, and the area is not closed but covered with a sterile dressing (Soud et al, 1992). Such dressings are changed routinely, and analgesics may be administered. Ongoing evaluation of neurovascular and motor function is essential for detecting and preventing compartmental syndrome.

H. CHILD MALTREATMENT

1. **Etiology and incidence**
   a. Child maltreatment consists of child physical abuse, sexual abuse, neglect, and emotional abuse. In 1992, more than three children died from child maltreatment daily in the United States. Of these deaths, 87% occurred in children younger than 5 years of age (Hymel, 1994).
   b. Child abuse reports have increased on average 6% annually over the past 7 years (Hymel, 1994). Parental, child, and societal factors are associated with child maltreatment. Parental factors include using corporal punishment for discipline, history of maltreatment as a child, low self-esteem, social isolation, lack of child development knowledge, unrealistic expectations for the child, depression, substance abuse, marital unrest and violence, and perhaps membership in a fringe group, cult, or sect (Davis and Zitelli, 1995; Hymel, 1994; Kelley, 1994a). Risk factors are young age (younger than 3 years), prematurity, multiple births, any special needs, prenatal drug exposure, single mother with transient paramours, or any temperament or other personality factors the parent perceives to be different or difficult (Davis and Zitelli, 1995; Hymel, 1994; Kelley, 1994a). Societal factors include poverty, unemployment, and other stressors; however, maltreatment can occur in all socioeconomic strata.
   c. Reporting of suspected child maltreatment by nurses and health care professionals is mandated by law. Critical care nurses who suspect child maltreatment are required to report their suspicions to their local child abuse hotline. Reporting is made in good faith, and follow-up by the local child welfare agency is required within a specified time period. No litigation can be brought against a nurse for filing a suspected child maltreatment report in good faith.

2. **History of the injury**
   a. Child physical abuse is suspected based on the physical findings and the history surrounding the injury. The physical findings speak for themselves. The history, however, is what differentiates intentional from unintentional injury.
   b. The history of the injury is elicited first by the nurse. Characteristics of the history that are consistent with child abuse include the following: the history is inconsistent with the injury; the caretaker denies any knowledge of how the injury occurred; the caretaker is reluctant to divulge information or changes the story; the child is developmentally incapable of the injury; there is a delay in seeking treatment; the child has prior hospitalizations or injuries; the caretaker's response is inappropriate to the level of injury; and there is a history of previous placement in foster care or with a child protective agency (Davis and Zitelli, 1995; Kelley, 1994a). All communication is documented using the child's and caretaker's own words.
   c. *Physical abuse* occurs from excessive force applied to the child from an adult caretaker. The abuse is manifested in cutaneous lesions (bruises, bite marks, burns), internal organ injuries, long bone fractures, and head trauma.

3. **Cutaneous Injuries**
   a. *Bruises* commonly occur in young children as they run and play. Normally, bruises are small, few in number, and found on the extensor surfaces, such as the shins, elbows, chin, and knees. Bruises indicative of physical abuse are found on the face and head. Black eyes are especially suspicious for maltreatment if they are bilateral or attributed to falls when other signs of trauma to the nose or superior orbital ridge are absent (Richardson, 1994). Bruises found on the chest, abdomen, thighs, buttocks, and back are also suspicious for physical abuse. These bruises are usually in various stages of healing and are numerous. Bruises that have the appearance of an object, such as a belt buckle, hand imprint, or looped electrical cord, are always treated as abuse.
      • In infants, bruises may be seen near the mouth, lips, and frenulum, when the caretaker repeatedly attempts to force feed a bottle into the infant's mouth. Bruises or rope burns may be found around the neck, wrists, or ankles and indicate that the child was restrained. Blistering and abrasions may be present, which may indicate the child's struggle against the restraints. The restraints can be made of rope, cloth, strap, or chain (Richardson, 1994). In infants and young children, paired oval bruises or pinch marks may be found on the cheeks, arms, earlobes, and other areas (Hymel, 1994).
      • School-age children who have repeatedly been subjected to beatings and bruising prefer to wear long-sleeved and long-legged clothing, even in warm weather, to hide the marks.
      • Any bruises must be evaluated in light of the plausibility of the injury event as stated by the caretaker, the child's past health history, the child's level of development, the presence of other injuries, and laboratory data (Richardson, 1994).
   b. *Bite marks* are highly indicative of child abuse. Adult bite marks are differentiated from child bite marks by measuring the maxillary intercanine distance; a distance greater than 3 cm indicates that an adult bit the child (Hymel, 1994).
   c. *Burns* occur from scalding liquids and contact with hot objects. Flame burns can be implicated in child abuse, such as in arson. An unintentional scald

burn can occur if the young child pulls a crock pot or pot of hot liquid onto himself or herself. The intensity of the burn would be greatest about the head, with the depth of burn tapering off as it reaches the chest. An intentional scald injury has a circumscribed area of injury that is full thickness.

- In young children who may have soiled themselves during toilet training, the caretaker may dunk the child's buttocks into a tub of hot water. The resulting scald injury is isolated to the perineum and buttocks. A donut-shaped scarring to the buttocks may be present if the child's buttocks were held against the tub itself. In contrast, a child who inadvertently fell into a tub would have burns about the head or side of the body.
- A curious child may suffer an unintentional hand burn by submerging the hand into a bucket of water. The resulting burn would be irregular, partial thickness in depth, and circumferential, as the pain response causes the child to quickly withdraw the hand. In the child who suffers an intentional burn, the caretaker holds the child's hands or feet in hot water. The resultant burn is circumferential, full thickness, and has a clear line of demarcation at the wrists or ankles. The flexion creases are spared from the burn.
- An unintentional contact burn can result when a young child bumps against a hot iron, holds a curling iron, or touches a kerosene heater. The resulting burn is irregular in shape and partial thickness in depth. An intentional contact burn is suspected when the shape of the burning item, such as the iron or electric stove burner, is observed on the child's body and the burn is full thickness in depth. Cigarette burns that are unintentional are noncircular and irregular, whereas intentional cigarette burns are circular and full thickness.
- Any burn that is found in an unlikely place, such as the soles of the feet, buttocks, or perineum, must be treated as an intentional injury and investigated accordingly.

4. **Internal organ injuries**
   a. Internal organ injuries occur from blunt forces applied to the children as they are struck, kicked, punched, beaten, thrown, or stabbed by caretakers. The manifestations of internal organ injury are the same in unintentional and intentional trauma. Liver lacerations, splenic rupture, pulmonary and cardiac contusions, as well as brain injury can occur through child maltreatment. The type and severity of internal injuries sustained from child maltreatment are more severe than those from pedestrian motor vehicle crashes (Chadwick et al, 1994).
   b. Children who sustain child maltreatment tend to be younger and preverbal, thus unable to verbalize how the injury occurred. These children are usually brought in for treatment because of worsening signs of injury, such as abdominal distention, vomiting, or other vague parental history or complaints. Children also may be brought for treatment with signs of fever or infection, which progresses to sepsis or hypovolemic shock (Chadwick et al, 1994). When rib fractures are present, a significant force was applied to the chest, and maltreatment must be suspected and investigated. Inflicted abdominal injury should be suspected when there are (1) clear signs of abdominal trauma; (2) unexplained shock; (3) unexplained cardiac arrest; (4) unconsciousness with suspected inflicted head injury; and (5) unexplained unconsciousness (Chadwick et al, 1994). Treatment for inflicted

abdominal and chest trauma is the same as for unintentional injury. As in cutaneous lesions, the history of the injury is important to ascertain (see section on History of the Injury).

5. **Long bone fractures**
   a. Maltreated children sustain long bone fractures, as their extremities are twisted and pulled by caretakers or from being thrown or beaten. Fracture patterns are consistent with the applied blunt forces and include transverse and greenstick fractures due to bending or direct impact from a caretaker's hand or blunt object, spiral and oblique fractures from twisting of the extremity, and metaphyseal fractures from shaking (Merten et al, 1994). The young child is brought for treatment because of inability to use an arm or to bear weight on a leg. The injured extremity appears deformed, painful, and swollen, as in unintentional musculoskeletal trauma.
   b. Diagnostic tests consist of radiographs to include the joints above and below the suspected fracture as well as radiographs of the opposite extremity. Such comparison views allow for the detection of previous healing fractures that the caretaker may not have divulged. Radiographic review determines the fracture's type, location, and age. Radiologic guidelines for estimating fracture age are that a soft callus forms in 14 to 21 days, a hard callus forms in 21 to 42 days, and remodeling occurs at 1 year (Mayeda, 1994). A skeletal survey is a radiographic review of all bones, including the skull, spine, chest, and upper and lower extremities. Treatment includes investigation of child maltreatment and operative or nonoperative management as indicated.

6. **Head trauma**
   a. Head trauma from child abuse is the most common cause of child abuse–related death and can also result in brain damage, psychologic dysfunction, and physical impairments (Levitt et al, 1994). Head trauma occurs from blunt forces (impact, shaking), penetrating forces (bullet), and lack of oxidation (asphyxia). Impact injury occurs when the child is struck by a caretaker's hand or object or the child is thrown against an unyielding surface. Resulting injuries include brain insults, skull fractures, facial fractures, and possible eye and ear injuries. Penetrating injuries occur from bullets, knives, or other objects projected at the child. Again, direct injuries to the brain, head, and face occur. Asphyxia from gagging or choking the child can lead to ischemia and brain damage; placing young children in gas ovens to "quiet them down" also leads to hypoxia and brain injury (Levitt et al, 1994). In *Munchausen syndrome by proxy,* the parent fabricates or induces symptoms in the child and may occlude the child's airway to induce apnea.
   b. Probably the most well-known form of child abuse is *shaken impact syndrome.* This syndrome occurs in infants and young children where the child is held by the chest, facing the caretaker, and the chest is compressed during the shaking episode; this shaking does not cause bruising to the chest or arms, but rib or humeral fractures may occur (Levitt et al, 1994). This violent shaking, which lasts for approximately 20 seconds with as many as 40 to 50 shakes (Levitt et al, 1994), leads to subdural hematoma formation, metaphyseal chip fractures, and retinal hemorrhages. High spinal cord injury can occur as well. The shaken infant may display lethargy, poor sucking ability, irritability, rhythmic eye opening and deviation, decerebrate or decorticate posturing, seizures, and alterations in muscle tone and responsiveness to voice, touch, or pain. The fontanelle may or may not be full (Davis and Zitelli, 1995). The child presents for treatment either seizing, in cardiac arrest, or with a history of a seizure. The definitive finding in

shaken impact syndrome is the presence of retinal hemorrhages; therefore, careful ocular examinations are imperative in any young child with a vague history who has seizures or cardiac arrest.

    c. Treatment is initiated based on the extent of the injuries. Surface bruises are photographed, and these photographs are placed in the child's medical record. The child protective agency is contacted. The caretaker or parent is informed of the suspicion for child maltreatment. Their reactions may range from relief to anger. It is best to have this information given to the family by the physician, with a nurse or social worker in attendance. The hospital's security officers may need to be nearby in the event that the family reacts violently. Abused children may be placed in foster care, and legal action may be taken against the family.

    d. In the ICU, abused children may die of their injuries. Because the nurse is in the position to support both the child and family, it may be very difficult to support suspected perpetrators who inflicted the life-threatening injuries. Furthermore, should the child die of the injuries, homicide charges may be filed. Nurses who care for such children should seek support from their hospital's ethics committee or peer support within their hospital.

7. **Sexual abuse**

    a. Sexuality is a part of human life, and children are naturally curious about sex. Normal sexual activity in childhood involves consenting, developmentally appropriate activities that are mutually motivated by curiosity and pleasure; peers who possess the same cognitive level are involved (Finkel and DeJong, 1994). Sexual abuse occurs when the child is pressured or coerced into contact and is involved in developmentally inappropriate sexual contact among nonpeers. The motivation is from a participant's needs or an outside influence (Finkel and DeJong, 1994). Children are incapable of giving their informed consent to participate in such activities, and they are not aware of the moral, legal, emotional, and physical consequences of sexual activity with adults or older children (Kelley, 1994b). Sexual abuse includes exhibitionism; voyeurism; fondling; digital penetration of the rectum or vagina; orogenital or vaginal-penile contact; vaginal penile or rectal penile penetration; insertion of foreign bodies into the urethra, vagina, or rectum; pornography; and prostitution (Kelley, 1994b).

    b. Like physical abuse, sexual abuse involves a host of family, child, and societal factors. Incest, for example, is allowed to continue in families who do not protect their children or who fail to have appropriate caretakers available. Children and adolescents who have unmet emotional needs are easy targets for child sex offenders. According to Finkel and DeJong (1994), a child is targeted for sexual abuse by the perpetrator. A nonsexual, supportive relationship is developed, and the sexualization occurs gradually over time. The child's participation is coerced, usually by the child's need to have a sense of worth and value. As the abuse goes on, the child is helpless to resist or complain, and secrecy is maintained through threats or rewards. The child feels guilty and betrayed as he or she continues in the relationship. If the child does come forward, the child's story may be discounted, allowing the abuse to continue.

    c. Sexual abuse occurs to children of both genders, all ages, and socioeconomic strata. Poverty, drug abuse, alcoholism, an unhappy family life, and living in a family without one or both natural parents may make the child vulnerable to this abuse (Finkel and DeJong, 1994).

    d. Sexual assault (rape) occurs in children and adolescents and is the forcible act of intercourse.

e. Young children who are victims of sexual abuse tend to act out sexually with their peers, siblings, and adults. They exhibit precocity in sexual remarks or questions that demonstrate their increased awareness of sexual behavior, and frequent and compulsive masturbation may be present (Kelley, 1994b). Extreme fears, hysteria during examination of the genitalia, refusing to sleep alone, and locking or barricading the bedroom door are also indicators of sexual abuse (Kelley, 1994b). These children become obsessed with cleanliness to remove blood or secretions and to avoid "feeling dirty." They have a preoccupation with genital references and may even draw them, a finding that is not common in children without sexual abuse. Adolescents may become runaways, develop depression and eating disorders, and engage in prostitution.

f. *Treatment:* The child with suspected sexual abuse may be brought for treatment by a caretaker. The caretaker may state that abuse is known, or the caretaker may state that the child has a vaginal or penile discharge or dysuria. Herpetic lesions to the mouth may be another complaint for treatment. Sexual abuse should be suspected in pregnant, young adolescents (10 years to 14 years of age), especially if the pregnancy is concealed, or with vaginal or penile discharge, foreign bodies, sexually transmitted diseases, or rectal or vaginal pain (Kelley, 1994b).

- *The sexually abused or assaulted child must undergo a physical examination and interview.* Experienced professionals in the care of these children must conduct these examinations to avoid contamination of evidence and to allow the child to tell the story only once. The *physical examination* may be deferred in the child with sexual abuse if the last episode occurred more than 72 hours before presentation (Finkel and DeJong, 1994). If the sexual abuse or assault occurred within 72 hours, the physical examination can be initiated.

- The physical examination may be done with a parent or caretaker present, provided that person is not the perpetrator. One nurse or rape crisis counselor assumes the role of support person, while another nurse assists with obtaining and labeling the specimens. The child can be placed on an adult's lap in the frog leg position or assume a knee-chest position on the examination table. The left lateral decubitus position allows for examination of the rectum. If at any point the child does not cooperate with the examination and becomes upset and fearful, the examination is stopped. An examination under anesthesia is then performed. The child is never restrained or forced to comply with the examination.

- The external genitalia are examined, and cultures for syphilis, gonorrhea, and chlamydia are obtained. Any lacerations, bruising, and bleeding are noted. A Wood's lamp is also used to observe for semen; a wet prep for sperm or semen detection is also obtained. In the adolescent female victim, a bimanual pelvic examination is indicated. In young females, a pediatric ear speculum may be used to visualize the cervix and cultures are again obtained. The rectal area is examined for bruising, bleeding, or tearing, and cultures are obtained. In the male child, similar cultures of the meatus and rectum are obtained, and both areas are observed for bruising, lacerations, or tearing.

- All evidence is obtained carefully and is secured in an assault kit that is usually provided by the local law enforcement agency. Such kits have prelabeled envelopes for specimen collection. Aside from the cultures, other specimens include a saliva sample, pubic hairs, a comb used to comb the hairs, finger nail scrapings, and blood specimens for VDRL, human immunodeficiency virus (HIV), hepatitis B, and human chorionic gonadotropin (HCG). Postmenarchal females are usually given the option to take a high dose of oral contraceptives to prevent pregnancy. Pharyngeal cultures are also obtained. The specimens are then sealed, and the collecting nurse's name is written on the outside of the collection box. The box is then hand delivered to the hospital police for safe keeping, who then sign for the box, or it is handed directly to the law enforcement agent, who signs for the box. This chain of evidence avoids potential evidence mishandling or tampering, either of which may jeopardize the legal process. The child's clothes are also obtained and placed in paper bags and given to law enforcement. Follow-up is completed through the hospital, rape crisis center, or regular health care professional.

- The examining professional carefully documents all the physical findings; the nurse documents the chain of evidence and the child's reaction to the examination.
- The *sexually abused or assaulted child is interviewed* by a trained professional. The parent or caretaker and child are interviewed separately. The child is not asked any leading questions and is simply asked to talk about what happened. The child may use puppets or dolls to demonstrate what occurred; using paper and crayons for drawing allows the nonverbal or preverbal child to depict the situation.
- The child is told that he or she did the right thing by coming forward with the story and that the child did not do anything wrong. Such statements decrease the sense of stigmatization, embarrassment, and isolation (Finkel and DeJong, 1994).

8. **Neglect**
   a. Neglect is the most prevalent type of child maltreatment and involves omitting the child's basic needs, including food, shelter, clothing, health care, and a safe environment (Kelley, 1994b). Neglect may go undetected as it may be associated with poverty. However, neglect should be considered based on what the family should be doing, as opposed to what they are economically capable of doing (Kelley, 1994b).
   b. Indicators for neglect include malnutrition and failure to thrive, unsanitary or unsafe living conditions, lack of proper immunizations, poor hygiene and inappropriate clothing for the weather, extensive dental caries, frequent absences from school, and abandonment (Kelley, 1994b).
   c. Neglected children may be brought for treatment by law enforcement authorities who respond to a complaint from a neighbor. Although it is unlikely that a child will enter the ICU for neglect alone, signs of neglect should be observed for in children who are admitted for possible child maltreatment, ingestions, or drug overdoses.

9. **Emotional abuse:** Emotional abuse occurs usually with other maltreatment forms. In this instance, the caretakers or parents do not provide a nurturing environment. These caretakers berate, belittle, verbally abuse, threaten, and expose their children to domestic violence (Kelley, 1994b). Signs of emotional abuse include sleep and feeding disorders, hyperactivity, developmental delays, and excessively passive or aggressive behavior. Again, although admission to the ICU is not warranted for emotional abuse, these behaviors may be observed in children who are in the ICU for other reasons. Such behaviors should be brought to the attention of the physician and social worker, so investigations into the child's home life can be made.

TOXICOLOGY   ROSE ANN GOULD SOLOWAY

The vast majority of poison exposures in children can and should be handled safely at home with the guidance of the poison center. However, critical care nurses must recognize, consult with the poison center about, and treat those exposures that are most likely to cause serious injury, illness, or death, and therefore those most likely to require treatment in an ICU.

DEFINITIONS

A. **POISONING VS. OVERDOSE**

The term *poison* is often used to refer to nonpharmaceutical substances and *overdose* is used for pharmaceuticals. However, any substance that enters the body and causes harm is a poison, and therefore the term *poisoning* is used in this chapter to describe the consequences of any exposure resulting in injury, illness, or death.

B. **POISON EXPOSURE**

Poison exposure means some type of inappropriate contact with a potentially harmful substance. Such exposure can be through ingestion, inhalation, ocular or dermal contact, or parenteral injection.

C. **ROUTES OF EXPOSURE**

The manner in which a potentially toxic substance enters the body can influence the time of onset, intensity, and duration of toxic effects. Statistically, most poisonings occur by ingestion. However, never overlook the importance of other routes of exposure: for example, inhalation and dermal routes for organophosphate insecticides; inhalation, nasal, and parenteral routes for drugs of abuse; ocular, dermal, oral, and inhalation for caustic chemicals; inhalation for gases, fumes, and vapors; and parenteral for envenomations. Except for those chemical exposures whose effects are confined to the site of exposure, the effects of a poison exposure are determined by the degree of absorption of the substance into the blood stream, the extent of metabolism to a less toxic or more toxic substance, distribution to target organs, and ultimate elimination from the body.

D. **ACUTE VS. CHRONIC EXPOSURE**

Most poison exposures in children are the result of acute ingestion. Chronic overdoses, or an acute overdose of a drug also taken for a long period of time, are possible for children who require therapeutic drugs for medical conditions. Chronic exposures are also possible for those abusing drugs, for victims of child abuse, and for victims of Munchausen syndrome by proxy. Kinetics, toxic blood levels, and clinical manifestations of poisoning may differ with acute and chronic administration of a drug.

ROLE OF THE POISON CENTER

The poison center is the source of expert clinical toxicology information. Twenty-four hours a day, 7 days a week, the physicians, nurses, and pharmacists at the poison center can assist in a number of ways. Staff provide expert advice about poisoning by drugs (legal, illegal, foreign, veterinary), household products, industrial chemicals, hazardous materials, environmental toxins, snakes, spiders, plants, mushrooms, and pill identification. Staff assist in determining if a complex of symptoms could be caused by poisoning. Poison centers locate sources for unusual antidotes (e.g., botulinum antitoxin), treatments, and laboratory studies. Staff perform clinical and epidemiologic research. Each patient becomes an anonymous part of a national database, which collectively identifies actual and in some cases previously unsuspected hazards. Data are used to reformulate or repackage products or to require removal of products from the market. The Joint Commission on Accreditation of Healthcare Organizations requires that the poison center phone number be posted in every health care facility. Phone stickers and posters are available from the poison center serving each area.

EPIDEMIOLOGY AND ETIOLOGY

A. EPIDEMIOLOGY
   1. The most comprehensive source of information about poison exposures in the United States is the Annual Report of the American Association of Poison Control Centers Toxic Exposure Surveillance System, published each September in *The American Journal of Emergency Medicine*. It allows differentiation between common but relatively benign poison exposures and those with serious consequences.
   2. In 1995, there were 2,023,089 poison exposures reported to 67 poison centers in the United States. More than 90% of these exposures occurred in a residence. In 72.1% of reported cases the poison exposures were managed over the telephone, without the patient's needing to seek hands-on medical care. A summary of the number of pediatric exposures and fatalities is in Table 9–9.
   3. The most common poison exposures in children during 1995 are listed in Table 9–10. Table 9–11 lists those substances associated with the most fatalities in all ages. It is clear that those substances most often involved with poison exposures and those most commonly associated with fatalities do not necessarily coincide, and a closer look at data is indicated. By combining records for the years 1983 through 1990, the American Association of Poison Control Centers was able to identify even uncommon poison exposures that posed the most danger to children under the age of 6, those most vulnerable to unintentional poisoning (Table 9–12).

B. RISK FACTORS
   All ages are vulnerable to iatrogenic poisonings (e.g., incorrect drugs or routes of administration in a health care setting); environmental poisons (e.g., carbon monoxide, pesticides, contaminated water); inadvertent ingestion of poisonous substances that were transferred into food containers such as baby bottles, milk containers, and soft drink bottles; and idiosyncratic reactions. Children of any age

Table 9–9.   NUMBER OF PEDIATRIC POISON EXPOSURES, 1995

AGE	NUMBER OF EXPOSURES	PERCENT OF ALL EXPOSURES	NUMBER OF FATALITIES	PERCENT OF ALL FATALITIES
Younger than 6	1,070,497	52.9	20	2.8
6–12	136,711	6.8	6	0.8
13–19	151,448	7.5	40	5.5

From Litovitz TL, Felberg L, White S, Klein-Schwartz W. 1995 annual report of the American Association of Poison Control Centers Toxic Exposure Surveillance System. *Am J Emerg Med.* 1996;14(5):487–537.

Table 9–10. MOST COMMON POISON EXPOSURES IN CHILDREN, 1995*

Younger Than Age 6	Ages 6–19
Cosmetics and personal care products	Analgesics
Cleaning substances	Bites and envenomations
Analgesics	Cleaning substances
Plants	Cough and cold preparations
Cough and cold preparations	Cosmetics and personal care products
Foreign bodies	Stimulants and street drugs
Topical medicines	Plants
Antimicrobials	Foreign bodies
Vitamins	Food products and food poisoning
Gastrointestinal tract medications	Antidepressants

*Listed from most common to least common.
From Litovitz TL, Felberg L, White S, Klein-Schwartz W. 1995 annual report of the American Association of Poison Control Centers Toxic Exposure Surveillance System. *Am J Emerg Med.* 1996;14(5):487–537.

Table 9–11. TEN MOST COMMON CAUSES OF POISON-RELATED FATALITIES, ALL AGES, 1995

Analgesics
Antidepressants
Cardiovascular drugs
Stimulants and street drugs (most, but not all, deaths were associated with illegal drugs)
Sedatives, hypnotics, and antipsychotic drugs
Alcohols
Gases and fumes
Asthma therapies
Insecticides, pesticides, rodenticides
Automotive products

From Litovitz TL, Felberg L, White S, Klein-Schwartz W. 1995 annual report of the American Association of Poison Control Centers Toxic Exposure Surveillance System. *Am J Emerg Med.* 1996;14(5):487–537.

may be victims of child abuse or Munchausen syndrome by proxy. In addition, there are some age-related physiologic and behavioral factors that may predispose to, exacerbate, or mitigate poison exposures.

1. **Infants** are poisoned when parents misread or disregard medication labels, when potentially harmful substances are left within an infant's grasp, or when older siblings "feed" or "help with" infants. Immature GI tract flora predispose infants to infant botulism and to methemoglobinemia from ingestion of foods

Table 9–12. MOST COMMON UNINTENTIONAL INGESTION FATALITIES IN CHILDREN YOUNGER THAN AGE 6, 1983–1990

Pharmaceuticals	Nonpharmaceuticals
Iron	Pesticides
Antidepressants	Hydrocarbons
Cardiovascular drugs	Alcohols
Salicylates	Gun bluing
	Cleaning substances

Data from Litovitz R, Manoguerra A. Comparison of pediatric poisoning hazards: an analysis of 3.8 million exposure incidents—a report from the American Association of Poison Control Centers. *Pediatrics.* 1992;89(6):999–1006.

or well water high in nitrites. Immature nervous systems exacerbate the risk of exposure to any CNS toxin. Rapid respiratory and metabolic rates increase the risk of carbon monoxide poisoning. Immature hepatic and renal systems may or may not increase the risk of poison exposures, depending on specific mechanisms for metabolism and excretion. An infant's small body weight increases the potential for danger if an infant is envenomated by snakes or spiders.

2. **Toddlers** are poisoned when potentially poisonous substances are left within reach. As consequences of normal growth and development, children grab or climb to reach anything that seems attractive, put everything in their hands into their mouths, and imitate adult behavior, including the taking of medicines. Children are unable to distinguish medicines and household products from benign look-alikes such as candy and soft drinks. Physiologically, toddlers face the same risks as infants in terms of the nervous, hepatic, and renal systems, respiratory rate and metabolic rate, and body weight.

3. **School-age children** may not be able to read or may misinterpret label instructions on products and medicines, succumb to "dares" of classmates, and may not be able to predict the consequences of their actions. Because of wide variability in normal growth and development, it is difficult to generally predict physiologic effects of many poison exposures.

4. **Preteens and teenagers** may misinterpret label instructions on products and medicines, succumb to "dares" of classmates, explore more widely outside the home and school environment, and may abuse drugs or attempt suicide. After about age 10, children metabolize acetaminophen in the adult fashion (i.e., generate increased amounts of the hepatotoxic metabolite). As they near the upper end of the teenage range, physiologic responses approach, then equal, expected adult responses.

NURSING DIAGNOSES

Toxicology is a complex discipline. Caring for a poisoned child requires knowledge of virtually every body system and the ability to anticipate needs and interventions, based on characteristics of the poison involved. The following list of nursing diagnoses is offered as a partial list of those that might be appropriate to the care of a poisoned child. The reader is referred to preceding chapters for those specific system interventions and outcomes that relate to symptomatic and supportive care for victims of poisoning.

❖ CAREGIVER ROLE STRAIN OR PARENTING ALTERATION RELATED TO CRITICAL ILLNESS, LACK OF SUPERVISION, OR GUILT

❖ IMPAIRMENT IN GAS EXCHANGE RELATED TO INEFFECTIVE AIRWAY CLEARANCE, HIGH RISK FOR ASPIRATION, INEFFECTIVE BREATHING PATTERN, OR INABILITY TO SUSTAIN SPONTANEOUS VENTILATION

❖ HYPOTENSION OR DECREASED CARDIAC OUTPUT RELATED TO TOXIC DOSE OF CARDIODEPRESSANT MEDICATIONS OR SUBSTANCES

❖ NUTRITION ALTERATION RELATED TO CONSTIPATION, DIARRHEA, INCONTINENCE, ORAL MUCOUS MEMBRANE ALTERATION, OR SWALLOWING IMPAIRMENT

❖ FLUID VOLUME DEFICIT OR FLUID VOLUME EXCESS RELATED TO INGESTION OF TOXIC SUBSTANCES

❖ PERIPHERAL NEUROVASCULAR DYSFUNCTION RELATED TO NEUROTOXICITY

❖ KNOWLEDGE DEFICIT RELATED TO APPROPRIATE DOSING OR SAFETY

❖ ALTERED LEVEL OF CONSCIOUSNESS RELATED TO IMPAIRMENT IN GAS EXCHANGE, DECREASED CARDIAC OUTPUT, OR NEUROLOGIC TOXICITY

MANAGEMENT OF PATIENTS WITH POISON EXPOSURES

A. **HISTORY**

1. Usually, the basic information is known: children spill things, brag about taking medicine or "helping mommy," or act guilty about having done something "forbidden."

2. In the absence of history, a high index of suspicion is required to determine if a poison exposure has occurred. Suspect a poison exposure when there is a sudden onset of illness; unexplained symptoms, findings, or laboratory values; an unusual complex of symptoms; exposure to a fire (carbon monoxide, cyanide); or psychiatric treatment in the child, a family member, or caretaker and therefore access to psychotropic drugs. In older children who are trauma victims, suspect drug or alcohol use as a precipitating factor. Also, previously undiagnosed medical conditions (e.g., glucose-6-phosphate dehydrogenase [G6PD] deficiency) may predispose to poisoning by some agents (naphthalene mothballs, dapsone), and the poison center can help identify such conditions.

3. To determine if a poison exposure may have occurred, ask about medicines and products in the home; whether there have been visitors in the home or if the child has visited elsewhere; if herbal medicines, home remedies, or foreign preparations have been used or are available; or if the child has been breast-feeding. To assess environmental factors, ask if anyone else is ill, for example, or if there have been any home improvement projects or new appliances installed.

4. In addition to ascertaining the nature of any symptoms, determine when they started and in what order they occurred. These can be valuable clues in determining what the poison is or if the available history is accurate.

B. **ASSESSMENT**

1. **Clinical assessment** in cases of poison exposure is no different from physical assessment for any other medical emergency. Characteristic complexes of symptoms, physical findings, and laboratory findings may assist with assessment of exposure to unknown poisons (Table 9–13).

2. The need for laboratory assessment depends on whether the poison is known and, if so, what the poison is; whether knowledge of test results will affect medical care, prognosis, or disposition of the patient; and, in some cases, whether there are medicolegal considerations.

   a. For many poisonings with anticipated systemic effects, baseline electrolytes; renal and hepatic functions; respiratory, cardiovascular, and hematologic parameters; and arterial blood gas (ABG) analysis are necessary.

   b. For some poisons, quantitative measurement in urine or serum determines whether treatment is needed.

   c. In other cases, laboratory studies may confirm the presence of particular substances but do not alter patient care (e.g., tricyclic antidepressants).

   d. At other times, laboratory values cannot be returned in enough time to influence patient care (e.g., cyanide).

   e. In some cases, the length of time between exposure and collection of the laboratory specimen influences the interpretation of laboratory results (e.g., acetaminophen, aspirin, and carbon monoxide).

   f. When a poisoning is suspected but not known, a comprehensive toxicology screen may be helpful in identifying the agent. How "comprehensive" such a screen is varies from facility to facility; it is essential to know what was tested for before declaring such a screening result to be "negative."

Table 9–13. TOXICOLOGIC SYNDROMES (TOXIDROMES)

Toxin	Vital Signs	Mental Status	Symptoms	Clinical Findings	Laboratory Findings
Acetaminophen	Normal (early)	Normal	Anorexia, nausea, vomiting	Right upper quadrant tenderness, jaundice (late)	Abnormal results from LFTs
Amphetamines	Hypertension, tachycardia, tachypnea, hyperthermia	Hyperactive, agitated, toxic psychosis	Hyperalertness	Mydriasis, hyperactive bowel sounds, flush, diaphoresis	Increased CPK level
Anticholinergics	Hypotension, hypertension, tachycardia, hyperthermia	Altered (agitation, lethargy to coma), hallucinations	Blurred vision	Dry mucous membranes, mydriasis, diminished bowel sounds, urinary retention	ECG abnormalities
Arsenic (acute)	Hypotension, tachycardia	Alert to coma	Abdominal pain, vomiting, diarrhea, dysphagia	Dehydration	Renal failure, abnormal findings from abdominal radiograph; dysrhythmias
Arsenic (chronic)	Normal	Normal to encephalopathy	Abdominal pain, diarrhea	Melanosis, hyperkeratosis, sensory motor neuropathy, hair loss, Mees' lines, skin cancer	Pancytopenia, proteinuria, hematuria, abnormal results from LFTs
Barbiturates	Hypotension, bradypnea, hypothermia	Altered (lethargy to coma)	Slurred speech, ataxia	Dysconjugate gaze, bullae, hyporeflexia	Abnormal results from ABG analysis
β-Adrenergic antagonists	Hypotension, bradycardia	Altered (lethargy to coma)	Dizziness	Cyanosis, seizures	Hypoglycemia, ECG abnormalities
Botulism	Bradypnea	Normal unless hypoxia	Blurred vision, dysphagia, sore throat, diarrhea	Ophthalmoplegia, mydriasis, ptosis, cranial nerve abnormalities	Normal
Carbamazepine	Hypotension, tachycardia, bradypnea, hypothermia	Altered (lethargy to coma)	Hallucinations, extrapyramidal movements, seizures	Mydriasis, nystagmus	ECG abnormalities
Carbon monoxide	Often normal	Altered (lethargy to coma)	Headache, dizziness, nausea, vomiting	Seizures	Elevated carboxyhemoglobin level, ECG abnormalities, metabolic acidosis
Clonidine	Hypotension, hypertension, bradycardia, bradypnea	Altered (lethargy to coma)	Dizziness, confusion	Miosis	Normal

ABG, arterial blood gas; *CPK*, creatine phosphokinase; *ECG*, elecrocardiogram; *LFT*, liver function test; *PT*, prothrombin time; *PTT*, partial thromboplastin time; *RBC*, red blood cell.
Modified from Goldfrank LR, Flomenbaum NE, Lewin NA, et al. *Goldfrank's Toxicologic Emergencies.* 5th ed. Norwalk, Conn: Appleton & Lange; 1994:144–145.

Table 9–13. **TOXICOLOGIC SYNDROMES (TOXIDROMES)** *(Continued)*

Toxin	Vital Signs	Mental Status	Symptoms	Clinical Findings	Laboratory Findings
Cocaine	Hypertension, tachycardia, hyperthermia	Altered (anxiety, agitation, delirium)	Hallucinations, paranoia	Mydriasis, tremor, perforated nasal septum, diaphoresis, seizures, active bowel sounds	ECG abnormalities, increased CPK level
Cyclic antidepressants	Hypotension, tachycardia, hyperthermia	Altered (lethargy to coma)	Confusion, dizziness	Mydriasis, dry mucous membranes, distended bladder, flush, seizures	Prolonged QRS complex, cardiac dysrhythmias
Digitalis	Hypotension, bradycardia	Normal to altered, visual hallucinations	Nausea, vomiting, anorexia, visual disturbances	None	Hyperkalemia, ECG abnormalities, increased digoxin level
Disulfiram, ethanol	Hypotension, bradycardia	Normal to altered; visual hallucinations	Nausea, vomiting, headache, vertigo	Flush, diaphoresis, tender abdomen	Abnormal ECG findings (ventricular dysrhythmias)
Ethylene glycol	Tachypnea	Altered (lethargy to coma)	Abdominal pain	Slurred speech, ataxia	Anion gap acidosis, osmolar gap, crystalluria, hypocalcemia, QT prolongation, renal failure
Iron	Hypotension (late), tachycardia (late)	Normal unless hypotensive, lethargy	Nausea, vomiting, diarrhea, abdominal pain, hematemesis	Tender abdomen	Hyperglycemia (child), leukocytosis (child), heme-positive stool or vomitus, metabolic acidosis, radiopaque material on abdominal radiograph
Isoniazid (INH)	Often normal	Normal or altered (lethargy to coma)	Nausea, vomiting	Seizures	Anion gap metabolic acidosis
Isopropyl alcohol	Hypotension, bradypnea	Altered (lethargy, irritability to coma)	Nausea, vomiting	Hyporeflexia, breath odor of acetone	Ketonemia, ketonuria, absence of glycosuria or acidosis
Lead	Hypertension	Altered (lethargy to coma)	Irritability, abdominal pain (colic), nausea, vomiting, constipation	Peripheral neuropathy, seizures, gingival pigmentation	Anemia, basophilic stippling, radiopaque material on abdominal radiograph, proteinuria

Table continued on following page

Table 9–13.   TOXICOLOGIC SYNDROMES (TOXIDROMES) *(Continued)*

Toxin	Vital Signs	Mental Status	Symptoms	Clinical Findings	Laboratory Findings
Lithium	Hypotension (late)	Altered (lethargy to coma)	Diarrhea, tremor	Weakness, tremor, ataxia, myoclonus, seizures	Leukocytosis, ECG abnormalities, renal abnormalities (diabetes insipidus)
Mercury	Hypotension (late)	Altered (psychiatric disturbances)	Salivation, diarrhea, abdominal pain	Stomatitis, ataxia, tremor	Proteinuria, renal failure
Methanol	Hypotension, tachypnea	Altered (lethargy to coma)	Blurred vision, blindness, abdominal pain	Hyperemic discs	Anion gap metabolic acidosis, increased osmolar gap
Opioids	Hypotension, bradycardia, bradypnea, hypothermia	Altered (lethargy to coma)	Slurred speech, taxia	Miosis, absent bowel sounds	Abnormal results from ABG analysis
Organophosphates, carbamates	Hypotension, bradycardia and tachycardia, bradypnea and tachypnea	Altered (lethargy to coma)	Diarrhea, abdominal pain, blurred vision, vomiting	Salivation, diaphoresis, lacrimation, urination, defecation, miosis, fasciculations, seizures	Depressed RBC and plasma cholinesterase activity
Phencyclidine (PCP)	Hypertension, tachycardia, hyperthermia	Altered (agitation, lethargy to coma)	Hallucinations	Miosis, diaphoresis, myoclonus, blank stare, nystagmus, seizures	Myoglobinuria, leukocytosis, increased CPK level
Phenothiazines	Hypotension, tachycardia, hypothermia, hyperthermia	Altered (lethargy to coma)	Dizziness	Miosis or mydriasis, decreased bowel sounds, dystonia	Abnormal ECG findings, abnormal abdominal radiograph findings
Salicylates	Hyperthermia, tachypnea	Altered (agitation, lethargy to coma)	Tinnitus, nausea, vomiting	Diaphoresis, tender abdomen	Anion gap metabolic acidosis; respiratory alkalosis; abnormal results from LFTs, PT and PTT; positive $FeCl_3$
Sedative-hypnotics	Hypotension, bradypnea, hypothermia	Altered (lethargy to coma)	Slurred speech, ataxia	Hyporeflexia, bullae	Abnormal findings from ABG analysis
Theophylline	Hypotension, tachycardia, tachypnea, hyperthermia	Altered (agitation)	Nausea, vomiting, diaphoresis	Diaphoresis, tremor, seizures, dysrhythmias	Hypokalemia, hyperglycemia, metabolic acidosis, abnormal ECG findings

g. It is usual, and desirable, to "treat the patient, not the laboratory." However, when caring for a poisoned patient, the exact opposite is sometimes necessary to prevent devastating consequences. In some common, potentially fatal poisonings, metabolites are responsible for toxic effects, and ideally the patient would be treated before toxic metabolites are generated and while the patient is still asymptomatic. In cases of acetaminophen, ethylene glycol, and methanol poisoning, laboratory studies do guide therapy.

C. INTERVENTIONS

1. **Prevention of absorption:** Decontamination is the initial step. This may refer to removal from contaminated air, irrigation of exposed eyes and skin, or GI tract decontamination.

   a. *Ocular exposure* is treated by copious irrigation, at least 15 to 20 minutes for acidic substances and 30 minutes for alkaline substances. Irrigation has been sufficient when a pH strip gently touched to the cul-de-sac indicates a neutral pH. Ocular irrigation in children is difficult at best, and the best method is the one that can be initiated quickly and then maintained! Ocular irrigation in teens can be performed as in adults, with a Morgan lens.

   b. *Dermal exposure* is also treated by copious irrigation for the times specified above. For older children, a shower is ideal. Protect staff from exposure to harmful substances, initiate irrigation, and remove contaminated clothing.

   c. *GI tract decontamination* includes gastric emptying with ipecac syrup, gastric lavage, or whole bowel irrigation, adsorbing remaining ingested substances with activated charcoal, then hastening evacuation of the charcoal complex with a cathartic.

      - *Ipecac syrup* induces vomiting by causing gastric irritation and through central mechanisms. While there has been a general movement in emergency departments away from the use of ipecac syrup, it is still an important drug. Some oral dosage forms are too large to be retrieved through gastric lavage tubes, and not all poisons are adsorbed to activated charcoal, including iron, one of the most dangerous poisonings in children. Ipecac syrup should also be kept and used at home with poison center guidance.

        ○ The dose of ipecac syrup follows: 6 to 11 months, 10 ml; 12 months to 45 kg (100 lb; approximately 10 to 12 years), 15 ml; teen or adult dose, 30 ml. Follow with half a glass of liquid for young children, a glass for older children. (The liquid need not be water.) Vomiting is expected within 20 to 30 minutes; if not, the dose may be repeated once. If vomiting has not occurred in 1 hour, the decision to pursue other means of gastric emptying depends on the absorption time of the substance in question.

        ○ Contraindications to ipecac include patients unable to protect the airway (younger than 6 months old, decreased level of consciousness, seizures); patients who may rapidly develop seizures or loss of consciousness (e.g., after ingestion of such substances as tricyclic antidepressants, calcium channel blockers, clonidine, and strychnine); ingestion of caustic substances; ingestion of foreign bodies; ingestion of most hydrocarbons, unless they contain another toxic substance such as a pesticide or heavy metal; history of a recent myocardial infarction; and third trimester of pregnancy.

      - *Gastric lavage* is difficult at best in young children. The efficacy of gastric lavage is limited by the respective sizes of the child, the tube, and the tablets. It is indicated in patients who have or could develop seizures and decreased level of consciousness and for ingestions in which administration of activated charcoal should rapidly follow gastric emptying.

- ○ Secure the airway and warm NS for instillation. The largest possible orogastric tube should be used, usually a 16- to 32-gauge French. Instill 50 to 100 ml of warm NS at a time, then allow it to remain in the stomach for a few minutes and drain by gravity. Repeat until lavage fluid is clear. Activated charcoal and cathartic can be administered before the lavage tube is withdrawn.
- ○ Gastric lavage is contraindicated for ingestions of caustic substances and hydrocarbons. However, careful lavage with a soft tube is sometimes used within 1 hour of an acid ingestion. If removal of a hydrocarbon is needed, ipecac-induced emesis is preferred, as there is a lower risk of aspiration.

- *Whole bowel irrigation* is sometimes used to treat poisonings when the amount of substance ingested is extremely dangerous or potentially fatal and when there are no effective treatments. Examples include iron, some sustained-release drugs such as calcium channel blockers, and sometimes ingested packets of illegal drugs such as cocaine and heroin. The general procedure is the same as for bowel preparations. Secure the airway if necessary and administer a polyethylene glycol–electrolyte solution until the rectal effluent is clear. The dose is 0.5 L/h for young children and 1 to 2 L/h for older children and adults.

- *Activated charcoal* is processed so that each molecule contains multiple binding sites. Activated charcoal adsorbs, or binds to, most clinically important drugs and poisons. This prevents absorption from the GI tract into the blood stream. Activated charcoal does not absorb metals (e.g., iron and lithium), caustic substances, or ethanol. When these substances are ingested, activated charcoal may still be indicated because of coingestants.

  - ○ The usual dose of activated charcoal is 0.5 to 1 g/kg for young children, 25 to 50 g for older children, and 50 g per dose for teenagers and adults.
  - ○ Activated charcoal should not be mixed with ice cream, syrups, or other items intended to improve palatability. The charcoal adsorbs most of these agents and would therefore be ineffective.
  - ○ Single doses of activated charcoal are indicated for most serious poison exposures because it decreases the amount of toxic substance available for absorption into the blood stream.
  - ○ Multiple doses of activated charcoal (every 2 to 6 hours) are useful in lowering toxic blood levels and shortening the course of poisoning from some substances that undergo enterohepatic or enterogastric recirculation. Some drugs are partially metabolized in the liver, then active drug is secreted into bile and deposited in the small bowel. Subsequent doses of activated charcoal adsorb the drug as this occurs. This is true regardless of the route of exposure. *"Intestinal dialysis"* takes advantage of concentration gradients. As drug is adsorbed to charcoal in the GI tract, previously absorbed, unmetabolized drug moves from receptor sites and intracellular spaces into the GI tract. As this occurs, it too is adsorbed by subsequent doses of activated charcoal. Among the drugs for which multiple doses of activated charcoal are indicated are aspirin, digitalis, carbamazepine, theophylline, PCP, phenobarbital, and the tricyclic antidepressants.
  - ○ *Cautions:* Always check for active bowel sounds before administering a

dose of charcoal to prevent a charcoal impaction. When multiple doses of activated charcoal are given, it is essential that a cathartic be administered no more than once, or occasionally twice, per day to prevent electrolyte imbalance and dehydration. Errors have occurred when charcoal suspension in sorbital has been mistakenly administered instead of charcoal in an aqueous suspension. It is also essential that the patient have active bowel sounds. Always check before administering the next dose of charcoal.

- *Cathartics:* Sorbitol and magnesium citrate are the most common cathartics used to treat poisoning.
  - *Sorbitol* may be combined with charcoal or administered afterward. It should be administered no more than once per day. The pediatric dose is 0.5 g/kg; for older teens and adults, 1 g/kg.
  - *Magnesium citrate* may be combined with charcoal or administered afterward. It should be administered no more than once per day. The dose is 4 ml/kg.

2. **Enhancement of elimination:** The means and possibility of enhancing elimination depend on a substance's volume of distribution and usual elimination.

   a. *Diuresis* may be useful for substances that have a small volume of distribution, at least initially, and are eliminated renally. The issue of volume overload in small children must always be considered. For substances that cause increased capillary permeability, pulmonary edema must also be considered.

   b. *Ion-trapping* is useful for some drugs that are more rapidly eliminated in an alkaline environment; examples include salicylates and phenobarbital. In these cases, administering sodium bicarbonate to alkalinize the urine enhances excretion. (Some drugs are more easily eliminated by acidifying the urine, but this is not recommended; precipitation of myoglobin and renal failure may occur.)

   c. *Extracorporeal measures* to enhance elimination of toxins may be useful in certain dangerous poisonings by substances that can be retrieved from the vascular compartment. Depending on the child's age, hemodialysis can be used for salicylates, lithium, methanol, and ethylene glycol, among others; hemoperfusion may be used for theophylline; and exchange transfusion is sometimes used to treat "gray baby syndrome" induced by chloramphenicol.

3. **Administration of antidotes:** There are few pharmacologic antidotes available. Most poisonings are treated by decontamination followed by symptomatic and supportive care. If a specific antidote is indicated, it is described as part of the treatment for poisonings considered below.

4. **Provision of supportive care:** Provision of symptomatic and supportive care for poisoning ranges from such simple measures as fluids and positioning for hypotension to invasive measures to support cardiovascular, respiratory, and hematologic functioning. Descriptions of individual poisons indicate if one particular drug (e.g., antiarrhythmic, anticonvulsant, or vasopressor) is preferred. Increasing or recurrent symptoms may be expected with some poisonings and occur unexpectedly in others. See Table 9–14 for possible reasons.

5. **Prevention of future episodes:** Circumstances contributing to iatrogenic poisonings must be considered. For young children, age- and development-specific poison prevention teaching may be required. Suspicions of abuse require legal and social service involvement. Drug abuse prevention and treatment programs and psychiatric intervention may be required for older children and teens.

Table 9–14.   CAUSES OF INCREASING OR RECURRING SYMPTOMS AND DRUG LEVELS

Incomplete gastrointestinal tract decontamination: Virtually any solid dosage form

Drug concentration or bezoar: aspirin, iron, meprobamate

Enterohepatic recirculation: amitriptyline, digoxin, phencyclidine

Ingestion of anticholinergic drug, or drug with anticholinergic properties: antihistamines, atropine, tricyclic antidepressants, glutethimide

Exposure to especially lipid-soluble substances: some organophosphate insecticides, anesthetic agents, ethchlorvynol

Incorrect or incomplete history

Incorrect laboratory values

Reexposure in the hospital

POISONINGS BY PHARMACEUTICAL AGENTS

A. ACETAMINOPHEN

Acetaminophen is found in hundreds of prescription and nonprescription analgesics, alone and in combination with other analgesics, including opioids; in combination with antihistamines in over-the-counter sleeping preparations; and in combination with decongestants, antihistamines, antitussives, expectorants, and analgesics in products to treat coughs, colds, and allergies. Most preparations are oral, but the drug also is available as rectal suppositories.

1. Acetaminophen is rapidly absorbed from the GI tract, but food or coingestion of an anticholinergic drug may delay peak absorption until about 4 hours after ingestion.

2. Acetaminophen is metabolized in the liver. Over about the age of 10 years, approximately 5% to 10% of the drug is metabolized by a hepatotoxic metabolite that is normally detoxified by the enzyme glutathione. In overdose the body's glutathione stores are depleted, causing the liver damage characteristic of acetaminophen overdose. In children younger than 10 years a different metabolic pathway is followed, presumably providing some degree of hepatic protection. This relative protection is not entirely reliable, and infants and young children can also die of hepatic injury after acetaminophen overdose. There is some renal metabolism of acetaminophen; therefore, renal injury, although not as common as hepatic injury, is possible.

3. The **toxic dose** of acetaminophen is related to body weight (or ideal body weight, in the case of markedly obese individuals); ingestions of unknown amounts or greater than 150 mg/kg require laboratory assessment of absorbed acetaminophen to predict toxicity.

4. Because the toxic effects of acetaminophen overdose are due to metabolites, **symptoms** of toxicity are delayed. Only rarely, after massive overdose, does a patient develop mental status changes, significant GI tract symptoms, and acidosis within hours after ingestion. Often there are no symptoms of overdose for 6 to 14 hours after ingestion. The earliest symptoms are nausea and vomiting. Within 24 to 48 hours after ingestion, hepatic enzymes rise. The patient may experience increasing GI tract symptoms and right upper quadrant pain, or the patient may feel relatively well. Within 72 to 96 hours after an untreated, severe overdose, hepatic encephalopathy with coagulopathies and hyperglycemia may ensue, followed rapidly by hepatic failure and death.

5. **Assessment**

   a. History should include the name of the drug; amount ingested; time of ingestion; and whether ingestion was acute, chronic, or both; and the type, onset, duration, or absence of symptoms.

  b. Draw a serum acetaminophen level at least 4 hours after ingestion. Also draw baseline hepatic, renal, and hematologic studies if the level is toxic or if ingestion was large or chronic by history or occurred more than 8 to 12 hours earlier.

6. **Treatment** of acetaminophen poisoning is straightforward and successful if the antidote is initiated within 8 to 12 hours after ingestion. Later administration has some utility. The specific antidote is N-acetylcysteine (NAC), which serves as a glutathione precursor and substitute to prevent NAPQI-induced hepatocellular injury. Indications for NAC include a toxic acetaminophen level in blood drawn 4 hours or more after ingestion and toxic ingestion by history or suspicion when laboratory results cannot be returned by 8 hours after ingestion.

  a. The loading dose is NAC 140 mg/kg administered PO, followed by 70 mg/kg every 4 hours for 17 doses—a total of 18 doses. Dilute the drug three-to-one in juice or a beverage palatable to the patient. In an alert patient offer the diluted drug over ice in a covered container. The entire course of therapy must be administered to every patient with an acute ingestion and a toxic acetaminophen level, even if the plasma acetaminophen level becomes negative. NAC is being used to treat effects of the toxic metabolite, not the parent compound.

  b. Administration of NAC is often complicated by vomiting induced by the poisoning and NAC itself. If a dose of NAC is vomited within 1 hour of administration, the dose must be repeated. If an antiemetic is required, use metoclopramide or another antiemetic that does not require hepatic metabolism. If necessary for successful NAC administration, a duodenal tube may be passed with fluoroscopic placement.

  c. *Other treatment* includes daily monitoring of hepatic enzymes and symptomatic and supportive care.

7. **Special considerations** include the need for a high index of suspicion. Acetaminophen poisoning is perfectly treatable if recognized early but potentially fatal if untreated. Those who recover and have no clinical or laboratory evidence of hepatic injury are not expected to experience sequelae. Those who develop liver failure from this poisoning may undergo successful liver transplantation.

B. ANESTHETICS FOR TOPICAL USE

Anesthetics for topical use contain benzocaine, dibucaine, and lidocaine. They are found in prescription and nonprescription remedies, including teething lotions, first-aid creams, and drugs infiltrated into wounds prior to suturing. Children have died rapidly after ingestion of dibucaine.

1. Children experience the rapid onset of dysrhythmias, seizures, and methemoglobinemia after ingestion or absorption of these drugs. As little as several milligrams are sufficient for toxic effects to occur.

2. **Suspect methemoglobinemia** in patients who are cyanotic and do not respond to oxygen. Tentative diagnosis can be made by inspection of the blood. A drop of the patient's blood on a piece of filter paper appears brown next to a drop of "normal" blood. Laboratory confirmation reports a percent of methemoglobin, the amount of normal hemoglobin that has been converted to methemoglobin and therefore cannot transport oxygen.

3. **Specific treatment** for methemoglobinemia is the IV administration of methylene blue. Treatment for other toxic manifestations is symptomatic and supportive.

C. TRICYCLIC ANTIDEPRESSANTS

Tricyclic antidepressants include amitriptyline, clomipramine, desipramine, doxepin, imipramine, nortriptyline, and others, both singly and in combination with other psychotropic agents. There are no therapeutic indications and no safe doses for these drugs in very young children, who may have access to drugs belonging to an older sibling or other family member. Imipramine is used in the treatment of nocturnal enuresis in older children. The tricyclic antidepressants are used to treat depression in preteens and teenagers.

1. In general, these drugs are rapidly absorbed. In large ingestions, sufficient drug may be absorbed for its anticholinergic properties to inhibit gastric motility, therefore significant amounts of unabsorbed drug may remain within the GI tract. These drugs are widely distributed and highly protein bound.

2. Tricyclic antidepressants have several effects: anticholinergic, responsible for dry mouth, early hypertension, and the hallucinations that sometimes accompany overdose; delayed uptake of norepinephrine, accounting for these drugs' therapeutic utility and for some CNS and cardiac effects of overdose; membrane-depressant effects on the heart, resulting in conduction delays and dysrhythmias; and α-adrenergic blocking properties, resulting in the significant hypotension characteristic of this poisoning.

3. The **toxic dose** cannot be predicted with certainty. Any amount is potentially dangerous for infants, toddlers, and young children. For teenagers and adults the toxic amount is variable. Ambulance transport, GI tract decontamination, and at least 6 hours of emergency department evaluation are required for every ingestion in a young child and ingestions larger than a therapeutic dose in older children. A patient who develops any clinical signs of toxicity within the 6-hour observation period requires admission to a monitored bed until the patient has been asymptomatic for 24 hours.

4. A **classic presentation** of tricyclic antidepressant poisoning includes the rapid onset of grand mal seizures and coma, perhaps within 30 minutes of ingestion; hypotension; metabolic acidosis; and numerous dysrhythmias, especially ventricular dysrhythmias and conduction delays. Common electrocardiogram (ECG) findings are numerous and include prolonged PR and QRS intervals.

5. When **assessing the patient,** anticipate the need for intubation if the patient is still conscious. The most useful laboratory study is ABG analysis. Symptomatic patients are likely to develop acidosis that is resistant to correction. Laboratory measurement of drug and metabolite levels correlates loosely with expected toxicity but are not necessary for patient care because they are not used to determine treatment.

6. **Treatment** includes GI tract decontamination, maintaining serum pH between 7.45 and 7.55, cardiac monitoring, and treatment of hypotension, seizures, and dysrhythmias.

    a. Administer activated charcoal every 4 hours until the patient is asymptomatic.

    b. Sodium bicarbonate is the drug of choice to treat tricyclic antidepressant poisoning. Although hyperventilation is sometimes used to correct acidosis, sodium bicarbonate is preferred, since it appears to have therapeutic effects in addition to the correction of acidosis.

    c. Lidocaine is indicated for dysrhythmias unresponsive to a normalized pH. Diazepam may be used for seizures.

    d. Hypotension must be treated aggressively and may require invasive support if fluids, positioning, and norepinephrine are ineffective.

7. **Amoxapine** is a cyclic antidepressant that causes few cardiovascular effects after overdose, but is often associated with status epilepticus. An overdose of amoxapine requires aggressive seizure control, often including intubation and muscular paralysis.

D. **BENZODIAZEPINES**

Benzodiazepines are used as adjuncts to anesthesia and as anticonvulsants. Young children may have access to these drugs if taken therapeutically by family members. They may also be abused or self-administered in suicide attempts. In general, overdoses of these drugs can be successfully treated with respiratory support and, sometimes, the antidote flumazenil. (Flumazenil effectively reverses respiratory depression associated with benzodiazepine overdose, but there are contraindications [see below].) However, combining a benzodiazepine with ethanol or another CNS depressant significantly increases the risk of death.

1. Commonly prescribed benzodiazepines include alprazolam, oxazepam, diazepam (Valium), and chlordiazepoxide (Librium). Midazolam (Versed) is used as an adjunct to anesthesia.

2. Benzodiazepines act by enhancing the effects of γ-aminobutyric acid (GABA), an inhibitory neurotransmitter in the brain. The many types of drugs within the class make it impossible to generalize about absorption and elimination. Some of those prescribed for therapeutic use in the outpatient setting (e.g., diazepam) have a long half-life, therefore significant and prolonged respiratory depression should be anticipated in someone who abused the drug or took a large quantity.

3. **Effects of overdose** include respiratory and CNS depression. In an uncomplicated overdose, there are no specific drug-related laboratory values of use. In a potential mixed overdose, determination of coingestants is important.

4. **Flumazenil (Romazicon)** is the specific antidote. A test dose may be used to help determine if respiratory depression is caused by a benzodiazepine overdose, although it should not be used to maintain wakefulness. Caution must be used to avoid precipitating withdrawal in a patient dependent on a benzodiazepine. Flumazenil should never be used if the patient has also overdosed on a tricyclic antidepressant, as an increased risk of seizures has been associated with this use. Likewise, flumazenil should not be used if the patient is known to have a seizure disorder.

5. **Treatment** includes symptomatic and supportive care. If the patient is habituated to the drug, withdrawal symptoms may occur. A protocol to prevent acute withdrawal and accomplish gradual withdrawal must be implemented.

E. CALCIUM CHANNEL BLOCKERS

Calcium channel blockers include diltiazem, nicardipine, nifedipine, verapamil, and others, in regular and sustained-release preparations. As indications for their use in cardiovascular disease and other conditions have increased, poison exposures and fatalities in children have also increased. No antidote or universally effective treatment exists. Aggressive GI tract decontamination and vigorous supportive care are required.

1. Calcium channel blockers are easily absorbed from the GI tract. Elimination rates vary but can be prolonged for days after an overdose.

2. Most simply stated, calcium is required for cellular contraction. These drugs, therapeutically and in overdose, slow the influx of calcium through calcium channels into the intracellular space of cardiac nodal tissue, myocardial tissue, and vascular (especially arteriolar) tissue. The result is conduction delays, diminished cardiac output, and hypotension.

3. The **toxic dose** is variable but small. A single nifedipine tablet was thought responsible for the death of a 12-month-old child. The ingestion of any amount of any of these drugs should be considered potentially fatal in a child.

4. **Physical assessment** must be comprehensive. There are multiple mechanisms for hypotension (decreased cardiac output, diminished peripheral vascular resistance), hypoxia and apnea (bradydysrhythmias, heart block, decreased cardiac output), and metabolic acidosis (hypoperfusion, hypoxia). Also common are CNS depression, seizures, possibly hypoxic seizures, headache and

flushing, perhaps due to vasodilation, and hyperglycemia (calcium channel blockers inhibit insulin release). Electrolyte monitoring, ABG analysis, and continuous assessment of respiratory and cardiovascular status are needed.

5. **Treatment** begins with aggressive GI tract decontamination. Although gastric lavage and charcoal-cathartic administration are part of emergency department treatment, consider whole bowel irrigation for ingestion of multiple tablets or sustained-release preparations. IV calcium chloride or calcium gluconate is indicated, although it is not always effective. In a patient with stable electrolyte and acid-base status, calcium chloride is preferred, as it contains a higher concentration of calcium. (Extravasation of calcium chloride can cause tissue necrosis, so placement and patency of peripheral IV lines must be checked before each administration by this route.) Glucagon may be used to increase the heart rate and conduction velocity, although it too is not always effective. Otherwise, treatment is symptomatic and supportive.

6. Serum calcium levels, especially, must be monitored closely while treatment continues. No absolute change in the quantity of the patient's calcium stores occurs. A change in the distribution of calcium stores occurs.

F. **CHLOROQUINE**

Chloroquine is used widely to prevent and treat malaria and rarely for other medical conditions such as rheumatoid arthritis. It is rapidly absorbed and has a narrow therapeutic margin. Exposures are unintentional in children, suicidal in adults, and a result of therapeutic error in all ages (i.e., taking the drug daily rather than weekly, as indicated). Overdoses are infrequent, but hypotension, seizures, cardiorespiratory collapse, and death can occur within 30 to 60 minutes after ingestion. There is no antidote.

1. The **toxic dose** of chloroquine overlaps the therapeutic dose. Children have died after ingestion of less than 1 g.

2. If a patient survives to reach the ICU, **treatment** includes activated charcoal and a cathartic, if not already administered, and vigorous symptomatic and supportive respiratory, cardiac, and neurologic care. Epinephrine and diazepam are the drugs of choice for cardiac effects and seizures. Close monitoring of electrolytes is necessary. Patients are often hypokalemic.

G. **DIGITALIS**

Digitalis overdoses in the pediatric population are usually acute, although chronic intoxication may occur. Children may have access to their own drugs or those of family members. Pediatric therapeutic doses must be carefully calculated and measured, and blood levels must be carefully monitored. Some plants contain cardiac glycosides with digitalis-like effects if ingested, including foxglove *(Digitalis purpurea)* and oleander *(Nerium oleander)*. Poisoning by these plants is treated as for digitalis poisoning.

1. Digitalis is usually rapidly absorbed and is excreted renally.

2. The **toxic effects** of digitalis are exacerbations of therapeutic effects. Digitalis interferes with the Na^+-K^+-ATPase pump, found in smooth muscle and abundantly in cardiac tissue. Therapeutically, this maintains the correct proportions of intracellular and interstitial sodium, potassium, and calcium necessary for cellular contraction and nodal conduction. When the Na^+-K^+-ATPase pump is poisoned by toxic concentrations of digitalis, intracellular calcium levels rise, intracellular potassium is depleted, and serum potassium levels become markedly elevated. (However, when digitalis is administered for a long period of time in conjunction with diuretics, patients may present with hypokalemia.) Any and every dysrhythmia can result. Atrial dysrhythmias, bradycardia, and heart block are most common, along with ventricular irritability and hypotension.

3. A **toxic dose** can be estimated by history, but there is no substitute for laboratory

evaluation of serum levels and careful evaluation of the patient. The therapeutic range is 0.5 to 2 ng/ml, but toxicity can occur within this range.

4. **Clinical effects of acute overdose** are GI and cardiovascular: nausea, vomiting, hypotension, bradycardia, and dysrhythmias. In chronic overdose, visual changes are also described, especially yellow or green "haloes" or "hazes." Laboratory evaluation of electrolytes, especially potassium, and renal function is needed, along with the serum digitalis level. Continuous cardiac monitoring is essential.

5. **Treatment of digitalis overdose** includes prevention of absorption, intensive monitoring, administration of the antidote, and symptomatic and supportive care.

   a. GI tract decontamination is indicated, with administration of multiple doses of activated charcoal to enhance clearance of digitalis.

   b. Usual measures are indicated to treat bradycardia and other dysrhythmias, hypotension, and hyperkalemia.

   c. Administration of the antidote Digibind, digoxin immune Fab fragments, quickly reverses severe hyperkalemia and life-threatening dysrhythmias. IV administration of 40 mg of digoxin immune Fab fragments (1 vial) binds 0.6 mg of digitalis. The poison center can help make other dose determinations if the amount of ingested digitalis is not available. Patients in renal failure may need dialysis to remove the digoxin immune Fab fragment complex.

   d. If the antidote is not available, standard but aggressive treatment is needed to treat hyperkalemia (insulin, glucose, and sodium bicarbonate), support blood pressure, and treat dysrhythmias. Patients in renal failure require dialysis to remove digitalis.

   e. Monitoring serum digitalis levels can be confusing after antidote administration, as some laboratory methods measure and report a concentration that includes both free digitalis and that bound to Fab fragments. It is necessary to know if reported digitalis levels are of free digitalis only. (This is especially important for patients treated therapeutically with digitalis who must remain digitalized.)

H. DIPHENOXYLATE AND ATROPINE

Diphenoxylate-atropine combinations (e.g., Lomotil) are used to treat diarrhea in adults. There is no safe amount of this drug for young children. The combination of powerful opioid and anticholinergic effects is the reason for both its therapeutic usefulness in adults and its danger in children.

1. The **anticholinergic effects** of atropine cause this drug to be retained in the GI tract for prolonged periods of time. The onset of opioid effects can be delayed for as long as 24 hours after ingestion.

2. Every child who ingests any amount of this drug must be monitored in an ICU for 24 hours.

3. **Treatment** includes GI tract decontamination, symptomatic and supportive care, and careful monitoring for the onset of CNS and respiratory depression induced by diphenoxylate, the opioid component of this drug. Naloxone is effective for symptoms of opioid overdose.

I. ORAL HYPOGLYCEMIC AGENTS

Oral hypoglycemic agents, including glyburide and glipizide, can cause the delayed onset of significant hypoglycemia in children, even in single-tablet ingestions. Every young child who swallows even one of these pills requires GI tract decontamination and admission, with frequent serum glucose determinations, for 24 hours. If hypoglycemia occurs, treat with IV glucose. Glucagon may be ineffective because small children have little stored glycogen.

J.   IMIDAZOLINE DERIVATIVES

Imidazoline derivatives are available to children in the form of clonidine, an antihypertensive, and such ocular and nasal vasoconstrictors as tetrahydrozoline, naphazoline, and oxymetazoline. All are α_2-agonists with mixed central and peripheral effects. A single tablet of clonidine, inadvertent application of even a used clonidine patch, and just several drops of the other drugs can cause the onset of coma, respiratory depression, and hypotension within 30 minutes of ingestion (or topical application, for liquid vasoconstrictors and decongestants). GI tract decontamination is indicated for solid dosage forms. Symptomatic and supportive care is required for 24 to 36 hours, and recovery is expected.

K.   IRON

Iron in the form of adult-strength supplements and prenatal vitamins with iron is a leading cause of poisoning death in children younger than 6 years of age. These preparations typically contain 60 to 65 mg of elemental iron per tablet, although some contain more than 100 mg of elemental iron. Iron supplements are sometimes used in suicide attempts by others, especially pregnant teenagers. (Overdoses of children's chewable multiple vitamin with iron preparations may cause iron and vitamin A toxicity, but have not been associated with iron-related fatalities in children.) The use of deferoxamine, a specific antidote, is important but may be limited in serious iron poisoning because of side effects, especially hypotension.

1. In **overdose,** iron causes significant corrosive injury to the GI tract. Absorption of iron is thus enhanced. Circulating free iron injures blood vessels and damages hepatocytes. As iron is metabolized, free hydrogen is released; in concert with other events, this produces metabolic acidosis.

2. **Mild symptoms** may occur with ingestion of more than 20 mg/kg of essential iron. Significant toxicity or death is possible with ingestions of more than 60 mg/kg; this amount of iron can be ingested by a 10-kg child who swallows just 10 typical adult-strength preparations. The amount of essential iron in each iron salt varies, and the potential risk is calculated by determining the iron salt and the amount of essential iron in each preparation, the number of pills missing, and the child's body weight. Actual risk is determined by serum iron levels and the presence or absence of symptoms.

3. The **course of severe iron poisoning** is described in steps, although it must be remembered that individual patients may not follow this outline precisely:

   a. *Phase I,* about 30 minutes to 2 hours after ingestion: GI tract symptoms, possibly severe, include hemorrhagic gastritis, vomiting, hematemesis, diarrhea, lethargy, and pallor.

   b. *Phase II,* about 2 to 10 or 12 hours after ingestion, is a latent phase during which the patient is asymptomatic. The systemic insults described above occur during this asymptomatic phase, and the patient abruptly enters phase III.

   c. *Phase III,* about 12 to about 48 hours after ingestion, involves a rapid onset of cardiovascular collapse. Hypotension, increasing lethargy and coma, seizures, pulmonary edema, hepatorenal failure with coagulopathies, and hypoglycemia, occur. Death may occur rapidly or after days or weeks of complications, including intestinal necrosis.

   d. *Phase IV,* about 6 weeks after exposure: Patients who survive the acute episode may require surgery for severe pyloric scarring.

4. **Assessment** of these patients includes careful evaluation of physical findings and laboratory results. Determine the nature of any symptoms and the time of onset compared with time of ingestion.

   a. *Initial laboratory studies* include serum iron level drawn 2 hours or more after ingestion, total iron binding capacity (though there is some disagreement about the utility of this measure in serious iron poisoning, as it can become falsely elevated), complete blood count (CBC), and electrolytes. Patients with more than mild GI tract symptoms also require ABG analysis, determination of electrolyte status, and baseline hepatic and renal function studies. Typing and crossmatch are indicated if there is frank bleeding or guaiac-positive stools.

   b. Iron tablets (not pediatric chewable vitamins with iron) are radiopaque. An abdominal flat plate may permit counting of tablets in the child's GI tract. (A flat plate demonstrating negative findings cannot be used to rule out iron ingestion.)

5. **Treatment** of the iron-poisoned child includes GI tract decontamination, chelation with deferoxamine, and symptomatic and supportive care.

   a. GI tract decontamination may begin with ipecac syrup if available in the home. Otherwise, gastric lavage and whole bowel irrigation are indicated. If an abdominal x-ray examination demonstrates iron pills in the intestinal tract, whole bowel irrigation is called for until the appropriate number of pills are counted in the rectal effluent or until a repeat x-ray examination documents that the pills have been removed. Iron is not adsorbed to activated charcoal.

   b. *Chelation* is required if the serum iron level is greater than 350 µg/dl in the presence of symptoms, or if the serum iron is greater than 500 µg/dl. Deferoxamine is administered intravenously. (Although the drug may be administered intramuscularly, this is inappropriate for the iron-poisoned child who is likely to be hypovolemic and hypotensive.) The usual dose of deferoxamine is 15 mg/kg/h. Higher doses are sometimes used, but may be associated with hypotension. "Vin rosé"–colored urine, if it occurs, is a marker for elimination of deferoxamine-iron chelate, but this does not always appear and cannot be relied on. Serum iron levels are more accurate.

   c. Serum iron levels must be repeated until it is certain that levels are dropping and that there is not a concretion, or clump, of iron tablets being slowly absorbed from the GI tract.

   d. Symptomatic and supportive care is otherwise required, but such measures must be aggressive to stop GI tract bleeding, treat hypovolemia and hypotension, and treat coagulopathies and other consequences of hepatic failure.

   e. There are two special dangers associated with iron poisoning. Parents and health care providers alike often think of iron as "just" a vitamin and are ignorant of the fact that quite small amounts of this essential element can cause fatalities in children. The asymptomatic latent phase of iron poisoning fools parents and health care providers who misinterpret the absence of symptoms as absence of risk.

L. ISONIAZID

Isoniazid (INH) is used to treat tuberculosis. Young children may have access to the drug, and it is used in suicide attempts by teenagers.

1. Isoniazid, given therapeutically or taken in overdose, depletes the body of pyridoxine (vitamin B_6). Pyridoxine is a cofactor in numerous enzymatic reactions, including those responsible for the generation of GABA. GABA is an inhibitory neurotransmitter in the CNS; depletion of GABA leads to seizures.

2. An **overdose** of INH precipitates the onset of grand mal seizures, perhaps within 30 minutes of ingestion, and the subsequent development of significant acidosis.

3. The only effective **treatment** for INH-induced seizures is IV pyridoxine. If the dose of INH is known, the dose of pyridoxine is a milligram-per-milligram

equivalent. If the dose is unknown, pyridoxine, 5 g IV, should be administered. Diazepam is an effective adjunct, as it enhances the action of GABA, but it cannot assist with synthesis of GABA and is not a substitute for pyridoxine.

4. Once seizures are controlled, GI tract decontamination can be carried out. Acidosis often corrects itself once seizures are controlled, but is amenable to the usual therapies. Treatment otherwise is symptomatic and supportive.

M. OPIOIDS

Opioids are found in a variety of prescription preparations and street drugs. Because the ICU nurse is familiar with the administration of opioid analgesics and antitussives, this section simply emphasizes a few points related to overdose.

1. The **classic triad of symptoms** (miosis, respiratory depression, and coma) may be masked by concomitant administration of other drugs. Abusers of stimulant drugs such as cocaine and amphetamines frequently use an opioid or other depressant simultaneously. Opioids may be abused inadvertently when drug dealers substitute them for or combine them with other drugs.

2. Young children can be markedly sensitive to some opioids. Dangerous situations may occur when parents both administer a codeine-containing antitussive or when the older sibling of a teething infant helps himself—or the infant—to paregoric (tincture of opium).

3. Some opioids are associated with **clinically significant differences:**
   a. Meperidine (Demerol) use or abuse is not necessarily associated with pin-point pupils. Also, normeperidine, the first metabolite of meperidine, is a CNS stimulant; chronic use or abuse is therefore associated with seizures.
   b. Propoxyphene (Darvon) and pentazocine (Talwin) may require up to 10 mg of naloxone to reverse the respiratory depression they induce, much higher than the usual naloxone dose of 0.01 mg/kg.
   c. Methadone has a half-life of about 24 hours, much longer than other opioids, and requires sustained doses of naloxone, by IV drip, to prevent respiratory depression until the methadone is eliminated. (Nalmefene hydrochloride, a newer opioid antagonist, has a longer half-life than naloxone, but its use in children has not yet been evaluated.)

N. SALICYLATE POISONING

Salicylate poisoning is most often due to aspirin. However, most fatal salicylate poisoning in children is from ingestion of methyl salicylate, a rapidly-absorbed liquid also known as oil of wintergreen. Another common source of salicylate ingestion in children is GI tract preparations containing bismuth subsalicylate. Older children and teenagers take aspirin in suicide attempts.

1. Aspirin is rapidly absorbed. In therapeutic doses, it has a small volume of distribution and much is bound to serum proteins. It undergoes hepatic metabolism and renal excretion. With chronic administration, receptors are saturated and free salicylate accumulates rapidly.

2. The **actions of salicylate in overdose** are complex and interdependent. Stimulation of the central respiratory drive causes respiratory alkalosis and metabolic acidosis. Interference with carbohydrate and lipid metabolism generates organic acids. Increased metabolic demands result in hypoglycemia, both in the serum and the CNS. Uncoupling of oxidative phosphorylation leads to hyperthermia. Direct CNS toxicity can cause tremor, agitation, seizures, and coma. Sequence and exact clinical effects depend on size, timing, and acuity of ingestion and the age and health of the patient. A careful evaluation of each patient's status and history is essential.

3. **Acute toxicity** generally correlates with ingested dose. Greater than 150 mg/kg by history may be associated with mild toxicity, greater than 300 mg/kg with greater toxicity, and greater than 500 mg/kg with fatality. More specific

determination is based on a serum salicylate level drawn 6 or more hours after ingestion.

4. In the absence of history, suspect salicylate poisoning in a patient who presents with tachypnea, tachycardia, hyperthermia, diaphoresis, mental status changes, respiratory alkalosis, metabolic acidosis, or mixed acid-base abnormalities. If present, tinnitus is an important clue, as is frank or occult GI tract bleeding.

5. **Treatment** includes gastric evacuation followed by multiple doses of activated charcoal administered every 4 hours with a cathartic once in 24 hours. Hydration is essential, but must be controlled to avoid precipitating pulmonary edema. Potassium supplementation is often needed. Administer sufficient amounts of sodium bicarbonate to correct acidosis and achieve a urine pH of about 8; this enhances renal excretion of salicylate. Hemodialysis is indicated for salicylate levels above about 100 mg/dl in acute ingestions (lower in patients with chronic ingestions) and seriously symptomatic patients. Otherwise, treatment must be aggressive but is symptomatic and supportive.

6. **Special considerations**
   a. Aspirin tablets readily clump together in the stomach, forming concretions that may be slowly absorbed over a prolonged period of time. If a large ingestion is suspected, it is essential to measure serial salicylate levels to avoid the delayed onset of fatal effects. Ingestion of sustained-release forms of aspirin also can cause the delayed onset of symptoms. Again, it is essential to monitor serial salicylate levels.
   b. Because the time between ingestion and death from salicylate poisoning can often be measured in just hours, a high index of suspicion and aggressive management are essential to prevent serious CNS effects and fatalities.

O. SYMPATHOMIMETICS

Sympathomimetic drugs are represented by both legal and illegal agents in the pediatric age group: cocaine is a legal, useful topical vasoconstrictor and a widely abused street drug; amphetamines are used as weight control agents, to treat hyperactivity disorders, and as the street drug "speed"; legal decongestants and appetite suppressants such as phenylpropanolamine are sold as "street speed" or amphetamine look-alikes. Children are poisoned by ingesting appetite suppressants or an overdose of cough, cold, or allergy preparations containing decongestants and by swallowing available street drugs. Teenagers are poisoned by taking overdoses of appetite suppressants, by abusing street drugs, or by attempting to avoid arrest by swallowing illicit drugs. The intended use, route of administration, and duration of action of these drugs may differ, but the acute clinical effects are indistinguishable, and treatment of acute effects is essentially the same. (Discussion of the numerous known medical consequences of cocaine and amphetamine abuse is beyond the scope of this review.)

1. The **toxic dose** is variable. Response to phenylpropanolamine may be idiosyncratic, with amounts above 50 mg associated with hypertension in some children. In street drugs, the actual amount of drug, as opposed to adulterants, is unknown.

2. **Clinical effects** are as expected for any sympathomimetic agent: tachycardia, hypertension, diaphoresis, mydriasis, agitation and tremulousness, and central vasoconstriction—including cardiac, cerebral, and visceral. In significant poisoning, ventricular dysrhythmias, seizures, hyperthermia, and coma may develop.

3. **Clinical assessment and laboratory evaluation** are straightforward. When possible, identification of the drug involved helps predict duration of effects: a few hours for cocaine unless complicated by cardiac, cerebral, or other events

caused by vasoconstriction, hyperthermia, or seizures; 18 to 24 hours for amphetamines, with the same caveat; variable for the other drugs, and dependent to some extent on whether they are sustained-release preparations. Although x-ray examinations are not generally indicated in poisoning by sympathomimetic drugs, in the case of swallowed illegal drugs they may help visualize the number and location of the packets.

4. **Treatment** of these poisonings includes GI tract decontamination where indicated, then symptomatic and supportive care. A single dose of activated charcoal with a cathartic is indicated unless drug packets (e.g., vials, condoms, balloons, or foil) have been swallowed. In these cases, multiple doses of activated charcoal are indicated until the packets pass.

P. **THEOPHYLLINE**

Theophylline, a drug with a very narrow therapeutic index, is available in standard and sustained-release preparations. Any overdose is potentially dangerous, but chronic overdoses and acute overdoses in a patient receiving long-term therapy are especially dangerous, with symptoms occurring at lower serum levels than in acute ingestions.

1. The **mechanisms of toxicity** of theophylline are not all understood. Among theophylline's actions are alterations in electrolyte balance, especially intracellular vs. extracellular potassium concentrations and resultant dysrhythmias; increased amounts of circulating endogenous catecholamines; and cardiovascular effects, including a decrease in peripheral vascular resistance.

2. There is **individual variability in toxic doses,** and a blood level is much more useful. A therapeutic level is 10 to 20 µg/ml. In some patients, symptoms of toxicity may occur at the upper end of that range. Levels above 40 µg/ml predict moderate toxicity after an acute overdose but may be associated with much more serious symptoms in a long-term user. Dangerous or fatal effects are associated with levels of 100 µg/ml after acute overdose and at lower levels with long-term use.

3. **Clinical effects** include nausea and vomiting, anxiety, tremor, tachycardia, and sometimes other dysrhythmias. Some patients may present with seizures and hypotension in the absence of significant prodromal signs. Expected laboratory abnormalities include hypokalemia, hyperglycemia, and metabolic acidosis in severe poisonings.

4. **Treatment** must be aggressive to prevent CNS and cardiovascular effects.
   a. Gastric emptying should be thorough if the patient presents soon enough after an acute overdose. In the ICU, monitor for increasing blood levels, which may indicate that a drug concretion has not been removed or that sustained-release tablets are in the bowel.
   b. Multiple doses of activated charcoal lower the serum theophylline level, even if the level is elevated because of iatrogenic overdose of IV theophylline or if no pills remain in the bowel.
   c. Hemodialysis is indicated for acute overdoses with levels greater than 80 µg/ml, chronic overdoses with levels greater than 40 to 60 µg/ml, and patients who are seriously symptomatic (e.g., with seizures, acidosis, and coma), regardless of the level.
   d. Hypokalemia must be corrected gently, as the problem is distribution of potassium between the intracellular and interstitial spaces, not absolute hypokalemia. Hydration must be maintained.
   e. Other treatment is symptomatic and supportive.

5. **Special consideration:** Patients receiving maintenance theophylline therapy can easily develop toxicity. Suspect theophylline toxicity in anyone taking the drug who develops symptoms after beginning a new drug, changing drug regimens, or becoming ill.

POISONING BY NONPHARMACEUTICAL AGENTS

A. **CARBON MONOXIDE**

Carbon monoxide is a colorless, odorless, tasteless, nonirritating gas—a product of incomplete combustion. The most common residential sources are house fires, exhaust from automobiles and gas-powered equipment, furnaces, space heaters, wood- and coal-burning stoves and fireplaces, and gas ovens and hot water heaters. Methylene chloride, found in paint strippers, is metabolized to carbon monoxide after ingestion, inhalation, or dermal absorption.

1. Carbon monoxide has an affinity for hemoglobin 200 times greater than that of oxygen. Besides displacing oxygen at hemoglobin receptor sites, it inhibits the release of oxygen from hemoglobin. Therefore, inadequate amounts of oxygen are circulating, and that which is circulating is less available to tissues.

2. The **effects of carbon monoxide poisoning** are related to hypoxemia; the greater the amount of carboxyhemoglobin, the more severe the symptoms. Direct cellular toxicity also occurs. A carboxyhemoglobin level of about 10% is associated with headache, nausea, and lethargy. As the carboxyhemoglobin level increases, GI tract and CNS symptoms increase. At a level of 50% the patient is unconscious, and victims of carbon monoxide exposure die at levels of about 70% or greater. Symptoms of chronic carbon monoxide exposure (e.g., due to malfunctioning furnaces or clogged chimneys), are often mistaken for a viral or flulike illness.

3. **Evaluating** victims of carbon monoxide poisoning requires close attention to symptoms experienced at any time since exposure, not just at the time of evaluation. The carboxyhemoglobin level at the time of presentation may have declined markedly since the patient was exposed. After an acute exposure to carbon monoxide, those who have lost consciousness, even if they are now awake, and fetuses are at greatest risk.

4. The **initial treatment** for carbon monoxide poisoning is 100% oxygen. Hyperbaric oxygen is indicated for those who were or are unconscious, pregnant women, those who remain symptomatic after oxygen administration, and those with recurrent symptoms.

5. **Psychometric testing** should be arranged for teenagers who have had significant exposures. (These studies generally are not conducted in young children. Wide variability in normal development makes them difficult or impossible to interpret.)

6. Other treatment is symptomatic and supportive.

7. **Special considerations**
   a. Children and household pets are at greatest risk for carbon monoxide poisoning because of their rapid respiratory and metabolic rates. When a family is poisoned by carbon monoxide, children are generally more seriously ill.
   b. *Aggressive treatment* is required because long-term neuropsychiatric sequelae have been documented in adults with carbon monoxide exposure. Because of the difficulty or impossibility of conducting and interpreting such tests in children, long-term sequelae are postulated but not documented.
   c. Consider carbon monoxide poisoning in any family or gathering in which a number of people become ill with GI tract and CNS complaints.
   d. Unless the source of carbon monoxide is known (e.g., suicide attempt with automobile exhaust, house fire) or remedied (e.g., repair of a faulty furnace), patients and their families may not return to a possibly contaminated environment.
   e. Encourage the installation of carbon monoxide detectors.

B. Caustic Substances

Caustic substances are those which can cause chemical burns. Young children are injured by unintentional contact with household substances, whereas older children may ingest these substances in suicide attempts. Occasionally, children are exposed when they attempt unsupervised experiments. Strongly acidic and alkaline substances can cause chemical burns. While the sources and mechanisms of injury are different, treatment and nursing care for both are essentially the same. The single exception is hydrofluoric acid, which is considered separately.

1. **Sources**
    a. *Acids* such as sulfuric acid, hydrochloric acid, and muriatic acid (dilute hydrochloric acid) are found in homes in toilet bowl cleaners, swimming pool chemicals, metal cleaners, and concrete and masonry cleaners. These products tend to be liquids and are associated with greater injury to the stomach than to the esophagus after ingestion.
    b. *Alkaline substances* are liquids or solids found in wet cement, drain openers, oven cleaners, laundry detergent, and automatic dishwasher detergent. Examples include sodium hydroxide, potassium hydroxide, calcium hydroxide, sodium carbonate, and some phosphates. Children who bite into ammonia capsules are likely to develop an alkaline burn to the tip of the tongue.

2. **Mechanism of injury**
    a. Acids precipitate proteins and dehydrate tissues; exposure causes vascular thrombosis and the rapid formation of eschar. This hard crust helps limit further penetration of acid into tissue. In general, serious injury is associated with exposure to products with a pH lower than 2.
    b. Alkaline substances cause vascular thrombosis and liquefaction necrosis. They disrupt cell walls and combine with lipids. This accounts for the soapy appearance of tissue and provides no protection whatever from further penetration of the chemical into tissue. In general, serious injury is associated with products with a pH higher than 12.

3. The **degree of injury** is determined by several factors. In addition to pH, the physical form of the substance may influence toxicity: liquid products transit the oropharynx and esophagus quickly and may cause the greatest injury to the stomach. However, a very viscous liquid may cause significantly higher injury. Solids and crystals are associated with injury to the lips, mouth, oropharynx, and esophagus. Duration of contact with tissue also influences the extent of injury. The presence of food and liquid in the stomach minimizes the amount and duration of contact between the caustic substance and the gastric mucosa.

4. **Ocular and dermal exposure** to caustic substances require copious irrigation with saline or water as indicated earlier in this chapter. If there are any symptoms after irrigation, ocular exposures to caustic substances require ophthalmologic consultation. After initial irrigation, dermal exposures to caustic substances are treated as thermal burns of similar degree.

5. After **ingestion of a caustic product,** there is no strict correlation between presence or absence of symptoms (including pain) and presence, location, or degree of injury.
    a. Mild effects of inflammation and irritation, similar to a first-degree thermal burn, require only symptomatic and supportive care.
    b. Partial- or full-thickness injuries are the equivalent of second- and third-degree thermal injuries. With ingestion of an acid (generally a liquid), there is risk of gastric perforation within about 3 days of ingestion. Otherwise, the risk of perforation is greatest during the granulation phase, perhaps up to

2 weeks. Then, the development of scar tissue and esophageal stricture commences.

  c. Initial pain may be oral, substernal, or epigastric.

6. **Assessment of the patient** includes visual inspection of exposed tissue, evaluation of acid-base and fluid and electrolyte status, determination of hemoglobin and hematocrit, and perhaps x-ray examinations to determine the presence or absence of free air.

7. **Treatment**

  a. Dilution with a small volume of water helps minimize contact between the caustic substance and tissue. Large volumes are not indicated because that would increase the risk of vomiting, with esophageal reinjury and the possibility of aspiration.

  b. Observe for respiratory distress. Soft tissue swelling and aspiration of caustic material can contribute to respiratory difficulty. If significant edema is present, oral or nasotracheal intubation is dangerous, and a tracheotomy or cricothyrotomy is needed.

  c. Observe for signs of fluid and electrolyte imbalance to evaluate loss of fluids or third-spacing of fluids.

  d. Observe for acidosis if the patient has ingested a large quantity of an acid, as may occur in a suicide attempt. Although direct injury is generally confined to points of contact with the chemical, acidosis is one possible systemic manifestation associated with acid ingestion.

  e. Esophagoscopy may be performed within a few hours or within the first 2 days. If the initial injury is thought to be severe or if circumferential burns are found on esophagoscopy, additional surgical procedures may be indicated. Gastrostomy may be performed to remove necrotic tissue, place a string or stent in the esophagus, or place a gastric feeding tube. Esophagectomy and colonic interposition (removing the esophagus and replacing it with a length of the patient's own colon) may also be performed.

  f. The use of steroids is controversial and depends on the preference and experience of individual gastroenterologists and surgeons. Steroids may decrease formation of restrictive scar tissue after circumferential burns but may also weaken tissue and predispose the patient to infection.

  g. Antibiotics are prescribed for patients taking steroids and for patients with specific indications.

  h. Observe the patient for signs of perforation and sepsis. Perforation may be accompanied by abdominal distention and a change in the amount or character of the patient's pain.

  i. Analgesics are indicated.

  j. Patients must remain NPO until esophagoscopy is performed.

8. **Special considerations**

  a. Until the patient is decontaminated, health care providers must avoid contact with caustic material.

  b. If the patient has sustained a serious injury, psychosocial considerations for the patient and the family come to the forefront. Ocular and dermal exposures may cause significant disfigurement, and ocular exposures may result in permanent blindness. Ingestion with significant injury means that the patient may require permanent tracheostomy or gastrostomy or both, major surgery and follow-up for esophagectomy and colonic interposition, or regular esophageal dilation for many years to come. Also, the risk of developing cancer at the site of the injury, although delayed for decades, is greater than in the general population.

9. **Hydrofluoric acid** is different from other acids, and indeed from other caustic

agents, in that it is absorbed dermally, even through intact skin, and can cause both local and systemic effects. It is used industrially to etch glass and computer chips, as a cleaning agent for metals and air-conditioning units, and as a rust remover. Products with low (but potentially dangerous) concentrations of hydrofluoric acid are sold for home use. Hydrofluoric acid is toxic by all routes of exposure, but dermal exposure is the most common and is discussed here.

a. In concentrations above 50%, hydrofluoric acid causes immediate local tissue injury along with significant pain. In concentrations between 20% to 50%, the onset of local injury and pain can be delayed for 8 hours or longer. In concentrations lower than 20%, effects of exposure may not be evident for 24 hours.

b. Hydrofluoric acid is absorbed through the skin and precipitates both calcium and magnesium. The result is intense pain at the site of the exposure. With significant exposure, systemic hypocalcemia, hypomagnesemia, hyperkalemia, and possibly fatal ventricular dysrhythmias are present.

c. Initial treatment is copious irrigation with running water, even in the absence of local effects. With exposure to the hands, subungual concentrations of hydrofluoric acid may be difficult to remove and often necessitate removal or splitting of the nails or injection of calcium (discussed below).

d. Treatment of local pain can be initiated with submersion in an iced magnesium sulfate solution (25% solution). A calcium gluconate gel, prepared by mixing 3.5 g of calcium gluconate powder in 5 oz of water-soluble gel (Goldfrank et al, 1994), is applied to painful areas until the pain subsides. When pain recurs, additional gel is applied. The patient should apply the gel liberally at home if pain recurs and return for further care if the gel ceases to be effective.

e. More serious exposures may be treated with intradermal injection or intraarterial infusion of calcium gluconate. Even minimal dermal exposure to high concentrations of hydrofluoric acid may cause systemic hypocalcemia. These patients must be admitted to monitored beds, and serial calcium levels must be closely monitored until it is certain the patient is out of danger.

C. **CYANIDE**

Cyanide is thought of as a fast-acting lethal poison, but there are circumstances when a slower onset of symptoms is possible. Treatment involves supportive care and the rapid administration of the antidote, the Taylor Pharmaceuticals Cyanide Antidote Package.

1. There are many **potential sources** of cyanide poisoning. Victims of fires may develop cyanide poisoning along with carbon monoxide poisoning. A number of plant seeds (apples, peaches, plums, pears, nectarines, and cherries) contain amygdalin, which generates hydrogen cyanide after ingestion. Laetrile, an ineffective treatment for cancer, is derived from apricot kernels and has caused death due to cyanide poisoning. Cyanide is a metabolite of nitroprusside; rapid or prolonged treatment can cause symptoms of cyanide poisoning. (Cyanide and thiocyanate levels should be monitored.) Nonoccupational cyanide poisoning in adults and teenagers is likely to result from suicidal ingestion of laboratory or photographic chemicals. Children have died rapidly after swallowing professional jewelry cleaning solutions containing cyanide. Acetonitrile, which is metabolized to cyanide, is found in liquids used to dissolve artificial fingernail glue; delayed onset of symptoms and death have occurred when this product was swallowed.

2. Cyanide interferes with the action of cytochrome oxidase and therefore with aerobic metabolism and cellular utilization of oxygen. It is likely that other enzyme systems are affected as well.

3. The **toxic dose** depends on the form of the chemical and route of administration. Small amounts of cyanide salts can cause rapid loss of consciousness and death. Substances that are metabolized to cyanide (e.g., amygdalin glycosides, acetonitrile, and nitroprusside) have a delayed onset of action, and the toxic dose is variable.

4. **Clinical effects** are related to hypoxia and typically progress within minutes from dizziness and headache to coma and death. Acidosis and hypotension are prominent. Patients with lesser exposures and those exposed to substances that must be metabolized have a less precipitous onset of symptoms.

5. **ABGs** must be followed closely. Cyanide can be measured in serum, but levels cannot be returned in time to be useful for acutely poisoned patients.

6. **Antidotal treatment** is with the three-part Taylor Pharmaceuticals Cyanide Antidote Package. First, methemoglobin is induced with nitrites; cyanmethemoglobin is formed as cyanide is thus removed from cytochrome oxidase. Administration of sodium thiosulfate results in the formation of relatively nontoxic thiocyanate.

   a. Amyl nitrite ampules are broken, placed in a cloth, and held in front of the patient's mouth for 15 out of 30 seconds, then repeated. This permits the formation of about 5% methemoglobin. This step may be skipped in favor of immediate administration of IV sodium nitrite.

   b. Sodium nitrite induces the formation of additional methemoglobin. The desired level of methemoglobin is 20% to no more than 40%. In children, the amount of sodium nitrite is calculated according to body weight and titrated to actual hemoglobin levels. Doses must be carefully calculated, since inducing too high a level of methemoglobinemia worsens hypoxia. High levels cannot be treated with methylene blue, as that would liberate free cyanide!

   c. Sodium thiosulfate in the presence of cyanmethemoglobin results in the formation of thiocyanate, which is eliminated renally.

   d. *Treatment* also includes respiratory support and symptomatic and supportive care.

7. **Special considerations**

   a. Too high a level of methemoglobin can itself be fatal. Pediatric doses of nitrites must be carefully calculated, and methemoglobin levels must be monitored.

   b. Brain-dead victims of cyanide poisoning may be considered as organ donors.

D. ENVENOMATIONS

Envenomations by snakes and spiders cannot be considered in depth in this book. Always consult the poison center when treating a patient with a snake or spider bite. All venoms are extremely complex mixtures, and any bite resulting in symptoms indicates a serious poisoning with the potential for multisystemic effects. Children are at greater risk than adults because of their small body size in relationship to the amount of venom injected.

1. The **venom of the Crotalidae** (rattlesnakes, copperheads, and cottonmouths [water moccasins]) can cause the rapid onset of life-threatening effects, although this is not expected with bites of copperheads and cottonmouths. Action at numerous venom receptors results in hypotension, increased capillary permeability resulting in local ecchymosis and edema, pulmonary edema, local tissue injury, myocardial injury, and bleeding and clotting disorders. Local wound care and intensive supportive care are both essential. Definitive antidotal treatment is the administration of polyvalent crotalid antivenin. There is no substitute for administration of sufficient quantities of antivenin in a patient poisoned by a rattlesnake. Common treatment errors include withholding

antivenin in a patient with a life- or limb-threatening envenomation for fear of allergic reactions and performing fasciotomy in lieu of administering sufficient antivenin in patients with peripheral edema.

2. The **venom of the Elapidae** (the coral snakes) can cause fatal poisoning by its neuromuscular effects, specifically, respiratory muscle paralysis. Onset of symptoms is delayed for 6 to 8 hours after envenomation. Fortunately, such fatalities are extremely rare. Treatment includes the administration of antivenin and respiratory support.

3. The **venom of the black widow spider** (*Lactrodectus mactans*) also can cause paralysis of respiratory muscles, although this is not usual. More common effects are immediate, intense pain at the site of the bite (which can be identified by two tiny fang marks, about 0.5 cm [¼ in] apart); muscle weakness, ataxia, and ptosis, especially in children; and intensely painful muscle contractions, across the abdomen for lower extremity bites and across the back and shoulders for upper extremity bites. Treatment includes administration of calcium and a muscle relaxant, typically methocarbamol. Antivenin is available, but its use is usually required only for very young children and the elderly.

E. ETHANOL

Ethanol is found in alcoholic beverages, mouthwash, and cosmetics such as perfumes, tonics, and hair spray. It is used therapeutically as the antidote for ethylene glycol and methanol poisoning. Young children are poisoned unintentionally or by adults who give them alcoholic beverages. Preteens and teenagers may indulge in binge drinking and may be alcohol dependent. In these cases, they are as vulnerable as adults to atrial dysrhythmias following binges and to medical and behavioral consequences of alcoholism.

1. Ethanol is rapidly absorbed and widely distributed. It is well known as a CNS depressant. In children, ethanol's hypoglycemic effects are significant; the immature liver does not maintain sufficient glycogen stores to counteract ethanol-induced hypoglycemia.

2. **Symptoms** related to ethanol-induced CNS depression are lethargy, ataxia, respiratory depression, hypothermia, and coma. These effects may begin within an hour of ingestion, followed within a few hours by hypoglycemic seizures, coma, and death. Metabolic acidosis may be present in large ingestions.

3. **Toxicity** may occur with an ethanol ingestion of 1 g/kg. This may be roughly estimated as the amount of alcoholic product ingested multiplied by the percent of ethanol in the product divided by the body weight of the patient (in kilograms). A fatal dose in children is approximately 3 g/kg; the fatal dose in teenagers and adults is widely variable.

4. **Physical assessment** is straightforward. Laboratory studies required include serum ethanol level, electrolytes, glucose, and ABG analysis.

5. **Treatment:** Gastric emptying is not useful more than 1 hour after ingestion. Activated charcoal does not adsorb ethanol. Careful monitoring and correction of serum glucose is essential. Other treatment is symptomatic and supportive. Ethanol is removed by hemodialysis, and this may be indicated for serious or potentially fatal ingestions.

6. **Special consideration:** Even preteens and young teenagers may be alcohol dependent. Be alert for signs of impending withdrawal: tremors, agitation, hallucinations, and seizures. Benzodiazepines are usually indicated for initial management of alcohol withdrawal.

F. ETHYLENE GLYCOL

Ethylene glycol is the ingredient in automobile antifreeze, the most common source of glycol poisoning in the pediatric population. Unintentional ingestions are the norm in young children, whereas adolescents drink antifreeze in suicide attempts or as an ethanol surrogate. This is a dangerous poisoning because ethylene glycol is sweet but is extremely toxic in small amounts. Effects are due to metabolites and are therefore delayed. Parents or victims mistakenly believe that absence of early symptoms indicates absence of toxicity.

1. Ethylene glycol is rapidly absorbed from the GI tract and is widely distributed. During the several steps in its metabolism, glycolic acid, lactic acid, and a number of other organic acids are generated, leading to the metabolic acidosis characteristic of this poisoning. Oxalic acid precipitates with calcium, leading to the deposition of calcium oxalate crystals in soft tissue (including the kidney) and renal failure.

2. The **toxic dose** is variable but small; the potential fatal dose is 1 to 1.5 ml/kg.

3. **Toxic effects** are delayed for as long as 12 to 24 hours; early effects resemble alcoholic inebriation. As the poisoning progresses, nonspecific symptoms of lethargy and GI tract complaints evolve into ataxia, seizures, coma, and renal failure. In the absence of specific history, ethylene glycol poisoning should be suspected in any patient who presents with or develops both coma and metabolic acidosis.

4. A **serum ethylene glycol level** is most useful but not always easily obtained. Presence or absence of an anion gap metabolic acidosis is more easily ascertained and is extremely useful. ABG analysis is required. A few hours after ingestion, the urine can be examined for the presence of calcium oxalate crystals. A serum ethanol level should be drawn in anticipation of antidotal therapy with ethanol.

5. **Treatment** includes prevention of absorption (if possible), prevention of metabolism to toxic metabolites, and enhanced elimination.
   a. Gastric emptying is useful only within 1 hour of ingestion.
   b. The specific antidote to ethylene glycol poisoning is ethanol. Both substances are metabolized by alcohol dehydrogenase, which preferentially metabolizes ethanol. The goal of antidotal treatment with ethanol, "ethanol blocking," is to saturate the enzyme, thus preventing metabolism of ethylene glycol until the ethylene glycol can be eliminated renally or removed by hemodialysis. The desired ethanol blood level is 100 mg/dl. The initial dose is calculated according to age, whether ethanol is already present, and whether the patient is habituated to ethanol. Subsequent doses are titrated to the serum ethanol level and must be adjusted if the patient is hemodialyzed. To prevent ethanol-induced hypoglycemia, serum glucose must be carefully monitored and, if necessary, corrected.
   c. Hemodialysis is indicated if the ethylene glycol level is greater than 50 mg/dl.
   d. Serial ethylene glycol levels should be determined until they are less than 10 mg/dl. Metabolism of ethylene glycol to nontoxic metabolites is enhanced by administration of pyridoxine and thiamine.
   e. Renal function and acidosis must be aggressively monitored and corrected.

6. **Special considerations:** A high index of suspicion is necessary because ethylene glycol is toxic in extremely small quantities and the most effective time to initiate treatment is before metabolism and symptoms occur. Aggressive treatment is necessary, not only to prevent renal damage and death but to minimize risks of peripheral nervous system damage in survivors.

G. METHANOL

Methanol is the ingredient in windshield washer solution. It is also found in gas line additives, fuel for chafing dishes and model airplanes, and deicing compounds. It is extremely toxic in small amounts, has a sweet taste, and, in the case of windshield washer solutions, resembles blue soft drinks, especially when transferred to beverage containers. It is also used as an ethanol surrogate and in suicides. The metabolites of methanol are responsible for its toxicity.

1. Methanol is rapidly absorbed from the GI tract. It is metabolized briefly to formaldehyde, then to formic acid. Generation of organic acids accounts for metabolic acidosis, and generation of formic acid accounts for optic nerve damage.

2. The **toxic dose** is variable but small, with permanent blindness associated with an ingestion of perhaps 10 ml of methanol and fatality associated with just a few milliliters more.

3. Because **toxicity** is due to metabolites, there may be no symptoms for 10 to 24 hours. The early nonspecific symptoms include inebriation, GI tract complaints, and lethargy. As formic acid is generated, ocular complaints begin. They have been described variously as double vision, dim vision, like being in a snowstorm, and actual blindness. The patient progresses to seizures and coma.

4. Since the area of **physical assessment** requiring unusual attention is examination of the optic disc for hyperemia and the retina for edema, ophthalmologic consultation should be secured promptly. Methanol levels are ideal but often difficult to obtain. Presence or absence of an anion gap metabolic acidosis is critical information, as is knowledge of ABGs. An ethanol level should be determined in anticipation of antidotal therapy with ethanol.

5. **Treatment** includes prevention of absorption (if possible), prevention of metabolism to toxic metabolites, and enhanced elimination.
   a. Gastric emptying is useful only within 1 hour of ingestion.
   b. The specific antidote to methanol poisoning is ethanol. Both chemicals are metabolized by alcohol dehydrogenase, which preferentially metabolizes ethanol. The goal of antidotal treatment with ethanol, "ethanol blocking," is to saturate the enzyme, thus preventing metabolism of methanol, until the methanol can be eliminated renally or removed by hemodialysis. The desired ethanol blood level is 100 mg/dl. The initial dose is calculated according to age and weight, whether ethanol is already present, and whether the patient is habituated to ethanol. Subsequent doses are titrated to the serum ethanol level and must be adjusted if the patient is hemodialyzed. Serum glucose must be carefully monitored during ethanol therapy to prevent hypoglycemia.
   c. Hemodialysis is indicated if the methanol level is greater than 50 mg/dl.
   d. Serial methanol levels should be determined until they are less than 10 mg/dl. Eventual metabolism of methanol to carbon dioxide and water is enhanced by administration of folate, if the patient is already symptomatic. If the patient is still asymptomatic, leucovorin may be given instead.
   e. Ocular status must be monitored. Acidosis must be aggressively monitored and corrected. Other treatment is symptomatic and supportive.

6. **Special considerations:** A high index of suspicion is necessary because methanol is toxic in extremely small quantities and the most effective time to initiate treatment is before metabolism occurs. Aggressive treatment is necessary, not only to prevent blindness and death but to minimize risks of peripheral nervous system damage in survivors.

H. GUN BLUING

Gun bluing is a product used to maintain the metal portion of some weapons. The most dangerous ingredient is selenious acid, which in addition to caustic effects causes the rapid onset of cardiovascular collapse. Poisonings are uncommon but are expected to be fatal. There is no antidote and no specific useful treatment. Patients who survive to reach the ICU require aggressive cardiorespiratory support and treatment for caustic injuries.

I. **HYDROCARBONS**

Hydrocarbons may be categorized in many ways: by chemical composition, intended purpose, volatility, and toxic effects. Some hydrocarbons are of particular danger to the pulmonary tract if aspirated, although not usually damaging to the GI tract if ingested. These includes gasoline, kerosene, lamp oil, mineral spirits, mineral seal oil, and other substances used as fuels, lighter fluids, lubricants, and polishes.

1. When **ingested,** these liquids may be irritating and cause nausea, diarrhea, and eructation. However, they are not absorbed from the GI tract and are not expected to cause systemic effects.

2. **Aspiration** of any amount of hydrocarbon is dangerous; when it occurs, pneumonitis is likely. Depending on the exact substance and its viscosity, expected effects include airway irritation, disruption of surfactant, and impaired oxygen exchange. The victim experiences hypoxia, cyanosis, and perhaps alveolar collapse. Chest x-ray findings may range from isolated basilar infiltrates to "whiting out," especially after aspiration of such low-viscosity hydrocarbons as charcoal lighter fluid. Bacterial pneumonia may follow.

3. **Relevant history** includes a history of coughing or choking after ingestion of a hydrocarbon; in these cases, aspiration is likely, and the victim must be assessed in a health care facility. Physical assessment should focus on pulmonary findings and CNS abnormalities secondary to hypoxia. Laboratory studies are necessary to determine status of oxygenation. A chest x-ray examination should be taken quickly if the patient is severely symptomatic on arrival at the health care facility; otherwise, it should be deferred until 2 hours after exposure to permit detection of changes.

4. **Treatment** of patients with hydrocarbon aspiration may need to be aggressive but is symptomatic and supportive. In general, steroids are not indicated, and antibiotics are indicated only if bacterial pneumonia develops.

J. **MUSHROOMS**

Mushrooms of many varieties can be poisonous and even fatal when ingested by the unwary. Children may eat wild mushrooms unintentionally, as they do many other things. More dangerous is the situation where an adult identifies wild mushrooms incorrectly, then cooks and serves them. In these cases, much more of the material is ingested. Mycologists divide mushrooms into numerous species; toxicologists divide them into several groups based on symptoms. The poison center can help you narrow the group of mushroom (thus treatment) on the basis of symptoms and can identify a mycologist for positive identification of wild mushrooms and their spores. (Any available mushroom specimen must be wrapped in waxed paper and refrigerated—safely—until it can be transported for identification or until it can be determined that specific identification is not necessary.) There are a few situations in which mushroom ingestion precipitates an ICU admission.

1. In the United States, there are two types of mushrooms that are inherently sufficiently toxic to cause fatalities. Both are differentiated by the delayed onset of GI tract symptoms. Sometimes, people do not associate nausea, vomiting, and diarrhea with mushrooms eaten hours or even the day before.

   a. *Amanita phalloides, A. verna,* and *A. virosa* are hepatotoxic. The onset of significant GI tract symptoms occurs 8 or more hours after ingestion. Death from hepatic and renal failure may occur in about 5 days. There are no antidotes and no universally effective treatments. If ingestion is recognized early enough, GI tract decontamination is necessary. Hemodialysis may remove hepatotoxic metabolites.

   b. *Gyromitra esculenta* is sometimes mistaken for the edible morel, with hepatotoxic consequences. Vigorous GI tract decontamination is required if the ingestion is recognized early enough. Ingestion of *Gyromitra* species results in monomethylhydrazine poisoning, similar to INH. Treatment is as for INH poisoning, including pyridoxine 25 mg/kg.

2. Other toxic mushrooms in the United States cause the rapid onset of GI tract and perhaps other symptoms, typically within 30 minutes to 2 hours. Numerous mushrooms can cause cholinergic, anticholinergic, or hallucinogenic effects. Treatment includes GI tract decontamination, then symptomatic and supportive care. Numerous mushrooms can cause the rapid onset of GI tract symptoms with associated fluid and electrolyte imbalances. Treatment may include GI tract decontamination, then symptomatic and supportive care with an emphasis on monitoring and replacing fluids and electrolytes.

K. ORGANOPHOSPHATE INSECTICIDES

Organophosphate insecticides are absorbed via ingestion, inhalation, and dermal contact. Highly toxic organophosphates such as Sarin, Tabun, and Soman are used as nerve gas agents in warfare and terrorist events; less toxic organophosphates include malathion, dursban, and diazinon, used in household settings. Children can be exposed by household exterminations (e.g., for fleas and termites), garden applications, and exposure to agricultural sprays and adolescents by occupational exposure and in suicide attempts.

1. Organophosphate insecticides are acetylcholinesterase inhibitors. By binding to acetylcholinesterase, organophosphate insecticides prevent acetylcholine from being hydrolyzed to choline and acetic acid. There is continued stimulation of acetylcholine receptors in the CNS and at muscarinic and nicotinic sites in the autonomic nervous system. Expected effects of exposure thus are referable to the CNS and to the autonomic nervous system. Onset of symptoms is variable: rapid for nerve gas agents and "typical" household pesticides, delayed and prolonged for extremely fat-soluble agents and those that must first be metabolized to toxic agents (e.g., fenthion).

    a. *Muscarinic symptoms* can be remembered by the mnemonic *sludge: s*alivation, *l*acrimation, *u*rination, *d*efecation, *g*astrointestinal effects (e.g., nausea), and *e*yes (e.g., pinpoint pupils).

    b. *Nicotinic effects* can be remembered by the mnemonic *mtwthf: m*ydriasis, muscle twitching, and cramps; *t*achycardia; *w*eakness; *(t)h*ypertension; and *f*asciculations.

    c. CNS effects include tremor, agitation, confusion, ataxia, lethargy, seizures, and coma.

2. The **greatest threat** to the patient is respiratory distress, both from bronchorrhea and from weakness or even paralysis of the respiratory muscles. The greatest threat to the health care provider is poisoning by being exposed to a patient who has not been decontaminated.

3. **Physical assessment** of the patient must necessarily be thorough, since acetylcholinesterase inhibition has broad and diverse systemic effects. The specific laboratory study required is measurement of red blood cell (RBC) cholinesterase. (Often, the more easily measured plasma cholinesterase level is measured; this is not as useful because it can be affected by many things other than organophosphate insecticide poisoning.) The range of normal varies, but a significant decrease from the expected normal is indicative of cholinesterase inhibition and organophosphate insecticide poisoning.

4. If not already carried out, a patient with dermal exposure must be decontaminated. Protect staff with impermeable gowns and gloves to minimize or prevent dermal exposure, remove and isolate contaminated clothing, and wash the patient thoroughly (twice with copious amounts of soap and water). Even vomitus of patients who have ingested these compounds can be hazardous to staff members.

5. **Atropine** is administered to occupy muscarinic receptors and alleviate muscarinic effects. The necessary dose is titrated to symptoms, especially bronchorrhea. The pediatric dose is 0.05 mg/kg, repeated every 5 to 10 minutes until bronchial secretions are controlled; atropine by IV drip may be required for hours or days, depending on the amount of insecticide absorbed and its duration of effects.

6. **Pralidoxime (2-PAM)** is administered to cleave the organophosphate-acetylcholinesterase bond before it "ages," or becomes permanent within 24 hours after exposure. It is used in severe organophosphate insecticide poisoning, and may be administered concurrently with atropine. Like atropine, it is administered until the patient remains asymptomatic.

7. Otherwise, care is symptomatic and supportive, with aggressive respiratory care.

8. **Special considerations:** Patients are often undertreated because care providers are reluctant to administer the necessarily high and prolonged doses of atropine or pralidoxime. Permanent neurologic effects have been associated with exposure to some organophosphate insecticides. Young children are especially susceptible to the effects of these insecticides.

9. **Carbamate insecticides** have the same acute toxic effects as organophosphate insecticides. However, pralidoxime is not usually used for poisoning by carbamate insecticides, as they are not thought to form permanent bonds with acetylcholinesterase.

PSYCHOSOCIAL CONSIDERATIONS

Parents often feel guilty about a poisoning episode. Although it is objectively true that most such incidents can be anticipated and avoided, the reality is that young children are extremely curious and move very fast. Even the most vigilant parent must blink her eyes, turn his back, tend to another child, or experience a momentary lapse in concentration. Most parents realize what they could have done differently to prevent the poisoning. It probably is most productive for health care providers to focus on what parents did right: recognized a dangerous situation; sought emergency assistance; cooperated with health care providers who attempted to elicit a history, identify the drug or product, and reconstruct the scenario; and provided support to the poisoned child and other family members during recovery. This can be followed by specific poison prevention information, which can be obtained from the poison center.

For older children or teens whose poisoning represented self-destructive or sociopathic behavior, psychiatric or social service consults are required.

If there is any suspicion of child abuse or Munchausen by proxy, there may be legal requirements to be fulfilled in addition to the need for psychiatric and social services referrals for the parents.

SEPTIC SHOCK   CATHY ROSENTHAL-DICHTER

A. **DEVELOPMENTAL ANATOMY AND PHYSIOLOGY**
1. **Immunity** of the young child is not equal to that of the developmentally mature host. Several aspects of the infant and young child's first, second, and third lines of defense are immature (see the developmental distinctions noted in

Chapter 8). The healthy infant and young child is not immunocompromised but immunologically inexperienced.

2. **Cardiac output regulation:** See Chapter 3 on maturational differences in the cardiac output and its associated components (heart rate, stroke volume, preload, contractility, and afterload). Changes in the child's cardiac output accompany the child's growth and development. Cardiac output is highest at birth (200 ml/kg/min) and then decreases throughout childhood to adolescence (100 ml/kg/min; Hazinski, 1989). The decrease in cardiac output is related to two events (Alyn and Baker, 1992): (1) a decrease in fetal hemoglobin and (2) an increase in adult hemoglobin and less oxygen requirements secondary to a changing surface area. In the young child, cardiac output is directly proportional to heart rate (Hazinski, 1992).

3. **Oxygen consumption:** Oxygen consumption is the volume of oxygen consumed by the tissues per unit of time. Oxygen consumption is the product of the cardiac output and the amount of oxygen extracted from each milliliter of blood; expressed as ml/kg/min. Changes in the child's oxygen consumption accompany the child's growth and development. As with cardiac output, oxygen consumption decreases throughout childhood. Normal values in the fetus are 8 ml/kg/min (Alyn and Baker, 1992), in the infant are 10 to 14 ml/kg/min, and in the child are 7 to 11 ml/kg/min (Hazinski, 1992).

B. ETIOLOGY

1. An infectious process, such as septic shock, occurs as a result of the following (Grimes, 1991):
   a. *Susceptible host:* As compared to the adult, the child admitted to the PICU is intrinsically more susceptible to infection because of age, the presenting clinical condition, and associated therapeutic interventions and monitoring devices.
   b. An *infectious organism* is able to illicit symptoms by one or both of the microorganism's direct actions or the host's physiologic responses to eradicate the microorganism.
   c. The *environment* permits the transmission of the organism to the host.

2. All microorganisms may lead to septic shock including bacteria, viruses, fungi, rickettsiae, spirochetes, protozoa, mycoplasmas, chlamydiae, and parasites.

3. Causative microorganisms often vary with the following:
   a. Patient's age: Risk of infection with certain microorganisms is age related.
   b. Immunocompetence: In immunocompromised patients the usual source of infection is the patient's endogenous flora. In immunocompetent patients the usual source is exogenous flora with some evidence that patients may benefit from protective isolation against ICU-acquired microorganisms (Maki, 1995).
   c. Location: In hospital-acquired (nosocomial) infection the etiologic organism is usually specific to the individual unit and institution and geographic region. Community-acquired infection comprises a significant proportion of infections in the PICU. In one study the PICU had nearly twice as many community-acquired infections as the adult medical-surgical ICU (Brown, 1985).
   d. Site of infection: In nosocomial infections, lower respiratory tract infection, bacteremia, urinary tract, and cutaneous and surgical infections are most common in the infant and child (Centers for Disease Control [CDC], 1984). Community-acquired infections are usually lower respiratory tract infection, genitourinary tract, and cerebrospinal fluid infections.

C. EPIDEMIOLOGY

1. **Incidence**
   a. Septic shock is the most common cause of death in the ICU (Natanson et al,

1995; Parillo et al, 1990). It is difficult to ascertain exact incidence of septic shock, since it does not have an International Classification of Diseases (ICD) code. Sepsis does have an ICD code and represents a significant risk to the infant and young child, representing the ninth leading cause of death for children aged 1 to 4 years and the 13th leading cause of death for children of all ages.

b. The incidence is increasing because of the more common use of and advances in medical technology; increased numbers of patients with impaired immune function, such as patients experiencing transplantations, oncologic conditions, and acquired immunodeficiency syndrome (AIDS); increased survival of vulnerable patients, such as neonates; and infections caused by antibiotic-resistant organisms (Natanson et al, 1995).

2. **Risk factors**

a. Susceptible patients are those with extremes in age (neonates and children younger than 3 years of age), noncompliance with immunization schedules, malnourishment or failure to thrive, chronic illness, malignancy, immuno-suppressive therapy (e.g., malignancy or transplant recipient), primary immunodeficiency, asplenia, AIDS, and congenital heart disease.

b. Aggressive microorganisms have changing resistance patterns.

c. Conducive environments such as the PICU increase risk. The infant or young child in the PICU has a significant risk of nosocomial infection, heavily influenced by the length of stay and exposure to invasive devices (e.g., endotracheal tubes, central venous and other intravascular lines, urinary catheters; Maki, 1995; Merritt, 1992).

D. PATHOPHYSIOLOGY

1. Septic shock, the most common form of distributive shock, is caused by a systematic activation of the inflammatory response as a result of infection, which results in profound vasodilation and disturbances in cardiovascular and other organ system functioning (Kumar and Parrillo, 1995).

2. All surfaces of the body exposed in any way to the external environment serve as the **first line of defense.** When the microorganism breeches any of these barriers, it gains access to the body's internal environment.

3. The inflammatory-immune response, the **second line of defense,** is then triggered in an effort to eliminate or neutralize the microorganism and its toxins, contain microorganism invasion, prevent access to the body's systemic environment (blood stream), and promote rapid healing of involved tissues.

4. When the microorganism overwhelms the second line of defense, it invades the body's tissues, and the microorganism and its toxins are released systemically into the blood stream (Natanson et al, 1995).

a. With systemic release of the microorganism and its toxins, there is an activation and release of various mediators and cytokines, referred to as a systemic inflammatory response syndrome (SIRS). SIRS is the body's systemic inflammatory-immune and hormonal response to severe injury or illness originating from a variety of sources, such as infection, hemorrhage, trauma, pancreatitis, and thermal injuries (American College of Chest Physicians [AACP] and Society for Critical Care Medicine [SCCM] 1992). SIRS is not dependent on an infection. For instance, experimental immunotherapy stimulates SIRS in patients in hopes of enhancing defense against many insults such as tumor cells (Byram, 1989). The presence of SIRS accompanied by an infectious process is referred to as sepsis (ACCP and SCCM, 1992). Sepsis represents a continuum of clinical states in which the patient displays varying degrees of severity, specifically with regard to hypoperfusion, organ dysfunction(s), and hypotension.

b. The degree and severity of SIRS or sepsis depends on the condition of the patient and the nature and severity of the infection (Ackerman, 1994; Natanson et al, 1995).

   c. Mechanisms within the inflammatory response and SIRS are the same, with the difference in the extent and magnitude of the response. Events or mechanisms of the inflammatory response serve protective functions, whereas SIRS causes deleterious outcomes (Table 9–15).

5. The activation and release of various mediators result from two sources: exogenous and endogenous.

   a. Exogenous mediators are released by the invading microorganism. Microorganism mediators include but are not limited to endotoxin (released from gram-negative bacteria), exotoxin (released from gram-positive bacteria), and mennan (released from fungal cell walls).

     • Endotoxin, a lipopolysaccharide that is an integral part of the outer membrane of all gram-negative bacteria, is the most commonly studied toxin in sepsis. Endotoxin is shed as bacteria multiply or die. The core lipid A chain of the lipopolysaccharide is identical in every gram-negative organism. Antibodies for the core lipid A have been developed and have been investigated in several clinical studies. Results of these studies have failed to conclusively support their use in the treatment of septic shock (Natanson et al, 1995). Endotoxin administration to normal adult human volunteers (Suffredini et al, 1989) and animals (Natanson et al, 1989) results in cardiovascular changes similar to those seen with sepsis.

     • Endotoxin levels have been correlated to the incidence of lactic acidosis, adult respiratory distress syndrome (ARDS), renal insufficiency, and myocardial dysfunction in adults (Danner et al, 1991) and severity of disease and outcomes in children (Brandtzaeg et al, 1989; Mertsola et al, 1991).

   b. Endogenous mediators are synthesized or activated by the host in response to an insult or invading microorganism (exogenous mediators). Endog-

Table 9–15. INFLAMMATION VS. SYSTEMIC INFLAMMATORY RESPONSE SYNDROME (SIRS): COMMON EVENTS BUT DIFFERENT OUTCOMES

EVENT	ROLE IN INFLAMMATION	ROLE IN SIRS, SEPSIS, AND SEPTIC SHOCK
Vasodilation	Nutrient delivery / Cellular access	Maldistribution of blood flow
Microvascular permeability	Nutrient delivery / Cellular access	Imbalance of oxygen supply and demand
Cellular activation	Phagocytosis	Diffuse mediator release
	Microorganism elimination	Cardiac dysfunction
Coagulation	Limit injury	Microvascular thrombi
	Prevent blood loss	Endothelial damage
		Tissue ischemia

Modified from Huddleston VB. The inflammatory/immune response: Implications for the critically ill. In: Huddleston VB, ed. *Multisystem Organ Failure: Pathophysiology and Clinical Implications*, 2nd ed. St Louis, Mo: Mosby–Year Book Inc; 1996.

enous mediators play an important role in the *normal* inflammatory-immune response, but an exaggerated activation results in life-threatening events, such as cardiovascular instability (Natanson et al, 1995).

c. Exogenous mediators (e.g., endotoxin) initiate an amplified, exaggerated activation of a myriad of host physiologic processes (Carcillo, 1993; Huddleston, 1992b) including plasma enzyme cascades, cellular responses, and biochemical mediators.

- Plasma enzyme cascade activation (Huddleston, 1992b) involves complement (see Chapter 8 for background information), which in SIRS results in excessive inflammation and excessive cellular activation with associated mediator release; coagulopathy, which in SIRS, results in excessive intravascular coagulation with endothelial damage, microvascular obstruction, and altered tissue perfusion; fibrinolysis, which in SIRS results in hemorrhage; and kallikrein-kinin (bradykinin) acting to enhance margination of neutrophils, which in SIRS results in massive vasodilation, increased capillary permeability, excessive inflammation, excessive cellular activation with associated mediator release, and bronchoconstriction.

- Cellular responses induce recruitment of all types of white blood cells (WBCs), platelets, mast cells, fibroblasts, and endothelial cells to participate (Huddleston, 1992b).

- Several types of *biochemical mediators* are released as a result of exaggerated recruitment and activation of the aforementioned cells:

  ○ Cytokines are hormonelike substances that serve as physiologic communicators between cells participating in the inflammatory immune response (see Table 8–4). These include interleukins, interferons, tumor necrosis factor (TNF), and colony-stimulating factors (CSFs).

  ○ Lipid mediators are arachidonic acid metabolites (prostaglandins, leukotrienes, and thromboxane) and platelet activating factor. Arachidonic acid is a normal constituent of cell membranes that is released from the walls of injured WBCs and metabolized through two pathways (lipoxygenase and cyclooxygenase) and result in lipid mediators. The lipoxygenase pathway results in the formation of thromboxane, prostacyclin, and prostaglandin, subsequently affecting vascular tone and permeability. The cyclooxygenase pathway results in the formation of leukotrienes, subsequently causing vascular and airway constriction and increased capillary permeability. Platelet activating factor is produced by endothelial cells, WBCs, and others and normally participates in the activation of platelets and other cells in inflammation and coagulation. In SIRS platelet activating factor triggers exaggerated mediator release, subsequently resulting in hemodynamic changes, endothelial damage, and excessive coagulation (Secor, 1994).

  ○ Toxic oxygen metabolites (oxygen-derived free radicals) are produced by numerous sources including xanthine oxidase systems, activated phagocytes, mitochondria, and arachidonic acid pathways. Normally, the metabolites are produced in small amounts during oxidative metabolism in a localized area and metabolized through numerous innate enzyme systems or membrane antioxidants (Huddleston, 1992a) and have bactericidal activity. In SIRS the metabolites damage cell membranes of endothelial cells and other tissues, which results in increased permeability, edema, and exaggerated inflammation. Toxic oxygen metabolites are thought to play a significant role in organ damage seen during septic shock (Huddleston, 1992a).

○ Proteolytic enzymes (proteases) are produced by numerous phago-cytic cells, such as neutrophils and macrophages. The enzymes assist the phagocyte in the digestion of bacteria and other foreign material, participate in wound healing, and serve as enzymatic catalysts for the enzyme cascades (e.g., complement, coagulation, fibrinolysis, and kallikrein-kinin) (Huddleston, 1992a). In SIRS proteolytic enzymes cause vascular and tissue damage, increased permeability, and edema.

○ Nitric oxide is thought to be an endothelium-derived relaxant factor that serves as a potent modulator of vascular tone and permeability.

d. Three of the most influential mediators of gram-negative septic shock include endotoxin, TNF, and interleukin-1 (IL-1; Secor, 1994). TNF is produced by monocytes and macrophages. It results in enhanced inflammatory-immune responses and promotes adhesion of neutrophils to endothelial cells and release of other mediators. Clinical manifestations include body temperature changes, tachypnea, alveolar thickening, tachy-cardia, increased vascular permeability, hypotension, metabolic acidosis, and altered blood distribution to organs, such as the kidney and gut (Secor, 1994). IL-1 is produced by lymphocytes, macrophages, and en-dothelial cells and released in response to TNF. It results in many of the same findings as TNF, as well as further release of TNF, platelet activating factors, and other mediators, such as IL-2 (Secor, 1994). Many of the clinical manifestations of IL-1 and TNF overlap, and actions of TNF and IL-1 are synergistic (Secor, 1994).

6. The mechanisms of each of the mediators vary, *but* the overall result of the exaggerated release of exogenous and endogenous mediators includes a distributive shock state characterized by maldistribution of blood volume, cardiac dysfunction, imbalance of oxygen supply and demand, and metabolic alterations (Fig. 9–2).

a. *Maldistribution of blood volume* results from (Robins, 1992) neuroendocrine activation including the release of catecholamines, glucagon, glucocorti-coids, aldosterone, renin, and angiotensin. Release of catecholamines results in vasoconstriction and redistribution of blood flow. Biochemical mediator release results in reduced peripheral resistance or increased peripheral vasodilation leading to blood pooling in the peripheral vascula-ture and increased microvascular permeability leading to leakage of inter-stitial fluid from the vascular space. Direct endothelial damage also leads to increased microvascular permeability. Coagulation activation leads to de-

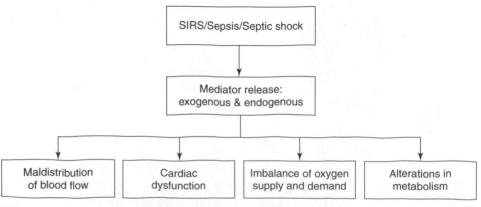

Figure 9–2. Outcomes of mediator release in systemic inflammatory response syndrome (SIRS), sepsis, and septic shock.

creased blood flow and microthrombi formation secondary to increased platelet aggregation and increased margination and chemotaxis of neutrophils (Fig. 9–3).

b. *Cardiac dysfunction* (Gates, 1992): There is inconclusive evidence of decreased coronary artery blood flow as the cause of cardiac dysfunction in sepsis and septic shock (Natanson et al, 1995). Sympathetic nervous system responsiveness alterations result in changes in contractility and cardiac output and cardiac index, which are normally enhanced through the sympathetic nervous system stimulation of myocardial β-adrenergic receptors. In early sepsis, there is enhanced β-adrenergic stimulation. Later in the continuum the myocardium becomes less sensitive to circulating catecholamines, and contractility declines (Gates, 1992).

- Mediator release is thought to be the culprit for cardiac dysfunction in sepsis and septic shock. Myocardial depressant factor is thought to be released by the pancreas during hypoperfusion and ischemia. Endotoxin's mechanism of action on the myocardium is unclear but is thought to be either a direct effect or an indirect effect through the stimulation of other mediators that reduce cardiac contractility (Gates, 1992). Many other mediators (e.g., IL-2, thromboxane, prostaglandin, leukotriene, and TNF) continue to be investigated with respect to their effect on various aspects of hemodynamics, including cardiac contractility (Gates, 1992). The hemodynamic profile characterized by low systemic vascular resistance (SVR) and profound tachycardia contributes to diminished coronary artery perfusion and further cardiac dysfunction (Carcillo, 1993).

c. *Imbalance of oxygen supply and demand*

- Hypoxemia is usually the result of respiratory failure and pulmonary edema secondary to mediator release and increased permeability (Hazinski et al, 1993). Maldistribution of blood flow exacerbates hypoxemia and may lead to ventilation perfusion abnormalities and intrapulmonary shunting. Imbalance of oxygen supply and demand with SIRS and septic shock is due to the decrease in the maximum oxygen delivery secondary to myocardial dysfunction and the decrease in the tissue's ability to extract the oxygen.

- In normal circumstances with healthy tissues and normal or increased oxygen transport, oxygen consumption is maintained at a constant. In other words, oxygen consumption is independent of oxygen transport. More oxygen is normally delivered to the tissues than is normally consumed. Delivering more oxygen does not change the amount consumed by the tissue (Mims, 1992). As oxygen availability to the tissues decreases, consumption is initially maintained by increasing the oxygen extraction ratio. When oxygen availability falls to a critical level, oxygen consumption falls (Fig. 9–4).

- The relationship between oxygen transport and oxygen consumption is altered in clinical conditions such as sepsis, ARDS, and multiple-organ dysfunction syndrome (MODS; Mims, 1992). Oxygen consumption is dependent on oxygen transport. The amount consumed is related to the amount delivered and is referred to as *supply dependency* or *pathologic supply dependency*. The cause of supply-dependent oxygen consumption in sepsis is through cellular defect (some evidence of impaired oxidative metabolism), maldistribution of blood flow at the microcirculatory level, or impaired oxygen diffusion (tissue inflammation and edema widens the diffusion distance between the capillary and cells; Mims, 1992).

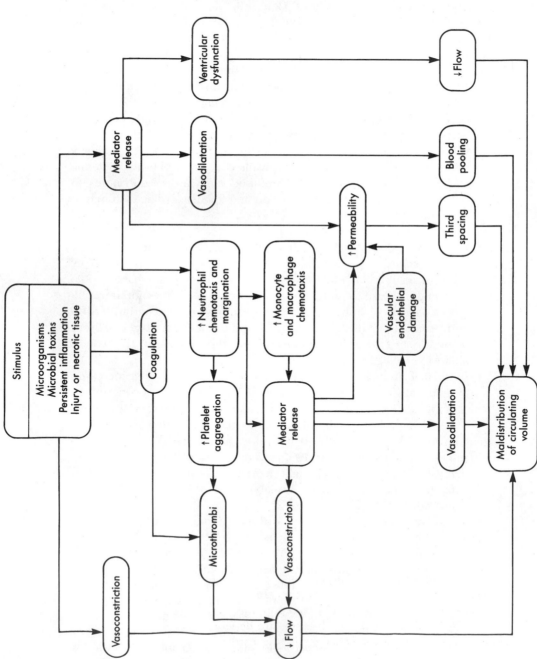

Figure 9–3. Processes leading to maldistribution of circulating volume. (From: Robins EV. Maldistribution of circulating volume. In: Huddleston VB, ed. *Multisystem Organ Failure: Pathophysiology and Clinical Implications*, 2nd ed. St Louis, Mo: Mosby–Year Book Inc; 1996.)

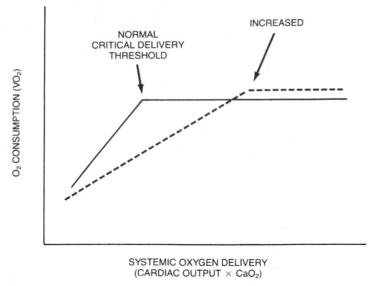

O₂ CONSUMPTION (VO₂)

NORMAL
CRITICAL DELIVERY
THRESHOLD

INCREASED

SYSTEMIC OXYGEN DELIVERY
(CARDIAC OUTPUT × CaO₂)

Figure 9–4. Relationship between oxygen delivery and oxygen consumption. (From Schumaker PT, Samuel RW. Oxygen delivery and uptake by peripheral tissues. *Crit Care Clin.* 1989;5:259.)

- The outcome is inadequate tissue perfusion. Adenosine triphosphate (ATP) is generated through increased glycolysis, which results in the by-product pyruvate and subsequently lactate and causes metabolic acidosis (Mims, 1992). If tissue demand is greater than supply, cellular injury occurs.

d. *Alteration in metabolism* (Kimbrell, 1992)

- Initially, metabolic alterations serve as compensatory mechanisms aimed at meeting the body's increased needs (Kimbrell, 1992). These alterations result from neurohormonal responses primarily mediated by the sympathetic nervous system and initially characterized by hypermetabolism (increase in resting energy expenditure, increase in cardiac output, increase in oxygen consumption and carbon dioxide production), hyperglycemia, and hypercatabolism.

- Inadequate substrate metabolism occurs. In carbohydrate metabolism, glycogen stores are depleted, usually in less than 12 hours. The liver initiates gluconeogenesis, while glucose utilization by cells decreases, glucose transport into the cells decreases, and serum glucose concentration increases. In lipid metabolism, catecholamine and decreased insulin lead to catabolism of triglycerides to free fatty acids and ketones for energy (from adipose tissue) with the potential for lipemia or hypertriglyceridemia. In protein metabolism, amino acids are needed for gluconeogenesis. The primary sites of amino acids include skeletal muscle, connective tissue, and unstimulated gut. Therefore, autocannibalism occurs with rapid loss of skeletal muscle to provide amino acids. In combination with decreased protein synthesis, there is an eventual deficiency of essential amino acids.

7. Compensatory responses to shock are mechanisms to increase tissue perfusion and prevent cellular, tissue, and vital organ injury in the presence of all shock states. Most compensatory mechanisms are dependent on various "sensing" mechanisms to recognize changes in the cardiac output or arterial blood pressure.

a. *Compensatory mechanisms* are sequentially stimulated in an effort to maintain perfusion.

- *Stretch receptors* (in the right atrium and pulmonary artery) sense volume changes, either from decreased circulating volume or in the case of septic shock from increased venous capacitance. Stimulation of these receptors results in an increase in sympathetic discharge to the medullary vasomotor center.

- Baroreceptors within the renal juxtaglomerular apparatus are stimulated by reduced renal afferent arteriolar pressure. The reduction in pressure causes activation of the renin-angiotensin-aldosterone system, which results in vasoconstriction of arterioles (and to a lesser extent veins), increased renal tubular reabsorption of sodium and water, and stimulation of the adrenal cortex. The stimulation of the adrenal cortex increases production of aldosterone, causing retention of renal sodium, thus expanding extracellular fluid volume (DeAngelis, 1991). A drop in MAP or pulse pressure close to physiologic range results in the decreased stretching of arterial baroreceptors (in aortic arch, carotid bodies, and splanchnic vessels) and loss of their inhibitory effect on the vasomotor center (baroreceptor reflex). Sympathetic vasomotor stimulation causes norepinephrine release from nerve endings and widespread vasoconstriction. Once MAP falls below 80 mm Hg for the aortic arch and 60 mm Hg for the carotid bodies, the activity of these baroreceptors is eliminated (Kumar and Parrillo, 1995).

- Norepinephrine-epinephrine vasoconstrictor reflex: Sympathetic vasomotor stimulation causes stimulation of the adrenal medulla and the release of epinephrine primarily, although some norepinephrine is secreted as well. This reflex accentuates and prolongs vasoconstrictive effects throughout the body including constriction of afferent and efferent arterioles of the kidney resulting in decreased glomerular filtration, decreased urine output, and increased sodium retention (DeAngelis, 1991).

- Vascular chemoreceptors are sensitive to changes in Po_2, Pco_2, and decreased pH (increased hydrogen ion concentration) and are activated when the blood pressure is less than approximately 80 mm Hg. On activation there is a substantial increase in sympathetic tone. The chemoreceptors have a limited role during normal physiologic homeostasis but an active role during shock (Kumar and Parrillo, 1995).

- CNS ischemia reflex serves as the most powerful stimulus to sympathetic tone in severe shock (Kumar and Parrillo, 1995). Medullary chemoreceptors are sensitive to increased carbon dioxide associated with decreased cerebral perfusion and to blood pressure lower than 60 mm Hg (Kumar and Parrillo, 1995).

CLINICAL ASSESSMENT

A. NURSING HISTORY

1. **Chief complaint:** The nursing history is guided by the child's chief complaint. The chief complaint is noted in the patient's or the primary caretaker's own words.

2. **History of the present illness** includes the date of onset, mode of onset, course, duration, and exposure to infectious agents including contact with infectious persons, animal (domestic or wild) bites, ingestion of contaminated food

or water, and foreign travel. Signs and symptoms to be noted include the following:

    a.   General: Fatigue, change in level of activity, chills, fever, weight loss, change in feeding, night sweats, malaise

    b.   Mental status: Confusion, restlessness, syncope, irritability, somnolence

    c.   Skin: Rash, petechiae, pallor, lesions, ulcers, rhinitis (see Table 9–16)

    d.   Lymph nodes: Enlargement (adenopathy), tenderness

    e.   Respiratory: Tachypnea, respiratory tract infection, respiratory distress, dyspnea, orthopnea, cough, hemoptysis, sputum, chest pain

    f.   Cardiovascular: Tachycardia, flushed skin

    g.   Abdomen: Anorexia, altered bowel sounds, diarrhea, constipation, melena, vomiting, hematemesis, protuberant abdomen (not age appropriate), abdominal pain, masses, hepatosplenomegaly

    h.   GU tract: Hematuria, number of voids or diapers per day

3. **Past medical history**

    a.   Aspects that alter the child's resistance to infection include recent injury, diet and nutrition, and immunization history.

    b.   Aspects that increase the child's risk of infection include prolonged antibiotic therapy, previous surgeries (e.g., thymectomy, splenectomy), liver or spleen disorders (functional splenectomy), metabolic and immune disorders (diabetes, renal disease, primary immunodeficiency, and allergies or hypersensitivities), malignancy, and a transplantation.

    c.   Previous infections, including childhood infectious diseases, should be noted.

4. **Family history** should note familial diseases that may increase the child's risk of infection.

5. **Medication history** should include those that increase the child's risk of infection.

6. **Social-cultural history and habits** include psychosocial history, environmental exposures such as radiation (either inadvertent exposure or radiation therapies [total or localized]) or chemical (inadvertent exposure to benzene, lead, etc.), and recent travel.

B. NURSING EXAMINATION OF THE PATIENT

1. **Inspection** includes level of consciousness, level of activity, general appearance, and respiratory rate, rhythm, and effort. Skin and mucous membranes should be examined for color and consistency, presence of lesions, and the presence of generalized or localized edema, which is usually periorbital or sacral. Pedal edema may occur after the child begins to walk. Characteristics of fontanelles and jugular venous distention are noted to assess hydration status. Precordial activity (sometimes referred to as sternal bulging) is noted and is due to hypertrophy of the right ventricle causing the lower end of the sternum and ribs to project forward. Although the point of maximal intensity (PMI) may be visible in some children, especially those that are thin, a prominent or heaving precordium may be an indication of cardiac dysfunction.

2. **Palpation**

    a.   Skin and mucous membranes are palpated for moisture, texture, refill, and temperature (note any demarcation in temperature from distal to proximal extremities and extremities vs. trunk). With cardiac dysfunction, blood is circulated at an insufficient rate, and compensatory vasoconstriction occurs in the extremities to shunt blood toward vital organs. Normal capillary refill is ≤2 seconds. The presence and intensity of peripheral pulses is noted. Also note proximal vs. distal pulse quality, since this is reflective of perfusion status.

b. The level at which the normal liver border may be palpable is related to age. In the infant the liver is normally felt up to 3 cm below the right costal margin; in the 1-year-old, up to 2 cm below the right costal margin; and in the 4- to 5-year-old, up to 1 cm below the right costal margin. The presence of hepatomegaly may indicate cardiac dysfunction, tumor, or hepatitis. An enlarged liver may also indicate fluid overload, since the liver may act as a sponge and become engorged when central venous pressure (CVP) increases.

3. **Auscultation:** Presence and quality of breath sounds is noted. Respiratory rate and heart rate should be evaluated within the context of the child's age, clinical condition, and other external factors, such as fever. Apical heart rate and rhythm are auscultated. In the infant and young child, cardiac output is directly proportional to heart rate, since stroke volume is small (Hazinski, 1989). Blood pressure is a late sign of decompensation but is still obtained. Blood pressure should be evaluated in the context of the child's age, clinical condition, and other parameters reflective of perfusion.

4. **Phases and clinical manifestations of septic shock** (Table 9–16):

Table 9–16. PHASES AND CLINICAL MANIFESTATIONS OF SEPTIC SHOCK

ORGAN SYSTEM	SEPSIS	HYPERDYNAMIC SEPTIC SHOCK*	HYPODYNAMIC SEPTIC SHOCK†
CNS	Change in activity Change in feeding Change in response	Clouded sensorium Irritability Disorientation Lethargy	Disorientation Lethargy Obtundation
Cardiovascular	Sinus tachycardia Bounding pulses	Sinus tachycardia Bounding pulses Warm, dry, flushed skin Widened pulse pressure ± Diminished perfusion ↑↓ Capillary refill ± Mottled extremities Generalized edema Relative hypovolemia Progressive hypotension	Sinus tachycardia Weak, thready pulse Dysrhythmias Narrowed pulse pressure Diminished perfusion ↓ Capillary refill Mottled extremities Generalized edema Hypotension
Pulmonary	Tachypnea	Tachypnea Progressive hypoxemia	Pulmonary edema
Metabolic	Fever or hypothermia Respiratory alkalosis	Fever or hypothermia Hyperglycemia or hypoglycemia Progressive metabolic acidosis	Fever or hypothermia Hyperglycemia or hypoglycemia Severe metabolic acidosis
Hematology-Immunology	Leukocytosis or leukopenia ↑ Immature neutrophils (bands)	Leukocytosis or leukopenia ↑ Immature neutrophils (bands)	Leukocytosis or leukopenia
Renal		↓ UOP	↓ UOP

*Hyperdynamic septic shock is characterized by increased cardiovascular findings and seemingly "good" perfusion; the body's demands are still not adequately met.
†Hypodynamic septic shock may be accompanied by early signs and symptoms of deteriorating organ dysfunction(s).
CNS, central nervous system; *UOP,* urine output.
Data from Carcillo JA. Management of pediatric septic shock. In: Holbrook PR, ed. *Textbook of Pediatric Critical Care.* Philadelphia, Pa: WB Saunders Co; 1993:114–142; and Robins EV. Maldistribution of circulating volume. In: Huddleston VB (ed.). *Multisystem Organ Failure: Pathophysiology and Clinical Implications.* St Louis, Mo: Mosby–Year Book Inc; 1992:85–108.

Stages may be identified in the clinical progression of septic shock in *some* children (Hazinski, 1992). During the hyperdynamic compensated phase, blood pressure is maintained. In the later, hyperdynamic uncompensated phase, blood pressure begins to fall. Hypodynamic state essentially appears congruent to cardiogenic shock.

5. **Correlating clinical findings with ACCP and SCCM proposed terminology (1992)**
   a. *Infection* is a microbial phenomenon characterized by an inflammatory response to the presence of microorganisms or the invasion of normally sterile host tissue by those organisms.
   b. *Bacteremia* is the presence of viable bacteria in the blood.
   c. *SIRS* is the acute development of two or more of the following (ACCP and SCCM, 1992):
      - Fever (>38° C) or hypothermia (<36° C)
      - Tachycardia (age related)
      - Tachypnea (age related)
      - Leukocytosis (WBC >12,000/mm^3), leukopenia (WBC <4000/mm^3), or greater than 10% bands
   d. *Sepsis* is the systemic response to infection; sepsis is diagnosed by the presence of SIRS associated with an infectious process and characterized by two or more of the aforementioned findings for SIRS. Documented bacteremia is not necessary for the diagnosis of sepsis.
   e. *Severe sepsis* is the presence of sepsis associated with organ dysfunction, hypoperfusion, or hypotension. Hypoperfusion and perfusion abnormalities may include but are not limited to acute alteration in mental status, lactic acidosis, or oliguria.
   f. *Septic shock* is the presence of severe sepsis associated with hypotension and hypoperfusion despite fluid resuscitation.
   g. *MODS* is characterized by organ function maintained *only* with supportive therapy.

C. INVASIVE AND NONINVASIVE DIAGNOSTIC STUDIES
   1. **Laboratory**
      a. *Serum hematologic studies* include the following:
         - CBC
         - WBC count (Chapter 8, Table 8–6): Total WBC count is generally considered to be normal at 5000 to 10,000/mm^3 but is age specific. Leukocytosis occurs in all forms of shock due to the demargination of neutrophils (Kumar and Parrillo, 1995). Leukopenia occurs in late septic shock *or* in infants and young children who are less able to repeatedly replace neutrophils in the face of an overwhelming infection. The WBC differential measures the five subcategories of circulating WBCs and is reported as a percentage. Neutropenia may be seen. An increased percentage (>10%) of bands (immature neutrophils) is seen when there is an increased demand for or decreased supply of neutrophils in the presence of an overwhelming infection (shift to the left). Lymphocytosis may be seen with viral infection. Absolute granulocyte or neutrophil counts (AGC or ANC) may be low. An ANC lower than 1000/mm^3 carries a moderate risk for infection, and an ANC lower than 500/mm^3 carries a high risk for infection.
         - Hemoglobin is variably affected. Usually with the extravasation of intravascular water there is erythrocytosis.
         - Platelet count increases acutely, but may be followed by thrombocytopenia with progressive septic shock.

- Other serum tests of inflammation that may be helpful include erythrocyte sedimentation rate (ESR) and C-reactive protein, which are elevated secondary to an infectious process.

  b. *ABG analysis* (DeAngelis, 1991): Respiratory alkalosis occurs early in the course of septic shock. Initial respiratory alkalosis occurs as a compensatory mechanism to reduce carbon dioxide, in the presence of increasing lactic acidosis from decreased perfusion. As septic shock progresses and respiratory reserves fail, metabolic acidosis develops. The body is unable to compensate for the increasing acid buildup. An anion gap acidosis is present because of the elevated levels of lactic acid.

  c. *Routine chemistries:* Electrolytes, sodium, potassium, chloride, and bicarbonate, are required to assess an anion gap. BUN and creatinine levels initially appear normal. Lactate should be followed serially, since it is a marker of tissue oxygen debt and supply-dependent oxygen consumption. It is a late marker of tissue hypoperfusion, but one of the few available means of estimating tissue oxygenation. Arterial lactate levels higher than 2 mEq/L are associated with increased mortality in the adult population.

  d. *Blood cultures* may identify causative microorganism. Aerobic and anaerobic cultures are usually obtained. Obtaining blood cultures is a *simultaneous* priority with administering broad-spectrum antibiotic coverage. Attempt to obtain blood cultures prior to the administration of antibiotics, but *never "hold" antibiotic administration to obtain blood cultures.*
    - The timing of culture results is dependent on the type of microorganism and the stage of the illness (Grimes, 1991). Results from cultures for common microorganisms such as streptococci, staphylococci, and *Enterobacter* are available in 24 to 48 hours. Results from a pneumococcal culture are available in 3 to 4 days.
    - Results from blood cultures may be negative. Some microorganisms, such as *Mycobacterium tuberculosis,* shed intermittently, causing negative results from cultures. This is common in patients with active tuberculosis (Grimes, 1991). In these instances, serial cultures may be required. Some patients, especially those who have received antibiotics, may also yield negative results from blood cultures.

  e. *Other specimens and cultures*
    - Sputum specimens from the lower respiratory tract vs. oropharyngeal secretions may be helpful.
    - Fecal cultures are used to find organisms that are not a part of the normal bowel flora or to determine normal flora that become pathogenic (e.g., *Clostridium difficile* or *Escherichia coli*).
    - Urine specimens with bacterial counts of less than 10,000/ml of urine are considered free of infection. Bacterial levels between 10,000 to 100,000/ml in urine cultures are inconclusive and require a second specimen. Bacterial counts greater than 100,000/ml of urine represent a definitive urinary tract infection.
    - Cerebrospinal fluid: Lumbar puncture is rarely indicated in septic shock (Carcillo, 1993). Gram stains are particularly useful with cerebrospinal fluid infections for the purpose of selecting antibiotics.

2. **Radiologic:** *Routine chest radiograph* is useful for ruling out pneumonia as the source of infection. Abdominal panels may be useful for suspected intra-abdominal processes, although such processes are usually clinically apparent (Kumar and Parrillo, 1995). Radiographic studies of other areas of the body are indicated by the child's history and physical examination.

3. **Invasive hemodynamic monitoring**
    a. All patients with suspected shock should have an indwelling *arterial catheter* to serially monitor blood pressure. Blood pressure assessment via manual sphygmomanometer or automatic noninvasive oscillometric techniques may be inaccurate in patients in shock secondary to marked peripheral vasoconstriction.
    b. *CVP* is most often used to manage the child with uncomplicated septic shock to trend intravascular volume status and response to therapy.
    c. A *pulmonary artery catheter* is helpful in managing the child in florid septic shock. It provides continuous monitoring of cardiac filling pressures (CVP and pulmonary artery wedge pressure [PAWP], an estimate of left ventricular end-diastolic pressure [LVEDP] and volume [LVEDV]), cardiac flow (cardiac output per cardiac index [CO/CI]), cardiac contractility (stroke volume, stroke volume index, stroke work index), and afterload (SVR, systemic vascular resistance index [SVRI]). It also allows for withdrawal of blood from the pulmonary artery catheter to determine oxygen consumption: pulmonary artery oxygen content and mixed venous oxygen saturation ($\overline{S}vo_2$).
4. **Hemodynamic parameters accompanying various shock states** (Table 9–17)

D. NURSING AND COLLABORATIVE DIAGNOSES
    ❖ FLUID VOLUME DEFICIT RELATED TO RELATIVE HYPOVOLEMIA, VASODILATION, CAPILLARY PERMEABILITY, DECREASED INTAKE, AND POTENTIAL INADEQUATE FLUID RESUSCITATION

Table 9–17. HEMODYNAMIC PARAMETERS ACCOMPANYING VARIOUS SHOCK STATES

PARAMETER	HYPOVOLEMIC SHOCK	CARDIOGENIC SHOCK	HYPERDYNAMIC SEPTIC SHOCK	HYPODYNAMIC SEPTIC SHOCK
Heart rate	Increased		Increased*	
MAP	Normal ~Compensated~ → Decreased ~Decompensated~†			
CO/CI	Decreased	Decreased	Increased then deceased‡	
CVP	Decreased	Increased	Normal to decreased *or* Decreased then increased	
PAWP	Decreased	Increased	Normal to decreased *or* Decreased then increased	
PVRI	Increased			
SVRI	Increased		Decreased then increased§	

*Adult patients: Patients who survived had increased heart rate but progressed toward normalcy after 24 h, whereas nonsurvivors displayed persistent increased heart rate.
†Adult patients: Nonsurvivors displayed unresponsive blood pressure secondary to low SVR and only small percentage secondary to low CO/CI.
‡Adult patients: Patients who survived had increased CO/CI but progressed towards normalcy after 24 hours, whereas nonsurvivors displayed persistent increased CO/CI.
§Adult patients: Patients who survived had decreased SVR/SVRI but progressed toward normalcy after 24 hours, whereas nonsurvivors displayed persistent decreased SVR/SVRI.
CO, cardiac output; *CI,* cardiac index; *CVP,* central venous pressure; *MAP,* mean arterial pressure; *PAWP,* pulmonary artery wedge pressure; *PVRI,* pulmonary vascular resistance index; *SVR,* systemic vascular resistance; *SVRI,* systemic vascular resistance index.
Modified from Curley MAQ. Shock. In: Curley MAQ, Smith J, Moloney-Harmon P, eds. *Critical Care Nursing of Infants and Children.* Philadelphia, Pa: WB Saunders Co; 1996:883.

❖ ALTERATION IN TISSUE PERFUSION RELATED TO MALDISTRIBUTION OF BLOOD FLOW SECONDARY TO SYSTEMIC INFLAMMATORY RESPONSE, CAPILLARY PERMEABILITY, VASODILATION, VASOCONSTRICTION, AND MICROVASCULAR THROMBI

❖ INADEQUATE CARDIAC OUTPUT DUE TO INCREASED ENERGY EXPENDITURES AND MYOCARDIAL DYSFUNCTION SECONDARY TO MEDIATOR RELEASE AND ACIDOSIS

❖ IMPAIRED GAS EXCHANGE RELATED TO VASOCONSTRICTION, INCREASED CAPILLARY PERMEABILITY, AND ALTERATIONS IN PULMONARY ENDOTHELIAL CELLS

❖ HYPERTHERMIA OR HYPOTHERMIA RELATED TO INFECTIOUS PROCESS, MEDIATOR RELEASE, AND INCREASED BASAL METABOLIC RATE

❖ ALTERATION IN NUTRITION, LESS THAN BODY REQUIREMENTS, RELATED TO HYPERMETABOLISM SECONDARY TO MEDIATOR RELEASE AND INADEQUATE NUTRITIONAL SUPPORT

E. **GOALS AND DESIRED PATIENT OUTCOMES**
   1. Prevention and early recognition of children with sepsis or septic shock
   2. Early, accurate, and complete administration of antibiotics
   3. Early and aggressive fluid resuscitation until improved perfusion is observed as evidenced by improved mental status, diminished tachycardia, capillary refill of less than 2 seconds, warm extremities, strong pulses, increased urine output, and restoration and maintenance of normal blood pressure (Carcillo, 1993)
   4. Restoration of optimal balance of oxygen supply and demand and thus tissue perfusion as indicated by arterial oxygen saturation of 92% or higher, hemoglobin concentration of 10 g/dl or greater, CI between 3.4 and 4.5 L/min/m^2 BSA, oxygen delivery (Do_2) between 500 and 600 ml/min/m^2, normal oxygen consumption ($\dot{V}o_2$); infants, oxygen 10 to 14 ml/kg/min; children, oxygen 7 to 11 ml/kg/min), and normalization of serum lactate of less than 2 mEq/L
   5. Early nutritional support
   6. Minimization of the risk and extent of organ dysfunction

F. **PATIENT CARE MANAGEMENT**
   1. Recognize that each specific intervention has a place in the overall treatment perspective (Bone, 1993; Natanson et al, 1995). Essential treatment *must* include both *definitive treatment* including identification, localization, and eradication of the source of infection with antibiotic administration **and** *advanced life support treatment* including oxygenation, ventilation, and circulation with fluid and inotropic administration. *Controversial treatments* are those with conflicting results or undetermined efficacy such as steroids and morphine antagonists. *Futuristic treatments* are those currently under investigation or scheduled for investigation in the future such as passive immunization and monoclonal antibody administration. Controversial and futuristic treatments often fall into one of two approaches, which include either neutralizing microbiologic toxins or modulating host inflammatory-immune responses.
   2. **Identify those patients at risk** for the development of sepsis or septic shock. Early recognition of sepsis or septic shock can be challenging, since either may be subtle and insidious, especially in younger patients such as neonates and infants and patients undergoing treatments or interventions that alter inflammatory-immune response, including glucocorticoid administration. The *classic presentation of fever, tachycardia,* and *vasodilation* with warm flushed skin is seen in the majority of children with innocuous viral and bacterial infection (tachypnea accompanies a respiratory source of infection) but also in children whose infection progresses to septic shock (Carcillo, 1993). Monitor ongoing changes in the patient or the patient's response(s) such as behavior, temperature patterns (e.g., fever), and WBC count.
   3. **Initial resuscitation**
      a. *Assessment of airway, breathing, and circulation (ABCs):* Rapid cardiopulmonary assessment, proposed by the American Heart Association Pediatric Ad-

vanced Life Support (PALS) Program (Table 9–18), includes a primary survey of life-threatening conditions followed by a secondary survey. Approximately 80% of children with septic shock require intubation and mechanical ventilatory support within 24 hours of admission (Carcillo et al, 1991). Obtain vascular access using PALS guidelines (Chameides and Hazinski, 1994). Central access and two IV access lines are preferred. Once the ABCs are ensured, the child should receive, as required, antibiotic administration, volume resuscitation, and vasoactive agents.

b. *Antibiotic administration:* Blood culture specimens should be obtained prior to the administration of antibiotics, but antibiotics should never be withheld to obtain a culture. *Administering antibiotics and obtaining cultures are a concomitant priority.* Empiric administration of antibiotics with the presence of bacterial septic shock is presumed in all patients (Carcillo, 1993). The American Academy of Pediatrics Committee on Infectious Disease recommendations include the following:

- *Outpatient sepsis*
  - Patients younger than 2 months: Ampicillin and gentamicin or ampicillin and cefotaxime or ceftriaxone
  - Patients older than 2 months: Cefotaxime or ceftriaxone or cefotaxime or ceftriaxone with a combination of ampicillin and chloramphenicol
- Nosocomial sepsis requires therapy that is specific to the individual hospital and ICU. Once the results of the cultures are known, the antibiotic regimen may be refined:
  - *Staphylococcus* and gram-negative organisms are common: Vancomycin and an aminoglycoside
  - Hospitals with significant methicillin-resistant *Staphylococcus aureus:* Vancomycin
  - Hospitals with significant gentamicin-resistant *Pseudomonas* or *Klebsiella:* Antibiotic with sensitivity toward these strains

c. *Volume resuscitation:* In a child with septic shock, an aggressive approach is taken: 20 ml/kg fluid bolus with subsequent boluses of 20 ml/kg to a total of 60 ml/kg in the first hour of resuscitation (Carcillo, 1993). Boluses are preceded and followed by systematic and repeated assessments of clinical parameters of perfusion and are administered until perfusion improves. *Some children require more than 60 ml/kg of fluid within the first hour of presentation.* Fluid boluses for volume resuscitation should be administered via IV push and within 20 minutes of presentation (Carcillo, 1993). The type of fluid initially is isotonic crystalloid fluid (LR or 0.9% NaCl).

d. *Vasoactive agents* (Table 9–19): If volume resuscitation fails to restore perfusion or severe hypotension is present, vasoactive agents are indicated. A mixed α- and β-adrenergic agent, such as dopamine (5 μg/kg/min), is usually initiated. If perfusion remains inadequate, dopamine is increased to β-adrenergic concentrations (10 μg/kg/min). If perfusion continues to be decreased, inotropic agents are added. In the presence of hypotension, the drug of choice is epinephrine. An example of a septic shock resuscitation protocol incorporating the use of fluids and vasoactive substances is as follows (Parillo, 1990):

- Fluid resuscitation until PAWP is 15 to 18 mm Hg: For the infant and young child, a more age-appropriate PAWP value is 12 to 15 mm Hg.
- Dopamine to raise the MAP to at least 60 mm Hg (age related)
- If the dopamine dose is greater than 20 μg/kg/min, norepinephrine or epinephrine is titrated to maintain the MAP ≥60 mm Hg. Dopamine is then decreased to renal doses (1 to 5 μg/kg/min).

Table 9–18. RAPID CARDIOPULMONARY ASSESSMENT OF A HEALTHY AND DECOMPENSATING CHILD

ASSESSMENT PARAMETER	HEALTHY CHILD	DECOMPENSATING CHILD
Airway Patency	Able to maintain independently	Maintainable with interventions such as head positioning, suctioning, adjuncts; unmaintainable requiring intubation
Breathing		
Respiratory rate	Within age-appropriate limits*	Tachypnea or bradypnea as compared to age-appropriate limits* *Note:* Warning parameter: >60 breaths/min
Chest movement (presence)	Chest rise and fall with each respiration	Minimal to no chest movement with respiratory effort
Chest movement (quality)	Silent and effortless respirations; chest rise concomitant with abdomen with each breath	Evidence of labored respirations with retractions; asynchronous movement between chest and abdomen with respirations
Air movement (presence)	Air exchange bilaterally in all lobes	Despite movement of chest, minimal or no air exchange is noted on auscultation
Air movement (quality)	Breath sounds of normal intensity and duration per auscultation assessment	Nasal flaring, grunting, stridor, or wheezing
Circulation		
Heart rate (presence)	Apical beat within age-appropriate limits*	Absent heart rate, bradycardia or tachycardia as compared to age-appropriate limits* *Note:* Warning parameters: Infant: <80 bpm Child <5 y: >180 bpm Child >5 y: >150 bpm
Heart rate (quality)	Heart rate regular with a normal sinus rhythm	Irregular, slow, or very rapid rate; common dysrhythmias include supraventricular tachycardia, bradyarrhythmias, and asystole
Skin	Warm, pink extremities with capillary refill ≤2 s; peripheral pulses present bilaterally with normal intensity	Pallor, cyanotic, or mottled skin; cool to cold extremities; capillary refill time >2 s; peripheral pulses weak or absent; central pulses weak
Cerebral perfusion	Alert to and interested in surroundings; recognizes parents; responsive to fear and pain; normal muscle tone	Irritable, lethargic, obtunded or comatose; minimal or no reaction to pain; loose muscle tone (e.g., floppy)
Blood pressure	Within age-appropriate limits	A fall in blood pressure from age-appropriate limits, a *late sign of decompensation* *Note:* A fall of 10 mm Hg systolic pressure is significant. Lower systolic blood pressure limit: infant ≤1 mo: 60 mm Hg; infant ≤1 y: 70 mm Hg; child ≥1 y: 70+ mm Hg (2 × age in y)

*All vital signs are interpreted within the context of age, clinical condition, and other external factors, such as the presence of fever.

Modified from Moloney-Harmon P, Rosenthal CH. Nursing care modifications for the child in the adult ICU. In: Stillwell S, ed. *Critical Care Nursing Reference Book*. St Louis, Mo: Mosby–Year Book, Inc; 1992:615–616.

Table 9–19. INOTROPIC AND VASOACTIVE AGENTS USED IN THE TREATMENT OF SEPTIC SHOCK

AGENT	DOSE* (μg/kg/min)	EFFECT	INDICATIONS AND CAUTIONS
Dopamine	1–20	1–5 μg/kg/min: Dopaminergic effects; primarily increase GFR and UOP 2–10 μg/kg/min: Dopaminergic effects persist with β_1-Adrenergic effects including chronotropy and inotrophy >10 μg/kg/min: α-Adrenergic effects including vasoconstriction	First-line choice Watch for tachyarrhythmias
Epinephrine	0.01–0.3 or higher	0.01–0.05 μg/kg/min: β_1-Adrenergic effects including chronotropy and inotropy >0.05 μg/kg/min: Increasing α-adrenergic effects producing vasoconstriction	Choice for patients unresponsive to dopamine
Dobutamine	2–20	Selective β-adrenergic effects including inotropy and chronotropy; β_2 adrenergic effects produce vasodilation	At doses >10 μg/kg/min may widen pulse pressure Watch for tachyarrhythmias and hypotension
Isoproterenol	0.05–0.1	β_1-adrenergic and β_2-adrenergic agonist β_1-adrenergic effects produce chronotropy β_2-adrenergic effects produce peripheral vasodilation	May be helpful with pulmonary hypertension May increase pulmonary shunting Watch for tachyarrhythmias and hypotension Will increase myocardial oxygen consumption
Norepinephrine	0.1–1 or higher	Excellent α-adrenergic agonist with β-adrenergic agonist activity Potent peripheral and renal vasoconstriction	Watch for tachyarrhythmias Will increase myocardial work, oxygen consumption
Phenylephrine		Partial α-adrenergic agonist	Agent for use in combination with β-adrenergic agonist
Nitroglycerin	1–20	1–3 μg/kg/min: Pulmonary vasodilation >3 μg/kg/min: Systemic vasodilation	Excellent vasodilator
Sodium nitroprusside	0.5–10	Systemic and pulmonary artery and venous dilator	Premier afterload reducing agent Frequently requires simultaneous administration of volume bolus Long-term use may be associated with cyanide toxicity

*There are some individual differences in the dose-to-response effect. Optimal dosing is through individual titration at the patient's bedside using serial and systematic assessment of clinical and hemodynamic parameters.
GFR, glomerular filtration rate; *UOP*, urine output.

(*Note:* Protocols should be used *only* as guides to therapy. Vasoactive support should be evaluated using consistent clinical criteria rather than numeric values only.)

4. **Cardiovascular management**

   a. *Support and optimize cardiac output:* Cardiac output may be within the normal range or increased at times in the continuum of septic shock, but it is still inadequate to meet the body's demands. Normal or increased cardiac output is often accompanied by low blood pressure and SVR, thus affecting perfusion and oxygen transport. Recommendations for each of the constituents of cardiac output serve *only* as a guideline. Each patient should be evaluated individually with regard to age, clinical context (including the changing continuum of septic shock), and total hemodynamic profile.

   b. *Increase preload with early, aggressive fluid therapy* (isotonic crystalloids first and colloids later): Volume administration is used to treat hypoperfusion, hypotension, and decreased preload due to increased capillary permeability, vasodilation, and maldistribution of blood flow. Fluid resuscitation in excess of 40 ml/kg to pediatric patients during the first hour after presentation was associated with improved survival, decreased occurrence of persistent hypovolemia, and no increase in the risk of cardiogenic pulmonary edema or ARDS (Carcillo et al, 1991). Aggressive fluid administration stops progression in approximately 50% of adult septic shock patients (Parrillo et al., 1990). Monitor the response to volume administration through repeated, systematic assessment of clinical parameters (Table 9–16). Serial measurements of cardiac filling pressures (CVP, pulmonary capillary wedge pressure [PCWP]) and ventricular performance (CO/CI, SVR) are useful in monitoring recommended CVPs of 5 to 8 mm Hg or PAWPs of 12 to 15 mm Hg.

   c. *Maximize contractility:* In sepsis the dysfunctional myocardium results in less cardiac output for a given LVEDV (Carcillo, 1993). Inotropic agents (e.g., dopamine, dobutamine, epinephrine) may be indicated for the improvement of contractility (Table 9–19).

   d. *Manipulate afterload* (SVR): Persistent hypotension may occur even in the presence of aggressive volume administration and is often related to mediator release and vasodilation rather than low CO/CI. Vasopressors may be indicated and larger doses may be required over time because of continuing mediator release, capillary leakage, and decreased responsiveness of α- and β-adrenergic receptors. Hypodynamic shock is characterized by increased SVR, low CO/CI, and high LVEDP. Vasodilators (e.g., nitroprusside, nitroglycerin) may be indicated. The goal for vasodilation therapy is to reduce afterload while increasing contractility, CO/CI, and tissue perfusion. Manipulation of afterload most often occurs in combination with an inotropic agent. The inotropic agent maintains the blood pressure and enhances contractility, whereas the vasodilator reduces the afterload and cardiac filling pressures.

   e. *Support and optimize heart rate:* Various inotropic and vasoactive agents may result in tachyarrhythmias and worsen the clinical and hemodynamic picture. Tachycardia may be significant, since two thirds of coronary artery perfusion occurs during diastole and is primarily determined by aortic diastolic pressure and duration of diastole. Manipulation of heart rate may require manipulation of CI, SVR, or *both* (Carcillo, 1993).

5. **Respiratory management**

   a. The *goal of respiratory management is to balance oxygen delivery with the individual patient's tissue oxygenation requirements* rather than normalizing hemodynamic parameters and laboratory values to age-appropriate values (Mims, 1992).

b. *Assess and maximize tissue oxygenation* (See Chapter 2). Support airway and ventilation. Position the child to support maximal airway patency. Provide supplemental oxygen. Anticipate intubation, since the majority of children with septic shock require intubation and mechanical ventilation.

c. *Assess tissue oxygenation* using parameters such as ABG analysis, oxygen saturation, and oxygen content. Normal PaO_2 is 80 to 100 mm Hg on room air. With supplemental oxygen, the lower limit of the normal PaO_2 expected for a given FIO_2 is estimated by multiplying the FIO_2 by 5. Hypoxemia is present if the hemoglobin saturation is less than 90%. *Oxygen content (CaO_2)* is the quantity of oxygen in each 100 ml of blood and includes both the amount dissolved in the plasma and carried in the hemoglobin. Normal oxygen content is 18 to 20 ml/dl of blood.

$$CaO_2 = [Hgb\ (g/dl) \times 1.36\ ml\ O_2/g\ Hgb \times SaO_2] + (0.003 \times PaO_2)$$

d. *Assess oxygen utilization* using the parameters of oxygen delivery and oxygen consumption.

- *Oxygen transport or delivery (DO_2)* is the volume of oxygen delivered to the tissues each minute and reflects the quantity of oxygen available to the tissues.

$$DO_2\ (ml/min/m^2) = CI \times Arterial\ O_2\ content$$

- *Oxygen consumption ($\dot{V}O_2$)* is the amount of oxygen consumed by the tissues per minute and reflects an overall index of total body metabolism. $\dot{V}O_2$ in infants and children, which ranges from 5 to 14 ml O_2/kg/min, can be measured, estimated, or calculated:

$$\dot{V}O_2 = CO \times [(SaO_2 - S\bar{v}O_2) \times (Hgb\ concentration \times 1.36\ ml/g)] \times 10$$

- *Oxygen extraction ratio* is determined by dividing oxygen consumption by oxygen transport or delivery with the normal value, around 20% to 25%, usually <25%.

$$O_2\ Extraction\ ratio = \frac{\dot{V}O_2}{\dot{D}O_2} = \frac{CaO_2 - CvO_2}{CaO_2}$$

- *Mixed venous oxygen saturation ($S\bar{v}O_2$)* is a continuous reflection of the balance between oxygen supply and oxygen demand, with the normal range between 60% and 80%.

e. *Optimize oxygen delivery:* See Chapters 2 and 3.

f. *Minimize oxygen demand:* Minimize states that increase metabolic rate such as seizures, cold stress, rigors, shivering, pain, fear, and agitation. Control fever with acetaminophen (Mims, 1992). Although acetaminophen is often cited as the drug of choice, clinical experience indicates the need for monitoring serum levels in patients with prolonged sepsis, since there may be an increased risk for toxicity. Aspirin is contraindicated with viral illness; it also inhibits prostaglandin synthesis and decreases renal blood flow. Avoid reducing fever below 37° C, since it will cause a shift of the oxyhemoglobin dissociation curve to the left, thereby impairing oxygen extraction (Mims, 1992).

6. **Minimize iatrogenic complications** (MacIntyre, 1993)

a. *Minimize the risk of and assess for barotrauma* by minimizing or avoiding excessive airway pressures and using the lowest required inspired oxygen concentrations.

    b. *Minimize the risk of and assess for further cardiac dysfunction* by monitoring electrolytes and watching for tachyarrhythmias secondary to vasoactive and inotropic agents or electrolyte imbalance.

    c. *Minimize the risk of and assess for aspiration* by placing a nasogastric tube, ensuring the tube's patency and function, and elevating the head of the bed 30 degrees if tolerated.

    d. *Minimize the risk of and assess for renal toxicity* by optimizing tissue perfusion, administering dopamine (at renal doses), and judiciously using medications that are toxic to the kidneys.

7. **Supportive and investigational therapies**

    a. *The best management is prevention:* Good hand washing is essential. The hands of health care personnel spread most nosocomial organisms from patient to patient (Maki, 1995). Research documents the infrequency of hand washing by health care personnel before and after patient contact as usually less than one third of the time (Albert and Condie, 1981; Davenport, 1992; Donowitz, 1987; Graham, 1990; McLane et al, 1983). All team members should wash their hands *before* and *after* every patient contact. Simple protective isolation (gown and gloves) for the care of high-risk children, particularly those who require prolonged (>7 days) ICU care has proven beneficial in reducing the incidence of nosocomial infection (Klein et al, 1989). Patients with severe neutropenia or high-dose corticosteroid therapy are at risk for infection from endogenous microorganisms and airborne fungi (e.g., *Aspergillus*). The risk of *Aspergillus* infection is directly related to counts of airborne fungi. Outbreaks of fungemias are usually linked to building construction or dysfunction in air control systems. Placement of patients in positive pressure rooms with sporefree HEPA-filtered air reduces this risk.

    b. The *GI tract normally serves as an effective barrier* by preventing contents of the bowel from entering the body and by preventing body contents from leaking into the intestinal lumen (Phillips and Olsen, 1993). Gram-negative bacteria, normally present within the intestinal lumen, are isolated from the body's internal environment by GI tract mucosa impermeability to gram-negative bacteria, GI tract lymphoid tissue preventing invasion of gram-negative bacteria, and anaerobic bacteria (commensal bacteria) preventing overgrowth of gram-negative bacteria (Hazinski, 1994).

- *Translocation* is the egress of bacteria or their by products across the mucosal barrier and into the lymphatics or portal circulation (O'Neill, 1992). It is important to minimize or prevent conditions thought to increase the risk for translocation (Hazinski, 1994; O'Neill, 1992). Compromised host defenses (first, second, or third line of defense) that increase the risk for translocation include changes in GI tract pH, thermal or traumatic injury, radiation therapy, immunosuppression, nutritional compromise, and liver dysfunction (altered Kupffer's cell function). Alteration in normal GI tract flora (through viral or bacterial infection, reduction or impairment of motility, or antibiotic administration) and alteration in gut membrane permeability (related to decreased perfusion [e.g., shock] or GI tract mucosal injury) also increase the risk for translocation.

- *Assess for evidence of GI tract compromise.* Monitor and report changes in stool, since this may be an indication of mucosal injury and facilitate a movement of plasma and blood into the intestinal lumen (O'Neill, 1992). Note the amount and consistency of diarrhea, guaiac-positive stools (or more obvious GI tract bleeding), and bacterial counts; stool cultures may indicate bacterial overgrowth. Increases in gastric output may be caused by numerous factors but may serve as an early indicator of GI tract compromise. Abdominal distention is also an early indicator of GI tract compromise. Mucosal pH can be measured indirectly via a balloon-tipped catheter (gastric tonometry). Normal pH reflects adequate perfusion, whereas an acidotic pH reflects tissue hypoxia. Ileus is a late sign of GI tract compromise.

- *Supportive GI tract therapies* include stress ulcer prophylaxis. Antacid therapy was once thought to protect the stomach and duodenum by maintaining a neutral pH but is now recognized to promote bacterial growth (O'Neill, 1992). Histamine receptor antagonists (H$_2$ blockers) are an alternative or adjunct to antacids, as they reduce acid secretion, although histamine is not the only stimulus to acid secretion. H$_2$ blockers may also contribute to bacterial growth. Sucralfate is a nonabsorbable aluminum salt that has minimal to no effect on gastric acid secretion. Actions include antibacterial properties; trophic effects on the gastric mucosa; coating of existing ulcers with a protective layer; prevention of ulcers by stimulating release of bicarbonate, mucus, and prostaglandin; and stimulation of mucus cell renewal (O'Neill, 1992).

- *Selective digestive decontamination (SDD)* is based on the belief that many infections in the critically ill are caused by endogenous bacteria in the GI tract that are either aspirated into the lungs or translocated across the mucosal barrier into the systemic circulation (O'Neill, 1992). The effect of decontamination on pneumonia and other nosocomial infections is inconclusive (Maki, 1995). A metaanalysis revealed that SDD had a significant reduction in the incidence of ventilator-associated pneumonias but no improvement in patient survival (Selective Decontamination, 1993). There appears to be a risk for increased colonization and infection with antibiotic-resistant microorganisms (Webb, 1992).

c. *Nutritional support* should include enteral feedings, since they prevent intestinal atrophy by stimulating mucosal cell turnover, stimulating hormones that have a trophic effect on the gut mucosa, and assisting in the sloughing of mucosal cells and promotion of new cell growth (O'Neill, 1992). Enteral feedings also enhance immune functions of the GI tract (Ackerman et al, 1994). The effects of the amount and type of feeding on bacterial translocation remains under investigation.

- *Glutamine* is an important nutrient thought to play an integral role in maintaining gut integrity (O'Neill, 1992). Glutamine is the primary fuel source for the enterocyte. As enterocytes use glutamine for fuel, glucose is spared for the organs that prefer glucose. The enteral route is thought to be more optimal than the parenteral route (Ackerman et al, 1994).

d. *CSFs:* See Chapter 8. An increased incidence of infection is associated with both severity and duration of neutropenia (ANC ≤1000/mm^3). Increased survival rates were noted in experimental newborn animal models of sepsis with the use of CSFs (Cairo et al, 1992; Cairo, Mauss, et al, 1990; Cairo, Plunkett, et al, 1990) through their ability to increase the number of circulating neutrophils and to augment the effectiveness of neutrophils and macrophages in killing microorganisms (Gillan et al, 1993). Administration of granulocyte colony-stimulating factor (G-CSF) has appeared to correct, in part, both neutropenia and neutrophil dysfunction observed in neonates during sepsis in phase I clinical trials (Gillan et al, 1992). Further clinical trials are currently underway.

e. *Prophylactic antibiotics:* Penicillin prophylaxis is recommended for patients with splenic dysfunction (sickle cell anemia) or who have had a splenectomy to prevent pneumococcal infection. Rifampin prophylaxis is recommended for those who have had close contact with *Haemophilus influenzae* or meningococcal disease.

f. *Vaccines:* Recent changes in the immunization program have the potential to significantly affect the incidence of community-acquired sepsis. *H. influenzae* type B vaccine is recommended for all 2-month-old to 4-year-old children. Hepatitis B vaccine is now initiated at birth and is being given to other ages as well. Meningococcal vaccine is recommended for high-risk patients. The measles-mumps-rubella (MMR) booster program was initiated to reduce the incidence of acute measles-related illness in adolescents (Slota, 1993).

G. **RELEVANT PHARMACOLOGY**

1. **Inotropic and vasoactive agents:** See Table 9–19.
2. **Ibuprofen** is a cyclooxygenase inhibitor that can block arachidonic acid metabolism through the cyclooxygenase pathway. Clinical trials show reduced morbidity and mortality from sepsis in animals with the use of prospective administration of ibuprofen (Balk et al, 1988).

COMPLICATIONS OF SEPTIC SHOCK

A. **IMPLICATIONS FOR OTHER SYSTEMS**

Given the complexity of the immune system, it is not surprising that a systemic inflammatory response and septic shock influence many body organs and systems. Many body systems are affected, and organ-specific dysfunction may result. Complications of septic shock include ARDS (see Chapter 2), disseminated intravascular coagulation (DIC; see Chapter 8), acute renal failure (see Chapter 5), and MODS.

B. **MULTIPLE-ORGAN DYSFUNCTION SYNDROME (MODS)**

MODS causes 97% of the deaths that occur within the PICU (Wilkinson et al, 1986). Sepsis is the cause of MODS in approximately 47% of the cases in one study (Wilkinson et al, 1987). Criteria for pediatric patients with MODS are detailed in Table 9–20 (Wilkinson et al, 1987).

1. **Frequency** of specific organ involvement in children experiencing MODS:
   a. Respiratory system (88%)
   b. Cardiovascular (44%)
   c. Neurologic (24%)
   d. Hematologic (7%)
   e. Renal (5%)

2. The **mortality** associated with MODS is related to the number of organ systems involved in the dysfunction process, but these estimates are not sensitive enough to be used as criteria for withholding therapy (Wilkinson et al, 1986 and 1987):
   a. One system is associated with 1% mortality.
   b. Two systems are associated with 11% to 26% mortality.
   c. Three systems are associated with 50% to 62% mortality.
   d. Four systems are associated with 75% mortality.

3. Children with **simultaneous organ dysfunction** have higher mortality rates than those children with progressive or sequential dysfunction (even with the same number of organs involved in dysfunction; Moloney-Harmon and

Table 9–20. CRITERIA FOR INFANTS AND CHILDREN WITH MULTIPLE-ORGAN DYSFUNCTION SYNDROME (MODS)

ORGAN SYSTEM	CRITERIA
Respiratory	Respiratory rate >90/min (infants <12 mo)
	Respiratory rate >70/min (children ≥12 mo)
	Pao_2 <40 mm Hg (in absence of cyanotic heart disease)
	$Paco_2$ >65 mm Hg
	Pao_2/Fio_2 <250 mm Hg
	Mechanical ventilation (>24 h if postoperative)
	Tracheal intubation for airway obstruction or acute respiratory failure
Cardiovascular	MAP <40 mm Hg (infants <12 mo)
	MAP <50 mm Hg (children ≥12 mo)
	Heart rate <50 bpm (infants <12 mo)
	Heart rate <40 bpm (children ≥12 mo)
	Cardiac arrest
	Continuous vasoactive drug infusion for hemodynamic support
Neurologic	Glasgow coma scale <5
	Fixed, dilated pupils
	Persistent (>20 min) increased ICP (>20 mm Hg or requiring therapeutic intervention)
Hematologic	Hemoglobin <5 g/dl
	WBC <3000/mm^3
	Platelets <20,000/mm^3
	DIC (PT >20 s or aPTT >60 s in presence of positive results from FSP assay)
Renal	BUN >100 mg/dl
	Serum creatinine >2 mg/dl
	Dialysis
GI tract	Blood transfusion >20 ml/kg in 24 h because of GI tract hemorrhage (endoscopic confirmation optional)
Hepatic	Total bilirubin >5 mg/dl and AST or LDH more than twice normal value (without evidence of hemolysis)
	Hepatic encephalopathy ≥grade II

AST, aspartate aminotransferase; *BUN,* blood urea nitrogen; *DIC,* disseminated intravascular coagulation; *FSP,* fibrin split products; *GI,* gastrointestinal; *ICP,* intracranial pressure; *LDH,* lactate dehydrogenase; *MAP,* mean arterial pressure; *PT,* prothrombin time; *aPTT,* activated partial thromboplastin time; *WBC,* white blood cell.
From Wilkinson JD, Pollack MM, Glass NL, Kanter RK, Katz RW, Steinhart CM. Mortality associated with multiple organ system failure and sepsis in pediatric intensive care. *J Pediatr.* 1987;111:324–328.

Czerwinski, 1992). One study (Proulx et al, 1994) found three independent risk markers for death. These risk markers were the maximum number of simultaneous organ system failures during the PICU stay, age ≤12 months, and the pediatric risk of mortality score (PRISM) on the day of admission.

4. **Sepsis** is not as strongly associated with MODS in children as in the adult population as more than 50% of pediatric critical care patients developed MODS in the absence of sepsis in one study (Wilkinson et al, 1987). Another study (Proulx et al, 1994) found that sepsis did not increase the risk for death in children.

BURNS   PAULA DICKERSON, MARY D. GORDON, and PAM WALTER

Burns in the pediatric patient introduce diagnostic and therapeutic difficulties related to correct estimation of burn size and depth, fluid resuscitation and maintenance, airway management, vascular access, and thermal maintenance. Children present with age-related limitations of physiologic reserve making it difficult for them to respond to an extensive burn injury. Recognition of the physiologic and psychosocial needs of children is paramount to providing optimal burn care.

A. INCIDENCE

1. Each year in the United States, 2 million people seek medical treatment for burn injuries. From 30% to 40% of patients hospitalized for burn injuries are younger than 15 years of age; with approximately twice as many boys injured (Herndon et al, 1993). The greatest portion of pediatric burn injuries occurs in infants and toddlers (Saffle et al, 1995).

2. In the home, burns and fires are the leading cause of pediatric injury-related deaths. Outside the home, burns and fires rank just behind motor vehicle crashes, falls, and drowning as a cause of unintentional injury-related death (Baker et al, 1992).

3. Among small children, scalds are the predominant burn injury, with a progressive increase in contact and flame burns with advancing age (Fig. 9–5; Saffle et al, 1995).

4. Ten percent of all burns in children admitted to burn centers in the United States are caused by abuse (Purdue and Hunt, 1991b).

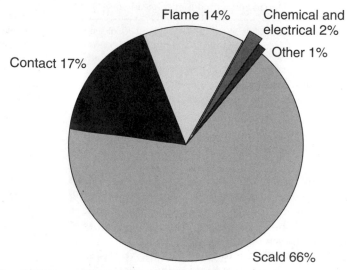

Figure 9–5.   Etiology of burn injuries in children 1 to 4 years old. (Data from Saffle JR, Davis B, Williams P, et al. Recent outcomes in the treatment of burn injury in the United States: a report from the American Burn Association patient registry. *J Burn Care Rehabil.* 1995;16[3, pt 1]:219–232.)

ANATOMY AND PHYSIOLOGY OF THE SKIN

A. STRUCTURE

1. **Depth:** Skin thickness varies, depending on the age and sex of the individual and location on the body. Proportionally, skin thickness in each body area is similar in children and adults, although infant skin thickness in each specific area may be less than half that of adult skin. The skin does not reach adult thickness until approximately 5 years of age (Heimback et al, 1992).

2. **Layers**

   a. *Epidermis:* The outermost (protective) layer consists mostly of epithelial cells. The epidermis contains keratin, which limits fluid loss, and melanin (Kahn et al, 1991), which contributes to the basic color of the skin. The deepest layers are on the palms of the hands and the soles of the feet. The innermost layer is responsible for the reproduction of new epithelial cells that migrate toward the surface to replace the outer layers. It has a high capacity for regeneration after damage, provided that the basal layer is intact or that the appendages are still present.

   b. *Dermis:* The dermis lies below the epidermis and is composed of connective tissue, elastic fibers, blood and lymph vessels, and nerves. It provides mechanical strength because of its high proportion of collagen and elastic fibers, and it also provides a reservoir of defensive and regenerative elements capable of combating infection and repairing deep wounds. The dermis contains portions of hair follicles, sebaceous glands, and ducts of sweat glands. The walls of the hair follicle are composed of epithelium and connective tissue. The sebaceous gland sac is lined with epithelial cells from the basement membrane. Because of the epithelial lining, the sweat glands and hair follicles serve in the reepithelialization of partial-thickness wounds.

   c. The *hypodermis* (also called the subcutaneous tissue) is composed of fat, smooth muscle, and connective tissue. It varies in thickness from one part of the body to another and is anchored by connective tissue originating in the dermis.

B. FUNCTIONS

1. **Protective barrier:** The skin is the primary barrier against damage from microorganisms, desiccation, and mechanical factors.

2. **Thermal regulation:** Heat exchange is regulated with the environment. Excretion and absorption also occur through the skin.

3. **Touch:** Skin receptors modulate sensory impulses, pain, temperature, and pressure.

4. **Appearance of the skin:** Skin contributes to body image.

PATHOPHYSIOLOGY OF THERMAL INJURY

A. CLINICAL COURSE

1. The **emergent phase** (1 to 3 days after the burn) begins with the initial hemodynamic response to thermal injury and lasts until capillary integrity is restored and fluid replacement is completed. IV fluid resuscitation is initiated in burns covering 10% to 15% total body surface area (TBSA) or greater in children (Herndon et al, 1993) and greater than 20% TBSA in adults.

2. The **acute phase** (3 days to weeks after the burn) begins with the onset of

diuresis of edema fluid mobilized from the interstitial space and continues through closure of the burn wound.

3. The **rehabilitative phase** begins on admission to the ICU and comprises prevention of functional deficits and psychosocial support. As wounds heal, correction of functional deficits begins with ongoing psychosocial support.

B. CLASSIFICATION OF CELLULAR INJURY

1. The local burn wound is the result of heat necrosis of cells and results in coagulation necrosis of tissue that has both breadth and depth (i.e., surface area and depth or degree).

2. The extent of cellular destruction depends on the intensity of the heat, duration of exposure, and the tissue involved. When absorption of heat energy exceeds the ability of the tissue to dissipate the absorbed heat, cellular injury results in varying depths.

3. The pathology of a cutaneous injury can be viewed in two ways.

a. *Functional classification:* Classification of the burn injury based on functional changes considers the extent and depth of the burn and defines more precisely the pathology (Fig. 9–6).

- The zone of hyperemia is the most superficial area. It is considered viable tissue and recovers in a matter of days. The injury is analogous to the erythema in first-degree burns (i.e., sunburn).
- The zone of stasis is less superficial and central to the zone of hyperemia. It is caused by vascular damage and the inflammatory response, resulting in compromised tissue perfusion. Over the ensuing 2 to 3 days after the burn, part or all the zone of stasis may evolve into a deeper injury. If resuscitation promptly restores compromised tissue blood flow, this tissue typically survives.
- The zone of coagulation is the area having the most intimate contact with the heat source and therefore the most damage. Since it is characterized by cellular death, coagulation necrosis is the result of most burn injury in this zone.

b. *Descriptive classification:* A descriptive classification is based on the destruction of the skin layers. This classification indicates which layer of skin has been injured and uses the familiar terminology of first-, second-, and third-degree burns (Fig. 9–7).

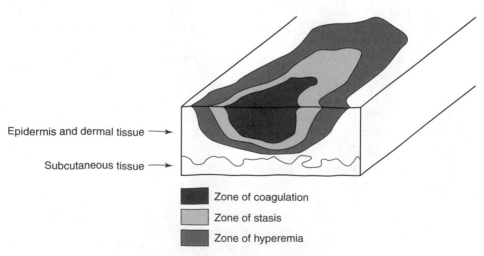

Epidermis and dermal tissue →
Subcutaneous tissue →

■ Zone of coagulation
■ Zone of stasis
■ Zone of hyperemia

Figure 9–6. Zones of tissue injury.

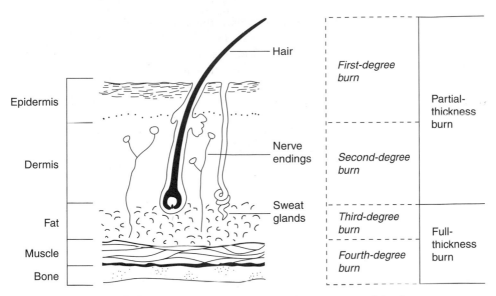

Figure 9–7.   Schematic cross-sectional representation of the skin.

C. SYSTEMIC RESPONSE TO THERMAL INJURY

1. An extensive burn affects all organ systems and is manifested by a biphasic pattern of early hypofunction (i.e., decreased cardiac output, increased capillary permeability) followed by hyperfunction (i.e., hypermetabolism).

2. The events, magnitude, and duration of the systemic manifestations of burn shock are proportional to the extent of burn injury and plateau at approximately 50% to 60% burn surface area (Pruitt and Goodwin, 1990).

3. Although the exact cause of burn shock is not totally understood, characteristic fluid volume shifts and hemodynamic changes that accompany burn shock have been identified.

    a. *Cardiovascular response:* The initial response to a large burn injury is characterized by a decrease in cardiac output and increased peripheral vascular resistance. An uncharacterized factor present in circulation following massive burns has been implicated in this myocardial depression (Morehouse et al, 1992). The increased peripheral vascular resistance develops as an initial physiologic response to hypovolemia, decreased cardiac output, and the release of vasoactive mediators from the stress response following injury.

    • Cardiac output returns to normal 18 to 24 hours after the burn. Peripheral vascular resistance returns to normal as cardiac output improves. As cardiac output improves, it exceeds normal values as the characteristic hyperdynamic state develops. Tachycardia develops as a physiologic response to hypovolemia, decreased cardiac output, and elevated catecholamine levels.

    • Microvasculature changes in the cell wall result in the disruption of normal capillary barriers separating the intravascular and interstitial compartments. This results in free exchange of fluid and plasma. This increased permeability permits essentially all elements of the vascular space, except blood cells and platelets, to escape, creating a relative hypovolemia. The fluid requirement necessary to restore and maintain tissue perfusion is directly related to the burn size. Capillary leak and edema following small burns are localized to the burn wound. Injury greater than 30% burn surface area produces not only localized burn wound edema but also a systemic capillary permeability and general body edema. The rate of progression of tissue edema is dependent on the adequacy and volume of fluid resuscitation. The maximal amount of edema occurs 8 to 12 hours after injury in small burns but up to 24 hours after injury in large burns. Capillary integrity is restored approximately 18 to 24 hours after the burn. Large burns may take up to 30 hours to regain capillary integrity.

b. *Hematologic response:* Within several hours of injury, as edema forms, the fluid shift and intravascular volume deficit results in hemoconcentration. The hematocrit increases secondary to loss of circulating plasma volume. Blood viscosity also increases.

- The characteristic anemia associated with burn injuries has multiple causes. Only about 10% of the RBC mass is lost to hemolysis during the burning process or by the extravasation of RBCs into the wound (Monafo and Bessey, 1992). Heat-injured RBCs have a shortened half-life and increased clearance. The ongoing postburn RBC hemolysis has been attributed to the release of inflammatory mediators (i.e., oxygen radicals, lipid peroxides) (Youn et al, 1992). Although the exact nature is not known, there is an impaired production of new RBCs by the bone marrow with a shortened RBC life span. Additionally, there is an ongoing effective blood loss related to daily wound care and multiple surgical procedures.
- Initially, there is a depression in serum clotting factors with a concomitant rise in fibrinogen degradation products, followed by a postresuscitation rise in increased levels of coagulation components. Platelet alterations include an increase in adhesiveness and shortened survival time.

c. *Pulmonary response:* In large burns without an inhalation injury, early alterations in pulmonary function occur indirectly through the release of inflammatory mediators (i.e., thromboxane) and intravascular hypoproteinemia, resulting in a transient hydrostatic pulmonary edema with a mild derangement in oxygenation (Sharar and Heimbach, 1991). A decrease in lung compliance may be related to chest wall edema, circumferential burns to the chest wall, smoke inhalation injury, preexisting lung disease, or fluid volume overload.

d. *GI tract response:* Decreased GI tract activity, caused by decreased tissue perfusion, is the by-product of hypovolemia and the neuroendocrine responses to injury. Risk for the development of a burn-stress-related ulceration (Curling's) and the incidence of ulceration have been greatly reduced by the routine use of antacid or H_2 receptor antagonist therapy. With adequate fluid resuscitation, GI tract activity returns to normal within 24 to 48 hours.

e. *Renal response:* With decreased intravascular volume there is a decrease in renal plasma flow and glomerular filtration rate (GFR), resulting in low urine output. If fluid resuscitation is inadequate or if resuscitation is delayed, oliguria ensues leading to acute renal failure. As the capillary integrity is restored, interstitial fluids are pulled back into the intravascular compartment, and diuresis occurs.

f. *Metabolic response:* With increased catecholamine and glucagon production, there is a mobilization of hepatic glycogen stores, coupled with a relative decrease in insulin production that commonly results in high serum glucose levels in the early postburn period. Within 24 to 48 hours after the burn, there is an increase in metabolism directly related to the severity of the injury. This hypermetabolic state is characterized by increases in oxygen consumption and heat production, with an increase in both core and skin temperatures. Severe injury accelerates nitrogen flow. Both protein synthesis and breakdown are increased. In patients not meeting nutritional goals, breakdown rates exceed synthesis, resulting in a negative nitrogen balance. As capillary integrity is restored, electrolyte replacement therapy becomes an ongoing process and continues until wound closure is achieved. As the wounds heal, either spontaneously or by skin grafting, the metabolic rate gradually returns to normal levels. The decrease in metabolic requirements is a gradual process. Metabolic requirements return to normal when the burn wound is fully mature, which may require up to 1 year or more after wound closure.

g. *Inflammatory-immune response:* Although the exact mechanisms of the inflammatory-immune response are not known, characteristic pathophysiologic activities are being recognized as a result of the burn injury. Alteration in the skin's protective function provides opportunity for invasion of microorganisms and primes the defensive mechanisms of the inflammatory and immune systems. It is hypothesized that a massive systemic inflammatory response is caused by the local trauma of a burn. It appears that a burn is a mediator-induced injury; although the local effects occur immediately, the systemic response to the mediators produced within a burn progresses and peaks 5 to 7 days after the injury (Youn et al, 1992). It is unclear if the immunosuppression after a burn injury is the result of biochemical substances (i.e., oxidants, histamine, prostaglandins, arachidonic acid metabolites) liberated from the burn itself or is produced in response to the burn (Kravitz, 1993). Additionally, postburn immunologic abnormalities during the clinical course of burn therapy are emphasized by the immunosuppressive effects of anesthetic agents, surgical procedures, multiple transfusions, and the use of systemic antibiotics.

h. *Hypothermia:* Children are more prone to the development of hypothermia because of their increased BSA-to-mass ratio (McCarthy and Surpure, 1990). Because of the increased BSA, children have greater evaporative water loss and greater heat loss from evaporation and convection. Hypothermia remains a major problem until the wounds have been skin grafted or healed. Hypothermia alone, without any injuries, can cause apnea, progressive metabolic acidosis, and ventricular arrhythmias (Purdue and Hunt, 1991a).

CAUSES OF BURN TRAUMA

A. **THERMAL INJURY**
   1. Thermal injuries result from direct heat, exposure to caustic chemicals, or contact with an electrical current. Radiation burns are rare.
   2. Thermal injuries may be further subdivided into flame-flash burns, scalds (caused by hot liquids such as water, grease, and tar), and contact burns (caused by hot solid objects).

B. **CHEMICAL BURNS**
   1. Chemical burns occur when the victim comes in direct contact with caustic chemicals, such as acids, alkalies, or petroleum-based products. Severity is related to the agent, its concentration, volume, and duration of contact.
   2. Prompt measures to remove the chemical ensures the most optimal result. Delay in treatment permits continued tissue damage. Search for a neutralizing agent wastes valuable time, but more importantly, the increased heat of the neutralizing reaction may cause further tissue damage (*Advanced Burn Life Support Course,* 1994).
   3. Initial treatment consists of removing all the patient's clothing, brushing the

skin if the caustic agent is a powder, and irrigating the involved area with copious amounts of tap water or placing the patient in a shower. Irrigation should continue from the time of the injury through evaluation in the hospital. Alkalies may require longer irrigation because they have a high binding affinity with the tissue and thus are more difficult to remove. Alkalies frequently cause greater damage than the acidic compounds.

4. Chemical injury to the eye deserves special attention because of the potential for permanent damage to the cornea. The eye should be flushed immediately and continuously until an ophthalmologic consultation is obtained. Irrigate with NS or a balanced salt solution. Tap water can be used if NS is not available.

5. Beside irrigation, specific treatment modalities for chemical agents (i.e., hydrofluoric acid, phenol, and phosphorus) can be determined by contacting a regional poison control facility, the hazardous materials division of the fire department, or the chemical manufacturer.

C. **ELECTRICAL INJURY**

1. Since amperage and resistance are variable, classification of this injury can be made according to voltage. Distinguishing electrical burns with significant soft tissue damage from those without can generally be done by arbitrarily dividing electrical burns into high-voltage (>1000 V) and low-voltage injuries (Purdue and Hunt, 1991b). Household voltages are generally 110 and 220 (*Advanced Burn Life Support Course,* 1994).

2. Most electrical burns in children are low-voltage accidents and generally occur in the home. The injury is usually a minor cutaneous burn and minimal to no soft tissue damage. Burns of the lip, mouth, and tongue are the most common form of electrical burn injury in small children; the mechanism of injury is suspected to be a combination of electric arc, flash burn, and contact burn. Most of these injuries are due to biting or sucking on an electrical cord or placing the tongue or lips on an electrical outlet. Typically, contact points occur at one or both angles of the mouth, resulting in coagulation necrosis of the oral commissure (Hunt, 1992).

3. Electrical injuries due to contact with high-voltage electricity are of two general types caused by the following mechanisms:

   a. The electrical current passes through the skin, causing cutaneous and deep tissue injury both locally and distant from the contact sites and often producing extensive underlying tissue (muscle or bone) damage. Contact points are often dry, circumscribed, and depressed. Deep tissue damage may result in extensive subfascial edema and tissue necrosis. A fasciotomy may be indicated to reduce pressure within the muscle compartment, thus maintaining blood flow to injured muscles. Associated complications may include the following:

      • Neurologic complications (secondary to the electrical current itself) may include cerebral complaints such as loss of consciousness, headaches, seizures, decreased memory, emotional liability, or learning impairment and peripheral complaints such as sensorimotor loss, paresthesias, paralysis, or paresis (Grube et al, 1990).

      • Renal complications may include acute tubular necrosis and acute renal failure related to hemochromogens (myoglobinuria and hemoglobinuria) released following muscle necrosis.

      • Cardiac arrhythmia and arrest can occur when the current disrupts the heart's conduction system.

      • Skeletal injuries (i.e., fractures, spinal cord injuries) may be related to powerful tetanic contractions by the muscle or a fall from a height after contact with high-voltage electrical current.

    b. The electrical current arcs external to the body, causing cutaneous injury. Heat may cause ignition of clothing and environmental objects. If clothing is ignited, a large surface area may sustain deep soft tissue burns due to the very high temperature. There may be no actual current damage. These wounds are the flash-flame type.

D. INHALATION INJURY

1. An inhalation injury may be the most important determinant of mortality in burn patients, having a greater effect than either TBSA burn or age. Inhalation injury exists in approximately 10% to 20% of hospitalized burn patients (Sharar and Heimbach, 1991). Over 50% of burn center mortalities are attributed to the pulmonary complications of inhalation injury (Demling, 1993).

2. Advances in fluid resuscitation, metabolic support, and wound management have increased the survival rate of burn patients but little progress has been made in the survival rate of the burn patient with inhalation injury (Sobel et al, 1992).

3. Respiratory failure during the first few hours to days after burn injury can be caused by asphyxia, upper airway obstruction, or chemical injury to the airway. The resulting injury can occur alone or in combination.

4. **Classification of injury**

    a. *Acute asphyxia related to hypoxia and carbon monoxide excess*

- The process of combustion involves consumption of oxygen; therefore, air inspired by fire victims has considerably lower than normal oxygen concentration, particularly when the fire occurs in a closed space. In a fire, as oxygen is consumed during combustion, carbon monoxide is released, since it is a basic by-product of incomplete combustion.

- Carbon monoxide causes toxicity by three mechanisms: formation of carboxyhemoglobin, shifting of the oxygen-hemoglobin dissociation curve to the left, and binding to other heme-containing proteins, namely cytochrome enzymes and myoglobin. Carbon monoxide is a colorless, tasteless, odorless, nonirritating gas with an affinity for hemoglobin 200 times greater than that of oxygen. As carbon monoxide is transported across the alveolar membrane, it preferentially binds with hemoglobin, in place of oxygen, to form carboxyhemoglobin. Carbon monoxide impedes the dissociation of oxygen from hemoglobin, shifting the oxygen-hemoglobin dissociation curve to the left, thereby impairing oxygen unloading at the tissue level. The result is a major impairment in oxygen delivery. Ninety-seven percent of oxygen is carried to the tissues on hemoglobin. Carboxyhemoglobin also interacts with the myoglobin of cardiac muscle and the cytochrome system, further interfering with oxygen utilization. In victims with preexisting coronary disease, hypoxia of the myocardium may precipitate angina, dysrhythmias, or cardiac arrest. Cerebral hypoxia may lead to cerebral edema. Even if victims recover, neurologic symptoms may persist when damage is severe.

- Tachypnea and cyanosis may be absent, since the partial pressure of oxygen in arterial blood (PaO_2) as perceived by the peripheral chemoreceptors (carotid body and aortic arch) is normal. The peripheral chemoreceptors controlling respiratory drive respond to changes in the PaO_2 and not to changes in the arterial oxygen saturation (SaO_2) even in the presence of high carboxyhemoglobin levels (Carrougher, 1993). Standard pulse oximeters are unable to distinguish between hemoglobin molecules saturated with oxygen (oxyhemoglobin) and those saturated with carboxyhemoglobin, producing a false elevation in oxygen saturation in victims with significant carbon monoxide toxicity (Carroll, 1993).

- Carbon monoxide toxicity is evaluated by measuring the arterial carboxyhemoglobin level. Elevated levels of carboxyhemoglobin serve as indirect evidence for exposure to combustion products. Multiple signs and symptoms have been associated with carboxyhemoglobin levels (Table 9–21; Demling, 1993; Sharar and Heimbach, 1991). A low carboxyhemoglobin level does not indicate minimal exposure. Administration of 90% to 100% oxygen displaces some, if not all, the carboxyhemoglobin before arrival to the emergency department or before an ABG analysis can be performed. Carbon monoxide has a constant half-life and is reduced by 50% in 4 hours at room air (in less than 1 hour if an oxygen concentration of 100% is used). Hyperbaric oxygen decreases the carbon monoxide concentration by 50% in 30 minutes (Sharar and Heimbach, 1991).

b. *Airway injury related to edema or obstruction:* Heat injury, from inhaling hot air, is limited to the upper airways (above the glottis) and may cause sufficient edema to produce mechanical obstruction. Direct thermal injury to the lower tracheobronchial tree and alveoli is rare because of the protective reflex closure of the glottis and the heat-dissipating capacity of the upper airway. Mucosal damage may result from both the heat and the chemical components of smoke. Mechanical obstruction of the airway is not limited to those with inhalation injury. The edema that accompanies scalds or even grease burns to the face and neck can be associated with enough edema to cause external airway compromise.

c. *Airway injury related to smoke inhalation:* Airway injury due to smoke is essentially a chemical injury caused by inhalation of the by-products of combustion and is related to the composition (i.e., benzene from plastics) and duration of the inhaled smoke. When the toxic material is inhaled, it adheres to the mucous membranes, producing a chemical burn to the tracheobronchial mucosa or as far down as the particles descend into the lung. Diagnosing the severity of the injury may be based more on the clinical course of the disease process than on initial physical findings. Generally, admission chest x-ray examinations underestimate the severity of lung damage because the injury is usually initially confined to the airways (Coblentz et al, 1990).

5. **Clinical assessment** (Table 9–22): The onset of symptoms is unpredictable, and a patient with possible inhalation injury must be observed closely. Many patients demonstrate minimal symptoms early after injury, and only when airway edema develops do symptoms become evident. Because of relatively small airways, upper airway obstruction in the pediatric patient may occur early and rapidly. Securing the endotracheal tube is a particular problem in the presence of burn injury. Facial edema coupled with wounds, secretions, and topical creams increase the difficulty of securing and maintaining proper tube placement.

Table 9–21. **CARBOXYHEMOGLOBIN LEVEL AND ASSOCIATED SIGNS AND SYMPTOMS**

CARBOXYHEMOGLOBIN LEVEL (%)	SIGNS AND SYMPTOMS
0–5	Normal value
<15	Often found in smokers
15–20	Headache, mild dyspnea, confusion
20–40	Disorientation, fatigue, nausea, syncope
>50	Coma, seizures, respiratory failure, death

Table 9–22. CLINICAL ASSESSMENT: INHALATION INJURY

History
"Closed space" injury
Exposure to noxious gases or smoke
Duration of exposure
Unconsciousness
CPR
Alcohol or drug abuse
Underlying disease
Were others involved
Accidental or intentional

Initial Diagnostic Findings
ABG: Within normal limits or hypoxemia and acidosis
Carboxyhemoglobin: Within normal limits or increased
Chest x-ray examination: Admission usually clear
Bronchoscopy
   Mucosal edema or sloughing
   Erythema
   Ulceration
   Carbonaceous material

Initial Physical Findings
Burns: Chest, face, neck, head
Edema: Face, neck, head
Singed: Nasal or facial hair, eyebrows
Soot: Mouth, pharynx, naris
Ulcerations: Mouth, pharynx
Carbonaceous sputum
Tachypnea
Dyspnea or stridor
Cyanosis
Bronchorrhea
Hoarseness
Wheezing, crackles, rhonchi
Retractions
Nasal flaring
CNS signs and symptoms: With decreased
    level of consciousness assess for
   Hypoxemia
   Hypovolemia
   Elevated carboxyhemoglobin

ABG, arterial blood gas; *CNS,* central nervous system; *CPR,* cardiopulmonary resuscitation.

DETERMINING THE SEVERITY OF A BURN INJURY

A. INTRODUCTION
1. Severity of a burn injury and its morbidity and mortality are determined by the type of burn; size, depth, and anatomic location of the wound; the patient's age; and any preexisting illness or associated trauma.
2. Major and minor burns are differentiated the same way for adults and children. Patients with a minor burn injury can usually be treated on an outpatient or non-burn-center basis. The American Burn Association (ABA) has identified burn injuries usually requiring referral to a burn center (Table 9–23).

B. DETERMINING THE DEPTH OF A BURN
1. Descriptive classification: See Table 9–24 and Figure 9–7.
2. Burns may be more severe (deeper) than they initially appear in the very young (and elderly) because of their thin skin.
3. Depth of injury is often very difficult to accurately estimate in the first 24 hours after the burn; wounds must be reevaluated on a daily basis to provide a more accurate determination of depth.
4. Characteristically in immersion scalds the underlying burn tissue initially appears red and dry. The red discoloration under these circumstances is due to hemoglobin fixed in the tissues. Immersion scald burns in children are usually full thickness (*Advanced Burn Life Support Course,* 1994; Demling, 1995; Purdue and Hunt, 1991c).

C. DETERMINING THE EXTENT OF A BURN
The extent of a burn is calculated as a percentage of TBSA. Various methods are available to determine the extent of burn surface area.
1. In the **rule of ones or hand rule,** the palm of an individual's hand represents approximately 1% of the TBSA. Therefore, using the victim's hand as a guideline, the extent of a small burn or one with an irregular outline or distribution can easily be estimated.

Table 9–23.   AMERICAN BURN ASSOCIATION: BURN CENTER REFERRAL CRITERIA

1. Second- and third-degree burns greater than 10% TBSA in patients younger than 10 or older than 50 years of age.
2. Second- and third-degree burns greater than 20% in other age groups.
3. Second- and third-degree burns that involve the face, hands, feet, genitalia, perineum, and major joints.
4. Third-degree burns greater than 5% TBSA in any age group.
5. Electrical burns including lightning injury.
6. Chemical burns.
7. Burn injury with inhalation injury.
8. Burn injury in patients with preexisting medical disorders that could complicate management, prolong recovery, or affect mortality.
9. Any patients with burns and concomitant trauma (i.e., fractures) in which the burn injury poses the greatest risk. The patient may be treated initially in a trauma center until stable before being transferred to a burn center. Physician judgment will be necessary in such situations and should be in concert with the regional medical control plan and triage protocols.
10. Hospitals without qualified personnel or equipment for the care of children should transfer children with burns to a burn center with these capabilities.
11. Burn injury in patients who will require special social-emotional or long-term rehabilitative support, including cases involving suspected child abuse, substance abuse, etc.

From American Burn Association. Hospital and prehospital resources for optimal care of patients with burn injury: guidelines for operation and development of burn centers. *J Burn Care Rehabil.* 1990;11(2):97–104.

Table 9–24.   DEPTH AND DEGREE OF BURN

DEPTH	DEGREE	CHARACTERISTICS
Superficial	First	Local pain and erythema
		Dry; without blisters
		Heals in 3–5 d
		Example: Sunburn
Partial thickness	Second	Appears red to pale ivory
Superficial partial thickness		Moist or with blisters
		Very painful
		Heals in 14–28 d with variable amount of scarring
		Caused by flash burns, scalds, or brief contact with hot objects
Deep partial thickness		Mottled; areas of waxy white injury
		Dry surface
		May be clinically indistinguishable from full-thickness burns
		Heals spontaneously in about 15–40 d unless infection converts it to full-thickness injury
Full thickness	Third	Elasticity of dermis destroyed
		Appears white, cherry red, brown, or black
		Appears dry, hard, or leathery
		Painless
		May require escharotomies if circumferential
		Caused by flame burns, chemical burns, electrical burns, or prolonged contact with source of heat
	Fourth	Involves the fat, fascia, muscle, or bone
		Seen in electrical and deep thermal burns

2. The **rule of nines** measures the percentage of burn surface area by dividing the body into multiples of nine. In the infant or child the rule is adjusted because the child's head has a larger proportional percentage of the TBSA.
3. The **Berkow** (Fig. 9–8) or **Lund and Browder nomogram** allows for a more accurate assessment that takes into account differences in BSA related to age and divides the body into smaller areas (i.e., foot, lower leg, and thigh).
4. Other methods use a standard **height and weight nomogram** to calculate the body surface area burned in square meters (m^2).

FLUID RESUSCITATION THERAPY

A. **GOALS**
1. Fluid resuscitation should be initiated in infants with burns covering ≥10% TBSA and in older children with burns ≥15% TBSA (Herndon et al, 1993).
2. The primary goal of fluid resuscitation is first to restore and then maintain intravascular volume at a level ensuring adequate tissue perfusion to vital organs. It is a balance between avoiding organ ischemia and preserving heat-injured but still viable tissues, while avoiding the complications of inadequate or excessive therapy. The volume infused should be continually titrated to avoid both underresuscitation and overresuscitation. Constant reevaluation of the patient's clinical course is essential.
3. In children, resuscitation therapy must be more exact, owing to limited physiologic reserves (especially those younger than 3 years of age). Because of their greater surface area in relation to body mass, children require more fluid for burn resuscitation than an adult with a similar size burn. Thus, provision for daily maintenance fluids in addition to the fluid requirements dictated by burn size must be emphasized (Herndon et al, 1993; Morehouse et al, 1992).
B. **CALCULATING RESUSCITATION FLUIDS FOR THE FIRST 24-HOUR POSTBURN PERIOD**
1. The quantity of fluid given is based on the extent of burn surface area and the weight of the patient.
2. A number of effective formulas have been developed for calculating fluid resuscitation for burn patients. All formulas use an electrolyte solution and a colloid, and all formulas include large volumes of sodium as the primary volume expander. The formulas differ in the amounts of free water given and the time each is administered after the burn. Most formulas advocate the use of crystalloid solutions, commonly LR because of its similar composition to fluid being lost. Ultimately, any formula used for fluid replacement is a starting point and serves only as a guide to clinical resuscitation.
C. **EXAMPLE FOR CALCULATING FLUID REPLACEMENT NEEDS USING THE PARKLAND FORMULA**
1. The volume calculated by the resuscitation formula is administered over the first 24 hours following injury. Calculations are based on the time of injury and not on the time of the patient's arrival at the hospital.
2. Half the calculated volume is given over the first 8 hours after the burn, and the remainder is given over the next 16 hours. The rationale for administering proportionately more fluid during the first 8 hours after the burn is to compensate for the plasma loss. Because most of the loss is resolved within 12 hours, the subsequent 16 hours generally call for less fluid.
3. Accurately weigh the patient on admission to the ICU to permit accurate determination of fluid replacement needs.

Parkland Memorial Hospital
Dallas, Texas

Burn Record
To be completed on admission

Name_____

Age_____ Date of Birth_____

Admit Date_____

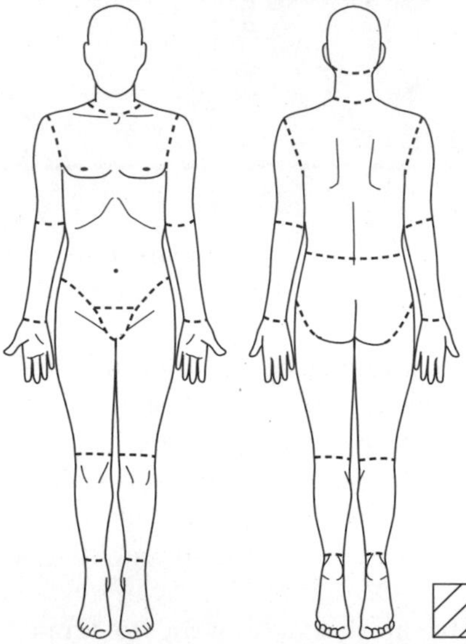

Date of Burn _____ Time of Burn _____

Weight (kg)_____ Height _____

2°_____ + 3°_____ = _____%

First 8 hrs

Second 8 hrs

Third 8 hrs

Albumin

Maintenance

Partial thickness

Full thickness

Percent Surface Area Burned (Berkow Formula)

Area	1 y	1–4 y	5–9 y	10–14 y	15 y	Adult	2°	3°
Head	19	17	13	11	9	7		
Neck	2	2	2	2	2	2		
Ant trunk	13	13	13	13	13	13		
Post trunk	13	13	13	13	13	13		
R buttock	2½	2½	2½	2½	2½	2½		
L buttock	2½	2½	2½	2½	2½	2½		
Genitalia	1	1	1	1	1	1		
RU arm	4	4	4	4	4	4		
LU arm	4	4	4	4	4	4		
RL arm	3	3	3	3	3	3		
LL arm	3	3	3	3	3	3		
R hand	2½	2½	2½	2½	2½	2½		
L hand	2½	2½	2½	2½	2½	2½		
R thigh	5½	6½	8	8½	9	9½		
L thigh	5½	6½	8	8½	9	9½		
R leg	5	5	5½	6	6½	7		
L leg	5	5	5½	6	6½	7		
R foot	3½	3½	3½	3½	3½	3½		
L foot	3½	3½	3½	3½	3½	3½		
						Total		

Figure 9–8. Burn Record: The Berkow Formula is used to calculate the total area of burn. (Courtesy Parkland Memorial Hospital, Dallas, Texas.)

Table 9–25.   CALCULATION OF MAINTENANCE FLUIDS IN CHILDREN BASED ON CHILD'S BODY WEIGHT

DAILY MAINTENANCE FLUID REQUIREMENTS	
CHILD'S WEIGHT	**DAILY FLUID REQUIREMENTS**
Up to 10 kg	100 ml/kg/24 h
11–20 kg	1000 ml for the first 10 kg
	plus 50 ml/kg for each kg more than 10 kg
21–30 kg	1500 ml for the first 20 kg
	plus 25 ml/kg for each kg more than 20 kg
31–40 kg	1750 ml for the first 30 kg
	plus 10 ml/kg for each kg more than 30 kg

4. Calculate basal fluid needs for normal daily maintenance requirements (Table 9–25).
5. Calculate fluid replacement based on burn size (Table 9–26).

D. MONITORING FLUID RESUSCITATION

1. Adequate resuscitation is reflected by normal mentation, stable vital signs, and urine output of 1 ml/kg/h in children weighing less than 30 kg and 30 to 50 ml/h for children weighing more than 30 kg (Rue, 1991). Using urine output as an indirect measurement of cardiac output has been found to be a generally reliable guide to adequacy of resuscitation, as maintenance of renal blood flow usually reflects adequate perfusion to other organs as well (Morehouse et al, 1992). Place an indwelling bladder catheter for accurate urinary output measurements and document hourly for all age groups. Begin at the rate calculated for burn resuscitation and adjust hourly (or every 30 minutes in infants) as necessary to achieve adequate urine output. A decreased urine output is most frequently the result of inadequate fluid administration. Assess and treat glycosuria; it may be difficult to accurately assess resuscitation and perfusion due to an osmotic diuresis, which further depletes the intravascular volume (Inaba and Seward, 1991).

Table 9–26.   EXAMPLE OF CALCULATING FLUID RESUSCITATION IN CHILDREN

Parkland Burn Resuscitation Formula

First 24 h After the Burn

4 ml LR* × Weight (in kg) × % Burn Surface Area

Give half the calculated amount in the first 8 hours after the burn and the remaining amount over the next 16 hours, *plus* daily maintenance volume as needed to maintain appropriate urine output.

10-kg Child With 50% Burn Surface Area

4 ml × 10 kg × 50% Burn Surface Area = 2000 ml LR* over 24 h

First   8 h = 1000 ml LR
Second   8 h =   500 ml LR
Third   8 h =   500 ml LR

Second 24 h After the Burn

Albumin 25% 0.1 ml × Weight (in kg) × % Burn Surface Area

D_5W† 1 ml × Weight (in kg) × % Burn Surface Area

Plus daily maintenance volume as needed to maintain appropriate urine output.

*Titrate LR and D_5LR based on serum glucose levels.
†D_5¼NS for infants and small children.
D, dextrose; *LR*, lactated Ringer's (solution); *NS*, normal saline; *W*, water.

2. Monitor serum glucose levels every 1 to 2 hours. Infants are at risk for hypoglycemia because of limited glycogen reserves that may become rapidly depleted when stressed, as in trauma or sepsis (Hazinski, 1992). In the early postburn period, blood glucose levels may drop rapidly rather than increase as with older children or adults. Titrating LR and D_5LR together during the first 24 hours after the burn may be necessary to avoid either hypoglycemia or hyperglycemia.

E. **FLUID MANAGEMENT AFTER RESUSCITATION (SECOND 24 HOURS AFTER THE BURN)**

1. As capillary integrity is restored, the plasma volume deficit is replaced with colloid-containing fluids in an attempt to replace the protein loss, restore plasma oncotic pressure, and minimize the volume requirements.

2. Postresuscitation urine output and replacement for evaporative water loss are maintained by infusion of 5% dextrose based on daily basal fluid requirements (see Table 9–25). Very young children, especially infants, are more sensitive to acute changes in serum sodium concentrations. The use of hypotonic solutions may lead to a severe hyponatremia, and rapid shifts in serum sodium concentrations may produce cerebral edema, intracranial bleeding, or seizures (Hazinski, 1992). Thus, salt-containing solutions in combination with 5% dextrose (i.e., $D_5\frac{1}{2}NS$; $D_5\frac{1}{4}NS$) should be used in infants or very young children.

F. **FLUID MANAGEMENT AFTER 48 HOURS**

Following the initial 48 hours, gradual reabsorption of edema fluid and diuresis occur. Fluid administration during this time is based on need, using electrolyte status and nutritional requirements.

INITIAL ASSESSMENT AND MANAGEMENT OF THE BURN VICTIM

A. **PRIMARY ASSESSMENT AND MANAGEMENT**

1. Assess the airway and breathing.

a. Airway management for the burn patient should be managed as for any trauma victim, including performing basic life support measures if indicated, providing 100% FIO_2 via face mask, assessing respirations for adequacy of rate and depth, and assessing for bilateral breath sounds.

b. Special considerations: The upper airway is susceptible to edema and obstruction as a result of exposure to heat and smoke. Because of relatively small airways in children, upper airway obstruction may occur early and rapidly. Circumferential full-thickness burns to the neck or chest may restrict ventilation.

2. Assess for associated injuries: The burn is often the most obvious injury, but other trauma or life-threatening injuries may be present in approximately 5% to 10% of burn patients (i.e., fractures, soft tissue injury, head injury, thoracic trauma, and abdominal injury). The burn injury may be compounded with blunt trauma from explosions, motor vehicle crashes, jumping to escape further injury, or falling from a height. Associated injuries should be identified and appropriately managed in the same manner as for any trauma patient (Weigelt, 1991).

3. Identify the type of burn: Although appropriate initial interventions often occur before arrival at the emergency department, never assume this step has been completed (i.e., chemical burns).

a. Eliminate the source and stop the burning process. The most important first-aid treatment is minimizing burn wound depth and extent.

b. After the burning agent is eliminated, cover the burns with clean, dry linen. Measures to conserve body heat are essential for all burn victims and particularly for the infant and young child. Wet compresses may be applied to small wounds but not to large injuries. Water increases body heat loss through the wound, a principal concern in small children. Wet dressings also promote hypothermia, which may accentuate the shock state, causing a further decrease in tissue perfusion, cardiac output, and perfusion to vital organs. Ice or ice water should never be used directly on the skin because of the potential for cold injury or for conversion of a lesser burn to a deeper injury (due to vasoconstriction).

4. Assess circulation.

a. Determine the extent and depth of the burn. Children with burns covering ≥10% TBSA require circulatory volume support.

b. Establish IV access for fluid resuscitation if indicated. Place two peripheral large-bore IV catheters, appropriate for the size of the child. The peripheral percutaneous route is the method of choice for immediate initial access; if the only accessible veins have overlying burned skin, do not hesitate to use them (*Advanced Burn Life Support Course*, 1994; *Advanced Trauma Life Support Course*, 1993). Unless indicated by other associated injuries, first-responders need not start an IV line if the primary hospital or burn center is less than 30 to 45 minutes away from the scene of injury (Pruitt and Goodwin, 1990). Cannulating small veins may be difficult in any infant or child but is even more so in a child with severe vasoconstriction. Maintaining venous access is a major priority. All IV catheters should be sutured. Adhesive tape is ineffective in securing IV catheters to burned tissue and may compromise blood flow in edematous extremities if applied circumferentially.

c. Evaluate skin color, sensation, peripheral pulses, and capillary refill. Circumferential third-degree burns of the extremities may impair circulation as a result of edema formation. Remove all clothing, rings, watches, and other jewelry. Jewelry on injured extremities may create a tourniquet effect, restricting blood flow. Insert a urinary catheter to monitor the effectiveness of fluid resuscitation.

5. Assess neurologic status: Use the GCS with a modified verbal score for children younger than 4 years of age (*Advanced Trauma Life Support Course*, 1993). Typically, the burn victim is initially alert and oriented (*Advanced Burn Life Support Course*, 1994). For a decreased level of consciousness, consider an associated injury, substance abuse, hypoxia, or preexisting medical condition.

B. **SECONDARY ASSESSMENT AND MANAGEMENT**

1. Obtain a history of the burn injury: Initial management and definitive care are guided by the mechanism, duration, severity, and time of the injury. As much information as possible should be obtained regarding the incident:

a. Cause of burn?

b. Did the injury occur in a closed space?

c. Time of injury?

d. Were harmful chemicals involved?

e. Were others involved?

f. Assess for intentional injury (possible child abuse; Table 9–27):

• Deliberate injury by burning is often an unrecognized and unappreciated component of thermal injury. The evaluating team must be aware of the possibility of abuse in any child who incurs a burn injury, particularly a child younger than 2 years of age. Tap water scald injuries are more likely to represent child abuse than other types of burn injuries (Purdue and Hunt, 1991c). Inflicted burns are frequently manifested by characteristic patterns of injury. Table 9–27 outlines characteristic patterns of unintentional and intentional burn injuries. Additionally, the mortality of abused children is higher than accidentally burned children (Purdue and Hunt, 1991c).

Table 9–27. ETIOLOGY AND CHARACTERISTIC PATTERNS OF INTENTIONAL AND UNINTENTIONAL BURN INJURIES IN CHILDREN

TYPE OF BURN	ETIOLOGY	UNINTENTIONAL CHARACTERISTIC WOUND PATTERN	INTENTIONAL CHARACTERISTIC WOUND PATTERN
Scalds			
Spill or Splash	Hot liquids		
Occur when a hot liquid falls from above the victim	Water Tea Coffee Soups Grease Tar	"Arrowhead" appearance Irregular margins Nonuniform depth The liquid cools as it flows downward producing a deeper burn in the topmost area with the depth becoming progressively more shallow and narrower as the fluid flows downward	Essentially the same as unintentional
or by throwing or pouring hot liquids on the victim			
Immersion	Mostly water		
Occur when the victim falls into a container of hot liquid	Hot tap water or boiling water	Splash marks Varying depth of burn Indistinct borders between burned and nonburned skin Multiple areas of burn as the patient struggles to get out of the hot liquid	Absence of splash marks Burn depth uniform Unvaried appearance Well-demarcated "waterlines," burns vs. nonburn margins Bilateral symmetric burns of the extremities, a "stocking and glove" distribution Burns of the buttocks or perineum Sparing of the flexor creases in both the groins and popliteal spaces Usually full-thickness
or is placed ("forced") into a container of hot liquid			
Flame Burns	Fire		Extreme depth of injury and relatively circumscribed areas compared to unintentional burns
Contact Burns	Hot solids	Usually one sided Lack of apparent pattern caused by patient movement	Faithfully depicts the outline of the hot object (i.e., grate/grill pattern) Uniform in all directions

- Management principles: Inconsistencies between the burn history and the injuries sustained, their appearance, pattern and depth of the burn, and length of time from injury to evaluation should alert the evaluating team to a potential child abuse situation. Evaluate all burned children for motor development and muscle coordination consistent with the mechanism of injury. Physical examination also includes careful evaluation for evidence of nonburn trauma (e.g., bruises, slap or whip marks, fractures, head trauma, or evidence of sexual abuse). When child abuse is suspected, a radiographic skeletal survey should be performed, and the appropriate authorities should be notified.

2. Obtain medical history: Underlying medical conditions frequently complicate burn management and prolong recovery. Determine the presence of preexisting disease or associated illness; medications, alcohol, or drugs; allergies or sensitivities; recent exposure to communicable diseases (i.e., varicella, tuberculosis); status of tetanus immunization (burn wounds are tetanus prone wounds and immunizations should be consistent with the recommendations of the American College of Surgeons); and status of other immunizations.

3. Obtain baseline diagnostic studies: Baseline laboratory studies are essential to evaluate the patient's subsequent progress. Evaluate ABGs and carboxyhemoglobin (if indicated), hematocrit and hemoglobin, electrolytes, albumin, urinalysis, BUN, chest x-ray examination, and 12-lead ECG (with electrical injury, ectopy or history of underlying cardiovascular disease).

4. Initial wound care: Wound care is not considered a component of emergency care except in chemical burns, in which immediate removal of the agent is essential (see Chemical Burns). Substantial wound care such as excessive manual debridement or application of topical antimicrobials (in the field or primary hospital) is not necessary if the patient will be transferred to a burn care facility.

C. METABOLIC AND NUTRITIONAL SUPPORT

1. Burn injury is one of the greatest insults the body can sustain and requires caloric and protein needs exceeding those of any other traumatic injury (Gottschlich et al, 1990). Energy expenditure in adult patients with large burns may be increased by as much as two times the basal metabolic rate (Ireton-Jones, 1991).

2. Providing aggressive nutritional support to patients with major burns to meet energy requirements, replace protein losses, promote wound healing and strengthen the immune system is a well-recognized aspect of burn therapy. Children normally require greater caloric and protein requirements per kilogram of body weight than an adult. For the pediatric burn patient the nutritional demands required by the hypermetabolic state of the burn injury superimposed on those for growth may result in a compromise in growth with little net weight gain for the duration of the recovery period (Cunningham et al, 1990).

3. Whenever possible, providing nutrition by the enteral route is preferred to use the absorptive mechanism of the GI tract and preserve mucosal integrity which may in turn minimize bacterial translocation from the GI tract (Gottschlich et al, 1990). The concepts of early and immediate feeding, particularly by the enteral route, are a major foci of ongoing investigations in patients following a burn injury. The tendency to initiate enteral tube feedings within 24 hours after the injury can accomplish adequate nutritional support (Hansbrough and Hansbrough, 1993; Herndon et al, 1993).

4. Parenteral nutrition is necessary for those unable to meet nutritional goals through the enteral route.

D. PHARMACOLOGY

1. **Topical antimicrobials**

   a. The moist, protein-rich avascular eschar (burn-injured tissue) provides an excellent culture medium for microorganisms. Within 1 week after the injury, bacteria are consistently present on any remaining eschar. Additionally, the thermal thrombosis that renders the eschar avascular prevents easy penetration by parenteral antibiotics and impedes delivery of the cellular components of the host defense system to the microorganisms (Pruitt and McManus, 1992). Consequently, parenteral antibiotics exert little effect on the rapid colonization of the burn wound.

   b. A better understanding of the pathogenesis of burn wound infection has led to the development of effective topical antimicrobial agents. The development of topical antimicrobials has reduced the use of prophylactic systemic antibiotics in the treatment of burn patients (Mozingo et al, 1993). Topical antimicrobials can temporarily control but not eradicate bacterial growth in necrotic or ischemic tissue, but the potential for invasive burn wound infection in any burn-injured patient remains. Patients with extensive burns in whom timely excision and grafting cannot be accomplished are those in which burn wound infection occurs with the greatest frequency.

   c. Factors affecting the choice of an antimicrobial agent include the depth, extent, and location of the burn; wound culture results; and current status of the wound (i.e., eschar intact, autograft).

   d. Advantages and disadvantages of specific topical agents: See Table 9–28.

2. **Medications**

   a. Multiple factors may affect the pharmacokinetics of drugs administered after a burn injury. Alterations to some drugs are due to hypermetabolism, increased renal blood flow, and GFR (Boucher et al, 1992). Additionally,

Table 9–28. TOPICAL ANTIMICROBIAL AGENTS

AGENT	ADVANTAGES	DISADVANTAGES
Silver sulfadiazine 1% (Silvadene, SSD, Thermazene)	Broad-spectrum antimicrobial activity Painless on application Readily available Minimal sensitivity May be used with open or closed dressing technique Most commonly used topical agent Moderate eschar penetration	Transient leukopenia
Mafenide acetate cream (Sulfamylon)	Penetrates through burn eschar and cartilage Effective gram-negative coverage	Painful on application May cause a metabolic acidosis (Alternating Sulfamylon and Silvadene application may diminish this effect)
Povidone-iodine ointment (Betadine)	May be applied prior to surgical excision to dry and toughen eschar, aiding its removal	Very painful on application Absorption of iodine may be a concern with impaired renal function
Silver nitrate solution 0.5%	Excellent antibacterial spectrum	Requires dressing Messy May cause electrolyte imbalances (hyponatremia and hypochloremia)

changes in plasma protein binding may influence the measured volume of distribution of some antibiotics.

b. In the early postburn period, changes in fluid volume and circulation prevent the use of the intramuscular or subcutaneous route for some drugs (i.e., morphine sulfate) because absorption by these routes is erratic.

E. **POTENTIAL COMPLICATIONS**

1. **Infection**

    a. Use of topical antimicrobial agents and early excision of burn wounds, coupled with early wound closure, have reduced the incidence of serious wound infections that complicate burn injuries (Pruitt and McManus, 1992).

    b. Although infection remains the most common cause of morbidity and mortality in burn patients, the infected site is now more often the lungs rather than the burn wound, with pneumonia as the predominant type of infection (Gross et al, 1990). Sepsis remains a major cause of death in the burn patient and has been reported to occur more often in those with an inhalation injury than in those with only cutaneous injury.

2. **Vascular compromise**

    a. Full-thickness circumferential extremity burns may compromise blood flow; a partial-thickness circumferential burn in a small child may result in vascular compromise.

    b. As edema develops under eschar, it can result in a tourniquet effect, compromising distal blood flow. It initially obstructs lymphatic flow, then venous return, and finally arterial flow. If not corrected, tissue ischemia and necrosis occur. An escharotomy (incision through the eschar) may be indicated to restore adequate circulation.

3. **Hypertrophic scars and contractures**

    a. Young children tend to scar and develop contractures more easily because of their thin skin (Warden, 1992). The natural tendency of scars to contract and the normal growth of a child combine to accelerate contracture deformities. Without reconstruction, contractures can lead to permanent skeletal and functional deformities. Thus, for contracture release and cosmetic reasons, multiple reconstructive procedures are more likely than a single reconstructive procedure. Lack of movement due to pain also contributes to the development of contractures. The younger the child, the less understanding the child has regarding the importance of improving functional outcome with proper positioning and range of motion exercises.

    b. Prevention begins with therapeutic positioning (i.e., placement of extremities in functional positions and splinting when necessary) on admission to the ICU.

F. **PSYCHOSOCIAL MANAGEMENT OF THE BURNED CHILD**

1. Several factors complicate the psychosocial sequelae of the burn-injured child. Circumstances surrounding the accident generate feelings of guilt, helplessness, despair, and anger from families. Disfigurement is frequently associated with a burn injury and severe and lengthy episodes of pain are common. There are increased risks of numerous medical and surgical complications during hospitalization. Because of the roller-coaster ride of good days and bad days, progress is made very slowly. Hospitalizations are lengthy, and even longer periods of rehabilitation follow discharge. Burn care may precipitate a financial disaster for the family. Since burn care requires a team approach, there are many people, procedures, and tasks the child must become familiar with each day.

2. The psychologic response of fear and anxiety is caused by multiple factors,

including fear of the unknown; separation from parents, family, and friends for extended periods of time; multiple invasive procedures during hospitalization; inability to communicate with mechanical ventilation and chemical paralyzation; altered sleep patterns and increased activities during the day and night; unfamiliar surroundings, equipment, and people; and pain.

3. Interventions to relieve anxiety
   a. Antianxiety medications are given prior to painful procedures.
   b. Allow frequent visiting for families. Encourage the family to bring items from home to remind the child of family life before the injury. Organize care into routines similar to home (i.e., a time to sleep, eat, play, dressing changes, and visitors).
   c. Provide the patient and family with frequent opportunities for education about the burn injury and care regimens required for optimal recovery. Support the family to be involved in daily activities and develop a partnership with the parents. Develop a trusting relationship with the patient and family. Provide honest but positive information.
   d. Promote restful time periods for the patient during the day and night and promote a quiet environment.
   e. Financial concerns are real because the expense of burn care is enormous. Provide for early social work involvement to facilitate financial assistance for the family if needed.

4. Pain
   a. The burn injury itself is the source of continuous (background) pain. Loss of the epidermal and partial loss of the dermal layer leave nerve endings exposed, creating a painful wound. This type of pain begins from the time of injury until wound healing is well advanced.
   b. Acute pain, or procedural pain, is associated with the multiple procedures required during the clinical course of the burn injury such as dressing changes (which are typically twice a day), surgical excision and grafting (donor sites; contracture release), daily physical therapy, and ambulating.
   c. Pain scales are useful to quantify painful episodes and to evaluate if medication is sufficient. When appropriate, develop strategies to give the patient some control over painful encounters. Allow the family to help when appropriate. Adequate pain management alleviates anticipatory pain and anxiety.

5. Fear of body image changes: Fear of not being accepted by their friends and of being different and wondering how people in general will treat them is common in burn patients. The fear usually occurs as the time for discharge comes closer. Planning for discharge begins on admission to the ICU. Encourage burn-injured patients to vent concerns. Psychologic counseling for patient and family is helpful. School reentry programs facilitate a successful return to school.

6. Anger, depression, and withdrawal are common sequelae of burn injury and require intervention through education and psychologic support. The goal is to assist the child in developing positive coping skills.

G. **NURSING DIAGNOSES, OUTCOMES, AND INTERVENTIONS**
   ❖ TISSUE PERFUSION ALTERED; CEREBRAL, CARDIOVASCULAR, RELATED TO INCREASED CAPILLARY PERMEABILITY; DECREASED INTRAVASCULAR FLUIDS; INCREASED EVAPORATIVE LOSSES
   1. **Expected outcomes**
      a. Appropriate sensorium
      b. Vital signs within expected parameters based on age, injury, and medical history; blood pressure adequate in relation to pulse and urine output

    c. Cardiac output within normal limits by the later part of postburn day 1; hyperdynamic level beginning postburn day 2

2. **Interventions**

    a. Assess the level of consciousness hourly. (Use the GCS adapted for children.) Burn injuries do not directly affect the sensorium, and patients should be awake and alert. A child with a decreased level of consciousness should be assessed for hypoxemia, hypovolemia, and carbon monoxide toxicity (carboxyhemoglobin level).

    b. Calculate resuscitation fluids for 24 hours, titrate fluid administration, and monitor response according to desired volume of urine output. Calculate and administer maintenance fluids in conjunction with resuscitation fluids.

    c. Monitor vital signs every hour. Monitor electrolytes and hematocrit every 8 to 12 hours. Closely monitor serum glucose, acid-base balance, and calcium levels. Observe CVP and pulmonary artery pressure if indicated.

    d. Observe nonburned tissue for evidence of decreased tissue perfusion (skin mottling, prolonged capillary refill, cool extremities, and pallor).

    e. Maintain body heat with use of over-the-bed heaters; cover the child's head if indicated.

❖ POTENTIAL TISSUE PERFUSION ALTERED, RENAL, RELATED TO DECREASED URINE OUTPUT; PRESENCE OF URINARY HEMOCHROMOGENS

1. **Expected outcome**

    a. Absence of renal failure

    b. Negative findings from urine glucose and acetone determinations

    c. Clear urine: If urinary hemochromogens are present, the urine is pink to port wine in color. The color of the urine is directly proportional to the pigment load, which is related to the volume of muscle damaged—the darker the color of the urine, the greater the pigment load.

2. **Interventions**

    a. Maintain urine output at 1 ml/kg/h for children weighing less than 30 kg and 30 to 50 ml/h for those weighing more than 30 kg. Monitor intake and output every hour and evaluate trends. Perform urine glucose and acetone determinations every 1 to 2 hours. Children may require increased hourly IV flow rates to flush hemochromogens through the kidneys. Monitor for an increase or decrease in urine pigmentation.

    b. Mannitol may be given to enhance hemochromogen excretion by establishing immediate urinary diuresis.

    c. Sodium bicarbonate may be given to alkalinize initial urinary output to minimize precipitation.

❖ INJURY, HIGH RISK FOR VASCULAR INSUFFICIENCY; PERIPHERAL, RELATED TO IMPAIRED VASCULAR PERFUSION IN EXTREMITIES WITH CIRCUMFERENTIAL BURNS, ELECTRICAL INJURY, AND STRESS RESPONSE TO INJURY

1. **Expected outcomes**

    a. Presence of adequate arterial perfusion to all extremities with deep burns, circumferential burns, or electrical injury

    b. No evidence of decreased joint function

2. **Interventions**

    a. Remove all jewelry and constrictive clothing. Maintain continuous elevation of the burned extremities. Monitor extremities hourly for signs and symptoms of limited blood flow. Monitor arterial pulses hourly for 24 to 48 hours on all extremities with deep burns, circumferential burns, or electrical burns. Use an ultrasonic flow device if pulses are not palpable.

    b. Escharotomies should be performed at the earliest sign of circulatory compromise (decreased pulse and complaints of deep aching muscle pain).

❖ GAS EXCHANGE, IMPAIRED, RELATED TO CARBON MONOXIDE POISONING OR INHALATION INJURY, INEFFECTIVE AIRWAY CLEARANCE RELATED TO TRACHEAL EDEMA

1. **Expected outcomes**
   a. Unlabored respirations appropriate for age
   b. P_{O_2} greater than 60 mm Hg, P_{CO_2} less than 50 mm Hg, oxygen saturation greater than 90%
   c. Clear bilateral breath sounds
   d. Ability to mobilize secretions
2. **Interventions**
   a. Assess and document breath sounds, chest excursion, respiratory rate, rhythm, and depth every 2 hours. Turn the patient and encourage the patient to cough and deep breathe every 2 hours. Administer humidified oxygen therapy as ordered. Elevate the head of the bed 30 to 45 degrees if not contraindicated. Monitor oxygen saturation hourly, evaluate ABGs as needed. Suction secretions every 1 to 2 hours as needed. Assess and document pulmonary secretions after suctioning.
   b. Monitor for indications of impending airway obstruction (i.e., stridor, wheezing, rales, hoarseness, tachypnea, use of accessory muscles for breathing, oxygen desaturation, head bobbing, or nasal flaring). Prepare for possible endotracheal intubation and mechanical ventilation. Because of relatively small airways in children, upper airway obstruction may occur early and rapidly.
   c. Check carboxyhemoglobin levels if the history of injury and signs and symptoms support the suspicion. Administer 100% F_{IO_2} if carbon monoxide is present.
   d. Observe for erythema or blistering around nose and mouth, soot in sputum, or tracheal tissue in pulmonary secretions.

❖ INFECTION, HIGH RISK FOR, RELATED TO IMPAIRED SKIN INTEGRITY FROM BURNS, IMPAIRED IMMUNE RESPONSE, AND NUMEROUS INVASIVE PROCEDURES

1. **Expected outcomes**
   a. Appropriate sensorium
   b. Adequate urine output
   c. Negative cultures
   d. Temperature 37.2° to 38.3° C (99° to 101° F) rectal
   e. Absence of infection
2. **Interventions**
   a. Cover wounds with a clean, dry sheet during transfer of the patient.
   b. Administer tetanus toxoid prophylaxis as ordered.
   c. Continually monitor temperature with soft rectal probe.
   d. Use aseptic technique during all aspects of patient care. Use sterile technique when performing invasive procedures. Change invasive lines and tubing according to unit policy.
   e. Remove dressings, wash wounds (in hydrotherapy or at bedside), apply topical antimicrobial agents, and reapply antimicrobial agents and dressings at least twice daily. Observe wounds for local signs of infection. Document wound condition and care.
   f. Observe for signs of sepsis or systemic inflammatory response. Perform cultures as ordered.
   g. Daily clean all equipment around the bedside, including the bed, with a germicidal solution.

❖ PAIN, RELATED TO ACUTE BURN INJURY

1. **Expected outcomes**
   a. The patient communicates or demonstrates increased level of comfort.
   b. Stable vital signs follow narcotic administration.

2. **Interventions**
   a. Assess the patient's need for analgesia as evidenced by verbal statements of pain (use age-appropriate assessment tools), changes in vital signs, or increased state of agitation.
   b. Assess for hypoxemia or hypovolemia as the cause of agitation prior to giving pain medication.
   c. After fluid resuscitation has been started and the patient is physiologically stable begin administering small incremental IV doses of opioids for procedural and breakthrough pain. Around-the-clock pain medication may be given. Consider the use of a patient-controlled analgesia (PCA) pump for children older than 7 years. Monitor and document patient response. Closely monitor the patient for procedural pain after administration of opioids; when the stimulus is removed, the patient could begin to appear oversedated. Anxiolytics are usually a helpful adjunct to opioids to reduce anxiety associated with a procedure.
   d. Reduce the patient's anxiety level through explanation of procedures and talking to the patient while performing nursing interventions.

❖ ALTERED NUTRITIONAL STATUS, LESS THAN BODY REQUIREMENTS RELATED TO HYPER-METABOLISM AND ALTERED GI TRACT FUNCTION

1. **Expected outcomes**
   a. The patient's weight remains within 10% of the patient's usual preburn weight (American Burn Association [ABA], 1995).
   b. The patient tolerates PO or enteral tube feedings.
   c. There is no evidence of GI tract bleeding.
2. **Interventions**
   a. Determine nutritional goals using one of the various formulas for estimating the energy requirements in pediatric burn patients. Maintain daily calorie count record.
   b. Children who are unable to consume the required amount of calories to meet their nutritional goals need enteral tube feedings. Assess gastric residuals every 2 to 4 hours with enteral tube feedings and assess GI tract function every 4 hours. Note the presence of abdominal distention and diarrhea.
   c. Assess electrolyte status every 8 to 12 hours. Weigh the patient daily and maintain strict input and output.
   d. Administer antacids or H_2 blockers as ordered. Assess for GI tract bleeding every 2 to 4 hours.

REFERENCES

Multiple Trauma

Acute Pain Management Guideline Panel. *Acute Pain Management: Operative or Medical Procedures and Trauma. Clinical Practice Guideline.* Rockville, Md: Agency for Health Care Policy and Research; 1992. Public Health Service, US Depart Health and Human Services. AHCPR publication No 92-0032.

Agran P, Winn D, Anderson C. Differences in child pedestrian injury events by location. *Pediatrics.* 1994;93(2):284–288.

American Academy of Pediatrics. Guidelines for monitoring and management of pediatric patients during and after sedation for diagnostic and therapeutic procedures. *Pediatrics.* 1992;89(6):1110–1115.

Barkin R, Rosen P. Environmental emergencies. In: Barkin R, Rosen P, eds. *Emergency Pediatrics.* 4th ed. St Louis, Mo: Mosby–Year Book Inc; 1994:309–317.

Bernardo LM, Trunzo R. Pediatric trauma. In: Kitt S, Selfridge-Thomas J, Proehl J, Kaiser J, eds. *Emergency Nursing: A Physiologic and Clinical Perspective.* 2nd ed. Philadelphia, Pa: WB Saunders Co; 1995:428–454.

Bernardo L, Waggoner T. Pediatric trauma. In: Sheehy S, ed. *Emergency Nursing: Principles and Practice.* 3rd ed. St Louis, Mo: Mosby–Year Book Inc; 1992:683–690.

Centers for Disease Control and Prevention. Air-bag-associated fatal injuries to infants and children riding in front passenger seats—United States. *MMWR.* 1995;44(45):845–847.

Chadwick D, Chin S, Salerno C, Landsverk J, Kitchen L. Deaths from falls in children: how far is fatal? *J Trauma.* 1991;31(10):1353–1355.

Chadwick D, Merten D, Reece R. Thoracic and abdominal injuries associated with child abuse. In: Reece R, ed. *Child Abuse: Medical Diagnosis and Management.* Philadelphia, Pa: Lea & Febiger; 1994:54–68.

Chameides L, Hazinski M. *Textbook of Pediatric Advanced Life Support.* Dallas, Tex: American Heart Association, American Academy of Pediatrics; 1994.

Chase D. Maxillofacial injuries. In: Buntain W, ed. *Management of Pediatric Trauma.* Philadelphia, Pa: WB Saunders Co; 1995:201–218.

Chiaviello C, Christoph R, Bond G. Infant walker-related injuries: a prospective study of severity and incidence. *Pediatrics.* 1994;93(6):974–976.

Committee on Injury and Poison Prevention. Firearm injuries affecting the pediatric population. *Pediatrics.* 1992;89(4):788–790.

Committee on Injury and Poison Prevention. Skateboard injuries. *Pediatrics.* 1995;85(4):612–613.

Committee on Trauma, American College of Surgeons. *Advanced Trauma Life Support Course for Physicians.* Chicago, Ill: American College of Surgeons; 1989:75–77.

Corriere J. Urinary tract injuries. In: Ford EG, Andrassy RJ, eds. *Pediatric Trauma.* Philadelphia, Pa: WB Saunders Co; 1994:223–243.

Creel J. Mechanisms of injuries due to motion. In: Campbell J, ed. *Basic Trauma Life Support: Advanced Prehospital Care.* 2nd ed. Englewood Cliffs, NJ: Prentice-Hall; 1988:1–20.

Davis H, Zitelli B. Childhood injuries: accidental or inflicted? *Contemp Pediatr.* 1995;12(1):94–112.

Digeronimo R, Mayes T. Near-hanging injury in childhood: a literature review and report of three cases. *Pediatr Emerg Care.* 1994;10(3):150–156.

Division of Injury Control, Center for Environmental Health and Injury Control, Centers for Disease Control. Childhood injuries in the United States. *Am J Dis Child.* 1990;144:627.

Donnellan W. Pediatric trauma. In: Kitt S, Selfridge-Thomas J, Proehl J, Kaiser J, eds. *Emergency Nursing: A Physiologic and Clinical Perspective.* 2nd ed. Philadelphia, Pa: WB Saunders Co; 1990:545–574.

Emergency Nurses Association. Position statement on family presence during resuscitation. Chicago, Ill: The Association; 1994.

Finkel M, DeJong A. Medical findings in child sexual abuse. In: Reece R, ed. *Child Abuse: Medical Diagnosis and Management.* Philadelphia, Pa: Lea & Febiger; 1994:185–247.

Gershman K, Sacks J, Wright J. Which dogs bite? A case-control study of risk factors. *Pediatrics.* 1994;93:913–917.

Goldstein B, Powers K. Head trauma in children. *Pediatr Rev.* 1994;15(6):213–219.

Grabb P, Pang D. Magnetic resonance imaging in the evaluation of spinal cord injury without radiographic abnormality in children. *Neurosurgery.* 1994;35(3):406–414.

Graham C, Kittredge D, Stuemky J. Injuries associated with child safety seat misuse. *Pediatr Emerg Care.* 1992;8(6):351–353.

Guidelines for cardiopulmonary resuscitation and emergency cardiac care. *JAMA.* 1992;268(16):2262–2275.

Gussack G, Simpson L. Ear, nose, and throat injuries. In: Buntain W, ed. *Management of Pediatric Trauma.* Philadelphia, Pa: WB Saunders Co; 1995:219–237.

Guyer B, Ellers B. Childhood injuries in the United States. *Am J Dis Child.* 1990;144:649–652.

Hall J, Reyes H, Meller J, Loeff D, Dembek R. The new epidemic in children: penetrating injuries. *J Trauma.* 1995;39(3):487–491.

Halpern J. Mechanisms and patterns of trauma. *J Emerg Nurs.* 1989;15:380.

Hoover D, Belinger M. Genitourinary trauma. In: Ehrlich F, Heldrich F, Tepas J, eds. *Pediatric Emergency Medicine.* Rockville, Md: Aspen Publishers; 1987:307–313.

Horowitz JR, Andrassy RJ. Considerations unique to children. In: Ford EG, Andrassy RJ, eds. *Pediatric Trauma.* Philadelphia, Pa: WB Saunders Co; 1994:3–19.

Hymel K. Child abuse. In: Ford EG, Andrassy RJ, eds. *Pediatric Trauma.* Philadelphia, Pa: WB Saunders Co; 1994:41–92.

Johnston C, Rivara F, Soderberg R. Children in car crashes: analysis of data for injury and use of restraints. *Pediatrics.* 1994;93(6):960–965.

Kelley S. Child abuse and neglect. In: Kelley S, ed. *Pediatric Emergency Nursing.* 2nd ed. Norwalk, Conn: Appleton & Lange; 1994a:89–107.

Kelley S. Sexual abuse. In: Kelley S, ed. *Pediatric Emergency Nursing.* 2nd ed. Norwalk, Conn: Appleton & Lange; 1994b:109–123.

Levitt C, Smith W, Alexander R. Abusive head trauma. In: Reece R, ed. *Child Abuse: Medical Diagnosis and Management.* Philadelphia, Pa: Lea & Febiger; 1994:1–22.

Li G, Baker S, Fowler C, DiScala C. Factors related to the presence of head injury in bicycle-related pediatric trauma patients. *J Trauma.* 1995;38(6):871–875.

Lobe T, Gore D, Swischuk L. Urinary tract injuries. In: Buntain W, ed. *Management of Pediatric Trauma.* Philadelphia, Pa: WB Saunders Co; 1995:371–382.

Ludwig S, Loiselle J. Anatomy, growth and development: impact on injury. In: Eichelberger M, ed. *Pediatric Trauma.* St Louis, Mo: Mosby-Year Book Inc; 1993:39–58.

Lynch J, Albanese C, Gardner M. Blunt urogenital trauma in prepubescent female patients: more than meets the eye! *Pediatr Emerg Care*. 1995;11(6):372–375.

Mayeda D. Orthopedic injuries: management principles. In: Barkin R, Rosen P, eds. *Emergency Pediatrics*. 4th ed. St Louis, Mo: Mosby Year Book Inc; 1994:476–482.

McKenna P, Welsh D, Martin L. Pediatric bicycle trauma. *J Trauma*. 1991;31(3):392–394.

Merten D, Cooperman D, Thompson G. Skeletal manifestations of child abuse. In: Reece R, ed. *Child Abuse: Medical Diagnosis and Management*. Philadelphia, Pa: Lea & Febiger; 1994:23–53.

Mofensen H, Greensher J. Accident prevention. In: Hoekelman RA, Friedman SB, Nelson NM, Seidel H, Weitzman ML, eds: *Primary Pediatric Care*. 2nd ed. St Louis, Mo: Mosby; 1992:260–284.

Mosenthal A, Livingston D, Elcavage J, Merritt S, Stucker S. Falls: epidemiology and strategies for prevention. *J Trauma*. 1995;38(5):753–756.

Nakayama D. *Pediatric Surgery: A Color Atlas*. Philadelphia, Pa: JB Lippincott Co; 1991.

Nakayama D, Gardner M, Rogers K. Disability from bicycle-related injuries in children. *J Trauma*. 1990;30(11):1390–1394.

Nakayama D, Pasieka K, Gardner M. How bicycle-related injuries change bicycling practices in children. *Am J Dis Child*. 1990;144(8):928–929.

Nakayama D, Venkataraman S, Orr R, Thompson A. Emergency airway management in pediatric trauma. *Trauma Q*. 1992;8(3):22–34.

Nakayama D, Waggoner T, Venkataraman S, Gardner M, Lynch J, Orr R. The use of drugs in emergency airway management in pediatric trauma. *Ann Surg*. 1992;216(2):205–211.

Nayduch D, Moylan J, Ruttledge R, Baker C, Meredith W, Thomason M. Comparison of the ability of adult and pediatric trauma scores to predict pediatric outcome following major trauma. *J Trauma*. 1991;31(4):452–458.

Nichols D, Yaster M, Lappe D, Buck J, eds. *Golden Hour: The Handbook of Advanced Pediatric Life Support*. St Louis, Mo: Mosby–Year Book Inc; 1991:340.

Olney B, Toby E. Musculoskeletal injuries. In: Buntain W, ed. *Management of Pediatric Trauma*. Philadelphia, Pa: WB Saunders Co; 1995:394–427.

Pang D, Pollack I. Spinal cord injury without radiographic abnormality in children—the SCIWORA syndrome. *J Trauma*. 1989;2(9):654–664.

Pang D, Wilberger J. Spinal cord injury without radiographic abnormalities in children. *J Neurosurg*. 1982;57:1114–1129.

Pautler M, Henning J, Buntain W. Mechanisms and biomechanics of traffic injuries. In: Buntain W, ed. *Management of Pediatric Trauma*. Philadelphia, Pa: WB Saunders Co; 1995:10–27.

Phelan A. Musculoskeletal trauma. In: Kelley SJ, ed. *Pediatric Emergency Nursing*. 2nd ed. Norwalk, Conn: Appleton & Lange; 1994:323–334.

Pollack I, Pang D. Spinal cord injury without radiographic abnormality (SCIWORA). In: Pang D, ed. *Disorders of the Pediatric Spine*. New York, NY: Raven Press Publishers; 1995:509–516.

Ray L, Yuwiler J. *Child and Adolescent Fatal Injury Databook*. San Diego, Calif: Children's Safety Network; 1994.

Reynolds M. Pulmonary, esophageal, and diaphragmatic injuries. In: Buntain W, ed. *Management of Pediatric Trauma*. Philadelphia, Pa: WB Saunders Co; 1995:238–247.

Richardson A. Cutaneous manifestations of abuse. In: Reece R, ed. *Child Abuse: Medical Diagnosis and Management*. Philadelphia, Pa: Lea & Febiger; 1994:167–184.

Rivara F. Child pedestrian injuries in the United States. *Am J Dis Child*. 1990;144:692–696.

Robertson L. Motor vehicles. *Pediatr Clin North Am*. 1985;32:87–94.

Schafermeyer R. Pediatric trauma. *Emerg Med Clin North Am*. 1993;11(1):187–205.

Scully T, Luerssen T. Spinal cord injuries. In: Buntain W, ed. *Management of Pediatric Trauma*. Philadelphia, Pa: WB Saunders Co; 1995:189–199.

Semonin-Holleran R. Trauma in childhood. In: Neff J, Kidd P, eds. *Trauma Nursing: The Art and Science*. St Louis, Mo: Mosby–Year Book Inc; 1992:527–553.

Senturia Y, Christoffel K, Donovan M. Children's household exposure to guns: a pediatric practice-based survey. *Pediatrics*. 1994;93(3):469–475.

Sheikh A, Brogan T. Outcome and cost of open- and closed-chest cardiopulmonary resuscitation in pediatric cardiac arrests. *Pediatrics*. 1994;93:392–398.

Soud T, Pieper P, Hazinski M. Pediatric trauma. In: Hazinski M, ed. *Nursing Care of the Critically-Ill Child*. 2nd ed. St Louis, Mo: The CV Mosby Co; 1992:829–873.

Templeton J. Mechanisms of injury: biomechanics. In: Eichelberger M, ed. *Pediatric Trauma*. St Louis, Mo: Mosby–Year Book Inc; 1993:20–36.

Tepas J. Abdominal injury. In: Ehrlich F, Heldrich F, Tepas J, eds. *Pediatric Emergency Medicine*. Rockville, Md: Aspen Publishers; 1987:229–237.

Ward J. Craniocerebral injuries. In: Buntain W, ed. *Management of Pediatric Trauma*. Philadelphia, Pa: WB Saunders Co; 1995:177–188.

Zavoski R, Lapidus G, Lerer T, Banco L. A population-based study of severe firearm injury among children and youth. *Pediatrics*. 1995;96(2):278–282.

Toxicology

Behrman RI, Kliegman RM, Nelson WE, Vaughan VC III, eds. *Nelson Textbook of Pediatrics.* 14th ed. Philadelphia, Pa: WB Saunders Co; 1992.

Cooney DO. *Activated Charcoal in Medical Applications.* New York, NY: Marcel Dekker Inc; 1995.

Ellenhorn MJ, Barceloux DG. *Medical Toxicology—Diagnosis and Treatment of Human Poisoning.* New York, NY: Elsevier; 1988.

Hardman JG, Limbird LE, eds. *Goodman and Gilman's The Pharmacological Basis of Therapeutics.* 9th ed. New York, NY: McGraw-Hill, 1996.

Goldfrank LR, Flomenbaum NE, Lewin NA, et al. *Goldfrank's Toxicologic Emergencies.* 5th ed. Norwalk, Conn: Appleton & Lange; 1994:1255–1266.

Lampe KF, McCann MA. *AMA Handbook of Poisonous and Injurious Plants.* Chicago, Ill: American Medical Association; 1985.

Sparks SM, Taylor CM. *Nursing Diagnosis Reference Manual.* 2nd ed. Springhouse, Pa: Springhouse Corporation; 1993.

Spoerke DG, Rumack BH. *Handbook of Mushroom Poisoning—Diagnosis and Treatment.* Boca Raton, Fla: CRC Press; 1994.

Septic Shock

American College of Chest Physicians (ACCP) and Society for Critical Care Medicine (SCCM). Consensus conference: definitions for sepsis and organ failure and guidelines for the use of innovative therapies in sepsis. *Crit Care Med.* 1992;20(6):864–874.

Ackerman MH. The systemic inflammatory response, sepsis, and multiple organ dysfunction. *Crit Care Nurs Clin North Am.* 1994;6(2):243–264.

Ackerman MH, Evans NJ, Eckland MM. Systemic inflammatory response syndrome, sepsis, and nutritional support. *Crit Care Nurs Clin North Am.* 1994;6(2):321–340.

Albert RK, Condie F. Handwashing patterns in medical intensive care units. *N Engl J Med.* 1981;304:1465.

Alyn IB, Baker LK. Cardiovascular anatomy and physiology of the fetus, neonate, infant, child, and adolescent. *J Cardiovasc Nurs.* 1992;6(3):1–11.

Balk RA, Jacobs RF, Tryka AF, Walls RC, Bone RC. Low dose ibuprofen reverses the hemodynamic alterations of canine endotoxin shock. *Crit Care Med.* 1988;16:1128.

Bone RC. Sepsis, the systemic inflammatory response syndrome, and multiple organ dysfunction syndrome: recent advances. *Sepsis and Septic Shock: Current Issues and Recent Development—Abstract Brochure.* Anaheim, Calif: National Teaching Institute, AACN; 1993.

Brandtzaeg P, Kierulf P, Gaustad P, et al. Plasma endotoxin as a predictor of multiple organ failure and death in systemic meningococcal disease. *J Infect Dis.* 1989;159:195–204.

Brown RB, Hosmer D, Chen HC, et al. A comparison of infections in different ICUs within the same hospital. *Crit Care Med.* 1985;13:472–476.

Byram D. Future expectations for critical care nurses: competence in immunotherapy. *Crit Care Clin North Am.* 1989;1:797–806.

Cairo M, Mauss D, Kommareddy S, et al. Prophylactic or simultaneous administration of recombinant human granulocyte colony stimulating factor in the treatment of group B streptococcal sepsis in neonatal rats. *Pediatr Res.* 1990;27:612–616.

Cairo M, Plunkett J, Mauss D, et al. Seven day administration of recombinant human granulocyte colony-stimulating factor to newborn rats: modulation of neonatal neutrophilia, myelopoiesis, and group B streptococcus sepsis. *Blood.* 1990;76:1788–1794.

Cairo M, Plunkett J, Nguyen A, et al. Effect of stem cell factor with and without granulocyte colony-stimulating factor on neonatal hematopoiesis: in vivo induction of newborn myelopoiesis and reduction of mortality during experimental group B streptococcal sepsis. *Blood.* 1992;80:96–101.

Carcillo JA. Management of pediatric septic shock. In: Holbrook PR, ed. *Textbook of Pediatric Critical Care.* Philadelphia, Pa: WB Saunders Co;1993:114–142.

Carcillo JA, Davis AI, Zaritsky A. Role of early fluid resuscitation in pediatric septic shock. *JAMA.* 1991;226(9): 1242–1245.

Centers for Disease Control. Nosocomial infection surveillance, 1984. *Centers for Disease Control Surveillance Summaries.* 1986;35:1SS,17SS–29SS.

Chameides L, Hazinski MF, eds. *Textbook of Pediatric Advanced Life Support.* Dallas, Tex: American Heart Association; 1994.

Curley MAQ. Challenges in pediatric critical care: shock. In: *AACN National Teaching Institute Proceedings Book.* Aliso Viejo, Calif: AACN; 1992:265.

Danner RL, Elin RJ, Hosseini JM, et al. Endotoxemia in humans. *Chest.* 1991;99:169.

Davenport SE. Frequency of handwashing by registered nurses caring for infants on radiant warmers and in incubators. *Neonat Network.* 1992;11:21–24.

DeAngelis R. Cardiovascular system. In: AACN (American Association of Critical Care Nursing). *Core Curriculum for Critical Care Nursing.* 4th ed. Philadelphia, Pa: WB Saunders Co; 1991:132–314.

Donowitz LG. Hand-washing techniques in a pediatric ICU. *Am J Dis Child.* 1987;141:683–685.

Frank MM. Complement and kinin. In: Stites DP, Terr AI, eds. *Basic and Clinical Immunology.* 7th ed. Norwalk, Conn: Appleton & Lange; 1991:161–174.

Gates DM. Myocardial dysfunction in sepsis and multisystem organ failure. In: Huddleston VB, ed. *Multisystem Organ Failure: Pathophysiology and Clinical Implications.* St Louis, Mo: Mosby–Year Book Inc; 1992:178–203.

Gillan E, Plunkett M, Cairo MS. Colony-stimulating factors in the modulation of sepsis. *New Horizons.* 1993;1(1):96–109.

Gillan E, Suen Y, Christensen R, et al. A comparison of G-CSF expression and production between newborn and adults and preliminary results of a randomized placebo controlled trial of rhG-CSF in newborns with presumed sepsis. *Exp Hematol.* 1992;29:773A. Abstract.

Graham M. Frequency and duration of handwashing in an intensive care unit. *Am J Infect Control.* 1990;18:77.

Grimes DE. *Infectious Diseases.* St Louis, Mo: Mosby–Year Book Inc; 1991.

Hazinski MF. Hemodynamic monitoring of children. In: Daily EK, Shroeder JS, eds. *Techniques in Bedside Hemodynamic Monitoring.* 4th ed. St Louis, Mo: The CV Mosby Co; 1989:247–315.

Hazinski MF. *Nursing Care of the Critically Ill Child.* 2nd ed. St Louis, Mo: Mosby–Year Book, Inc; 1992.

Hazinski MF. Mediator-specific therapies for the systemic inflammatory response syndrome, sepsis, severe sepsis, and septic shock: present and future approaches. *Crit Care Nurs Clin North Am.* 1994;6(2):309–319.

Hazinski MF, Iberti TJ, MacIntyre NR, et al. Epidemiology, pathophysiology and clinical presentation of Gram-negative sepsis. *Am J Crit Care.* 1993;2(3):224–235.

Huddleston VB. Inflammatory mediators and multisystem organ failure. In: Huddleston VB, ed. *Multisystem Organ Failure: Pathophysiology and Clinical Implications.* St Louis, Mo: Mosby–Year Book Inc; 1992a:37–56.

Huddleston VB. The inflammatory/immune response: implications for the critically ill. In: Huddleston VB, ed. *Multisystem Organ Failure: Pathophysiology and Clinical Implications.* St Louis, Mo: Mosby–Year Book Inc; 1992b:16–36.

Jafari HS, McCracken GH. Sepsis and septic shock: a review for clinicians. *Pediatr Infect Dis J.* 1992;11:739–749.

Kimbrell JD. Alterations in metabolism. In: Huddleston VB, ed. *Multisystem Organ Failure: Pathophysiology and Clinical Implications.* St Louis, Mo: Mosby–Year Book Inc; 1992:125–139.

Klein BS, Perloff WH, Maki DG. Reduction of nosocomial infection during pediatric intensive care by protective isolation. *N Engl J Med.* 1989;3210:1714.

Kumar A, Parrillo JE. Shock: classification, pathophysiology, and approach to management. In: Parrillo JE, Bone RC, eds. *Critical Care Medicine: Principles of Diagnosis and Management.* St Louis, Mo: Mosby–Year Book, Inc; 1995:291–339.

MacIntyre NR. Conventional therapy for the septic patient. *Sepsis and Septic Shock: Current Issues and Recent Developments.* Abstract Brochure: Symposium at the American Association of Critical Care Nurses 1993 National Teaching Institute. 1993:33–35.

Maki DG. Nosocomial infection in the intensive care unit. In: Parrillo JE, Bone RC, eds. *Critical Care Medicine: Principles of Diagnosis and Management.* St Louis, Mo: Mosby–Year Book Inc; 1995:893–954.

McLane C, Chenelly S, Sylvestrak ML, et al. A nursing practice problem: failure to observe aseptic technique. *Am J Infect Control.* 1983;11:178.

Merritt WT. Nosocomial infections in the pediatric intensive care unit. In: Rogers MC, ed. *Textbook of Pediatric Intensive Care.* 2nd ed. Baltimore, Md: Williams & Wilkins; 1992:976–1008.

Mertsola J, Kennedy WA, Waagner D, et al. Endotoxin concentration in cerebrospinal fluid correlate with clinical severity and neurologic outcome of *Haemophilus influenzae* type b meningitis. *Am J Dis Child.* 1991;145:1099–1103.

Mims BC. Imbalance of oxygen supply and demand. In: Huddleston VB, ed. *Multisystem Organ Failure: Pathophysiology and Clinical Implications.* St Louis, Mo: Mosby–Year Book Inc; 1992:109–124.

Moloney-Harmon P, Czerwinski SJ. The pediatric patient. In: Huddleston VB, ed. *Multisystem Organ Failure: Pathophysiology and Clinical Implications.* St Louis, Mo: Mosby–Year Book Inc; 1992:265–292.

Natanson C, Eichenholz PW, Danner RL, et al. Endotoxin and tumor necrosis factor challenges in dogs stimulate the cardiovascular profile of human septic shock. *J Exp Med.* 1989;169:823.

Natanson C, Hoffman WD, Parrillo JE. Septic shock and multiple organ failure. In: Parrillo JE, Bone RC, eds. *Critical Care Medicine: Principles of Diagnosis and Management.* St Louis, Mo: Mosby–Year Book Inc; 1995:355–374.

O'Neill PI. Gastrointestinal system: target organ and source. In: Huddleston VB, ed. *Multisystem Organ Failure: Pathophysiology and Clinical Implications.* St Louis, Mo: Mosby–Year Book Inc; 1992:158–177.

Parrillo J, Parker MM, Natanson C, et al. NIH conference: septic shock in humans—advances in the understanding of pathogenesis, cardiovascular dysfunction, and therapy. *Ann Intern Med.* 1990;113(3):227–242.

Philichi LM. Multiple system organ failure in the pediatric population. *Crit Care Nurse Q.* 1994;16(4):96–105.

Phillips MC, Olsen LR. The immunologic role of the gastrointestinal tract. *Crit Care Clin North Am.* 1993;5(1):107–120.

Proulx F, Gauthier M, Nadeau D, Lacroix J, Farrell CA. Timing and predictors of death in pediatric patients with multiple organ system failure. *Crit Care Med.* 1994;22(6):1025–1030.

Robins EV. Maldistribution of circulating volume. In: Huddleston VB, ed. *Multisystem Organ Failure: Pathophysiology and Clinical Implications.* St Louis, Mo: Mosby–Year Book Inc; 1992:85–108.

Saez-Llorenz X, McCracken GH. Sepsis syndrome and septic shock in pediatrics: current concepts of terminology, pathophysiology, and management. *J Pediatr.* 1993;123(4):497–508.

Secor VH. The inflammatory/immune response in critical illness: role of the systemic inflammatory response syndrome. *Crit Care Nurs Clin North Am.* 1994;6(2):251–264.

Selective Decontamination of the Digestive Tract Trialist's Collaborative Group. Meta-analysis of randomized controlled trials of selective decontamination of the digestive tract. *Br Med J.* 1993;307:525.

Slota MC. The cutting edge of pediatric critical care. *Crit Care Nurse.* June 1993;(suppl):22–23.

Suffredini AF, Fromm RE, Parker MM, et al. The cardiovascular response of normal humans to the administration of endotoxin. *N Engl J Med.* 1989;321:280.

Webb CH. Antibiotic resistance associated with selective decontamination of the digestive tract. *J Hosp Infect Control.* 1992;22:1.

Weber DJ, Gammon WR, Cohen WS. The acutely ill patient with fever and rash. In: Mandell GL, Douglas RG, Bennett JE, eds. *Principles and Practice of Infectious Diseases.* 3rd ed. New York, NY: Churchill Livingstone; 1990:479–489.

Wilkinson JD, Pollack MM, Glass NL, et al. Mortality associated with multiple organ system failure and sepsis in pediatric intensive care. *J Pediatr.* 1987;111:324–328.

Wilkinson JD, Pollack MM, Ruttiman UE, Glass NL, Yeh TS. Outcome of pediatric patients with multiple organ system failure. *Crit Care Med.* 1986;14:271–274.

Burns

Advanced Burn Life Support Course. Lincoln, Neb: National Burn Institute; 1994.

American College of Surgeons Committee on Trauma. *Advanced Trauma Life Support Course: Injuries Due to Burns and Cold* (instructor manual). 5th ed. Chicago, Ill: The College; 1993.

American Burn Association. Burn care outcomes and indicators. In: Proceedings from the Committee On The Organization and Delivery of Burn Care presented at the 27th annual meeting of the American Burn Association; April, 1995; Albuquerque, NM.

American Burn Association. Hospital and pre-hospital resources for optimal care of patients with burn injury: guidelines for operation and development of burn centers. *J Burn Care Rehabil.* 1990;11(2):97–104.

Baker SP, O'Neill B, Ginsburg MJ, et al. *The Injury Fact Book.* New York, NY: Oxford University Press; 1992.

Bernardo L, Sullivan K. Care of the pediatric patient with burns. In: Trofino R, ed. *Nursing Care of the Burn-Injured Patient.* Philadelphia, Pa: FA Davis Co; 1991.

Boucher BA, Kuhl DA, Hickerson WL. Pharmacokinetics of systemically administered antibiotics in patients with thermal injury. *Clin Infect Dis.* 1992;14(2):458–463.

Buntain WL. *Management of Pediatric Trauma.* Philadelphia, Pa: WB Saunders Co; 1995.

Carroll P. Clinical application of pulse oximetry. *Pediatr Nurs.* 1993;19(2):150–151.

Carrougher GJ. Inhalation injury. In: Kravitz M, ed. *AACN Clinical Issues in Critical Care Nursing: Burn Care.* Philadelphia, Pa: JB Lippincott Co; 1993.

Clark WR. Inhalation injury. In: Rylah LTA, ed. *Critical Care of the Burned Patient.* New York, NY: Cambridge University Press; 1992.

Coblentz C, Chiles C, Putnam C. Radiologic evaluation. In: Haponik E, Munster A, eds. *Respiratory Injury: Smoke Inhalation and Burns.* New York, NY: McGraw-Hill Book Co; 1990.

Cunningham JJ, Lydon MK, Russell WE. Calorie and protein provision for recovery from severe burns in infants and young children. *Am J Clin Nutr.* 1990;51:553–557.

Demling RH. Smoke inhalation injury. *New Horizons.* 1993;1(3):422–434.

Demling RH. Use of Biobrane in management of scalds. *J Burn Care Rehabil.* 1995;16(3):329–330.

George A, Hancock J. Reducing pediatric burn pain with parent participation. *J Burn Care Rehabil.* 1993;14(1):104–107.

Gottschlich M, Alexander JW, Bower RH. Enteral nutrition in patients with burns or trauma. In: Rombeau JL, Caldwell MD, eds. *Clinical Nutrition: Enteral and Tube Feeding.* 2nd ed. Philadelphia, Pa: WB Saunders Co; 1990.

Gross PA, Neu HC, Aswapokee P, et al. Deaths from nosocomial infections: experience in a university hospital and a community hospital. *Am J Med.* 1990;68:219.

Grube BJ, Heimbach DM, Engrav LH, et al. Neurologic consequences of electrical burns. *J Trauma.* 1990;30(3):254–258.

Hansbrough WB, Hansbrough JF. Success of immediate intragastric feeding of burned patients. *J Burn Care Rehabil.* 1993;(14)5:512–516.

Hazinski MF. *Nursing Care of the Critically Ill Child.* St Louis, Mo: The CV Mosby Co; 1992.

Heimbach D, Engrav L, Gruba B, et al. Burn depth: a review. *World J Surg.* 1992;16(1):10–15.

Herndon DN, Rutan RL, Rutan TC. Management of the pediatric patient with burns. *J Burn Care Rehabil.* 1993;14(1):3–9.

Hunt JL. Soft tissue patterns in acute electric burns. In: Lee RC, Cravalho EG, Burke JF, eds. *Electrical Trauma: The Pathophysiology, Manifestations and Clinical Management.* New York, NY: Cambridge University Press; 1992.

Inaba AS, Seward PN. An approach to pediatric trauma: unique anatomic and pathophysiologic aspects of the pediatric patient. In: Burkle FM, Wiebe RA, eds. *Emerg Med Clin North Am.* 1991;9(3):523–548.

Ireton-Jones C, Baxter CR. Nutrition for adult burn patients: a review. *Nutr Clin Pract.* 1991;6(1):3–10.

Kahn AM, Cohen MJ, Kaplan L. Treatment for depigmentation resulting from burn injuries. *J Burn Care Rehabil.* 1991;12(5):468–473.

Kravitz M. Immune consequences of burn injury. In: Kravitz M, ed. *AACN Clinical Issues in Critical Care Nursing: Burn Care.* Philadelphia, Pa: JB Lippincott Co; 1993.

McCarthy DL, Surpure JS. Pediatric trauma: initial evaluation and stabilization. *Pediatr Ann.* 1990;19:585–596.

Monafo WW, Bessey PQ. Pathophysiology of burn shock. In: Rylah LTA, ed. *Critical Care of the Burned Patient.* New York, NY: Cambridge University Press; 1992.

Morehouse JD, Finkelstein JL, Marano MA, et al. Resuscitation of the thermally injured patient. *Crit Care Clin.* 1992;8(2):355–365.

Mozingo DW, McManus AT, Pruitt BA. Appropriate use of parenteral antibiotics in managing burns. *Surgical Infections: Index and Reviews.* 1993;1(1):16–19.

Pain management of the burn patient, part 2. *J Burn Care Rehabil.* 1995;16(3, suppl).

Pruitt BA Jr, Goodwin CW Jr. Thermal and environmental injury. In: More EE, ed. *Early Care of the Injured Patient.* Philadelphia, Pa: BC Decker Inc; 1990.

Pruitt BA Jr, McManus AT. The changing epidemiology of infection in burn patients. *World J Surg.* 1992;16(1):57–67.

Purdue GF, Hunt JL. Hypothermia and frostbite. In: Mancini ME, Klein J, eds. *Decision Making in Trauma Management: A Multidisciplinary Approach.* Philadelphia, Pa: BC Decker Inc; 1991a.

Purdue GF, Hunt JL. Inhalation injuries and burns in the inner city. *Surg Clin North Am.* 1991b;71(2):385–397.

Purdue GF, Hunt JL. Pediatric burn trauma. In: Mancini ME, Klein J, eds. *Decision Making in Trauma Management: A Multidisciplinary Approach.* Philadelphia, Pa: BC Decker Inc; 1991c.

Rue LW, Cioffi WG. Resuscitation of thermally injured patients. *Crit Care Nurs Clin North Am.* 1991;3(2):181–189.

Saffle JR, Davis B, Williams P, et al. Recent outcomes in the treatment of burn injury in the United States: a report from the American Burn Association patient registry, part 1. *J Burn Care Rehabil.* 1995;16(3):219–232.

Sharar SR, Heimbach DM. Inhalation injury: current concepts and controversies. *Adv Trauma Crit Care.* 1991;6:213–230.

Sobel JB, Goldfarb W, Slater H, et al. Inhalation injury: a decade with progress. *J Burn Care Rehabil.* 1992;13(5):573–575.

Warden GD. The pediatric burn patient: issues in wound management. *Burn Management Report.* 1992;1(2):1–11.

Watkins P. Psychological stages in adaptation following burn injury: a method for facilitating psychological recovery of burn victims. *J Burn Care Rehabil.* 1988;9(4):376–384.

Weigelt JA, Klein J. Mechanism of injury. In: Mancini ME, Klein J, eds. *Decision Making in Trauma Management: A Multidisciplinary Approach.* Philadelphia, Pa: BC Decker Inc; 1991.

Youn Y-K, LaLond C, Demling R. The role of mediators in the response to thermal injury. *World J Surg.* 1992;16(1):30–36.

Appendix
Case Studies

Each of the system-based chapters presented an overview of developmental anatomy and physiology and the pathophysiology involved in various conditions commonly encountered in children hospitalized in pediatric critical care units. To facilitate analysis of clinical signs and symptoms and problem solving related to patient care, the following case studies are presented for further review of selected patient problems.

Case Study A

David, a 19-day-old, 4 kg male born to a 17-year-old gravida 1, para 1 mother, was discharged on day 2 of life. Five- and ten-minute Apgar scores were 6 and 8. Examination at discharge was without detectable pathology. Two days before presentation, David was noted to be eating poorly. One day before, he was lethargic. The morning of presentation he was difficult to arouse, refused to eat, had marked respiratory effort, and was pale.

In the emergency room, initial vital signs were heartrate (HR) of 60 bpm, respiratory rate (RR) of 90/min with marked retractions, flaring, and grunting, right arm blood pressure of 40/19, and afebrile. The infant was immediately intubated and placed on mechanical support with an FIO_2 of 100%. Initial arterial gases were SaO_2 65%, PO_2 30 mm Hg, PCO_2 38 mm Hg, pH 6.9, base deficit (BD) -15. Resuscitation was continued following placement of femoral central venous access. Following the infusion of albumin, initiation of dopamine and dobutamine drips, and repeated administration of bicarbonate, the saturation remained at 70%, blood pressure was 45/20, and the HR was 200 bpm in normal sinus rhythm (NSR). Prostaglandin E_1 infusion was initiated, and in 10 minutes, saturation rose to 80%, pH was 7.30, and BD was -5. Blood pressure rose to 60/35, and the infant began producing urine.

Echocardiogram examination revealed mitral and aortic atresia, a hypoplastic aortic arch, severe coarctation, a diminutive nonapex forming left ventricle, and a restrictive patent ductus arteriosus (PDA) with bidirectional flow.

1. What physiologic event precipitated the initial patient decompensation?

    Physiologic closure of the PDA decreases perfusion to the aorta below the area of obstruction with acidosis and shock resulting.

2. Discuss the significance of four limb blood pressures in this situation.

    When the ductus is open, all four pressures will be equal because perfusion is maintained distally. In severe low output, all pressures will be diminished because of poor distal perfusion. During good perfusion a closed ductus results in a blood pressure differential between upper and lower extremities.

3. When correcting acidosis in a neonate, what precautions are necessary?

    Rapid repletion of bicarbonate or repletion with hypertonic bicarbonate can cause fluid shifts in the brain. It should be replaced slowly in a central line and diluted with normal saline.

4. Following this degree of shock, what further patient evaluation is necessary before surgery?

Full evaluation for end-organ insults should be performed and should include renal function studies, liver function tests, and cranial ultrasound.

Four days later, with normal kidney and liver function and a normal cranial ultrasound, a Norwood operation with a 3.5 mm Blalock-Taussig (BT) shunt was performed without incident. Initial blood gases and vital signs in the ICU were Sao_2 86%, Po_2 48 mm Hg, Pco_2 26 mm Hg, pH 7, BD -19, HR 195 bpm in junctional rhythm, blood pressure 50/30 on Fio_2 of 80%. Urine output was scant, extremities cool, and pulses not palpable. The infant was on dopamine, fentanyl, and epinephrine drips.

5. Explain the relationship between the oxygen saturation, heart rate, blood pressure, and blood gases.

Saturation was high. Thus most of the cardiac output was directed to the lungs, resulting in hypotension, tachycardia, and acidosis. Junctional rhythm is most likely a response to the acidosis and low cardiac output. Oxygen should be weaned rapidly to 21% to 30% to decrease pulmonary vasodilatation. Bicarbonate can be used to treat the metabolic acidosis, and the ventilatory rate can be decreased to achieve a slight relative respiratory acidosis.

6. What significance does the junctional tachycardia have in relation to cardiac output? List three treatment options.

Junctional tachycardia (JT) often results from low cardiac output, catecholamine release, fever, or exogenous pressors and can be detrimental to cardiac output in infants. JT can be treated with pacing or antiarrhythmics or treatment of underlying conditions.

Chest tube output was 40 ml/h for the first 3 hours after surgery and has stopped. The baby remains oliguric, hypotensive, tachycardic, and acidotic.

7. What are the potential causes of this hemodynamic state? What assessment parameters are necessary to confirm suspicions? What is your treatment plan?

The infant may be hypovolemic, requiring volume resuscitation. Or the acute bleeding may have resulted in a clot formation in the atrium or chest tube itself, which may be causing tamponade. If so, a chest x-ray study would demonstrate a widened mediastinum. An echogram may show fluid, a clot behind the heart, or an underfilled ventricle. Pulsus paradoxus may be present. If cardiac output is severely compromised, the chest needs to be opened to evacuate the clot or blood. If bleeding is ongoing, a return to the operating room is necessary. Other supportive measures include volume and calcium replacement and treatment of acidosis.

The infant survives and is being prepared for discharge. His parents tell you they wish to have more children. They want to know why this happened and what the risks are for future pregnancies. In preparation for discharge, you are reviewing current health needs and the need for future surgery.

8. How would you counsel this family in regard to risk, infant nutrition, caloric need, and growth and development?

A family history is necessary to evaluate for other congenital heart diseases (CHD). The risk is higher in families with more than one child with CHD. In hypoplastic left heart syndrome (HLHS) the actual recurrence risk may be higher than the quoted increased risk of 2% to 4%. A genetic evaluation may be desired.

Growth will be slower than normal. Development is often within the expected range, although there may be some lags in gross motor skills with severe cyanosis or failure. Caloric demands are greater than requirements for the general pediatric population, and with failure, requirements of 130 to 150 kcal/kg/d may be required.

9. What is the next operation this child will need and what are the expected benefits?

The second stage is the hemi-Fontan or bidirectional Glenn. The benefit of the second stage is to reduce the pressure and volume overload on the ventricle by removing the systemic-to-pulmonary shunt (which would become relatively smaller anyway). This procedure may increase energy and growth but may not significantly increase saturation. It does provide for stable saturation until the final procedure, however.

10. Discuss the potential long-term problems and outlook for this and any infant following physiologic palliation with the Fontan procedure.

Long-term problems associated with the Fontan procedure include ventricular dysfunction (sometimes requiring transplant), protein-losing enteropathy, dysrhythmias, recurrent effusions and ascites, arteriovenous malformations (more common after the second stage), and exercise limitations.

Case Study B

A 3-year-old boy was found with an open bottle of his mother's prenatal vitamins with iron. The color of the tablet coating is seen inside the child's mouth. Twenty-five tablets are unaccounted for.

1. Following ingestion of iron, gastrointestinal (GI) decontamination may include all of the following *except:*
   a. Ipecac syrup
   b. Gastric lavage
   c. Activated charcoal
   d. Whole bowel irrigation

   c: *activated charcoal.* Iron is not adsorbed to activated charcoal.

2. For the next several hours it is important to observe this child for the development of any of the following *except:*
   a. GI bleeding
   b. Coma
   c. Acute tubular necrosis
   d. Metabolic acidosis
   e. Coagulopathies

   c: *acute tubular necrosis.* In overdose, iron causes significant corrosive injury to the GI tract. Circulating free iron injures blood vessels and damages hepatocytes. As iron is metabolized, free hydrogen is released and in concert with other events produces metabolic acidosis. GI tract symptoms, lethargy, cardiovascular collapse, seizures, pulmonary edema, hepatorenal failure with coagulopathies, and hypoglycemia may occur.

3. The child experienced vomiting, diarrhea, and abdominal pain for about 3 hours and then gradually fell into an undisturbed sleep. The most likely explanation is:
   a. The iron tablets have been eliminated from the GI tract, and the child is out of danger.
   b. The child is now in the asymptomatic latent phase, during which iron is being absorbed and metabolized.
   c. Since the child's symptoms are not characteristic of iron poisoning, he probably has a GI virus or food poisoning.
   d. These symptoms are characteristic of an allergic reaction to vitamin supplements and were precipitated by the large amounts of vitamins in these adult-strength supplements.

   b: *the child is now in the asymptomatic latent phase, during which iron is being absorbed and metabolized.* This occurs between 2 and 10 or 12 hours after ingestion. Systemic insults occur during this phase, and then the child abruptly enters the third phase with a rapid onset of cardiovascular collapse.

4. The most effective definitive therapy for acute iron intoxication is:
   a. Deferoxamine
   b. Volume expanders
   c. Hemodialysis
   d. Resin hemoperfusion
   e. Exchange transfusion

   a: *deferoxamine.* Deferoxamine is an iron-chelating agent administered intravenously.

Case Study C

Suzy, a 5-year-old girl, was hit by a car while crossing the street. Paramedics arrived at the scene within 10 minutes of the accident. She was found to have labored, irregular breathing and a heart rate of 50 bpm.

She was intubated immediately, and hyperventilation was initiated. On arrival at the emergency department she was being manually ventilated and cardiac compressions were in progress. She was stabilized following a brief resuscitation period. Rapid neurologic assessment revealed enlarged but reactive pupils, fluid draining from the left ear, bruising over the left mastoid bone, and decorticate posturing. She was given a bolus of mannitol (Osmitrol) and furosemide (Lasix) and sent to radiology for a CT scan. CT results revealed a skull fracture, small cerebral laceration, and diffuse cerebral swelling. She was taken to the operating room for a ventricular intracranial pressure (ICP) catheter followed by admission to the pediatric intensive care unit (PICU).

1. Based on the clinical examination, Suzy most likely has which of the following types of skull fractures?
   a. Growing skull fracture
   b. Basilar skull fracture
   c. Right frontal bone skull fracture
   d. Depressed skull fracture

   b: *basilar skull fracture.* Basilar fractures present with specific symptoms related to a break in the basilar portion of the skull bones. Battle's sign represents postauricular hematoma and swelling from damage to the sigmoid sinus temporal bone. Rhinorrhea represents cerebrospinal fluid (CSF) leakage into the middle ear cavity with drainage through the eustachian tube. Otorrhea represents CSF leakage from the ear canal related to a tear of the dura mater.

2. In most patients the most effective way to acutely lower ICP is by:
   a. Administering furosemide
   b. Hyperventilation
   c. Hyperoxygenation
   d. Administering a barbiturate

   b: *hyperventilation.* Although intervention needs to be individualized for each patient, a lower $PaCO_2$ causes the pH to increase (decreased H^+ concentration) and decreases cerebral tissue acidosis. Precapillary arterioles constrict in response to decreased H^+ concentration. Cerebral blood flow, cerebral blood volume, and ICP decrease. Adequate cerebral perfusion pressure must be maintained.

   On the second day of admission, Suzy's ICP acutely increased to 55 mm Hg and remained there for 6 minutes and then returned to its baseline. During this period the mean arterial blood pressure was 90 mm Hg, the right pupil was dilated and fixed, and she had decerebrate posturing.

3. Suzy's waveform is best described as:
   a. C wave
   b. P1 wave
   c. A wave
   d. B wave

   c: *A wave.* A waves (plateau) are spontaneous, rapid, irregular increases in ICP to 50 to 100 mm Hg lasting 5 to 20 minutes. A waves are frequently associated with dilated pupil(s), vomiting, abnormal posturing, decreased level of consciousness, widened pulse pressure, dysrhythmias, and decreased respirations. They represent impaired cerebral blood flow and occur most often with decreases in blood pressure associated with hypovolemia.

4. Which of the following nursing interventions is indicated at this time?
   a. Elevate the head of bed 45 degrees
   b. Administer lidocaine
   c. Administer oxygen
   d. Open the ventriculostomy drain

   d: *open the ventriculostomy drain:* CSF drainage will promote displacement of excess cerebral volume. CSF drainage by clamping and unclamping of the drainage device is controlled by physician order.

5. During the acute period of ICP elevation, Suzy's cerebral perfusion pressure (CPP) was:
   a. 15 mm Hg
   b. 90 mm Hg
   c. 35 mm Hg
   d. 40 mm Hg

c: *35 mm Hg.* CPP calculation: CPP = MAP (mean arterial pressure) – ICP
Normally CPP is greater than 50 mm Hg in the child and greater than 60 mm Hg in the adolescent.

6. If a child with a closed head injury develops polyuria, hypernatremia, and serum hyperosmolality, the nurse suspects:
   a. Diabetes mellitus
   b. Diabetes insipidus (DI)
   c. Syndrome of inappropriate antidiuretic hormone (SIADH)
   d. Thyrotoxicosis

   b: *diabetes insipidus.* DI can result from head trauma. It is a clinical condition characterized by a decrease in urine concentration and water conservation, resulting in excessive diuresis, urine osmolality less than 200 mOsm/kg, specific gravity (SG) less than 1.005, serum sodium greater than 145 mmol/L, serum osmolality greater than 300 mOsm/kg, tachycardia, and dehydration. This may be an ominous sign in head trauma.

   Suzy's ICP is stabilized by the fourth day. Follow-up CT demonstrated blood in the subarachnoid space.

7. Suzy is most at risk for which of the following complications?
   a. Obstructive hydrocephalus
   b. Epidural hematoma
   c. Blindness
   d. Motor paralysis

   a: *obstructive hydrocephalus.*

Case Study D

A 10-month-old girl, Sara, is admitted to the PICU with acute mental status changes. One of Sara's siblings died of suspected liver failure. Sara's laboratory studies include the following results: total bilirubin 5.2 mg/dl, aspartate aminotransferase (AST) 4268 IU/L, ammonia 220 μmol/L, albumin 3.2 g/dl, platelets 180,000/mm³, white blood cell count (WBC) 8.2 × 10⁹/L, and prothrombin time (PT) 33 seconds. She is on 0.5 L of oxygen per nasal cannula, is lethargic, and does not respond to stimuli.

1. Which of the following assessment findings would you observe?
   a. Jaundice
   b. Kernicterus
   c. Polysplenia
   d. Situs inversus

   a: *jaundice.* An accumulation of yellow pigment in the skin and other tissues, jaundice is evident when total bilirubin is greater than 3 mg/dl. Kernicterus is the presence of yellow pigment in the basal ganglia of the brain. Dark-colored urine and pale-colored stool may occur.

2. Which of the following blood products would best treat Sara's coagulopathy?
   a. Platelets
   b. Packed red blood cells
   c. Fresh frozen plasma (FFP)
   d. 25% albumin

   c: *fresh frozen plasma.* Coagulopathy in liver disease is related to the liver's abnormal production of prothrombin and other clotting factors and its ineffective removal of activated clotting factors. FFP contains the necessary clotting factors.

3. The rationale for administering lactulose enemas is to:
   a. Promote ammonia excretion
   b. Provide supplemental glucose
   c. Promote intestinal reabsorption of ammonia
   d. Prevent intestinal translocation

   a: *promote ammonia excretion.* A diseased liver may be unable to remove toxic metabolites (such as ammonia) normally formed during the degradation of proteins, amino acids, and blood.

Ammonia accumulation may contribute to the encephalopathy that occurs. Lactulose (Cephulac) acidifies colonic flora and promotes ammonia elimination.

4. The family consents to a liver biopsy to assist with her diagnosis. The postbiopsy interventions by the nurse caring for Sara would include:
   a. Left-side-lying positioning, vital signs every 15 minutes for 1 hour, monitoring of gastric pH
   b. Prone positioning, vital signs hourly for 1 hour, monitoring of serial hematocrits
   c. Right-side-lying positioning, vital signs every 15 minutes for 1 hour, monitoring of serial hematocrits
   d. Left-side-lying positioning, vital signs every 15 minutes for 1 hour, monitoring of gastric pH

   c: *right-side-lying position* (to apply pressure to the biopsy site), *vital signs every 15 minutes for 1 hour* (to monitor for bleeding and hypotension), and *monitoring of serial hematocrits* (to monitor for bleeding).

5. Sara's change in neurologic status can be attributed to:
   a. Jaundice
   b. Esophageal varices
   c. Asterixis
   d. Hepatic encephalopathy

   d: *hepatic encephalopathy.* Monitoring for signs of increased ICP should be frequent. Placement of an ICP monitoring device may be contraindicated in the presence of coagulopathy. Other measures may be used to monitor and treat intracranial hypertension.

Case Study E

Jennifer, a 6-year-old girl, is admitted to the PICU following a history of fever and rash for 2 days. On admission to the emergency department, she was manually ventilated with a bag-valve-mask device. Her heart rate and blood pressure were normal, and her temperature was 39° C. Neurologically she responded appropriately to pain, and her pupils were equal and reacted to light (PERL). Her trunk had a fine petechial rash. She rapidly deteriorated in the emergency department, requiring advanced life support. Routine laboratory tests, chest x-ray film, and lumbar puncture (CSF analysis) were obtained before admission to the unit. The tentative diagnosis was bacterial meningitis.

1. On the basis of the clinical examination the pathogen most likely responsible for her meningitis is:
   a. *Haemophilus influenzae* type b
   b. *Neisseria meningitidis*
   c. *Escherichia coli*
   d. Enterovirus

   b: *Neisseria meningitidis.* Petechial rash may occur with *N. meningitidis. N. meningitidis* is a prominent organism causing bacterial meningitis in children over 2 months of age.

2. Jennifer has a positive Brudzinski sign, which is best described as:
   a. Extension of upper and lower extremities
   b. Pupil constriction with neck flexion
   c. Back pain and resistance after passive extension of the lower legs
   d. Flexion of hip and knees after passive flexion of the neck

   d: *flexion of the hips and knees after passive flexion of the neck.* Bacterial meningitis is also characterized by nuchal rigidity (stiff neck), Kernig's sign (back pain and resistance with passive extension of the lower legs), photophobia (abnormal tolerance of light), fever, vomiting, lethargy, headache, and alteration in consciousness.

3. Which of the following interventions has highest priority?
   a. Ordering a kinetic bed to prevent skin breakdown
   b. Administering intravenous broad-spectrum antibiotics
   c. Transferring to radiology for a CT scan
   d. Assisting with insertion of an ICP catheter

   b: *administering intravenous broad-spectrum antibiotics.* Antimicrobial therapy is the mainstay of bacterial meningitis treatment. Chemoprophylaxis is also given to close contacts of patients with *N. meningitidis* and *H. influenzae.*

4. Typical CSF characteristics following bacterial meningitis include:
   a. Elevated WBC, decreased glucose, elevated protein, positive Gram stain
   b. Normal WBC, normal glucose, elevated protein, positive Gram stain
   c. Elevated WBC, increased glucose, decreased protein, positive Gram stain
   d. Decreased WBC, increased glucose, increased protein, negative Gram stain

   a: *elevated WBC* (polymorphonuclear cells predominate; may be normal in neonates), *decreased glucose* (should be compared to serum glucose; may be normal in neonates), *elevated protein* (normal 10 to 30 mg/dl in children; 20 to 170 mg/dl in neonates), and *positive Gram stain.* In addition, the organism culture will be positive, and the fluid is usually turbid or cloudy.

5. Jennifer develops a urine output of 0.3 ml/kg/h. Laboratory studies reveal serum sodium of 125 mmol/L; serum osmolality of 256 mOsm/kg; urine specific gravity (SG) of 1.025; urine sodium of 45 mmol/d, and urine osmolality of 600 mOsm/kg. What would the appropriate therapeutic intervention be?
   a. Fluid bolus of normal saline
   b. Furosemide 1 mg/kg
   c. Fluid restriction
   d. Observation

   c: *fluid restriction.* The SIADH is associated with meningitis. Symptoms include a serum osmolality of less than 280 mOsm/kg, urine osmolality elevated inappropriately in relation to serum osmolality, serum sodium less than 135 mmol/L, urine sodium greater than 30 mmol/d, and urine SG greater than 1.020. Usually fluid restriction to insensible losses is sufficient to decrease blood volume and increase serum sodium. Serum sodium should be normalized over 24 to 48 hours to prevent neurologic sequela.

Case Study F

A 5-year-old girl was admitted to the PICU following craniotomy for excision of a suprasellar tumor. Approximately 12 hours after admission the following were noted: decreased level of consciousness, tachycardia, hypotension, and a urine output of 15 ml/kg/h with an SG of 1.003. Laboratory studies revealed serum sodium 160 mmol/L, serum osmolality 340 mOsm/kg, and urine sodium 20 mmol/d. The diagnosis of DI was made. Initial treatment was urine replacement (ml/ml) with 0.5 normal saline (NS). Twenty-four hours later her level of consciousness improved, urine output remained at 10 to 15 ml/kg/h with a low SG, serum sodium was 150 mmol/L, and serum osmolality was 305 mOsm/kg.

Desmopressin (DDAVP) 5 µg/kg intranasally was begun. Within 2 hours her urine output had dropped to 3 ml/kg/h with an SG of 1.010. IV replacement of urinary losses was discontinued, and maintenance fluids were continued. Urine output and SG were monitored every hour. When urine output exceeded 2 ml/kg/h and SG fell below 1.010, another intranasal dose of desmopressin was administered. Two days later the IV was discontinued, and the DI was managed with twice daily doses of desmopressin and ad lib oral intake.

1. This child would require correction over a period of 48 hours to prevent cerebral:
   a. Dehydration and hemorrhage
   b. Edema and herniation
   c. Hemorrhage and edema
   d. Dehydration and herniation

   b: *edema and herniation.* Slow correction of a hyperosmolar state is necessary to prevent cerebral edema and possible herniation. A rapid decrease in serum osmolality causes water to move into the cells (which were previously at equilibrium with the serum osmolality), precipitating cellular swelling.

2. The cardiovascular signs and symptoms of DI primarily are due to:
   a. Decreased preload
   b. Decreased afterload
   c. Decreased contractility
   d. Decreased conduction

   a: *decreased preload.* Intravascular volume loss is secondary to the absence of ADH with unchecked free water loss by the kidney. Treatment with exogenous ADH increases water reabsorption by the kidney, maintaining blood volume.

3. Desmopressin is synthetic:
   a. ADH
   b. Renin
   c. Aldosterone
   d. Insulin

   a: *ADH.* Desmopressin is a form of ADH replacement therapy for the treatment of DI. The primary pathophysiologic abnormality in DI is ADH deficiency.

Case Study G

Rob, a 13-year-old boy with a history of leukemia, received a bone marrow transplant 80 days ago. He was admitted to the intensive care unit in septic shock.

1. Which of the following indicate an attempt by the kidneys to compensate for the changes in the child's condition?
   a. Increased serum bicarbonate, vasoconstriction of arterioles, secretion of renin
   b. Decreased serum bicarbonate, vasoconstriction of arterioles, secretion of renin
   c. Increased sodium excretion, vasodilation of arterioles, secretion of renin
   d. Increased sodium reabsorption, vasodilation of arterioles, secretion of renin

   a: *increased serum bicarbonate, vasoconstriction of arterioles, secretion of renin.* In an effort to correct acidosis, the kidney increases the bicarbonate in the serum to increase uptake of the hydrogen ions. The arterioles constrict to compensate for decreased perfusion and decreased renal blood flow. The kidneys release renin in response to sympathetic stimulation. Renin is converted to angiotensin I, which is converted to angiotensin II, which causes vasoconstriction and secretion of aldosterone. To maintain adequate volume, sodium reabsorption is increased.

2. On day 2, Rob's blood urea nitrogen (BUN) increased to 75 mg/dl, and the creatinine remained at 2.4 mg/dl. The increase in BUN may be an indication of worsening acute renal failure (ARF) and acute tubular necrosis (ATN).
   a. True
   b. False

   b: *false.* An increase in BUN without an increase in creatinine is most likely an indication of dehydration, decreased renal perfusion, or high catabolic state. An indication of ATN would be a rising BUN *and* creatinine level.

3. Rob gained 5 kg during the first 24 hours. This volume was largely the result of volume given during the fluid resuscitation. Rob received regular doses of furosemide (Lasix). After several days of high-dose diuretics, Rob's urine output increased to 7 ml/kg/h, and his weight decreased. The team began to notice a rising serum phosphorus level. This was most likely the result of:
   a. Dehydration
   b. Muscle wasting
   c. Hypocalcemia
   d. Hyperkalemia

   c: *hypocalcemia.* Alterations in calcium balance are often related to the use of loop diuretics, which block tubular reabsorption of calcium and may cause hypocalcemia. As serum calcium decreases, phosphorus increases. Since the mechanism for excretion of phosphate is primarily generated by the kidneys, patients in renal failure are at high risk for hyperphosphatemia.

4. Rob's serum phosphorus level remained greater than 9 mg/dl despite calcium administration. Options for further treatment of the hyperphosphatemia should include:
   a. Hemodialysis or continuous renal replacement therapy (CRRT)
   b. Increasing the dose of furosemide
   c. Administration of magnesium
   d. All of the above

   a: *hemodialysis or CRRT.* Increasing the dose of furosemide may lead to further hypocalcemia and resultant hyperphosphatemia. The administration of magnesium will not decrease the serum phosphate level.

Case Study H

Angie, an 18-month-old toddler, lives with her mother and 10-year-old sister. At noon Angie pulled the electrical cord to a crock pot of boiling beans, spilling the contents over her face, trunk, and arms. At 12:30 PM Angie's mother brought Angie to the emergency department. Angie is crying and restless. Angie's temperature is 36.5° C (rectal), HR 110 bpm and regular, blood pressure 100/80, respirations 30/min and nonlabored. Angie weighs 11 kg.

1. Most pediatric burn injuries occur in:
   a. Newborns
   b. Infants and toddlers
   c. School-age children
   d. Adolescents

   b: *infants and toddlers.* Most burns occur in the very active and curious age group of infants and toddlers. Among small children, scalds are the predominant burn injury.

2. The extent of cellular destruction within the burn wound depends on:
   a. Duration of exposure
   b. Intensity of the heat
   c. Tissue involved
   d. All of the above

   d: *all of the above.* Duration of exposure, intensity of heat, and the tissue involved all determine the extent of destruction. When absorption of heat energy exceeds the ability of the tissue to dissipate the absorbed heat, cellular injury in varying depths results.

3. A burn injury in which the entire integument is destroyed can be described as a:
   a. First-degree burn
   b. Second-degree burn
   c. Third-degree burn
   d. Fourth-degree burn

   c: *third-degree burn.* First- and second-degree burns are partial-thickness burns. A third-degree burn destroys all the layers of skin. Fourth-degree burns involve fat, fascia, muscle, and bone as well.

4. The initial hemodynamic response to a large burn injury includes:
   a. Increase in cardiac output and decrease in peripheral vascular resistance
   b. Increase in cardiac output and peripheral vascular resistance
   c. Decrease in cardiac output and increase in peripheral vascular resistance
   d. Decrease in cardiac output and peripheral vascular resistance

   c: *decrease in cardiac output and increase in peripheral vascular resistance.* An uncharacterized factor present in circulation following massive burns has been implicated in this myocardial depression. The increased peripheral vascular resistance develops as an initial physiologic response to hypovolemia, decreased cardiac output, and the release of vasoactive mediators from the stress response following injury. Cardiac output returns to normal 18 to 24 hours after the burn, and peripheral vascular resistance returns to normal after cardiac output improves.

Angie has mostly large fluid-filled blisters on her trunk and arms. The blisters on her face have ruptured, and the underlying tissue is wet and pink. With the burn record the extent and depth of Angie's burn is calculated to be 21%.

5. In the first 8 hours the amount calculated for burn fluid resuscitation (using Table 9–26) is:
   a. 924 ml
   b. 462 ml
   c. 223 ml

   b: *462 ml:* 4 ml × 11 kg × 21% ÷ 2

6. The amount calculated for maintenance fluid requirements per 24 hours (using Table 9–25) is:
   a. 1000 ml
   b. 1050 ml

c. No daily maintenance fluids needed

b: *1050 ml/24 h.*

7. To determine the adequacy of fluid resuscitation, the minimum desired urine output for Angie would be:
   a. 30 ml/h
   b. Three wet diapers per shift
   c. 11 ml/h

   c: *11 ml/h.*

8. In the emergent period of care the primary cause of shock related to the burn injury is:
   a. Cardiogenic
   b. Hypovolemic
   c. Neurogenic
   d. Septic

   b: *hypovolemic.* The first and primary goal is fluid resuscitation aimed at restoring and then maintaining intravascular volume at a level adequate for tissue perfusion to vital organs. Septic and cardiogenic shock may occur later.

9. With a large burn the patient may experience a decrease in lung compliance related to:
   a. Fluid volume overload
   b. Restrictive burns to the chest
   c. Smoke inhalation injury
   d. All of the above

   d: *all of the above.* A decrease in lung compliance may be related to chest wall edema, circumferential burns to the chest wall, smoke inhalation injury, preexisting lung disease, or fluid volume overload.

10. Immediate initial treatment of a chemical burn includes:
    a. Removing all patient clothing and locating a neutralizing agent
    b. Removing all patient clothing, brushing a powdered chemical from the skin, and locating a neutralizing agent
    c. Removing all patient clothing, brushing a powdered chemical from the skin, and copious irrigation of the wound with tap water

    c: *removing all patient clothing, brushing a powdered chemical from the skin, and copious irrigation of the wound with tap water.* Prompt measures to remove the chemical ensures the best response. Delay in treatment permits continued tissue damage. Search for a neutralizing agent wastes valuable time. In some cases the increased heat of the neutralizing reaction may further damage tissue.

11. The one best initial treatment for a burn-injured patient with suspected carbon monoxide toxicity is:
    a. Fresh air
    b. Administration of 100% O_2
    c. Hyperbaric oxygenation

    b: *administration of 100% O_2.* Administration of 100% O_2 will displace some if not all the carboxyhemoglobin before the patient's arrival at the emergency department. Carbon monoxide has a constant half-life and is reduced by 50% in 4 hours at room air, in less than 1 hour in 100% O_2, and in 30 minutes when hyperbaric oxygenation is used.

12. In an assessment of suspected child abuse the physical examination should document:
    a. If the distribution of the burn injury is consistent with the history of the injury
    b. If there are characteristic patterns of intentional injury, such as "stocking and glove" distribution
    c. If there is a delay in seeking medical attention
    d. All of the above

    d: *all of the above.* All these assessments are important in determining intentional injury. Deliberate injury by burning is often an unrecognized and unappreciated component of thermal injury. The evaluating team must be aware of the possibility of abuse in any child who incurs a burn injury, especially in children less than 2 years of age.

13. The preferred route of drug administration in the early postburn period is:
   a. IM
   b. IV
   c. SC

   b: *IV.* In the early postburn period, changes in fluid volume and circulation prevent the use of the IM or SC route for some drugs since absorption by these routes may be erratic.

Case Study I

James, a 2-month-old boy with a large ventricular septal defect (VSD), is admitted to the emergency department for symptoms of respiratory distress. He has a history of 3 days of low-grade fever, coughing, and congestion and a 3-year-old sibling with an upper respiratory tract infection. The parents note that he has eaten poorly for the last 24 hours and has had only 2 wet diapers. Admitting HR is 194 bpm, RR is 90/min, temperature is 38.2° C, blood pressure is 68/50, and Sao_2 is 84%. James is dusky with mottled extremities and is irritable, retracting, and grunting. Audible wheezing and crackling is noted on auscultation. Admitting diagnosis is probable respiratory syncytial virus (RSV) bronchiolitis.

When James' respiratory condition continues to deteriorate in the PICU, endotracheal intubation and mechanical ventilation are required. Intravenous fluids are initiated. James is then noted to be resting comfortably with a HR of 152 bpm, RR of 36/min on synchronized intermittent mandatory ventilation (SIMV) with an Fio_2 of 0.4, blood pressure of 80/62, normal arterial blood gases, and Sao_2 of 98%.

1. Which diagnostic test is most definitive for RSV bronchiolitis?
   a. Lung biopsy
   b. Pulse oximetry
   c. Fluorescent antibody test
   d. Arterial blood gas analysis

   c: *fluorescent antibody test.* Rapid fluorescent antibody test for RSV may be used to test nasopharyngeal secretions. Direct isolation of the virus is possible through nasopharyngeal washing but may require 2 weeks for positive culture results. The diagnosis is based primarily on clinical observations. Chest radiography may demonstrate hyperinflation, atelectasis, and peribronchial thickening in about half of infected patients. Arterial blood gas analysis may demonstrate hypoxemia or hypercarbia. Pulse oximetry may demonstrate hypoxemia.

2. Prevention of spread of the RSV can be enacted with:
   a. Restriction of visiting
   b. Good handwashing
   c. Strict gown and glove isolation
   d. Transfer to a rehabilitation facility

   b: *good handwashing.* This is required to prevent spread of the virus to other patients and families, particularly high-risk patients. Patients at high risk for RSV infection include immunosuppressed patients and children with congenital heart disease, bronchopulmonary dysplasia (BPD), cystic fibrosis, prematurity, and other chronic illnesses.

3. Medications often used during endotracheal intubation of infants and children include:
   a. Steroids and NSAIDs
   b. Barbiturates, antiemetics, and neuromuscular blockers
   c. Benzodiazepines, neuromuscular blockers, and steroids
   d. Neuromuscular blockers, sedatives, and anticholinergics

   d: *neuromuscular blocking agents, sedatives, and anticholinergics.* Such medications are frequently used during the intubation procedure. Rapid sequence intubation is used when there are concerns about regurgitation and aspiration.

4. Which of the following statements concerning airway pressures in children who are mechanically ventilated is *not* correct?
   a. The greater the lung compliance, the higher the peak inspiratory pressure (PIP).
   b. Positive end expiratory pressure (PEEP) tends to "stent" open the airways, which might otherwise collapse at end expiration.
   c. Continuous positive airway pressure (CPAP) provides positive airway pressure sustained throughout spontaneous respiratory cycles.

d. Mean airway pressure is influenced by a variety of mechanisms including tidal volume, PEEP, and PIP.

a: *incorrect.* Compliance is the relationship of volume to pressure within a closed space. Lung compliance is determined by the elasticity of lung tissue and the presence of surfactant in the alveoli. Therefore greater compliance will enable *lower* PIPs.

5. Which of the following statements concerning ventilator modes in children is true?
   a. Intermittent mandatory ventilation (IMV) does not allow the patient to breath spontaneously.
   b. SIMV incorporates a sensor that recognizes spontaneous breaths and retimes delivery of the next ventilator breath.
   c. During pressure support ventilation (PSV) a lower pressure limit will provide greater support for the patient.
   d. The trigger is the mechanism that terminates inspiration.

   b: *SIMV incorporates a sensor that recognizes spontaneous breaths and retimes delivery of the next ventilator breath.* The spontaneous breaths are not regulated by the preset parameters. IMV delivers a preset number of breaths at preset parameters, but the patient *can* breathe spontaneously from the circuit. PSV allows the patient to breathe spontaneously, triggering ventilator support with a pressure sensor. When spontaneous effort is sensed, gas flow is delivered until the airway pressure reaches a preset minimum limit. The *higher* the pressure limit, the greater the support for the patient. The trigger is the mechanism that *initiates* inspiration.

The nurse caring for James notes a sudden decrease in SaO_2 from 98% to 82%.

6. What is the first priority for nursing interventions?
   a. Administer a sedative agent
   b. Increase the FIO_2 and ventilator rate
   c. Reposition the endotracheal tube
   d. Assess the patency of the endotracheal tube

   d: *assess the patency of the endotracheal tube.* This should be done first. Auscultate the chest to assess for presence and equality of breath sounds. Repositioning the tube may be required if it is demonstrated that there are diminished breath sounds on one side of the chest either through auscultation or radiographic examination. Most of the time when this occurs in children, the tube is in the right main stem bronchus. Endotracheal tube suctioning may be required if auscultation reveals increased secretions or a blocked tube. If atelectasis or edema of the small airways has progressed, increased FIO_2 or increased ventilatory support may be required. Sedative agents should not be administered until all other potential causes of hypoxemia have been ruled out.

7. Evaluate the following arterial blood gases:
   pH 7.42, PO_2 92 mm Hg, PCO_2 42 mm Hg, base deficit (BD) −1
   a. Metabolic alkalosis
   b. Within normal limits
   c. Metabolic acidosis
   d. Respiratory alkalosis

   b: *within normal limits.*

8. Evaluate the following arterial blood gases:
   pH 7.28, PO_2 74 mm Hg, PCO_2 59 mm Hg, BE 0
   a. Compensated metabolic acidosis
   b. Uncompensated metabolic alkalosis
   c. Compensated respiratory alkalosis
   d. Uncompensated respiratory acidosis

   d: *uncompensated respiratory acidosis.*

9. The concept of permissive hypercarbia is a strategy that allows:
   a. A higher PCO_2 with normal oxygenation, pH >7.15, and no evidence of cerebral dysfunction
   b. A higher PCO_2 with a minimum PO_2 of 50 mm Hg, pH >7, and a normal mental status
   c. A respiratory alkalosis with a PO_2 in the normal range.

    d. A respiratory acidosis with P_{CO_2} ranging from 80 to 100 mm Hg.

    a: *a higher P_{CO_2} with normal oxygenation, pH >7.15, and no evidence of cerebral dysfunction.* Permissive hypercarbia is a strategy for guiding ventilator manipulations that allow hypercarbia to exist with normal oxygenation, pH >7.15, P_{CO_2} between 45 and 80 mm Hg, and no evidence of cerebral dysfunction. Over time, physiologic compensation normalizes the pH. The benefit is that it allows minimal volume ventilation, which reduces the risk of lung injury.

Case Study J

    Janet, a 6-month-old infant, has been admitted to the emergency room with a fever of 102° F and a history of cold and flu symptoms over the last 24 hours. The infant is lethargic. Heart rate is 190 bpm. Respiratory rate is 50/min. Blood pressure is 80/45. Temperature is 102° F. The infant has a sunken fontanelle and has not had a wet diaper in more than 18 hours.

1. Which signs and symptoms would indicate dehydration?
    a. Urine output <0.5 ml/kg/h, decreased urine sodium content, urine osmolarity <300 mOsm/L
    b. Urine output <0.5 ml/kg/h, decreased urine sodium content, urine osmolarity >500 mOsm/L
    c. Urine output >1 ml/kg/h, increased urine sodium content, urine osmolarity >500 mOsm/L
    d. Urine output >1 ml/kg/h, decreased urine sodium content, urine osmolarity <300 mOsm/L

    b: *urine output <0.5 ml/kg/h, decreased urine sodium content, urine osmolarity >500 mOsm/L.* In the event of decreased fluid balance the kidneys attempt to compensate by increasing sodium reabsorption, which decreases sodium excretion and decreases urine output. As a result, urine osmolarity increases.

2. The most important priority for this patient is to:
    a. Obtain blood cultures
    b. Place a Foley catheter
    c. Obtain vascular access
    d. Intubate and start mechanical ventilation

    c: *obtain vascular access.* Vascular access to begin fluid replacement and restore adequate circulation would be the first priority. Establishing an airway and breathing are always the first priorities in resuscitation; however, the history of this child did not indicate the need to assist airway or breathing. It would be important to obtain necessary tests; however, this would come after adequate vascular access has been established.

3. Normal urine output for an infant would be expected to be greater than or equal to:
    a. 0.5 ml/kg/h
    b. 1 ml/kg/h
    c. 1 to 3 ml/kg/h
    d. 3 to 5 ml/kg/h

    c: *1 to 3 ml/kg/h:* An infant's normal urine output is between 1 and 3 ml/kg/h. A child would be expected to have a urine output greater than or equal to 1 to 2 ml/kg/h.

4. Water is conserved or eliminated by the kidneys in response to which of the following:
    a. Urine sodium concentration
    b. Serum potassium concentration
    c. Level of ADH
    d. Presence of aldosterone

    c: *level of ADH:* Vasopressin, or ADH, plays a role in water balance. The distal convoluted tubule and collecting ducts are impermeable to water, so water may be excreted as dilute urine. If ADH is present, the distal tubule and collecting ducts become permeable, water is reabsorbed, and the urine is more concentrated. A rise in the solute concentration of the extracellular fluids and blood plasma stimulates cells in the hypothalamus to increase production and release of ADH from the posterior pituitary. ADH brings the message to the kidneys to retain water and decrease the solute concentration. Decreased solute concentration causes decreased ADH, which causes dilute urine. Increased solute concentration causes increased ADH, which causes concentrated urine.

Case Study K

Chip, a 13-year-old boy, has been admitted to the emergency room with a history of a fall from the monkey bars at a playground. The child has a large bruise over the abdominal region. Initial blood tests reveal a serum potassium level of 8.6 mg/dl.

1. First priority for the treatment of hyperkalemia would be:
   a. Initiation of continuous venovenous hemodialysis (CVVH)
   b. Normal saline fluid bolus
   c. Administer glucose and insulin
   d. Administer sodium bicarbonate

   c: *administer glucose and insulin.* The first priority for the treatment of severe hyperkalemia would be the administration of insulin and glucose. CVVH would not be appropriate. Intermittent hemodialysis would be the more appropriate extracorporeal therapy for initial treatment and rapid potassium removal. CVVH may be used at a later time in the course of this child's treatment.

2. Serious clinical manifestations of hyperkalemia may include:
   a. Metabolic alkalosis
   b. Metabolic acidosis
   c. Hypocalcemia
   d. Hypertension

   b: *metabolic acidosis.* Acidosis is a common clinical manifestation of hyperkalemia.

Case Study L

A child presents to the PICU with lethargy, polyuria, serum glucose of 550 mg/dl, a blood pH of 7.25, glycosuria, and ketonuria.

1. Hyperglycemia is present in the child with uncontrolled diabetic ketoacidosis (DKA) due to:
   a. Decreased tissue utilization of glucose and increased counterregulatory hormones
   b. Increased counterregulatory hormones and Increased tissue utilization of glucose
   c. Increased tissue utilization of glucose and decreased counterregulatory hormones
   d. Decreased counterregulatory hormones and decreased tissue utilization of glucose

   a: *decreased tissue utilization of glucose and increased counterregulatory hormones.* In the absence of insulin, stored substrates are mobilized and cellular uptake of glucose is inhibited. An increase in counterregulatory hormones contributes to increased glucose production and hyperglycemia.

2. Appropriate therapeutic intervention would be:
   a. Regular insulin IV or SC bolus of 0.1 U/kg followed by continuous infusion of regular insulin
   b. NPH insulin IV bolus of 0.1 U/kg followed by continuous infusion of regular insulin
   c. Regular insulin SC of 0.1 U/kg followed by maintenance IV fluids
   d. NPH insulin SC of 0.1 U/kg followed by maintenance IV fluids

   a: *regular insulin IV or SC bolus of 0.1 U/kg followed by continuous infusion of regular insulin.* Volume expansion is administered as boluses of normal saline during the first 1 to 2 hours. Additional fluid boluses are given as needed to treat poor perfusion. Dextrose 5% is added to IV fluids when the blood glucose falls below 250 mg/dl.

Case Study M

A 15-year-old girl was found unconscious; a bottle of her mother's amitriptyline was found next to her. She had a grand mal seizure in the ambulance en route to the emergency department.

1. The toxicity of tricyclic antidepressants significantly contributes to which of the following effects:
   a. Drooling and respiratory distress

b. Agitation and restlessness
c. Prolonged, accelerated hypertension
d. Numerous dysrhythmias

d: *numerous dysrhythmias.* Tricyclic antidepressants have the following effects: anticholinergic (resulting in dry mouth, early hypertension and hallucinations), delayed uptake of norepinephrine (resulting in some CNS and cardiac effects), membrane depressant effects on the heart (resulting in numerous dysrhythmias, especially ventricular disorders and conduction delays), and alpha adrenergic blockade (resulting in the hypotension characteristic of this poisoning).

2. The single most important drug in the management of tricyclic antidepressant overdose is:
a. Dopamine
b. Glucagon
c. Lidocaine
d. Phenytoin
e. Sodium bicarbonate

e: *sodium bicarbonate.* Symptomatic patients are likely to develop acidosis that is resistant to correction. Although hyperventilation is sometimes used to correct acidosis, sodium bicarbonate is preferred, since it appears to have therapeutic effects in addition to the correction of acidosis.

3. In cases of intentional drug overdose it is especially important to obtain laboratory evaluation of which potential coingestant:
a. Acetaminophen
b. Cocaine
c. Ethanol
d. Heroin
e. Salicylates

a: *acetaminophen.*

4. After tricyclic antidepressant overdose, death is usually due to:
a. Cardiac dysrhythmias
b. Disrupted neurotransmission in the central nervous system
c. Hepatotoxicity
d. Profound hypotension
e. Refractory seizures

a: *cardiac dysrhythmias.* The toxic dose cannot be predicted with certainty. Any amount is potentially dangerous in children. At least 6 hours of emergency department evaluation is required for every ingestion in young children and for ingestions larger than the therapeutic dose in older children. Patients who become symptomatic in the 6-hour observation period require admission to a monitored bed until they have been asymptomatic for 24 hours.

Index

Note: Page numbers in *italics* refer to illustrations; page numbers followed by t refer to tables.

A

Abdomen, acute, 439, 446–447
  auscultation of, 427
  in renal system assessment, 361
  in trauma assessment, 572
  inspection of, 427
  palpation of, 427–428
  percussion of, 428
  protuberance of, 427
  trauma to, 431–435, 582
    blood volume in, 433, 433t
    blunt, 431–432
    diagnosis of, 432, 432t
    imaging of, 432
    in child abuse, 590–591
    nursing diagnoses in, 432
    penetrating, 432
    signs and symptoms of, 432
    treatment of, 432–433
Abdominal reflex, 299
Abducens nerve, 291t, 302t, 305t
ABO blood group, 490–491
  in platelet transfusion, 503–504
Absent breath sounds, 48
Absolute refractory period, of cardiac muscle, 157
Acetaminophen, for pain, 14
Acetaminophen poisoning, 600t, 606–607
Acetazolamide (Diamox), in acute renal failure, 380
N-Acetyl cysteine, in acetaminophen poisoning, 607
Acetylcholine, in blood flow regulation, 152
  in cardiac regulation, 153
Acid, 369
Acid burns, 618–620
Acid-base balance, 369. See also *Acidosis; Alkalosis; Diabetic ketoacidosis.*
Acidosis, metabolic, in acute renal failure, 375, 375t
    in asthma, 113
    in septic shock, 640
  potassium excretion in, 368
  renal response to, 369, 375t
Acoustic nerve, 291t, 302t, 306t
Acquired immunodeficiency syndrome (AIDS), 526–533
  cardiomyopathy in, 533

Acquired immunodeficiency syndrome (AIDS)
    (Continued)
  cell-mediated immunity in, 529
  central nervous system infection in, 533
  clinical categories of, 527, 527t
  definition of, 526
  diagnosis of, 538–529
  etiology of, 526–527
  humoral immunity in, 528–529
  lymphocytic interstitial pneumonitis in, 532–533
  management of, 529–533
    zidovudine in, 529–530
  nursing diagnoses in, 529
  pathophysiology of, 526
  Pneumocystis carinii pneumonia in, 530–532
    prophylaxis for, 532
  pulmonary lymphoid hyperplasia in, 532–533
  respiratory dysfunction in, 533
  risk factors for, 526–527
  signs and symptoms of, 527–528
Acrocyanosis, in cardiovascular system assessment, 159
Action potential, of cardiac muscle cells, 158
  of neuron, 286, 287
Activated charcoal, in poisoning management, 604–605
Activated clotting time, 490
Activated partial thromboplastin time, 489–490
Active transport, in renal system, 362
Acute chest syndrome, in sickle cell disease, 520
Acute tubular necrosis, 371–372, 378. See also *Renal failure, acute.*
  definition of, 371
  diuretic phase of, 371–372
  ischemic, 371
  nephrotoxic, 371
  oliguric phase of, 371
  onset of, 371
  pathophysiology of, 371
  recovery phase of, 372
  vs. acute renal failure, 372, 372t
Addison's disease, 401
Adenosine (Adenocard), cardiovascular effects of, 180–181
Adenovirus, in pneumonia, 104t

Adolescent, as parents, 5
  communication with, 16
  development of, 3
  fears of, 7
  pain management in, 13t
  play opportunities for, 18
  stress response of, 6
  working with, 3–4
Adrenal cortex, 400
  abnormalities of, 401
  development of, 402
  hormones of, 389t, 400–401
Adrenal gland, 400–402
  autonomic nerve stimulation of, 295t
  cells of, 400
  development of, 402
  hormones of, 389t–390t
  location of, *388*, 400
Adrenal insufficiency, 401
Adrenal medulla, 400
  abnormalities of, 402
  development of, 402
  hormones of, 390t, 401–402
β-Adrenergic agonists, in bronchopulmonary
        dysplasia, 133–134
β-Adrenergic antagonist poisoning, 600t
Adrenocorticotropic hormone (ACTH), 389t, 396
Adrenocorticotropic hormone (ACTH) stimulation
        test, 405, 408
Adult respiratory distress syndrome (ARDS), 115–121
  clinical presentation of, 117
  complications of, 120–121
  definition of, 115
  diagnosis of, 117
  etiology of, 117
  management of, 117–121
    goals of, 117–118
    infection surveillance in, 120
    mechanical ventilation in, 118–119, *119*
    nutritional support in, 119–120
    patient monitoring in, 118
  pathophysiology of, 115–117, *115, 116*
Advanced cardiac life support, 184–186
Adventitious breath sounds, 48
Afterload, 154
β-Agonists, in pulmonary disorders, 66
Air bags, in vehicle-related trauma, 561
Air leak syndromes, 90–94, *90, 92, 93*. See also
        Pneumothorax.
Airway. See also *Lungs; Respiratory system.*
  antigen resistance of, 472
  developmental anatomy of, 35–37
  edema of, in laryngotracheobronchitis, 102, *103*
  in asthma, 106–115. See also *Asthma.*
  in burn injury, 674
  in cardiopulmonary failure, 184–185, 186
  in trauma assessment, 568–569
  in trauma treatment, 574–575
Airway resistance, 38, 74, 75
Alagille syndrome, liver transplantation in, 457
Alanine aminotransferase, reference values for, 450t
Albumin, reference values for, 451t
  transfusion of, 506
Albuterol, in asthma, *112,* 113, 114t

Aldosterone, 389t, 400
  in volume homeostasis, 367
Alkaline burns, 618–620
Alkaline phosphatase, reference values for, 407t, 450t
Alkalosis, potassium excretion in, 368
  renal response to, 369, 375t
  respiratory, in septic shock, 640
Allen test, 174–175
Allergens, skin testing of, 492
Allergic reactions, with transfusions, 507
Allergy. See also *Anaphylaxis.*
  skin testing for, 492
Alpha cells, 387–388, *390*
Alpha-fetoprotein, in brain tumor, 337
  in neural tube defects, 353
Aluminum hydroxide (Amphojel), 429
Alveolar pores of Kohn, 37
Alveolar stage, of pulmonary embryology, 33, *34*
Alveolar ventilation, 73t, 74
Alveolus(i), *35,* 37
  postnatal development of, 33
Amanita poisoning, 625
γ-Aminobutyric acid, in hepatic encephalopathy, 453
Aminophylline, in asthma, *112,* 113, 114t
  in bronchopulmonary dysplasia, 134
Amitriptyline poisoning, 607–608
  case study of, 695–696
Ammonia, in hepatic encephalopathy, 453
  reference values for, 451t
Amoxapine poisoning, 608
Amphetamines, maternal use of, fetal cardiac
        anomalies and, 160t
Amphetamine poisoning, 600t, 615–616
Amphojel (aluminum hydroxide), 429
Amphotericin B, contraindication to, 501
Amputation, 587–588
Amrinone lactate (Inocor), cardiovascular effects of,
        178
Amyl nitrite, in cyanide poisoning, 621
Anaphylaxis, 514, 515t
  with intravenous immunoglobulin administration,
        502
Androgens, 389t–390t
Anemia, 465–466, 509–510
  hemolytic, 466
  iatrogenic, 510
  in acute renal failure, 375–376
  in burn injury, 656
Anesthesia, general, in status epilepticus, 327
Aneurysm, intracranial, 329–330
Angiography, 170–171, *171*
  in neurologic assessment, 310–311
  in pulmonary assessment, 52
  in respiratory distress, 52
Animal bites, prevention of, 559t
Anterior cord syndrome, 345
Antiarrhythmic agents, 180–182
Antibiotics, in aspiration pneumonitis, 88
  in asthma, *112,* 113
  in burn injury, 670, 670t
  in CNS infection, 334–335
  in pneumonia, 106
  in septic shock, 643
  prophylactic, in septic shock prevention, 649

Antibody(ies), platelet, 536–537
  production of, 475–476, 477t
Anticholinergic agents, antagonistic action of, 63
  in acute respiratory failure, 72t
  in asthma, *112,* 113, 114t
  in bronchopulmonary dysplasia, 134
Anticholinergic poisoning, 600t
Anticoagulants, 469–470
Anticoagulation, in continuous renal replacement
      therapy, 383
  natural, 480–481
Anticonvulsant agents, in status epilepticus, 326–327,
      327t
  long-term side effects of, 327
  maternal use of, fetal cardiac anomalies and, 160t
Antidepressant poisoning, 601t, 607–608
  case study of, 695–696
Antidiuretic hormone, 389t, 394–395
  in central diabetes insipidus, 421–422, 422t
  in water balance, 366–367, 694
  inappropriate secretion of, 417–419. See also
      *Syndrome of inappropriate antidiuretic hormone
      secretion.*
  serum osmolality and, 395
Antidote, 605
  in acetaminophen poisoning, 607
  in cyanide poisoning, 621
  in digitalis poisoning, 611
  in ethylene glycol poisoning, 623
  in methanol poisoning, 624
  in opioid poisoning, 614
  in organophosphate poisoning, 627
  in snake bite, 621–622
Antigen. See also *Immunity.*
  airway response to, 472
  chemical barriers to, 471
  complement activation by, 473
  cutaneous barrier to, 471–472
  gastrointestinal tract response to, 472
  inflammatory response to, 472–473
  mechanical barriers to, 471
  ophthalmologic response to, 472
  phagocytosis response to, 473
  physical barriers to, 471
Antigens, epitopes of, 470
  skin testing of, 492
Antiglobulin test, 488
Antihemophilic factor, 505
Antihypertensive agents, 182–183
Antiinflammatory agents, in asthma, *112,* 113, 114t
  in bronchopulmonary dysplasia, 134
  in pulmonary disorders, 66
Antilymphocyte globulin, for therapeutic
      immunosuppression, 496
Antithrombin III, 469
Antithrombin system, 481
Antithymocyte globulin, for therapeutic
      immunosuppression, 496
α₁-Antitrypsin deficiency, liver transplantation in, 456
Anxiety, after burn injury, 671–672
Aorta, coarctation of, 234–236, *235, 237*
  end-to-end anastomosis of, in coarctation of aorta,
      236, *237*
  trauma to, 95, 96, 96t

Aortic arch, anatomy of, *235*
  interruption of, 234–236
Aortic body, in cardiac regulation, 153
Aortic stenosis, 227–230, *228*
  supravalvular, 229–230
  valvular, 227–229, *228*
Aortic valve, 147–148, *147*
Aortoplasty, in coarctation of aorta, 236, *237*
Aortopulmonary shunt, in tricuspid atresia, 249
Aplasia, of stem cells, 462
Aplastic crisis, in sickle cell disease, 519–520
Apneustic respiration, *46,* 300, 307t
Apresoline (hydralazine), cardiovascular effects of, 183
AquaMEPHYTON (phytonadione), 428
Arachidonic acid, metabolites of, in septic shock, 631
Arachnoid, 278, 283
  in cerebrospinal fluid circulation, 279, *279*
Arrhythmias. See *Dysrhythmias.*
Arsenic poisoning, 600t
Arterial pressure, 155
  monitoring of, 173–174, *174, 175*
  regulation of, 155
Arterial switch operation, in transposition of great
      vessels, 246–247, *247*
Arterial vascular access, in cardiopulmonary failure,
      185
Arteriography, in renal trauma, 385
Arteriohepatic dysplasia, liver transplantation in, 457
Arterioles, 148
Arteriovenous malformation, intracranial, 328–329
Artery(ies), 148
  autonomic nerve stimulation of, 294t
  coronary, 149, *149*
Arthropathy, in hemophilia, 540
Ascites, in hepatic failure, 454, 456
Aspartate aminotransferase, reference values for, 450t
Aspergillus, in septic shock, 647
Asphyxia, 659–660
Aspiration, foreign body, 88–90. See also *Foreign body
      aspiration.*
  prevention of, 557t
Aspiration pneumonitis, 86–88. See also *Pneumonitis,
      aspiration.*
Aspirin, for pain, 14
  platelet effects of, 497
Aspirin poisoning, 614–615
Assist-control ventilation, 76, *79*
Asterixis, in hepatic failure, 455
Asthma, 106–115
  cellular mediators of, 106, *107*
  chest radiography in, 110
  clinical evaluation score for, 111t
  clinical presentation of, 107–110, 108t
  complications of, 113
  definition of, 106
  diagnostic evaluation of, 110
  differential diagnosis of, 109–110
  gas exchange in, 107
  laboratory tests in, 110
  management of, 110–113, 111t, 114t
    intubation in, 111
    mechanical ventilation in, 111–113
    medications in, *112,* 113, 114t
    supportive care in, 113

Asthma *(Continued)*
  metabolic acidosis in, 113
  mild, 109t
  moderate, 109t
  mortality and, 115
  neurogenic factors in, 106
  pathophysiology of, 106–107, *107*
  patient history in, 107–108
  physical examination in, 108–109
  prognosis for, 113, 115
  pulmonary function in, 107
  pulmonary function tests in, 110
  severe, 109t
  severity of, 109, 109t
Asymmetric tonic neck response, 298
Ataxic respiration, *46*, 300, 307t
Atelectasis, during mechanical ventilation, 85
  in asthma, 107
Atherosclerosis, genetic factors in, 211
Atracurium, in acute respiratory failure, 72t
Atria, 146, *146*, *147*
  electrical depolarization of, 158
Atrial fibrillation, 202t, 203
Atrial flutter, 201, 202t, 203
Atrial pathways, internodal, 155, *156*
Atrial septal defect, 218–219
Atrioventricular block, first-degree, 204, *205*
  second-degree, 204–205, *205*
  third-degree (complete), 205–206, *205*
Atrioventricular nodal reentry, 202t
Atrioventricular node, 155, *156*, 157
  conduction disorders of, 204–206, *205*
  dysrhythmias of, 201, *201*, 202t
Atrioventricular septal defect, 222–223
Atrioventricular valves, 147, *147*
  development of, 146
Atropine, 430
  cardiovascular effects of, 181
  in organophosphate poisoning, 627
  in pulmonary disorders, 64t
Atropine poisoning, 611
Atropine sulfate, in acute respiratory failure, 72t
Atrovent (ipratropium bromide), in asthma, 114t
  in bronchopulmonary dysplasia, 134
Aura, of seizure, 325
Auscultation, during mechanical ventilation, 82
  for breath sounds, 47–48
  in cardiovascular system assessment, 163–164
  in respiratory system assessment, 47–48
  in septic shock assessment, 638
  of abdomen, 427
  of fontanelles, 297
  of lungs, 47–48
  of skull, 297
Autoimmune disease, 514–515
Automaticity, of cardiac cells, 157
Autonomic dysreflexia, 347
Autonomic hyperreflexia, 347–348
Autonomic nervous system, 289, 291–292, *292*, *293*
  parasympathetic, 291, *292*
  sympathetic, 291, *292*
Axon, 277, *277*
Azathioprine (Imuran), for immunosuppression, 431,
    495–496

Azidothymidine (zidovudine), 529–530
  mechanism of action of, 494
  side effects of, 494
Azotemia, in acute renal failure, 374

B
Babinski's reflex, assessment of, 299
Bachmann's bundle, 155
Back, in trauma assessment, 573
Bacteremia, 639
Bacteria, in colon, 425
Bag-valve mask, in cardiopulmonary failure, 184–185
  in trauma treatment, 575
Bainbridge reflex, in cardiac regulation, 153
Balloon valvuloplasty, in aortic stenosis, 228
  in pulmonary valve stenosis, 241, *241*
Barbiturates, for pain, 14
  in pulmonary disorders, 62
Barbiturate coma, in status epilepticus, 327
Barbiturate poisoning, 600t
Bardet-Biedl syndrome, cardiac anomalies in, 160t
Baroreceptors, in blood flow regulation, 152
  in septic shock, 636
Baroreceptor reflex, in shock, 194
Barotrauma, during mechanical ventilation, 85
  in septic shock, 647
Barrel chest, 45, *45*
Basal ganglia, 280
Basal metabolic rate, 426–427
Base, definition of, 369
Basilar fracture, 340, 341
Basophils, 467
  differentiation of, *462*
Battle's sign, in basilar fracture, 341
  in trauma assessment, 572
Behavior, in trauma assessment, 570–571
Benadryl (diphenhydramine), for pruritus, 64t
Benzocaine poisoning, 607
Benzodiazepines, for pain, 14
  in pulmonary disorders, 59–61, 60t
Benzodiazepine poisoning, 608–609
Bereavement, 28–29
Berkow nomogram, in burns, 663, *664*
Berry aneurysm, intracranial, 329–330
Beta cells, 387, *390*
Betadine (povidone-iodine ointment), in burn injury,
    670, 670t
Bicycle safety, 560t
Bicycle trauma, 562
Bilevel positive airway pressure, 82
Biliary atresia, liver transplantation in, 456
Biliary tree, 426
Bilirubin, reference values for, 450t–451t
Biomedicus ventricular assist device, 189t
Bites, animal, prevention of, 559t
  snake, 621–622
  spider, 621–622
Bite marks, in child abuse, 589
Black widow spider bite, 622
Bladder, autonomic nerve stimulation of, 295t
  catheterization of, in trauma treatment, 577
  disorders of, after bone marrow transplantation,
    544–545
  trauma to, 584

Blalock-Taussig shunt, in pulmonary atresia with intact ventricular septum, 255
  in tetralogy of Fallot, 243, *244*
Bleeding. See also *Hemorrhage.*
  hypovolemia with, 516–517
  in disseminated intravascular coagulation, 534
  occult, 435
  platelet levels and, 480
  with cardiac assist devices, 190
Bleeding time, 489
Blood. See also *Hematopoietic system.*
  typing of, 490–491
Blood flow, autoregulation of, 152
  cardiac, *151*
  cerebral, brain, 288–289
    in neurologic assessment, 315
  drug delivery and, 58–59
  fetal, 149–150, *150*
  in congestive heart failure, 192
  in hypoplastic left heart syndrome, 231
  in pulmonary atresia with intact ventricular septum, 254
  in tetralogy of Fallot, 242
  in total anomalous pulmonary venous return, 252–253
  in tricuspid atresia, 248
  in truncus arteriosus, 250
  metabolic hypothesis of, 152
  myogenic response hypothesis of, 152
  peripheral, regulation of, 152–153
  pulmonary, 39, *39*
  renal, 369–370
Blood gases, during mechanical ventilation, 82
  in asthma, 107, 110
  in bronchopulmonary dysplasia, 132, 133
  in pulmonary evaluation, 53t
Blood pressure, 256
  in cardiovascular system assessment, 163
  in neurologic assessment, 308
  regulation of, 369
Blood transfusion, 498–500
  after bone marrow transplantation, 541, 541t
  allergic reactions with, 507
  alloimmunization with, 508
  bacterial contamination of, 507–508
  complications of, 506–509
  febrile reactions with, 507
  graft-versus-host disease with, 509
  hemolytic reactions in, 506–507
  hypocalcemia with, 509
  hypothermia with, 509
  in sickle cell disease, 520
  iron overload with, 509
  metabolic complications of, 509
  packed red blood cells for, 499–500
  whole blood for, 498–499, 499t
Blood volume, 433t
  in septic shock, 632–633, *632*
  pulmonary, 37
Blood-brain barrier, 282–283
Blood-CSF barrier, 283
Body image, after burn injury, 672
Bone marrow, biopsy of, 491
  necrosis of, in sickle cell disease, 521–522

Bone marrow transplantation, 540–546
  acute complications of, 542–546
  allogeneic, 540–541
  autologous, 540
  blood product guidelines for, 541, 541t
  cardiac complications of, 544
  case study of, 689
  chronic graft-versus-host disease after, 546
  definition of, 540
  gastrointestinal tract dysfunction after, 542–543
  graft-versus-host disease after, 545–546, 545t
  hemorrhagic cystitis after, 544–545
  hepatic dysfunction after, 542
  indications for, 540
  infection after, 542
  management after, 541–542
  pulmonary complications of, 543–544
  renal dysfunction after, 543
  syngeneic, 540
Botulism, 600t
Bowel. See also *Gastrointestinal system.*
  infarction of, 439, 446–447
  irrigation of, in poisoning management, 604
  necrotizing disease of, 447–448, 448t
  perforation of, 439, 446–447
Bowman's capsule, 360, 366t
Brace, in scoliosis, 351
Bradycardia, in trauma assessment, 570
Bradycardia tachycardia syndrome, 199
Brain, biopsy of, 337
    in CNS infection, 334
  blood flow of, 288–289
  cerebrum of, 279–280, *280*
  embryogenesis of, 274–276, *276*
  glucose metabolism of, 288
  in trauma assessment, 570
  intermediate zone of, 276
  marginal zone of, 276
  metabolism of, 288
  oxygen metabolism of, 288
  subventricular zone of, 276
  trauma to, 339–342
    cardiovascular tissue perfusion in, 342
    etiology of, 340
    gas exchange in, 342
    in child abuse, 590, 591–592
    incidence of, 339–340
    management of, 342
    neurodiagnosis of, 341–342
    pathophysiology of, 340
    symptoms of, 340–341
  tumors of, 335–338
    chemotherapy for, 337–338
    diagnosis of, 337
    etiology of, 336
    incidence of, 336
    infratentorial, 336
    management of, 337–338
    pathophysiology of, 336
    radiation therapy for, 337
    supratentorial, 336–337
    symptoms of, 336–337
    tissue perfusion in, 338
  ventricular zone of, 276

Brain death, 308
Brain stem, 281–282, *281*
Brain stem auditory evoked responses, in neurologic
    assessment, 316
Breath, first, 33
Breath sounds, absent, 48
    adventitious, 48
    auscultation for, 47–48
    bronchial, 48
    bronchovesicular, 48
    diminished, 48
    vesicular, 48
Breathing, control of, 40–41, *40*
    evaluation of, 45, *46*
    in trauma assessment, 569
    in trauma treatment, 575–576
    mechanics of, 41
    nose, in infant, 35
    sensor monitoring of, 76
    work of, in respiratory failure, 184
Bretylium, cardiovascular effects of, 181
Bronchial breath sounds, 48
Bronchioles, *35, 37*
Bronchiolitis, 97–99, *98*
    clinical course of, 99
    clinical presentation of, 98–99
    complications of, 99
    definition of, 97
    diagnostic tests in, 99
    etiology of, 98
    management of, 99
    obliterative, after lung transplantation, 139
    outcomes of, 99
    pathophysiology of, 97
    patient history in, 98
    physical examination in, 98
    prevention of, 99
    supportive care for, 99
Bronchitis, *98*
Bronchoalveolar lavage, after lung transplantation, 138
    in *Pneumocystis carinii* pneumonia, 530
    in pneumonia, 105
Bronchoconstriction, in adult respiratory distress
        syndrome, 116
Bronchodilators, 65–66
    in asthma, *112*, 113
    in bronchopulmonary dysplasia, 133–134
Bronchopulmonary dysplasia, 131–135
    complications of, 135
    diagnostic tests for, 132–133
    etiology of, 131–132
    management of, 133–135
        anticholinergic agents in, 134
        antiflammatory agents in, 134
        bronchodilators in, 133–134
        diuretic therapy in, 134
        goals of, 133
        methylxanthines in, 134
        monitoring in, 134
        nutritional support in, 134
        oxygen supplementation in, 133
        ventilation in, 133
    nursing diagnoses in, 133
    outcome of, 135

Bronchopulmonary dysplasia *(Continued)*
    pathophysiology of, 132
    signs of, 132
    symptoms of, 132
Bronchovesicular breath sounds, 48
Bronchus(i), *35, 37*
    inadvertent intubation of, 575
    rupture of, 583t
    trauma to, 94, 97
Bronchus-associated lymphoid tissue, 464
Brown-Séquard's syndrome, 346
Bruises, in child abuse, 589
Bumetanide (Bumex), in acute renal failure, 379
Bundle branch block, 206
Bundle branch system, 156, *156*
Bundle of His, 156
Burns, 563, 652–675
    acute phase of, 653–654
    assessment of, 666–675
        airway evaluation in, 666
        associated injury in, 666
        medical history in, 669
        neurologic examination in, 667
        patient history in, 667–669, 668t
    Berkow nomogram in, 663, *664*
    cardiovascular response to, 655–656
    case study of, 690–692
    chemical, 618–620, 657–658
    classification of, 654, *654, 655*
    clinical course of, 653–654
    complications of, 671
    contact, 668t
    contractures after, 671
    depth of, 661, 662t
    descriptive classification of, 654, *655*
    electrical, 658–659
    emergent phase of, 653
    etiology of, 652, *652*, 657–660
    extent of, 661, 663, *664*
    first-degree, *655*, 662t
    flame, 668t
    fourth-degree, *655*, 662t
    full thickness, 662t
    functional classification of, 654, *654*
    gastrointestinal tract response to, 656
    hand rule in, 661
    hematologic response to, 656
    hypertrophic scars after, 671
    hypothermia with, 657
    immersion, 668t
    in child abuse, 589–590
    in infants, 552
    in preschoolers, 553
    in toddlers, 552
    incidence of, 652
    infection with, 671
    inflammatory-immune response to, 657
    inhalational, 659–660, 660t, 661t
    intentional, 590, 667–668, 668t
    Lund and Browder nomogram in, 663
    metabolic response to, 656–657
    nursing diagnoses in, 672–675
    partial thickness, 662t
    pathophysiology of, 653–657

Burns *(Continued)*
  prevention of, 555t, 559t
  pulmonary response to, 656
  radiant, 563
  rehabilitative phase of, 654
  renal response to, 656
  rule of nines in, 663
  rule of ones in, 661
  scald, 668t
  second-degree, *655,* 662t
  severity of, 661–663, 662t
  superficial, 662t
  systemic response to, 655–657
  third-degree, *655,* 662t
  treatment of, airway monitoring in, 674
    body image changes and, 672
    catheter access for, 667
    fluid therapy in, 663, 665–666, 665t, 673
    infection prevention in, 674
    medications in, 670–671
    nutritional support in, 669, 675
    pain management in, 672, 674–675
    psychosocial aspects of, 671–672
    topical antimicrobials in, 670, 670t
    urine output during, 673
    vascular monitoring in, 673
    wound care in, 669
  type of, 666–667
  unintentional, 590
  vascular compromise with, 671
BVS 5000 ventricular assist device, 189t

C

Caffeine, in acute renal failure, 380
Calcitonin, 389t, 399
Calcium, reference range for, 407t
  serum, 368
    in acute renal failure, 374
Calcium carbonate (Titralac), 429
Calcium channel blockers, in cardiomyopathy, 260
Calcium channel blocker poisoning, 609–610
Calcium gluconate, in acute renal failure, 374
Calcium gluconate gel, in hydrofluoric acid injury, 620
Calories, requirements for, 427t
Canalicular stage, of pulmonary embryology, 33, *34*
Canals of Lambert, 37
Candidiasis, oral, 512
Cannula, nasal, in acute respiratory failure, 70t
Capillaries, 148
Capillary filling time, in cardiovascular system
    assessment, 163
Captopril, cardiovascular effects of, 182
Carafate (sucralfate), 429
Carbamate poisoning, 602t, 627
Carbamazepine poisoning, 600t
Carbohydrates, metabolism of, in septic shock, 635
    insulin effects on, 391
Carbon dioxide, end-tidal, 55, 56t
  in respiratory failure, 184
  pulmonary diffusion of, 42
  transcutaneous monitoring of, 55
Carbon monoxide poisoning, 600t, 617, 659–660
Carboxyhemoglobin, in carbon monoxide poisoning,
    660, 660t

Cardiac arrest, trauma-related, 576–577
Cardiac assist devices, 187–190
  bleeding with, 190
  cardiac output with, 190
  infection with, 190
  multiorgan system dysfunction with, 190
  psychosocial issues with, 190
  thrombus with, 190
Cardiac catheterization, 170–171, *171*
  in aortic stenosis, 228
  in atrial septal defect, 219
  in atrioventricular septal defect, 223
  in bronchopulmonary dysplasia, 133
  in cardiac inflammation, 262
  in cardiomyopathy, 260
  in coarctation of aorta, 236
  in double outlet right ventricle, 224
  in Ebstein's anomaly, 226
  in hypoplastic left heart syndrome, 231
  in Kawasaki disease, 265, *265*
  in mitral stenosis, 238, 239
  in patent ductus arteriosus, 218
  in pulmonary atresia with intact ventricular septum,
    255
  in pulmonary valve stenosis, 240–241
  in supravalvular stenosis, 230
  in tetralogy of Fallot, 243
  in transposition of great vessels, 246
  in tricuspid atresia, 249
  in truncus arteriosus, 251
  in ventricular septal defect, 221
Cardiac center, in blood flow regulation, 152–153
Cardiac index, 153, 177
Cardiac life support, advanced, 184–186
Cardiac output, 153, 177
  during mechanical ventilation, 85
  in asthma, 107
  in burn injury, 655
  in congestive heart failure, 192
  in persistent pulmonary hypertension of newborn, 128
  in scoliosis, 352
  in septic shock, 628, 646
  in spinal cord injury, 349
  with cardiac assist devices, 190
Cardiac tamponade, 95, *95,* 96t, 268–269, *268*
  pericardiocentesis for, *96,* 97
Cardinal vein, 148
Cardioaccelerator center, in blood flow regulation,
    152–153
Cardiomyopathy, 258–260
  definition of, 258
  diagnosis of, 259–260
  dilated (congestive), 259
  etiology of, 259
  extracorporeal life support in, 187
  hypertrophic, 259
  in acquired immunodeficiency syndrome, 533
  management of, 260
  nursing diagnoses in, 260
  pathophysiology of, 258–259
  restrictive, 259
  signs and symptoms of, 259
Cardiopulmonary failure, 184
  airway maintenance in, 184–185

Cardiopulmonary failure *(Continued)*
  arterial vascular access in, 185
  central venous vascular access in, 185
  chest compressions in, 185, 186
  intraosseous vascular access in, 185
  pharmacologic support in, 185–186
Cardiovascular system, 144–155. See also *Cardiac;*
    Congenital heart disease; Heart and specific
    disorders.
  adenosine effects on, 180–181
  amrinone lactate effect on, 178
  angiographic evaluation of, 170–171, *171*
  atropine effects on, 181
  autonomic testing of, 169
  bretylium effects on, 181
  captopril effects on, 182
  cardiac catheterization evaluation of, 170–171, *171*
  chest x-ray examination of, 165–166, *165, 166*
  clinical assessment of, 158–164
    appearance in, 159
    auscultation in, 163–164
    blood pressure in, 163
    capillary filling time in, 163
    chest observation in, 161
    clubbed fingers in, 161, *161*
    family history in, 159, 160t
    heart sounds in, 163–164
    inspection in, 159–161, *161*
    lifts in, 162
    liver palpation in, 163
    medication history in, 159
    murmurs in, 164
    palpation in, 161–163, *162*
    patient history in, 158–159
    peripheral pulses in, 162–163
    physical examination in, 159–164, *161, 162*
    precordium observation in, 161
    psychosocial history in, 159
    skin color in, 159–161
    thrills in, 162
  diazoxide effects on, 182–183
  digoxin effects on, 179
  dobutamine effects on, 179
  dopamine effects on, 179
  echocardiographic assessment of, 169, *170*
  electrocardiographic evaluation of, 166–168, *167,*
    167t
    continuous, 172–173, *173*
  electrophysiologic studies of, 171–172
  epinephrine effects on, 179–180
  exercise stress testing of, 168–169
  fetal, 149–150, *150*
  hemodynamic monitoring of, 173–177, *174–177*
  Holter monitor evaluation of, 168
  hydralazine effects on, 183
  in burn injury, 655, 671, 673
  in congenital heart disease, 214–215
  in trauma assessment, 569–570
  isoproterenol effects on, 180
  laboratory assessment of, 165
  lidocaine effects on, 181
  magnetic resonance imaging of, 172, *172*
  multiple unit gated acquisition examination of, 172
  neonatal, 151–153

Cardiovascular system *(Continued)*
  nifedipine effects on, 183
  nitroglycerin effects on, 183
  nitroprusside effects on, 183
  norepinephrine bitartrate effects on, 180
  perfusion studies of, 172
  procainamide effects on, 181
  propranolol effects on, 181–182
  pulse oximetry assessment of, 165
  quinidine effects on, 182
  transitional, 150–151, *151*
  verapamil effects on, 182
Carotid arteries, 282
Carotid body, in cardiac regulation, 153
Catecholamines, 390t, 401–402
Cathartics, in poisoning management, 605
Catheterization, cardiac, 170–171, *171*. See also
    Cardiac catheterization.
  for intracranial pressure monitoring, 311–312
  in burn treatment, 667
  pulmonary artery, 54
    in bronchopulmonary dysplasia, 133
    in septic shock, 641
  urinary, contraindication to, 584
    in trauma treatment, 577
Cavopulmonary shunt, bidirectional, in hypoplastic
    left heart syndrome, 232–234
  in pulmonary atresia with intact ventricular septum,
    255
Central cord syndrome, 345
Central herniation, in intracranial pressure elevation,
    321–322, *321*
Central nervous system, 274–289. See also *Brain;*
    Neurologic system; Spinal cord.
  blood flow of, 288–289
  brain of, 279–282, *280, 281*
  cells of, 276–277, *277*
  developmental anatomy of, 274–286, *275–281,*
    284–286, 285t
  developmental physiology of, 286–289, *288*
  embryogenesis of, 274–276, *275, 276*
  extracerebral structures of, 277–279, *278, 279*
  in asthma, 107–108
  infection of, 332–335
    in acquired immunodeficiency syndrome, 533
  intracranial pressure dynamics of, 287, *288*
  metabolism of, 288
  spinal cord of, 283–286, *284–286,* 285t
Central venous access, in cardiopulmonary failure, 185
Central venous pressure, monitoring of, 174–175
Cephulac (lactulose), 430
Cerebellum, 282
  assessment of, 299–300
Cerebral blood flow, 288–289
  in neurologic assessment, 315
Cerebral edema, 320
  post-traumatic, 340
  with diabetic ketoacidosis, 413
Cerebral perfusion pressure, 289
Cerebral veins, 282
Cerebrospinal fluid, analysis of, in brain tumor, 337
  in hydrocephalus, 339
  in neurologic assessment, 316
  circulation of, 279, *279*

Cerebrospinal fluid (Continued)
  composition of, 279
  drainage of, in intracranial pressure elevation, 324
  in encephalitis, 334
  in meningitis, 333–334
  intracranial elevation of, 338–339
  production of, 278
Cerebrovascular accident, in sickle cell disease, 521
Cerebrum, circulation of, 282–283
  contusion of, 340, 341
  laceration of, 340
  post-traumatic swelling of, 340
Cervical spine, in trauma assessment, 568–569
  in trauma treatment, 575
  trauma to, 581–582
Charcoal, in poisoning management, 604–605
Chelation, in iron poisoning, 613
Chemical burns, 563, 618–620, 657–658. See also
      Burns.
Chemoreceptor reflex, in shock, 194
Chemoreceptors, in breathing control, 40–41, 40
  in cardiac regulation, 153
  in septic shock, 636
Chemotaxis, developmental aspects of, 473–474
  in inflammatory response, 472
Chemotherapeutic agents, hematologic side effects of,
      493
Chest, cylindric shape of, 34
  in cardiovascular system assessment, 161
  in trauma assessment, 569, 572
Chest compressions, in cardiopulmonary failure, 185,
      186
Chest pain, in pulmonary disease, 43
Chest physiotherapy, during mechanical ventilation, 84
Chest syndrome, in sickle cell disease, 520
Chest tube, in congenital diaphragmatic hernia, 125
  in hemothorax, 97
  in pneumothorax, 92, 93
Chest wall, compliance of, 74, 74
  developmental anatomy of, 37
  inspection of, 43–45, 44, 45
  percussion of, 47, 47
Chest x-ray, during mechanical ventilation, 83
  in adult respiratory distress syndrome, 118
  in aortic stenosis, 227
  in aspiration pneumonitis, 87
  in asthma, 110
  in atrial septal defect, 219
  in atrioventricular septal defect, 223
  in bronchopulmonary dysplasia, 132
  in cardiac inflammation, 262
  in cardiac trauma, 269
  in cardiomyopathy, 259
  in cardiovascular system assessment, 165–166, 165,
      166
  in coarctation of aorta, 236
  in double outlet right ventricle, 224
  in Ebstein's anomaly, 226
  in foreign body aspiration, 89
  in hypoplastic left heart syndrome, 231
  in infection, 491
  in laryngotracheobronchitis, 102
  in lymphocytic interstitial pneumonitis, 532
  in mitral stenosis, 238, 239

Chest x-ray (Continued)
  in patent ductus arteriosus, 218
  in Pneumocystis carinii pneumonia, 530
  in pneumonia, 105
  in pneumothorax, 91
  in pulmonary atresia with intact ventricular septum,
      254
  in pulmonary evaluation, 52
  in pulmonary valve stenosis, 240
  in respiratory distress, 52
  in septic shock, 640
  in shock, 195
  in supravalvular stenosis, 230
  in tetralogy of Fallot, 243
  in thoracic trauma, 96, 96t
  in total anomalous pulmonary venous return, 253
  in transposition of great vessels, 246
  in trauma treatment, 578
  in tricuspid atresia, 248
  in truncus arteriosus, 251
  in ventricular septal defect, 221
Cheyne-Stokes respiration, 46, 300, 307t
Chief cells, 399, 424
Child abuse, 588–594
  bite marks in, 589
  bruises in, 589
  burns in, 589–590, 667–668, 668t
  contact burns in, 668t
  cutaneous injury in, 589–590
  emotional abuse in, 594
  etiology of, 588
  flame burns in, 668t
  head trauma in, 591–592
  immersion burns in, 668t
  incidence of, 588
  internal injuries in, 590–591
  long bone fractures in, 591
  neglect in, 594
  patient history in, 589
  photographs of, 592
  reporting of, 588, 592
  scalding injury in, 668t
  sexual abuse in, 592–594
Chloral hydrate, for pain, 14
Chloramphenicol (Chloromycetin), hematologic side
      effects of, 494
  indications for, 494
  mechanism of action of, 494
Chloride, in fluid homeostasis, 367
Chloromycetin (chloramphenicol), 494
Chloroquine poisoning, 610
Choking, in infants, 552
  prevention of, 557t
Cholestasis, liver transplantation in, 456–457
Chordae tendineae, 145
Choroid plexus, 278
Cimetidine, 428–429
Cingulate herniation, in intracranial pressure
      elevation, 321, 322
Circulation. See Cardiovascular system.
Circumflex artery, 149, 149
Circumflex coronary artery, 149, 149
Citroma (magnesium citrate), 430
Clomipramine poisoning, 607–608

Clonidine poisoning, 600t

Clubbing, fingertip, 46

   in cardiovascular system assessment, 161, *161*

Cluster respiration, *46*

CNS ischemia reflex, in septic shock, 636

Coagulation, 470, 470t, 480–481, *481*

   dysfunction of, 534–535

   evaluation of, 489–490

   in burn injury, 656

   in disseminated intravascular coagulation, 534–535

   in inflammation, 630t

Coagulation factors, 470t, 480, *481*

   assay of, 490

   deficiency of, 537–540. See also *Hemophilia.*

   in disseminated intravascular coagulation, 535

Coarctation of the aorta, 234–236, *235, 237*

Cocaine poisoning, 601t, 615–616

Codeine, for pain, 15t

Cold agglutinins, 491

Cold injury, 563–564, 564t, 565t

Colon, 425, *425*

   trauma to, 435

Colony-stimulating factors, 478t

   in septic shock prevention, 648

Coma, 297–298, 297t, 308

Coma scale, 297–298, 297t

   in trauma assessment, 571t

Comfort, provision of, 18

Communication, during sedation, 16–17

   in trauma treatment, 579

   with children, 3–4, 8, 15–17, 18

   with family, 23

   with grieving family, 28–30

Compartment syndrome, 588

Complement, assays of, 488

   disorders of, 523–524

   in antigen response, 473

   serum levels of, 474

Compliance, in intracranial pressure dynamics, 287

   pulmonary, 38, 74, *74*

      dynamic, 56

      measurement of, 56–57

      static, 57

Computed tomography, in brain trauma, 341

   in brain tumor, 337

   in CNS infection, 334

   in hydrocephalus, 339

   in neurologic assessment, 309

   in pulmonary evaluation, 52

   in renal trauma, 385

   in respiratory distress, 52

   in spinal cord injury, 348

   in trauma evaluation, 578

   xenon, in neurologic assessment, 315

Concussion, brain, 340

Congenital heart disease, 211–255

   acyanotic physiology in, 216, 217–226. See also specific diseases.

   case study of, 682–684

   classification of, 216–217

   cyanotic physiology in, 217, 241–255. See also specific diseases.

   dysfunctional ventilatory weaning process in, 213–214

Congenital heart disease *(Continued)*

   etiology of, 211

   extracorporeal life support in, 186–187

   fluid volume excess in, 215–216

   genetic factors in, 211

   infection with, 211–212

   nursing diagnoses in, 211–216

   obstructive physiology in, 216, 226–241. See also specific diseases.

   pain in, 214

   patient knowledge deficit in, 212–213

   respiratory function in, 213–214

   tissue perfusion in, 214–215

Congestive heart failure, 191–193

   blood flow in, 192

   cardiac output in, 192

   clinical signs and symptoms of, 191–192

   definition of, 191

   diagnosis of, 192

   etiology of, 191

   management of, 192–193

   mechanical interventions for, 193

   nursing diagnoses in, 192

   pathophysiology of, 191

   surgical treatment of, 193

   systemic compensatory response to, 191

Consciousness, clouding of, 297

   in trauma assessment, 570–571, 571t

   level of, 297–298, 297t

Continuous arteriovenous hemofiltration, 382–384

Continuous positive airway pressure ventilation, 76, *79*

Continuous renal replacement therapy, 382–384

   anticoagulation in, 383

   extracorporeal circuit in, 384

   fluid balance in, 384

   hemodynamic stability in, 383–384

   thermoregulation in, 383

   vascular access site for, 383

Continuous venovenous hemofiltration, 382–384

Contractility, cardiac, 154–155

Contractures, after burn injury, 671

Contrast media, in nephrotic syndrome, 377–378

Controlled mandatory ventilation, 76, *78*

Contusion, cerebral, 341

   myocardial, 95, 97, 268–269

   pulmonary, 94

Conus medullaris, 346

Convective transport, in continuous renal replacement therapy, 383

Coombs test, 488

Copperhead snake bite, 621–622

Coral snake bite, 622

Corneal reflex, 305t

Coronary arteries, 149, *149*

Corpus callosum, 280

Corticosteroids, for immunosuppression, 431, 495

   in intracranial pressure elevation, 324

   in pulmonary disorders, 66

Corticotrophs, 394

Corticotropin-releasing hormone, 394t, 396

Cortisol, 389t, 400

Cottonmouth snake bite, 621–622

Cough, evaluation of, 50t, 51

   nighttime, 43

Coumadin (warfarin), 497–498
  administration of, 498
  mechanisms of action of, 498
  side effects of, 498
Crackles, 48
Cranial nerve(s), 289, 291t
  I (olfactory), 291t
    in child, 303t
    in infant, 301t
  II (optic), 291t
    in child, 304t
    in infant, 301t
  III (oculomotor), 291t
    in child, 304t, 305t
    in infant, 301t, 302t
  IV (trochlear), 291t
    in child, 305t
    in infant, 302t
  IX (glossopharyngeal), 291t
    in child, 306t
    in infant, 303t
  V (trigeminal), 291t
    in child, 305t
    in infant, 302t
  VI (abducens), 291t
    in child, 305t
    in infant, 302t
  VII (facial), 291t
    in child, 306t
    in infant, 302t
  VIII (acoustic), 291t
    in child, 306t
    in infant, 302t
  X (vagus), 291t
    in child, 307t
    in infant, 303t
  XI (spinal accessory), 291t
    in child, 307t
    in infant, 303t
  XII (hypoglossal), 291t
    in child, 307t
    in infant, 303t
C-reactive protein, 487
  in septic shock, 640
Creatine phosphokinase, in cardiac trauma, 269
Creatinine, in acute renal failure, 372
  production of, 370
Cremasteric reflex, assessment of, 299
Crepitus, 46
Cricoid cartilage, 35, 36
Cricothyrotomy, in trauma treatment, 575
Critical care unit, 8–10
  day-night cycle maintenance for, 17
  light levels of, 9
  noise levels of, 8, 9t, 17
  play in, 17–18
  privacy deprivation in, 9
  sensory deprivation in, 9
  sleep deprivation in, 9, 10t
  sound levels of, 8, 9t
  technology in, 9–10
Cromolyn sodium, in asthma, 112, 113
Crossmatching, of human leukocyte antigens, 487
Crotalidae bite, 621–622

Croup. See Laryngotracheobronchitis (croup).
Croup Score, in laryngotracheobronchitis, 103, 103t
Cryoprecipitate, 504–505
Culture, 512
  in pneumonia, 105
  in septic shock, 640
Cushing's reflex, in neurologic assessment, 308
Cushing's syndrome, 401
Cyanide poisoning, 620–621
Cyanosis, 46, 49, 50, 51
  in cardiovascular system assessment, 159–161
  in respiratory failure, 184
Cyclosporine (Sandimmune), 430–431, 495
Cystic fibrosis, lung transplantation in, 136, 140
Cystitis, hemorrhagic, after bone marrow
        transplantation, 544–545
Cytokines, 461–462
  in septic shock, 631
Cytomegalovirus, infection with, after lung
        transplantation, 139
    transfusion-acquired, 508

D

Damus Kaye Stanzel operation, in tricuspid atresia, 249
Darvon (propoxyphene) poisoning, 614
Day-night cycle, maintenance of, 17
ddC (dideoxycytidine), 530
ddI (dideoxyinosine), 530
D-dimer, 469
  assay of, 490
Dead space, physiologic, 73t
Dead space ventilation, 74
Decerebrate posturing, 299
Decorticate posturing, 299
Deep tendon reflexes, 285, 286
  evaluation of, 298–299
Defecation, in spinal cord injury, 350
Deferoxamine, in iron poisoning, 613
Delta cells, 388, 390
Demerol (meperidine), for pain, 15t
Demerol (meperidine) poisoning, 614
Dendrites, 276, 277
Depolarization, of neuron, 286
Dermatome, 289, 290
Dermis, 653, 655
Desipramine poisoning, 607–608
Development, assessment appropriate for, 3–5
  stages of, 2–3
Dexamethasone, in pulmonary disorders, 66
Diabetes insipidus, 419–422
  case study of, 688–689
  central, 420, 420
    treatment of, 421–422, 422t
  collaborative diagnoses in, 421
  complications of, 422
  diagnosis of, 420–421
  etiology of, 420
  monitoring for, 422
  nephrogenic, 420, 420
    treatment of, 422
  pathophysiology of, 419, 420
  signs and symptoms of, 420, 421t
  treatment of, 421–422
  water deprivation test in, 421

Diabetes mellitus, 408–413. See also *Diabetic ketoacidosis; Hyperglycemic, hyperosmolar, nonketotic syndrome.*
  insulin-dependent (type I), 408
  insulin-independent (type II), 408–409
  maternal, fetal cardiac anomalies and, 160t
Diabetic ketoacidosis, 409–413, *409*, 412t, 413t
  case study of, 695
  cerebral edema in, 413
  collaborative diagnoses in, 411
  complications of, 413
  diagnosis of, 411
  differential diagnosis of, 411
  electrolyte therapy in, 412
  etiology of, 410
  fluid therapy in, 412, 412t
  insulin therapy in, 412–413, 413t
  monitoring for, 413
  mucormycosis in, 413
  pathophysiology of, 409–410, *409*
  risk factors for, 410
  signs and symptoms of, 410–411, 410t
  treatment of, 411–413, 412t, 413t
  vs. hyperglycemic, hyperosmolar, nonketotic syndrome, 415, 415t
Diamox (acetazolamide), in acute renal failure, 380
Diapedesis, in inflammatory response, 472
Diaphragm, developmental anatomy of, 37
Diaphragmatic hernia, 445t
  congenital, 121–126
    cardiac abnormalities with, 123
    definition of, 121
    embryology of, 121, *122*
    gastrointestinal abnormalities with, 123
    incidence of, 122
    mortality with, 122
    operative repair of, 125
    pathophysiology of, 122–123
    postoperative care in, 125–126
    preoperative care in, 123–125
Diazepam (Valium), for pain, 15t
  in pulmonary disorders, 59–61, 60t
  in status epilepticus, 327t
Diazoxide (Hyperstat), cardiovascular effects of, 182–183
Dibucaine poisoning, 607
Dideoxycytidine (ddC), 530
Dideoxyinosine (ddI), 530
Diencephalon, 275, *275*, *276*, 280–281
Diffusion, in continuous renal replacement therapy, 383
DiGeorge syndrome, cardiac anomalies in, 160t
  truncus arteriosus in, 250, 251
Digibind, in digitalis poisoning, 611
Digitalis poisoning, 601t, 610–611
Digits, traumatic amputation of, 587–588
Digoxin (Lanoxin), cardiovascular effects of, 179
Diltiazem poisoning, 609–610
Diminished breath sounds, 48
Diphenhydramine (Benadryl), for pruritus, 64t
Diphenoxylate poisoning, 611
Direct Coombs test, 488
Disseminated intravascular coagulation, 534–535
  complications of, 535
  diagnosis of, 534–535

Disseminated intravascular coagulation *(Continued)*
  etiology of, 534
  management of, 535
  nursing diagnoses in, 535
  pathophysiology of, 534
  risk factors for, 534
  signs and symptoms of, 534
Disulfiram poisoning, 601t
Diuresis, in poisoning management, 605
Diuretic agents, in acute renal failure, 379–380
  in bronchopulmonary dysplasia, 134
  in cardiomyopathy, 260
  in congestive heart failure, 193
  in intracranial pressure elevation, 324
Dobutamine (Dobutrex), cardiovascular effects of, 179
  in septic shock, 645t
Do-not-resuscitate order, 26–27
Dopamine (Intropin), cardiovascular effects of, 179
  in acute renal failure, 380
  in septic shock, 645t
Double outlet right ventricle, 223–224
Down syndrome (trisomy 21), cardiac anomalies in, 160t
Doxepin poisoning, 607–608
Droperidol (Inapsine), for nausea, 64t
Drowning, 563
  in toddlers, 553
  prevention of, 558t, 560t
Drugs. See also specific drugs.
  absorption of, 58
  dosing strategies for, 59
  nephrotoxicity of, 377–378
Ductus arteriosus, closure of, 217
  constriction of, 151
  patent, 217–218
Duodenum, 424, *425*
Dura mater, 278, 283
Dying, stages of, 28
Dying children, 26–30
  care for, 27–28
  organ donation from, 27
  pain management of, 26
  treatment withdrawal from, 26–27
Dysreflexia, autonomic, 347
Dysrhythmias, 196–206
  atrial activity of, 197
  classification of, 196–197
  extracorporeal life support in, 187
  in diabetic ketoacidosis, 410t
  interpretation of, 197
  physiology of, 196
  precipitation of, 197
  QRS complex in, 197
  rate of, 197
  rhythm of, 197
  supraventricular, 197–203, *197*, *200*, 202t. See also specific dysrhythmias.
  ventricular, 203–204, *203*. See also specific dysrhythmias.

E

Ears, in trauma assessment, 572
Ebstein's anomaly, 224–226, *225*

Echocardiography, 169, *170*
  in aortic stenosis, 227–228
  in atrial septal defect, 219
  in atrioventricular septal defect, 223
  in bronchopulmonary dysplasia, 133
  in cardiac inflammation, 262
  in cardiac trauma, 269
  in cardiomyopathy, 260
  in coarctation of aorta, 236
  in double outlet right ventricle, 224
  in Ebstein's anomaly, 226
  in hypoplastic left heart syndrome, 231
  in Kawasaki disease, 264
  in mitral stenosis, 238, 239
  in patent ductus arteriosus, 218
  in persistent pulmonary hypertension of newborn,
    127
  in pulmonary atresia with intact ventricular septum,
    255
  in pulmonary valve stenosis, 240
  in rheumatic fever, 263
  in shock, 195
  in tetralogy of Fallot, 243
  in total anomalous pulmonary venous return, 253
  in transposition of great vessels, 246
  in tricuspid atresia, 248
  in truncus arteriosus, 251
  in ventricular septal defect, 221
Ectoderm, 274
Edema, cellular, 320
  cerebral, 320
    post-traumatic, 340
    with diabetic ketoacidosis, 413
  in adult respiratory distress syndrome, 116, *116*
  in burn injury, 655–656
  in inhalational injury, 660
  in laryngotracheobronchitis, 102, *103*
  interstitial, 320
  vasogenic, 320
Edward's syndrome (trisomy 18), cardiac anomalies in,
    160t
Ehlers-Danlos syndrome, cardiac anomalies in, 160t
Eisenmenger's syndrome, 219
Elapidae bite, 622
Elastance, in intracranial pressure dynamics, 287
Elbow, fracture of, 586–587
Electrical injury, 563, 658–659. See also *Burns.*
Electrocardiography, continuous, 172–173
  heart rate on, 168
  in acute renal failure, 373
  in aortic stenosis, 227
  in atrial septal defect, 219
  in atrioventricular septal defect, 223
  in bronchopulmonary dysplasia, 132
  in cardiac inflammation, 262
  in cardiac trauma, 269
  in cardiomyopathy, 259
  in cardiovascular system assessment, 166–168, *167,*
    167t
  in coarctation of aorta, 236
  in double outlet right ventricle, 224
  in Ebstein's anomaly, 226
  in hypoplastic left heart syndrome, 231
  in Kawasaki disease, 264

Electrocardiography *(Continued)*
  in mitral stenosis, 238, 239
  in patent ductus arteriosus, 218
  in pulmonary atresia with intact ventricular septum,
    254
  in pulmonary valve stenosis, 240
  in rheumatic fever, 263
  in supravalvular stenosis, 230
  in tetralogy of Fallot, 243
  in total anomalous pulmonary venous return, 253
  in transposition of great vessels, 246
  in tricuspid atresia, 248
  in truncus arteriosus, 251
  in ventricular septal defect, 221
  interpretation of, 168
  leads for, 168
  P wave on, 167, *167*
  pacemaker on, 208
  paper for, 166, *167*
  PR interval on, 167, *167,* 167t
  QRS interval on, *167,* 168
  QT segment on, *167,* 168
  ST segment on, *167,* 168
  T wave on, *167,* 168
Electroencephalography, in CNS infection, 334
  in neurologic assessment, 315–316
  in seizures, 325, 326t
Electrolytes, 367–369
  during mechanical ventilation, 83
  in asthma, 110
  in CNS infection, 335
  in diabetic ketoacidosis, 412
  in encephalopathy, 345
ELISA, for human immunodeficiency virus antibody,
    528
Ellis–van Creveld syndrome, cardiac anomalies in,
    160t
Embolism, fat, in sickle cell disease, 521–522
Embolization, of arteriovenous malformation, 329
Embryology, of larynx, 36
  of lung, 33, *34*
  of nose, 35
  of pharynx, 36
  of pulmonary circulation, 37
  of trachea, 36
Emotional abuse, 594. See also *Child abuse.*
Emotional support, 18–19
  in trauma treatment, 578–579
Empty heart syndrome, 576–577
Encephalitis, 332–335
  cerebrospinal fluid analysis in, 334
  clinical symptoms of, 333
  etiology of, 333
  incidence of, 332
  management of, 334–335
  pathophysiology of, 333
Encephalopathy, 342–345
  diagnosis of, 344
  etiology of, 343
  hepatic, 453, 454
    treatment of, 455
  pathophysiology of, 343
  treatment of, 344–345
Endocardial tube, formation of, 144

Endocarditis, 260–263
    diagnosis of, 262
    etiology of, 261
    management of, 262–263
    nursing diagnoses in, 262
    pathophysiology of, 261
    signs and symptoms of, 261–262
Endocardium, 145
Endocrine system, 387–422, *388*
    anatomy of, 387–388, 391–402. See also specific
        glands.
    assessment of, 402–408
        abdominal examination in, 404t, 405
        ACTH stimulation test in, 405, 408
        blood chemistries in, 405, 406t–407t
        cardiovascular examination in, 405
        chest examination in, 404t
        computed tomography in, 408
        diagnostic studies in, 405–408, 406t–407t
        electrocardiography in, 408
        family history in, 402
        genitourinary examination in, 404t, 405
        glucose tolerance test in, 405, 408t
        head and neck examination in, 403, 404t
        insulin tolerance test in, 405
        integumentary examination in, 404, 404t
        laboratory studies in, 405–408, 406t–407t
        magnetic resonance imaging in, 408
        musculoskeletal examination in, 404t, 405
        neonatal history in, 402
        neurologic examination in, 404–405, 404t
        past medical history in, 403
        patient history in, 402–403
        patient medication history in, 403
        physical examination in, 403–405, 404t
        prenatal history in, 402
        pulmonary examination in, 405
        radiologic tests in, 408
        TRH stimulation test in, 405
        ultrasound in, 408
        urine tests in, 405
    integrated functioning of, 387
Endoderm, 274
Endotoxin, in septic shock, 630
Endotracheal intubation, in acute respiratory failure,
        69–70, 70t, *71*, 71t, 72
    in trauma treatment, 574–575
Endotracheal tube, in cardiopulmonary failure, 185
End-tidal carbon dioxide, 55, 56t
Enteral nutrition, in adult respiratory distress
        syndrome, 119–120
Enterocolitis, necrotizing, 447–448, 448t
Envenomations, 621–622
Eosinopenia, 467
Eosinophils, 467
    differentiation of, *462*
    reference values for, 485t
Eosinophilia, 467
Epicardium, 145
Epidermis, 653, *655*
Epidural space, tumor invasion of, 516
Epiglottis, *35*
Epiglottitis, acute, 99–102
    clinical presentation of, 100

Epiglottitis *(Continued)*
    complications of, 102
    definition of, 99, *100*
    diagnostic tests in, 100
    differential diagnosis of, 100, 101t
    etiology of, 100
    management of, 101–102
    outcome of, 102
    pathophysiology of, 99–100
    physical examination in, 100
    prevention of, 101
    supportive care for, 101–102
Epilepsy, 326–327, 327t. See also *Seizures.*
    electroencephalography in, 315–316
Epinephrine, 390t
    cardiovascular effects of, 179–180
    effects of, 401
    in asthma, *112,* 113, 114t
    in septic shock, 645t
    regulation of, 401
    synthesis of, 401
Epithalamus, 280–281
Epithelium, pulmonary, *34*
Epstein-Barr infection, after liver transplantation,
        458
Erythrocyte(s), 465–466
    differentiation of, *462*
    function of, 470
    leukocyte-poor, 500
    sickled, 517–522. See also *Sickle cell disease.*
Erythrocyte sedimentation rate, 487
    in septic shock, 640
Erythropoiesis, 465–466
    cyanosis and, 160–161
Erythropoietin, 461
    in hematopoiesis, 465
    indications for, 492
    mechanisms of action of, 493
    production of, 370
    recombinant, 370
    side effects of, 493
Escharotomy, in burn injury, 671
Escherichia coli, in hemolytic uremic syndrome, 377
Esophageal varices, 438–439, *438*
    complications of, 439
    sclerotherapy in, 438–439
    Sengstaken-Blakemore tube in, 438, *438*
    transjugular intrahepatic portal-systemic shunt in,
        439, *439*
Esophagitis, 512
Esophagoscopy, in chemical burns, 619
Esophagus, *35,* 424, *425*
    dorsal mesentery of, 121
Ethanol, in ethylene glycol poisoning, 623
    in methanol poisoning, 624
Ethanol poisoning, 601t, 622
Ethylene glycol poisoning, 601t, 622–623
Exchange transfusion, in gray baby syndrome, 605
Exercise stress testing, 168–169
    contraindications to, 169
    in aortic stenosis, 227
Expiration, in newborn, 33
Extracorporeal life support, 186–190, *188,* 189t
    in congenital heart disease, 186–187

Extracorporeal life support (*Continued*)
    indications for, 186–187
    nursing diagnoses in, 190
Extracorporeal membrane oxygenation, 81, 188, *188,*
    189t
    in persistent pulmonary hypertension of newborn,
        128
Extremities, in trauma assessment, 573
    traumatic amputation of, 587–588
Eyes, antigen resistance of, 472
    autonomic nerve stimulation of, 294t
    chemical burn of, 618–620
    in trauma assessment, 572
    irrigation of, 603, 658
    testing of, in child, 304t–305t
        in infant, 302t–303t

F

Face, in trauma assessment, 571–572
    testing of, in child, 305t–306t
    trauma to, 580–581
Facial nerve, 291t, 302t, 306t
Factor IX, assay for, 538
    in hemophilia A, 539
Factor VIII, assay for, 538
    in hemophilia A, 505, 539
Falls, 554
    case study of, 695
    in infants, 552
    in school-age children, 553
    in toddlers, 552
    prevention of, 555t–556t
Falx cerebelli, 278
Falx cerebri, 278
Family, 19–26
    assessment of, 20–22
    bereaved, 28–29
    care planning with, 23–24
    communication with, 23
    cultural traditions of, 21
    financial concerns of, 22
    in trauma treatment, 579
    parental role support for, 22
    physical needs of, 21
    psychologic needs of, 20
    sibling support for, 24
    spiritual considerations of, 21–22
    stresses on, 20
        responses to, 20–21
    support system for, 21
    transfer anxieties of, 24–25
    trust development with, 23
    visiting privileges for, 25–26
Famotidine (Pepcid), 429
Fat, body, 393
Fat embolism, in sickle cell disease, 521–522
Fats, metabolism of, insulin effects on, 391
Febrile reactions, with blood transfusion, 507
Femur, fracture of, 587
Fentanyl, for pain, 15t
    in pulmonary disorders, 60t, 61
Fetal alcohol syndrome, cardiac anomalies in, 160t
Fetor hepaticus, 455
Fetus, circulation of, 149–150, *150*

Fever, with blood transfusion, 507
    with infection, 511–512
Fibrin degradation products, measurement of, 490
Fibrin split products, measurement of, 490
Fibrinogen, measurement of, 490
Fibrinolytic agents, 498
Fibrinolytic system, 481
Filter replacement fluid, in continuous renal
        replacement therapy, 384
Filtration fraction, in continuous renal replacement
        therapy, 382–383
Fingers, clubbing of, 46
        in cardiovascular system assessment, 161, *161*
    traumatic amputation of, 587–588
Finger-to-nose test, 300
Firearm injury, 562–563
Firearm safety, 560t
Fires. See *Burns.*
Fistula, tracheoesophageal, 444t–445t
Flaccidity, 299
Flail chest, 91, 92
Fluid(s), during mechanical ventilation, 83
    in adult respiratory distress syndrome, 119
    in asthma, 110, 113
    in burn treatment, 663, 665–666, 665t, 667, 673
    in cardiomyopathy, 260
    in CNS infection, 335
    in congenital diaphragmatic hernia, 124, 125
    in congestive heart failure, 193
    in continuous renal replacement therapy, 384
    in diabetic ketoacidosis, 412, 412t
    in encephalopathy, 345
    in hyperglycemic, hyperosmolar, nonketotic
        syndrome, 415
    in hypovolemia, 516
    in septic shock, 646
    in shock, 196
    in tracheoesophageal fistula, 130, 131
    in trauma treatment, 576
    renal tubule reabsorption by, 364–365
Fluid volume excess, in congenital heart disease,
        215–216
Flumazenil (Romazicon), antagonistic action of, 64t,
        65
    in benzodiazepine poisoning, 609
Fluoroscopy, in pulmonary evaluation, 52
    in respiratory distress, 52
Follicle-stimulating hormone, 389t, 397
    reference range for, 406t
Follicle-stimulating hormone–releasing factor, 394t
Fontan procedure, 683–684
    in hypoplastic left heart syndrome, 234
    in tricuspid atresia, 249
Fontanelles, 277–278, *278*
    auscultation of, 297
    in trauma assessment, 570
    palpation of, 296–297
Foramen of Magendie, 278
Foramen ovale, patent, 218–219
Foramina of Luschka, 278
Forced expiratory volume, in asthma, 110
Forced expiratory volume in first second (FEV_1), 57
Forced vital capacity, *57*
    in asthma, 110

Foreign body aspiration, 88–90
  clinical course of, 89
  clinical presentation of, 88–89, *89*
  complications of, 90
  diagnostic tests for, 89
  emergency care for, 89–90
  etiology of, 88
  management of, 89–90
  pathophysiology of, 88
  patient history in, 88
  physical examination in, 88–89
  prevention of, 89
  respiratory care for, 90
  supportive care for, 90
  vs. aspiration pneumonitis, 87
Fracture(s), 584–587, *585*, 586t
  basilar, 340, 341
  displaced, 585
  elbow, 586–587
  femoral, 587
  in child abuse, 591
  Le Fort, 581
  mandibular, 580
  midfacial, 581
  nasal, 581
  nondisplaced, 585
  open, 586, 586t
  physeal, 586, 586t
  radiography of, 578
    in child abuse, 591
  rib, 94, 96t, 97, 583t
  Salter-Harris classification of, 586, 586t
  skull, 340
  spinal, 345–350, 575. See also *Spinal cord, injury to.*
  treatment of, 577–578
  types of, 585, *585*
Free radicals, in septic shock, 631
Fremitus, 46
Fresh frozen plasma, 504, 505t
Friction rubs, in cardiovascular system assessment, 162
Friedreich's ataxia, cardiac anomalies in, 160t
Frontal lobe, 279, *280*
Frostbite, 564, 565t
Full liquid ventilation, 81
Functional residual capacity, 41, *41, 57*, 73t, 74
Fungal infection, in septic shock, 647
Funnel chest, 45, *45*
Furosemide, in acute renal failure, 379
Fusiform aneurysm, intracranial, 329–330

G

Gait, observation of, 300
Gallbladder, *425*, 426
  autonomic nerve stimulation of, 295t
Ganciclovir, 494–495
  after lung transplantation, 139
  mechanisms of action of, 494
  side effects of, 495
Gas exchange, in asthma, 107
  in spinal cord injury, 349
  respiratory, 41–43, *42*
Gastric emptying, 424
Gastric lavage, in poisoning management, 603–604
Gastrointestinal system, 424–458
  anatomy of, 424–426, *425*

Gastrointestinal system *(Continued)*
  antigen resistance of, 472
  atresia of, 442t–443t
  atropine effects on, 430
  chemical burn of, 618–620
  cimetidine effects on, 428–429
  clinical assessment of, 427–428
  congenital abnormalities of, 123, 440t–445t
  decontamination of, 603–605
  development of, 426–427
  drug absorption in, 58
  drug effects on, 428–431
  dysfunction of, after bone marrow transplantation, 542–543
  famotidine effects on, 429
  gastroschisis of, 441t
  glycopyrrolate effects on, 430
  hemorrhage of, 435–439, 436t, *438, 439*
    diagnosis of, 437
    gastric pH in, 438
    imaging studies in, 437
    laboratory studies in, 437
    signs and symptoms of, 435–436, 436t
    treatment of, 437–438
  in burn injury, 656
  in congenital diaphragmatic hernia, 123
  in graft-versus-host disease, 545, 546
  in pulmonary disease, 43
  in septic shock, 647–648
  in trauma treatment, 577
  intussusception of, 443t
  ischemia of, 447–448
  lactulose effects on, 430
  magnesium citrate effects on, 430
  magnesium hydroxide and aluminum hydroxide effects on, 429
  magnesium hydroxide effects on, 430
  malrotation of, 442t
  motility of, 426
  omeprazole effects on, 429
  omphalocele of, 440t
  perforation of, 439, 446–447
  physiology of, 424–426, *425*
  propranolol effects on, 428
  ranitidine effects on, 429
  somatostatin effects on, 428
  sucralfate effects on, 429
  trauma to, 431–435. See also *Abdomen, trauma to.*
  vasopressin effects on, 428
  vitamin K_1 effects on, 428
  volvulus of, 442t
Gastroschisis, 441t
Gastrostomy tube, in tracheoesophageal fistula, 130
Gate theory, of cardiac conduction system, 157
Genitourinary system. See also *Renal system.*
  in trauma treatment, 577
  trauma to, 584
Germ cell layers, 274
Giant aneurysm, intracranial, 329–330
Giant cell hepatitis, 453
Gingivitis, 513t
Glands, endocrine, 387–402, 389t–390t. See also *Endocrine system* and specific glands.
  exocrine, 387
Glandular stage, of pulmonary embryology, 33, *34*

Glasgow Coma Scale, 297–298, 297t
Glipizide poisoning, 611
Glomerular filtration rate, 362–364, 363t
  in fluid homeostasis, 367
  regulation of, 362–363, 363t
  shock and, 363, 364t
Glomerulonephritis, acute, acute renal failure in, 377
Glomerulus, 361, 366t
Glossopharyngeal nerve, 291t, 303t, 306t
Glucagon, 390t, 392
Glucocorticoids, 389t
  in asthma, 114t
  in pulmonary disorders, 66
Glucose, cerebral metabolism of, 288
  in acute renal failure, 373
Glucose intolerance, in acute renal failure, 374
Glucose tolerance test, 405, 408t
Glucosuria, in diabetic ketoacidosis, 410t
Glutamine, in septic shock prevention, 648
γ-Glutamyl transpeptidase, reference values for, 450t
Glyburide poisoning, 611
Glycopyrrolate (Robinul), 430
Gonadotrophs, 394
Gonadotropin-releasing hormone, 394t
Gortex patch, in tetralogy of Fallot, 243–244
Graft-versus-host disease, acute, 545–546
  after bone marrow transplantation, 545–546, 545t
  chronic, 546
  clinical stages of, 545t
  with transfusion, 509
Granulocytes, 466–467
  absolute count of, 486
Granulocyte colony-stimulating factor, 478t
  indications for, 493
  mechanisms of action of, 493
Granulocyte transfusion, 500–502
Granulocyte-macrophage colony-stimulating factor, 478t
  indications for, 493
  mechanisms of action of, 493
Gray matter, of spinal cord, 283, *285*
Grief, 28–29
  stages of, 28–29
Growth, in pulmonary disease, 43
Growth hormone, 389t, 396
  reference range for, 406t
Growth hormone–inhibiting hormone, 394t
Growth hormone–releasing hormone, 394t, 396
Grunting, in respiratory failure, 184
Gun bluing poisoning, 624
Gunshot wounds, abdominal, 582
Gut-associated lymphoid tissue, 465
Gyromitra esculenta poisoning, 625–626

H

Haemophilus influenzae type B vaccine, in septic shock prevention, 649
Halothane, in asthma, *112*, 113, 114t
Hanging, trauma with, 563
Head, in trauma assessment, 571
  inspection of, 296
  trauma to, 579–580
    in child abuse, 591–592
    mild-to-moderate, 579
    severe, 579–580

Head hood, in acute respiratory failure, 70t
Hearing, testing of, in child, 306t
  in infant, 303t
Heart, abnormalities of, in congenital diaphragmatic hernia, 123
  angiographic evaluation of, 170–171, *171*
  arteries of, 149, *149*
  atria of, 146, *146, 147*
  autonomic nerve stimulation of, 294t
  blood flow of, *151*
  borders of, evaluation of, 165, *165*
  catheterization of, 170–171, *171*. See also *Cardiac catheterization.*
  conduction system of, 155–156, *156*
    electrophysiology of, 156–158
    gate theory of, 157
  contractility of, 154–155
  contusion of, 268–269, *268*, 583t
  electrophysiology of, 156–158
  embryologic development of, 144–149
    days 15–23, 144
    days 22–35, 145, *146*
    days 23–28, 144–145, *145*
    days 27–45, 145–146
    days 32–33, 146
    days 34–36, 146–148, *147*
    weeks 4–7, 148
  in acute renal failure, 378
  in trauma assessment, 569–570
  infection of, 260–266, 264t
  inflammatory diseases of, 260–266, 264t, *265*. See also specific diseases.
  internodal atrial pathways of, 155, *156*
  pacemaker cells of, 157
  parasympathetic stimulation of, 153
  refractoriness of, 157
  resting membrane potentials of, 156
  rupture of, 268–269, *268*
  septa of, embryologic development of, 145–146
  size of, evaluation of, 165
  sympathetic stimulation of, 153
  threshold potentials of, 157
  transplantation of, 266–268
    in cardiomyopathy, 260
  trauma to, 95, *95*, 268–269, *268*
    in child abuse, 590
  valves of. See also specific valves.
    embryologic development of, 147–148, *147*
  ventricles of, 146, *147*
    depolarization of, 158
    double inlet, 248
    embryologic development of, 145, *146*
    function of, 153–155, *154*
    isometric relaxation of, 158
    repolarization of, 158
Heart disease, congenital, 211–255. See also *Congenital heart disease* and specific diseases.
  myocardial, 258–260. See also *Cardiomyopathy.*
Heart failure, after bone marrow transplantation, 544
  congestive, 191–193. See also *Congestive heart failure.*
  in acquired immunodeficiency syndrome, 533
Heart loop, formation of, 144–145, *145*
Heart rate, in septic shock, 646
  on electrocardiography, 168

Heart sounds, in aortic stenosis, 227
  in cardiovascular system assessment, 163–164
  in Ebstein's anomaly, 226
  in hypoplastic left heart syndrome, 231
  in mitral stenosis, 238
  in pulmonary atresia with intact ventricular septum, 254
  in total anomalous pulmonary venous return, 253
  in transposition of great vessels, 245–246
  in trauma assessment, 570
  in tricuspid atresia, 248
  in truncus arteriosus, 250
  in ventricular septal defect, 221
  S_1, 163
  S_2, 163–164
  S_3, 164
  S_4, 164
Heart transplantation, 266–268
  in cardiomyopathy, 260
Heart tube, formation of, 144
Heartmate ventricular assist device, 189t
Heat cramps, 565, 566t
Heat exhaustion, 565, 566t
Heat loss, in trauma evaluation, 571
Heat stroke, 565, 566t
Heel-shin test, 300
Hematemesis, 435
Hematochezia, 435
Hematocrit, 484, 485t
  blood transfusion effect on, 499t
  reference values for, 485t
Hematologic system, 461–546
  antilymphocyte globulin effects on, 496
  antithymocyte globulin effects on, 496
  assessment of, 482–492
    absolute cell counts in, 486–487
    activated clotting time in, 490
    activated partial thromboplastin time in, 489–490
    antiglobulin test in, 488
    biopsies in, 491–492
    bleeding time in, 489
    blood typing in, 490–491
    bone marrow biopsies in, 491
    chest x-ray in, 491
    chief complaint in, 482
    cold agglutinins in, 491
    complement assays in, 488
    complete blood count in, 484–487, 485t
    Coombs test in, 488
    C-reactive protein in, 487
    D-dimer assay in, 490
    delayed hypersensitivity skin testing in, 492
    differential white blood count in, 485t, 486
    erythrocyte sedimentation rate in, 487
    family history in, 482
    fibrin split products assay in, 490
    fibrinogen assay in, 490
    hematocrit in, 484, 485t
    hemoglobin in, 484, 485t
    histocompatibility testing for, 487–488
    immediate hypersensitivity skin testing in, 492
    immunoglobulin levels in, 488
    lymph node biopsies in, 491–492
    lymphocyte count in, 486–487

Hematologic system (*Continued*)
    monoclonal antibodies in, 488–489
    neutrophil count in, 486
    patient health history in, 482–483
    patient medication history in, 483
    patient social-cultural history in, 483
    peripheral smear in, 484
    physical examination in, 483–484
    platelet count in, 489
    prothrombin time in, 489
    red blood count in, 484, 485t
    reticulocyte count in, 484
    skin testing in, 492
    thromboplastin time in, 490
    total immunoglobulin level in, 488
    total white blood count in, 484, 485t, 486
  azathioprine effects on, 495–496
  cells of, 465–469. See also specific cells.
  chemotherapeutic agent effects on, 494
  chloramphenicol effects on, 494
  corticosteroid effects on, 495
  cyclosporine A effects on, 495
  development of, 461–465, *462, 464*
  diagnostic tests of, 484–492, 485t
  erythropoietin effect on, 492–493
  functions of, 470–481. See also *Coagulation; Immunity.*
  ganciclovir effects on, 494–495
  granulocyte colony-stimulating factor effect on, 493
  granulocyte-macrophage colony-stimulating factor effect on, 493
  heparin effects on, 497
  interleukin-3 effect on, 493
  muromonab-CD3 effects on, 496
  plasma factors of, 469–470, 470t
  streptokinase effect on, 498
  suppression of, 493–498
  thrombopoietin effect on, 493
  tissue-type plasminogen activator effect on, 498
  trimethoprim-sulfamethoxazole effects on, 494
  urokinase effect on, 498
  warfarin effects on, 497–498
  zidovudine effects on, 494
Hematoma, epidural, 341
  extradural, 340
  in hemophilia, 539
  subdural, 341
Hematopoiesis, 461–465, *462*
  sites of, 462–465
Hematuria, trauma-related, 584
Hemodialysis, 381–382
  in methanol poisoning, 624
  in poisoning management, 605
  in theophylline poisoning, 616
Hemoglobin, 484, 485t
  blood transfusion effect on, 499t
  decrease in, 509–510
  in septic shock, 639
  reference values for, 485t
  synthesis of, 465
Hemoglobin A, 465
Hemoglobin AS, 517
Hemoglobin F, 465
Hemoglobin S, 465

Hemoglobin SC, 517

Hemoglobin SS, 517–522. See also *Sickle cell disease.*

Hemoglobinuria, 466

Hemolysis, 466

   in burn injury, 656

   with blood transfusion, 506–507

Hemolytic anemia, 466

Hemolytic-uremic syndrome, acute renal failure in, 376–377

   vs. idiopathic thrombocytopenic purpura, 537

Hemophilia, 537–540

   complete blood count in, 538

   complications of, 539–540

   diagnosis of, 538

   etiology of, 538

   factor IX assay in, 538

   factor VIII assay in, 538

   factor VIII in, 505

   management of, 539

   nursing diagnoses in, 539

   pathophysiology of, 537–538

   prothrombin time in, 538

   risk factors for, 538

   signs and symptoms of, 538

   x-ray in, 538

Hemorrhage. See also *Bleeding.*

   hypovolemia with, 516–517

   intracranial, 328–332. See also *Intracranial hemorrhage.*

   of gastrointestinal tract, 435–439, 436t, *438, 439.* See also *Gastrointestinal system, hemorrhage of.*

   trauma-related, 576

Hemorrhagic cystitis, after bone marrow transplantation, 544–545

Hemostasis, 479, *479*

   procoagulants in, 480

   secondary, 480

Hemothorax, 95, 96, 96t, 583t

   chest tube placement for, 97

   definition of, *90*

Hemotympanum, in basilar fracture, 341

Heparin, in disseminated intravascular coagulation, 535

   indications for, 497

   mechanisms of action of, 497

   side effects of, 497

Hepatic failure, 449, 452–456. See also *Liver failure.*

Hepatitis, 449, 452–453

   clinical presentation of, 452

   giant cell, 453

   icteric stage of, 452

   posticteric stage of, 452

   preicteric stage of, 452

Hepatitis A virus, 449

Hepatitis B virus, 452

   transfusion-acquired, 508

Hepatitis C virus, 452

   transfusion-acquired, 508

Hepatitis D virus, 452

Hepatoblastoma, liver transplantation in, 457

Hepatocellular carcinoma, liver transplantation in, 457

Hepatorenal syndrome, 378

Hepatosplenomegaly, in hepatic failure, 454, 456

Hernia, diaphragmatic, 445t

   congenital, 121–126. See also *Diaphragmatic hernia, congenital.*

High-frequency jet ventilation, 77

High-frequency oscillatory ventilation, 77, 79

High-frequency ventilation, 77, 79

Histocompatibility testing, 487–488

Holter monitoring, 168

Homicide, adolescent, 554

Honesty, with children, 3

Hormones, 387, 389t–390t. See also *Endocrine system and specific glands and hormones.*

Hospitalization, 6–8

   fear of, 6–7

   play opportunities during, 17–18

   psychosocial supports for, 18–19

   separation stress with, 7–8

Human chorionic gonadotropin, in brain tumor, 337

Human immunodeficiency virus (HIV), immune response to, 528–529

   infection with, 527, 527t. See also *Acquired immunodeficiency syndrome (AIDS).*

      intravenous immunoglobulin in, 501–502

      transfusion-acquired, 508

   p24 antigen of, 528

   testing for, 528–529

   transmission of, 527, 533

Human leukocyte antigens, 470–471

   class I, 471

   class II, 471

   class III, 471

   compatibility testing of, 487–488

Humidification, during mechanical ventilation, 84

Hunter's syndrome, cardiac anomalies in, 160t

Hurler's syndrome, cardiac anomalies in, 160t

Hydralazine (Apresoline), cardiovascular effects of, 183

Hydrocarbon poisoning, 625

Hydrocephalus, 338–339

   acquired, 338

   communicating, 338

   congenital, 338

   noncommunicating, 338

   normal-pressure, 338

Hydrocephalus ex vacuo, 338

Hydrochlorothiazide, in acute renal failure, 379

Hydrofluoric acid injury, 619–620

17-Hydroxyprogesterone, reference range for, 406t

Hyperbilirubinemia, 448–449

   laboratory studies in, 450t–451t

   signs and symptoms of, 450t–451t

   treatment of, 449

Hypercarbia, permissive, 694

   during mechanical ventilation, 82–83

Hyperglycemia, 409–410, *409.* See also *Ketoacidosis, diabetic.*

Hyperglycemic, hyperosmolar, nonketotic syndrome, 414–416

   collaborative diagnoses in, 415

   complications of, 416

   diagnosis of, 414–415, 415t

   differential diagnosis of, 415, 415t

   etiology of, 414

   fluid therapy in, 415

Hyperglycemic, hyperosmolar, nonketotic syndrome (*Continued*)
  monitoring for, 416
  pathophysiology of, 414
  risk factors for, 414
  signs and symptoms of, 414, 415t
  treatment of, 415–416
Hyperkalemia, in acute renal failure, 373
Hyperlipoproteinemia, genetic factors in, 211
Hypermagnesemia, in acute renal failure, 374
Hypermetabolism, in burn injury, 656–657
Hyperosmolality, in diabetic ketoacidosis, 410t
Hyperparathyroidism, 399
Hyperphosphatemia, 368
  in acute renal failure, 373–374
Hyperpnea, in diabetic ketoacidosis, 410t
Hypersensitivity reaction. See also *Anaphylaxis.*
Hypersensitivity reactions, delayed, 515t
  immediate, 514, 515t
  skin testing for, 492
Hyperstat (diazoxide), cardiovascular effects of, 182–183
Hypertension, definition of, 256
  intracranial, 320–328. See also *Intracranial pressure, elevation of.*
  malignant, 256
  portal, in liver failure, 455–456
  pulmonary, in adult respiratory distress syndrome, 116
Hypertensive crisis, 256–258
  assessment of, 257
  clinical presentation of, 257
  definition of, 256
  diagnosis of, 257
  etiology of, 256–257
  hypotension with, 258
  interventions for, 257–258
  nursing diagnoses for, 258
  pathophysiology of, 256
  patient history in, 257
Hyperthermia, in neurologic assessment, 300, 308
  with infection, 511–512
Hyperthyroidism, 399
Hypertrophic scar, after burn injury, 671
Hyperventilation, in asthma, 107
  in intracranial pressure elevation, 323
  neurogenic, central, *46*, 300, 307t
Hypnotic poisoning, 602t
Hypocalcemia, in acute renal failure, 374
  with transfusion, 509
Hypodermis, 653, *655*
Hypoglossal nerve, 291t, 303t, 307t
Hypoglycemia, acute, 416–417
  diagnosis of, 416–417
  etiology of, 416
  pathophysiology of, 416
  risk factors for, 416
  signs and symptoms of, 416
  treatment of, 417
  in newborn, 393
  with diabetic ketoacidosis, 413
Hypokalemia, in theophylline poisoning, 616
  with diabetic ketoacidosis, 413
Hypoparathyroidism, 399

Hypopharynx, *35*, 36
Hypoplasia, of stem cells, 462
Hypoplastic left heart syndrome, 230–234, *230, 233*
Hypotension, in septic shock, 646
  in trauma assessment, 569
  trauma-related, 576
Hypothalamic-pituitary complex, 393–397, *393*
Hypothalamus, 281, 393, *393*
  cells of, 393–394
  development of, 397
  functions of, 394, 394t
  hormones of, 394t
Hypothermia, 563–564, 564t, 565t
  in burn injury, 657
  with transfusion, 509
Hypothyroidism, 398–399
Hypovolemia, 516–517
  in adult respiratory distress syndrome, 116
  in tracheoesophageal fistula, 131
Hypoxemia, in septic shock, 633
Hypoxia, in tetralogy of Fallot, 242–243
  in tricuspid atresia, 248
Hypoxic-ischemic encephalopathy, 342–345
  diagnosis of, 344
  etiology of, 343
  management of, 344–345
  pathophysiology of, 343

I

Iatrogenic anemia, 510
Ibuprofen, for pain, 14
  in septic shock, 649
Idiopathic thrombocytopenic purpura, 536–537
  vs. hemolytic-uremic syndrome, 537
Ileum, 424–425, *425*
Imidazoline poisoning, 612
Imipramine poisoning, 607–608
Immune system, 470–471, 474–477. See also *Hematologic system.*
  antigens in, 470–471
  in acquired immunodeficiency syndrome, 528–529
  in burn injury, 657
  in cardiac transplantation, 266
  in septic shock, 629–635, *632, 634, 635*
  major histocompatibility complex in, 470–471
Immunity, acquired, 474–477, 475t, *476*
  cell-mediated, 474–475, 475t, *476*
    skin testing of, 492
  humoral, 474, 475–476, 475t, *476*, 477t
Immunodeficiency, acquired, 526–533. See also *Acquired immunodeficiency syndrome (AIDS).*
  combined, severe, 524–526. See also *Severe combined immunodeficiency.*
  congenital, 522–524
  definition of, 522
  secondary, 533
Immunoglobulin(s), 475, 477–478, 477t
  in pulmonary evaluation, 53t
  intravenous, 501–502
  measurement of, 488
Immunoglobulin A, 477t, 479t
  deficiency of, 523
Immunoglobulin D, 477t, 479t
  in pulmonary evaluation, 53t

Immunoglobulin E, 477t, 479t
  in asthma, 106, *107*
  in pulmonary evaluation, 53t
Immunoglobulin G, 477t, 478, 479t
  in pulmonary evaluation, 53t
Immunoglobulin M, 477t, 479t
  in pulmonary evaluation, 53t
Immunosuppression, 522
Immunosuppressive therapy, 430–431, 495–496
  azathioprine for, 431
  corticosteroids for, 431
  cyclosporine for, 430–431
  for lung transplantation, 138
  muromonab-CD3 for, 431
  tacrolimus for, 430
Imuran (azathioprine), for immunosuppression, 431,
    495–496
Inapsine (droperidol), for nausea, 64t
Incest, 592
Inderal (propranolol), 428
  cardiovascular effects of, 181–182
Indirect Coombs test, 488
Infants, communication with, 15
  development of, 2
  fears of, 6
  pain management in, 11t
  play opportunities for, 18
  stress response of, 5
  working with, 3
Infection, 510–511, 639
  after bone marrow transplantation, 542
  after liver transplantation, 458
  after lung transplantation, 138, 139
  cardiac, 260–266, 264t
  culture for, 512
  hyperthermia with, 511–512
  in burn injury, 671, 674
  in congenital heart disease, 211–212
  in neural tube defects, 354
  in septic shock, 628. See also *Septic shock.*
  in sickle cell disease, 519
  intravenous immunoglobulin in, 501
  nosocomial, in adult respiratory distress syndrome,
    120
    in congenital diaphragmatic hernia, 126
    in persistent pulmonary hypertension of
      newborn, 128
    in tracheoesophageal fistula, 130
  of central nervous system, 332–335
  oral, 512–514, 513t–514t
  prevention of, 511
  transfusion-acquired, 507–508
  vs. inflammation, 510, 511
  with cardiac assist devices, 190
Inflammation, 472–473, 510–511
  in burn injury, 657
  myocardial, 260–266, 264t, *265*
  systemic, 511
  vs. infection, 510, 511
Influenza, in pneumonia, 104t
Infratentorial herniation, in intracranial pressure
    elevation, 322
Inhalational injury, 659–660, 660t. See also *Burns.*
  assessment of, 660, 661t

Inocor (amrinone lactate), cardiovascular effects of,
    178
Inotropic agents, 178–180
  in cardiomyopathy, 260
  in congestive heart failure, 193
Insecticide poisoning, 626–627
Inspiration, first, 33
Inspiratory flow, 73t, 75
Inspiratory pressure, 74
Inspiratory time, 73t
Insulin, 390t
  biosynthesis of, 388
  deficiency of, 409–413, *409.* See also *Ketoacidosis,*
    diabetic.
  in acute renal failure, 373
  in diabetic ketoacidosis, 412–413, 413t
  in hyperglycemic, hyperosmolar, nonketotic
    syndrome, 415–416
  metabolic effects of, 391–392
  reduction of, 391–392
  regulation of, 388, *391,* 392t
Insulin tolerance test, 405
Insulin-like growth factor, reference range for, 406t
Interferon alfa, 478t
Interferon beta, 478t
Interferon gamma, 478t
Interleukin-1, 478t
  in septic shock, 632
Interleukin-2, 478t
Interleukin-3, 478t
  indications for, 493
  mechanisms of action of, 493
Interleukin-4, 478t
Interleukin-5, 478t
Intermittent mandatory ventilation, 76, *78*
  synchronized, 76, *78*
Interstitial pneumonitis, after bone marrow
    transplantation, 543–544
Intestine, 424–425. See also *Gastrointestinal system.*
  atresia of, 442t–443t
  autonomic nerve stimulation of, 295t
  trauma to, 435
Intraaortic balloon pump, 187
Intracranial hemorrhage, 328–332
  catastrophic, 331
  imaging of, 331
  in aneurysm, 329–330
  in arteriovenous malformation, 328–329
  intraventricular, 330–332
  periventricular, 330–332
  saltatory, 331
  silent, 331
  tissue perfusion in, 331–332
  vasospasm in, 332
Intracranial pressure, 287, *288*
  elevation of, 320–328
    acute, 322
    central herniation in, 321–322, *321*
    cerebral edema in, 320
    chronic, 322
    cingulate herniation in, *321,* 322
    etiology of, 320
    in basilar fracture, 341
    infratentorial herniation in, 322

Intracranial pressure *(Continued)*
    management of, 322–324
        midbrain compression in, 322
        pathophysiology of, 320–322, *321*
        pontine compression in, 322
        supratentorial herniation in, 321–322, *321*
        symptoms of, 322
        uncal herniation in, 321, *321*
    monitoring of, 311–315, *314*
        A wave in, 314, *314*
        B wave in, 314, *314*
        C wave in, 314–315, *314*
        epidural, 312
        external fiberoptic transducer for, 312
        fiberoptic catheters for, 311–312
        fluid-filled systems for, 311, 313
        in brain trauma, 342
        infection control for, 313
        insertion site care for, 313
        intraparenchymal, 312–313
        intraventricular, 312
        subarachnoid, 312
        subdural, 312
        waveform analysis during, 313–315, *313, 314*
Intracranial volume, 287
Intraosseous vascular access, in cardiopulmonary
        failure, 185
Intravenous immunoglobulin, 501–502
    in idiopathic thrombocytopenic purpura, 537
    indications for, 501–502
    reactions to, 502
Intropin (dopamine), cardiovascular effects of, 179
    in acute renal failure, 380
    in septic shock, 645t
Intubation, communication during, 16
    in asthma, 111
    in congenital diaphragmatic hernia, 123–124
    in persistent pulmonary hypertension of newborn,
        127
Intussusception, 443t
Inverse-ratio ventilation, 77
Iodine, metabolism of, 398
Iodine starch test, in trauma evaluation, 587
Ion-trapping, in poisoning management, 605
Ipecac syrup, in poisoning management, 603
Ipratropium bromide (Atrovent), in asthma, 114t
    in bronchopulmonary dysplasia, 134
Iron overload, with chronic blood transfusion, 509
Iron poisoning, 601t, 612–613
    case study of, 384
Islets of Langerhans, 387–388, *390*
Isoniazid poisoning, 601t, 613–614
Isopropyl alcohol poisoning, 601t
Isoproterenol (Isuprel), cardiovascular effects of, 180
    in septic shock, 645t
Isoptin (verapamil), cardiovascular effects of, 182
Isuprel (isoproterenol), in septic shock, 645t

J
Jaundice, 448–449
    in hepatic failure, 454
Jaw, testing of, 305t
Jejunum, 424, *425*
Jones criteria, in rheumatic fever, 263, 264t

K
Kawasaki disease, 264–266, *265*
    diagnosis of, 264–265, *265*
    etiology of, 264
    extracorporeal life support in, 187
    management of, 265–266
    nursing diagnoses in, 265
    pathophysiology of, 264
    signs and symptoms of, 264
Kayexalate enema, in acute renal failure, 373
Kehr's sign, 433
    in abdominal trauma, 582
Kernicterus, 449
Ketamine, for pain, 14
    in asthma, *112,* 113, 114t
    in pulmonary disorders, 60t, 62
Ketoacidosis, diabetic, 409–413, *409,* 412t, 413t. See
        also *Diabetic ketoacidosis.*
Ketonuria, in diabetic ketoacidosis, 410t
Kidney(s). See also *Renal failure; Renal system.*
    anatomy of, 360–361
    antidiuretic hormone effects on, 395
    arteries of, 360
    biopsy of, in acute renal failure, 372
    dysfunction of, after bone marrow transplantation,
        543
    in acid-base balance, 369
    in burn injury, 656, 673
    in erythropoietin production, 370
    in hepatic encephalopathy, 453–454
    in hepatic failure, 454, 455
    transplantation of, 384–385
    trauma to, 385–386, 584
Knee-jerk reflex, *286*
Knife trauma, 563
Kohn, alveolar pores of, 37
Konno procedure, in aortic stenosis, 228–229
Kupffer's cells, 465, 468
Kyphoscoliosis, thoracic, 45, *45*

L
Lacrimal glands, autonomic nerve stimulation of, 295t
Lactotrophs, 394
Lactulose (Cephulac), 430
Ladd procedure, in congenital diaphragmatic hernia,
    125
Lambert, canals of, 37
Lanoxin (digoxin), cardiovascular effects of, 179
Laplace's law, 148
Laryngotracheobronchitis (croup), *98,* 102–104
    airway edema in, 102, *103*
    clinical presentation of, 102
    definition of, 102
    differential diagnosis of, 101t
    etiology of, 102
    management of, 102–104, 103t
    pathophysiology of, 102, *103*
    severity of, 103, 103t
    supportive care for, 103–104, 103t
Larynx, *35*
    embryology of, 36
Latrodectus mactans bite, 622
Laurence-Moon syndrome, cardiac anomalies in, 160t
Lavage, peritoneal, in trauma evaluation, 578

Le Fort fractures, 581
Leads, for continuous electrocardiography, 173, *173*
    for electrocardiography, 168
Lead poisoning, 601t
Left atrial monitoring, 177, *177*
Left bundle branch system, 156, *156*
Left coronary artery, 149, *149*
Left heart syndrome, hypoplastic, 230–234, *230, 233*
Leukocytes, 466–469. See also specific types.
    function of, 470–478
    hyperactivity of, 514–516
    hypoactivity of, 510–511
    reference values for, 485t
Leukocytosis, in septic shock, 639
Leukopenia, in septic shock, 639
Leukotrienes, in septic shock, 631
Levophed (norepinephrine bitartrate), cardiovascular
    effects of, 180
Lidocaine, cardiovascular effects of, 181
Lidocaine poisoning, 607
Life-sustaining treatment, withdrawal of, 26–27
Lifts, in cardiovascular system assessment, 162
Light, in critical care unit, 9
Light touch, evaluation of, 299
Limbic system, 280
Lips, care for, 513t
Liquid ventilation, 81
Lithium, maternal use of, fetal cardiac anomalies and,
    160t
Lithium poisoning, 602t
Liver, *425, 426,* 465
    autonomic nerve stimulation of, 295t
    development of, 426
    in graft-versus-host disease, 545
    palpation of, 427, 483–484
        in cardiovascular system assessment, 163
        in septic shock, 638
    trauma to, 434
        in child abuse, 590
    venoocclusive disease of, after bone marrow
        transplantation, 542
Liver failure, 449, 452–456
    acute, 454
    ascites in, 456
    case study of, 686–687
    chronic, 454–455
    coagulopathy in, 454, 455
    collaborative diagnoses in, 455
    complications of, 456
    drug-induced, 453
    encephalopathy of, 453, 454
        treatment of, 455
    fulminant, 453
    hematologic pathophysiology of, 454
    hepatitis in, 449, 452–453
    hepatosplenomegaly in, 456
    hypersplenism in, 454
    kidneys in, 455
    pathophysiology of, 453–454
    portal hypertension in, 455–456
    renal pathophysiology of, 453–454
    treatment of, 455–456
Liver transplantation, 456–458
    contraindications to, 457

Liver transplantation *(Continued)*
    Epstein-Barr infection after, 458
    in Alagille syndrome, 457
    in biliary atresia, 456
    in hepatoblastoma, 457
    in hepatocellular carcinoma, 457
    in intrahepatic cholestasis, 456–457
    in metabolic diseases, 456
    infection after, 458
    lymphoproliferative disease after, 458
    nursing diagnoses in, 457
    preparation for, 457
    rejection of, 458
    treatment of, 457–458
Loop diuretics, in acute renal failure, 379
Loop of Henle, 366t
Lorazepam, in pulmonary disorders, 59–61, 60t
    in status epilepticus, 327t
Lumbar puncture, in neurologic assessment, 316
Lungs. See also *Airway; Respiratory system.*
    auscultation of, 47–48
    autonomic nerve stimulation of, 294t
    biopsy of, in pneumonia, 105
    compliance of, 38, 74, *74*
        measurement of, 56–57
    contusion of, 583t
    developmental anatomy of, 36–37
    embryology of, 33, *34*
    function of, after bone marrow transplantation,
        543–544
        in burn injury, 656
    gas exchange of, 41–43, *42*
    infection of, 104–106. See also *Pneumonia.*
        in spinal cord injury, 350
    injury to, during mechanical ventilation, 85
    physiologic function of, 38–43, *39–41*
    postnatal development of, 33–34, *35*
    resistance of, 38
    trauma to, 94
        in child abuse, 590
Lung transplantation, 135–140, 267–268
    complications of, 139–140, 139t
    definition of, 135
    donor evaluation for, 137
    evaluation for, 136–137
    immunosuppression for, 128
    in cystic fibrosis, 140
    indications for, 135–136, 136t
    infection prophylaxis in, 128
    lymphoproliferative disease after, 140
    nursing diagnoses in, 137
    nutritional monitoring in, 128–139
    outcomes of, 137–138, 140
    rejection of, 128, 139, 139t
Lung volumes, 41, *41,* 73–76, 73t
    postnatal development of, 33–34
Lupus erythematosus, maternal, fetal cardiac
        anomalies and, 160t
Luteinizing hormone, 389t, 397
    reference range for, 406t
Lymph, 463
Lymph nodes, 463–464, *464*
    biopsy of, 491–492
    palpation of, 483

Lymphatic system, 463–464, *464*
Lymphatics, pulmonary, 37–38
Lymphoblast, 461, *462*
Lymphocytes, 468–469
    absolute count of, 486
    B, 468
        disorders of, 522–523
    differentiation of, *462*
    memory, 469
    reference values for, 485t
    T, 468
        CD4, 468
            count of, 486
        CD8, 468
            count of, 487
        disorders of, 523, 524
        suppressor, 468
Lymphocytic interstitial pneumonitis, in acquired
        immunodeficiency syndrome, 532–533
Lymphocytosis, 468
    in septic shock, 639
Lymphopenia, 468
Lymphoproliferative disease, after liver
        transplantation, 458
    after lung transplantation, 140

M

Maalox (magnesium hydroxide and aluminum
        hydroxide), 429
Macewen's sign, in hydrocephalus, 339
Macrophages, 468
    differentiation of, *462*
Macrophage colony-stimulating factor, 478t
Mafenide acetate cream (Sulfamylon), in burn injury,
        670, 670t
Magnesium, serum, 369
    in acute renal failure, 374
Magnesium citrate, in poisoning management, 605
Magnesium citrate (Citroma), 430
Magnesium hydroxide (Milk of Magnesia), 430
Magnesium hydroxide and aluminum hydroxide
        (Maalox), 429
Magnesium sulfate, in asthma, 114t
Magnesium sulfate solution, in hydrofluoric acid
        injury, 620
Magnetic resonance imaging, 341–342
    in brain tumor, 337
    in CNS infection, 334
    in hydrocephalus, 339
    in neurologic assessment, 309–310
    in pulmonary evaluation, 52
    in respiratory distress, 52
    in spinal cord injury, 348
    of cardiovascular system, 172, *172*
Major histocompatibility complex, 470–471
Malnutrition, in hepatic failure, 454–455
Mandible, fracture of, 580
Mannitol (Osmitrol), in intracranial pressure
        elevation, 323–324
Manometry, pressure, 56
Marfan syndrome, cardiac anomalies in, 160t
Margination, in inflammatory response, 472
Mast cells, in asthma, 106, *107*
Maxilla, trauma to, 580–581

Mean airway pressure, 75
Mean arterial pressure, 155
Mean corpuscular volume, reference values for, 485t
Mechanical ventilation, 73–86. See also *Ventilation,*
        mechanical.
    in trauma treatment, 576
Mechanoreceptors, in breathing control, 40, *40*
Medulla, vasomotor center of, 152–153
Medulla oblongata (myelencephalon), *276*, 281–282,
        281
Megakaryoblast, 461, *462*
Megakaryocytes, 469
Megakaryocyte colony-stimulating factor, 493
Melena, 435
Memory cells, 469
Meninges, 278
Meningitis, 332–335
    case study of, 687–688
    cerebrospinal fluid analysis in, 333–334
    clinical symptoms of, 333
    etiology of, 332
    incidence of, 332
    management of, 334–335
    pathophysiology of, 333
Meningocele, 353
Meningococcal vaccine, in septic shock prevention,
        649
Meperidine (Demerol), for pain, 15t
Meperidine (Demerol) poisoning, 614
Mercury poisoning, 602t
Mesencephalon (midbrain), 275, *276*, 281, *281*
Mesoderm, 274
Metabolic acidosis, in asthma, 113
Metabolic rate, basal, 426–427
Metencephalon (pons), *276*, 281, *281*
Methadone, for pain, 15t
    in pulmonary disorders, 60t
Methadone poisoning, 614
Methanol poisoning, 602t, 623–624
Methemoglobinemia, 607
Methylprednisolone (Solu-Medrol), for
        immunosuppressive therapy, 431
    in asthma, 114t
    in pulmonary disorders, 66
    in spinal cord injury, 348–349
Methylxanthines, in asthma, *112*, 113
    in bronchopulmonary dysplasia, 134
Metoclopramide (Reglan), for nausea, 64t
Metolazone, in acute renal failure, 379
Midaxillary line, *44*
Midazolam (Versed), for pain, 15t
    in pulmonary disorders, 59–61, 60t
    in status epilepticus, 327t
Midbrain (mesencephalon), 275, *276*, 281, *281*
Midbrain compression, in intracranial pressure
        elevation, 322
Midclavicular line, *44*
Midfacial fractures, 581
Military antishock trousers, 187
    in trauma, 433
Milk of Magnesia (magnesium hydroxide), 430
Minute ventilation, 73t, 74
Mitral insufficiency, congenital, 238–239
Mitral stenosis, 236, 238

Mitral valve, 147, *147*
Mitral valve disease, 236, 238
Mixed venous oxygen saturation, 54
Monoblast, 461, *462*
Monoclonal antibodies, diagnostic use of, 488–489
    for therapeutic immunosuppression, 496
Monocytes, 467
    reference values for, 485t
Monocytopenia, 468
Monocytosis, 467
Monosynaptic reflex arc, 285, *286*
Moro reflex, evaluation of, 298
Morphine, for pain, 15t
    in pulmonary disorders, 60t, 61
Motor vehicle crashes, 552, 554, 561–562
    adolescent injury in, 554
    air bag–related injury in, 561
    case study of, 384–386
    infant injury in, 552
    patient history in, 565–566
    pedestrian injury in, 561–562
    preschooler injury in, 553
    prevention of, 557t–558t, 559t
    restraining device–related injury in, 561
    school-age children injury in, 553
    toddler injury in, 553
Mouth, care guidelines for, 513t–514t
    infection of, 512–514
Mucocutaneous lymph node syndrome, 264–266, *265*.
        See also *Kawasaki disease.*
Mucolytics, in asthma, *112*, 113
Mucormycosis, with diabetic ketoacidosis, 413
Mucosa-associated lymphoid tissue, 464–465
Mucositis, 512–514, 513t–514t
Mucus plugs, in asthma, 107
Multimodality evoked responses, in neurologic
        assessment, 316
Multiorgan system dysfunction, 639
    in sickle cell disease, 522
    with cardiac assist devices, 190
    with septic shock, 650–651, 651t
Munchausen syndrome by proxy, in child abuse, 591
Murmurs, 164
    diastolic, 164
    holosystolic, 164
    in Ebstein's anomaly, 226
    in transposition of great vessels, 245–246
    in tricuspid atresia, 248
    in truncus arteriosus, 250
    in ventricular septal defect, 221
    midsystolic, 164
    systolic, 164
Muromonab-CD3 (Orthoclone OKT3), for
        immunosuppressive therapy, 431
    for therapeutic immunosuppression, 496
Muscle, cardiac, 144
Mushroom poisoning, 625–626
Mustard-Senning operation, in transposition of great
        vessels, 246
Mycotic aneurysm, intracranial, 329–330
Myelencephalon (medulla oblongata), *276*, 281–282,
        281
Myeloblast, 461, *462*
Myelodysplasia, 352–354

Myelography, in spinal cord injury, 348
Myelomeningocele, 353
Myocardial contusion, 95, 97, 268–269
Myocardial depressant factor, in shock, 194
Myocarditis, 260–263
    diagnosis of, 262
    etiology of, 261
    extracorporeal life support in, 187
    management of, 262–263
    nursing diagnoses in, 262
    pathophysiology of, 260–261
    signs and symptoms of, 261
Myocardium, 145. See also *Heart.*
    contusion of, 95, 97, 268–269
    disease of, 258–260. See also *Cardiomyopathy.*

N

Nalbuphine (Nubain), for pain, 15t
    for pruritus, 64t
Naloxone (Narcan), antagonistic action of, 63–65, 64t
Narcotics, for pain, 14, 15t
Nasal cannula, in acute respiratory failure, 70t
Nasopharyngeal airway, in trauma treatment, 574
Nasopharyngeal glands, autonomic nerve stimulation
        of, 295t
Nasopharynx, *35*, 36
Natural killer cells, 468–469
Neck, in trauma assessment, 572
Necrotizing enterocolitis, 447–448, 448t
Needle thoracentesis, in pneumothorax, 92, *93*
Negative inspiratory force, 56
Negative pressure ventilation, 81
Neglect, 594. See also *Child abuse.*
Nephron, anatomy of, 360–361
    cortical, 360–361
    juxtaglomerular, 361
    tubular components of, 361
    vascular components of, 361
Nephrotic syndrome, acute renal failure in, 377–378
Nerves, cranial, 289, 291t. See also *Cranial nerve(s).*
    impulse conduction by, 286–287
    traumatic injury to, 587
Neural crest, *275*
Neural groove, 274, *275*
Neural plate, 274
Neural tube, 274, *275*, 276
Neural tube defects, 352–354
    infection in, 354
Neuroendocrine system, 393–397, *393*
Neurofibromatosis, cardiac anomalies in, 160t
Neuroglia, 277
Neurologic system, 274–354. See also specific
        neurologic disorders.
    assessment of, 293, 296–308
        angiography in, 310–311
        blood pressure in, 308
        cerebellar function in, 299–300
        cerebral blood flow in, 315
        computed tomography in, 309
        consciousness level in, 297–298, 297t
        cranial nerve function in, 300, 301t–307t
        deep tendon reflexes in, 298–299
        electroencephalography in, 315–316
        evoked potentials in, 316

Neurologic system (*Continued*)
  family history in, 296
  fontanelle palpation in, 296–297
  fundoscopic examination in, 300
  gait in, 300
  Glasgow Coma Scale in, 297–298, 297t
  intracranial devices in, 317–320, *317, 319*
  intracranial pressure monitoring in, 311–315,
    313, 314
  lumbar puncture in, 316
  magnetic resonance imaging in, 309–310
  motor function in, 298–299
  motor response in, 299
  patient history in, 296
  physical examination in, 296–308, 297t,
    301t–307t
  primitive reflexes in, 298
  pulse in, 308
  radioisotope scan in, 311
  respiratory patterns in, 300, 307t
  sensory function in, 299
  skull auscultation in, 297
  skull examination in, 296–297
  skull percussion in, 297
  social history in, 296
  superficial reflexes in, 299
  temperature in, 300, 308
  transcranial Doppler ultrasound in, 315
  vital signs in, 300, 307t
  xenon computed tomographic scan in, 315
  x-rays in, 309
 central, 274–289. See also *Central nervous system.*
 neurodiagnostic monitoring of, 309–316
 peripheral, 289–293. See also *Peripheral nervous
    system.*
 radiography of, 309
Neuromuscular blocking agents, communication
    during, 16–17
 for pain, 14
 in pulmonary disorders, 59, 72t
Neuron, 276–277, *277*
 in impulse conduction, 286–287
Neurotoxins, in hepatic encephalopathy, 453
Neurotransmitters, 292
 in hepatic encephalopathy, 453
Neurulation, 274, *275*
Neutropenia, 467, 474
 in septic shock, 639, 648
Neutrophils, 466–467
 absolute count of, 486
 development of, 473–474
 differentiation of, *462*
 in adult respiratory distress syndrome, 115–116, *115*
 reference values for, 485t
 storage of, 474
Neutrophilia, 467
Nicardipine poisoning, 609–610
Nifedipine (Procardia), cardiovascular effects of, 183
Nifedipine (Procardia) poisoning, 609–610
Ninhydrin print test, in trauma evaluation, 587
Nipride (nitroprusside), cardiovascular effects of, 183
Nitric oxide, in congenital diaphragmatic hernia, 124
 in persistent pulmonary hypertension of newborn,
    128

Nitric oxide (*Continued*)
 in pulmonary disorders, 65
 in septic shock, 632
Nitroglycerin, cardiovascular effects of, 183
 in septic shock, 645t
Nitroprusside (Nipride), cardiovascular effects of, 183
Nodal escape beat, 201, *201*
Nodal premature beat, 201, *201*
Nodal (junctional) tachycardia, 201, *201,* 202t
Noise, critical care unit levels of, 8, 9t, 17
 minimization of, 17
Noninvasive phasic augmentation device, 187
Nonsteroidal anti-inflammatory agents, platelet effects
    of, 497
Norepinephrine, 390t, 401–402
 effects of, 401–402
 in blood flow regulation, 152
 in cardiac regulation, 153
 in septic shock, 645t
 synthesis of, 401
Norepinephrine bitartrate (Levophed), cardiovascular
    effects of, 180
Norepinephrine-epinephrine vasoconstrictor reflex, in
    septic shock, 636
Nortriptyline poisoning, 607–608
Norwood operation, in hypoplastic left heart
    syndrome, 232, *233*
Nose, embryology of, 35
 fractures of, 581
 in trauma assessment, 572
Novacor ventricular assist device, 189t
Nubain (nalbuphine), for pain, 15t
 for pruritus, 64t
Nutrition, after lung transplantation, 138–139
 during mechanical ventilation, 83
 in adult respiratory distress syndrome, 119–120
 in bronchopulmonary dysplasia, 134
 in burn injury, 669, 675
 in congenital diaphragmatic hernia, 125, 126
 in persistent pulmonary hypertension of newborn,
    128
 in septic shock prevention, 648
 in tracheoesophageal fistula, 130

O

Obliterative bronchiolitis, after lung transplantation,
    139
Obtundation, 297
Occipital lobe, 280, *280*
Oculomotor nerve, 291t, 301t, 302t, 304t, 305t
Olfactory nerve, 291t, 301t, 303t
Omeprazole (Prilosec), 429
Omphalocele, 440t
Ondansetron (Zofran), for nausea, 64t
Opioid poisoning, 602t, 614
Optic nerve, 291t, 301t, 304t
Oral care guidelines, 513t–514t
Oral cavity, 424, *425*
 in trauma assessment, 572
 infection of, 512–514, 513t–514t
Organ donation, from dying children, 27
Organophosphate poisoning, 602t, 626–627
Oropharyngeal airway, in trauma treatment, 574
Oropharynx, *35, 36*

Orthoclone OKT3 (muromonab-CD3), for immunosuppressive therapy, 431
  for therapeutic immunosuppression, 496
Orthotic brace, in scoliosis, 351
Osmitrol (mannitol), in intracranial pressure elevation, 323–324
Osmolality, serum, antidiuretic hormone release and, 395
Osmotic diuretics, in acute renal failure, 380
Osteogenesis imperfecta, cardiac anomalies in, 160t
Ostium primum defect, 218–219
Ostium secundum defect, 218–219
Ovaries, location of, *388*
Overdose, vs. poisoning, 595
Oximetry, pulse, 54
Oxygen, cerebral metabolism of, 288
  consumption of, in septic shock, 628, 633, 635, *635*, 647
    in trauma assessment, 569
  diffusion of, in lungs, 41–42
  transcutaneous monitoring of, 54
  transport of, 42
Oxygen imbalance, in septic shock, *632,* 633, 635, *635*
Oxygen therapy, in acute respiratory failure, 69–70, 70t, 71t, 72
  in adult respiratory distress syndrome, 118–119
  in bronchopulmonary dysplasia, 133
  in congenital diaphragmatic hernia, 123
  in septic shock, 646–647
  in tracheoesophageal fistula, 130
  in trauma treatment, 575, 577
Oxygen toxicity, during mechanical ventilation, 85
Oxygenation, in intracranial pressure elevation, 323
Oxyhemoglobin dissociation curve, 42–43, *42*
Oxyphil cells, 399
Oxytocin, 389t, 395–396

P

p24 antigen, of human immunodeficiency virus, 528
P wave, on electrocardiography, 167, *167*
Pacemaker(s), 206–211
  asynchronous mode of, 207
  bleeding with, 208
  capabilities of, 207
  complications of, 208, 210t
  components of, 206
    problems with, 208
  demand (inhibited) mode of, 207–208
  emboli with, 208
  epicardial leads for, 207
  esophageal, 207
  fixed mode of, 207
  in cardiomyopathy, 260
  indications for, 206
  inhibited mode of, 208
  insertion of, 208
  modes for, 207–208
  nomenclature for, 208, 209t
  noncapture by, 210t
  on electrocardiography, 208
  oversensing by, 210t
  permanent, 207, *207*
    nursing intervention for, 208, 2100

Pacemaker(s) *(Continued)*
  temporary, 207
    nursing intervention for, 208
  transthoracic, 207
  transvenous lead for, 207, *207*
  triggered mode of, 208
  undersensing by, 210t
Pacemaker cells, of heart, 157
Pain, in burn injury, 672, 674–675
  in congenital heart disease, 214
  in hydrofluoric acid injury, 620
  in scoliosis, 352
  in tracheoesophageal fistula, 130
  management of, developmental stage and, 10–14, 11t–13t
    nonpharmacologic, 10–14, 11t–13t
    pharmacologic, 14, 15t
  misconceptions about, 7, 7t
  trauma-related, 578
Pain sensation, evaluation of, 299
Painful vasoocclusion crisis, in sickle cell disease, 520–521
Palate, *35*
Palmar grasp, evaluation of, 298
Palpation, during mechanical ventilation, 82
  in cardiovascular system assessment, 161–163, *162*
  in respiratory system assessment, 46–47
  in septic shock, 638
  in ventricular hypertrophy, 161
  of abdomen, 361, 427–428
  of chest, 46–47
  of fontanelles, 296–297
  of liver, 427, 483–484, 638
  of lymph nodes, 483
  of spleen, 483–484
Pancreas, 387–388, 391–393, 425–426, *425*
  autonomic nerve stimulation of, 295t
  cells of, 387–388, *390*
  development of, 392–393
  glucagon of, 392
  hormones of, 390t
  insulin release from, 388, *391*
  insulin synthesis by, 388
  location of, 387, *388*
  somatostatin of, 392
Pancrease, trauma to, 434–435
Pancuronium, in acute respiratory failure, 72t
Panda sign, in basilar fracture, 341
Papillary muscles, 145
Parachute reflex, evaluation of, 298
Parainfluenza virus, in pneumonia, 104t
Paraldehyde, in status epilepticus, 327
Parasympathetic nervous system, 291, *292*
  in blood flow regulation, 152
  in cardiac regulation, 153
Parathyroid glands, 399–400
  cells of, 399
  development of, 399–400
  hormones of, 389t
  location of, *388,* 399
Parathyroid hormone, 389t, 399
  in calcium metabolism, 368
  serum phosphate levels and, 368
Parents. See *Family.*

Parietal cells, 424
Parietal lobe, 280, *280*
Partial liquid ventilation, 81
Partial spinal cord syndrome, 346
Passive transport, in renal system, 362
Patau's syndrome (trisomy 13), cardiac anomalies in, 160t
Patch aortoplasty, in coarctation of aorta, 236, *237*
Patent ductus arteriosus, 217–218
Patent foramen ovale, 218–219
Peak inspiratory pressure, 75
Pectus carinatum, 45, *45*
Pectus excavatum, 45, *45*
Pediatric Coma Scale, in trauma assessment, 571t
Pediatric Trauma Score, 573–574
Pelvis, fracture of, 587
   in trauma assessment, 573
Penicillin, prophylactic, in septic shock prevention, 649
Penis, in sickle cell disease, 522
Pentamidine isethionate, in *Pneumocystis carinii* pneumonia, 531
Pentazocine (Talwin) poisoning, 614
Pepcid (famotidine), 429
Percussion, of abdomen, 428
   of chest wall, 47, *47*
   of skull, 297
     in hydrocephalus, 339
Perflugon ventilation, 81
Perfusion studies, of cardiovascular system, 172
Pericardial tamponade, 583t
Pericardiocentesis, *95,* 97
   in cardiac inflammation, 262
Pericarditis, 260–263
   diagnosis of, 262
   etiology of, 261
   management of, 262–263
   nursing diagnoses in, 262
   pathophysiology of, 261
   signs and symptoms of, 262
Pericardium, 145
Peripheral cyanosis, in cardiovascular system assessment, 159–160
Peripheral nervous system, 289–293. See also *Central nervous system; Neurologic system.*
   afferent fibers of, 289
   autonomic, 289, 291–292
     neural transmission in, 292
     neurotransmitters of, 292
     systemic effects of, 292, 294t–295t
   cranial nerves of, 289, 291t. See also *Cranial nerve(s).*
   developmental anatomy of, 289–291, *290*
   dorsal root of, 289
   efferent fibers of, 289
   spinal nerves of, 289, *290*
   ventral root of, 289
Peripheral pulses, in cardiovascular system assessment, 162–163
Peripheral smear, 484
Peripheral vascular resistance, 177
   regulation of, 369
Peritoneal dialysis, 380–381
   complications of, 381
Peritoneal lavage, in trauma evaluation, 578

Permissive hypercarbia, 694
Persistent pulmonary hypertension of newborn, 126–128
   clinical presentation of, 127
   definition of, 126
   diagnosis of, 127
   etiology of, 126
   family support in, 128
   in congenital diaphragmatic hernia, 124
   infection control in, 128
   management of, 127–128
   nutrition in, 128
   pathophysiology of, 127
pH, gastric, development of, 472
   in gastrointestinal tract hemorrhage, 438
Phagocytes, mononuclear, 467–468
Phagocytosis, 473, 474
   disorders of, 523
Pharynx, embryology of, 36
   testing of, 306t–307t
Phencyclidine poisoning, 602t
Phenobarbital, in status epilepticus, 327t
Phenothiazine poisoning, 602t
Phenylephrine, in septic shock, 645t
Phenylketonuria, cardiac anomalies in, 160t
Phenylpropanolamine poisoning, 615–616
Phenytoin, in status epilepticus, 327t
Pheochromocytoma, 402
Phosphate, serum, 368
   in acute renal failure, 373–374
Phosphorus, reference range for, 407t
Physical abuse, 589. See also *Child abuse.*
Physical restraints, 8
Phytonadione (AquaMEPHYTON), 428
Pia mater, 278, 283
Pigeon chest, 45, *45*
Pilocarpine iontophoresis, in pulmonary evaluation, 53t
Pineal gland, location of, *388*
Pitressin, 428
Pituitary gland, anterior (adenohypophysis), 393, *393*
   cells of, 394
   hormones of, 389t
   development of, 397
   hormones of, 389t
   posterior (neurohypophysis), 393, *393*
   hormones of, 389t
Placing reflex, evaluation of, 298
Plasma factors, 469–470, 470t
Plasma protein fraction (Plasmanate), transfusion of, 506
Plasma transfusion, after bone marrow transplantation, 541, 541t
Plasminogen, 469
Platelet(s), 469, 479–480
   antibodies to, 536–537
   aspirin effects on, 497
   differentiation of, *462*
   hemostatic response to, 479, *479*
   medication effects on, 480
   nonsteroidal anti-inflammatory agent effects on, 497
   suppression of, 496–497
Platelet activating factor, in septic shock, 631

Platelet count, 489
  in septic shock, 639
Platelet transfusion, 502–504
  ABO compatibility in, 503–504
  after bone marrow transplantation, 541, 541t
  alloimmunization with, 508
  in idiopathic thrombocytopenic purpura, 537
  indications for, 503, 504t
  results of, 503
  Rh compatibility in, 503
Play, facilitation of, 17–18
Plebostatic axis, 174, *174*
Pleural fluid examination, in pneumonia, 105
Pleuroperitoneal membranes, in diaphragm
        development, 121
Pneumatic antishock garment, 187
  in trauma treatment, 576
Pneumocystis carinii pneumonia, in acquired
        immunodeficiency syndrome, 530–532
  prophylaxis against, 532
Pneumonia, *98*, 104–106
  clinical presentation of, 105–106
  definition of, 104
  diagnostic tests in, 105–106
  during mechanical ventilation, 85
  etiology of, 104, 104t
  management of, 106
  pathophysiology of, 105
  patient history in, 105
  physical examination in, 105
Pneumonitis, aspiration, 86–88
    clinical course of, 87
    clinical presentation of, 86–87
    definition of, 86
    diagnostic tests for, 87
    differential diagnosis of, 87
    etiology of, 86, 86t
    management of, 87–88
    pathophysiology of, 86
    prevention of, 87–88
    supportive care in, 88
  interstitial, after bone marrow transplantation,
        543–544
Pneumothorax, 94–95, 96t, 583t
  chest tube placement for, 92–94, *93*
  clinical presentation of, 91–92, *92*
  definition of, 90, *90*
  diagnostic tests in, 91–92
  etiology of, 91
  management of, 92–94
  needle thoracentesis for, 92, *93*
  open, 91, *92*
  patient history in, 91
  physical examination in, 91
  prevention of, 92
  supportive care for, 93–94
  tension, 91, *92*, 94, 95–96, 96t
    in congenital diaphragmatic hernia, 124
  trauma-related, 576
Poison Center, 595–596
Poisoning, 595
  acetaminophen, 600t, 606–607
  acute, 595
  β-adrenergic antagonist, 600t

Poisoning *(Continued)*
  amitriptyline, 607–608
  amoxapine, 608
  amphetamine, 600t, 615–616
  anticholinergic, 600t
  antidepressant, 601t, 607–608
    case study of, 695–696
  arsenic, 600t
  aspirin, 614–615
  assessment of, clinical findings in, 599–603,
        600t–602t
    laboratory tests in, 599–603, 600t–602t
    patient history in, 599
  atropine, 611
  barbiturate, 600t
  benzocaine, 607
  benzodiazepine, 608–609
  botulism, 600t
  calcium channel blocker, 609–610
  carbamate, 602t, 627
  carbamazepine, 600t
  carbon monoxide, 600t, 617, 659–660
  chloroquine, 610
  chronic, 595
  clomipramine, 607–608
  clonidine, 600t
  cocaine, 601t, 615–616
  cyanide, 620–621
  cyclic antidepressant, 601t
  desipramine, 607–608
  dibucaine, 607
  digitalis, 601t, 610–611
  diltiazem, 609–610
  diphenoxylate, 611
  disulfiram, 601t
  doxepin, 607–608
  epidemiology of, 596, 596t, 597t
  ethanol, 601t, 622
  ethylene glycol, 601t, 622–623
  glipizide, 611
  glyburide, 611
  gun bluing, 624
  hydrocarbon, 625
  hypnotic, 602t
  imidazoline, 612
  imipramine, 607–608
  in adolescents, 598
  in infants, 597–598
  in school-age children, 598
  in toddlers, 598
  iron, 601t, 612–613
  isoniazid, 601t, 613–614
  isopropyl alcohol, 601t
  lead, 601t
  lidocaine, 607
  lithium, 602t
  management of, 599–606
  meperidine, 614
  mercury, 602t
  methadone, 614
  methanol, 602t, 623–624
  mushroom, 625–626
  nicardipine, 609–610
  nifedipine, 609–610

Poisoning (*Continued*)
  nortriptyline, 607–608
  nursing diagnoses in, 598
  opioid, 602t, 614
  organophosphate, 602t, 626–627
  pentazocine, 614
  phencyclidine, 602t
  phenothiazine, 602t
  phenylpropanolamine, 615–616
  prevention of, 605
  propoxyphene, 614
  psychosocial considerations in, 627
  recurrence of, 605, 606t
  risk factors for, 596–598
  salicylate, 602t, 614–615
  sedative, 602t
  selenious acid, 624
  substances in, 596, 597t
  sympathomimetic, 615–616
  theophylline, 602t, 616
  treatment of, 603–605
    activated charcoal in, 604–605
    antidotes in, 605
    cathartics in, 605
    diuresis in, 605
    extracorporeal measures in, 605
    gastric lavage in, 603–604
    gastrointestinal tract decontamination in, 603–605
    ion-trapping in, 605
    ipecac syrup in, 603
    ocular irrigation in, 603
    supportive care in, 605
    whole bowel irrigation in, 604
  tricyclic antidepressant, 601t, 607–608
    case study of, 695–696
  verapamil, 609–610
  vs. overdose, 595
Polycythemia, cyanosis and, 160–161
Polyhydramnios, in tracheoesophageal fistula, 130
Polysynaptic reflex arc, 285
Pons (metencephalon), *276*, 281, *281*
Pontine compression, in intracranial pressure elevation, 322
Pores of Kohn, 37
Portal hypertension, in liver failure, 455–456
Positive end-expiratory pressure (PEEP), 75
  in adult respiratory distress syndrome, 118, *119*
  in asthma, 111–112
  physiologic, 75
Positive pressure ventilation, 76–77, *78–80*
  noninvasive, 81–82
Posterior cord syndrome, 345
Postsynaptic membrane, 287
Potassium, serum, 367–368, 410
  in acute renal failure, 373
  in diabetic ketoacidosis, 410t
Potassium-sparing diuretics, in acute renal failure, 379–380
Povidone-iodine ointment (Betadine), in burn injury, 670, 670t
PP cells, 388
PR interval, on electrocardiography, 167, *167*, 167t
Pralidoxime, in organophosphate poisoning, 627

Preacinar arteries, of pulmonary circulation, 37
Precordium, in cardiovascular system assessment, 161
Prednisone, for immunosuppressive therapy, 431
  in asthma, 114t
  in lymphocytic interstitial pneumonitis, 532–533
Preload, 153–154
Premature ventricular contraction, *203*
Preschoolers, communication with, 16
  development of, 2
  fears of, 6–7
  pain management in, 12t
  play opportunities for, 18
  stress response of, 5–6
  working with, 3
Pressoreceptors, in blood flow regulation, 152
Pressure support ventilation, 76–77
Presynaptic membrane action potential, 287
Priapism, in sickle cell disease, 522
Prilosec (omeprazole), 429
Privacy, absence of, 9
Procainamide (Pronestyl), cardiovascular effects of, 181
Procardia (nifedipine), cardiovascular effects of, 183
Procardia (nifedipine) poisoning, 609–610
Procoagulants, 469, 480
Proerythroblast, 461, *462*, 465
Prograf (tacrolimus), 430
Progressive familial intrahepatic cholestasis, liver transplantation in, 456–457
Prolactin, 389t, 397
Prolactin-inhibiting factor, 394t
Prolactin-releasing factor, 394t
Pronestyl (procainamide), cardiovascular effects of, 181
Propofol, in pulmonary disorders, 60t, 62–63
Propoxyphene (Darvon) poisoning, 614
Propranolol (Inderal), 428
  cardiovascular effects of, 181–182
Proprioception, evaluation of, 299
Prosencephalon, *276*
Prostaglandins, in renal blood flow, 369–370
  in septic shock, 631
Prosthetic cardiac valve, in aortic stenosis, 229
Proteases, in septic shock, 632
Proteins, drug binding to, 58
  metabolism of, insulin effects on, 391
Protein C, 469
Protein S, 469
Prothrombin time, 489
  reference values for, 451t
  vitamin K deficiency and, 517
Pruritus, in hepatic failure, 455
Pseudomonas cepacia, pulmonary infection with, 136
Psychosocial supports, 18–19
Pulmonary artery, evaluation of, 165–166, *166*
  monitoring of, 175–177, *176*
Pulmonary artery banding, in tricuspid atresia, 249
Pulmonary artery catheterization, 54
  in bronchopulmonary dysplasia, 133
  in septic shock, 641
Pulmonary artery wedge pressure, monitoring of, 175, 177
Pulmonary atresia with intact ventricular septum, 254–255, *255*

Pulmonary atresia with ventricular septal defect, 244, *245*

Pulmonary capillary wedge pressure, 177

Pulmonary circulation, developmental anatomy of, 37–38

  developmental physiology of, 38–39, *39*

Pulmonary contusion, 94

Pulmonary edema, in adult respiratory distress syndrome, 116, *116*

Pulmonary function tests, 56–57, *57*

  in asthma, 110

  in bronchopulmonary dysplasia, 133

Pulmonary hypertension, in adult respiratory distress syndrome, 116

Pulmonary lymphoid hyperplasia, in acquired immunodeficiency syndrome, 532–533

Pulmonary pressure, intravascular, 39

Pulmonary system, 33–140. See also *Airway; Lungs; Respiratory system.*

Pulmonary valve, 147, *147*

Pulmonary valve stenosis, 239–241, *240, 241*

Pulmonary vascular resistance, 39–40

  in adult respiratory distress syndrome, 116

Pulmonary veins, anomalous return of, 251–254, *252*

Pulse, in cardiovascular system assessment, 162–163

  in neurologic assessment, 308

  in trauma assessment, 570

Pulse oximetry, 54

  in cardiovascular system assessment, 165

  in trauma assessment, 573

  in trauma treatment, 575

Pulse pressure, 155

Pulsus paradoxus, 163

Purkinje system, 156

Pyridoxine, in isoniazid poisoning, 613–614

Q

QRS interval, on electrocardiography, *167,* 168

QT segment, on electrocardiography, *167,* 168

Quinidine, cardiovascular effects of, 182

R

Raccoon sign, in basilar fracture, 341

Radiocontrast dye, in nephrotic syndrome, 377–378

Radionucleotide scan, in acute renal failure, 372

  in neurologic assessment, 311

  in renal trauma, 385

Ranitidine (Zantac), 429

Rastelli operation, in transposition of great vessels, 247

Rattlesnake bite, 621–622

Reactive airway disease, bronchodilators in, 65–66

Rectum, *425*

  trauma to, 435

Red blood cells, 465–466. See also *Erythrocyte(s).*

Red blood count, 484, 485t

Reflexes, evaluation of, 298–299

Reflex arc, 285, *286*

Refractory period, of cardiac muscle, 157

Reglan (metoclopramide), for nausea, 64t

Relative refractory period, of cardiac muscle, 157

Remembrance packet, for family, 30

Renal arteries, 360

Renal clearance, 363–364

Renal collecting ducts, 361, 366t

Renal failure, acute, 370–380

  anemia in, 375–376

  clinical manifestations of, 373–379, 375t, 376t

  continuous renal replacement therapy in, 382–384

  definitions of, 370–371

  diagnosis of, 372, 372t

  glucose intolerance in, 374

  hemodialysis in, 381 382

  hyperkalemia in, 373

  hypermagnesemia in, 374

  hyperphosphatemia in, 373–374

  hypocalcemia in, 374

  in acid-base balance, 375, 375t

  in acute glomerulonephritis, 377

  in cardiac failure, 378

  in hemolytic-uremic syndrome, 376–377

  in hepatorenal syndrome, 378

  in nephrotic syndrome, 377–378

  in tumor lysis syndrome, 378

  intrarenal, 371–372, 378

    clinical source of, 371–372

    definition of, 371

    etiology of, 371

    ischemic, 371

    nephrotoxic, 371

    pathophysiology of, 371

  management of, 378–380

    renal replacement therapy in, 380–384

  multisystem complications of, 376, 376t

  peritoneal dialysis in, 380–381

  postrenal, 370

  prerenal, 370, 378

    vs. acute tubular necrosis, 372, 372t

  uremia in, 374–375

Renal system, 360–386. See also *Kidney(s); Renal failure.*

  active transport mechanisms of, 362

  anatomy of, 360–361

  assessment of, 361–370

    acid-base balance in, 369

    arterial blood pressure regulation in, 369

    clearance measurement in, 363–364

    creatinine production in, 370

    electrolyte balance in, 367–369

    erythropoietin production in, 370

    glomerular filtration rate in, 362–364, 363t

    physical, 361

    renal blood flow in, 369–370

    sodium concentration in, 367

    tubular reabsorption in, 364–365

    tubular secretion in, 365

    urea production in, 370

    uric acid production in, 370

    urine concentration in, 365

    urine formation in, 362–365

    vasopressin in, 366–367

    water balance in, 365–367

  filtration process of, 362–365, 363t, 366t

  passive transport mechanisms of, 362

  transport mechanisms of, 362

  trauma to, 385–386, 584

Renal transplantation, 384–385

Renal tubules, 366t. See also *Acute tubular necrosis.*

  countercurrent mechanism of, 365–366

Renal tubules *(Continued)*
  fluid reabsorption by, 364–365
  secretory processes of, 365
Renin-angiotensin system, in shock, 194
Renin-angiotensin-aldosterone system, in arterial
        pressure regulation, 155
  in peripheral vascular resistance, 369
Repolarization, of neuron, 286
Residual volume, 41, *41*
Resistance, airway, 74, 75
Respiration. See also *Respiratory system; Ventilation,
        mechanical.*
  in CNS infection, 335
  in neurologic assessment, 300, 307t
  in scoliosis, 351–352
  in spinal cord injury, 349
  in trauma assessment, 569
Respiratory center, 40, *40*
Respiratory cyanosis, in cardiovascular system
        assessment, 159
Respiratory distress syndrome. See also *Adult
        respiratory distress syndrome.*
  surfactant in, 65
Respiratory effort, 45, *46*
Respiratory failure, 184
  acute, 67–73
    clinical course of, 69
    clinical presentation of, 68–69
    definition of, 67
    diagnostic tests in, 69
    management of, 69–73, 70t, *71,* 71t, 72t
      complications of, 73
      medications in, 60t, 72, 72t
      outcomes of, 73
      rapid-sequence intubation in, 72
      supplemental oxygen in, 69, 70t, 71t, 72
    nonpulmonary causes of, 67–68
    pathophysiology of, 67–68, 67t, *68*
    patient history in, 68
    physical examination in, 68–69
    prevention of, 69
    pulmonary causes of, 67
  in acquired immunodeficiency syndrome, 533
  in bronchopulmonary dysplasia, 134
Respiratory frequency, 73t
Respiratory insufficiency, 45, *46*
Respiratory rate, 75
  in respiratory failure, 184
Respiratory reflex, in cardiac regulation, 153
Respiratory syncytial virus, case study of, 692–694
  in pneumonia, 104t
  intravenous immunoglobulin prophylaxis against,
        502
Respiratory system. See also *Airway; Lungs.*
  anatomy of, comparative, 67, 67t, *68*
    developmental, 33–38, *34, 35*
  angiography of, 52
  anticholinergic drug effects on, 63, 64t
  clinical assessment of, 43–51
    auscultation in, 47–48
    cough in, 50t, 51
    cyanosis in, 49, *50,* 51
    inspection in, 43–46, *44–46*
    palpation in, 46–47

Respiratory system *(Continued)*
    patient history in, 43
    percussion in, 47, *47*
    physical examination in, 43–51, *44–47,* 49t, *50,*
        50t
    stridor in, 48–49, 49t
  compliance monitoring of, 56–57
  computed tomography of, 52
  developmental physiology of, 38–43, *39–42*
  disorders of. See also specific disorders, e.g.,
        Respiratory failure.
    β-agonist medications for, 66
    antiflammatory agents for, 66
    barbiturates for, 60t, 62
    benzodiazepines for, 59–61, 60t
    bronchodilators for, 65–66
    corticosteroids for, 66
    diagnostic studies in, 51–53, 53t
    ketamine for, 60t, 62
    neuromuscular blocking agents for, 59, 72t
    nitric oxide for, 65
    opiates for, 60t, 61
    propofol for, 60t, 62–63
    surfactant for, 65
  drug effects on, 57–66, 58t, 60t, 64t. See also
        specific drugs.
    blood flow and, 58–59
    body fluid distribution and, 58, 58t
    dosing strategies and, 59
    enteral absorption and, 58
    protein binding and, 58
    remedial agents for, 63–66, 64t
  end-tidal carbon dioxide monitoring of, 55, 56t
  flumazenil effects on, 64t, 65
  fluoroscopy of, 52
  in congenital heart disease, 213–214
  laboratory evaluation of, 51–53, 53t
  magnetic resonance imaging of, 52
  mixed venous oxygen saturation monitoring of, 54
  monitoring of, 54–57, 56t, *57*
  naloxone effects on, 63, 64t, 65
  pressure manometer monitoring of, 56
  pulse oximetry monitoring of, 54
  radiologic evaluation of, 52
  spirometry monitoring of, 56, *57*
  transcutaneous carbon dioxide monitoring of, 55,
        56t
  transcutaneous oxygen monitoring of, 54
  ventilation-perfusion scan of, 52
  volume loops evaluation of, 57
  x-ray of, 52
Resting membrane potential, cardiac, 156, 157
  neuronal, 286
Reticular formation, 282
Reticulocytes, 465
  reference values for, 485t
Reticulocyte count, 484
Retinal hemorrhage, in child abuse, 592
Retinoic acid, maternal use of, fetal cardiac anomalies
        and, 160t
Revised Trauma Score, 573–574
Reye's syndrome, 342–345
  diagnosis of, 344
  etiology of, 343

Reye's syndrome *(Continued)*
  incidence of, 343
  management of, 344
  pathophysiology of, 343
  progression of, 343–344
Rh blood group, 491
  in platelet transfusion, 503
Rheumatic fever, 263–264, 264t
  diagnosis of, 263
  etiology of, 263
  management of, 264
  nursing diagnoses in, 263
  pathophysiology of, 263
  signs and symptoms of, 263, 264t
Rhinorrhea, in basilar fracture, 341
Rhombencephalon, *276*
Ribs, fracture of, 94, 96, 96t, 97, 583t
Rickets, in hepatic failure, 455
Rifampin, prophylactic, in septic shock prevention, 649
Right bundle branch system, 156, *156*
Right coronary artery, 149, *149*
Robinul (glycopyrrolate), 430
  in acute respiratory failure, 72t
Rocuronium, in acute respiratory failure, 72t
Romazicon (flumazenil), antagonistic action of, 64t, 65
  in benzodiazepine poisoning, 609
Rooting reflex, evaluation of, 298
Ross procedure, in aortic stenosis, 229

S
Saccular aneurysm, intracranial, 329–330
Salicylate poisoning, 602t, 614–615
Salivary glands, 424
  autonomic nerve stimulation of, 295t
Salter-Harris fracture classification, 586, 586t
Sandimmune (cyclosporine), 430–431, 495
Scalding, 590, 668t
Scalp, 277
Scar, after burn injury, 671
School-age children, communication with, 16
  development of, 2–3
  fears of, 7
  pain management in, 12t–13t
  play opportunities for, 18
  stress response of, 6
  working with, 3
Scimitar syndrome, cardiac anomalies in, 160t
SCIWORA (spinal cord injury without radiographic abnormalities), 581
Scoliosis, 350–352
  cardiac output in, 352
  congenital, 351
  diagnosis of, 351
  idiopathic, 351
  management of, 351–352
  neuromuscular, 351
  pain in, 352
  pathophysiology of, 351
  respiration in, 351–352
  spinal cord injury in, 352
Sedation, communication during, 16–17
  in congenital diaphragmatic hernia, 124
  in persistent pulmonary hypertension of newborn, 127

Sedative poisoning, 602t
Seizures, 324–327
  aura of, 325
  classification of, 324–325
  definition of, 324
  etiology of, 324
  generalized (convulsive or nonconvulsive), 325, 326t
  in antidepressant poisoning, 608
  in isoniazid poisoning, 613–614
  incidence of, 324
  management of, 325–327, 327t
  motor symptoms of, 325
  neurodiagnostic findings in, 325, 326t
  partial (focal, local), 324–325, 326t
  pathophysiology of, 325
  postictal phase of, 325
  prodromal period of, 325
  systemic effects of, 325
Selective digestive decontamination, in septic shock prevention, 648
Selenious acid poisoning, 624
Semilunar valves, 147–148, *147*
  development of, 147
Sengstaken-Blakemore tube, in esophageal varices, 438, *438*
Sensory deprivation, in critical care unit, 9
  interventions for, 17
Sensory overload, interventions for, 17
Sepsis, 639. See also *Septic shock.*
Septic shock, 627–651, *634*
  arachidonic acid metabolites in, 631
  assessment of, ABG analysis in, 640
    auscultation in, 638
    blood culture in, 640
    cerebrospinal fluid examination in, 640
    chemistry tests in, 640
    chest x-ray in, 640
    fecal cultures in, 640
    hematologic studies in, 639–640
    hemodynamic monitoring in, 641, 641t
    laboratory tests in, 639–640
    radiologic examination in, 640
    sputum cultures in, 640
    urine specimen in, 640
  baroreceptors in, 636
  blood volume distribution in, 632–633, *632, 634*
  carbohydrate metabolism in, 635
  cardiac dysfunction in, *632,* 633
  cardiac output and, 628
  cellular responses in, 630t, 631
  chemoreceptors in, 636
  clinical assessment of, 636–650
    family history in, 637
    inspection in, 637
    liver palpation in, 638
    medication history in, 637
    nursing history in, 636–637
    palpation in, 637–638
    past medical history in, 637
    social-cultural history in, 637
  clinical manifestations of, 638–639, 638t
  CNS ischemia reflex in, 636
  compensatory responses to, 635–636

Septic shock *(Continued)*
  complications of, 650–651, 651t
  cytokines in, 631
  developmental aspects of, 627–628
  endogenous mediators of, 630–631
  endotoxin in, 630
  epidemiology of, 628–629
  etiology of, 628
  exogenous mediators of, 630
  extracorporeal life support in, 187
  free radicals in, 631
  hyperdynamic, 638–639, 638t
  hypodynamic, 638–639, 638t
  hypoxemia in, 633
  immune system in, 629–635, *632, 634, 635*
  incidence of, 628–629
  interleukin-1 in, 632
  mediator release in, *632,* 633
  metabolic alterations in, 635
  multiple-organ dysfunction syndrome with, 650–651, 651t
  nitric oxide in, 632
  norepinephrine-epinephrine vasoconstrictor reflex in, 636
  nursing diagnoses in, 641–642
  oxygen consumption and, 628
  oxygen imbalance in, *632,* 633, 635, *635*
  pathophysiology of, 629–636
    blood volume distribution in, 632–633, *632*
    cardiac dysfunction in, *632,* 633
    cytokines in, 631
    endogenous mediators in, 630–631
    endotoxin in, 632
    exogenous mediators in, 630
    free radicals in, 631
    interleukin-1 in, 632
    lipid mediators in, 631
    metabolic changes in, 635
    nitric oxide in, 632
    oxygen supply and demand in, 633–635, *634, 635*
    proteases in, 632
    systemic inflammatory response syndrome in, 629–630, 631t
    tumor necrosis factor in, 632
  plasma enzyme cascade activation in, 631
  prevention of, 647
  proteases in, 632
  risk factors for, 629
  stretch receptors in, 636
  treatment of, 642–650
    ABCs in, 642–643, 644t
    antibiotics in, 643
    barotrauma with, 647
    cardiac output in, 646
    cardiovascular therapy in, 645t, 646
    dobutamine in, 645t
    dopamine in, 645t
    epinephrine in, 645t
    fluid therapy in, 646
    goals of, 642
    heart rate optimization in, 646
    isoproterenol in, 645t
    nitroglycerin in, 645t
    norepinephrine in, 645t

Septic shock *(Continued)*
    oxygen in, 646–647
    phenylephrine in, 645t
    precautions with, 647–648
    respiratory therapy in, 646–657
    resuscitation in, 642–644, 644t, 646
    sodium nitroprusside in, 645t
    supportive therapy in, 648–650
    vasoactive agents in, 643, 645t, 646
    vasodilators in, 646
    vasopressors in, 646
    volume resuscitation in, 643
  tumor necrosis factor in, 632
Septum, ventricular, pulmonary atresia with, 254–255, *255*
Septum transversum, in diaphragm development, 121
Severe combined immunodeficiency, 524–526
  complications of, 526
  diagnosis of, 524–525
  etiology of, 524, 525
  management of, 525–526
  nursing diagnoses in, 525
  pathophysiology of, 524
  signs and symptoms of, 524
Sex hormones, maternal use of, fetal cardiac anomalies and, 160t
Sexual abuse, 592–594. See also *Child abuse.*
  interview in, 594
  physical examination in, 593–594
  treatment of, 593–594
Sexual assault (rape), 592
Shaken impact syndrome, 591–592
Shock, 193–196
  cardiogenic, 194
  cellular changes in, 194
  compensatory mechanisms in, 194
  compensatory phase of, 195
  definition of, 193–194
  diagnosis of, 195
  etiology of, 194–195
  glomerular filtration rate and, 363, 364t
  hypovolemic, 194
  in diabetic ketoacidosis, 410t
  management of, 195–196
  metabolic changes in, 194–195
  nursing diagnoses in, 195
  pathophysiology of, 194–195
  progressive phase of, 195
  refractory phase of, 195
  septic, 627–651. See also *Septic shock.*
  signs and symptoms of, 195
Shoulders, testing of, 307t
Shunt, ventricular, 318–320, *319*
Siblings, working with, 24
Sick sinus syndrome, 199
Sickle cell disease, 517–522
  acute chest syndrome in, 520
  aplastic crisis in, 519–520
  bone marrow necrosis in, 521–522
  cerebrovascular accident in, 521
  complications of, 519–522
    prevention of, 518
  diagnosis of, 518
  etiology of, 517

Sickle cell disease *(Continued)*
  fat embolism in, 521–522
  infection in, 519
  management of, 518–519
  multiorgan dysfunction syndrome in, 522
  pain management in, 518–519
  pathophysiology of, 517
  priapism in, 522
  risk factors for, 517
  signs and symptoms of, 518
  splenic sequestration crisis in, 519
  vasoocclusive crisis in, 520–521
Sickle cell–β-thalassemia, 517
Sieving coefficient, in continuous renal replacement
     therapy, 382
Silver nitrate solution 0.5%, in burn injury, 670,
     670t
Silver sulfadiazine, in burn injury, 670, 670t
Sinoatrial block, 198
Sinoatrial node, 155, *156*, 157
  conduction disorders of, 198, *205*
Sinoatrial pause, 198
Sinus arrhythmia, *197*
  respiratory reflex in, 153
Sinus bradycardia, *197*, 198–199, *205*
Sinus dysrhythmia, 197–198
Sinus pause, *197*, 201, *201*
Sinus rhythm, *197*
Sinus tachycardia, *197*, 198, *205*
Skateboard trauma, 562
Skin, antigen barrier of, 471–472
  autonomic nerve stimulation of, 295t
  burns of, 652–675. See also *Burns.*
  care of, during mechanical ventilation, 83–84
  chemical burn of, 618–620
  color of, in cardiovascular system assessment,
     159–161
  cyanosis of, 46
  functions of, 653
  hydrofluoric acid injury to, 619–620
  in graft-versus-host disease, 545, 546
  in spinal cord injury, 349–350
  irrigation of, 603
  organophosphate exposure of, 626–627
  structure of, 653, *655*
Skin testing, 492
Skin-associated lymphoid tissue, 464
Skull, 277
  fracture of, 340
  inspection of, 296
  percussion of, 297
     in hydrocephalus, 339
  volume of, 287, *288*
  x-ray of, 309
     in brain trauma, 342
     in hydrocephalus, 339
Sledding safety, 560t
Sleep, in pulmonary disease, 43
Sleep deprivation, in critical care unit, 9, 10t
  interventions for, 17
Smell, testing of, in child, 303t
  in infant, 302t
Smoke inhalation, 660. See also *Burns.*
Snake bites, 621–622

Sodium, in fluid homeostasis, 367
  serum, 368, 410
     in diabetic ketoacidosis, 410t
Sodium bicarbonate, in metabolic acidosis, 368
Sodium nitrite, in cyanide poisoning, 621
Sodium nitroprusside, in septic shock, 645t
Sodium thiosulfate, in cyanide poisoning, 621
Solu-Medrol (methylprednisolone), for
     immunosuppressive therapy, 431
  in asthma, 114t
  in pulmonary disorders, 66
  in spinal cord injury, 348–349
Somatomedin C, reference range for, 406t
Somatosensory evoked responses, in neurologic
     assessment, 316
Somatostatin, 392, 428
Somatotrophs, 394
Sorbitol, in poisoning management, 605
Sound, critical care unit levels of, 8, 9t, 17
Spider bites, 621–622
Spina bifida, 352–354
Spina bifida cystica, 353
Spina bifida occulta, 353
Spinal accessory nerve, 291t, 303t, 307t
Spinal cord, 283–286, *285*, 285t
  embryogenesis of, 276
  hemorrhage of, 347
  injury to, 345–350, 581–582
     autonomic hyperreflexia in, 347
     cardiac output in, 349
     complete, 345
     concussion in, 346
     contusion in, 346
     diagnosis of, 348
     elimination in, 350
     etiology of, 346
     gas exchange in, 349
     in scoliosis, 352
     incidence of, 346
     incomplete, 345–346
     laceration in, 346
     management of, 348–349
     pathophysiology of, 346–347
     pulmonary infection in, 350
     respiratory function in, 349
     shock in, 347
     skin integrity in, 349–350
     temperature regulation in, 350
     transection in, 346, 347
     without radiographic abnormality, 346
  tracts of, 285, 285t
  tumor compression of, 516
Spinal cord injury without radiographic abnormalities
     (SCIWORA), 581
Spinal dysraphism, 352–354
Spinal nerves, 289, *290*
Spinal shock, 347
Spine, 283, *284*
  circulation of, 286
  congenital abnormalities of, 352–354
  curvature of, 350–352. See also *Scoliosis.*
  decompression of, in spinal cord injury, 348
  fractures of, 345–350, 575. See also *Spinal cord,
     injury to.*

Spine (*Continued*)
  fusion of, in scoliosis, 351–352
  immobilization of, in spinal cord injury, 348
  surgical fixation of, in spinal cord injury, 348
  x-ray of, 309
    in spinal cord injury, 348, 575
Spirometry, 56, *57*
Splanchnic circulation, 426
Spleen, in hematopoiesis, 463
  palpation of, 483–484
  trauma to, 433–435
    in child abuse, 590
Splenectomy, in idiopathic thrombocytopenic
    purpura, 537
  in trauma, 434
Splenomegaly, in sickle cell disease, 519
Splenorrhaphy, in trauma, 434
Sports, adolescent injury during, 554
Sputum examination, in *Pneumocystis carinii*
    pneumonia, 530–531
  in pneumonia, 105
  in pulmonary evaluation, 53t
ST segment, on electrocardiography, *167*, 168
Staff, psychological support for, 30
Status epilepticus, 326–327, 327t
Stem cells, 461, *462*
  aplasia of, 462
  hypoplasia of, 462
Steroids, in idiopathic thrombocytopenic purpura, 537
  in lymphocytic interstitial pneumonitis, 532–533
  in *Pneumocystis carinii* pneumonia, 531
Stomach, 424, *425*
  acidity of, 472
  autonomic nerve stimulation of, 294t
  trauma to, 435
Stomatitis, 512
Strangulation, prevention of, 557t
Streptokinase, 498
Stress, coping response to, 5–6
  family, 19–26. See also *Family.*
    assessment of, 20–22
    interventions for, 22–26
  fears and, 6–7
  interventions for, 10–19
    communication as, 15–17
    emotional support as, 18–19
    environmental measures as, 17
    pain management as, 10–14, 11t–13t, 15t
    play as, 17–18
  pain in, 7–8, 7t
  physiologic responses to, 5
  sensory deprivation and, 9, 10t
  sensory overload and, 8–9, 10t
  sleep deprivation and, 9
  technology and, 9–10
Stretch receptors, in blood flow regulation, 152
  in cardiac regulation, 153
  in septic shock, 636
Stridor, 48–49, 49t
  differential diagnosis of, 101t
Stroke, in sickle cell disease, 521
Stroke volume, 153–155, *154*
Stupor, 297
Subaortic stenosis, discrete, 229
Subthalamus, 281

Succinylcholine, in acute respiratory failure, 72t
Sucking, testing of, 303t
Sucralfate (Carafate), 429
Sufentanil, for pain, 15t
Suffocation, in infants, 552
Suicide, adolescent, 554
Sulfamylon (mafenide acetate cream), in burn injury,
    670, 670t
Superior mediastinal syndrome, 516
Supernormal period, of cardiac muscle, 157
Supratentorial herniation, in intracranial pressure
    elevation, 321–322, *321*
Supraventricular dysrhythmias, 197–203, *197, 200,*
    202t. See also specific dysrhythmias.
Supraventricular tachycardia, 199–200, *200*
Surfactant, in respiratory distress syndrome, 65
Sutures, cranial, 277, *278*
  in trauma assessment, 570
Svo$_2$ monitoring, 178
Swallowing, testing of, 303t, 306t
Sweat chloride test, in pulmonary evaluation, 53t
Sympathetic nervous system, 291, *292*
  in blood flow regulation, 152
  in cardiac regulation, 153
Sympathomimetic drug poisoning, 615–616
Synapse, 277
  in impulse conduction, 286–287
Syndrome of inappropriate antidiuretic hormone
    secretion, 417–419
  collaborative diagnoses in, 419
  complications of, 419
  diagnosis of, 418–419
  differential diagnosis of, 418–419
  during mechanical ventilation, 85
  etiology of, 417–418
  pathophysiology of, 417
  signs and symptoms of, 418, 418t
  treatment of, 419
Systemic inflammatory response syndrome, 511,
    629–630, 630t, 639. See also *Septic shock.*
Systemic vascular resistance, 154, 177

T

T wave, on electrocardiography, *167,* 168
Tachycardia, in trauma assessment, 569–570
Tacrolimus (Prograf), 430
Talwin (pentazocine) poisoning, 614
Taste, testing of, 306t
Taylor Pharmaceuticals Cyanide Antidote Package, 621
Tearing, 472
Technology, in critical care unit, 9–10
Teeth, care guidelines for, 514t
  traumatic loss of, 580
Telangiectasis, in hepatic failure, 455
Telencephalon, 275, *275, 276,* 279–280, *280*
Temperature, body, in neurologic assessment, 300, 308
    in spinal cord injury, 347, 350
    with infection, 511–512
Temporal lobe, 279–280, *280*
Tendons, injury to, 588
Tension pneumothorax, 91, *92,* 94, 95–96, 96t, 583t.
    See also *Pneumothorax.*
  in congenital diaphragmatic hernia, 124
Tentorium cerebelli, 278
Terbutaline, in asthma, 114t

Terminally ill child, 26–30
　care for, 27–28
　organ donation from, 27
　pain management of, 26
　treatment withdrawal from, 26–27
Testes, trauma to, 584
Tetralogy of Fallot, 242–244, *244*
　anatomy of, 242, *242*
Thalamus, of diencephalon, 281
Thalidomide, maternal, fetal cardiac anomalies and,
　　160t
Theophylline, in bronchopulmonary dysplasia, 134
Theophylline poisoning, 602t, 616
Thermoregulation, in continuous renal replacement
　　therapy, 383
Thiazide diuretics, in acute renal failure, 379
Thiopental, in pulmonary disorders, 60t
Thirst, 367
Thoracentesis, in pneumothorax, 92, *93*
　in trauma treatment, 576
Thoratec ventricular assist device, 189t
Thorax, contours of, 44, *44*
　developmental anatomy of, 37
　inspection of, 43–45, *44, 45*
　percussion of, 47, *47*
　trauma to, 94–97, *95*, 576, 582, 583t
　　clinical presentation of, 95–96
　　complications for, 97
　　diagnostic tests for, 96, 96t
　　etiology of, 94
　　outcomes of, 97
　　pathophysiology of, 94–95
　　patient history of, 95
　　physical examination in, 95–96
　　supportive care for, 97
Threshold potential, of cardiac muscle cell, 157
Thrombocytes, 469
Thrombocytopenia, 480
　in septic shock, 639
Thrombocytopenic purpura, idiopathic, 536–537
　vs. hemolytic-uremic syndrome, 537
Thromboplastin time, 490
Thrombopoietin, 461
Thrombosis, heparin for, 497
Thromboxane, in septic shock, 631
Thrombus, with cardiac assist devices, 190
Thymus gland, in hematopoiesis, 463
　location of, *388*
Thyroglobulin, 397–398
Thyroid gland, 397–399
　cells of, 397–398
　development of, 399
　dysfunction of, cardiac anomalies in, 160t
　hormones of, 389t
　iodine metabolism of, 398
　location of, *388*, 397
Thyroid-stimulating hormone, 389t, 396
　reference range for, 407t
Thyrotrophs, 394
Thyrotropin. See *Thyroid-stimulating hormone.*
Thyrotropin-releasing hormone, 394t, 396
Thyroxine (T_4), 389t, 398
　abnormalities of, 398–399
　reference range for, 406t
Tidal volume, 73, 73t, 75

Tissue plasminogen activator, 498
Tissue typing, of human leukocyte antigens, 487
Titralac (calcium carbonate), 429
Toddlers, communication with, 15–16
　development of, 2
　fears of, 6
　pain management in, 11t
　play opportunities for, 18
　stress response of, 5
　working with, 3
Toes, traumatic amputation of, 587–588
Toe-to-heel walking, 300
Tongue, testing of, in child, 306t, 307t
　in infant, 303t
Total anomalous pulmonary venous return, 251–254,
　　252
Total lung capacity, 41, *41*, 73t
Touch, evaluation of, 299
　sensitivity to, 29
Tours, of hospital, 18
Toxicology, 595–627. See also *Poisoning.*
Trachea, *35*
　aspiration of, in pulmonary evaluation, 53t
　embryology of, 36
　rupture of, 583t
　trauma to, 94, 97
Tracheitis, *98*
　differential diagnosis of, 101t
Tracheoesophageal fistula, 128–131, 444t–445t
　clinical presentation of, 130
　definition of, 128
　diagnosis of, 130
　embryology of, 128–129, *129*
　incidence of, 129
　operative management of, 130
　postoperative care in, 130–131
　preoperative care in, 130
　tracheomalacia with, 129
Tracheomalacia, in tracheoesophageal fistula, 129
Tracheostomy, in trauma treatment, 575
Transcutaneous carbon dioxide monitoring, 55
Transcutaneous oxygen monitoring, 54
Transjugular intrahepatic portal-systemic shunt, in
　　esophageal varices, 439, *439*
Transplantation. See *Bone marrow transplantation; Liver,
　　transplantation of; Lung(s), transplantation.*
Transport, in renal system, 362
Transposition of great vessels, 245–247, *247*
Trauma, 551–594
　abdominal, 431–435, 582. See also *Abdomen, trauma
　　to.*
　acceleration-deceleration forces in, 562
　AMPLE history in, 567
　amputation, 587–588
　animal bite–related, 562
　　prevention of, 559t
　assessment of, abdomen examination in, 572
　　airway evaluation in, 568–569
　　back examination in, 573
　　cervical spine evaluation in, 568–569
　　chest examination in, 572
　　chest x-ray in, 578
　　circulatory evaluation in, 569–570
　　computed tomography in, 578
　　ear examination in, 572

Trauma *(Continued)*
  exposure evaluation in, 571
  extremity examination in, 573
  eye examination in, 572
  face examination in, 571–572
  head examination in, 571
  neck examination in, 572
  nerve evaluation in, 587
  neurologic evaluation in, 570–571, 587
  nose examination in, 572
  patient health history in, 567
  patient history in, 565–567
  pelvis examination in, 573
  peritoneal lavage in, 578
  primary, 568–571
  pulse oximetry in, 573
  respiratory evaluation in, 569
  resuscitation after, 565–574
  secondary, 571–573, 571t
  trauma scoring in, 573–574
  vital signs in, 573
  AVPU evaluation in, 570
  bicycle, 562
    prevention of, 560t
  brain, 339–342. See also *Brain, trauma to.*
  burns in, 552, 563, 652–675. See also *Burns.*
  by developmental stage, 552–554
  cardiac, 268–269, *268*
  cardiac arrest with, 576–577
  chemical, 563
  choking in, 552
    prevention of, 557t
  cold-related, 563–564, 564t, 565t
  consciousness evaluation in, 577
  crush, 562
  drowning in, 553, 563
    prevention of, 558t, 560t
  electrical, 563
  epidemiology of, 551–552, 551t
  extremity, 587–588
  falls in, 552, 553, 554
    prevention of, 555t–556t
  firearm-related, 562–563
  genitourinary tract, 584
  hanging-related, 563
  head, 579–580
  heat-related, 565, 566t
  homicide-related, 554
  in infants, 552
  in toddlers, 552–553
  incidence of, 551–552, 551t
  knife, 563
  maxillofacial, 580–581
  mechanisms of, 554, 561–565
    by developmental stage, 552–554
    in adolescents, 554
    in infants, 552
    in preschoolers, 553
    in school-age children, 553
    in toddlers, 552–553
    kinetic forces in, 554, 561–563
  musculoskeletal, 584–587, *585*, 586t
  nerve, 587
  of child abuse, 588–594. See also *Child abuse.*

Trauma *(Continued)*
  pain management in, 578
  patient health history in, 567
  patient history of, 565–567
  Pediatric Coma Scale in, 571t
  penetrating, 562–563
  prevention of, 555t–560t
  radiant, 563
  renal, 385–386, 584
  resuscitation after, 565
  shear, 562
  skateboard, 562
  spinal cord, 345–350, 581–582. See also *Spinal cord, injury to.*
  sports-related, 554
  suffocation in, 552
  suicide-related, 554
  thermal, 563
  thoracic, 94–97, *95*, 576, 582, 583t. See also *Thorax, trauma to.*
  treatment of, 574–578
    airway procedures in, 574–575
    body part preservation in, 577
    circulation procedures in, 576–577
    compartment syndrome with, 588
    crystalloid fluids in, 576
    emotional support in, 578–579
    fracture immobilization in, 577
    gastric tube insertion in, 577
    intravenous access for, 576
    laboratory tests in, 576
    pain management in, 578
    respiration procedures in, 575–576, 577
    urinary catheter in, 577
    warming procedures in, 577
  vehicle-related, 552, 554, 561–662
    adolescent injury in, 554
    air bags in, 561
    case study of, 384–386
    infant injury in, 552
    patient history in, 565–566
    pedestrian injury in, 561–562
    preschooler injury in, 553
    prevention of, 557t–558t, 560t
    restraining devices in, 561
    school-age children injury in, 553
    toddler injury in, 553
Trauma Score, 573–574
Traumatic aneurysm, intracranial, 329–330
TRH stimulation test, 405
Tricuspid atresia, 247–249
Tricuspid valve, 147, *147*
  in Ebstein's anomaly, 224–226, *225*
Tricyclic antidepressant poisoning, 601t, 607–608
  case study of, 695–696
Trigeminal nerve, 291t, 302t, 305t
Triiodothyronine (T$_3$), 389t, 398–399
  reference range for, 406t
Trills, in cardiovascular system assessment, 162
Trimethadione, maternal use of, fetal cardiac anomalies and, 160t
Trimethoprim-sulfamethoxazole, in *Pneumocystis carinii* pneumonia, 531
  side effects of, 494

Trisomy 13 (Patau's syndrome), cardiac anomalies in, 160t

Trisomy 18 (Edward's syndrome), cardiac anomalies in, 160t

Trisomy 21 (Down syndrome), cardiac anomalies in, 160t

Trochlear nerve, 291t, 302t, 305t

Truncus arteriosus, 249–251, *250*
  classification of, 249, *250*
  division of, 146
  extracardiac anomalies in, 250

Tumors, brain, 335–338. See also *Brain, tumors of.*
  complications of, 515–516
    spinal cord compression with, 516
    superior mediastinal syndrome with, 516
    tumor lysis syndrome with, 515–516

Tumor lysis syndrome, 515–516
  acute renal failure in, 378

Tumor necrosis factor, 478t
  in septic shock, 632

Turner's syndrome, cardiac anomalies in, 160t

Twitch monitoring, during mechanical ventilation, 83

Tyrosinemia, liver transplantation in, 456

U

Ulcers, in burn injury, 656
  treatment of, in septic shock prevention, 648

Ultrafiltration, in continuous renal replacement therapy, 383

Ultrasound, in acute renal failure, 372
  in neurologic assessment, 315
  in renal trauma, 385

Umbilical vein, 148

Uncal herniation, in intracranial pressure elevation, 321, *321*

Urea, production of, 370

Uremia, in acute renal failure, 374–375
  platelet function and, 480

Ureter, autonomic nerve stimulation of, 295t

Urethra, trauma to, 584

Uric acid, production of, 370

Urinalysis, in acute renal failure, 372
  in trauma evaluation, 584

Urinary catheterization, contraindication to, 584
  in trauma treatment, 577

Urination, in spinal cord injury, 350

Urine, analysis of, in acute renal failure, 372
  in trauma evaluation, 584
  blood in, 584
  concentration of, 365
  formation of, 362–365
  output of, in burn injury, 673

Urokinase, 498

Uterus, autonomic nerve stimulation of, 295t

V

V receptors, for antidiuretic hormone, 395

Vaccines, in septic shock prevention, 649

Vagus nerve, 291t, 303t, 307t

Valium (diazepam), for pain, 15t
  in pulmonary disorders, 59–61, 60t
  in status epilepticus, 327t

Valves, cardiac. See also specific valves.
  embryologic development of, 146–148, *147*

Valvuloplasty, in aortic stenosis, 228, *228*

Varices, esophageal, 438–439, *438*

Vasoconstriction, in inflammatory response, 472
  in shock, 194

Vasoconstrictor reflex, in septic shock, 636

Vasodilation, 152
  in inflammation, 472, 630t

Vasodilators, in congestive heart failure, 193

Vasomotor center, in blood flow regulation, 152–153

Vasoocclusion crisis, in sickle cell disease, 520–521

Vasopressin. See *Antidiuretic hormone.*

Veins, 148
  autonomic nerve stimulation of, 294t

Venoconstriction, 152

Venous switch operation, in transposition of great vessels, 246

Ventilation, alveolar, 73t, 74
  in intracranial pressure elevation, 323
  mechanical, 73–86
    acute lung injury with, 85
    arterial blood gases during, 82–83
    assessment of, 82
    atelectasis with, 85
    barotrauma with, 85
    cardiac output with, 85
    case study of, 692–693
    chest physiotherapy during, 84
    complications of, 85–86
    disease-specific requirements for, 80t
    flow delivery patterns for, 77, *80*
    fluid monitoring during, 83
    high-frequency, 77, 79
    in acute respiratory failure, 69–70, 70t, 71t, 72
    in adult respiratory distress syndrome, 118, *119*
    in asthma, 111–113
    in bronchopulmonary dysplasia, 133
    in congenital diaphragmatic hernia, 123–124
    in persistent pulmonary hypertension of newborn, 127
    in *Pneumocystis carinii* pneumonia, 531
    in tracheoesophageal fistula, 130
    in trauma treatment, 576
    inverse-ratio, 77
    liquid, 81
    management of, 82–86
    monitoring of, 82–83
    negative pressure, 81
    nutrition during, 83
    objectives of, 73
    oxygen toxicity with, 85
    performance specifications for, 75–76
    phase variables in, 77, *79, 80*
    physiologic principles of, 73–76, 73t, *74*
    pneumonia with, 85
    positive pressure, 76–77, *78–80*
      noninvasive, 81–82
    psychologic aspects of, 84
    SIADH with, 85
    skin care during, 83–84
    supportive care during, 83–84
    trigger mechanism in, 77, *79*
    twitch monitoring during, 83
    weaning from, 84–85
      in congenital heart disease, 213–214

Ventilation-perfusion matching, 39
Ventilation-perfusion mismatch, in adult respiratory
   distress syndrome, 117
   in bronchopulmonary dysplasia, 132
Ventilation-perfusion scan, in pulmonary evaluation,
   52
   in respiratory distress, 52
Ventricles, cardiac, 146, *146, 147*
   depolarization of, 158
   double inlet, 248
   embryologic development of, 145, *146*
   function of, 153–155, *154*
   hypertrophy of, 161
   isometric relaxation of, 158
   repolarization of, 158
   intracranial, 278
      external drainage of, 317–318, *317*
      internal drainage of, 318–320, *319*
Ventricular assist device, 188, 189t
Ventricular dysrhythmias, 203–204, *203.* See also
   specific dysrhythmias.
Ventricular fibrillation, *203*
Ventricular septal defect, 220–222, *220*
   in double outlet right ventricle, 223–224
   pulmonary atresia with, 244, *245*
Ventricular septal myotomy, in cardiomyopathy, 260
Ventricular septum, pulmonary atresia with, 254–255,
   255
Ventricular shunt, 318–320, *319*
Ventricular tachycardia, 203–204, *203*
Venules, 148
Verapamil (Isoptin), cardiovascular effects of, 182
Verapamil poisoning, 609–610
Vercuronium, in acute respiratory failure, 72t
Versed (midazolam), for pain, 15t
   in pulmonary disorders, 59–61, 60t
   in status epilepticus, 327t
Vertebrae, 283, *284.* See also *Spine.*
   congenital abnormalities of, 352–354
Vertebral arteries, 282
Vertebral line, *44*
Vertigo, in basilar fracture, 341
Vesicular breath sounds, 48
Vibration sense, evaluation of, 299
Vision, testing of, in child, 304t–305t
   in infant, 302t–303t
Visiting privileges, 25–26
Visual evoked responses, in neurologic assessment,
   316
Vital capacity, 41, *41,* 73t, 74
Vital signs, in trauma assessment, 573

Vitamin D, in phosphate metabolism, 368
Vitamin K, deficiency of, 517
Vitamin K$_1$ (AquaMEPHYTON), 428
Vitelline vein, 148
Vocal cords, 36
Volume loops, evaluation of, 57
Volume resuscitation, in septic shock, 643
Volvulus, 442t
Vulnerable period, of cardiac muscle, 157

W

Warfarin (Coumadin), 497–498
   administration of, 498
   mechanisms of action of, 498
   side effects of, 498
Warming, passive, in trauma treatment, 577
Water, body, 58, 58t
Water balance, 365–367
   antidiuretic hormone in, 366–367, 694
Water deprivation test, in diabetes insipidus, 421
Water moccasin snake bite, 621–622
Water safety, 560t
Western blot, for human immunodeficiency virus
   antibody, 528
Wheezing, 48. See also *Asthma.*
   differential diagnosis of, 109–110
   in respiratory failure, 184
White blood cell count, in pulmonary evaluation, 53t
White blood cells, 466–469. See also *Leukocyte(s)* and
   specific types.
White blood count, 484, 485t, 486
   differential, 485t, 486
   total, 484, 486
White matter, of spinal cord, 283–285, *285*
Williams' syndrome, cardiac anomalies in, 160t
Wilson's disease, liver transplantation in, 456
Wolff-Parkinson-White syndrome, 200
Wrinkle test, in trauma evaluation, 587

X

Xanthomas, in hepatic failure, 455
Xenon computed tomography, in neurologic
   assessment, 315
   in trauma evaluation, 578

Z

Zantac (ranitidine), 429
Zidovudine (azidothymidine, AZT), 529–530
   mechanism of action of, 494
   side effects of, 494
Zofran (ondansetron), for nausea, 64t